The Comprehensive Textbook of Healthcare Simulation

Adam I. Levine • Samuel DeMaria Jr.
Andrew D. Schwartz • Alan J. Sim
Editors

The Comprehensive Textbook of Healthcare Simulation

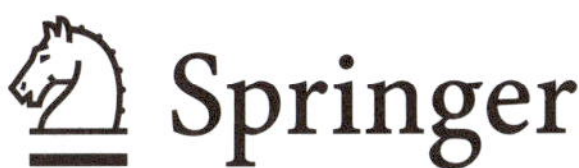

Editors
Adam I. Levine, MD
Departments of Anesthesiology
Otolaryngology, and Structural & Chemical Biology
Icahn School of Medicine at Mount Sinai
New York, NY
USA

Samuel DeMaria Jr., MD
Department of Anesthesiology
Icahn School of Medicine at Mount Sinai
New York, NY
USA

Andrew D. Schwartz, MD
Department of Anesthesiology
Icahn School of Medicine at Mount Sinai
New York, NY
USA

Alan J. Sim, MD
Department of Anesthesiology
Icahn School of Medicine at Mount Sinai
New York, NY
USA

ISBN 978-1-4614-5992-7 ISBN 978-1-4614-5993-4 (eBook)
DOI 10.1007/978-1-4614-5993-4
Springer New York Heidelberg Dordrecht London

Library of Congress Control Number: 2013940777

Printed on acid-free paper

Springer is part of Springer Science+Business Media (www.springer.com)

I dedicate this book to my remarkable wife, Robin, and my beautiful daughter, Sam, whose love, support, and devotion have been unwavering.

–Adam I. Levine, MD

For the love of my life, Tara.

–Samuel DeMaria Jr., MD

To my wife, Pam, and our three beautiful children, Sammy, Kai, and Kona.

–Andrew Schwartz, MD

For my parents, Maria and Al, and my brother, Andrew.

–Alam J. Sim, MD

Foreword

While simulation in general is probably prehistoric and a recent review traces crude elements of simulation for healthcare purposes back thousands of years, in many respects the modern era of simulation in healthcare is only about 25–30 years old. Much has happened in those years. There are no definitive metrics for growth of this endeavor. In fact, experts still debate aspects of terminology, and even what qualifies as a "simulation" differs greatly among those in the field. Looking just at the last decade's growth of the Society for Simulation in Healthcare (SSH) is instructive of what has happened in this period. Whereas in 2004 the SSH had just under 200 members, in 2012 it has over 3,000 members. Similar growth has occurred in the attendance at the International Meeting on Simulation in Healthcare (IMSH) and other simulation meetings (nearly 3,000 attendees at the 2012 IMSH conference). There has been rapid expansion of industries connected to healthcare simulation: the primary industries of those who manufacture simulators or part-task/procedural trainers and the secondary and tertiary industries of those providing services to the primary manufacturers or to the educators and clinicians who utilize simulators to do their work. Similarly, simulation has spawned a variety of new jobs and job types from new gigs for working actors (as standardized "patients," "family members," or other) to "simulationists" or "simulation technicians" to "simulation educators."

Just, say, 15 years ago (let alone 25 years ago), there was only a smattering of publications about simulation in healthcare as we now think of it. Knowledge and experience about the topic were largely in the heads of a few pioneers, and both the published and unpublished knowledge dealt only with a handful of clinical domains. Things are very different today. Information about simulation is exploding. There are thousands of papers, thousands of simulation groups and facilities, and thousands of experts. Besides the flagship peer-reviewed, indexed, multidisciplinary journal *Simulation in Healthcare* (of which I am the founding and current Editor-in-Chief), papers on simulation in healthcare are published in other peer-reviewed journals in specific disciplines or about specific clinical domains. No one can keep track of all the literature any more. It is thus of great importance to have textbooks on the topic. Some textbooks are aimed at the novice. Other textbooks aim to be what I would call a "reference textbook"; they are intended to serve as a benchmark for the field, providing a comprehensive and in-depth view for all, rather than a cursory look for the beginner. Using a reference textbook, a serious individual new to the field can get up to speed, while those already experienced can find material about subfields not their own as well as new or different views and opinions about things they thought they knew. Drs. Levine, DeMaria Jr., Schwartz, and Sim should be commended; *The Comprehensive Textbook of Healthcare Simulation* is a reference textbook. The book aims to be comprehensive, and clearly it addresses just about every arena of simulation and every adjunctive technique and issue. It is indeed a place where anyone can find detailed information on any aspect of the full spectrum of the field. The authors represent many of the best-known simulation groups in the world. I am proud to say that many authors are on the editorial board of *Simulation in Healthcare*; some are Associate Editors. A number of authors are current or former members of the SSH Board of Directors. I should disclose that I myself am an author or coauthor of two contributions to this textbook.

The field of simulation in healthcare is very broad, and while it has matured somewhat in the last quarter century, it is still a very young field. As with every textbook—especially a multiauthored one—anyone with experience in the field will find much herein to agree with and some things about which they disagree. Agreement may lead to wider adoption of good ideas. The disagreements should lead to further innovation and research exploring the nuances and the limits of this powerful set of techniques. Whenever any of those outcomes transpires, it will be a testament to the power of the book to inspire others.

Stanford, CA, USA David M. Gaba, MD

Contents

Part II Simulation Modalities and Technologies

Part III Simulation for Healthcare Disciplines

Contributors

Kathryn E. Adams, BS Department of Continuing Education, Society for Simulation in Healthcare, Minneapolis, MN, USA

Rajesh Aggarwal, PhD, MA, MRCS Division of Surgery, Department of Surgery and Cancer, Imperial College London, London, UK

Department of Surgery, Perelman School of Medicine, University of Pennsylvania, Philadelphia

St. Mary's Hospital, Imperial College NHS Trust, London, UK

Ali Alaraj, MD Department of Neurosurgery, University of Illinois at Chicago and University of Illinois Hospital and Health Science Systems, Chicago, IL, USA

Pamela Andreatta, PhD Department of Obstetrics and Gynecology, University of Michigan, Ann Arbor, MI, USA

Kivanc Atesok, MD, MSc Faculty of Medicine, Institute of Medical Science, University of Toronto, Toronto, ON, Canada

Tamika C. Auguste, MD Department of Obstetrics and Gynecology, Georgetown University School of Medicine, Washington, DC, USA

Department of OB/GYN Simulation, Women's and Infants' Services, Washington Hospital Center, Washington, DC, USA

Najib T. Ayas, MD, MPH Department of Medicine, University of British Columbia, Vancouver, BC, Canada

Thomas J. Benedetti, MD, MHA Department of Obstetrics and Gynecology, University of Washington, Seattle, WA, USA

Haim Berkenstadt, MD Department of Anesthesiology and Intensive Care, Sackler Faculty of Medicine, Tel Aviv University, Tel Aviv, Israel

Department of Anesthesiology, Sheba Medical Center, Ramat Gam, Israel

Farhan Bhanji, MD, MSc Department of Pediatrics, Richard and Sylvia Cruess Faculty Scholar in Medical Education, McGill University, Montreal, QC, Canada

Divisions of Pediatric Emergency Medicine and Pediatric Critical Care, Montreal Children's Hospital, Montreal, QC, Canada

Daniel M. Birk, MD Department of Neurosurgery, University of Illinois at Chicago and University of Illinois Hospital and Health Science Systems, Chicago, IL, USA

Victoria Brazil, MBBS, FACEM, MBA School of Medicine, Bond University, Gold Coast, QLD, Australia

Department of Emergency Medicine, Royal Brisbane and Women's Hospital, Brisbane, QLD, Australia

Judith A. Buchanan, MS, PhD, DMD School of Dentistry, University of Minnesota, Minneapolis, MN, USA

Fady T. Charbel, MD Department of Neurosurgery, University of Illinois at Chicago and University of Illinois Hospital and Health Science Systems, Chicago, IL, USA

Adam Cheng, MD, FRCPC, FAAP Department of Research and Development, KIDSIM-ASPIRE Simulation, Alberta Children's Hospital and Pediatrics, University of Calgary, Calgary, AB, Canada

Sam Clarke, MD Department of Emergency Medicine, Harbor-UCLA Medical Center, Torrance, CA, USA

Paul D. Colavita, MD Department of Gastrointestinal and Minimally Invasive Surgery, Carolinas Medical Center, Charlotte, NC, USA

Department of General Surgery, Carolinas Medical Center, Charlotte, NC, USA

Colleen Y. Colbert, PhD Office of Medical Education, Evaluation & Research Development, Department of Internal Medicine, Texas A&M HSC College of Medicine/ Scott & White Healthcare, Temple, TX, USA

Office of Medical Education, Evaluation & Research Development, Department of Internal Medicine, Scott & White Healthcare, Temple, TX, USA

James M. Cooke, MD Department of Family Medicine, University of Michigan, Ann Arbor, MI, USA

Thomas Corrado, MD Department of Anesthesiology, Stony Brook University, Stony Brook, NY, USA

Paula Craigo, MD Department of Anesthesiology, College of Medicine, Mayo Clinic, Rochester, MN, USA

Shad Deering, MD, LTC MIL, USA, MEDCOM, MAMC Department of Obstetrics/ Gynecology, Uniformed Services University of the Health Sciences, Bethesda, MD, USA

Department of Obstetrics/Gynecology, Madigan Army Medical Center, Tacoma, WA, USA

Samuel DeMaria Jr., MD Department of Anesthesiology, Icahn School of Medicine at Mount Sinai, New York, NY, USA

Ellen S. Deutsch, MD, FACS, FAAP Department of Anesthesia and Critical Care, Center for Simulation, Advanced Education, and Innovation, The Children's Hospital of Philadelphia, Philadelphia, PA, USA

Yue Dong, MD Departments of Pulmonary and Critical Care Medicine, Multidisciplinary Simulation Center, Mayo Clinic, Rochester, MN, USA

Bonnie Driggers, RN, MS, MPA Department of Nursing, Oregon Health and Science University, Portland, OR, USA

Jonathan P. Duff, MD, FRCPC Division of Critical Care, Department of Pediatrics, University of Alberta, Edmonton, AB, Canada

Edmonton Clinic Health Academy (ECHA), Edmonton, AB, Canada

William F. Dunn, MD, FCCP, FCCM Division of Pulmonary and Critical Care Medicine, Mayo Clinic Multidisciplinary Simulation Center, Mayo Clinic, Rochester, MN, USA

Kenneth A. Egol, MD Department of Orthopaedic Surgery, NYU Hospital for Joint Diseases, New York, NY, USA

Orit Eisenberg, PhD MAROM Unit, Assessment and Admissions Centers, National Institute for Testing and Evaluation, Jerusalem, Israel

Assessment and Measurement Unit, Israel Center for Medical Simulation, Jerusalem, Israel

Chad Epps, MD Departments of Clinical and Diagnostic Services and Anesthesiology, University of Alabama at Birmingham, Birmingham, AL, USA

Jason H. Epstein, MD Department of Anesthesiology, Icahn School of Medicine at Mount Sinai, New York, NY, USA

James I. Fann, MD Department of Cardiothoracic Surgery, Stanford University, Palo Alto, CA, USA

Stanford University Medical Center, Palo Alto, CA, USA

VA Palo Alto Health Care System, Palo Alto, CA, USA

Department of Cardiothoracic Surgery, CVRB, Stanford, CA, USA

Ruth M. Fanning, MB, MRCPI, FFARCSI Department of Anesthesia, Stanford University School of Medicine, Stanford, CA, USA

Richard H. Feins, MD Department of Thoracic Surgery, University of North Carolina, Chapel Hill, NC, USA

Rosemarie Fernandez, MD Division of Emergency Medicine, Department of Medicine, University of Washington School of Medicine, Seattle, WA, USA

David M. Gaba, MD Department of Immersive and Simulation-Based Learning, Stanford University, Stanford, CA, USA

Department of Anesthesia, Simulation Center, VA Palo Alto Health Care System, Anesthesia Service, Palo Alto, CA, USA

Maria F. Galati, MBA Department of Anesthesiology, Icahn School of Medicine at Mount Sinai, New York, NY, USA

Christopher J. Gallagher, MD Department of Anesthesiology, Stony Brook University, Stony Brook, NY, USA

Kathleen Gallo, PhD, MBA, RN, FAAN Center for Learning and Innovation/Patient Safety Institute, Hofstra North Shore-LIJ School of Medicine, North Shore-LIJ Health System, Lake Success, NY, USA

Jesika S. Gavilanes, Masters in Teaching Statewide Simulation, Simulation and Clinical Learning Center School of Nursing, Oregon Health and Science University, Portland, OR, USA

Matthew T. Gettman, MD Department of Urology, Mayo Clinic, Rochester, MN, USA

Kenneth Gilpin, MD, ChB, FRCA Department of Anaesthesia, Cambridge University, Cambridge, UK

Anaesthetic Department, Cambridge University Hospital, Little Eversden, Cambridge, UK

Andrew Goldberg, MD Department of Anesthesiology, Icahn School of Medicine at Mount Sinai, New York, NY, USA

Elizabeth Goldfarb, BA Department of Psychology, New York University, New York, NY, USA

Sara N. Goldhaber-Fiebert, MD Department of Anesthesia, Stanford University School of Medicine, Stanford, CA, USA

Michael Good, MD Administrative Offices, College of Medicine, University of Florida, Gainesville, FL, USA

Wanda S. Goranson, MSN, RN-BC Department of Clinical Professional Development, Iowa Health – Des Moines, Des Moines, IA, USA

James A. Gordon, MD, MPA MGH Learning Laboratory, Division of Medical Simulation, Department of Emergency Medicine, Massachusetts General Hospital, Boston, MA, USA

Gilbert Program in Medical Simulation, Harvard Medical School, Boston, MA, USA

Tristan Gorrindo, MD Division of Postgraduate Medical Education, Massachusetts General Hospital, Boston, MA, USA

Department of Psychiatry, Massachusetts General Hospital, Boston, MA, USA

Riki N. Gottlieb, DMD, FAGD Virtual Reality Simulation Laboratory, International Dentist Program, Virginia Commonwealth University School of Dentistry, Richmond, VA, USA

Department of General Practice, Admissions, Virginia Commonwealth University School of Dentistry, Richmond, VA, USA

Derek A. Gould, MB, ChB, FRCP, FRCR Department of Medical Imaging, Royal Liverpool University Hospital, Liverpool, UK

Department of Radiology, Royal Liverpool University NHS Trust, Liverpool, UK

Faculty of Medicine, University of Liverpool, Liverpool, UK

Lori Graham, PhD Office of Medical Education, Internal Medicine, Texas A&M HSC College of Medicine, Bryan, TX, USA

Vincent J. Grant, MD, FRCPC Department of Paediatrics, University of Calgary, Calgary, AB, Canada

KidSIM Human Patient Simulation Program, Alberta Children's Hospital, Calgary, AB, Canada

Gregory Hall, BA Department of Orthopaedic Surgery, NYU Langone Medical Center Hospital for Joint Diseases, New York, NY, USA

Basil Hanss, PhD Department of Medicine, Icahn School of Medicine at Mount Sinai, New York, NY, USA

Rose Hatala, MD, MSc Department of Medicine, University of British Columbia, Vancouver, BC, Canada

Department of Medicine, St. Paul's Hospital, Vancouver, BC, Canada

Emily M. Hayden, MD, MHPE MGH Learning Laboratory, Division of Medical Simulation, Department of Emergency Medicine, Massachusetts General Hospital, Boston, MA, USA

Gilbert Program in Medical Simulation, Harvard Medical School, Boston, MA, USA

Bonnie An Henderson, MD Department of Ophthalmology, Harvard Medical School, Boston, MA, USA

Ophthalmic Consultants of Boston, Waltham, MA, USA

George L. Hicks Jr., MD Division of Cardiothoracic Surgery, University of Rochester Medical Center, Rochester, NY, USA

Lisa D. Howley, MEd, PhD Department of Medical Education, Carolinas HealthCare System, Charlotte, NC, USA

Luv R. Javia, MD Department of Otorhinolaryngology/Head and Neck Surgery, Perelman School of Medicine at the University of Pennsylvania, Philadelphia, PA, USA

Department of Pediatric Otolaryngology, Children's Hospital of Philadelphia, Philadelphia, PA, USA

Laith M. Jazrawi, MD Division of Sports Medicine, Department of Orthopaedic Surgery, NYU Langone Medical Center Hospital for Joint Diseases, New York, NY, USA

Kanav Kahol, PhD Affordable Health Technologies, Public Health Foundation of India, New Delhi, India

Joel A. Kaplan, MD Department of Anesthesiology, University of California San Diego, San Diego, CA, USA

Daniel Katz, MD Department of Anesthesiology, Icahn School of Medicine at Mount Sinai, New York, NY, USA

Yury Khelemsky, MD Department of Anesthesiology, Icahn School of Medicine at Mount Sinai, New York, NY, USA

Amrita Kumar, MD, BSc, MBBS, MSc, FRCR Department of Medical Imaging, Royal Liverpool University Hospital, Liverpool, UK

Department of Imaging, University College Hospital London, London, UK

Kim Leighton, PhD, RN, CNE Department of Educational Technology, Center for Excellence in Clinical Simulation, Bryan College of Health Sciences, Lincoln, NE, USA

Staci Leisman, MD Department of Medicine, Icahn School of Medicine at Mount Sinai, New York, NY, USA

Adam I. Levine, MD Departments of Anesthesiology, Otolaryngology, and Structural and Chemical Biology, Icahn School of Medicine at Mount Sinai, New York, NY, USA

Ronald S. Levy, MD, DABA Patient Simulation Center, Departments of Anesthesiology/ Neuroscience and Cell Biology, University of Texas Medical Branch at Galveston, Galveston, TX, USA

Jenifer R. Lightdale, MD, MPH Department of Pediatrics, Harvard Medical School, Boston, MA, USA

Department of Gastroenterology and Nutrition, Children's Hospital Boston, Boston, MA, USA

Jay D. Mabrey, MD, MBA Department of Orthopaedics, Baylor University Medical Center, Dallas, TX, USA

Brian P. Mahoney, MD Department of Anesthesiology, Ohio State Wexarn Medical Center, Boston, MA, USA

Jennifer Manos, RN, BSN Center for Simulation and Research, Cincinnati Children's Hospital Medical Center, Cincinnati, OH, USA

Juli C. Maxworthy, DNP, MSN, MBA, RN, CNL, CPHQ, CPPS School of Nursing and Health Professions, University of San Francisco, San Francisco, CA, USA

WithMax Consulting, Orinda, CA, USA

James McKinney, MD, MSC Department of Cardiology, University of British Columbia, Vancouver, BC, Canada

Steven A. McLaughlin, MD Department of CME and Simulation, University of New Mexico, Albuquerque, NM, USA

Department of Emergency Medicine, University of New Mexico, Albuquerque, NM, USA

Shekhar Menon, MD Division of Emergency Medicine, Northshore University Healthsystem, Evanston, IL, USA

Curtis Mirkes, DO Department of Internal Medicine, Scott & White Healthcare/Texas A&M HSC College of Medicine, Temple, TX, USA

Deborah D. Navedo, PhD, CPNP, CNE Center for Interprofessional Studies and Innovation, MGH Institute of Health Professions, Boston, MA, USA

MGH Learning Laboratory, Massachusetts General Hospital, Boston, MA, USA

Thomas P. Noeller, MD, FAAEM, FACEP Department of Emergency Medicine, Case Western Reserve University School of Medicine, Cleveland, OH, USA

Department of Emergency Medicine, MetroHealth Stimulation Center, MetroHealth Health Medical Center, Cleveland, OH, USA

Lou Oberndorf, MBA/MS METI, Sarasota, FL, USA

Oberndorf Family Foundation, Sarasota, FL, USA

Oberndorf Holdings LLC, Sarasota, FL, USA

John M. O'Donnell, RN, CRNA, MSN, DrPH Nurse Anesthesia Program, University of Pittsburgh School of Nursing, Pittsburgh, PA, USA

Department of Anesthesiology, Peter M. Winter Institute for Simulation, Education and Research (WISER), Pittsburgh, PA, USA

Department of Acute/Tertiary Care, University of Pittsburgh School of Nursing, Pittsburgh, PA, USA

Thomas A. Oetting, MS, MD Department of Ophthalmology and Visual Sciences, University of Iowa Hospitals and Clinics, Iowa City, IA, USA

Surgical Service Line, Department of Ophthalmology, Veterans Medical Center, UIHC-Ophthalmology, Iowa City, IA, USA

Paul Edward Ogden, MD Department of Internal Medicine, Academic Affairs, Texas A&M University System – HSC College of Medicine, Bryan, TX, USA

Yasuharu Okuda, MD Department of Emergency Medicine, SimLEARN, Simulation Learning Education & Research Network, Veterans Health Administration, Orlando, FL, USA

Timothy Ryan Owens, MD Department of Neurological Surgery, Duke University Medical Center, Durham, NC, USA

Susan J. Pasquale, PhD Department of Administration, Johnson and Wales University, Providence, RI, USA

Adam D. Peets, MD, MSc (Med Ed) Department of Critical Care Medicine, University of British Columbia, Vancouver, BC, Canada

Tiffany Pendergrass, BSN, RN, CPN Center for Simulation and Research, Cincinnati Children's Hospital Medical Center, Cincinnati, OH, USA

Marjolein C. Persoon, MD Department of Urology, Catharina Hospital Eindhoven, Eindhoven, The Netherlands

Department of Surgery, Jeroen Bosch Ziekenhuis, 's-Hertogenbosch, Noord-Brabant, The Netherlands

Paul E. Phrampus, MD Department of Anesthesiology, Peter M. Winter Institute for Simulation, Education and Research (WISER), Pittsburgh, PA, USA

Department of Emergency Medicine, UPMC Center for Quality Improvement and Innovation, University of Pittsburgh, Pittsburgh, PA, USA

Rajesh Reddy, MD Department of Anesthesiology, Icahn School of Medicine at Mount Sinai, New York, NY, USA

Gina M. Rogers, MD Department of Ophthalmology and Visual Sciences, University of Iowa Hospitals and Clinics, Iowa City, IA, USA

Kathleen Rosen, MD Department of Anesthesiology, Cleveland Clinic Lerner College of Medicine, Case Western Reserve University, Cleveland, OH, USA

Department of Anesthesiology, Cleveland Clinic, Cleveland, OH, USA

Jenny W. Rudolph, PhD Center for Medical Simulation, Boston, MA, USA

Department of Anesthesia, Critical Care and Pain Medicine, Massachusetts General Hospital, Boston, MA, USA

Robert M. Rush Jr., MD, FACS Department of Surgery and the Andersen Simulation Center, Madigan Army medical Center, Tacoma, WA, USA

Central Simulation Committee, US Army Medical Department, Andersen Simulation Center, Madigan Army Medical Center, Tacoma, WA, USA

Department of Surgery, University of Washington, Seattle, WA, USA

Department of Surgery, USUHS, Bethesda, MD, USA

Ross J. Scalese, MD, FACP Division of Research and Technology, Gordon Center for Research in Medical Education, University of Miami Miller School of Medicine, Miami, FL, USA

Barbara M.A. Schout, MD, PhD Urology Department, VU University Medical Center, Amsterdam, Noord Holland, The Netherlands

Andrew D. Schwartz, MD Department of Anesthesiology, Icahn School of Medicine at Mount Sinai, New York, NY, USA

Howard A. Schwid, MD Department of Anesthesiology and Pain Medicine, University of Washington School of Medicine, Seattle, WA, USA

Michael Seropian, MD Department of Anesthesiology, Oregon Health and Science University, Portland, OR, USA

Megan R. Sherman, BA Department of Surgery, Institute for Simulation and Interprofessional Studies (ISIS), University of Washington, Seattle, WA, USA

Jeffrey H. Silverstein, MD Department of Anesthesiology, Icahn School of Medicine at Mount Sinai, New York, NY, USA

Alan J. Sim, MD Department of Anesthesiology, Icahn School of Medicine at Mount Sinai, New York, NY, USA

Robert Simon, EdD Department of Anesthesia, Harvard Medical School, Boston, MA, USA

Center for Medical Simulation, Cambridge, MA, USA

Pramudith V. Sirimanna, MBBS, BSc (Hons) Division of Surgery, Department of Surgery and Cancer, Imperial College London, London, UK

St. Mary's Hospital, Imperial College NHS Trust, London, UK

Michael D. Smith, MD, FACEP Department of Emergency Medicine, Case Western Reserve University, MetroHealth Medical Center, Cleveland, OH, USA

Dimitrios Stefanidis, MD, PhD, FACS, FASMBS Department of General Surgery, University of North Carolina–Charlotte, Charlotte, NC, USA

Department of General Surgery, Carolinas HealthCare System, Charlotte, NC, USA

Christopher G. Strother, MD Departments of Emergency Medicine and Pediatrics, Mount Sinai Hospital, New York, NY, USA

Demian Szyld, MD, EdM Department of Emergency Medicine, The New York Simulation Center for the Health Sciences, New York, NY, USA

Department of Emergency Medicine, New York University School of Medicine, New York, NY, USA

Jeffrey M. Taekman, MD Department of Anesthesiology, Duke University School of Medicine, Durham, NC, USA

Department of Anesthesiology, Human Simulation and Patient Safety Center, Duke University Medical Center, Durham, NC, USA

David D. Thiel, MD Department of Urology, Mayo Clinic Florida, Jacksonville, FL, USA

Matthew K. Tobin, BS College of Medicine, University of Illinois at Chicago, Chicago, IL, USA

Nancy Tofil, MD, MEd Department of Pediatrics, Division of Critical Care, Pediatric Simulation Center, University of Alabama at Birmingham, Birmingham, AL, USA

Laurence C. Torsher, MD Department of Anesthesiology, College of Medicine, Mayo Clinic, Rochester, MN, USA

Alexander J. Towbin, MD Department of Radiology, Radiology Informatics, Cincinnati Children's Hospital Medical Center, Cincinnati, OH, USA

Ankeet D. Udani, MD Department of Anesthesia, Stanford University School of Medicine, Stanford, CA, USA

Kathleen M. Ventre, MD Department of Pediatrics/Critical Care Medicine, Children's Hospital Colorado/University of Colorado, Aurora, Denver, CO, USA

J. Marjoke Vervoorn, PhD, DDS Educational Institute, Academic Centre for Dentistry Amsterdam (ACTA), Amsterdam, The Netherlands

Courtney West, PhD Office of Medical Education, Internal Medicine, Texas A&M HSC College of Medicine, Bryan, TX, USA

Marjorie Lee White, MD, MPPM, MEd Department of Pediatrics and Emergency Medicine, Pediatric Simulation Center, University of Alabama at Birmingham, Birmingham, AL, USA

Robert I. Williams, MBA Department of Anesthesiology, The Mount Sinai Hospital, New York, NY, USA

Leslie A. Wimsatt, PhD Department of Family Medicine, University of Michigan, Ann Arbor, MI, USA

Amitai Ziv, MD, MHA Medical Education, Sackler School of Medicine, Tel Aviv University, Tel Aviv, Israel

Patient Safety and Risk Management, Israel Center for Medical Simulation (MSR), Chaim Sheba Medical Center, Tel Hashomer, Israel

Part I

Introduction to Simulation

Healthcare Simulation: From "Best Secret" to "Best Practice"

1

Adam I. Levine, Samuel DeMaria Jr., Andrew D. Schwartz, and Alan J. Sim

Introduction

Throughout history healthcare educators have used patient surrogates to teach, assess, and even conduct research in a safe and predictable environment. Therefore, the use of healthcare simulation is historically rooted and as old as the concept of healthcare itself. In the last two decades, there has been an exponential rise in the development, application, and general awareness of simulation use in the healthcare industry. What was once essentially a novelty has given rise to entire new fields, industries, and dedicated professional societies. Within a very short time, healthcare simulation has gone from "best secret" to "best practice."

Ambiguity, Resistance, and the Role of Simulation: Organization of this Book

So why do we need a comprehensive textbook of healthcare simulation? Although growth has been relatively rapid, in reality, the ambiguity of the field's vision, resistance of adoption by practitioners, and an ill-defined role for simulation in many healthcare arenas have characterized the recent history of simulation. Despite this fact, we are now at a place where clarity, acceptance, and more focused roles for simulation have begun to predominate. This transformation has spawned a rapidly evolving list of new terminologies, technologies, and teaching and assessment modalities. Therefore, many educators, researchers, and administrators are seeking a definitive, up-to-date resource that addresses solutions to their needs in terms of training, assessment, and patient safety applications.
Hence, we present this book *The Comprehensive Textbook of Healthcare Simulation*.

Most medical disciplines now have a collective vision for how and why simulation fits into trainee education, and some have extended this role to advanced practitioner training, maintenance of competency, and even as a vehicle for therapeutic intervention and procedural rehearsal. Regardless of the reader's background and discipline, this book will serve those developing their own simulation centers or programs and those considering incorporation of this technology into their credentialing processes. It will also serve as a state-of-the-art reference for those already knowledgeable or involved with simulation, but looking to expand their knowledge base or their simulation program's capability and target audience. We are proud to present to the reader an international author list that brings together experts in healthcare simulation in its various forms. Here you will find many of the field's most notable experts offering opinion and best evidence with regard to their own discipline's best practices in simulation.

Organization

The book is divided into five parts: Part 1: Introduction to Simulation, Part 2: Simulation Modalities and Technologies, Part 3: The Healthcare Disciplines, and Parts 4 and 5: on the practical considerations of Healthcare Simulation for Professional and Program Development.

In Part 1 the reader is provided with a historic perspective and up-to-date look at the general concepts of healthcare simulation applications. The book opens with a comprehensive review of the history of healthcare simulation (Chap. 2). The embedded memoir section ("Pioneers and Profiles") offers the reader a unique insight into the history of simulation through the eyes and words of those responsible for making it. These fascinating personal memoirs are written by people who were present from the beginning and who were

A.I. Levine, MD (✉)
Departments of Anesthesiology, Otolaryngology, and Structural and Chemical Biology, Icahn School of Medicine at Mount Sinai, New York, NY, USA
e-mail: adam.levine@mountsinai.org

S. DeMaria Jr., MD • A.D. Schwartz, MD • A.J. Sim, MD
Department of Anesthesiology, Icahn School of Medicine at Mount Sinai, New York, NY, USA

A.I. Levine et al. (eds.), *The Comprehensive Textbook of Healthcare Simulation*,
DOI 10.1007/978-1-4614-5993-4_1, © Springer Science+Business Media New York 2013

responsible for simulation's widespread adoption, design, and application. Here we are honored to present, for the first time, "the stories" of David Gaba, Mike Good, Howard Schwid, and several others. Drs. Gaba and Good describe their early work creating the Stanford and Gainesville mannequin-based simulators, respectively, while Dr. Schwid describes his early days creating the first computer-based simulators. Industry pioneer Lou Obendorf shares his experience with simulation commercialization including starting, expanding, and establishing one of the largest healthcare simulation companies in the world. Other authors' stories frame the early days of this exciting field as it was coming together including our own involvement (The Mount Sinai Story) with simulation having acquired the first simulator built on the Gainesville simulator platform, which would ultimately become the CAE METI HPS simulator.

The rest of this section will prove invaluable to healthcare providers and is devoted to the application of simulation at the broadest levels: for education (Chaps. 3, 4, and 5), assessment (Chaps. 11 and 12), and patient safety (Chap. 9). The specific cornerstones of simulation-based activities are also elucidated through dedicated chapters emphasizing the incorporation of human factors' training (Chap. 8), systems factors (Chap. 10), feedback, and debriefing (Chaps. 6 and 7). Special sections are included to assist educators interested in enriching their simulation-based activities with the introduction of humor, stress, and other novel concepts.

The earlier opposition to the use of simulation by many healthcare providers has to a large degree softened due to the extensive work done to demonstrate and make simulation a rigorous tool for training and assessment. As the science of simulation, based in adult learning theory (Chap. 3), has improved, it has become more and more difficult for healthcare workers to deny its role in healthcare education, assessment, and maintenance of competence. Further, this scientific basis has helped clarify ambiguity and better define the role of simulation never before conceived or appreciated. Crisis resource management (Chap. 8), presented by the team who pioneered the concept, is a perfect example of evidence driving best practice for simulation. Two decades ago, one might have thought that simulation was best used for teaching finite psychomotor skills. We know now that teamwork, communication, and nontechnical human factors necessary to best manage a crisis are critical to assure error reduction and patient safety and can be a major attribute of simulation-based training. This scientific rigor has helped redefine and guide the role for simulation in healthcare.

In Part 2, we present the four major areas of modalities and technologies used for simulation-based activities. These can be found in dedicated chapters (Chap. 13 on standardized patient, Chap. 14 on computer- and internet-based simulators, Chap. 15 on mannequin-based simulators, and Chap. 16 on virtual reality and haptic simulators). Again, this group of fundamental chapters provides the reader with targeted and timely resources on the available technology including general technical issues, applications, strengths, and limitations. The authors of these chapters help to demonstrate how the technological revolution has further expanded and defined the role of simulation in healthcare. Each chapter in this section is written by experts and in many cases is presented by the pioneers in that particular technological genre.

Throughout this textbook, the reader will find examples to determine which way the "wind is blowing" in various medical disciplines (Part 3). Here we include a comprehensive listing of healthcare disciplines that have embraced simulation and have expanded the role in their own field. We have chosen each of these disciplines deliberately because they were ones with well-established adoption, use, and best practice for simulation (e.g., anesthesiology and emergency medicine) or because they are experiencing rapid growth in simulation implementation and innovation (e.g., psychiatry and the surgical disciplines). While many readers will of course choose to read the chapter(s) specific to their own medical discipline, we hope they will be encouraged to venture beyond their own practice and read some of the other discipline-specific chapters that may seem to have little to do with their own specialty. What the reader will find in doing so will most certainly interest them, since learning what others do, in seemingly unrelated domains, will intrigue, inspire, and motivate readers to approach simulation in different ways.

The book closes with Parts 4 and 5, wherein the authors present several facets of professional and program development in simulation (i.e., how to become better at simulation at the individual, institutional, and societal levels). We have organized the available programs in simulation training "up the chain" from medical students, resident and fellow, to practicing physicians and nurses as well as for administrators looking to start centers, get funding, and obtain endorsement or accreditation by the available bodies in simulation.

Welcome

This textbook has been a labor of love for us (the editors), but also for each one of the authors involved in this comprehensive, multinational, multi-institutional, and multidisciplinary project. We are honored to have assembled the world's authorities on these subjects, many of whom were responsible for developing the technology, the innovative applications, and the supportive research upon which this book is based. We hope the reader will find what he or she is looking for at the logistical and informational level; however, we have greater hope that what they find is a field still young but with a clear vision for the future and great things on the horizon. We as healthcare workers, educators, or administrators, in the end, have patients relying upon us for safe and intelligent care. This young but bustling technique for training and assessment, which we call simulation, has moved beyond "best secret" to "best practice" and is now poised for a great future.

2 The History of Simulation

Kathleen Rosen

Pioneers and Profiles

Personal Memoirs by Howard A. Schwid, David Gaba, Michael Good, Joel A. Kaplan, Jeffrey H. Silverstein, Adam I. Levine, and Lou Oberndorf

Introduction

Simulation is not an accident but the result of major advancements in both technology and educational theory. Medical simulation in primitive forms has been practiced for centuries. Physical models of anatomy and disease were constructed long before plastic or computers were even conceived. While modern simulation was truly borne out in the twentieth century and is a direct descendent of aviation simulation, current healthcare simulation is possible because of the evolution of interrelated fields of knowledge and the global application of systems-based practice and practice-based learning to healthcare.

Technology and the technological revolutions are fundamental to these advancements (Fig. 2.1). Technology can take two forms: enhanced technology and replacement technology. As the names imply, enhanced technology serves to improve existing technologies, while replacement technology is potentially more disruptive since the new technology serves to displace that which is preexisting. However, according to Professor Maury Klein, an expert on technology:

> Technology is value neutral. It is neither good nor evil. It does whatever somebody wants it to do. The value that is attached to any given piece of technology depends on who is using it and evaluating it, and what they do with it. The same technology can do vast good or vast harm [1].

The first technological revolution (i.e., the industrial revolution) had three sequential phases, each having two components. The power revolution provided the foundation for later revolutions in communications and transportation. It was these revolutions that resulted in the global organizational revolution and forever changed the way people relate to each other and to the world. The communications revolution was in the middle of this technology sandwich, and today simulation educators recognize their technology is powerless without effective communication (see Fig. 2.1).

K. Rosen, MD
Department of Anesthesiology, Cleveland Clinic Lerner College of Medicine, Case Western Reserve University, Cleveland, OH, USA

Department of Anesthesiology, Cleveland Clinic, Cleveland, OH, USA
e-mail: krr622@gmail.com

Overview

This overview of the history of healthcare simulation will begin with a review of the history of computers and flight simulation. These two innovations provide a context for and demonstrate many parallels to medical simulation development. The current technology revolution (information age) began in the 1970s as computer technology, networking, and information systems burst upon us. Computing power moved from large expensive government applications to affordable personal models. Instantaneous communication with or without visual images has replaced slower communication streams. During this same time period, aviation safety principles were identified as relevant to healthcare systems.

Previous "history of simulation narratives" exerted significant effort toward the historic justification of simulation modalities for healthcare education. The history and success of simulation in education and training for a variety of other disciplines was evidence for the pursuit of healthcare simulation. However, no other field questioned the ability of deliberate practice to improve performance. At long last, most healthcare professionals cannot imagine a world without simulation. It is time to thank simulation education innovators for their perseverance. An editorial in Scientific American in the 1870s declared erroneously that the telephone was destined to fail [1]. Similarly, simulation educators didn't stop when they were dismissed by skeptics, asked to prove the efficacy of simulation, or ridiculed for "playing with dolls."

A.I. Levine et al. (eds.), *The Comprehensive Textbook of Healthcare Simulation*,
DOI 10.1007/978-1-4614-5993-4_2, © Springer Science+Business Media New York 2013

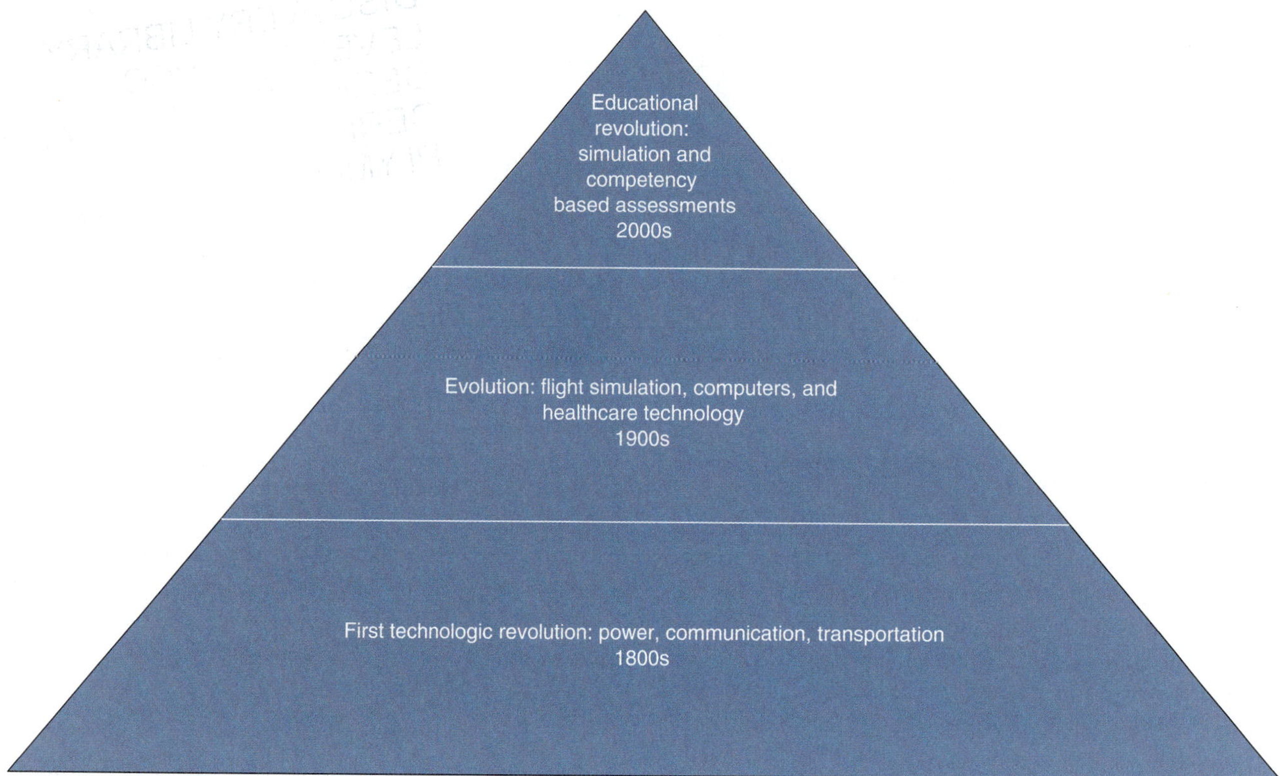

Fig. 2.1 Overview of the revolutions in technology, simulation, and medical education

The History of Computers

Man developed counting devices even in very primitive cultures. The earliest analog computers were designed to assist with calculations of astronomy (astrolabe, equatorium, planisphere), geometry (sector), and mathematics (tally stick, abacus, slide rule, Napier's bones). The Computer History Museum has many Internet-based exhibits including a detailed timeline of the history of computation [2–5]. One of the oldest surviving computing relics is the 2000-year-old Antikythera mechanism. It was discovered in a shipwreck in 1901. This device not only predicted astronomy but also catalogued the timing for the Olympic games [6].

During the nineteenth century, there was an accelerated growth of computing capabilities. During the 10-year period between 1885 and 1895, there were many significant computing inventions. The precursor of the keyboard, the comptometer, was designed and built from a macaroni box by Dorr E. Felt in 1886 and patented a year later [7]. Punch cards were introduced first by Joseph-Marie Jacquard in 1801 for use in a loom [8]. This technology was then applied to calculator design by Charles Babbage in his plans for the "Analytical Machine" [9].

Herman Hollerith's Electric Tabulating Machine was the first successful implementation of punch card technology on a grand scale and was used to tabulate the results of the 1890 census [10]. His innovative and successful counting solution earned him a cover story for Scientific American. He formed the Tabulating Machine Company in 1895. In 1885, Julius Pitrap invented the computing scale [11]. His patents were bought by the Computing Scale Company in 1891 [12]. In 1887, Alexander Dey invented the dial recorder and formed Dey Patents Company, also known as the Dey Time Register, in 1893 [13, 14]. Harlow Bundy invented the first time clock for workers in Binghamton, NY, in 1889 [15]. Binghamton turned out to be an important site in the history of flight and medical simulation during the next century. Ownership of all of these businesses would change over the next 25 years before they were consolidated as the Computing Tabulating Recording Corporation (CTR) in 1911 (see Fig. 2.2). CTR would change its name to the more familiar International Business Machines (IBM) in 1924 [16].

Interestingly, the word *computer* originally referred only to people who solved difficult mathematical problems. The term was first applied to the machines that could rapidly and accurately calculate and solve problems during World War II [17]. The military needs during the war spurred development of computation devices, and computers rapidly progressed from the mechanical-analog phase into the electronic digital era. Many of the advances can be traced to innovations by Konrad Zuse, a German code breaker, who is credited by many as the inventor of the first programmable computer [18]. His innovations included the introduction of binary processing with the Z1 (1936–1938). Ultimately, he would separate memory and processing and replace relays with vacuum tubes. He also developed the first programming language.

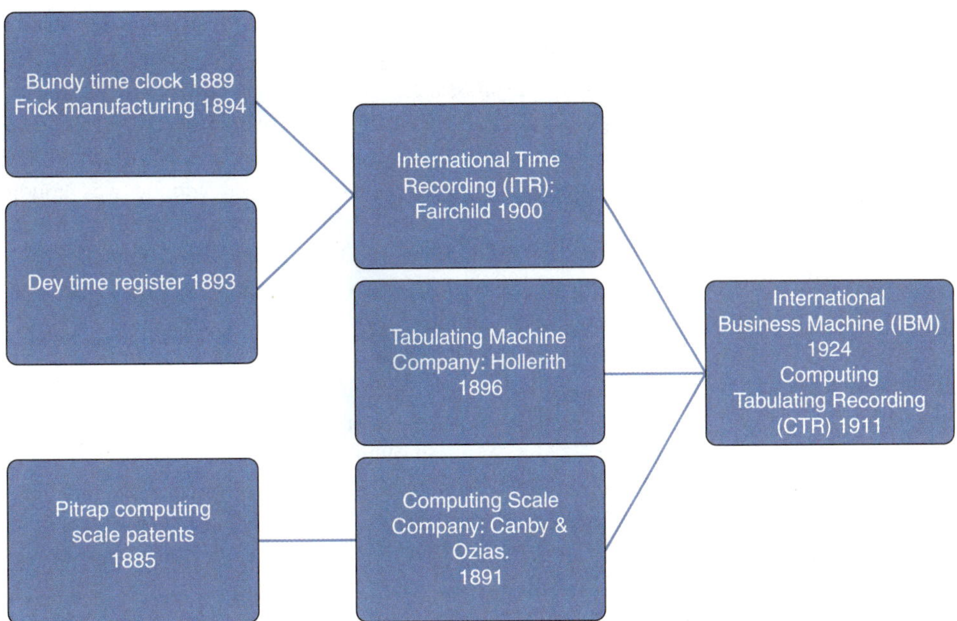

Fig. 2.2 Development of IBM

During the same time period (1938–1944) in the USA, the Harvard Mark 1, also known as the Automatic Sequence Controlled Calculator, was designed and built by Howard Aiken with support from IBM. It was the first commercial, electrical-mechanical computer. Years later, Aiken, as a member of the National Bureau of Standards Research Council, would recommend against J. Presper Eckert and John Mauchly and their vision for mass production of their computers [17].

In the 1950s, Remington Rand purchased the Eckert-Mauchly Computer Company and began production of the UNIVAC computer. This universal computer could serve both business and scientific needs with its unique alphanumeric processing capability [19]. Computers were no longer just for computing but became managers of information as well as numbers. The UNIVAC's vacuum tube and metallic tape design was the first to challenge traditional punch card models in the USA. Many of its basic design features remain in present-day computers. IBM responded to this challenge with the launch of a technologically similar unit, simply labeled 701. It introduced plastic tape and faster data retrieval. The key inventions of the latter part of the decade were solid-state transistor technology, computer disc storage systems, and magnetic core memory.

The foundation for modern computers was completed in the 1960s when they became entirely digital. Further developments and refinements were aimed at increasing computer speed and capacity while decreasing size and cost. The 1980s heralded the personal computer and software revolution, and the 1990s saw progressive increases in magnetic data storage, networking, portability, and speed. The computer revolution of the twenty-first century has focused on the client/server revolution and the proliferation of small multipurpose mobile-computing devices.

History of Flight Simulation

Early flight training used real aircraft, first on the ground and then progressing to in-flight dual-control training aircraft. The first simple mechanical trainers debuted in 1910 [20]. The Sanders trainer required wind to simulate motion. Instructors physically rocked the Antoinette Learning Barrel to simulate flight motions [21]. By 1912, pilot error was recognized as the source of 90% of all crashes [22]. Although World War I stimulated and funded significant developments in aviation training devices to reduce the number of noncombat casualties and improve aerial combat, new inventions stalled during peacetime until the innovations of Edwin A. Link.

Edwin Link was born July 26, 1904, less than a year after the first powered flight by the Wright brothers. His father started the Link Piano and Organ Company in 1910 in Binghamton, NY. He took his first flying lesson at the age of 16 and bought his first airplane in 1928. Determined to find a quicker and less expensive way to learn to fly, Link began working on his Blue Box trainer and formed the Link Aeronautical Corporation in 1929. He received patent # 1,825,462 for the Combination Training Device for Student Aviators and Entertainment on September 29, 1931 [23]. At first he was unable to convince people of its true value, and it became a popular amusement park attraction. National Inventor's Hall of Fame posthumously recognized Edwin Link for this invention in 2003 [24]. In the 1930s, the US Army Air

Corps became responsible for mail delivery. After experiencing several weather-related tragedies, the army requested a demonstration of the Link trainer. In 1934 Link successfully sold the concept by demonstrating a safe landing in a thick fog. World War II provided additional military funding for development, and 10,000 trainers were ordered by the USA and its allies.

Edwin Link was president of Link Aviation until 1953. He stayed involved through its 1954 merger with General Precision Equipment Corporation and finally retired in 1959. Link simulators progressed for decades in parallel with the evolution of aircraft and computers. Link began spaceflight simulation in 1962. The Singer Company acquired Link Aviation in 1968. Twenty years later, the flight simulation division was purchased by CAE Inc. [25]. This company would become involved with the commercial manufacture of high-fidelity mannequin simulators in the 1990s. By 2012, CAE expanded their healthcare simulation product line by acquiring Immersion Medical, a division of Immersion Inc. devoted to the development of virtual reality haptic-enabled simulators, and Medical Education Technologies Inc. (METI), a leading model-driven high-fidelity mannequin-based simulation company.

Pioneers of Modern Healthcare Education and Simulation

"The driving force of technology evolution is not mechanical, electrical, optical, or chemical. It's human: each new generation of simulationists standing on the shoulders - and the breakthroughs - of every previous generation" [26]. The current major paradigm shift in healthcare education to competency-based systems, mastery learning, and simulation took almost 50 years. This history of simulation will pay tribute to those pioneers in technical simulation, nontechnical simulation, and patient safety who dared to "boldly go where no man had gone before" [27, 28] and laid the foundation for medical simulation innovations of the 1980s and beyond.

The Legacy of Stephen J. Abrahamson, PhD

Stephen Abrahamson wrote a summary of the events in his professional life titled "Essays on Medical Education." It chronicles his 30-year path as an educator. Although chance meetings ("Abrahamson's formula for success: Dumb Luck") and coincidences play a role in his story, the accomplishments would not have occurred without his knowledge, persistence, and innovative spirit [29]. He was first a high school teacher and then an instructor for high school teachers before entering Temple University where he received his Master of Science degree in 1948 and his PhD in Education from New York University in 1951. His postdoctoral work at Yale focused on evaluation [30].

Abrahamson began his first faculty appointment at the University of Buffalo in 1952. His expertise was quickly recognized and he was appointed as head of the Education Research Center. His career in medical education began when he met George Miller from the School of Medicine who sought help to improve medical education with assistance from the education experts. This was indeed a novel concept for 1954. Dr. Abrahamson knew education, but not medical education, and adopted an ethnographic approach to gain understanding of the culture and process. After a period of observation, he received a grant for the "Project in Medical Education" to test his hypothesis that medical education would benefit from faculty development in educational principles. Two of his early students at Buffalo who assisted in this project achieved later significant acclaim in the field of medical education. Edwin F. Rosinski, MD, eventually became the Deputy Assistant Secretary for the Department of Health Education and Welfare and drafted legislation favoring research in medical education. Hillard Jason was a medical student who was also awarded a doctorate in education and would help to advance standardized patient evaluation.

This project held several seminars that were attended by medical school administrators. Three of the attendees from California would eventually figure prominently in Abrahamson's future. Dr. Abrahamson describes 1959 as the year his career in medical education began [30]. He accepted an invitation to serve as a visiting professor at Stanford in the capacity of medical consultant (1959–1960). His primary function was to provide expertise on student evaluation for their new curriculum.

The University of Southern California (USC) successfully recruited Dr. Abrahamson to become the founding leader of their Department of Medical Education in 1963. Howard Barrows, MD, attended a project seminar before he and Abrahamson would become colleagues at USC. In a 2003 interview, Abrahamson stated, "Howard is one of the most innovative persons I have ever met" [31]. He collaborated with Dr. Barrows on the development of "programmed patients" (see Barrows' tribute below) for medical education by writing a successful grant application to support the program and coauthored the first paper describing this technique [32].

The first computerized patient simulator, known as Sim One, was conceived during a "3-martini lunch" with medical colleagues in 1964 [33]. Dr. J. Samuel Denson, Chief of the Department of Anesthesiology, was a clinical collaborator. Denson and Dr. Abrahamson attempted to obtain funding from the National Institutes of Health (NIH) but received many rejections. Dr. Abrahamson's submitted a proposal to the United States Office of Education's Cooperative Research

Project and was awarded a $272,000 grant over 2 years to cover the cost of development. The group partnered with Aerojet General and unveiled Sim One on March 17, 1967. A pictorial overview of Sim One is available [34–36].

The team of researchers from USC (Stephen Abrahamson, Judson Denson, Alfred Paul Clark, Leonard Taback, Tullio Ronzoni) applied for a patent on January 29, 1968. The full name of the simulator on the patent was Anesthesiological Training Simulator. Patent # 3,520,071 was issued 2 years later on July 14, 1970 [37]. The patent is referenced in 26 future patents by the American Heart Association; the Universities of Florida, Miami, and Texas; and many companies including CAE-Link, MedSim-Eagle, Gaumard, Simbionix, Laerdal, Bausch & Lomb, Critikon, and Dragerwerk Aktiengesellschaft.

The opening argument for the patent may be the first documented discussion of using simulation to improve medical education and promote patient safety: "It has been considered possible to improve the efficacy of medical training and to reduce the potential hazards involved in the use of live patients during the teaching process by means of simulation techniques to teach medical skills."

The mannequin used for Sim One was an original construction and not a repurposed low-fidelity model. The mannequin was open at the back and bolted to the operating table to accommodate electric and pneumatic hardware. Interestingly the patent asserted that "mannequin portability is neither necessary nor desirable," a concept that was ultimately contradicted in the evolution of mannequin-based simulation.

There were a number of features in Sim One that are found in current high-fidelity mannequins. The mannequin could breathe "normally." The virtual left lung had a single lobe while the right had two. The lower right lobe contained two-thirds of the right lung volume. Temporal and carotid arteries pulses were palpable. Heart sounds were present. Blood pressure could be taken in the right arm, and drugs injected in the left via a coded needle that would extrapolate drug concentration. Ten drugs were programmed in the simulator including thiopental, succinylcholine, ephedrine, medical gases, and anesthetic vapors. Not only did the eyelids open and close but the closing tension was variable. Pupils were also reactive to light in a continuous fashion. The aryepiglottic folds could open and close to simulate laryngospasm. Similar to the early versions of Harvey®, The Cardiopulmonary Patient Simulator, Resusci Annie®, and PatSim, the mannequin did not extend below the hips.

Some of its capabilities have not yet been reproduced by modern mannequins. This mannequin could simulate vomiting, bucking, and fasciculations. In addition to eye opening, the eyebrows wrinkled. They moved downward with eye closing but upward with forehead wrinkling. Sophisticated sensors gauged endotracheal tube placement, proper mask fit (through magnets), and lip pinching. The jaw would open and close with slight extension of the tongue upon jaw opening. The jaw was spring loaded with a baseline force of 2–3 lb and capable of exerting a maximum biting force of 10–15 lb. A piano wire changed the position of the epiglottis when a laryngoscope was inserted. Sensors in the airway could also detect endobronchial intubation and proper endotracheal tube cuff inflation. Cyanosis was visible diffusely both on the face and torso and in the mouth. The color change was continuous from pink to blue to gray. Cyanosis was most rapidly visible on the earlobes and mucus membranes.

The project received a great deal of publicity. It was prominently featured by Time, Newsweek, and Life magazines. CBS news with Walter Cronkite interviewed Dr. Abrahamson. In 1969, the USC collaborators published two papers featuring Sim One. The first was a simple description of the technology [38]. The second paper described a prospective trial comparing acquisition of skill in endotracheal intubation by new anesthesia residents with and without simulation training. Mastery of this routine anesthesia procedure was achieved more rapidly by simulation trainees than controls [39]. Large interindividual variability and small sample size prevented portions of the results from achieving statistical significance. This article was rereleased in 2004 as a classic paper [40].

Considering the computing power of the day, it is impressive what this mannequin could do from a commercial computer model circa 1968. Sim One was lauded by some but was discounted by many despite this success, a theme common to most disruptive technology. Sim One was used to train more than 1,000 healthcare professionals before its "death" in 1975, as parts wore out and couldn't be replaced [31]. Abrahamson's forecast of mastery education and endorsement of standardized patients were equally visionary. His essays detail some of the obstacles, biases, and frustrations that the truly farsighted encounter. In the end, Sim One was likely too far ahead of its time.

The Legacy of Howard S. Barrows, MD

Howards Barrows is credited with two major innovations in medical education: standardized patients and the problem-based learning discussion (PBLD) [41, 42]. Both are now commonplace types of simulation. He completed his residency in neurology at Columbia and was influenced by Professor David Seegal, who observed each medical student on his service perform a complete patient examination [43]. This was considered rare in 1960. In that year, he joined the faculty at USC. Early in his career, he developed a passion for medical education that was influenced by attending one of the Project Medical Education Seminars hosted by Stephen Abrahamson.

Several unrelated events stimulated the birth of the first "programmed patient." Sam, a patient with syringomyelia for the National Board of Neurology and Psychiatry exam, related to Barrows that he was treated roughly by an examiner, so he falsified his Babinski reflex and sensory findings as repayment [44]. Stephen Abrahamson joined USC in 1962 and gave Barrows 8-mm single-concept film cartridges to document and teach the neurologic exam. Barrows hired Rose McWilliams, an artist's model, for the film lessons. He wanted an objective way to assess medical students' performance at the end of their neurology clerkship. As a result in 1963, he developed the first standardized patient case dubbed Patty Dugger. He taught Rose to portray a fictionalized version of a real patient with multiple sclerosis and paraplegia. He even constructed a checklist for Rose to complete. While Barrows was passionate about the technique, his critics far outnumbered the supporters, especially at USC. Standardized patients were discounted as "too Hollywood" and "detrimental to medical education by maligning its dignity with actors" [32, 44].

In spite of widespread criticism, Barrows persisted in using standardized patients (SPs) because he thought that it was valuable to grade students on actual performance with "patients" instead of the grooming or manners displayed to preceptors. He and coauthor Abrahamson published their experience in a landmark article [45]. Initially, they called the patient actors "programmed patients." Other terms used to describe early SPs are patient instructor, patient educator, professional patient, surrogate patient, and teaching associate. Barrows left to a more supportive environment, the brand new McMaster University, in 1971. He began working with nurse Robyn Tamblyn at McMaster. She transitioned from SP to writing her doctoral thesis about the SP education method and would later play a role in the development of the SP portion of the Canadian licensing exam.

In the 1970s Barrow's major project was to serve as founding faculty of McMaster University Medical School, the first school to employ an entirely PBLD based curriculum. During this time period, Barrows received support from the American Medical Association (AMA) to use SPs for continuing education seminars titled "Bedside Clinics in Neurology." The SPs not only portrayed neurology patients but also conference attendees to help challenge and prepare the faculty [46]. Another early supporter of the SP programs for medical schools was Dr. Hilliard Jason. He established the standardized patient program at Michigan State University after seeing a Patty Dugger demonstration at a conference. He developed four cases of difficult patients who presented social challenges in addition to medical problems. Jason advanced the concept with the addition of video recording of the interaction.

Barrows relocated once again to Southern Illinois University in 1981. There, his SP programs progressed from education and evaluation tools to motivations for curricular reform. The Josiah Macy Foundation provided critical support over the next two decades to complete the transition of SP methodology from Barrow's soapbox to the national standard for medical education and evaluation. Stephen Abrahamson was the recipient of a 1987 grant to develop education sessions for medical school deans and administrators and in the 1990s the Macy foundation supported the development of consortia exploring the use of SPs for high-stakes assessment.

Despite the early struggles, the goal to design and use national Clinical Performance Exams (CPX) was ultimately achieved. By 1993, 111 of 138 US medical schools were using standardized patients and 39 of them had incorporated a high-stakes exam [43]. The Medical Council of Canada launched the first national CPX in 1993. The Educational Commission for Foreign Medical Graduates (ECFMG) adopted their CPX in 1994 followed by the United Kingdom's Professional Linguistics Assessment Board in 1998. Finally in 2004, USMLE Step II Clinical Skills Exam became an official part of the US National Board of Medical Examiners licensing exam [47].

The Legacy of Ellison C. (Jeep) Pierce, MD

The Anesthesia Patient Safety Foundation (APSF) was the first organization to study and strive for safety in healthcare. The APSF recognizes Dr. Ellison (Jeep) Pierce as its founding leader and a true visionary whose work would profoundly affect the future of all healthcare disciplines. "Patients as well as providers perpetually owe Dr. Pierce a great debt of gratitude, for Jeep Pierce was the pioneering patient safety leader" [48]. Pierce's mission to eliminate anesthesia-related mortality was successful in large part because of his skills, vision, character, and passion, but a small part was related to Abrahamson's formula for success which John Eichhorn described in the APSF Newsletter as an original serendipitous coincidence [49]. His training in anesthesia began in 1954, the same year that the first and highly controversial paper describing anesthesia-related mortality was published [50]. This no doubt prompted much of his later actions. Would the same outcome have occurred if he remained in surgical training and not gone to the University of Pennsylvania to pursue anesthesia training? What if he didn't land in Boston working for Dr. Leroy Vandam at Peter Bent Brigham Hospital? Would another faculty member assigned the resident lecture topic of "Anesthesia Accidents" in 1962 have had the same global impact [50]?

Two Bostonian contemporary colleagues from the Massachusetts General Hospital, Arthur Keats and Jeffrey Cooper, challenged the 1954 conclusions of Beecher and Todd in the 1970s. Dr. Keats questioned the assignment of blame for anesthesia mortality to one individual of a group when three complex and interrelated variables (anesthesia, surgery, and patient condition) coexist [51]. Dr. Cooper stoked the anesthesia mortality controversy by suggesting that the process of errors needed to be studied, not mortality rates. His landmark paper applied critical incident analysis from military aviation to anesthesia [52]. Most of the critical events discovered were labeled "near misses." Cooper's group followed up with a multi-institutional prospective study of error, based on data learned from the retrospective analysis at their hospital [53, 54]. Pierce's department was one of the four initial collaborators. Many safety features of modern anesthesia machines can be traced to incidents described in these reports. Collection of this type of information would finally become a national initiative almost 30 years later with the formation of the Anesthesia Quality Institute (AQI). The AQI was chartered by the ASA House of Delegates in Oct 2008 [55]. Its central purpose is to collect and distribute data about clinical outcomes in anesthesiology through the National Anesthesia Clinical Outcomes Registry (NACOR).

By 1982, Pierce had advanced to the position of first vice president of the American Society of Anesthesiologists (ASA). Public interest in anesthesia safety exploded with the April 22 airing of the 20/20 television segment titled "Deep Sleep, 6,000 Will Die or Suffer Brain Damage." His immediate response was to establish the ASA Committee on Patient Safety and Risk Management. One accomplishment of this committee was the production of educational patient safety videotapes.

Dr. Pierce continued his efforts in the field of patient safety after becoming ASA president. He recognized that an independent entity was necessary because a global and multidisciplinary composition essential to a comprehensive safety enterprise was not compatible with ASA structure and regulations. In 1984, Pierce hosted the International Symposium on Anesthesia Morbidity and Mortality with Jeffrey Cooper and Richard Kitz. The major product of this meeting was the foundation of the APSF in 1985 with Pierce as its first leader. The APSF provided significant help to the simulation pioneers of the 1980s. One of the four inaugural APSF research grants was awarded to David Gaba, MD, and titled "Evaluation of Anesthesiologist Problem Solving Using Realistic Simulations" [50]. The APSF also organized and held the first simulation meeting in 1988 and a simulation curriculum meeting in 1989. The second significant product of this inaugural meeting was the start of the Anesthesia Closed Claims Project the following year [56]. Pierce was instrumental in persuading malpractice carriers to open their files for study. Early reports from this project spurred the adoption of respiratory monitoring as part of national standard [57].

Dr. Pierce was asked to present the 34th annual Rovenstine lecture at the annual ASA meeting in 1995. He titled that speech "40 Years Behind the Mask: Safety Revisited." He concluded the talk with this admonition: "Patient Safety is not a fad. It is not a preoccupation of the past. It is not an objective that has been fulfilled or a problem that has been solved. Patient safety is an ongoing necessity. It must be sustained by research, training, and daily application in the workplace" [50]. He acknowledged that economic pressures would bring a new era of threats to safety through production pressure and cost containment. His vision of the APSF as an agency that focuses on education and advocacy for patient safety endures, pursuing the goal that "no patient shall be harmed by anesthesia."

A *Partial* History of Partial Task Trainers and Partial Mannequins

The development and proliferation of medical task trainers is not as well chronicled in the medical literature as it is for high-fidelity simulators. The number of words devoted to each device reflects the amount of public information available about the products not their successes and value in medical education. The current vendors are summarized in Table 2.1. In part the military and World War II can be credited for an accelerated use and development of plastic and synthetic materials that are fundamental to the development

Table 2.1 Partial task trainer vendors

Company	Country of origin	Classic products	Founding date
Partial task trainer manufacturers			
3B Scientific	Germany	Various	1948
Adam Rouilly	UK	Various	1918
Cardionics	USA	Auscultation simulator	
Gaumard Scientific	USA	Birthing simulators	1949
Laerdal	Norway	Resusci Annie and family	1940s
Limbs and Things	UK	Various	1990
Schallware	Germany	Ultrasound	
Simulab	USA	Various	1994
SOMSO Modelle	Germany	Various	1876

of the current industry. Some of the vendors eventually transitioned to the manufacture of full-scale mannequins or haptic surgical trainers.

Adam Rouilly

Adam Rouilly was founded in London in 1918 by Mr. Adam and Monsieur Guy Rouilly [58]. The initial purpose of the business was to provide real human skeletons for medical education. M. Rouilly stated a preference for the quality of SOMSO (an anatomic model company founded 1876 in Sonneberg) products as early as 1927. These models are still commercially available today from Holt Medical. Their models were the only ones distributed by Adam Rouilly. The Bedford nursing doll was the result of collaboration between M. Rouilly and Miss Bedford, a London nursing instructor. This 1931 doll was life size with jointed limbs, a paper-mache head, real hair, and realistic glass eyes. This fabric model would be replaced by more realistic and durable plastic ones in the 1950s. In 1980, they launched the Infusion Arm Trainer for military training.

Gaumard Scientific

The British surgeon who founded Gaumard Scientific had experience with new plastic materials from the battlefield [59, 60]. In 1946, he discovered a peacetime use for them in the construction of task trainers, beginning with a skeleton. Gaumard released their first birthing simulator, the transparent obstetric phantom, in 1949. The product line was expanded in 1955 to include other human and animal 3D anatomic models. Their rescue breathing and cardiac massage mannequin debuted in 1960. It featured an IV arm, GU catheterization, and colonic irrigation. Their 1970 female nursing simulator added dilating pupils. Additional GYN simulators were added in 1975–1990 for basic physical exam, endoscopy, and laparoscopic surgery. In 2000, Gaumard entered the arena of full-scale electronic mannequin simulators with the birth of Noelle®. Although Gaumard offers a varied product line, their origin and unique niche centers on the female reproductive system (see Table 2.2).

Table 2.2 Evolution of mannequin simulation

	CAE-Link	Gaumard	Laerdal	METI	Other
1960			Resusci Annie®		
1967					Sim One
1968					Harvey®
1986	CASE 0.5				
1988	CASE 1.2			GAS	
1990					PatSim
1992	CAE-Link				Leiden
1993					Sophus
1994				Loral-GAS	ACCESS
1995	CASE 2.0	Code Blue III ®			
1996				METI HPS®	
1997	MedSim-Eagle				
1999	UltraSim®			PediaSim®	
2000		Noelle® Noelle® S560	SimMan®		
2001				ECS®	TraumaMan®
2002		PEDI®			
2003		Premie		ExanSim®	
2004		HAL® S3000		BabySim®	
2005					
2006		Noelle® S555 and S565	SimBaby®		
2007		Noelle® S575		iStan	
2008		PediatricHAL® PremieHAL®	SimMan 3G®		
2009			SimNewB® ALS PROMPT®	METIMan®	
2010		Susie® S2000			
2011	Acquires METI	HAL® S3201, S1030, and S1020	MamaNatalie® BabyNatalie® SimJunior®	iStan 2®	

Harvey®: The Cardiopulmonary Patient Simulator

Harvey® debuted at the University of Miami in 1968. Dr. Michael Gordon's group received two early patents for the Cardiac Training Mannequin. Gordon named the mannequin after his mentor at Georgetown, Dr. W. Proctor Harvey. Harvey was recognized as a master-teacher-clinician and received the James B. Herrick Award from the American Heart Association [61]. The first Harvey was patent # 3,662,076 which was entered on April 22, 1970 and granted on May 9, 1972 [62]. The arguments for the device included the haphazard and incomplete training afforded by reliance on patient encounters. The inventors desired to provide superior and predictable training with a realistic mannequin that could display cardiac diseases on command. Students could assess heart beat, pulses, and respirations. Multiple pulse locations were incorporated at clinically important locations including right ventricle, left ventricle, aorta, pulmonary artery, carotids, and jugular vein. Audible heart sounds were synchronized with the pulses. Michael Poylo received a separate patent 3,665,087 for the interactive audio system on May 23, 1972 [63]. A description of the development of the "Cardiology Patient Simulator" appeared in *The American Journal of Cardiology* a few months after the patent was issued [64]. Normal and abnormal respiratory patterns were later integrated.

The second Harvey was patent # 3,947,974 which was submitted on May 23, 1974 and granted on April 6, 1976 [65]. This patent improved the auscultation system and added a blood pressure measurement system. A special stethoscope with a magnetic head activated reed switches to initiate tape loops of heart sounds related to the stethoscope location. A representation of 50 disease states, natural aging, and papillary reaction was proposed. Six academic centers in addition to the University of Miami participated in the early testing of this simulator. Their experience with the renamed Harvey® simulator was reported in 1980 [66]. An early study documented the efficacy of Harvey® as a training tool. Harvey® would be progressively refined and improved over the next three decades. The impact of a supplemental comprehensive computer-based instructional curriculum, UMedic, was first described in 1990 [67]. Harvey's most recent patent was granted on Jan 8, 2008 [68]. The Michael S. Gordon Center for Research in Medical Education asserts that "Harvey® is the oldest continuous university-based simulation project in medical education" [69]. The current Harvey® Cardiopulmonary Patient Simulator is available from Laerdal.

The Laerdal Company

The Laerdal company was founded in the 1940s by Asmund S. Laerdal [70]. Initially their products included greeting cards, children's books, wooden and later plastic toys and dolls. In 1958, Laerdal became interested in the process of resuscitation after being approached by two anesthesiologists, Dr. Bjorn Lind and Dr. Peter Safar, to build a tool for the practice of airway and resuscitation skills [71]. Laerdal developed the first doll designed to practice mouth-to-mouth resuscitation that would become known worldwide as Resusci Annie. The inspiration for Resusci Annie's face came from a famous European death mask of a young girl who drowned in the Seine in the 1890s. When Resusci Annie was launched commercially in 1960, Laerdal also changed the company logo to the current recognizable image of the Good Samaritan to reflect the transition of Laerdal's focus and mission. The Laerdal company expanded their repertoire of resuscitation devices and trainers for the next 40 years. More sophisticated Resusci Annies were sequentially added to the line including Recording Resusci Annie, Skillmeter Resusci Annie, and the smaller personal-sized Mini Annie. The Laerdal Foundation for Acute Medicine was founded in 1980 to provide funds for research related to resuscitation. In 2000, Laerdal purchased Medical Plastics Laboratories and entered the arena of full-scale computerized simulation with the launch of SimMan®.

Limbs and Things

Margot Cooper, a medical illustrator from the UK, founded Limbs and Things in 1990 [72]. The company's first products were dynamic models of the spine and foot. Their first soft tissue models were launched the following year. Their first joint injection model (the shoulder) and their first hysteroscopy simulator debuted in 1992. The following year, Limbs and Things was granted its first patent for simulated skin and its method of casting the synthetic into shapes. In 1994, Dr. Roger Kneebone first demonstrated Limbs and Things products at a meeting of the Royal College of General Practitioners (RCGP) in London. That same year, the Bodyform laparoscopic trainer debuted and the company received its first Frank H. Netter Award for contributions to medical education. In 1997 Limbs and Things entered the realm of surgical simulation and progressively expanded their product line to include a complete basic surgical skills course package. A 1999 award-winning surgical trainer featured a pulsatile heart. The PROMPT® birthing simulator and training course first appeared in 2006 and was recognized with the company's second Netter Award in 2009. The Huddleston ankle/foot nerve block trainer was introduced in 2010.

There are four additional companies that design and manufacture medical trainers for which minimal historical data is publically available. Simulab Corporation was founded in 1994. It offers a large variety of trainers and simulators. Its best-known product, TraumaMan®, first appeared in 2001. It was quickly adopted as the standard for training in the national Advanced Trauma Life Support course replacing live animals. Cardionics markets itself as the "leader in auscultation." They offer digital heart and breath sound trainers and the Student Auscultation Mannequin (SAM II). SAM II is an integrated torso for auscultation using the student's own stethoscope.

Two smaller German companies are gaining notoriety for their trainer development. The modern 3B corporation was founded in 1948 in Hamburg by three members of the Binhold family. In 1993, 3B Scientific Europe acquired one of its predecessors known for manufacturing medical trainers for almost 200 years ago in Budapest, Hungary. The company transitioned into the world of simulation in 1997, and globalization is well underway. The newer Schallware company produces ultrasound training simulators. They offer three partial mannequins for imaging the abdomen, the pregnant uterus, and the heart.

The History of Mannequin Simulators or a Tale of Two Universities and Three Families of Mannequins

In the same time period that Dr. Barrows was revolutionizing medical education and evaluation and Dr. Cooper was injecting principles of critical incidents and human factors into the discussions of anesthesia safety, Dr. N. Ty Smith and Dr. Yasuhiro Fukui began to develop computer models of human physiology and pharmacodynamics. The first drug they modeled was the uptake and distribution of halothane. This early model used 18 compartments and 88 equations [73]. The effect of ventilation mode and CO_2 was studied in a second paper [74]. Addition of a clinical content and interface accompanied the modeling of nitroprusside [75]. These models were the basis for three future commercial simulation projects. Drs. Smith and Sebald described Sleeper in 1989 [76]. This product would evolve into body simulation product (BODY™) of the 1990s and beyond.

Dr. Schwid, one of Dr. Smith's fellows from UCSD, would simplify the models so that they could run on a small personal computer. An abstract from their 1986 collaboration describes the first software-based complete anesthesia simulator [77]. A crude graphic display of the anesthesia environment facilitated virtual anesthesia care. A more detailed report of this achievement appeared the next year in a computing journal not necessarily accessed by physicians [78]. Dr. Schwid introduced the precursor of the Anesoft line of software products, the Anesthesia Simulator Consultant (ASC), also in 1989. Early experience with ASC documented the efficacy of this tool for practicing critical incident management [79–81]. A detailed product review recommended the costly software but stated there were some difficulties with navigation and there was room for improvement of realism [82]. A review of Schwid's second product, the Critical Care Simulator, was not so flattering. The reviewer described many deficiencies and concluded that only the very inexperienced would find any benefit. He recommended that experienced doctors would get more value from the study of traditional textbooks [83]. Today the Anesthesia Simulator and the Critical Care Simulator are two of ten products offered by Anesoft, and over 400,000 units have been sold.

Pioneers and Profiles: A Personal Memoir by Howard A. Schwid

When I was 12 years old, an episode of the TV series Mission Impossible had a profound effect on me. In this episode the IMF team made a leader of a foreign country believe he was on a moving train by putting him in a train car-sized box that rocked back and forth, had movies of scenery playing through glass panels on the sides of the box, and had the appropriate sound effects. It was amazing to me that it was possible to create an artificial environment so real that someone would believe that they were in a moving train when in fact they were in a box in a warehouse. I was hooked on simulation.

A year later, one of the presents I received for my Bar Mitzvah was a radio kit. The kit contained three transistors, an inductor, and dozens of resistors and capacitors. I was fascinated by the concept that a bunch of inert components could be assembled into something that produced music and voices. I hoped to someday learn more about how it worked.

I was lucky to attend a high school in Glendale, Wisconsin, that offered computer programming. In 1972 I took my first programming course via modem time-share access to an early computer, the PDP 11. I quickly became lost in the possibilities. A friend and I spent an entire year teaching a computer to become unbeatable at Qubic, a four-in-a-row three-dimensional tic-tac-toe game. We didn't know the jargon but we were working on the fundamentals of artificial intelligence. Qubic wasn't quite as glamorous as chess but we learned a lot about representing and manipulating data to mimic logical thought processes. One teacher encouraged our efforts, providing us with access to the locked computer room on weekends. I had to hide the Qubic program from my parents because they thought game programming was a waste of time.

In 1974, I entered college at the University of Wisconsin–Madison; I was interested in biomedical engineering. At that time biomedical engineers had to choose electrical, mechanical, or chemical engineering for undergraduate studies. I chose electrical engineering because of my initial fascination with that radio kit and my interest in computers. I also took the required premed courses along with the engineering courses in case I decided to go to medical school. While my engineering friends took electives like geography, I took organic chemistry. And while my premed friends took the easiest electives they could find, I took electromagnetic fields and systems control theory. This is definitely not the easiest way to earn a GPA high enough to get into medical school.

Two college courses really stand out as having a formative effect on my career. The first was Nerve and Muscle Models taught by C. Daniel Geisler. I was fascinated with using the same electrical components I studied in electrical engineering to represent conduction of action potentials in axons. Since Professor Geisler was an auditory physiologist, we also covered mathematical descriptions of the motion of the cochlear membrane. The second course was Mathematical Models of Cardiovascular Physiology taught by Vincent Rideout. In this course we programmed a hybrid analog-digital computer to represent pressures and flows in the cardiovascular system. Much of the course was based on the multiple modeling method of Yasuhiro Fukui.

As a senior in college, I worked under Professor Geisler refining a model of transmission from inner ear hair cell motion to firing of action potentials in cochlear nerve fibers. In theory better understanding of the nonlinear properties of transduction could lead to improved design of cochlear implants. This project involved fine-tuning of model parameters to match observed physiological data, a skill I would later put to use.

I worked a couple summers as a junior electrical engineer designing filters for electronic music keyboards. The work was interesting, but I couldn't see myself working as an engineer for the rest of my career, so I applied to medical school. During the application process, one interview stands out. The interviewer explained to me that an electrical and computer engineer had no business going to medical school because computers had nothing to offer in medicine. I wish I had been better prepared to defend myself.

Fortunately other interviewers were more open-minded, and ultimately I was accepted to several medical schools. I decided to stay in Madison in order to continue work on the auditory physiology project. The first semester of medical school was especially difficult for me. Although I had taken all the prerequisite courses, electrical engineering had not prepared me well for medical school which required a completely different set of skills. To do well on tests, engineering required memorization of only a few key equations but a thorough understanding of the fundamental principles underlying the equations. The preclinical years of medical school, in contrast, emphasized memorization of large amounts of information, a skill I needed to quickly develop. Also, I felt I had learned the principles of cardiovascular physiology better in my engineering classes than in medical school physiology class. In the hybrid computer lab, we could actively manipulate heart rate, preload, afterload, and contractility and observe the results on blood pressures and flow. In medical school those same principles were addressed in lectures and a 2-hour dog lab where the professor demonstrated some of these principles which was unsatisfying by comparison. I thought it would be more useful and engaging for medical students to run their own experiments on a computer using a mathematical model of the cardiovascular system rather than passively observing a dog lab in a lecture hall.

Third year of medical school was the beginning of the clinical years. My first clinical rotation was cardiac surgery where I observed my first patient with an indwelling pulmonary artery catheter. I thought this is what medicine is all about: measure the complete status of the patient, manipulate the physiology, and fix the problem. I was still that naïve engineering student. Over the next few rotations, it became clear that things were more complicated. Physicians are seldom able to measure everything and are often unable to fix the problem.

Like all third-year students, I was trying to decide in a very short period of time and with very little information what area of medicine to pursue in residency. Otolaryngology may have allowed me to continue work on the auditory system, but I didn't have steady enough hands for delicate surgery. I found internal medicine unsatisfying because patients were often sent home with a medication for a problem and may not have follow-up for months. I wanted immediate feedback since my control theory class proved that delays make control difficult.

Fortunately for me, anesthesiology was a required rotation for all medical students at the University of Wisconsin which was not the case at other medical schools. Monitors, dials, infusions, multiple physiologic systems, pharmacology, and immediate feedback, I immediately recognized that I had found my place. I also discovered Eger's uptake and distribution, an area of medicine that could be described by a set of mathematical equations.

As an added bonus, I learned that Professor Rideout had built a uniquely close relationship between the University of Wisconsin Department of Electrical and Computer Engineering and the Department of Anesthesiology through Ben Rusy. In 1982, as a senior in medical school, I was able to start an independent study month developing a digital computer model, written in Fortran, of uptake and distribution of inhalation agents based on previous hybrid computer models of Yasuhiro Fukui and N. Ty Smith. Soon after, I became an anesthesiology resident at the University of Wisconsin, enabling me to continue to work on the model with Rideout and Rusy. By the end of residency, the model contained many of the important factors and interactions essential to delivering anesthesia: cardiovascular system with beating heart, flowing blood and control, respiratory system with gas exchange and control, and pharmacokinetics and dynamics of inhalation and intravenous agents. The model was the simulation engine capable of reasonably predicting simulated patient response to administration of anesthetic agents in a variety of pathophysiological conditions. Like the old Mission Impossible episode, the next step was to build the train car.

Professor Rideout introduced me to N. Ty Smith, the visionary anesthesiologist that added inhalation anesthetics to the Fukui cardiovascular model. In 1985, after completing my anesthesiology residency, I became Ty Smith's fellow at UCSD. We immediately started working with Rediffusion Simulation Incorporated, a flight simulator company that wanted to test the market for medical simulators. In the first months of my fellowship, I worked closely with Charles Wakeland of Rediffusion. We rewrote the physiologic-pharmacologic model in C++ and built a graphical user interface on a Sun workstation with an animated patient and physiological monitor. We created four case scenarios to demonstrate the simulator's capabilities. The simulator was awarded Best Instructional Exhibit at the 1985 New York State Society of Anesthesiologists Postgraduate Assembly.

To my knowledge, Rediffusion did not pursue medical simulation despite the warm reception to our prototype. During my fellowship year, I interviewed for full-time faculty positions which would allow me to continue the development of medical simulation. I met with the chairs of several highly respected academic anesthesiology departments. Most believed there was no future in medical simulation, and some even went so far as to counsel me to do something else with my career. Tom Hornbein, chair of the University of Washington Department of Anesthesiology and the first climber along with his partner to conquer the West Ridge of Mount Everest, explained that my chosen academic career path was riskier than many of the faculty he hired, but he agreed to give me a chance. I didn't see much risk because building the simulator was the main goal of my academic career. If I failed in this career path, I could have switched to private practice anesthesiology. Earlier that year, Charles Wakeland observed that I had the "fatal fascination": that I could not stop working on this project, no matter what the consequences. He was right. Luckily I had a supportive wife who also understood that I needed to complete the project. The difference in salary between academics and private practice was acceptable since academic practice would provide nonclinical time to get this idea out of my head.

In 1986 I became a full-time faculty member of the University of Washington. My research time was devoted to continuing development of the simulation program. I viewed long-term funding as the biggest hurdle. At that time I was unable to find any grants for medical simulation so I decided to generate money the old-fashioned way—earn it. Since I wanted to build a useful product, I would have the marketplace validate the significance of the project through sales of the final product. I decided to form a company which would market and sell my simulation programs. The funds generated would be used for further development. Discussions with my chair and the University of Washington Office of Technology Transfer were successful, and Anesoft Corporation was formed in 1987.

As it turned out, the prototype anesthesia simulator built with Rediffusion was not being used due to the large expense of Sun workstations. My next goal was to make the anesthesia simulator program work on existing personal computers with no added hardware, making it more affordable and opening it up to a wider audience. Anesoft initially started selling three educational programs for cardiovascular physiology and hemodynamic monitoring and operated under DOS. By 1988, with sales of Anesoft programs and the assistance of a grant from the Anesthesia Patient Safety Foundation, I was fortunate to be able to hire a programmer, Dan O'Donnell. Dan had just completed his master's work in computer graphics and had a previous doctorate in mathematics. Dan was exactly what was needed for the project at that time. In the next few years, we were able to add many new features to the anesthesia simulator program including finite-state machine programming to handle model discontinuities for critical incident simulation, automated case recording (Anesthesia Simulator-Recorder), and on-line help with automated debriefing and scoring (Anesthesia Simulator Consultant). Soon we dropped the word consultant and simply called the program Anesthesia Simulator.

In the early 1990s, sales of the Anesoft Anesthesia Simulator grew rapidly. The customer base was exactly the opposite of what we had expected. We thought medical schools would purchase the programs first, followed by residency training programs, followed by hospitals and individual anesthesiologists and nurse anesthetists. Interestingly, anesthesiologists and nurse anesthetists in private practice purchased the most copies. A number of hospitals purchased the software for their medical library for use by their clinicians, but few residency programs and even fewer medical schools made purchases.

Also in the early 1990s, another flight simulator company, CAE-Link, became interested in testing the medical simulation market. They combined their engineering expertise with David Gaba's CASE simulator from Stanford, some of our mathematical models, and Jeff Cooper's insight into human factors and anesthesia critical incidents. The result was a prototype mannequin with breathing, pulses, and appropriate cardiorespiratory responses to administrated drugs and fluids. Our main concern was to distinguish our computerized mannequin from Sim One, the first computer-controlled, full-scale patient simulator, developed by Abrahamson and Denson in 1969. Sim One was technically quite sophisticated, but its purpose was stated to be improvement of anesthesiology resident training concerning induction of anesthesia. We believed the reason that use of Sim One did not spread beyond its institution of development was that its stated scope of application was too narrow. We thought the broader purpose of training for the management of critical incidents would allow our simulator to succeed. We built the simulator with this purpose in mind. Ultimately the CAE-Link Patient Simulator lost out to the METI Human Patient Simulator originally developed by the team in Gainesville, Florida.

Meanwhile, Anesoft continues to grow with sales now totaling about 500,000 registered installations. The current product line includes ten screen-based simulation programs covering a wide variety of medical specialties containing almost 200 cases in the library of prewritten case scenarios contributed by dozens of medical experts. The programs have been translated into multiple languages and are in use in almost every country in the world. Anesoft now develops and sells medical simulation programs for multiple platforms including Windows computers, Macintosh computers, iPhone, iPad, Android phones and tablets, and Windows phones. Many of the programs operate on the web and are compatible with institutional learning management systems.

There are several factors that have contributed to Anesoft's success. First is the explosion of computer technology that has occurred since the company was formed in 1987. Remember that IBM did not introduce the PC until 1981. In 1987 it was still a fantasy to think that almost everyone would have a computer sitting on his desktop. In the 1990s came the internet with phenomenal growth of access to digital content. Now we are experiencing a tidal wave of mobile-computing capability with smartphones and tablets. The devices people now carry in their pockets are much more powerful than the desktop computers that ran our first version of the anesthesia simulator.

The second factor that contributed to Anesoft's growth is the overall expansion of the interest in simulation in the healthcare community. The Institute of Medicine report "To Err is Human" showed that errors are common, emphasizing improved training for teamwork and patient safety. The report supported the idea that medical simulation may reduce errors through improved training. Furthermore there are now new societies, journals, books, conferences, and even a few grants devoted to simulation in healthcare. It is a much better time to be in the healthcare simulation field than 1982 when I started working on the digital model of cardiovascular physiology.

Mannequins were under development in independent projects at two US universities in the late 1980s. Did the visionary developers from Stanford and the University of Florida at Gainesville realize that they were on the brink of launching disruptive technology and systems at that time? Now that healthcare simulation is past the tipping point, arguments for the noble cause of simulation are unnecessary. The developers of modern healthcare simulation recognized the power and potential of this new methodology decades before the general public. Dr. David Gaba reviewed the status of simulation in a 2004 article and delivers two possible versions of the future based on whether simulation actually reaches its tipping point [84]. See Table 2.2 for a timeline of the development of mannequin simulators.

In Northern California, the Comprehensive Anesthesia Simulation Environment (CASE) mannequin system prototype appeared in 1986 titled CASE 0.5. An updated version CASE 1.2 was used for training and research in 1987. This 1.2 prototype used a stock mannequin torso "Eddie Endo" from Armstrong Industries. The CASE 1.2 added physiologic monitoring which had not been available on Sim One partly because monitoring was not yet standard in that era. The physiologic simulators of ECG, invasive blood pressure, temperature, and oximetry displayed patient data on a Marquette monitor. Eddie had been modified to demonstrate metabolic production of CO_2. A mass spectrometer was used to measure output of CO_2 from the lungs. The simulator had breath sounds and produced clinically relevant pressures when ventilated with the Ohmeda Modulus II® anesthesia machine. Noninvasive blood pressure was emulated on a Macintosh computer to resemble the output of a Datascope Accutorr. Urine output and fluid infusion were also shown with inexpensive catheter systems [85]. An essential characteristic of this project was the staging of exercises in a real operating room to mimic all facets of critical incidents [86]. A variety of conditions and challenges were scripted from non-life-threatening minor equipment failures or changes in physiology to major physiologic aberrations or even critical incidents. This prototype was considered to be inexpensive in comparison to flight simulators, only $15,000. Many of the future applications of simulation in healthcare are accurately forecast by both Gaba and Gravenstein's accompanying editorials [86, 87]. They both acknowledge the power of the technology and the high cost of training. They predicted that personnel effort will cost much more over time than the initial investment in hardware and software.

Twenty-two residents and/or medical students participated in CASE 1.2 training exercises in this initial study [88]. Seventeen of 72 returned feedback about the experience. They rated the experience on a scale of 1–10 for realism. Items scored included case presentation, anesthesia equipment, instrument readings, response to drug administration, physiologic responses, simulated critical incidents, and mannequin. Most items received scores between 8 and 9 except for the mannequin. They downgraded the mannequin to 4.4 overall for being cold, monotone in color, lacking heart sounds, having no spontaneous ventilation/difficult mask ventilation, missing limbs, and therefore peripheral pulses.

The next generation of the Stanford's simulator CASE 2.0 would incorporate physiologic models from the ASC and a full-body mannequin. Dr. Gaba's interests in simulation, patient safety, human factors, and critical incident training converged when he took a sabbatical and brought CASE 2.0 and his innovative Anesthesia Crisis Resource Management (ACRM) curriculum to Boston for a series of seminars with Harvard faculty. ACRM extracted principles of Aviation Crew (Cockpit) Resource Management to the management of critical medical incidents. The ACRM concept was progressively refined and explained in detail in the 1994 textbook titled *Crisis Management in Anesthesiology* [89]. This collaboration led to the establishment of the first simulation center outside of a developing university in Boston in 1993. That early center in Boston has become the present-day Center for Medical Simulation (CMS) [90].

Pioneers and Profiles: A Personal Memoir by David Gaba

Over 26 years ago, I began my work on simulation in healthcare. The genesis of this work and its path may be of interest to some. I got into simulation from the standpoint of patient safety, not—initially—from the standpoint of education. First, I had a background in biomedical engineering, but my interests in engineering school trended toward what I labeled (for my custom-created area of specialization) "high-level information processing." This included studies in what then passed for "artificial intelligence" (including learning 2 arcane programming languages LISP and SNOBOL) as well as a course in human factors engineering. I also realized that my interests in biomedical engineering focused more on the clinical aspects than on the engineering aspects. Hence, I confirmed my desire to go to medical school rather than pursue an engineering PhD. Anesthesia was a natural home for engineers in medicine. Nonetheless, my MD thesis research was on the adverse effects of electric countershock (e.g., defibrillation) on the heart, and upon joining the faculty at Stanford, I quickly took up this same research thread in the animal lab. At the same time, I was interested in—like most anesthesiologists—how we could best safeguard our patients. The Anesthesia Patient Safety Foundation (APSF) was just being formed. In 1984 I read the book Normal Accidents [1] by Charles Perrow, who was the only social scientist (a Yale sociologist) on the Kemeny Commission that investigated the Three Mile Island nuclear power plant accident. Out of this experience, Perrow developed a theory of how accidents emerged from the banal conditions of everyday operations, especially in industries that combined tight coupling with complexity. As I read the book, with every turn of the page I said "this is just like anesthesia." I had my research fellow Mary Maxwell, MD, and my lab medical student, Abe DeAnda, read the book, and we talked about it. From that came a seminal paper applying some of Perrow's ideas and many of our own, to a discussion of Breaking the Chain of Accident Evolution in Anesthesia, published in 1987 in *Anesthesiology* [2]. Perrow had detailed many case studies of famous accidents, delineating

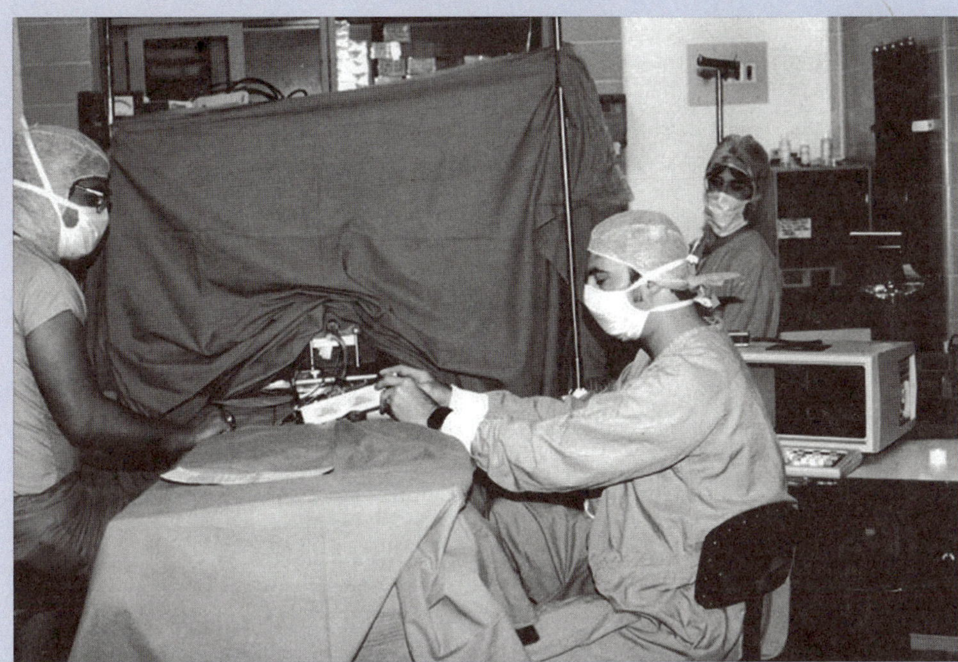

Fig. 1 The pre-prototype "CASE 0.5" simulator, May 1986. Dr. Gaba (*center right*) operates an off-the-shelf clinical waveform generator. The Compaq computer behind him is used to send information to the noninvasive blood pressure "virtual machine" created on a Macintosh 512K computer in the anesthesia work area. Dr. Mary Maxwell (research fellow) is the scenario "hot-seat" participant (*back right*). Medical student Abe DeAnda Jr. (*left*) assists Dr. Gaba with the scenario. © 1986, David M. Gaba, MD

the decisions made by the operators at various stages in the timeline. We were similarly interested in how anesthesiologists made decisions in the dynamic setting of the operating room. Working in the animal lab, we said, "hmm… maybe we can bring people here, make bad things happen [to the dog] and see how the anesthesiologists respond." But we thought that this would be hard to control; animals weren't cheap and it would take time to get them prepared for the experiments, and the animal rights people wouldn't like it (although the animals would already be anesthetized and wouldn't know a thing about it). So, we said "you know…. We need a simulator." I was familiar with simulators in concept from my love of aviation and space (I had audiotaped the TV coverage of all the Apollo missions). We looked around and there really were no simulators for anesthesia (not counting "Resusci Annie"). Without the Internet (in about 1985), it was difficult for us to search older literature. Thus, we were completely unaware about the developments in the late 1960s of a mannequin-based simulator at USC—Sim One—by Abrahamson and Denson [3, 4]. Since both Abe and I were engineers, instead of giving up we said, "well… maybe we can MAKE our own simulator." So, in 1985 that's what we set out to do.

We knew that biomedical engineers had waveform generators they used to test monitors, so we borrowed one. And, because the modern pulse oximeter had been developed nearby by former and current Stanford anesthesia faculty, we were able to cadge an oximetry test "stimulator" from Nellcor. For the noninvasive blood pressure, we had no idea of how to stimulate such a device, so we opted to create a virtual device (programmed in APL on a Macintosh 512K computer) that appeared to perform the NIBP function (complete with clicks as the cuff pressure descended to a new plateau on the stepped deflation). This was fed data in string form (e.g., "S101/D77/H75") typed into a Compaq ("sewing machine" style) portable computer. We borrowed an Ambu intubation trainer (the one with a cutaway neck so students could see the angles of the airway) and lengthened the trachea with an endotracheal tube and made a "lung" from a reservoir bag from an anesthesia breathing circuit kit. These parts were cobbled together to allow us to perform the first "pre-prototype" simulation scenario (Fig. 1).

Mary was the test anesthesiologist unaware of the scenario, which was a pneumothorax during general anesthesia for laparotomy. After a period of normal vital signs, we partially clamped the endotracheal tube "trachea" (raising the peak inspiratory pressures), began dropping the SaO_2 (with the Nellcor stimulator), progressively lowered the blood pressure (sending strings to the NIBP), and manipulated the waveform generator to increase the heart rate of the ECG. During all this, we recorded Mary's think-out-loud utterances with a portable tape recorder. Later we transcribed the tape and analyzed qualitatively the cognitive processes used to diagnose and treat the problem. So went the very first simulation in our work.

Fortunately at that time, the APSF announced its first round of patient safety grant funding. I applied, proposing not only to build a simulator based on this pre-prototype but also to conduct a study of the effect of fatigue on the performance of anesthesiologists—and all for only $35,000! The grant reviews were very positive (I still have a copy!) and we won a grant. We did make good on the first promise within a year, but the fatigue study had to wait another 10 years to finally happen.

The first real simulator was built in 1987 and 1988. It used an off-the-shelf mannequin with a head, neck, and thorax (and two elastic lung bags). We added tiny tubing to carry CO_2 into the lungs (with hand stopcocks and a manual flowmeter to control the flow) and placed a pulmonary artery catheter into each main-stem bronchus. Inflating the balloon would occlude the bronchus, allowing us to mimic pneumothorax and endobronchial intubation. We got a much more powerful waveform generator that provided ECG and all invasive pressures. More importantly, it was controlled from a keypad connected by an RS232 port. Thus, we could have our main computer tell it what to do. There was little control over the amplitude of the invasive pressures, so Abe hand built a 3-channel digitally controlled analog amplifier based on a design I found in a hobbyist book on electronics. This let us scale the basic invasive waveforms to our target values. The Nellcor stimulator could also be controlled over a serial port. We kept our virtual NIBP on the Mac 512K. We then wrote software (in a very arcane language ASYST) to control all the separate pieces and used a (novel for the time) serial port extender to allow us to address three different serial ports. Three clinical devices showed the heart rate—so any heart rate changes had to show up on all of them. Again, we fed data to the main computer as text strings. O98/H55/S88/D44 would make the O_2 sat 98%, the heart rate (on three devices) 55, and the BP 88/44 (on both the NIBP and arterial line—if one was present). In those days we had to keep the control desk with all the components and the main computer (a PC286) in the OR with the simulator mannequin and the participant. A tank of CO_2 at the end of the table fed the CO_2 to the mannequin's lungs. The anesthesiologist could perform most functions normally on the mannequin. Though the participant could easily see us controlling the simulator, it didn't seem to make much difference.

We needed a name for the simulator. After discarding some humorous risqué suggestions, we picked the acronym CASE for Comprehensive Anesthesia Simulation Environment. The first everyday system was called CASE 1.2. In 1988 we published a paper in *Anesthesiology* [5] describing CASE 1.2, providing questionnaire data from early participants, and—at the direction of the editor agreeing to provide a packet of design data—sketches and source code to any credible investigator who asked for it. A few did. At least one other simulator was created using elements of the information that we provided (but not the one that would turn out to be the main "competition"). Periodically I would see a simulator using exactly the same approach and components that we used—without attribution. Whether this was independent convergent evolution or idea theft was never determined.

Because of our interest in the problem solving of anesthesiologists, we first used CASE 1.2 not for education and training but rather to do a set of experiments with subjects of differing levels of experience in anesthesiology, each managing a standard test case in which multiple sequential abnormal events were embedded. We studied early first year residents (PGY1—in those days the residency was only 2 years), second year residents, faculty, and private practice anesthesiologists (Fig. 2).

Three papers came out of those experiments. This time *Anesthesiology* failed to grasp the importance of these studies; thus, all three papers appeared in *Anesthesia & Analgesia* [6–8]. The bottom line from these studies was that (a) different kinds of problems were easier or harder to detect or to correct, (b) more experienced people on the whole did better than less experienced people, but (c) the early PGY1s did pretty well and there was a least one case of a catastrophic failure in every experience group. This told us that both early learners and experienced personnel could use more training and practice in handling anomalous situations and also reinforced the notion that—like pilots—they could benefit from an "emergency procedures manual," a "cognitive aid."

We also began thinking more about the problem-solving processes in real cases. I looked at my mentors, faculty in my program who embodied the "cool in a crisis." At the same time, we discovered the fairly newly evolving story of Cockpit Resource Management training in commercial aviation, focusing not on "stick-and-rudder" skills of flying the airplane but on making decisions and managing all team and external resources. In February 1987, the PBS science show NOVA aired an episode called "Why Planes Crash." Not only did it have a simulator reenactment of an infamous airliner crash (Eastern 401), it also talked a lot about CRM and featured a NASA psychologist working at NASA's Ames Research Center—just down the road from us in Mountain View, CA. CRM's focus on decision making and teamwork seemed to be just what we could see we needed in anesthesiology. I went to talk to the Ames people and had a great discussion, and they gave some written materials [9]. From this was born our second grant application to

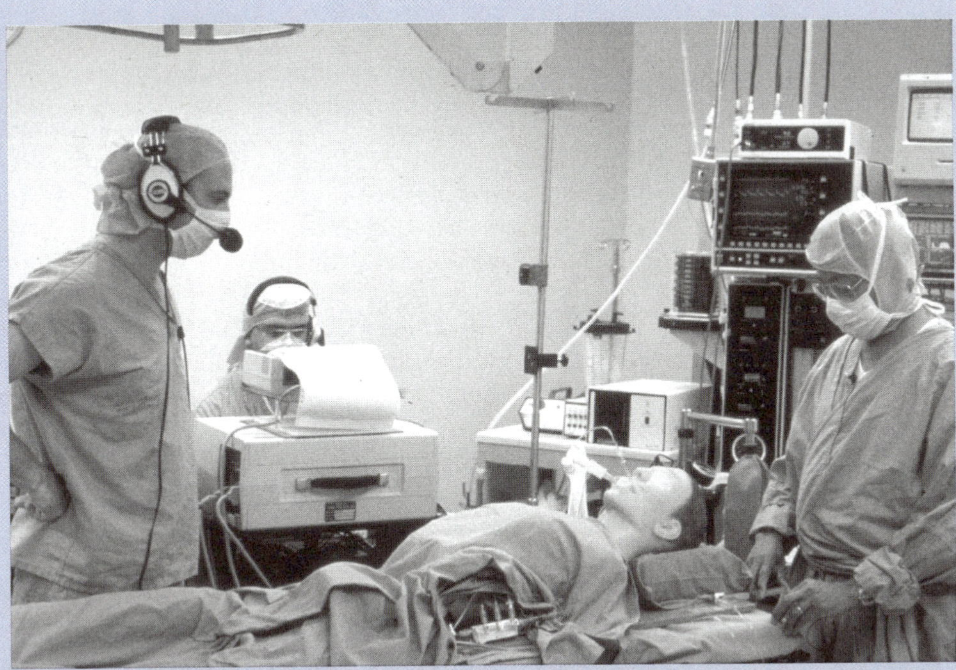

Fig. 2 The CASE 1.2 simulator in use, 1989. Dr. Gaba runs a scenario in the study of cognition of anesthesiologists at different levels of training with an attending anesthesiologist as the subject. Medical student Abe DeAnda Jr. operates the simulation equipment. © 1989, David M. Gaba, MD

APSF in which we proposed to develop an analog training course for anesthesiologists to be called Anesthesia Crisis Resource Management (ACRM—since no one in anesthesia knew what a "crew" was). This proposal was also successful. During 1989 and early 1990, we prepared a course syllabus, one component of which was a Catalog of Critical Incidents in Anesthesia—to mimic the pilots' manual of emergency procedures (this later grew into our textbook *Crisis Management in Anesthesiology* [10], published in 1994). We developed didactic materials and a set of four simulation scenarios. From aviation CRM, we learned that debriefing after simulation was important. As experienced clinical teachers, we figured we knew how to do that. Luckily, we turned out to be right.

We held the first ACRM course in September 1990 (more than 22 years ago!) for 12 anesthesia residents (CA2 residents as I recall). In those days we took the simulator to a real OR for the weekend (the first "in situ simulations"!). ACRM was a grueling 2-day affair. Day one was didactics and group work. Day two was simulations for three groups of four each, one group after the other. Each group did all four scenarios and then went off (with their videotape) to debrief with one of the three instructors. Besides me, I chose my two mentors Kevin Fish and Frank Sarnquist as the debriefers. That was a long day! The first evaluations were very positive. The second ACRM course was held in December 1990 for 12 experienced anesthesiologists—faculty and private practitioners. Even from this seasoned group, it got rave reviews (and as in our study before, a spectrum of performance good to bad even amongst anesthesia professionals).

Between 1990 and 1992, we started to create a second-generation patient simulator (CASE 2.0). John Williams, another medical student with an engineering background (BS and MS in Electrical Engineering from MIT), joined the team. John was a genius. Based on existing literature, he created a full cardiovascular model that moved mathematical blood around the body from chambers (with a volume and elastance) through various conduits (with a volume and conductance). The cardiovascular model iterated approximately 200 times per second (5-ms update time). Waveforms were generated in real time as the pressure could be inferred from the volume of mathematical blood in a chamber or conduit with a known elastance or conductance. The ECG was modeled from a rhythm library (although I myself started experimenting with network models that could generate different cardiac rhythms de novo). The CASE 2.0 simulator had the cardiovascular model running on a special chip—a "transputer"—hosted on a board in a Macintosh computer. Transputers were made for parallel processing—one could easily add additional transputers to speed processing, but in the end, this feature was never utilized.

Several events helped to foster and spread the ACRM paradigm and simulation. The APSF was petitioned by both our group and the University of Florida Gainesville group (Nik Gravenstein Senior, Mike Good, and Sem Lampotang et al. also working on simulation) for further support to sustain research and development of "anesthesia simulation" until commercial manufacturers for simulators could be found. The APSF Executive Committee made a site visit to each of these groups in 1991. The site visit to Stanford had the committee observe an actual ACRM course. Based on that experience, Jeff Cooper, PhD, took the concept to the (then five) Harvard anesthesia programs and formed a group to explore pursuing ACRM simulation training for residents from these sites. This led to a task force of anesthesiologists from the Harvard programs coming to VA Palo Alto (Stanford) to "take" an ACRM course in 1991. Based on a very positive experience, the decision was made for the Harvard anesthesia programs to sponsor me to come to Boston, with my simulator (there were no commercially available devices at that time), for 3 months in fall of 1992 during my first sabbatical. I taught (with assistance at the beginning from Steve Howard and John Williams) 18 ACRM courses for residents, faculty, and CRNAs and in the process trained a cadre of Harvard anesthesiologists (and Jeff) to be ACRM instructors [11]. This cadre went on to found the Boston Anesthesia Simulation Center (BASC) which later morphed into the Center for Medical Simulation (www.harvardmedsim.org) in Cambridge, MA.

We came back from Boston eager to establish a dedicated simulation center at Stanford. Initial attempts to find a physical site for the center at the Stanford School of Medicine or Stanford Hospital and Clinics proved unsuccessful, but thanks to the efforts of Richard Mazze, MD, then Chief of Staff (and former Chief of Anesthesia) at the VA hospital in Palo Alto—where I was a staff anesthesiologist and associate professor—we were able to obtain space in a modular building at the VA that had housed a temporary diagnostic radiology center. In 1995 the simulation center at VAPAHCS was born, and shortly thereafter we conducted the first instructor training course, using a syllabus designed jointly by personnel from BASC and from the simulation center at University of Toronto. This collaboration assisted each other in planning and conducting simulation training for a few years. My colleague Kevin Fish spent a sabbatical at University of Toronto as well.

In 1992 we began negotiations with representatives from CAE-Link, a division of CAE, a large Canadian conglomerate. CAE itself produced flight simulators for the civil market. CAE-Link produced only military flight simulators and was the descendent of the Link Corporation, the first manufacturer of commercial flight simulators (dating back to the late 1920s and early 1930s) (www.link.com/history.html). CAE-Link was looking for new markets after the collapse of the Soviet Union and the democratization of the countries of Eastern Europe. CAE-Link's files contained prior suggestions of the use of simulators for healthcare, but in 1992 they surveyed the literature in the field and found us. The deal was consummated that year. Originally, CAE-Link produced a nearly exact copy of CASE 2.0 for a Belgian client, but then they along with John Williams and me and Howard Schwid, assistant professor of anesthesia from University of Washington, combined forces to develop the software and hardware for the first commercial simulator from CAE-Link. Howard had developed on-screen simulators for anesthesia (and later other fields). CAE-Link used our cardiovascular model (and some of our other models), as well as model's from Schwid for the pulmonary system, other body systems, and pharmacokinetics and pharmacodynamics, as the basis for the math models of the CAE-Link Patient Simulator, which was introduced in 1995. I contributed a number of other design features of this device, especially in the instructor interface. This device was sold around the world. CAE-Link handed the product over to its CAE-Electronics subsidiary and then sold the product line and information to a small simulation company, Eagle Simulation. Eagle later merged with an Israeli company MedSim that already manufactured an ultrasound simulator. The MedSim-Eagle Patient Simulator competed very well on the market, but in the middle of the dot-com boom, the board of directors fired the existing management (which then included Dr. Amitai Ziv) and eventually abandoned the MedSim-Eagle Patient Simulator, probably because they were not making enough return on investment compared to the returns then available in the Internet bubble. This left the entire user community in the lurch with dozens of installed systems around the world. Although three groups (METI, Tokibo—the Japanese distributor—and a group of the Eagle employees) were interested in buying the product line, MedSim-Eagle never entered any serious negotiations, and the product was in fact abandoned by the manufacturer. Users tried to help each other maintain their units, and they bought up retired or abandoned (but functioning) units to acquire spare parts. As I write this, there are still some of these simulators in regular use, more than a decade after the manufacturer stopped supporting them. I contend that this is testament to the sound engineering and manufacturing of these devices. It was, however, a travesty for us financially (Medsim defaulted on license and royalty payments to the inventors) as well as for the simulation community because a really good simulator was lost to the market. For those who recently or still use (d) the CAE-Link/Eagle/MedSim Patient Simulator, can we imagine what it might be like today if it had a further 12 years of engineering development?

Because of this turn of events, my group, which had solely used the CAE-Link/Eagle/MedSim-Eagle simulator, then became a purchaser and user of simulators from many manufacturers. At one time we operated simulators from MedSim-Eagle, METI, and Laerdal simultaneously.

In the last 25 years, much has happened in simulation. The introduction in 2001 of what I call the "medium-capability" simulators that had about 70% of the features of the MedSim-Eagle Patient Simulator or the METI HPS did, but at 15% of the cost, was groundbreaking—qualifying as a "low end disruptive innovation" in the Clay Christensen model [12]—where a less capable but cheaper unit opened huge chunks of the market.

Looking back on it all, I believe there are a number of useful lessons for future investigators. First is that we were an example of a bunch of young engineer/clinicians (faculty and students) who "didn't know any better." At times I was counseled to get senior faculty involved, but they didn't really grasp the idea, and I felt that waiting to find a mentor would just waste time and effort. Perhaps had I joined an existing group of faculty and engineers, we could have accomplished things more systematically. However, my little band of students and I did everything on a shoestring, but we *did it* rather than thinking about it or planning it. We believe strongly in philosophy made famous in Nike advertising—"just do it." In fact, an enabling factor in our work was the opening of an electronics "supermarket" (Fry's Electronics) only a few miles from our lab. Rather than order everything from catalogues (and there was no Internet then), we could browse the aisles at Fry's for hardware! Living in Silicon Valley had some advantages.

Another important lesson was that we found meaningful parallels between our clinical world and those arenas where progress was being made. The original patient simulator, Sim One—technologically "years before its time"—never amounted to much, and it died out because no one knew what to do with it. It was used, frankly, only in rather banal applications [13]. There was no "killer app" in modern parlance. Thus, another unique achievement of my group was our connecting medicine and medical simulation to Cockpit (later Crew) Resource Management, which we first discovered in 1987, adapting it by September 1990 to become Anesthesia Crisis Resource Management. This was revolutionary, and it has had a lasting effect. This development launched simulation out of the consideration as a mere "toy" or something useful only for students and novices. The ACRM approach showed that simulation could be useful even for highly experienced personnel, and not just for addressing the nuts and bolts of medical work. Crisis Resource Management has now become a well-known catchphrase, and at least within the healthcare simulation community, it has achieved generic status much like other words in earlier eras (e.g., escalator, zipper, xerox) although we never trademarked ACRM or Crisis Resource Management.

Another lesson is that the most fertile ground for adopting an innovation is not always in one's own backyard. People talk of a "not-invented-here" phenomenon whereby things from the outside are never accepted in an organization. But the reverse is also sometimes true. In our case it was only after my successful sabbatical at the Harvard anesthesia programs and their initiative to create a simulation center that it became possible for me to get my local institution to develop a center for me as described earlier. We later occupied space (some of it purpose-built) in the brand new hospital building at VA Palo Alto. Small simulation centers followed at Stanford (CAPE and the Goodman Surgical Simulation Center), and in 2010 our flagship Goodman Immersive Learning Center (about 28,000 ft^2) opened at Stanford (see CISL.stanford.edu). Yet, to this day, I have not been able to implement many of my ideas at Stanford, while I have seen others adopt them, or invent them anew, elsewhere. Thus, innovators should not despair when their own house doesn't adopt their creations; if the ground is fertile elsewhere, go with it.

I and my group have long believed that we are doing this work not for our own glory or aggrandizement (though accolades are always welcome!) but rather to improve patient safety and outcomes and improve teaching and learning. Whether that occurs in Palo Alto, in Tuebingen, in Melbourne, in Shantou (China), or anywhere else doesn't much matter. There is a saying so profound that it appears both in the Jewish Mishnah (Sanhedrin 4.5) and in the Muslim Qur'an (Surah 5, Verse 32): "Whoever saves a life, it is as if he has saved the whole world." I believe that our work, through the growing community of simulation in healthcare around the world, has indeed led to many lives (and hearts and brains) saved and thus to saving the world a few times over. And that is indeed a nice thing to contemplate in the latter half of my career.

References

1. Perrow C. Normal accidents. New York: Basic Books; 1984.
2. Gaba D, Maxwell M, DeAnda A. Anesthetic mishaps: breaking the chain of accident evolution. Anesthesiology. 1987;66(5): 670.
3. Abrahamson S, Denson J, Wolf R. A computer-based patient simulator for training anesthesiologists. Educational Technol. 1969;9(10).
4. Denson J, Abrahamson S. A computer-controlled patient simulator. JAMA. 1969;208:504.
5. Gaba D, DeAnda A. A comprehensive anesthesia simulation environment: re-creating the operating room for research and training. Anesthesiology. 1988;69(3):387.

6. Gaba D, DeAnda A. The response of anesthesia trainees to simulated critical incidents. Anesth Analg. 1989;68:444.
7. DeAnda A, Gaba D. Unplanned incidents during comprehensive anesthesia simulation. Anesth Analg. 1990;71:77.
8. DeAnda A, Gaba D. The role of experience in the response to simulated critical incidents. Anesth Analg. 1991;72: 308.
9. Cockpit Resource Management Training. NASA conference publication 2455. Washington: National Aeronautics and Space Administration; 1986.
10. Gaba D, Fish K, Howard S. Crisis management in anesthesiology. New York: Churchill-Livingstone; 1994.
11. Holzman RS, Cooper JB, Gaba DM, Philip JH, Small SD, Feinstein D. Anesthesia crisis resource management: real-life simulation training in operating room crises. J Clin Anesth. 1995;7(896318130):675.
12. Christensen C. The innovator's dilemma. Boston: Harvard Business Review Press; 1997.
13. Hoffman K, Abrahamson S. The "cost-effectiveness" of sim one. J Med Educ. 1975;50:1127.

Commercialization of CASE 2.0 began in 1992–1993 when licenses were acquired and models were produced by CAE-Link [85]. The original name of the commercial product was the Virtual Anesthesiology™ Training Simulator System. The name was shortened to the Eagle Patient Simulator™ when the product was bought later by MedSim-Eagle Simulation Inc. These full-body mannequins had realistic and dynamic airways in addition to other original CASE 2.0 features. Eyes that opened and closed with pupils that could dilate added to the realism. In 1999, an article describing the incorporation of the groundbreaking new technology of transesophageal echocardiography into the MedSim mannequin was published [85]. Unfortunately, production of this simulator stopped when an Israeli company bought MedSim and decided to focus on ultrasound simulation independent of the mannequin. Although the CAE-Link simulator was the early commercial leader, its success was dwarfed by the Gainesville simulator by the late 1990s.

The Gainesville Anesthesia Simulator (GAS) was the precursor of current products by Medical Education Technologies Inc. (METI). Drs. Good and Gravenstein partnered with Loral Aviation in a similar but independent effort to develop mannequin simulation at the University of Florida in Gainesville in 1988. The philosophy and mission of these two simulation groups was distinct and different. The Stanford team was focused on team performance during critical events. Good and colleagues at Gainesville used their simulator to introduce residents to anesthesia techniques, common errors, and machine failures. The GAS simulator was a full-body model from the beginning. It demonstrated spontaneous ventilation and palpable pulses in its earliest stages. A complex model of gas exchange to demonstrate clinical uptake and distribution and a moving thumb that allowed assessment of neuromuscular blockade were two other unique features. The Gainesville group also progressed from vital sign simulators to developing their own models of physiology and pharmacology. After an initial abstract in anesthesiology, this group was not as prolific as the Stanford group in advertising their product and accomplishments in the traditional literature [91]. The two early reports describing the GAS simulator appeared in the *Journal of Clinical Monitoring* [92, 93].

Pioneers and Profiles: A Personal Memoir by Michael Good

How the University of Florida's Gainesville Anesthesia Simulator Became the Human Patient Simulator

Mastery is a powerful motivator of behavior [1]. Humans will practice tirelessly to master important skills, including those of physical performance and those of cognition. Consider the Olympic athlete or the chess master. And so begins the story of the University of Florida (UF)'s Gainesville Anesthesia Simulator, which later became the highly successful Human Patient Simulator. These sophisticated learning systems were developed to allow anesthesiologists—and, later, all healthcare professionals—to acquire important clinical skills, including those needed every day and those called into action only rarely, through realistic and repeated rehearsal. In short, these simulators were created to facilitate mastery.

Like most beginning anesthesiology resident physicians, my initial learning experiences took place in an operating room with a senior resident and an attending anesthesiologist. We provided anesthesia for two or three surgical patients each day. I had to learn many cognitive and psychomotor skills. Each task had to be completed in a precise manner and given order. Mastery was important early on. I remember commenting to my teachers that I wished we could perform 15 or more anesthetics a day and "skip" the lengthy "surgical interval" of each patient's care.

A year later, I became the more senior resident, now helping a beginner learn basic anesthesia skills. Two or three cases a day did not provide sufficient repetition. My own learning was now focused on how to recognize and treat uncommon complications in anesthesia, and for these, there was no method other than memory and chance encounter. I again commented to colleagues about the desire for additional practice opportunities within a more compressed and efficient time frame.

The magical "ah ha" moment actually occurred in the batting cage of the local sports complex in the fall of 1985. As I practiced my hitting skills, I realized the pitching machine that was repeatedly throwing softballs toward me was creating a realistic learning opportunity outside the context of an actual softball game. If softball hitters could practice their skills using a simulated pitcher, why couldn't anesthesiologists learn and practice their skills with a simulated patient?

Dr. Joachim S. "Nik" Gravenstein was a graduate research professor in the UF Department of Anesthesiology and well-known nationally and internationally for using advanced technology to assure the safety of patients receiving anesthesia. When I first approached Gravenstein with the notion of a patient simulator, he strongly embraced the concept as a needed advance in the profession. We began meeting regularly and plotting how to realize this dream. Armed with my bachelor's degree in computer science and Arthur Guyton's 1963 analog circuit of the human cardiovascular system, I began programming an early cardiovascular model as digital computer code on a portable minicomputer.

In the mid-1980s, Gravenstein worked with Dr. Jan Beneken, chair of medical electrical engineering at Eindhoven University of Technology in the Netherlands, to assemble an international research group of anesthesiologists, engineers, and graduate students informally known as the "Bain team" because their first project was to develop computer models of the Bain breathing circuit [2, 3]. In early 1987, Gravenstein connected me with Samsun "Sem" Lampotang, a member of that Bain team, who was completing his doctoral research in mechanical engineering as a graduate research assistant in the UF Department of Anesthesiology. Lampotang and collaborators had recently developed an innovative methodology to enhance a mechanical test lung with simulated carbon dioxide (CO_2) production and spontaneous breathing [4] and used it for validation work in the Bain project. Lampotang's lung model created realistic capnograms when connected to respiratory monitoring equipment, both during spontaneous breathing and when connected to mechanical ventilators and anesthesia delivery systems. This early hardware model of the human pulmonary system, which realistically interacted with unaltered monitoring equipment, would form the basis for the first physiologic system in the Gainesville Anesthesia Simulator and a design philosophy favoring physical over screen-based simulator designs.

Based on his experiences with the Bain project, Lampotang recommended and Gravenstein and I agreed that a real anesthesia delivery system and real respiratory gases should be used in creating the Gainesville Anesthesia Simulator. Because of the need for a real anesthesia delivery system, Gravenstein suggested that I seek help from manufacturer Ohmeda to develop a prototype anesthesia simulator. I wrote to Thomas Clemens, director of research and development at Ohmeda, requesting financial support for the project. At the same time, Lampotang was working to establish an industry externship for the summer of 1987 and had also written to Clemens. Serendipity prevailed as my letter and Lampotang's letter collided on Clemens' desk. When Lampotang arrived at Ohmeda, Clemens assigned him to develop the Gainesville Anesthesia Simulator as his summer externship project.

Version 1 of the Gainesville Anesthesia Simulator (GAS I) was created by Lampotang at Ohmeda between May and August 1987. The lung model was enhanced with computer-controlled adjustment of CO_2 production and lung compliance, and a series of computer-controlled actuators were concealed within the anesthesia delivery system to create machine fault scenarios such as CO_2 rebreathing or hypoxic inspired gas. Interestingly, e-mail, then still a novelty, proved to be a key ingredient in the success of the early simulator project. Lampotang was working at the Ohmeda facility in Madison, Wisconsin, while Gravenstein was in Gainesville, and I was on clinical anesthesia rotations in Jacksonville. We quickly realized the benefit of asynchronous e-mail communication and used it to achieve daily coordination and updates between the three developers who were in distant cities on different time zones and work schedules.

In August 1987, Lampotang and the simulator returned to Gainesville. Dr. Gordon Gibby, a UF anesthesiologist with a background in electrical engineering, assembled circuitry and software to allow computer control of the pulse rate and oxygen saturation reported by the pulse oximeter; the interface became known as "Mr. Desat." The Gainesville Anesthesia Simulator was unveiled as an exhibit at the 1987 Annual Meeting of the American Society of Anesthesiologists in Atlanta, Georgia, and was recognized with the first place award as Best Scientific and Educational Exhibit. For the first time, participants at a national meeting had the opportunity to experience hands-on simulation in anesthesia. The future would bring many more such opportunities. Following this public debut, the UF simulator team partnered further with Ohmeda and Dr. Gilbert Ritchie at the University of Alabama to build a lung model that physically consumed and excreted volatile anesthetic gases. The new lung model defined version 2 of the Gainesville Anesthesia Simulator (GAS II).

In addition to his many roles at UF, Gravenstein was also a member of the Anesthesia Patient Safety Foundation (APSF), including its executive committee. Because of the potential to improve safety, Gravenstein believed the APSF should invest in the development of patient simulation. Accordingly, Gravenstein instructed me to meet him in New York at the APSF executive committee meeting to review the patient simulation initiative at UF. Gravenstein was returning from Europe. On his flight to New York, his plane made an emergency landing in Newfoundland. The passengers were evacuated down inflatable slides and moved to a vacant hangar to await another aircraft. Gravenstein was impressed with the manner in which the flight attendants quickly and efficiently directed passengers through the aisles, out the plane door, and down the inflatable slides. In the hangar, Gravenstein commended the flight attendants and offered that their proficiency suggested they had led such evacuations before. One flight attendant replied that this was her first real-life emergent evacuation but that she and her team had practiced the drill many times before in the flight simulator. Later in New York, his face still somewhat pale from the experience, Gravenstein recounted the entire story to the APSF executive committee, which quickly agreed on the important role simulation could play in anesthesia patient safety.

Shortly thereafter, the APSF funded simulator projects at UF and at Stanford, with a focus on developing realistic clinical signs in the emerging patient simulators. This emphasis on clinical signs heralded a transition, from anesthesia simulation to Human Patient Simulator. Lampotang's keen engineering skills proved exceptionally valuable throughout the Human Patient Simulator's developmental life cycle and especially as clinical signs were incorporated. Palpable pulses synchronized with the cardiac cycle, a thumb twitch (which we named "Twitcher") responsive to neuromuscular blockade monitoring [5], sensors to detect the volume of injected intravenous medications, airway resistors, urinary systems, simulated hemorrhage, and the detection of therapeutic procedures such as needle thoracostomy all required eloquent engineering designs. The end result was and remains realistic physical interaction between learner and patient simulator, and Lampotang's many talents are in large part responsible for this success.

The timing of the APSF grant was crucial for the UF simulator development team, enabling us to hire Ron Carovano on a full-time basis. Carovano's initial connection with the simulator project was, again, serendipitous. Jack Atwater, a UF electrical engineering graduate turned medical student, advised Carovano on his senior engineering project. The growing number of simulator components that required high-speed computer instructions was rapidly outstripping the capabilities of the IBM XT desktop computer which Lampotang had claimed from Ohmeda. Atwater was working to create a series of single-board computers (dubbed by the simulator team as data acquisition and control system, or DACS, boards), to control the simulator hardware components and interface them with the physiologic models running on the XT computer. Carovano joined the team as a senior engineering student and worked initially with Atwater on the DACS board development and implementation.

In the spring of 1989, Carovano was accepted into UF's Masters of Business Administration (MBA) program for the fall semester. Carovano continued to work with the simulator development team on a part-time basis during his 2 years of MBA studies. As he approached graduation in the spring of 1991, UF received the APSF grant. That grant allowed the UF simulator team to employ Carovano on a full-time basis, with half his time devoted to continued engineering research and the other half of his assignment as business administrator, drawing on his newly acquired skills from his MBA program. Over the years, Carovano contributed to the success of the simulator project not only as an electrical engineer but also as a business administrator. The Gainesville Anesthesia Simulator development team was one of the first "research" teams on the UF campus to have a full-time business administrator, which proved to be a key component of the project's ultimate success.

By 1994, Carovano was working primarily on the business aspects of the simulator project. Because of his business expertise, the simulator team successfully competed for a large state grant from the Florida High Technology and Industry Council. As the Human Patient Simulator matured into a successful prototype, Lampotang spearheaded the team's efforts to secure patents for the novel technology that had been created [6]. In all, 11 patents were eventually awarded on the initial patient simulator technology developed at UF.

In November 1991, the UF team held its first simulator-based continuing medical education course. The course was designed to help anesthesiologists learn to recognize and treat rare complications in anesthesia, such as malignant hyperthermia, and malfunctions within the anesthesia delivery system. Attendees included Adam Levine from Mount Sinai and Gene Fried from the University of North Carolina, individuals and institutions that were soon to become early adopters of simulator-based learning.

The unparalleled realism achieved by the Human Patient Simulator results in large part from its dynamic and automated reactivity, which in turn is created by sophisticated mathematical models of human physiology and pharmacology running within the simulator software. The mastermind behind most of these models was, and remains today, Willem van Meurs, who joined UF's simulator development team in 1991. As van Meurs was completing his PhD defense in Toulouse, France, at the Paul Sabatier University in September 1991, jury president (defense committee chair) Dr. Jan Beneken shared with him the theses and reports from two Eindhoven master's students who had been working on the simulator project in Gainesville [7, 8]. Van Meurs was intrigued. Gravenstein, Beneken, van Meurs, and I agreed upon a plan in which van Meurs would begin working as a post-doctoral associate for UF, initially in Eindhoven under the direction of Beneken, and then move to Gainesville in 1992 as an assistant professor of anesthesiology to improve the cardiovascular and anesthetic uptake and distribution models for the Gainesville Anesthesia Simulator. This work elaborated on Beneken's past research as well as on van Meurs' PhD work on the modeling and control of a heart lung bypass machine.

Upon his arrival in Gainesville in September 1992, van Meurs worked with Lampotang to further advance the mechanical lung model by creating computer-controlled models of chest wall mechanics, airways resistance, and pulmonary gas exchange, including volatile anesthetic consumption [9–11]. The significantly enhanced lung was fully integrated with the cardiopulmonary physiologic models to create version 3 of the Gainesville Anesthesia Simulator (GAS III). We all have very fond memories of the first night (yes, the great discoveries and accomplishments were always at night) that the patient simulator started breathing on its own, automatically controlling its own depth and rate of breathing so as to maintain arterial CO_2 tension near 40 mmHg and to ensure sufficient arterial oxygen tension. We had the simulator breathe in and out of a paper bag, and it automatically began to hyperventilate as alveolar, then arterial, CO_2 tension increased. Several years later at a conference in Vail, Colorado, I was summoned to the exhibit hall early in the morning by the technical team because the patient simulator was breathing at a rate greater than its known baseline. A quick systems check revealed that the simulator, through its hybrid mechanical and mathematical lung model, was responding (appropriately!) to the lowered oxygen tensions encountered at the 8,000-ft altitude of the ski resort.

Beginning in 1994, van Meurs led the development of an original cardiac rhythm generator, which we then used to control overall timing in a mathematical model of the human cardiovascular system. With the addition of the sophisticated cardiovascular model and its integration with the pulmonary model, the patient simulator became so realistic and dynamic that it began replacing animals in hemodynamic monitoring learning laboratories for anesthesiology residents and a variety of learning sessions for medical students, including those focused on respiratory and cardiovascular physiology and pathophysiology [12, 13].

Van Meurs next turned his attention to pharmacology and in 1995 embarked upon a plan to incorporate pharmacokinetic, pharmacodynamic, and related physiologic control mechanisms such as the baroreceptor into the simulator models and software [14, 15]. At the same time, the well-functioning adult models of the cardiovascular and respiratory systems were further enhanced for pregnancy [16] and with age-specific parameter files for a child, an infant [17], and a neonate.

In 1993, UF accepted from Icahn School of Medicine at Mount Sinai Department of Anesthesiology its first purchase order for a Human Patient Simulator and then orders two and three from the State of Florida Department of Education. As interest and inquiries increased, the UF simulator development team quickly realized it needed an industry partner to professionally manufacture, sell, distribute, and service the emerging simulator marketplace. On April 22, 1993, I reviewed the UF simulator project in a presentation at the University of Central Florida's Institute for Simulation and Training. In the audience was Relf Crissey, a business development executive for defense contractor Loral Corporation. After the presentation, Crissey put me in contact with Louis Oberndorf, director of new business development for Loral. The UF team was already in technology transfer discussions with CAE-Link Corporation, a manufacturer of aviation simulators, but these discussions were not advancing. The UF simulator team worked with Oberndorf and others at Loral on the complex technology transfer process, and a UF-Loral partnership was announced in January 1994 at the annual meeting of the Society for Technology in Anesthesia in Orlando, Florida. The UF patient simulator technology was licensed to Loral in August 1994. Loral initially assigned the team of Ray Shuford, Jim Azukas, Beth Rueger, and Mark McClure at its manufacturing facility in Sarasota, Florida, to commercially develop UF's Human Patient Simulator.

Following the licensing agreement to Loral, the UF simulator development team supported product commercialization and continued work on enhancements, including additional drugs, clinical scenarios, and patient modules. In the summer of 1996, the UF and Loral team took the full simulator and a complete operating room mock-up to the World Congress of Anaesthesiologists in Sydney, Australia [18]. There, using the Human Patient Simulator, a randomized controlled trial of meeting participants was conducted, comparing the ability of anesthesiologists to detect problems during anesthesia with and without pulse oximetry and capnography [19].

In January 1996, Lockheed Martin acquired the defense electronics and system integration businesses of Loral [20] and then spun a number of these business units out to create L-3 Communications [21]. As these corporate changes were taking place, Oberndorf felt strongly that the Human Patient Simulator deserved a company focused entirely on its advancement and related medical educational technologies and that he personally was ready for this challenge. In August 1996, Oberndorf created his own company, Medical Education Technologies Inc. (METI), which then assumed the simulator licenses for the UF-patented Human Patient Simulator technology. Over the next decade, Oberndorf and METI created a highly successful company and helped to spawn a new commercial industry (see elsewhere in this chapter).

In the spring of 1997, Carovano became a full-time employee of METI coincident with METI receiving a large Enterprise Florida grant to develop patient simulators for community colleges. In 1998, van Meurs also joined METI, as director of physiologic model development, and in September 1998, he returned to Europe as an associate professor of applied mathematics at the University of Porto in Portugal, where he worked with collaborators to create an innovative labor and delivery patient simulator. He continues to consult with METI and CAE Healthcare, to advance mathematical modeling of human physiology [22] and pharmacology, and remains active in the patient simulation community. Lampotang has continued his academic career as a professor of anesthesiology and engineering at UF. He and his team continue to develop patient simulators and training systems, including the web-enabled Virtual Anesthesia Machine [23], and simulators that combine physical and virtual components for learning central venous catheterization [24] and ventriculostomy [25]. In 2011, CAE Healthcare acquired METI. That same year, Oberndorf and his wife Rosemary created the Oberndorf Professorship in Healthcare Technology at UF to assure the ongoing development of innovative learning technologies that improve healthcare.

Dr. Jerome H. Modell, chair of the department of anesthesiology from 1969 until 1993, deserves special mention. Without the tremendous support of Dr. Modell as our department chair, the simulator project would not have completed its successful journey. From examples too numerous to recount, consider that as the simulator team outgrew its development home in the anesthesiology laboratory, Modell, who was also a director of the medical school's faculty practice plan, became aware of residential property one block from the medical center that the faculty practice had acquired and was holding as a future office building site. Until the faculty practice was ready to build, Modell arranged for this residential unit to become the simulator development laboratory. The 3,000-ft^2 house became dedicated completely for the simulator development effort and affectionately became known as the "Little House on the Corner." Modell was also instrumental in providing critical bridge funding at a moment when the development team suffered the inevitable grant hiatus. The bridge funding brought us through the grant drought, to our next funded grant. Without Modell's bridge funding, the project's success and the eventual technology transfer to industry might never have happened. Modell, an avid horse enthusiast, also pioneered the use of the simulator technology to train veterinary students in the UF College of Veterinary Medicine [26].

Gravenstein continued to champion patient simulation until his death in January 2009. Words fail to adequately describe the quiet but very forceful and worldwide impact of J.S. Gravenstein on human patient simulation. At each intersection of decision along this incredible journey, whether it was simulator design, educational approach, structure of the grant application or draft manuscript, interactions with industry and foundations, study design, or countless other aspects of the project, Gravenstein provided strategically accurate advice and direction that never wavered from true north. We clearly owe our success to his immense wisdom.

And like so many aspects of life, my own story now comes full circle. As the UF simulator technology successfully transferred to industry in the 1990s, I became interested in health system leadership and, beginning in 1994, began accepting positions of increasing leadership responsibility within the Veterans Health Administration and then at UF. In 2009, I was asked to serve as the ninth dean of the UF College of Medicine. In the coming years, a key strategic goal for UF will be to build a new medical education building and, within it, an experiential learning center where healthcare learners of all disciplines will work together with patient simulators to achieve a most important goal: mastery.

Acknowledgment The author thanks simulator coinventors Samsun Lampotang, Ronald Carovano, and Willem van Meurs for their tremendous help in creating and reviewing this chapter and Melanie Ross and John Pastor for their editorial review.

References

1. Pink DH. Drive: the surprising truth about what motivates us. New York: Penguin Group (USA) Inc.; 2009.
2. Beneken JEW, Gravenstein N, Gravenstein JS, van der Aa JJ, Lampotang S. Capnography and the Bain circuit I: a computer model. J Clin Monit. 1985;1:103-13.
3. Beneken JEW, Gravenstein N, Lampotang S, van der Aa JJ, Gravenstein JS. Capnography and the Bain circuit II: validation of a computer model. J Clin Monit. 1987;3:165-77.
4. Lampotang S, Gravenstein N, Banner MJ, Jaeger MJ, Schultetus RR. A lung model of carbon dioxide concentrations with mechanical or spontaneous ventilation. Crit Care Med. 1986;14:1055-7.
5. Lampotang S, Good ML, Heijnen PMAM, Carovano R, Gravenstein JS. TWITCHER: a device to simulate thumb twitch response to ulnar nerve stimulation. J Clin Monit Comput. 1998;14:135–40.
6. Lampotang S, Good ML, Gravenstein JS, Carovano RG. Method and apparatus for simulating neuromuscular stimulation during medical surgery. US Patent 5,391,081 issued 21 Feb 1995.
7. Heffels JJM. A patient simulator for anesthesia training: a mechanical lung model and a physiologic software model, Eindhoven University of Technology Report 90-E-235; Jan 1990.
8. Heynen PMAM. An integrated physiological computer model of an anesthetized patient, Masters of Electrical Engineering, Eindhoven University of Technology; 1991.
9. Van Meurs WL, Beneken JEW, Good ML, Lampotang S, Carovano RG, Gravenstein JS. Physiologic model for an anesthesia simulator, abstracted. Anesthesiology. 1993;79:A1114.
10. Sajan I, van Meurs WL, Lampotang S, Good ML, Principe JC. Computer controlled mechanical lung model for an anesthesia simulator, abstracted. Int J Clin Monit Comput. 1993;10:194–5.
11. Lampotang S, van Meurs WL, Good ML, Gravenstein JS, Carovano RG. Apparatus for and method of simulating the injection and volatilizing of a volatile drug. US Patent 5,890,908, issued 1999.
12. Öhrn MAK, van Meurs WL, Good ML. Laboratory classes: replacing animals with a patient simulator, abstracted. Anesthesiology. 1995;83:A1028.
13. Lampotang S, Öhrn M, van Meurs WL. A simulator-based respiratory physiology workshop. Acad Med. 1996;71(5):526–7.
14. Van Meurs WL, Nikkelen E, Good ML. Pharmacokinetic-pharmacodynamic model for educational simulations. IEEE Trans Biomed Eng. 1998;45(5):582–90.
15. Van Meurs WL, Nikkelen E, Good ML. Comments on using the time of maximum effect site concentration to combine pharmacokinetics and pharmacodynamics [letter]. Anesthesiology. 2004;100(5):1320.
16. Euliano TY, Caton D, van Meurs WL, Good ML. Modeling obstetric cardiovascular physiology on a full-scale patient simulator. J Clin Monit. 1997;13(5):293–7.
17. Goodwin JA, van Meurs WL, Sá Couto CD, Beneken JEW, Graves SA. A model for educational simulation of infant cardiovascular physiology. Anest Analg. 2004;99(6):1655–64.
18. Lampotang S, Good ML, Westhorpe R, Hardcastle J, Carovano RG. Logistics of conducting a large number of individual sessions with a full-scale patient simulator at a scientific meeting. J Clin Monit. 1997;13(6):399–407.
19. Lampotang S, Gravenstein JS, Euliano TY, van Meurs WL, Good ML, Kubilis P, Westhorpe R. Influence of pulse oximetry and capnography on time to diagnosis of critical incidents in anesthesia: a pilot study using a full-scale patient simulator. J Clin Monit Comput. 1998;14(5):313–21.
20. Wikipedia. http://en.wikipedia.org/wiki/Loral_Corporation. Accessed 14 Apr 2012.
21. Wikipedia. http://en.wikipedia.org/wiki/L3_Communications. Accessed 14 Apr 2012.
22. Van Meurs W. Modeling and simulation in biomedical engineering: applications in cardiorespiratory physiology. New York: McGraw-Hill Professional; 2011.
23. Lampotang S, Dobbins W, Good ML, Gravenstein N, Gravenstein D. Interactive, web-based, educational simulation of an anesthesia machine, abstracted. J Clin Monit Comput. 2000;16:56–7.
24. Robinson AR, Gravenstein N, Cooper LA, Lizdas DE, Luria I, Lampotang S. Subclavian central venous access mixed reality simulator: preliminary experience. Abstract ASA 2011.
25. Lampotang S, Lizdas D, Burdick A, Luria I, Rajon D, Schwab W, Bova F, Lombard G, Lister JR, Friedman W. A mixed simulator for ventriculostomy practice. Simul Healthcare. 2011;6(6):490.
26. Modell JH, Cantwell S, Hardcastle J, Robertson S, Pablo L. Using the human patient simulator to educate students of veterinary medicine. J Vet Med Educ. 2002;29:111–6.

Dr. Good did inform the world of this new technology and the GAS training method through national and international conferences [94]. He began at an ASA education panel at the annual meeting in 1988 with a presentation titled "What is the current status of simulators for teaching in anesthesiology?" Both Drs. Good and Gaba contributed to the simulation conference cosponsored by the APSF and FDA in 1989. A few months later, Dr. Good presented "The use of simulators in training anaesthetists," to the College of Anaesthetists at the Royal College of Surgeons in London. Dr. Good gave simulation presentations for the Society of Cardiovascular Anesthesia, the Society for Technology in Anesthesia, and the World Congress of Anaesthesia. He would return to the World Congress in 1996. He was a visiting professor at the Penn State University–Hershey in 1992 and Mount Sinai Medical Center in 1994. All of this publicity preceded the commercial launch of the Loral/University of Florida simulator in 1994. In the spring of 1994, the first external Loral/Gainesville simulator was installed in the Department of Anesthesiology of the Icahn School of Medicine at Mount Sinai in New York City for a purchase price of $175,000. The Mount Sinai team included Drs. Jeff Silverstein, Richard Kayne, and Adam Levine.

Pioneers and Profiles: The Mount Sinai Story

A Personal Memoir by Joel A. Kaplan

Tell me, I'll forget
Show me & I may not remember
Involve me & I'll understand

—Chinese proverb

In the Beginning ...

During my academic career, I have been involved in many educational initiatives, but none has had the positive impact of the gradual transition to simulation-based education for healthcare providers. As a resident in anesthesiology at the University of Pennsylvania, I often heard the chairman, Dr. Robert Dripps, say that "every anesthetic is an experiment" in physiology and pharmacology. This certainly was a true statement in the early 1970s but often made me wonder why we could not learn this information without putting a patient at risk.

I arrived back in my hometown of New York City in July, 1983, to become chairman of the Department of Anesthesiology at the Mount Sinai Hospital and School of Medicine (MSSM). My primary goal was to develop the leading academic department in New York, recognized for its excellence in clinical care, education, and research, or as some called it "Penn East." The first 5 years were devoted to providing the best clinical care while training a new generation of anesthesiologists, many of whom would become subspecialists in the expanding areas of cardiothoracic anesthesia, neuroanesthesia, and clinical care medicine, all fields requiring extensive cardiovascular and respiratory monitoring of patients in the perioperative period. These complex patients would receive multiple anesthetic and cardiovascular drugs given by residents who had not used them routinely or seen their full effects in sick patients during or after major surgery. In addition, as a teacher and chairman, I was always looking for new ways to evaluate both our students and faculty.

At the time, Icahn School of Medicine at Mount Sinai had pioneered a standardized patient program for teaching medical students, and it was being used by all of the medical schools in the New York City area. I had explored options for teaching our residents, but it did not meet our needs except for preoperative evaluations. In addition, our faculty were lecturing in the physiology and pharmacology courses and were looking for new ways to introduce students to the anesthetic drugs. From my experiences in teaching cardiopulmonary resuscitation, I had some familiarity with the Stanford University simulator program, and the concept had great appeal as a possible new teaching technique in all areas of anesthesiology, which could meet many of my objectives for our department.

The residency program director at the time, Richard Kayne, MD, returned from a national meeting and told me about the University of Florida's (U of F) simulation program in Gainesville and his meeting with Michael Good, MD, the program director. I immediately told him to follow up because I had great interest in potentially developing a similar program at Mount Sinai to teach our residents and medical students in a simulated environment instead of by lectures and "see one, do one, teach one" methods in the operating room. In the early 1990s, after a few discussions with the U of F and the manufacturers of the early models of the Gainesville Simulator, we were fortunate to become the first beta test site for the first Loral simulator systems.

Under the leadership of Dr. Jeffrey Silverstein, Richard Kayne, and Adam Levine, we decided to set up a mock operating room (OR), with video equipment and teaching techniques similar to those used in the MSSM Standardized Patients Center. The plan was to use the mock OR to teach anesthesia residents the basics of anesthetic physiology and pharmacology and, via a series of case scenarios, progressively more serious cardiovascular and respiratory problems during surgical procedures. The only available OR at the time was at our affiliated Bronx VA Hospital, and thus, the first simulator was located there. It was fully developed using department funds from Mount Sinai and updated by Loral with the support of Louis Oberndorf, vice president of marketing and business and head of the project. It remained at the VA Hospital for about a year but never met our full goals because of the off-site location for most of our students and residents, inadequate technical support, and lack of full-time dedicated staff and faculty.

In the spring of 1995, we had the simulator moved to an available operating room at the Mount Sinai Hospital. Drs. Richard Kayne and Adam Levine continued to lead the project and took direct charge with technical support and additional departmental funds. U of F and Loral were very helpful at this time in programming the simulator with us and providing extra maintenance support. This led to the simulator program expanding rapidly and becoming very popular in the department and school of medicine. The major uses at this time were for new resident orientations, afternoon teaching sessions for first and second year residents, and weekly medical student sessions on cardiovascular and respiratory physiology. Eventually these physiology sessions were expanded and became a fundamental and integrated component of the very popular physiology course for first year medical students. These teaching programs were very successful, with many other faculty joining in the expanding new educational opportunity.

At one of our monthly staff meetings, after bragging about our success with the simulator, I decided to introduce another idea for its use. My thought was to develop a program of annual evaluation of the faculty's clinical skills, with documentation for the hospital and school of medicine, to demonstrate their expertise and the new role for simulation, analogous to the airline industry's use of cockpit simulators. I then asked for comments and there was nothing but dead silence. Obviously, this idea caused some concern with the faculty, and they just were not ready for it at the time. In fact, we never did develop this annual evaluation program in the department. It is good to see that some departments now use simulators for testing, and some even use them to help reduce malpractice insurance premiums. I still believe there is an important role for simulation in evaluation and certification of practitioners, and I am pleased to see that the American Board of Anesthesiology has introduced simulation as a part of the Maintenance of Certification in Anesthesiology (MOCA) program. It is a shame that anesthesiology did not do this much earlier, before other specialties, such as surgery, added simulation into their certifying programs.

The initial costs of the equipment, continued updates, and maintenance had been paid for out of departmental funds. This eventually became quite expensive, and I asked the faculty to develop programs with the simulator that could earn funds to pay for the maintenance and upkeep. Out of their plans and work came important programs that made the simulator self-sufficient. These programs included:

1. Pharmaceutical company training programs—Drug company representatives (6 per class for 2–3 days) would observe the effects of administering their new products in the simulator and then also be able to watch the use of the drugs in the OR. This was especially useful with the introduction of remifentanil and propofol.
2. Impaired physician programs—Multiple types of programs were developed under the leadership of Paul Goldiner, MD, and Adam Levine, MD, working with many other faculty. These included a 1-year simulation teaching fellowship in which former residents with chemical dependancy were allowed to transition back into teaching and clinical practice under intense supervision. This program was later expanded to help the New York State Society of Anesthesiologists evaluate clinical skills of practitioners before permitting them to return to practice.

These early programs eventually led to the large simulation center that now exists in the Mount Sinai Department of Anesthesiology. It is one of the 32 (at the time of this writing) American Society of Anesthesiologists' approved simulation centers throughout the United States, and the continued innovations by the faculty have made it one of the major strengths of the department's educational programs.

Upon leaving Mount Sinai in 1998, I had the opportunity to continue to fully develop a multidimensional simulation and standardized patients center as Dean of the University of Louisville (U of L) School of Medicine and Vice President of Health Affairs of the U of L Health Science Center (HSC). This center was started with a very generous gift from John Paris, MD, a graduate of the school of medicine, and was expanded by becoming the Alumni Simulation Center. With 4 METI-equipped simulation rooms and eight standardized patient rooms, it became the core of our new educational programs at the HSC, with the integrated teaching of students from the schools of medicine, nursing, dentistry, and public health. For the U of L, the home of the Flexner medical educational philosophy of endless lectures, this conversion to reality-based simulation education was a major change. The faculty pioneered new programs teaching basic sciences, general medical care, specialty care, and team care with providers from various healthcare fields. One of the most interesting educational programs took place shortly after 9/11 and the anthrax attacks in the Northeast, when the simulation center became one of the nation's earliest first-responder teaching centers, funded by the Federal and state governments, to train Kentucky's emergency response teams in conjunction with our emergency and trauma healthcare practitioners. Thus, what was started as a small simulator program at Mount Sinai eventually grew into a national model for team training and assessment performance.

A Personal Memoir by Jeffrey H. Silverstein

Early Days of Simulation

I was introduced to simulation during a visit to the University of Florida at Gainesville. I was visiting the Dr. Joachim Gravenstein to discuss further work on postoperative cognitive dysfunction. I had known Mike Good from some other ASA activities, and we took a short tour through the simulator they were developing. Sem Lampotang was the primary engineer on the project. The simulator that they had was quite large and fit on one large platform—basically a metal cart in which the mannequin lay on the top, sort of like a tall OR table with all of the mechanisms contained below the mannequin. For that time, the device was amazingly advanced. It had respiratory movement controlled by two bellows, one for each lung, and it expired CO_2. This was totally remarkable. The physiologic model was still relatively new and required manipulation from the computer screen. The appearance of the physiology on an anesthesia monitor was extremely realistic for the electrocardiogram and blood pressure tracings. Skipped beats were associated with a lack of pressure/perfusion.

At the time, Dr. Richard Kayne was the anesthesia residency program director at Mount Sinai. After some discussion, Richard suggested to Dr. Joel Kaplan, the chairman of the Department of Anesthesiology, that we look into being an early participant in this arena. With a good deal of enthusiasm, Richard and I took another trip to Florida to investigate the idea of becoming the beta test site for the Gainesville simulator. At the time, another simulator group also existed. The primary investigators/developers of that group were Dr. David Gaba at Stanford (currently the associate dean for immersive and simulation-based learning at the Stanford School of Medicine) and Dr. Jeffrey Cooper at Harvard. Their group had a very different approach to simulation. The group at Gainesville was primarily focused on the physiology and developing a model that acted and reacted as a human would to the various interventions involved in anesthesiology as well as various types of pathophysiology. The primary foci of the pathophysiology at the time were cardiac arrhythmias and blood pressure changes. The point of the simulation exercise was the demonstration and education in physiology. The Gaba and Cooper group were focused on group dynamics. They borrowed the term called Crew Resource Management from aviation simulation. The approach involved staffing a simulation of an event with a cadre of actors who would all behave in a prescribed manner to create specific stressful situations during the simulation. These simulations would involve loss of an airway or loss of power in the OR. The episodes were videotaped, and the primary learning forum was the debriefing after the incident in which all involved would discuss how the individual immersed in the simulation has behaved and what options they had for improving group interactions. As suggested by the title, the primary goal was interpersonal management of the crew involved. By contrast, the Gainesville group was primarily focused on the teaching of physiology as encountered in the operating room. The sessions would involve real-time discussions about what was going on and the underlying physiology. These were essentially bedside discussions and were not at all focused on group dynamics.

We investigated partnering with the Stanford/Harvard group including one visit to Dr. Gaba at the Stanford Veterans Administration Hospital. That group had already entered into a manufacturing agreement with CAE-Link, a company that was involved in the development and fabrication of aviation simulators. Gainesville was just starting their negotiations with manufacturers and was interested in having a beta test site for their unit. We decided to enter into this agreement and expected delivery of the unit in the Spring of 1994.

Initially, the simulator was installed at the Bronx Veterans Affairs Medical Center on Kingsbridge Road. We had a spare operating room, appropriate monitors, and a reasonably current anesthesia machine to dedicate to the project. The VA administration was excited and supportive of this project and contributed some funds for equipment. Dr. Kayne and Dr. Adam Levine would come up to run the simulator sessions for residents. My partner at the VA, Dr. Thomas Tagliente, and I would set up and run sessions for the four to five anesthesiology residents who rotated through the VA at that time as well as session including all members of the operating room staff.

Two large-scale simulations were the malignant hyperthermia drill and the complete loss of power in the operating room scenario. Malignant hyperthermia is a complicated emergency that many nurses and anesthesiologists never experience. Everyone in the ORs prepared for this drill. When we began, things started out sort of slowly, but eventually a sense of purpose carried into the scenario and everyone focused on performing their role. In this capacity, one of the nurses planned to insert a rectal tube for cold-water lavage. The mannequin did not have an orifice for the rectum, so the nurse simply lay the rectal tube on the metal frame that supported the mannequin, close to where an anus would have been. She then opened the bag holding the cold water and started to shower all of the electronics which were contained under the frame. This was completely unexpected, and we had to rapidly cut off the simulation and power everything down before it got wet. For the loss of power in the operating room scenario, we worked with engineering to identify the circuit breakers to cut off power to the OR where there simulator was living. They were most helpful. We trained everyone, made sure our flashlights were working, and started the simulation. I turned off the circuits and there was the briefest flash of lights, but everything kept working. We called engineering who discovered that the emergency generator had kicked in. They needed time to figure out how to temporarily disconnect that circuit. We rescheduled. After a few weeks, we tried again. This time the lights flickered a little more and everything came back on. The loss of power was enough to reset some of the digital clocks on some of the equipment, but it never got dark. The explanation for this was that a second generator kicked in and that they would work on disconnecting that one temporarily, but they were now getting concerned that we were turning off multiple circuits and needed to make sure that they would all get turned back on when we were through, as the backup generators were not just for one room but the entire OR suite. We finally rescheduled, got everyone in position, received confirmation from engineering that everything was ready, and turned off the circuit breakers in the OR. Nothing happened, the most demure of flickers if you were paying attention. The engineers were surprised to find out that a small third generator designed to power only the ICUs also included the OR (but not the recovery room). We gave up and never successfully ran the loss of power scenario.

Drs. Kayne and Levine decided to try a randomized trial of simulation by splitting the incoming class of residents into two groups, one of which had intense simulation multiple days per week while the other half had their standard in the operating room apprenticeship. Although I do not believe the results were ever published, my recollection was that there was no discernible difference between the groups, suggesting that new trainees could acquire basic skills in a simulated environment without exposing patients to new trainees during their steep learning curve.

We were also asked by Dr. Kaplan to use the simulator to assess the technical capabilities of some anesthesia assistants. Anesthesia assistant, as opposed to certified registered nurse anesthetists (CRNA), was a position that had been developed down south. Mount Sinai, which a that time had no CRNAs, was considering starting an anesthesia assistant program. The two individuals who came to be assessed out on the simulator could not have been more different. One was a large young man who loved the simulator. He thought it was so much fun, and everything that he did was well considered and well done. The other candidate was a woman who could never get beyond her own suspension of disbelief. The mannequin was plastic, not human. She has a very hard time performing regular anesthesia drills, such as induction and intubation. She kept stopping in disbelief. My conclusion to Dr. Kaplan was that the simulator was not an effective preemployment screening tool.

Traveling up to the VA to do simulation was impractical. Simulation was very time consuming, so Tom and I were doing more of this, even though we both were running a basic science laboratory as well as a clinical service. The decision to move the simulator to Sinai essentially ended my involvement with simulation in general. It sure was fun.

A Personal Memoir by Adam I. Levine

"Based on my first simulation experience I saved my patient's life."

It may be a little presumptive to invite myself to write my own story alongside pioneers like Mike Good and David Gaba. I do so with much gratitude and appreciation for both Mike and David for contributing to a field that has been the pillar of my own career. I also do so to both memorialize the "Mount Sinai Story" and highlight my own mentors who without their presence I could not imagine what I would be doing today or where I would be doing it.

Like many things in life, it's all about timing. I was fortunate to be at the right place at the right time. I graduated Icahn School of Medicine at Mount Sinai in 1989 and was excited to be starting my anesthesiology residency at Mount Sinai. When I began my education, I certainly had no plans to become an anesthesiologist, but the dynamic faculty of the anesthesiology department at Mount Sinai made the practice exciting and intriguing, and I was instantly hooked. I was also extremely fortunate to have met the then program director, Richard Kayne, MD. Looking back I can't tell you why, but I knew instantly upon meeting him that he was destined to be my mentor and the absolute reason I ranked Mount Sinai number one on my rank list. Boy did I get that right.

Instantly I found Richard's Socratic teaching style remarkably appealing for my own education and amazingly affective when I had the privilege of teaching more junior residents and medical students. Having such an amazing educational mentor, I knew I was going to stay in an academic center and devote my career to educating others. During my last year of training, I was fortunate to be chosen as a chief resident and even more fortunate that this role afforded me an opportunity to not only participate in further educational activities but also to have an administrative role, an experience I never would have appreciated otherwise. It was through these experiences that I knew I wanted to stay as a faculty member at Mount Sinai and that I wanted to be Richard's assistant helping to run the residency. The culmination of these experiences led next to amazing opportunities with simulation.

BS (Before Simulation)

As a resident I knew the department was looking to acquire the first simulator from the University of Florida and even joked about it during my chief resident roast at graduation (*the way things are going when we get the new simulator there will be an attending working with it by themselves*). It was during the early nineties and interest in anesthesia as a career choice for medical student was essentially nonexistent and the department was dramatically reducing the residency numbers causing many faculty to work by themselves.

I attended an early meeting in Florida to see the new device. I can remember Sem Lampotang conducting scenarios that focused on rare, life-and-death issues including machine failures (they had an ingenious way of remotely controlling machine mishaps) and the impossible airway. I also remember feeling incredibly anxious and tried to stay in the wings fearing that I might be selected to step in. As luck would have it, and I say that sarcastically, Sem picked me to step up to the head of the bed and save the dying patient who could not be intubated or ventilated. With little left to do, Sem suggested I perform a needle cricothyrotomy and then jet ventilate the patient. Having never actually done that and with step by step instruction from Sem, I picked up the 14-gauge angiocath, attached a 10-ml syringe, and with trepidation and trembling hands proceeded to perform the procedure successfully, only to be ultimately thwarted because I couldn't figure out how to jerry-rig a jet-ventilating device from random OR supplies (an important lesson that we still use to this day… if you need to jet ventilate someone you need a jet ventilator). Little did I know at the time that this first experience with simulation would be the reason I would be able to save one of my actual patient's life by performing that exact procedure during my first year of practice when my patient's airway became completely obstructed during an attempted awake fiberoptic intubation.

Preparing for Delivery

As a new attending and having established my interest in education, I was honored when Richard asked me if I wanted to be involved with the new simulation initiative at Mount Sinai. Dr. Joel Kaplan was my chairman, an innovative world famous cardiac anesthesiologist who established a department committed to education and prided itself on having the latest and greatest technology and being an early adopter of that technology, a legacy that lives on in the department to this day. It was Joel who wanted simulation at Mount Sinai and made sure to support it and allocated the necessary resources for the project to succeed. The plan was to install the simulator in an available operating room at the Mount Sinai Veterans Administration affiliate in Bronx, New York (BVA) (known now as the James J. Peters VA Medical Center). In preparation, I attended another early "simulation" meeting to see the version of the device we were about to receive. The meeting, whose theme was teaching with technology, was held in Orlando, Florida, at the end of January 1994 and conducted jointly by the Society for Technology in Anesthesia (STA) and the Society for Education in Anesthesia (SEA) sponsored by the Anesthesia Patient Safety Foundation (APSF). There again I met Mike and Sem, and once again Sem was conducting his simulation-based road show, which I again tried in vain to avoid being selected.

In addition to developing an acceptable OR site for the equipment, we also pieced together a working audio-video system with a mixing board capable of recording and playing back superimposed performances and physiologic data. We also assembled a team of faculty and conducted frequent *preparatory* meetings at Mount Sinai and the BVA to discuss and develop an entirely new method of teaching with simulation as we designed the new simulation-based curriculum, the importance of scenario building and debriefing, and planned to conduct an IRB-approved randomized study collaboratively with the University of Florida.

Planning to Study Simulation Training

In a previous study, Good et al. had demonstrated that new residents developed earlier acquisition of anesthesia skills from simulation training compared to those that learned anesthesia in a traditional manner. Here we planned to increase the number of participants and conduct a multicenter study where we would split our new July 1st anesthesia residents into two groups. One group (control) would learn anesthesia traditionally in a clinical apprenticeship; the other group (study) would have no real patient encounters and would learn basic anesthesia skills exclusively on a simulator during the first 2 weeks of training. The topics selected mirrored those being taught in Florida, induction of anesthesia, emergence from anesthesia, hypoxemia, hypotension, regional anesthesia, ACLS, and the difficult airway. Given the fact that the study residents would have no true patient encounters, we also creatively invented standardized patient encounters for preoperative evaluation training and mock anesthesia machine and room preparation sessions (much of these early experiences were incorporated into a lasting orientation curriculum we have conducted with all of our residents during July and August since 1995). Eventually we tested each resident individually with a simulation scenario that had one to two intraoperative events (hypotension/hypoxia) at 3 and 6 months time intervals. Although we oriented the control residents to the simulator and allowed them to use it prior to testing, I was never 100% comfortable with the study design; were we teaching residents to be better real anesthesiologists, or were we teaching people to be better anesthesiologists for a simulator (this study flaw still affects the validity with much of the simulation-based research today). Ultimately, we found no difference in performance between the two groups, admittedly I was incredibly disappointed. We put our hearts and souls into the curriculum and the education, and I thought we were creating a supergroup of anesthesiology residents capable of early independent care during the most challenging of intraoperative events. Interestingly, when discussing the results with Mike, he had a unique spin on it and thought this was an enormous success. Although we thought the simulated group would be superior, Mike anticipated that they would be behind the residents who learned on real patients. He thought that since we didn't see any deficits in the simulated group, this was remarkable proof that simulation-based education should be used during early training, so patients don't have to be subjected to the new resident's steep learning curve, and resident education does not have to be compromised. Unfortunately, we never published the results because I could never get over what I believed to be a major flaw in the study design.

Serial Number 1: Taking Delivery

At a cost of $175,000 dollars, bought with departmental funds, we officially took receipt and installed the very first Loral Human Patient Simulator during April 1994 (Loral licensed the rights from University of Florida). During the 2-week installation, Richard and I would spend the entire time at the VA, and it was during that time that I officially meet Lou Oberndorf, vice president of development for Loral; Jim Azukas, lead engineer from Loral; and Beth Rueger, the Loral project manager. It was also during that time that I worked side by side with Mike as the equipment was assembled and tested in OR 7, an actual working operating room at the BVA, making it a true first "in situ" simulator.

The simulator was an engineering marvel. It was essentially a patient façade, since the mannequin was mounted to the steel table. The mannequin was affectionately known as "bucket head" (Fig. 1), which accurately described its appearance. All computerized actuators and hardware were mounted below the device (Fig. 2). Interfacing with the existing anesthesia equipment and monitors was pos-

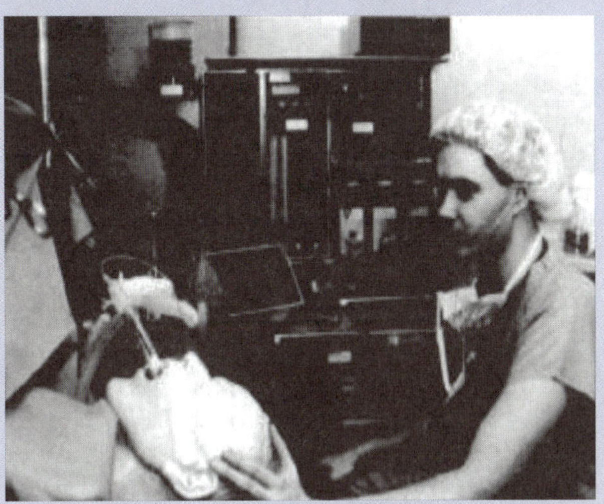

Fig. 1 Michael Good, MD, professor and dean of the University of Florida Gainesville, next to one of the original Gainesville Anesthesia Simulators (GAS) later known as the Loral Simulator or "bucket head," METI HPS, and now CAE/METI HPS

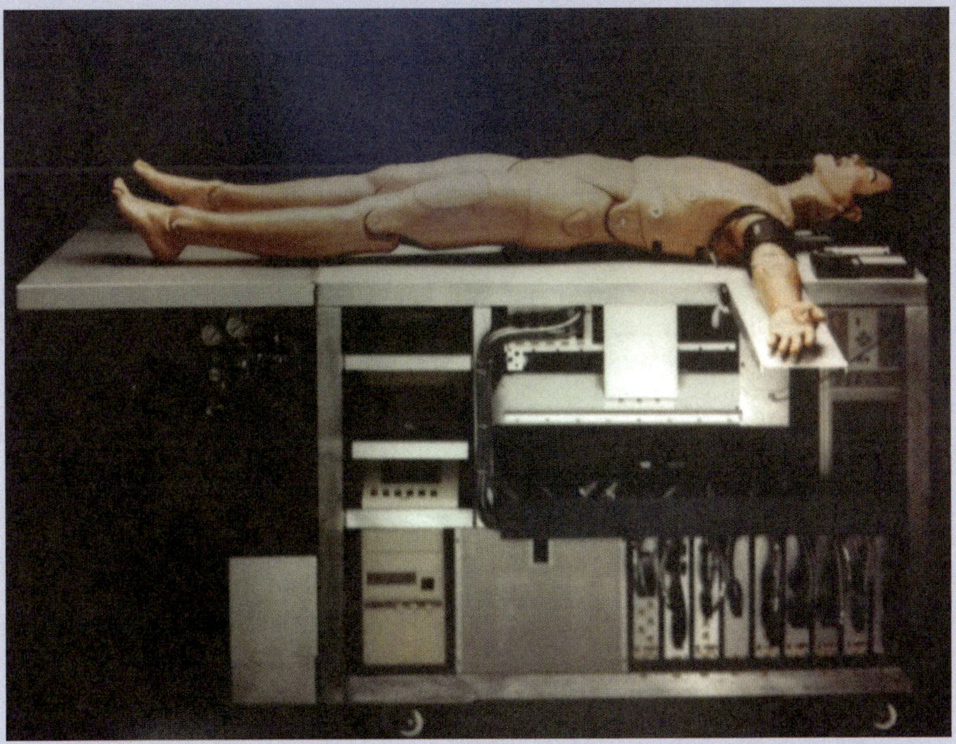

Fig. 2 One of the original table-mounted designs of the Loral Human Patient Simulator

sible and very realistic. Pistons effectively allowed airway changes dynamically and drove the lungs reliably. Remarkably, the device had physiologic oxygen consumption and exhaled actual carbon dioxide, which was detectable by our anesthesia gas analysis system. It also could detect inhaled anesthetics and oxygen via an embedded stand-alone mass spectrometer. We were like kids at FAO Schwarz playing with our new toy and checking out what it could do. We were fascinated when we gave the simulator a puff of albuterol, and it became apneic and died. The gas vehicle of albuterol is interpreted to be isoflurane, a potent inhaled anesthetic, by mass spectrometry, so the simulator behaved as if it was exposed to a massive overdose of anesthetic agent…AMAZING!!!!!

Even though it was remarkably sophisticated, the early version only recognized seven intravenous agents (succinylcholine, atracurium, thiopental, ephedrine, epinephrine, fentanyl, and atropine), ran on DOS software, and could not be easily programmed. In order to make the simulator behave a certain way, medications had to be administered through the computer interface. For example, if you wanted the simulator to stop breathing, either paralytic, fentanyl or thiopental had to be given. Interestingly there was no naloxone, but you could administer negative doses and subtract off the fentanyl as if a reversal agent was given. Although programming was not initially possible, Mike and Jim gave us access to the software code to the "shunt fraction." This allowed us to develop hypoxemia scenarios, and this therefore was the first physiologic parameter that was programmable.

Things weren't always smooth sailing during these early days. Apparently during the reengineering of the simulator, hardware substitutions created software and hardware incompatibilities, and occasionally the ECG and/or the pulse oximeter would go a little haywire, and the patient would spontaneously desaturate or become tachycardic. This was to be expected given the fact that this was a beta unit and the first one ever built. Occasionally we had internal flooding from the drug recognition system. At the time the barcode scanner was attached to the metal table. The syringe had to be manually scanned and then injected. The volume was collected in a bag inside a Lucite box sitting on top of a scale (during initial simulator booting, we had to tare the scale for drug dose accuracy). Every so often the bag would overflow and the box would leak internally—bad for computerized parts to say the least.

Although we had 3 months to get things in order and create the scenarios for the new residents and the study, we ended up needing every moment of that time to create the curriculum and develop cases with the existing technology. The lessons learned during the early days proved invaluable as the simulation technology improved and scenario building and programming became possible.

July 1, 1994

During the initial launch, we learned a lot about simulation, simulation-based education, and formative assessment (and debriefing as a whole). Richard and I were fascinated by the process and the prospect of introducing simulation to a broader audience and were convinced that this technology was hugely advantageous to medical educators and would naturally be part of all training programs. I can remember during the first week of the project, when one of our new residents, Mike Port, who induced anesthesia with a bolus of thiopental, had difficulty with the intubation and spontaneously turned on isoflurane and ventilated the patient with inhaled anesthetic. When asked why, Mike stated that he did not want the patient waking up while he worked through the airway issue (remember this resident had never given an anesthetic to an actual patient, and here he was managing the patient way beyond his level of education). Richard and I turned to each other and thought this was one of the most incredibly powerful environments for education and student self-discovery when we saw that. Another memorable event occurred during the testing phase, Kenneth Newman (Fig. 3), a study group resident, failed to place the pulse oximeter on the patient and conducted the entire anesthetic without saturation monitoring. Needless to say he never detected the hypoxic event, but to this day Ken has never forgotten about his mistake and brings it up frequently and every time we get together to conduct a PBL together at annual anesthesia meetings. Recognizing the power of mistakes, errors, and failure was born from such early experiences and has set the tone of our simulation scenarios and our research efforts to this day.

Lessons Learned

During the initial project launch and the early years, we were essentially inventing much of what we were doing with simulation. Although Mike, Sem, and the team from Florida served as phenomenal resources, much of what we did in those early years was created on the fly and allowed us to develop a style that was all our own and that worked for us. Although much of the curriculum from Florida revolved around tasks and simple maneuvers, we started developing elaborate scripts and scenarios that were developed to illustrate the topics to be covered. In addition to the primary topics like hypoxia and hypotension, much of the curriculum focused on team training and building, handoffs, error reduction, professionalism, and communication. It was also clear that residents in the

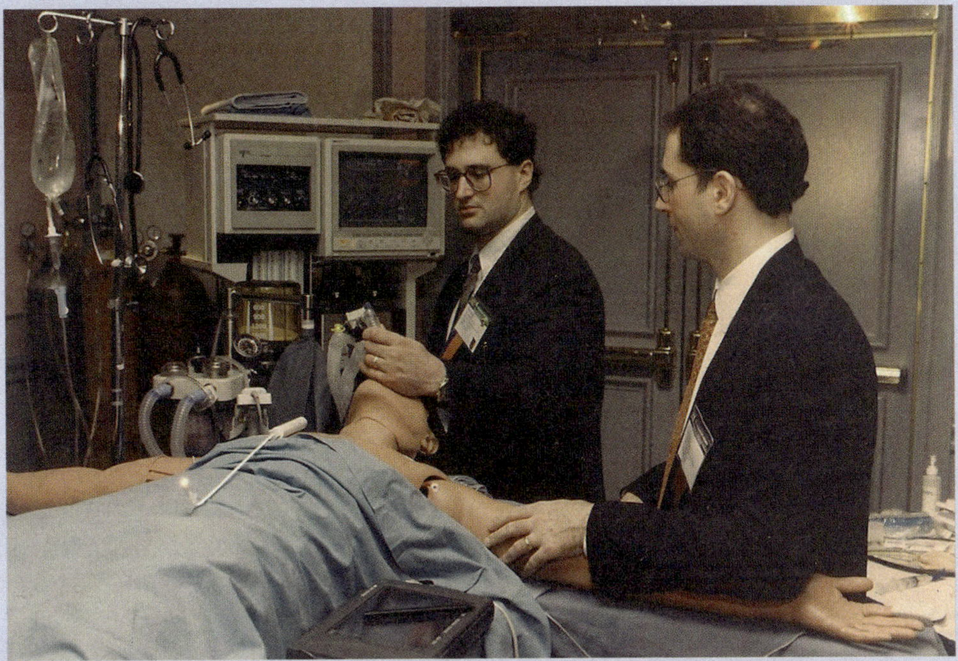

Fig. 3 Kenneth Newman, MD, using one of the original simulators during a Difficult Airway Workshop at the New York State Society of Anesthesiologist Postgraduate Assembly (Circa 1996)

simulator would become exceedingly cautious and hypervigilant; thus, the "pushy" surgeon was born, coaxing them to get going or the "bothersome" nurse creating distraction with frequent interruptions or introducing potential errors (drug swaps and blood incompatibilities). Scenarios too would be developed to create distraction; simulation participants knew something was coming and tried to predict the event based on the background story. Obviously the ability to anticipate events is an indispensible ability as an anesthesiologist, but it can cause a simulation to lose its educational power or to become derailed. Therefore, asthmatic patients rarely got bronchospastic, and difficult airway cases were always framed in another complex case like obstetrics or thoracic. As the scenarios became more and more elaborate, so too did our scenario programming. By the end of the DOS era, all of scenarios would cause the software to crash; thus, the adage that "no simulated patient would die" was instantly thrown out since all scenarios ultimately ended in asystole—it was then more likely that "no simulated patient would fail to die." From these experiences it was also apparent that our students themselves didn't wither and die from undue stress. In fact upon arrival to the simulator they would proudly proclaim "were her to kill another one", demonstrating an early benefit of "stress innovation" (Chap. 5).

It was clear that having the simulator off-site proved to be a logistic impossibility and neither faculty nor residents could make use of the technology, so we moved the equipment to the Mount Sinai campus during the spring of 1995 and installed it into an available operating room and continued with "in situ" simulation. On July 1 1995, we introduced a simulation-based education for all of our new anesthesiology residents during a unique 7-week simulation-based curriculum modeled after our study curriculum. We have conducted this course as part of our residents' anesthesia orientation every year since 1995. It was during this time that we also introduced the technology for medical student education and readily developed simulation-based physiology courses on the pulmonary, cardiovascular, and autonomic nervous system. These labs have also been conducted annually since their inception in 1996.

AS (After Simulation)

In 1995, Mike Good and Lou Oberndorf would come to Mount Sinai periodically to demonstrate the simulators to a variety of people. Initially I attended these meetings to simply turn the equipment on, but naturally I became the person they wanted to talk to and hear from. I had no financial connection with the company or the technology but spoke openly about the device and its use as an educator. Little did I know, these people were thinking of investing in a start-up company that would allow the simulation technology to live on. Fortunately for all of us, invest they did and in 1996, 2 years after serial number one arrived at Mount Sinai, Medical Education Technologies Inc. (METI) was born. As an early simulation expert, I would travel to other programs and give grand rounds and simulation demonstrations. Many of the people I met along the way have been lifelong friends and are thankfully contributing to this textbook. One memorable visit to Colorado (and one both Mike and I remember) really sticks out as to how truly amazing the equipment is. When I arrived for the simulation demonstration, several METI technicians were puzzled by the fact that the simulator was breathing at a rate of 22–24 per min (it was modeled to have a baseline respiratory rate of 12–14). I told them that I felt winded when I got off the plane, and the simulator, with its ability to sense the low oxygen tension, tried to improve its own oxygenation by increasing its respiratory rate. During this demonstration, we were also able to demonstrate that you can suffocate the simulator by placing a plastic bag over its head. The equipment desaturated; became hypercarbic, tachypneic, and tachycardic; developed ectopic cardiac beats; and ultimately arrested.

In 2000, as Mike became more involved with administrative responsibilities at the University of Florida, I was offered the role of associate medical director of METI, which I readily accepted and maintained from 2000 to 2002. It was a part-time consulting position but established at a time METI was developing its new mannequin, and I got to participate in its design. This was a memorable time for me and I looked forward to monthly meetings with Jim (Azukas) at a sculpting house in Manhattan to watch the progress and make technical recommendations as the mannequin sculpture took shape. The sculpture would ultimately serve as the mold for the rendering of the plastic mannequin. When I first saw the original form, I asked "why so large?" and was told this was because the plastic would shrink 9–10% in the curing process, and we (METI) want to have an adult male mannequin to be 5 ft 10 in., the average adult American male. Unfortunately, the plastic only shrunk 2% and the simulator ended up much bigger than anticipated; yup he's a big guy.

Although frustrating as the process could often be, I am still to this day very proud of the arterial track design, instead of the typical cut outs where one would feel pulses; the company went with my suggestion and created furrows in the arms allowing the arterial tubing to descend into the arm resulting in dissipating pulses as one progresses proximally.

During the last decade and a half, we have upgraded, added, and moved our simulators many times. We have had seven to eight generations of HPSs and no fewer sites to conduct simulation. In 2002 we established our permanent facility, the HELPS (Human Emulation, Education, and Evaluation Lab for Patient Safety and Professional Study) Center, located in our newly built office space.

We also achieved several milestones during that time. We became one of the first multi-simulator centers when we acquired our second METI HPS (along with one of the first pediatric simulators) in 1997. We did so in order to efficiently conduct simultaneous small group physiology labs for the expanding medical school. That same year we conducted one of the first interdisciplinary simulations. With the help of METI, we moved our simulator to our level 1 trauma center affiliate in Queens, NY, so we could create simulations for a NOVA special on head trauma. Gathering attendings and trainees from anesthesiology, neurosurgery, emergency medicine, and general surgery, along with respiratory therapists and ER nurses, we conducted an entire day of trial simulations before the actual filming scheduled for the following day. Early in the day, I witnessed a lot of missteps and miscommunication and poor follow-through. As expected the patients did poorly. Interestingly midday some of the participants turned to me and asked if I was making the scenarios easier, because the patients were doing better. I simply replied no; over the course of practicing, the team was simply working together more effectively with improved leadership, communication, and follow-through (closed-loop communication). Ironically or fortuitously or both, we did these simulation on the first of a month, and the trauma team had yet to work together in a real case, and the trauma team leader, the chief resident of general surgery, also never ran a trauma team before these simulations. Months later a medical student on his anesthesiology rotation told me soon after the filming, which he witnessed, the same team was called to a trauma and it was remarkably similar to one of the simulated scenario. He told me that the team and the patient did great and many commented that the simulations were invaluable. Based on these experiences, the city hospital purchased its own simulator. It's ironic to think that we were only planning for a TV spot and what we were actually doing was deliberate multidisciplinary team training in the simulator. In addition to a prime spot in a NOVA special, our program was highlighted on the cover of the New York Times, and CNN's Jeanne Moos did a nice and yes humorous piece about the program.

We pride ourselves in staying true to our roots; all simulations are run by physicians and conducted from our very modest (1,500-ft^2 center) yet technologically sophisticated HELPS center. We have developed a multidisciplinary simulation curriculum from our American Society of Simulation (ASA)-endorsed center and conduct MOCA courses as well as a multitude of educational products for a variety of audiences and learners. In addition we have developed unique simulation-based programs including our community service programs for local underprivileged elementary, middle school, and high school students, our very popular elective in simulation for medical students, and our clinical educator track for residents interested in clinical educational careers. I know Joel Kaplan wanted to start using simulation for faculty assessment when he was chair; in fact it was for this reason that Joel was particularly interested in acquiring simulation at Mount Sinai. Fortunately I managed to deflect its use for this purpose for several years and long enough for Joel to leave Mount Sinai to become the Dean of Louisville. Although at the time I never had to don a "black hood" and assess our own faculty, we now do so frequently and provide an exceedingly valuable reentry program of assessment and retaining for anesthesiologists seeking to maintain or regain competence, licensure, and their clinical practice. This idea is often surprising when we talk about it to others—but we had been planning to use the simulator for physician assessment before it even arrived in the 1990s.

I am currently blessed to be surrounded by wonderful collaborative colleagues like Drs. DeMaria, Sim, and Schwartz, who are my coeditors of this textbook. I attribute much of our center's recent research and academic success to Dr. Samuel DeMaria, who joined me as an elective student nearly 8 years ago and who himself has now become a mentor to an entire generation of students and residents interested in education and simulation.

I could not be happier and I am proud to dedicate this book and this memoir to all of my mentors and could not be more thrilled to assemble the world's simulation experts to contribute to a textbook that punctuates my lifelong career. We're involved in something great here, and mine is just another part of the interesting road this technology has taken to be where it is today.

Table 2.3 Gainesville Anesthesia Simulator patents

Patent #	Subject	Date awarded
5,391,081	Neuromuscular stimulation	2/21/1995
5,584,701	Self-regulating lung	12/17/1996
5,772,442	Bronchial resistance	6/30/1998
5,769,641	Synchronizing cardiac rhythm	6/30/1998
5,779,484	Breath sounds	7/14/1998
5,868,579	Lung sounds	2/9/1999
5,882,207	Continuous blood gases	3/16/1999
5,890,908	Volatile drug injection	4/6/1999
5,941,710	Quantifying fluid delivery	8/24/1999

Features of the early commercial model were interchangeable genitalia, programmable urine output, and an automatic drug recognition system that relied on weighing the volume of injectate from bar-coded syringes. Loral Data Systems later sold its interest in the GAS to Medical Education Technologies Inc., founded in 1996. This product was renamed the Human Patient Simulator (HPS). The Gainesville simulation group (S. Lampotang, W. van Meurs, M.L. Good, J.S. Gravenstein, R. Carovano) would receive nine patents on their new technology before the turn of the century (see Table 2.3) [95–103]. Cost limited the purchase of these mannequins to only a small portion of medical centers. The initial cost was ~$250,000 just for the mannequin and accompanying hardware and software. This did not include medical supplies such as monitors or anesthesia machines or disposable patient care products. METI released the first pediatric mannequin in 1999. It used the same computer platform as the HPS adult mannequin.

After the merger between Laerdal and Medical Plastics Laboratory (MPL), METI was not able to purchase MPL's models to be converted into their HPS mannequins. METI began a process of designing and manufacturing their own mannequins with progressively more realistic features including pliable skin, a palpable rib cage, and pulses that became less prominent as the arteries traveled up the extremities. Working in a sculpting house in Manhattan, the original human models were fashioned in clay, went through many iterations, and were intended to result in a male human form 5 ft 10 in. tall (due to a miscalculation in the curing process, the resulting mannequin turned out to be much larger). Then, METI responded to Laerdal's challenge with the development of the price competitive Emergency Care Simulator (ECS) in 2001. In 2003 METI released the first computerized pelvic exam simulator. Their first infant simulator, BabySim®, was released in 2005. PediaSim® transitioned to the ECS® platform in 2006. METI released iStan® as its first tetherless mannequin in 2007. The funding and impetus for the design and manufacture of iStan® came from the US military. They needed a training mannequin that was portable and durable enough to be dropped on the battlefield. METIMan®, a lower-cost wireless mannequin designed for nursing and prehospital care, was released in 2009. An updated version of iStan® and METI's new user Internet-based interface, MUSE®, were released in 2011. In August 2011, CAE Healthcare acquired METI® for $130 million. Their combined product line includes METI's mannequins and associated learning solutions and CAE Healthcare's ultrasound and virtual reality endoscopy and surgical simulators. METI has sold an approximate 6,000 mannequin simulators worldwide.

Pioneers and Profiles: A Personal Memoir by Lou Oberndorf

The Birth of a Healthcare Learning Revolution: The Development of the Healthcare Simulation Industry for an International Commercial Market

Most young people entering a healthcare profession today will save the life of a human patient simulator that pulses, bleeds, and breathes before they save a human life. They will engage in hours of intensive, hands-on learning that was unavailable to their counterparts just a generation ago. They will immerse themselves in more complex critical care scenarios than they might see in a lifetime of practice and will respond without any risk to a real patient. That is nothing short of a healthcare learning revolution—and it has occurred within the span of less than 15 years.

In 1994, I visited a young research team at the University of Florida that was working on the GAS—the Gainesville Anesthesia Simulator. Led by Dr. Joachim Stefan "J.S." Gravenstein, a world-renowned anesthesiologist and patient safety expert, they had obtained funding to develop a practice patient for anesthesia residents. Taking a lead from flight simulation, they wanted to be able to recreate rare, life-threatening events that could occur with an anesthetized patient. Their vision would require nothing less than engineering a three-dimensional model of a human being.

With funding from the Anesthesia Patient Safety Foundation, the Florida Department of Education, Enterprise Florida, and the University of Florida, Dr. Gravenstein had assembled an interdisciplinary team to build a human patient. The five-member team of inventors consisted of physicians, engineers, and a businessman—Dr. Gravenstein; Dr. Michael Good, who is currently dean of the University of Florida College of Medicine; Mathematical Modeler Willem Van Meurs; Biomedical Engineer Samsun "Sem" Lampotang; and Ron Caravano, who had recently completed his MBA.

I was the vice president of marketing and business development for Loral, a top-ten defense company based in New York City. In the early 1990s, Loral was the largest simulation training contractor in the defense industry. At the time, the industry had forecast a downturn in defense budgets, so companies were looking for ways to use their technologies in nondefense arenas. In my position, I sought out technologies that Loral could incubate to create new commercial businesses, and I managed an emerging markets portfolio.

My 10 years of experience in the United States Air Force and 20 years in the aerospace industry had taught me the value of simulation as a learning tool. While I did not have a background in patient safety or physiology, I understood the power of simulation to train professionals.

When I watched the GAS mannequin in a University of Florida lab for the first time, I was blown away. The inventors had created a cardiovascular, respiratory, and neurological system that was modeled after human physiology. I saw enormous possibility and the opportunity to create a business.

The team had worked on refining the model for several years. They had advanced the technology down the road and were representing an anesthesia patient very accurately. However, the GAS mannequin was tethered to a table, and it was not an easily reproduced piece of equipment.

At that time, in 1994, there was one other advanced patient simulator under development in the United States, at Stanford University in California. The international medical mannequin business consisted of task trainers and CPR dummies. Ray Shuford, an industrial engineer and vice president at Loral, and I negotiated a license with the University of Florida in 1994. Ray would oversee development of the patient simulator within Loral's plant in Sarasota, Florida.

Our first job was to industrialize the product—to create an assembly process, documentation, source material, and a business plan. We delivered Loral's first human patient simulator to Dr. Adam Levine of Icahn School of Medicine at Mount Sinai in April of 1994. The price was $175,000.

Over the next 2 years, Loral sold 13 human patient simulators, mostly to anesthesia departments in medical schools and often to people who knew of the inventors. Anyone who purchased the HPS was stepping out, taking a risk on a product that had never existed before. Dr. Takehiko *Ikeda, an anesthesiologist with Hamamatsu University* in Japan, was the first international buyer. Santa Fe Community College in Florida was also an early adopter, with the help of funding from the State of Florida Education Department.

While a number of aerospace and defense companies were interested in healthcare simulation, we had only one competitor in our specialized field. CAE, the flight simulation company based in Canada, licensed the Stanford University patient simulator, and we competed head-to-head in anesthesia departments for the first 2 years.

I participated in sales calls to witness firsthand the reaction of potential customers. We met with the early adopters, the risk takers who love technology. They were all academics and anesthesiologists. Their reactions confirmed my instincts that this could be a very effective medical training tool.

But after 2 years of trying to introduce a radical new way of teaching healthcare as a defense company, Loral had not progressed very far. The corporation decided they were going to close the doors on patient simulation and medical education as a business area.

I had seen the power of it, and I couldn't allow that to happen. At the end of 1995, I approached Loral with the proposition that I buy the licenses, assets, and documentation to spin off a new company. This would not be an enterprise underwritten by a large corporation with deep pockets—I raised the money by taking out a second mortgage on my house and securing one other private investor.

In 1996, with only $500,000 in working capital, five employees, and two systems worth of parts on the shelves, we spun the business off from Loral and founded METI—Medical Education Technologies Inc. Loral elected to keep a stake in the company, and we remained housed within their Sarasota plant.

Loral and CAE had sold more than 30 patient simulators in the United States. There was a toehold in the medical education market for both products. However, now that we were focused exclusively on patient simulation, we had to find a way to very quickly ramp up the number of simulators we were selling. Within the first year, we made strategic decisions that defined us as a company and opened the doors to rapid growth.

In our travels, I had learned that the biggest technology shortfall was that the simulator was anchored to the table. An early, driving philosophy and strategic goal was to make the simulator more flexible and more mobile. I wanted to take the technology to the learner, not make the learner come to the technology.

The table housed the computer, the lungs, the pneumatics, and the fluid for the simulator. We made the decision to take it off the table and put all of our initial research and development effort into having it ready to debut at an annual meeting of anesthesiologists. We bet the farm on it. Within 90 days, our engineering team had taken it off the table, and the newly renamed METI HPS premiered at the 1996 American Society of Anesthesiologists (ASA) annual conference.

We had disrupted the technology—something I didn't have the phrase for until years later, when I read *The Innovator's Dilemma* by Clay Christensen. Disruptive technologies, according to Christensen, are innovations that upset the existing order of things in an industry. We were determined from the start that we would always disrupt our own technology rather than have someone do it for us. That principle defined METI for many years and led ultimately to the creation of the world's first pediatric patient simulator, PediaSIM, and the first wireless patient simulator, known as the METI iStan.

We sold our first redesigned HPS model before the end of 1996. It was purchased by the National Health Trust learning center in Bristol, England. In a span of a few months, we had become a global company. At the time, there were approximately 120 schools of medicine in the United States. We knew our success would be dependent on reaching a wider audience. We decided to add two market segments—nursing education and combat medicine for the military. The academic medical community at the time didn't think nursing schools needed advanced patient simulation or that they could afford it. I was convinced they did need it and that patient simulation could bring about a learning revolution in all of healthcare.

We were fortunate to have political leaders in the state of Florida who agreed. We met with Florida's Governor Lawton Chiles and Secretary of Education Betty Castor, who was also in charge of workforce development. They wanted nursing students to have access to patient simulation and said they would provide matching funds for four simulators per year in Florida's community colleges. Subsequent governors and secretaries of education continued to support funding for our patient simulation.

In the military, we were immediately successful with simulation executives with the US Army in Orlando. Within months, we had established the framework that would define our growth in the following years—we sold to schools of medicine, schools of nursing, community colleges, and the military. We were a global company. And we were dedicated to relentless technological innovation.

Within a year or so of the launch of METI, we introduced PediaSIM, the first pediatric simulator. By 1997, METI was profitable. For the next 11 years, we grew revenues by an average of more than 25% each year. By 1998, CAE had exited the marketplace, and by 2000, we were the only company producing high-fidelity patient simulators.

Long before social marketing was a common practice, we adopted the concept of the METI family as a company value. As we were a start-up, everyone who made the decision to purchase a METI simulator in the early years was putting his or her career on the line. They didn't know if METI could survive and be counted on to be a true educational partner. From the beginning, we valued every customer.

In the late 1990s, we brought together 13 of our educators and faculty in a small conference room in Sarasota, Florida, to engage in dialogue about simulation, what they needed for their curriculum, and what we were producing to advance the industry. That was the launch of what is now the Human Patient Simulation Network (HPSN), an annual conference that attracts more than 1,000 clinicians and educators from around the world

When the United States Department of Defense initiated its Combat Trauma Patient Simulation program, we partnered to create a virtual hospital system that would simulate the entire process of patient care—from the point of injury or illness to medical evacuation to an aid station and then to a surgical center or hospital. On September 10, 2001, it was research and development project. On September 12, 2001, it was a capability whose time had come. The CTPS program was the foundation of our METI Live virtual hospital program.

In the early years, whenever we shipped an HPS, the inventors would travel with the simulator to help install it and provide basic training on the technology. Most of the faculty who purchased the simulators were young and very comfortable with technology, and they created their own curriculum with the authoring tool we delivered.

But at METI, we always had twin passions—innovation and education. As we grew, we realized we needed to build a library of curriculum for our patient simulators. We reached out to our family of educators and clinicians and partnered to develop what we now call simulated clinical experiences (SCEs) for critical care, nursing, disaster medical readiness, advanced life support, infant and pediatric emergencies, and respiratory education. Over the years, we created hundreds of SCEs that were validated by our education partners.

In 2001, we learned that the largest medical mannequin task trainer manufacturer in the world, Laerdal, would enter the patient simulation market with the launch of its mid-fidelity SimMan. Laerdal's entry both validated and challenged us. To compete on price, we pushed to launch our ECS Emergency Care Simulator, a more mobile and affordable version of the HPS. Our subsequent products retained the HPS physiology, but they were even more mobile, more affordable, and easier to operate.

Before we founded METI, there were 13 Human Patient Simulators in the world, and they were consigned to small departments in elite medical schools. Today, there are more than 6,000 METI simulators at healthcare institutions in 70 countries. Students and clinicians at all levels of healthcare have access to this technology, and more lives are saved each year because of it. We've been on an extraordinary journey and have been involved with changing the way healthcare education is delivered.

Several European centers developed their own economical designs of computerized simulation mannequins. Two European products would never become commercial and were instructor driven rather than model based. Stavanger College in Norway developed a realistic simulator named PatSim in 1990. This product did have some unique features. Hydraulic pressure waves in simulated arteries produced the arterial waveforms instead of electronic pulse generators. The mannequin had a visual display of cyanosis and was able to regurgitate [104]. The mannequin could breathe spontaneously and could display several potential incidents including laryngospasm, pneumothorax, and changes in lung compliance and airway resistance. The Anaesthetic Computer-Controlled Emergency Situation Simulator (ACCESS), designed at the University of Wales, was also described in a 1994 report [105]. This model was very inexpensive using simple resuscitation mannequins and a microcomputer to emulate the patient monitor. Experts performed better than junior trainees in managing medical crises. They had fewer patient deaths and resolved incidents in less time suggesting good validity. By 2001, the ACCESS simple model was used by ten different centers in the UK [85].

Two other European centers developed more sophisticated model-driven simulators. The Leiden Anaesthesia Simulator was launched at the 1992 World Congress of Anaesthesia. The Stanford group assisted in the formation of this product by sharing technical details of the CASE simulator [86]. This model used a commercial intubation mannequin with an electromechanical lung capable of spontaneous or controlled ventilation [106]. This group also demonstrated the efficacy of simulator training for residents in the management of a malignant hyperthermia critical incident [107]. This simulator would eventually incorporate physiologic models. The Sophus Anesthesia Simulator from Denmark debuted in 1993. Its development was chronicled in a booklet [108]. An updated version was described 2 years later [109]. The Sophus simulator was also adopted by the University of Basel, Switzerland. That group added animal parts to develop a mixed-media multidisciplinary team-training simulator known as Wilhelm Tell. This group's version of Crisis Resource Management was Team Oriented Management Skills (TOMS) [85, 110].

The growth of simulation centers was relatively slow in the early to mid-1990s. In the profile of cumulative growth, several waves of increased activity are visible (see Fig. 2.3). After the initial launch of commercial products in 1993–1994, simulation center expansion continued at a pace of approximately ten centers per year worldwide for 2 years. Although MedSim had a slight head start in commercialization, MedSim and METI had installed approximately equal number of units by 1996. Centers in Boston, Toronto, Pittsburgh, and Seattle in the USA and centers in Japan and Belgium featured the MedSim model. METI was in operation at US centers in NYC, Rochester NY, Augusta, Hershey, Nashville, and Chapel Hill and in Japan. New centers appeared at triple that rate for the next 2-year period from 1997 to 1998. Growth slowed again for the time period between1999 and 2000. METI developed stra-

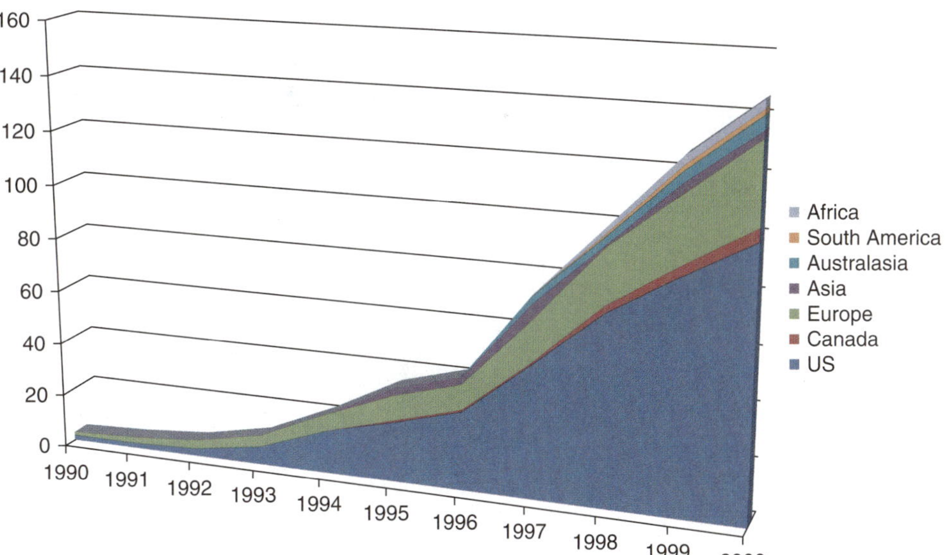

Fig. 2.3 Cumulative expansion of simulation centers in the 1990s

tegic alliances with the military and aimed marketing efforts at allied health training programs especially in Florida and international markets in Japan, Africa, and Australia. METI jumped into the lead by the start of the next century, and MedSim was out of the mannequin business completely.

In 2000, MedSim was gone but there were new products on the horizon. After a year of beta testing, Laerdal launched its first computerized commercial mannequin, SimMan®, in 2001. This product had most of the features of previous models at a fraction of the cost. It debuted for less than $50,000. SimMan® did not incorporate any computer modeling of physiology. The mannequin responses were driven by the instructor. The original SimMan® officially retired after 10 years of service and 6,000 units sold. He was replaced by the updated wireless version, SimMan Essential®. The wireless SimMan 3G was an intermediate step. In 2002, Laerdal began to work with Sophus to develop microsimulation and formally acquired Sophus the following year. Laerdal introduced two infant mannequins, SimBaby® and SimNewB®. Later they began selling PROMPT® birthing simulator from Limbs and Things. They then released a low-cost realistic trainer MamaNatalie® in 2011 for use in underdeveloped regions in an effort to decrease perinatal mortality. Laerdal also became the distributor for Harvey®, The Cardiopulmonary Patient Simulator, and the associated UMedic, a multimedia computer-based learning curriculum.

Gaumard also transitioned from task trainers to enter the arena of computerized mannequins with the introduction of Noelle® in 2000. In 2002 and 2003, Gaumard launched their PEDI® and Premie® models. The production of a cheaper, simpler lower-fidelity family of mannequins began with tetherless HAL® in 2004. Three pediatric HAL® models were added in 2008 (see Table 2.2). Gaumard introduced the first and only non-obstetric female computerized mannequin, Susie®, in 2010.

The sale of mannequins and founding of simulation centers exploded during 2000–2010 with two spikes of accelerated activity (see Figs. 2.4 and 2.5). The first peak, 2003–2005, coincided with the establishment of the Society for Simulation in Healthcare in 2004 and the introduction of new products by several vendors. The second burst, 2008–2009, may be related to the popularity of in situ simulation facilitated by the new wireless technology. A significant slowing of new development in 2010 is concerning. Hopefully, this is a temporary event and not a marker of decreased utilization of simulation.

Surgical Simulation

In the 1990s, four major forces stimulated development of computerized surgical simulation. The first was the rising acceptance and popularity of minimally invasive procedures as alternatives to traditional open operations. Early surgical simulators emphasized the development of eye-hand coordination in a laparoscopic environment. The simple Laparoscopic Training Box (Laptrainer) by US Surgical Corporation facilitated practice of precision pointing, peeling, knot tying, and precise movement of objects. The Society of American Gastrointestinal Endoscopic Surgeons (SAGES) was the first group to develop guidelines for laparoscopy training in 1991. Crude anatomic models were the first simple simulators [111]. The KISMET simulator appeared in 1993 and incorporated telesurgery. The Minimal Access Therapy Training Unit Scotland (MATTUS) was the first effort of national coordination of training in these procedures [112].

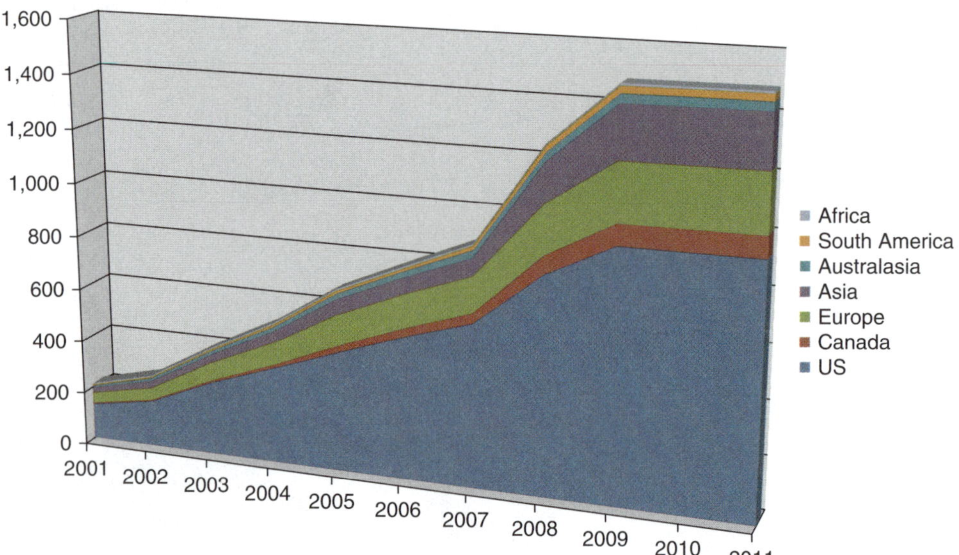

Fig. 2.4 Cumulative expansion of simulation centers in the 2000s

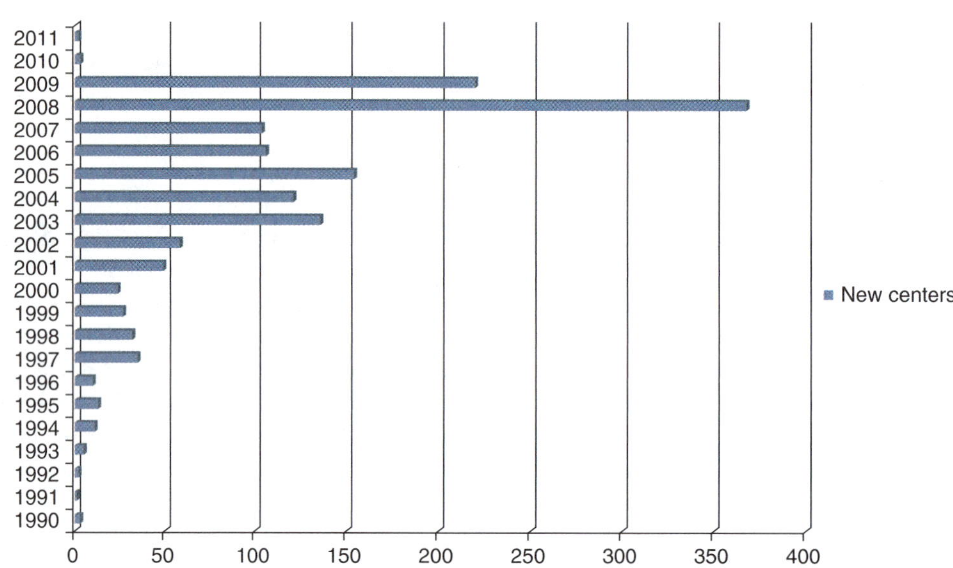

Fig. 2.5 Annual increases in simulation centers worldwide

The second force contributing to the development of surgical simulation was the progression of computing power that would allow increasingly realistic depiction of virtual worlds. The third critical event was the completion of the first Visible Human Project by the National Library of Medicine in 1996. This dataset, based on radiologic images from actual patients, enabled accurate three-dimensional reconstruction of anatomy. Finally, the transition of medical education from an apprenticeship format to competency-based training with objective assessment was key for the acceptance of simulation in surgery [113, 114].

Canadian pioneer Dr. Richard Reznick ignited the evolution of objective measurement of surgical skills with the Objective Structured Assessment of Technical Skills (OSATS) [115, 116]. Canadian colleagues also released the McGill Inanimate System for Training and Evaluation of Laparoscopic Skills (MISTELS) which formed the basis for the current golden standard in surgical training evaluation, the Fundamentals of Laparoscopic Surgery (FLS) [117]. FLS was validated by SAGES, and it is a joint program between SAGES and the American College of Surgeons (ACS). These programs are propelling surgical training down the path of criterion-based training (mastery education model) instead of the traditional time-based path. Training devices needed to evolve to support mastery education in surgery.

Three crude virtual reality trainers appeared in the 1987–1992 [118, 119]. The subjects of these prototypes that didn't progress beyond the investigation stage were limb movement, wound debridement, and general surgery. The first commercial unit was the Minimally Invasive Surgical Trainer (MIST-VR) [120, 121]. MIST-VR was felt to be an improvement over simpler models because it could accurately track performance, efficiency, and errors. Transfer of skills learned in the trainer to the operating room in the form of increased speed and reduced errors was reported [122, 123]. Similar benefits were described for the early Endoscopic Surgical Simulator (ESS), a collaboration between otolaryngologists and Lockheed Martin that prepared residents to perform sinus surgery [124]. The MIST trainer is currently available from Mentice Inc. Mentice was founded in 1999. Mentice launched the first endovascular simulator VIST in 2001 and later added a small compact version called the VIST-C. The FDA recognized the value of simulation training by requiring practice in a simulated environment before approval to use new carotid vessel stents. Mentice also acquired and markets the Xitact™ IHP and Xitact™ THP haptic laparoscopic devices.

HT Medical, founded in 1987 by Greg Merril, demonstrated its first virtual reality endoscopy simulator in 1992. Based on this success, HT Medical was acquired by Immersion in 2000, a company that focused on nonmedical haptic hardware and software for gaming and the automobile industry. The BMW iDrive was developed in collaboration with Immersion and represented one of the first computer/haptic interfaces in a motor vehicle. The new division that focused on haptic devices for healthcare training was named Immersion Medical Inc. They expanded their product line to include endovascular simulation, bronchoscopy simulation, ureteroscopy simulation, an intravascular catheter simulator (now Laerdal's Virtual IV ®), a robotic arm for orthopedic surgery, and the high-fidelity Touchsense® tactile and force feedback systems. An updated version of the endoscopy simulator is still in production today as the CAE Endoscopy VR Surgical Simulator [125]. CAE Healthcare also acquired Haptica's ProMIS™ surgical training system in 2011. The ProMIS™ is a unique hybrid trainer that uses real instruments with virtual and physical models and is the only trainer to allow practice through a single keyhole.

Simbionix entered the arena of procedural simulation in 1997 and released their first commercial product, GI Mentor™, in 2000. Their next product was the URO/Perc Mentor™. Simbionix launched the LAP Mentor™ laparoscopy trainer in 2003. They followed with the release of ANGIO Mentor™ for practice of endovascular procedures in 2004. In 2005 Simbionix partnered with eTrinsic. ETrinsic was recognized for web-based curriculum and evaluation development. This move brought Simbionix from simple technical systems to integrated educational solutions. More recently, Simbionix partnered in 2011with McGraw-Hill to bring AccessSurgery™ an on-line resource to customers of Simbionix's MentorLearn system. Simbionix continues to add surgical modules to their training hardware. The latest releases from 2010 to 2011 are TURP, nephrectomy, and pelvic floor repair. Surgical simulation by Simbionix has progressed to a concept of pre-practice using virtual representations of actual patient anatomy: "mission rehearsal." The first report of this type of surgical rehearsal appeared in 1987 when an orthopedic surgeon used an early virtual reality simulator of the leg developed at Stanford to assess the results of tendon repair by walking the leg [118]. Endovascular simulation was the next to adapt this technology to advance problem solving for complicated patients. In 2010, Simbionix received grant support to develop a hysterectomy module, obtained FDA approval for their PROcedure Rehearsal Studio™ software, and launched a mobile training app.

Three other recent developments may further refine and impact surgical simulation. The first is a proliferation of devices to track hand motion including Blue Dragon, Ascension Technology's Flock of Birds, Polhemus, and the Imperial College Surgical Assessment Device (ICSAD). Hand tracking may be used by itself or with the addition of eye tracking. Simulation has also become an integral part of robotic surgery. There are four current robotic simulators available [126]. One group cautions that while current simulators are validated in the acquisition of new skills, improvements in technology and realism are necessary before they can recommend routine use for advanced training or maintenance of certification [127]. Another group has helped to define the future priorities for surgical simulation [128]. One key priority is to extend the validation of simulation training to patient outcomes.

The American College of Surgeons (ACS) was the first group to offer official accreditation of simulation centers. In addition to mannequin-based simulation and team training, these sites must also offer simulation for minimally invasive surgery. Currently, over 60 centers worldwide have achieved this milestone (see Fig. 2.6). Expansion was almost linear for the first 4 years with the addition of ~10 approved centers each year [129]. The process stalled in 2010 similar to the data from Bristol Medical Simulation Center about the worldwide expansion of simulation centers but seemed to be recovering in 2011.

Conclusion

It is difficult to pinpoint the precise moment when simulation in healthcare reached the tipping point. As late as 2004, Dr. Gaba projected two possible scenarios for the future of simulation in healthcare. One version was a very bleak vision in which simulation did not achieve acceptance. It is now clear that simulation has experienced that "magic moment" similar in force and scope to a full-scale social revolution [130]. While technology facilitated this revolution in healthcare education, it was dependent on visionary

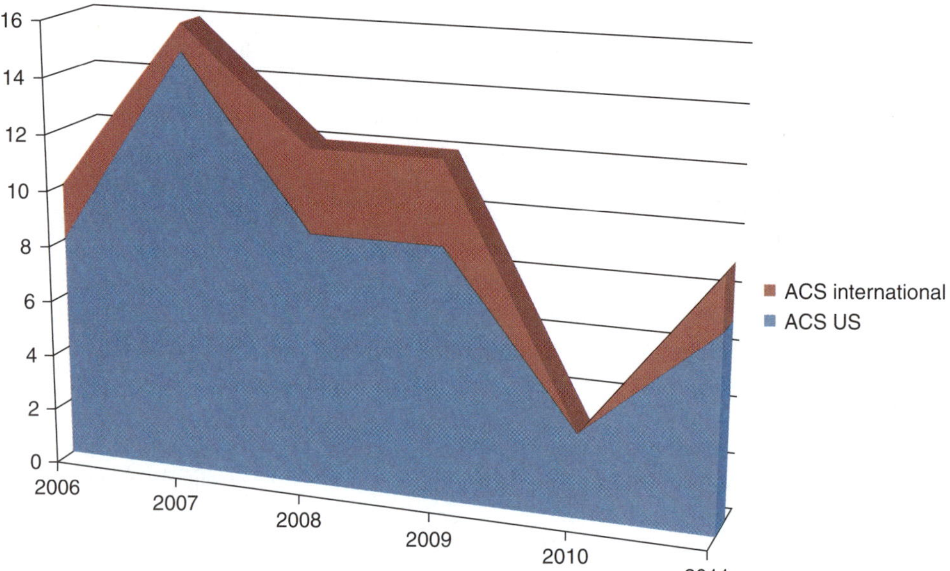

Fig. 2.6 ACS accreditation of simulation centers

people who implemented this technology in ways that will benefit many. There is more of the simulation story yet to be written. Despite beneficial and monumental changes in healthcare education and healthcare team performance, the incidence of medical error has not decreased and some believe that it is increasing [131]. Simulation has not yet demonstrated the desired effect on patient safety and outcomes. It is possible that it is too early to assess simulation's impact on patient safety. Alternatively, it is possible that additional change and innovation are necessary before this goal can be attained.

References

1. Maury K. The technological revolution. Foreign Policy Res Inst Newsl. 2008;13(18). [Serial online]. Available at: http://www.fpri.org/footnotes/1318.200807.klein.techrevolution.html. Accessed 4 Jan 2012.
2. Computer History Museum. Exhibits. Available at: http://www.computerhistory.org/exhibits/. Copyright 2013. Accessed 12 Mar 2013.
3. Computer History Museum. Revolution: Calculators. Available at: http://www.computerhistory.org/revolution/calculators/1. Copyright 1996–2013. Accessed 12 Mar 2013.
4. Computer History Museum. Revolution: Timeline. Available at: http://www.computerhistory.org/revolution/timeline. Copyright 1996–2013. Accessed 12 Mar 2013.
5. Computer History Museum. Computer History Timeline. Available at: http://www.computerhistory.org/timeline/. Copyright 2006. Accessed 12 Mar 2013.
6. Computer History Museum. A Classical Wonder: The Antikythera Mechanism. Available at: http://www.computerhistory.org/revolution/calculators/1/42. Copyright 1996–2013. Accessed 12 Mar 2013.
7. Computer History Museum. Introducing the Keyboard. Available at: http://www.computerhistory.org/revolution/calculators/1/55. Copyright 1996–2013. Accessed 12 Mar 2013.
8. Computer History Museum. The Punched Card's Pedigree. Available at: http://www.computerhistory.org/revolution/punched-cards/2/4. Copyright 1996–2013. Accessed 12 Mar 2013.
9. Computer History Museum. The Revolutionary Babbage Engine. Available at: http://www.computerhistory.org/babbage/. Copyright 1996–2013. Accessed 12 Mar 2013.
10. Computer History Museum. Making Sense of the Census: Hollerith's Punched Card Solution. Available at: http://www.computerhistory.org/revolution/punched-cards/2/2. Copyright 1996–2013. Accessed 12 Mar 2013.
11. IBM archives 1885. Available at: http://www-03.ibm.com/ibm/history/history/year_1885.html. Accessed 4 Jan 2012
12. IBM archives 1891. Available at http://www-03.ibm.com/ibm/history/history/year_1891.html Accessed 4 Jan 2012.
13. IBM archives 1880's. Available at: http://www-03.ibm.com/ibm/history/history/decade_1880.html. Accessed Jan 2012.
14. IBM archives 1893. Available at: http://www-03.ibm.com/ibm/history/history/year_1893.html. Accessed 4 Jan 2012.
15. IBM Archives 1889. Available at: http://www-03.ibm.com/ibm/history/history/year_1889.html. Accessed 4 Jan 2012.
16. IBM Archives 1920's. Available at: http://www-03.ibm.com/ibm/history/history/decade_1920.html. Accessed 4 Jan 2012.
17. Ceruzzi PE. The advent of commercial computing. A history of modern computing. Salisbury: MIT Press; 2003. p. 1–47.
18. Ceruzzi PE. Chapter 2: Computing comes of age, 1956–1964. In: A history of modern computing. Salisbury: MIT Press; 2003. p. 48–78.
19. Rojas R, Zuse K. Konrad Zuse internet archive. (German, 1910–1995). Available at http://www.zib.de/zuse/home.php/Main/KonradZuse. Accessed 4 Jan 2012.
20. Allerton D. Historical perspective. In: Principles of flight simulation. West Sussex: John Wiley & Sons; 2009. p. 1–9.
21. Greeneyer F. A history of simulation: part III-preparing for war in MS & T magazine 2008, issue 6. Available at: http://halldale.com/insidesnt/history-simulation-part-iii-preparing-war. Accessed 4 Jan 2012.
22. Greeneyer F. A history of simulation: part II-early days in MS & T magazine 2008, issue 5. Available at: http://halldale.com/insidesnt/history-simulation-part-ii-early-days. Accessed 4 Jan 2012.
23. Link EA, Jr. Combination training device for aviator students and entertainment. US Patent # 1,825,462. Available at: http://www.google.com/patents?id=CRJuAAAAEBAJ&pg=PA13&dq=edwin+link+1,825,462&hl=en&sa=X&ei=y0r_TvjuFOTk0QGz9dHCA

g&ved=0CDMQ6AEwAA#v=onepage&q=edwin%20link%20 1%2C825%2C462&f=false. Accessed 4 Jan 2012.
24. National Inventor's Hall of fame. Edwin A Link. Available at: http://www.invent.org/hall_of_fame/192.html. Copyright 2002. Accessed 4 Jan 2012.
25. Ledbetter MN. CAE-link corporation in airlift tanker: history of US airlift and tanker forces. Padukah: Turner Publishing; 1995. p. 76.
26. Greenyer F. A history of simulation: part I. in MS & T magazine 2008, issue 4. Available at: http://halldale.com/insidesnt/history-simulation-part-i. Accessed 4 Jan 2012.
27. Compton WD. Where no man has gone before: a history of Apollo lunar exploration missions in NASA special publication-4214 in the NASA History Series, 1989. Available at: http://history.nasa.gov/SP-4214/cover.html. Accessed 4 Jan 2012.
28. Star Trek Database. Where No Man Has Gone Before. Available at: http://www.startrek.com/database_article/where-no-man-has-gone-before. Copyright 1966. Accessed 12 Mar 2013.
29. Abrahamson S. Essays on medical education (S.A.'s on medical education). Lanham: University Press of America® Inc; 1996.
30. Simpson DE, Bland CJ. Stephen Abrahamson, PhD, ScD, Educationist: a stranger in a kind of paradise. Adv Health Sci Educ Theory Pract. 2002;7:223–34.
31. Guilbert JJ. Making a difference. An interview of Dr. Stephen Abrahamson. Educ Health. 2003;16:378–84.
32. Barrows HS, Abrahamson S. The programmed patient: a technique for appraising student performance in clinical neurology. J Med Educ. 1964;39:802–5.
33. Hoggett R. A history of cybernetic animals and early robots. Available at: http://cyberneticzoo.com/?tag=stephen-abrahamson. Accessed 12 Mar 2013.
34. YouTube. Sim one computerized dummy medical patient invention newsreel PublicDomainFootage.com. Available at: http://www.youtube.com/watch?v=dFiqr2C4fZQ. Accessed 4 Jan 2012.
35. YouTube. Future shock (1972) 3/5. Available at: http://www.youtube.com/watch?v=oA_7yWPlCYo. Accessed 4 Jan 2012.
36. Abrahamson S, Denson JS, Clark AP, Taback L, Ronzi T. Anesthesiological training simulator. Patent # 3,520,071. Available at: http://www.google.com/patents/US3520071. Accessed 4 Jan 2012.
37. Denson JS, Abrahamson S. A computer-controlled patient simulator. JAMA. 1969;208:504–8.
38. Abrahamson S, Denson JS, Wolf RM. Effectiveness of a simulator in anesthesiology training. Acad Med. 1969;44:515–9.
39. Abrahamson S, Denson JS, Wolf RM. Effectiveness of a simulator in anesthesiology training. Qual Saf Health Care. 2004;13:395–9.
40. Hmelo-Silver CE. In Memoriam: remembering Howard S. Barrows. Interdiscip J Probl Based Learn. 2011;5:6–8.
41. State Journal-Register: Springfield Illinois. Obituaries: Howard S Barrow. Available at: http://www.legacy.com/obituaries/sj-r/obituary.aspx?n=howard-s-barrows&pid=149766653. Copyright 2011. Accessed 12 Mar 2013.
42. Wallace P. Following the threads of innovation: the history of standardized patients in medical education. Caduceus. 1997;13:5–28.
43. Barrows HS. An overview of the uses of standardized patients for teaching and evaluating clinical skills. Acad Med. 1993;68:443–53.
44. Wallace J, Rao R, Haslam R. Simulated patients in objective structured clinical examinations: review of their use in medical education. APT. 2002;8:342–8.
45. Tamblyn RM, Barrows HS. Bedside clinics in neurology: an alternate format for the one-day course in continuing medical education. JAMA. 1980;243:1448–50.
46. Dillon GF, Boulet JR, Hawkins RE, Swanson DB. Simulations in the United States Medical Licensing Examination™ (USMLE™). Qual Saf Health Care. 2004;13:i41–5.
47. Eichhorn JH, Cooper JB. A tribute to Ellison C. (Jeep) Pierce, Jr., MD, the beloved founding leader of the APSF. APSF Newsletter fall 2011. [Serial online]. Available at: http://www.apsf.org/newsletters/html/2011/fall/02_pierce.htm. Accessed 4 Jan 2012.
48. Beecher HK, Todd DP. A study of deaths associated with anesthesia and surgery. Ann Surg. 1954;140:2–34.
49. Eichhorn JH. The APSF at 25: pioneering success in safety, but challenges remain. 25th anniversary provokes reflection, anticipation. APSF Newsl. Summer 2010;25(2). [Serial online]. Available at: http://www.apsf.org/newsletters/html/2010/summer/index.htm. Accessed 4 Jan 2012.
50. Pierce EC. The 34th Rovenstine lecture. 40 years behind the mask: safety revisited. Anesthesiology. 1996;84:965–75.
51. Keats AS. What do we know about anesthetic mortality? Anesthesiology. 1979;50:387–92.
52. Cooper JB, Newbower RS, Long CD, McPeek B. Preventable anesthesia mishaps: a study of human factors. Anesthesiology. 1978;49: 399–406.
53. Cooper JB, Long CD, Newbower RS, Phillip JH. Multi-hospital study of preventable anesthesia mishaps. Anesthesiology. 1979;51:s348.
54. Cooper JB, Newbower RS, Kitz RJ. An analysis of major errors and equipment failures in anesthetic management: considerations for prevention and detection. Anesthesiology. 1984;60:34–42.
55. Dutton RP. Introducing the anesthesiology quality institute: what's in it for you? ASA Newsl. 2009;73:40–1 [Serial online].
56. Cheney FW. The American Society of Anesthesiologists closed claims project: the beginning. Anesthesiology. 2010;115:957–60.
57. Eichhorn JW. Prevention of intraoperative anesthesia accidents and related severe injury through safety monitoring. Anesthesiology. 1989;70:572–7.
58. Adam Rouilly. Our history. Available at: http://www.adam-rouilly.co.uk/content/history.aspx. Copyright 2013. Accessed 12 Mar 2013.
59. Gaumard. Our History of Innovation. Available at: http://gaumardscientific.mybigcommerce.com/our-history/ Accessed 4 Jan 2012.
60. Gaumard. E-news November 2010. Available at http://www.gaumard.com/newsletter/nov-10/index.html. Accessed 4 Jan 2012.
61. March SK. W. Proctor Harvey: a master clinician teacher's influence on the history of cardiovascular medicine. Tex Heart Inst J. 2002;29:182–92.
62. Gordon MS, Messmore FB. Cardiac training manikin. Patent # 3,662,076. Available at: http://www.google.com/patents?id=NEovAAAAEBAJ&printsec=abstract&source=gbs_overview_r&cad=0#v=onepage&q&f=false. Accessed 4 Jan 2012.
63. Poylo MC. Manikin audio system. Patent # 3,665,087. Available at: http://www.google.com/patents?id=554yAAAAEBAJ&printsec=abstract&source=gbs_overview_r&cad=0#v=onepage&q&f=false. Accessed 4 Jan 2012.
64. Gordon MS. Cardiology patient simulator: development of an animated manikin to teach cardiovascular disease. Am J Cardiol. 1974;34:350–5.
65. Gordon MS, Patterson DG. Cardiological manikin auscultation and blood pressure systems. Patent # 3,947,974. Available at: http://www.google.com/patents?id=UwkvAAAAEBAJ&printsec=abstract&zoom=4&source=gbs_overview_r&cad=0#v=onepage&q&f=false. Accessed 4 Jan 2012.
66. Gordon MS, Ewy GA, DeLeon Jr AC, et al. "Harvey", the cardiology patient simulator: Pilot studies on teaching effectiveness. Am J Cardiol. 1980;45:791–6.
67. Sajid AW, Ewy GA, Felner JM, et al. Cardiology patient simulator and computer-assisted instruction technologies in bedside teaching. Med Educ. 1990;24:512–7.
68. Gordon MS et al. Cardiopulmonary patient simulator. Patent # 7,316,568. Available at: http://www.google.com/patents/US7316568?printsec=abstract&dq=7,316,568&ei=iy3-ToKaDqji0QGS0umRAg#v=onepage&q=7%2C316%2C568&f=false. Accessed 4 Jan 2012.

69. Michaels S Gordon Center for Research in Medical Education. The all new Harvey. Available at: http://www.gcrme.miami.edu/#/harvey-major-changes. Accessed 4 Jan 2012.
70. Laerdal. History: Laerdal Yesterday and Today. Available at: http://www.laerdal.com/us/doc/367/History. Copyright 2012. Accessed 12 Mar 2013.
71. Grenvik A, Schaefer J. From Resusci-Anne to Sim-Man: the evolution of simulators in medicine. Crit Care Med. 2004; 32(Suppl):S56–7.
72. Limbs and Things. Company History. Available at: http://limbsandthings.com/us/about/history/. Copyright 2002–2013. Accessed 12 Mar 2013.
73. Fukui Y, Smith NT. Interactions among ventilation, the circulation, and the uptake and distribution of halothane-use of a hybrid computer model: I. The basic model. Anesthesiology. 1981;54:107–18.
74. Fukui Y, Smith NT. Interactions among ventilation, the circulation, and the uptake and distribution of halothane-use of a hybrid computer model: II. Spontaneous vs controlled ventilation and the effects of CO2. Anesthesiology. 1981;54:119–24.
75. Mandel JE, Martin JF, Schneider AM, Smith NT. Towards realism in modelling the clinical administration of a cardiovascular drug. Anesthesiology. 1985;63:a504 [Abstract].
76. Smith NT, Sebald AV. Teaching vasopressors with sleeper. Anesthesiology. 1989;71:a990 [Abstract].
77. Schwid HA, Wakeland C, Smith NT. A simulator for general anesthesia. Anesthesiology. 1986;65:a475 [Abstract].
78. Schwid HA. A flight simulator for general anesthesia training. Comput Biomed Res. 1987;20:64–75.
79. Schwid HA, O'Donnell D. The anesthesia simulator-recorder: a device to train and evaluate anesthesiologist's response to critical incidents. Anesthesiology. 1990;72:191–7.
80. Schwid HA, O'Donnell D. Anesthesiologists management of critical incidents. Anesthesiology. 1992;76:495–501.
81. Schwid HA, O'Donnell D. The anesthesia simulator-consultant: simulation plus expert system. Anesthesiol Rev. 1993;20:185–9.
82. Gutierrez KT, Gross JB. Anesthesia simulator consultant. Anesthesiology. 1995;83:1391–2.
83. Kelly JS, Kennedy DJ. Critical care simulator: hemodynamics, vasoactive infusions, medical emergencies. Anesthesiology. 1996;84:1272–3.
84. Gaba DM. The future vision of simulation in health care. Qual Saf Health Care. 2004;13:i2–10.
85. Smith B, Gaba D. Simulators. In: Lake C, editor. Clinical monitoring: practical application for anesthesia and critical care. Philadelphia: W. B. Saunders; 2001. p. 26–44.
86. Gaba DM, DeAnda A. A comprehensive anesthesia simulation environment: re-creating the operating room for research and training. Anesthesiology. 1988;69:387–94.
87. Gravenstein JS. Training devices and simulators. Anesthesiology. 1988;69:295–7. [Editorial].
88. Gaba DM, DeAnda A. The response of anesthesia trainees to simulated critical incidents. Anesthesiology. 1988;69:A720. Abstract.
89. Gaba DM, Fish KJ, Howard SK. Crisis management in anesthesiology. Philadelphia: Churchill Livingston; 1994.
90. Center for Medical Simulation, 2009. History of medical simulation and the development of CMS. Available at: http://www.harvardmedsim.org/about-history.php. Accessed 4 Jan 2012.
91. Good ML, Gravenstein JS, Mahla ME, et al. Can simulation accelerate the learning of basic anesthesia skills by beginning anesthesia residents? Anesthesiology. 1992;77:a1133. Abstract.
92. Good ML, Lampotang S, Gibby GL, Gravenstein JS. Critical events simulation for training in anesthesiology, abstracted. J Clin Monit. 1988;4:140.
93. Good ML, Gravenstein JS, Mahla ME, et al. Anesthesia simulation for learning basic anesthesia skills, abstracted. J Clin Monit. 1992;8:187–8.
94. Michael L Good MD Curriculum Vitae. Available at: http://www.med.ufl.edu/about/employment-dean-search-cv-good.pdf. Accessed 4 Jan 2012.
95. Lampotang S, Good ML, Gravenstein JS, et al. Method and apparatus for simulating neuromuscular stimulation during medical simulation. Patent # 5,391,081. Available at: http://www.google.com/patents?id=sV0cAAAAEBAJ&printsec=frontcover&dq=5,391,081&hl=en&sa=X&ei=jfn_TtKOAurn0QGP5cWtAg&ved=0CDMQ6AEwAA. Accessed 4 Jan 2012.
96. Lampotang S, van Meurs W, Good ML, et al. Self regulating lung for simulated medical procedures. Patent # 5,584,701. Available at: http://www.google.com/patents?id=soweAAAAEBAJ&printsec=frontcover&dq=5,584,701&hl=en&sa=X&ei=qvn_Tp3mBsnV0QG2qvWPAg&ved=0CDMQ6AEwAA. Accessed 4 Jan 2012.
97. Lampotang S, van Meurs W, Good ML, et al. Apparatus and method for simulating bronchial resistance or dilation. Patent # 5,772,442. Available at http://www.google.com/patents?id=3C8cAAAAEBAJ&printsec=frontcover&dq=5,772,442&hl=en&sa=X&ei=xvn_Ts6hHML30gGrm8mMBA&ved=0CDMQ6AEwAA. Accessed 4 Jan 2012.
98. Lampotang S, van Meurs W, Good ML, et al. Apparatus and method for synchronizing cardiac rhythm related events. Patent # 5,769,641. Available at: http://www.google.com/patents?id=bV4nAAAAEBAJ&printsec=frontcover&dq=5,769,641&hl=en&sa=X&ei=_Pn_TuOpB6Xb0QHehdXIDQ&ved=0CDMQ6AEwAA. Accessed 4 Jan 2012.
99. Lampotang S, van Meurs W, Good ML, et al. Apparatus and method of simulating breath sounds. Patent # 5,779,484. Available at: http://www.google.com/patents?id=AuonAAAAEBAJ&printsec=frontcover&dq=5,779,484&hl=en&sa=X&ei=Evr_Tv7qH6jl0QHW9LX-Ag&ved=0CDMQ6AEwAA. Accessed 4 Jan 2012.
100. Lampotang S, van Meurs W, Good ML, et al. Apparatus and method for simulating lung sounds in a patient simulator. Patent # 5,868,579. Available at: http://www.google.com/patents?id=8OsXAAAAEBAJ&printsec=frontcover&dq=5,868,579&hl=en&sa=X&ei=J_r_ToT9I-PV0QHzxMyDAg&ved=0CDMQ6AEwAA. Accessed 4 Jan 2012.
101. Lampotang S, van Meurs W, Good ML, et al. Apparatus and method for quantifying fluid delivered to a patient simulator. Patent # 5,882,207. Available at: http://www.google.com/patents?id=rGcXAAAAEBAJ&printsec=frontcover&dq=5,882,207&hl=en&sa=X&ei=VPr_TvGtLKnX0QGRuamEAg&ved=0CDMQ6AEwAA. Accessed 4 Jan 2012.
102. Lampotang S, van Meurs W, Good ML, et al. Apparatus for and method of simulating the injection and volatizing of a volatile drug. Patent # 5,890,908. Available at: http://www.google.com/patents?id=qqMWAAAAEBAJ&printsec=frontcover&dq=5,890,908&hl=en&sa=X&ei=dfr_TuWgCefm0QHzz4HQDw&ved=0CDMQ6AEwAA. Accessed 4 Jan 2012.
103. Lampotang S, van Meurs W, Good ML, et al. Apparatus and method of simulation the determination of continuous blood gases in a patient simulator. Patent # 5,941,710. Available at: http://www.google.com/patents?id=Lw8ZAAAAEBAJ&printsec=frontcover&dq=5,941,710&hl=en&sa=X&ei=h_r_TqjaJunl0QH00IHMAg&ved=0CDMQ6AEwAA. Accessed 4 Jan 2012.
104. Arne R, Stale F, Petter L. Pat-Sim. Simulator for practicing anesthesia and intensive care. Int J Clin Monit Comput. 1996;13:147–52.
105. Byrne AJ, Hilton PJ, Lunn J. Basic simulations in anaesthesia: a pilot study of the ACCESS system. Anaesthesia. 1994;49:376–81.
106. Chopra V, Engbers FH, Geerts MJ, Filet WR, Bovill JG, Spierhjk J. The Leiden anaesthesia simulator. Br J Anaesth. 1994;73:287–92.
107. Chopra V, Gesnik B, DeJing J, Bovill JG, Spierdijk J, Brand R. Does training on an anaesthesia simulator lead to improvement in performance? Br J Anaesth. 1994;73:293–7.
108. Anderssen HB, Jensen PF, Nielsen FR, Pedersen SA. The anaesthesia simulator SOPHUS. Roskilde: Riso National Laboratory; 1993.

109. Christensen UJ, Andersen SF, Jacobsen J, Jensen PF, Ording H. The Sophus anaesthesia simulator v. 2.0. A windows 95 control-center of a full scalc simulatora. Int J Clin Monit Comput. 1997;14:11–6.
110. Cooper JB, Taquetti VR. A brief history of the development of mannequin simulators for clinical education and training. Qual Saf Health Care. 2004;13:i11–8.
111. Satava RM. Accomplishments and challenges of surgical simulation. Surg Endosc. 2001;15:232–41.
112. Cuschieri A, Wilson RG, Sunderland G, et al. Training initiative list scheme (TILS) for minimal access therapy: the MATTUS experience. J R Coll Surg Edinb. 1997;42:295–302.
113. Satava RM. Historical review of surgical simulation-a personal perspective. World J Surg. 2008;32:141–8.
114. Satava RM. The revolution in medical education-the role of simulation. J Grad Med Educ. 2009;1:172–5.
115. Faulkner H, Regher G, Martin J, Reznik R. Validation of an objective structured assessment of technical skill for surgical residents. Acad Med. 1996;71:1363–5.
116. Martin JA, Regehr G, Reznick R, MacRae H, et al. Objective structured assessment of technical skills (OSATS) for surgical residents. Br J Surg. 1997;84:273–8.
117. Fundamentals of Laparoscopic Surgery. Available at: http://www.flsprogram.org/. Copyright 2013. Accessed 12 Mar 2013.
118. Delp SL, Loan JP, Hoy MG, Zajac FE, Topp EL, Rosen JM. An interactive graphics-based model of the lower extremity to study orthopedic surgical procedures. Trans Biomed Eng. 1990;37:757–67.
119. Satava RM. Virtual reality surgical simulator: first steps. Surg Endosc. 1993;7:203–5.
120. Wilson MS, Middlebrook A, Sutton C, Stone R, McCloy RF. MIST VR: a virtual reality trainer for laparoscopic surgery assesses performance. Ann R Coll Surg Eng. 1997;79:403–4.
121. Taffinder NJ, Russell RCG, McManus IC, Darzi A. An objective assessment of laparoscopic psychomotor skills: the effect of a training course on performance. Surg Endosc. 1998; 12(5):493.
122. Darzi A, Smith S, Taffinder NJ. Assessing operative skill. BMJ. 1999;318:877–8.
123. Seymour NE, Gallagher AG, Roman SA, O'Brien MK, Bansal VK, Andersen DK, et al. Virtual reality improves operating room performance: results of a randomized double blind study. Ann Surg. 2002;236:458–63.
124. Edmond CV, Wiet GJ, Bolger B. Surgical simulation in otology. Otolaryngol Clin North Am. 1998;31:369–81.
125. Immersion. Medical Products. Available at: http://www.immersion.com/markets/medical/index.html. Copyright 2013. Accessed 12 Mar 2013.
126. Lallas CD, Davis JW. Robotic surgery training with commercially available simulation systems in 2011. A current review and practice pattern survey from the Society of Urologic Robotic Surgeons. J Endourol. 2011. [Serial online]. Available at: http://www.ncbi.nlm.nih.gov/pubmed/22192114. Accessed 4 Jan 2012.
127. De Visser H, Watson MO, Salvado O, Passenger D. Progress in virtual reality simulators for surgical; training and certification. Med J Aust. 2011;194:S38–40.
128. Stefanidis D, Arora S, Parrack DM, et al. Association for Surgical Education Simulation Committee. Research priorities in surgical simulation for the 21st century. Am J Surg. 2012;203:49–53.
129. American College of Surgeons: Division of Education. Listing of ACS Accredited Education Institutes. Available at: http://www.facs.org/education/accreditationprogram/list.html. Revised 10 Nov 2011; Accessed 4 Jan 2012.
130. Gladwell M. The tipping point. Boston: Back Bay Books; 2002. p. 3–132.
131. Adverse events in hospitals: national incidence among medicare beneficiaries. Department of Health and Human Services. Office of the Inspector General. 2010;1–74.

Education and Learning Theory

3

Susan J. Pasquale

Introduction

As the use of medical simulation in healthcare continues to expand, it becomes increasingly important to appreciate that our approach to teaching, and our knowledge of pedagogy and learning, will need to expand proportionately. It is this complementary expansion that will serve to provide an environment that optimally addresses basic and vital educational and patient care outcomes. Teaching and learning is fundamental to the use of medical simulation in healthcare. However, all too frequently, teaching and learning is circumvented only to have the focus on the technology or equipment without adequate preparation for the teaching or adequate reflection about the learning.

There are many theoretical perspectives of learning, including behaviorist, cognitivist, developmental, and humanist. There are learning theory perspectives offered such as Bruner's constructivist theory, Bandura's social learning theory, Kolb's experiential learning, Schon's reflective practice theory, and sociocultural theory that draws from the work of Vygotsky, to name a few, many of which intersect and overlap with each other. Mann [1] presents a review of theoretical perspectives that have influenced teaching in medical education. However, having knowledge of theory alone will not build the bridges needed to enhanced teaching and learning. It is how to operationalize the theory, how to put it into practice in a teaching and learning environment, that will make that connection.

It is important to make a distinction between theories of learning and theories of teaching. While "theories of learning deal with the ways in which an organism learns, theories of teaching deal with the ways in which a person influences an organism to learn" [2]. As such, it is presumed that "the learning theory subscribed to by a teacher will influence his or her teaching theory." Knowles et al. [3], make the distinction by noting that learning is defined as "the process of gaining knowledge and or expertise … and … emphasizes the person in whom the change is expected to occur, [while] education emphasizes the educator."

It is essential to possess at least a foundational understanding of learning theory to better understand the process of learning and the learner. That being said, the practice of most teachers is influenced by some philosophy of teaching or framework that guides their teaching, even if that theoretical orientation is not implicit or fully recognized by them. Therefore, the intent of this chapter is to begin to connect theory with practice by presenting the reader with practical, easy to use information that operationalizes aspects of educational theories and theoretical perspectives into approaches that are immediately applicable to learning in an educational environment focused on healthcare simulation and that will serve to guide teaching practices.

Perspectives on Teaching and Learning

The term "learning experience" refers to "the interaction between the learner and the external conditions in the environment to which they can react. Learning takes place through the active behavior of the student; it is what *he* does that he learns, not what the teacher does" [4].

Harden et al. [5], remind us that "educators are becoming more aware of the need to develop forms of learning that are rooted in the learner's practical experience and in the job they are to undertake as a professional on completion of training." The authors further make the point that development of critical reflection skills is essential to effectiveness in clinical healthcare.

The use of experiential learning enhances the learner's critical thinking, problem-solving, and decision-making skills, all goals of teaching with medical simulation. Experiential learning helps move the learner through stages

S.J. Pasquale, PhD
Department of Administration,
Johnson and Wales University,
8 Abbott Park Place, Providence, RI 02903, USA
e-mail: susan.pasquale@jwu.edu

A.I. Levine et al. (eds.), *The Comprehensive Textbook of Healthcare Simulation*,
DOI 10.1007/978-1-4614-5993-4_3, © Springer Science+Business Media New York 2013

that can strengthen the teaching and learning experience. Experiential learning operates with the principle that experience imprints knowledge more readily than didactic or online presentations alone. In experiential learning, learners build knowledge together through their interactions and experiences within a learning environment that engages the learner and supports the construction of knowledge.

"Simulation is a 'hands-on' (experiential learning) educational modality, acknowledged by adult learning theories to be more effective" [6], than learning that is not experiential in nature. Simulation offers the learner opportunities to become engaged in experiential learning. In a simulation learning environment, learning takes place between learners, between the teacher and learner, between the learner and content, and between the learner and environment.

In Dewey's experiential learning theory, knowledge is based on experiences that provide a framework for the information. Dewey asserts that it is important for learners to be engaged in activities that stimulate them to apply the knowledge they are trying to learn so as they have the knowledge and ability to apply it in differing situations. As such, "they have created new knowledge and are at an increased level of readiness for continued acquisition and construction of new knowledge" [7]. Experiential learning offers the learner the opportunity to build knowledge and skills. Learning to apply previously acquired knowledge and skills to new situations requires practice and feedback.

In Kolb's cycle of experiential learning, the learner progresses through a cycle consisting of four related phases: concrete experience (an event), reflective observation (what happened), abstract conceptualization (what was learned, future implications), and active experimentation (what will be done differently). Learners' prior experiences have a direct relationship to their future learning, thus reinforcing the importance of the four phases of the experiential learning process, in particular the reflective observation and abstract conceptualization aspects. Dewey stresses that opportunities for reflection are essential during an experience, in that they provide opportunities for the learner to make the connection between the experience and the knowledge they draw from the experience. As such, as learners move through the phases of experiential learning, they strengthen their ability to internalize the process as they continue to learn how to become better learners and how to be lifelong learners. Schon's "reflection on action," is "a process of thinking back on what happened in a past situation, what may have contributed to the … event, whether the actions taken were appropriate, and how this situation may affect future practice" [7]. As learners increasingly internalize this process of reflection on action, it is expected that it will be supplemented by "reflection in action," which occurs immediately, while the learning event is occurring.

There is a direct relationship between experiential learning theory and constructivist learning theory. In constructivism, learners construct knowledge as they learn, predicated on the meaning they ascribe to the knowledge based on their experience and prior knowledge. This points to a significant relationship between a learner's prior knowledge and experience and their process of constructing new knowledge. Within this constructivism paradigm, the learner is guided by the teacher to establish meaningful connections with prior knowledge and thus begins the process of constructing new knowledge for themselves.

In constructivism frameworks, the learner constructs knowledge through active engagement in the learning environment and with the content. Simulation is a common teaching-learning method within this framework, in which the learner constructs knowledge for application in real-world activities. This framework also gives the learner more responsibility for self-assessment, a component of the Kolb framework noted earlier. The role of the teacher is more of a guide or facilitator. Further, if the learner finds the learning task to be relevant, intrinsic motivation is more likely, leading to deeper learning with more links to prior knowledge, and a greater conceptual understanding. Simulation holds the potential to operationalize the constructivist framework, in that it provides active engagement with the content, coupled with application to real-world activities. Within constructivism, learners are provided the opportunity to construct knowledge from experiences. The theory also purports that an individual learns in relationship to what else he/she knows, meaning that learning is contextual.

Bruner's theory of instruction and interest in sequencing of knowledge is not unlike Kolb experiential learning cycle, in that it addresses "acquisition of new information …, manipulation of knowledge to make it fit new tasks…, and checking whether the manipulated information is adequate to the task" [3]. As such, it includes reflecting on what happened and what will be done differently next time.

Self-regulation theory, based on the work of Bandura, similarly to Kolb's cycle, can also be viewed as a cyclical loop, during which the learners "engage in an iterative process during which they use task-specific and metacognitive strategies, and continuously gather information about the effectiveness of these strategies in achieving their goals" [8]. Typically, the phases of the self-regulation process are preparation or forethought about what is to take place, the experience or performance itself, and self-reflection.

Situated learning, a perspective of sociocultural learning, asserts that "learning is always inextricably tied to its context and to the social relations and practices there; it is a transformative process that occurs through participation in the activities of a community" [1]. Mann notes that "situated learning can complement experiential learning by framing the…experience within a community of practice" [1].

Learning and Prior Knowledge

A goal of learning is to assimilate new information into an existing organization of information or memory. The more connections new information has to prior knowledge, the easier it is to remember. When new knowledge is linked with a learner's accurate and well-organized prior information, it is easier to learn in that it becomes a part of the connections that already exist and avoids becoming rote or memorized information [9]. Correspondingly, it is important to assess prior knowledge of the learner so that new knowledge acquired by the learner does not link to that inaccurate prior knowledge, in turn, building on an incorrect foundation of information. Consequently, it is important to recognize that the outcomes of student learning are influenced by the prior knowledge they bring to the learning experience.

Applying learning theory and our knowledge of teaching is vital to the success of the patient care and educational goals of medical simulation; it is therefore important to consistently look for incorrect prior knowledge in the learner. Assessment is a key element of the teaching process, in that teaching needs to begin with an analysis of what the learner needs. The needs and level of the learners are essential in helping the learners to build on prior knowledge and skills.

Research indicates that learners have differing cognitive styles or preferred ways of processing information. Further, learners have preferred variables that influence ways in which they prefer to learn. Those preferred variables include whether they prefer to learn independently, from peers, or teachers; whether they prefer to learn through auditory, tactile, kinesthetic, or visual inputs; whether they prefer more detail-oriented, concrete, abstract, or combinations of these; and what the characteristics are of the physical environment in which they prefer to learn.

Learning is also influenced by the learner's approach to learning, which encompasses their motivation for learning. Learners can employ three approaches to learning—surface, deep, and strategic. Entwistle [10], notes features and differences of these three approaches to learning (see Table 3.1).

Table 3.1 The features of three approaches to learning

Deep approach
Intention to understand
Motivated by intrinsic interest in learning
Vigorous interaction with content
Versatile learning, involving both:
Comprehension learning
Relate new ideas to previous knowledge
Relate concepts to everyday experience
Operational learning
Relate evidence to conclusions
Examine the logic of the argument
Confidence
Surface approach
Intention to reproduce or memorize information needed for assessments
Motivated by extrinsic concern about task requirement
Failure to distinguish principles from examples
Focus on discrete elements without integration
Unreflectiveness about purpose or strategies
Anxiety or time pressures
Strategic approach
Intention to obtain highest possible grades
Motivated by hope for success
Organize time and distribute effort to greatest effect
Ensure conditions and materials for studying appropriately
Use previous exam papers to predict questions
Be alert to cues about marking schemes

Motivation and Learning

Research points to a relationship between motivation to learning. Intrinsic motivation links to a deep approach to learning, where as extrinsic motivation links to a surface approach to learning. Mann endorses a relationship between motivation and learning, noting that motivation and learning are integrally related [11]. "A necessary element in encouraging the shift from extrinsic to intrinsic motivation appears to be the opportunity for learners to practice a skill/task until they gain competence; satisfaction with accomplishments and competence is itself motivating, and encourages in the learner further practice and the confidence to undertake new tasks" [12].

Mann points out that "the development of self-efficacy is essential to support and encourage motivation" [11]. Self-efficacy is defined as perception of one's "capabilities to produce designated levels of performance…." [12]. "Self-efficacy beliefs determine how people feel, think, motivate themselves and behave… People with high assurance in their capabilities approach difficult tasks as challenges to be mastered rather than as threats to be avoided. Such an efficacious outlook fosters intrinsic interest and deep engrossment in activities" [12].

Similar to Mann's perspectives about self-efficacy, Voyer and Pratt [13], comment that "the relationship between the evolving professional identify of the learner and the receipt of feedback either confirms or questions that evolving identity in the form of information about the person's competence." Thus, in that identity and competence are highly related, feedback on competence is interpreted as directly related to the learner's sense of self. As suggested by Mann [11] earlier, identity, competence, and self-efficacy all also directly influence a learner's motivation. That being said, it becomes clear that the reflective observation phase of Kolb's experiential learning cycle, and the feedback on performance inherent in that phase, is essential and a key link to the development of intrinsic motivation for further learning. Moreover, it is the reflective observation of what happened in the experience, and the abstract conceptualization of what was learned and what the implications are for future iterations of the same experience (i.e., what will be done differently next time), that facilitates the learner's progression of understanding through the five stages of Miller's triangle (i.e., knows what, knows how, shows how, does, and mastery) [14], as well as through Bloom's hierarchy of cognitive learning. Bloom's six levels of increasing difficulty or depth representing the cognitive domain are:

1. Knowledge
2. Understanding (e.g., putting the knowledge into one's own words)
3. Application (e.g., applying the knowledge)
4. Analysis (e.g., calling upon relevant information)
5. Synthesis (e.g., putting it all together to come up with a plan)
6. Evaluation (e.g., comparing and evaluating plans)

Self-Reflection and Learning

Reflection is "the process by which we examine our experiences in order to learn from them. This examination involves returning to experience in order to re-evaluate it and glean learning that may affect our predispositions and action in the future" [15].

"Reflection is a metacognitive (*thinking about thinking*) process that occurs before, during and after a situation with the purpose of developing greater understanding of both the self and the situation so that future encounters with the situation are informed from previous encounters" [16]. As such, it is critical for learners to develop metacognitive skills. However, learners may make metacognitive errors such as not recognizing when they need help in their learning. Such errors stress the need for regular feedback and reflection on learning experiences so as not to compromise a false sense of competence and self-efficacy while maintaining the learner's professional sense of self and motivation.

Reflective learning is grounded in experience. This "reflection on experience" was the aspect of reflection paid most attention to by Schon. However, it is "reflection in action" that has been deemed as essential in self-assessment. "Without a culture that promotes reflection…, learners may not consider their progress systematically and may not articulate learning goals to identify gaps between their current and desired performance" [17].

If the goal of teaching is to facilitate learning, then it is essential that teacher activities be oriented toward the process of learning process. A Learning-Oriented Teaching Model (LOT) "reflects an educational philosophy of internalization of teacher functions in the learner in a way that allows optimal independent learning…." [18]. The LOT model is not unlike Kolb's, with its use of reflective observation as a prerequisite for the learner's movement through his other phases. The only apparent difference being that the LOT model is a more longitudinally based model, with the ultimate internalization of learning the result of multiple cycles of the Kolb phases. The metacognitive skills needed by the learner for this reflective observation, so as to assess, identify, and alter deficits in knowledge, are not easy to acquire and may necessitate significant feedback and guidance. Learners may also need guidance on how to incorporate new knowledge and experience into existing knowledge and then apply it, thus application of the LOT model in support of constructivism and experiential learning theory.

Conclusion

It is clear that developing an increased awareness of the processes of learning is fundamental in guiding our teaching practice. This chapter has provided information on a number of teaching and learning perspectives, and on their commonalities and intersections, that are immediately applicable to the environment of healthcare simulation. It is expected that the reader will use the information to enhance their practice of teaching and, thus, the learning of those they teach.

References

1. Mann KV. Theoretical perspectives in medical education: past experience and future possibilities. Med Educ. 2011;45(1):60–8.
2. Gage NL. Teacher effectiveness and teacher education. Palo Alto: Pacific Books; 1972.
3. Knowles MS, Holton III EF, Swanson RA. The adult learner: the definitive class in adult education and human resource development. 5th ed. Houston: Gulf Publishing Co; 1973.
4. Tyler R. Basic principles of curriculum and instruction. Chicago: The University of Chicago Press; 1949.
5. Harden RM, Laidlaw JM, Ker JS, Mitchell HE. Task-based learning: an educational strategy for undergraduate, postgraduate and continuing medical education. AMEE medical education guide no. 7. Med Teach. 1996;18:7–13. Cited by: Laidlaw JM, Hesketh EA, Harden RM. Study guides. In: Dent JA, Harden RM, editors. A practical guide for Med Teach. Edinburgh: Elsevier; 2009.
6. Ziv A. Simulators and simulation-based medical education. In: Dent JA, Harden RM, editors. A practical guide for medical teachers. Elsevier: Edinburgh; 2009.
7. Kaufman DM. Applying educational theory in practice. In: Cantillon P, Hutchinson L, Wood D. editors. ABC of learning and teaching in medicine. London: BMJ Publishing Group; 2003.
8. Sandars J, Cleary TJ. Self-regulation theory: applications to medical education: AMEE guide no. 58. Med Teach. 2011;33(11): 875–86.
9. Svinicki M. What they don't know can hurt them: the role of prior knowledge in learning. Teach Excellence. A publication of The

Professional and Organizational Development Network in Higher Education. 1993–1994;5(4):1–2.
10. Entwistle N. A model of the teaching-learning process. In: Richardson JT, Eysenck MW, Piper DW editors. Student learning: research in education and cognitive psychology. The Society for Research into Higher Education and Open University Press. Cited by: Forster A. Learning at a Distance. Madison: University of Wisconsin-Madison; 2000.
11. Mann KV. Motivation in medical education: how theory can inform our practice. Acad Med. 1999;74(3):237–9.
12. Bandura A. Self-efficacy. In: Ramachaudran VS, editor. Encyclopedia of human behavior, vol. 4. New York: Academic Press; 1994. p. 71–81. (Reprinted in Friedman H, editor. Encyclopedia of mental health. San Diego: Academic Press; 1998.) http://www.uky.edu/~eushe2/Bandura/BanEncy.html. Accessed 8 Mar 2013.
13. Voyer S, Pratt DD. Feedback: much more than a tool. Med Educ. 2011;45(9):862–4.
14. Dent JA, Harden RM. A practical guide for medical teachers. Edinburgh: Elsevier; 2009.
15. Mann K, Dornan T, Teunissen P. Perspectives on learning. In: Dornan T, Mann K, Scherpbier A, Spencer J, editors. Medical education theory and practice. Edinburgh: Elsevier; 2011.
16. Sandars J. The use of reflection in medical education: AMEE guide no. 44. Med Teach. 2009;31(8):685–95.
17. Bing-You RG, Trowbridge RI. Why medical educators may be failing at feedback. JAMA. 2009;302(12):1330–1. Cited by: Hauer KE, Kogan JR. Realising the potential value of feedback. Med Educ. 2012; 46(2): 140–2.
18. ten Cate O, Snell L, Mann K, Vermunt J. Orienting teaching toward the learning process. Acad Med. 2004;79(3):219–28.

4 The Use of Humor to Enrich the Simulated Environment

Christopher J. Gallagher and Tommy Corrado

Introduction

> Nothing is less funny than talking about being funny.
>
> Someone must have said that.

"Take my mannequin, please!"

If you're looking for side-splitting humor to rope people into your simulator, then you have come to the right chapter. Roll out a few of our one-liners and you are sure to *close* your simulator center in no time.

What?

That's right, this chapter is more about "reining in" your humor than "burying the students in hilarity." Humor is a part of teaching in the simulator, but it's like chocolate—fine in small measures, but no one wants to be force-fed cappuccino truffles until they're comatose. So hop on board and we'll take you through a carefully titrated aliquot of humor to keep your sim sessions interesting without making them treacly sweet.

Here's how we're going to attack the entire question of humor in the simulator:

- Should you include humor?
- Should you study humor?
- Do you need to justify use of humor?
- Does the literature back up humor?
- And finally, what should you, the simulation educator, do about including humor in your simulation experiences?

Do You Need to *Include* Humor?

> Simulation is theater.
> All theater has comedy.
> Therefore all men are kings.
>
> Famous logician/simulator instructor

C.J. Gallagher, MD (✉) • T. Corrado, MD
Department of Anesthesiology,
Stony Brook University, 19 Beacon Hill Dr.,
Stony Brook, NY 11790, USA
e-mail: christopher.gallagher@stonybrook.edu

What is the best meeting to go to all year?

- American Society of Anesthesiology? Naa, too big.
- Comic-Con? Better, better, but still not the best.
- International Meeting for Simulation in Healthcare (IMSH)? Yes!

And why is that? Because that is where all the simulator people go. And simulator people all have two things in common:

1. Not good looking enough for Hollywood.
2. Not talented enough for Broadway.

That's right; a convention of simulator people is, in effect, a convention of *actors*. (D-listers, at best, but still.) Because simulation, with all the emphasis on mannequins and scenarios and checklists, is still *theater*. No one remembers which props Shakespeare used in *Macbeth*, and only archeologists can guess the width of the proscenium at the original Globe Theatre on the banks of the Thames, but we still remember the *characters* that Shakespeare created. We still focus on the *actors*. And at the IMSH you will meet the dramatis personae that populate the world's simulator "stages."

At the IMSH, you will meet nurse educators, anesthesiologists, emergency medicine, and internal medicine—nearly every specialty (I've never seen a pathologist at these meetings, only a matter of time, though). And everyone, every presentation, every talk, and every workshop is basically an attempt to create educational *stagecraft*:

- We'll show you how we create a believable scenario where a transfusion mix-up leads to a cardiac arrest.
- Attend our workshop where we'll show you how to create the makeup effects to generate a believable mass-casualty setting.
- Look over our creation, an LED display that makes it look like the patient is going into anaphylaxis.
- Would you like whipped cream with that? (Oops, you stepped up to the Starbucks®.)

The entire meeting focuses on stagecraft—creating a mini-drama where you teach your students how to handle a syringe swap or a respiratory arrest or a difficult airway or a multi-trauma victim.

A.I. Levine et al. (eds.), *The Comprehensive Textbook of Healthcare Simulation*,
DOI 10.1007/978-1-4614-5993-4_4, © Springer Science+Business Media New York 2013

Where does humor come in?

All stagecraft for all time has employed humor. So roll up your sleeve, shove your entire arm into that bag of history next to you, and let's take a look.

- What is the symbol we use for Greek theater? The two masks, one frowning, one smiling. The ancient Greeks always sweetened their tragedies with a dollop of humor.
- Opera may be a bit stuffy, but when Figaro belts out his funny song in *The Barber of Seville*, it cracked them up at La Scala Theater in Milan. Skip forward a few centuries, and Bugs Bunny is using the same song to make *us* laugh.
- Shakespeare killed off people left and right in *Hamlet* and dumped some hefty memorizing for legions of captive English students ("To be or not to be, that is [the assignment]"), but even here, he managed to squeak in a few humorous lines:

> Hamlet: "What's the news?"
> Rosencrantz: "None, my lord, but that the world's grown honest."
> Hamlet: "Then is doomsday near."
>
> Hamlet Act II, Scene 2

So what the heck, if it's good enough for them, it's good enough for us. Our "simulation stagecraft" should have a little humor in it too.

OK, but *how* do you do it?

Do You Need to *Study* Humor?

> Manager of The Improv in Miami, "I'll bet you tell funny stories at work, don't you?"
> Gallagher, scuffing his feet, "Yeah."
> Manager, smiling, "And you think that's going to work here, don't you?"
> Gallagher, looking down in an "Aw shucks" way, "Yeah."
> Manager, no longer smiling, "Well, it won't. You'll bomb and look like an idiot."
> Verbatim conversation three weeks before Gallagher's first stand-up performance "Injecting a Little Humor" at The Improv in Miami, 2005

Study humor? Doesn't that kind of, well, *kill* it? Doesn't humor just sort of "happen"? "Well up" from your witty self?

In the realm of stand-up comedy, the answer is "Yes, you DO need to study comedy!" as I discovered in my own first foray into that bizarre realm. The manager of The Improv saved me from certain disaster, by steering me in the right direction.

> Here's the deal," she said. "When you're up there in front of a bunch of strangers, you can't just weave a long shaggy dog story and hope they'll hang with you until you finally get to the funny part. You'll lose them, you've got to get to the point, and fast. Stand up is more like learning to play the violin than just 'standing there saying funny things,' so you get to the bookstore and pick up *Stand-Up Comedy: The Book*, by Judy Carter. You get that book and you study it like you're getting ready for finals. You do every single exercise in that book, just like she says. And you write your jokes just exactly the way she does. Do that, and you'll kill. Do it your own way, and you'll die out there.

I had a busy three weeks adapting to the "ways of stand-up." But it paid off. Here's what I learned and here's the take-home lesson for you, if you seek to inject some humor into your "simulator act":

- All stand-up is amazingly formulaic.
- *Straight line, second straight line, twist.*
- *Straight line, second straight line, twist.*
- Watch Leno or Letterman tonight, or watch any of the zillion stand-up comics on The Comedy Channel. Watch comedy monologues on YouTube or listen on a satellite radio station that specializes in comedy. It's ALWAYS THE SAME.
- Watch reruns of Seinfeld (especially his monologues at the end of the show) or Woody Allen on old *Tonight* shows. It will floor you when you realize that, whether it's X-rated humor from the street or highbrow humor from Park Avenue, the basic 1 – 2 – 3 of all stand-up jokes is identical.

You set up the situation, then you deliver the punch. Let's see if we can do this ourselves (yes, creating humor takes practice, just like playing an instrument).

As I sit here writing, it's July 11, 2011, 5:50 p.m., I'm sitting at my dining room table and I just pulled the New York Times front section over to me. Let's look at something on the front page and see if we can "create humor," using the formula:

- Straight line, second straight line.
- Twist.

OK, here's an article on the People Skills Test that a med school is using to see if aspiring doctors will be good team players.

A Medical School is using a People Skills Test on their applicants.

Good people skills should translate into good doctors, they guess.

Show up with parsley stuck in your teeth and there goes a career in brain surgery.

OK, Comedy Central will not be blocking out a three-hour special for me anytime soon, but you get the drift. You set it up with two factual statements (drawn from today's newspaper), and (this is the hard part, and why I make my living as an anesthesiologist and not a comedian) then you throw your own twist into the equation.

So that's how stand-up comedy's done. But does that mean you have to do stand-up comedy in your simulation center? Of course not. You're there to teach a lesson, not "grab the mike and bring the house down" with your rip-roaring wit. But I think it's worth the effort (especially if you're not a "natural" at snappy comebacks) to study a little bit of "comedy creation." Spend a few bucks and a few hours honing your humorous skills with the pros. The exercises in Judy Carter's book are actually pretty funny (surprise surprise, funny stuff in a book about comedy, who'd a thunk it?). And what the heck, if this simulation job doesn't work out, who knows, maybe you WILL be the next Jerry Seinfeld! They code the patient for 20 min, the simulated family members are going crazy, the sweat is dripping, and then you come in the room and say, "Oh, isn't this guy a DNR?" Everybody laughs, the scenario ends on a lighter note and you can foray right into the basics of systems-based- practice and checking simple things like DNR orders before keeping the heroics up for 20 min in real life.

Do You Need to *Justify* Humor?

> "Welcome to Journal Club, today we're looking at 'Humor in Medical Instruction'."
> Scowling face in the back, "I hope we have Level 1 Recommendations for it."
> Second scowling face, "Where was this double-blind, placebo-controlled, multi-center, sufficiently powered study done?"
> "Uh…"
> *My Life in Hell: Worst Moments from Journal Club*
> Christopher Gallagher, MD
> Born-Again Agnostic Press,
> expected pub'n date December 21, 2012

We justify what we do in medicine in one of two ways:

1. There is good evidence for it.
2. We make our best educated guess.

Thank God for good research, which, in its most rigorous form, uses proven techniques (double-blinding, placebo-controls, appropriate statistical analysis) to answer our many questions. Good evidence makes it easy to recommend the right drug/procedure/technique.

But plenty of times, we're stuck with our best educated guess. Moral issues prohibit us from doing a placebo control, or the complication is so rare that we cannot sufficiently power the study. And in the "soft" area of medical education, it becomes hard to design a "double-blinded" study.

Take humor.

Who out there will do the definitive study on whether "adding humor to simulation education" will improve patient outcomes?

- Funding? Who's going to pay for this? Billy Crystal? Chris Rock? Conan?
- Study design? How do you "double-blind" to humor? Tell crummy jokes to half the group, and slay the other half with top-notch hilarity?
- Statistics? Statistics and humor? "Three nonparametric data points stepped into a bar…"

So when it comes to justifying humor:

1. There is good evidence for it. NOT REALLY.
2. We make our best educated guess. YOUR GUT TELLS YOU, YES.

We have to go with (2) and make our best educated guess.

What's the Literature Say About Humor in Simulation Education?

First, let's look to textbooks and see about Humor in Simulation Education.

Clinical Simulation: Operations, Engineering and Management, Richard R Kyle, Jr, W. Bosseau Murray, editors, Elsevier, 2008. 821 pages, 10 pages of biographies of all the contributing authors (from all over the world, the only marginal contributor in the bunch being myself). This hefty tome (must be 5 lb if it's an ounce) has 22 topics fleshed out into 82 chapters and covers everything from soup to nuts in the simulation realm. Surely humor must be one of the:

- Topics? No.
- Chapters? No.
- Mentioned in the index? No.

Let's try something else. How about the book that I myself coauthored? Surely I must have mentioned humor in there somewhere? Let's peruse *Simulation in Anesthesia* (Chris Gallagher and Barry Issenberg, Elsevier, 2007). Although it's true there is humor in the book itself (mainly in the pictures), the subject of *using humor during instruction* somehow escapes the chapters, subheadings, and yes, the index. (Note to self, don't let that happen in the second edition.)

So the textbooks we're releasing don't seem to embrace humor in simulation instruction. Hmm. Where to next? The library!

A Trip to the Medical Library

"Yes, may I help you?" the librarian asks.

"Where is the card catalog?" I ask.

"The what?"

"The card catalog," I look askance at banks of computer terminals, this is not going well, "where you find out which books are on the shelves."

The librarian stares at me as you'd stare at a 12-armed extraterrestrial, just disgorged from a flying saucer. She assesses me as merely insane but too old to be sufficiently dangerous to warrant stirring the security guard from his slumber.

"What kind of books are you looking for?" she asks.

"Medical humor."

Click, click, click, click. Wait. Click click. "Try WZ 305."

"Thanks."

I walk past medical students with iPads in holders, iPods with earbuds, and thumbs in rapid-fire text mode. One of them looks up, takes the measure of my age, and takes a quick glance to the AED on the wall. Maybe this will be his big day to shine!

The stacks smell of old books, rarely read, and never checked out. (Why buy books when they're outdated by the time they're published?) WZ 305 coughs up a 1997 *The Best of Medical Humor* [1] and a 1998 *Humor for Healing* [2]. Well, humor is forever, so maybe the advice they have (no matter that it was written when Bill Clinton reigned over a country with a *surplus* [how quaint]) is still applicable?

Humor for Healing assures that humor has a long medical pedigree (p. 56–7):

- Laughter causes a "slackening body by the oscillation of the organs, which promotes restoration of equilibrium and has a favorable effect on health."
- Laughter "seems to quicken the respiratory and circulatory processes."
- Laughter also earned kudos for promoting "good digestion and heightening resistive vitality against disease."

Of course all these quaint and curious observations date back centuries. That is, the same people were *lauding* humor that were draining blood, applying poultices, giving clysters, and other "therapeutic" measures to *balance* our humors. So, consider the source.

OK, so humor is dandy for our health; what about humor in medical education? *The Best of Medical Humor* picks up on that, though nothing specifically mentions *simulation* education (we'll have to make that intellectual hopscotch ourselves). Articles like "Consultsmanship: How to Stay One-Up on Colleagues" and "Postmortem Medicine-An Essential New Subspecialty" assure us that humor has a welcome place in our ongoing education as doctors.

Other books have gained (infamous) cult status as "humor with a smidgeon of medical education thrown in":

- *Anesthesia for the Uninterested*, AA Birch, JD Tolmie, Aspen Publishers, Rockville, MD, 1976. In one fantastically politically incorrect picture, a scantily clad young lady stands near anesthetic apparatus in Playboy attire, with the label "The Ether Bunny."
- *House of God*, S Shem, Dell, New York, 1980. THE book for telling young doctors what life on the wards is actually like. Technology has changed, but the same machinations and madness hold sway in hospitals today, just like they did when Dr. Shem (a pseudonym, he knew better than to reveal his actual identity!) described them 30 years ago.
- *Board Stiff*, but wait, that's my book, let's not go there.

Suffice it to say, the marriage (however dysfunctional) of medical education to humor is here to stay.

Medical education *in the simulator* is medical education. Different, yes, in style. Augmented with mannequins, technology, and some additional techniques, but it is still medical education. So if humor works to:

- Aid the health of our students (*Humor in Healing*)
- Add spice to medical education (*The Best of Medical Humor*)
- Bend political correctness to educational ends (*Anesthesia for the Uninterested*)
- Show doctors-to-be the reality of hospital life (*House of God*) then humor has a welcome place in our simulators.

OK, we've looked at recent *textbooks*, we've made a trip to the *library* (how retro), now let's scour the *literature* and see what's up with humor in the simulator.

Crisp white coats and clipboards in hand, silent, stone-like faces veiling faint expressions of awe and fear, the Interns follow their Attending during rounds. No less a cliché, a bow tie peaks out from below his stringent scowl. As the group moves from bedside to bedside attention drifts between nervous looking patients and House Officers being lambasted for not knowing the subtleties of the most esoteric maladies. Then he speaks up. Hawaiian shirt collar visible where nobody else ventured more than a tasteful pastel. Hair unkempt, papers bulging from everywhere and an extremely pleasant smile on his face. His demeanor is disheveled yet pleasant as he is singled from the pack. All concern washes from the face of the terrified octogenarian they are discussing as he soothes her with his comical charms. The Attending, at first flabbergasted by his lack of reverence for tradition, soon learns how the simple gift of humor can be more potent than any man made elixir. Everyone present looks around approvingly and we in the audience feel a little better about the $12 we just spent on the movie ticket.

Actual doctors retch at this sap.

While the *Patch Adams* (Universal Studios, 1998, Robin Williams playing the insufferably cutesy doctor) perception of healthcare providers being dry, cold, and analytical may make for a great story line, it just doesn't seem to ring true in the real world. Most people are funny. We enjoy laughing and like making others do the same. "Did you see Letterman night?" or "I'm a little tired today, I stayed up watching Leno" seems a lot more common than "I just couldn't get myself to turn off CSPAN-2 yesterday." The major problem with humor is that just like sense of taste, every person's preference is a little different. Some people find the slapstick physical comedy of the Three Stooges or Chris Farley hysterical while others are drawn to the subtle, dry wit of a Mitch Hedberg or Stephen Wright. Keeping this in mind and with knowledge of your target audience, it's possible to use humor to give your simulations both flavor and flair.

Definition of Humor and Its Application

Humor, on the whole, is a difficult enough concept to define and understand, no less study. Merriam-Webster defines humor as something that is or is designed to be comical. To paraphrase Supreme Court Justice Potter Stewart's famous line from the 1964 case Jacobellis v. Ohio: "I know it when I see it" Howard J. Bennett, in his review article

"Humor in Medicine," provides a nice breakdown of the study of humor: humor and health, humor and patient-physician communication, humor in the healthcare professional, humor in medical education, and humor in the medical literature [3].

Humor in Medicine and Education

While review articles and essays on the role of humor in medicine and education have appeared in the literature for decades, a relative vacuum exists with respect to humor and simulation. Fortunately parallels that exist in the same principles can be applied with minimal modification.

In a 1999 editorial in the Medical Journal of Australia, Ziegler noted that 80% of the faculty at the Sydney Children's Hospital incorporated humor in their teaching sessions. They believed that the use of humor in teaching reduced stress, increased motivation, improved morale, enjoyment, comprehension, common interest, and rapport between students and faculty [4]. Humor can be employed as an educational tool as long as it is relative to the subject being taught.

In the 1996 article "Humor in Medicine" in the journal *Primary Care*, Wender notes that humor is playing an increasingly apparent role in medicine [5]. Matters such as the expression of frustration and anger, discussion about difficult matters, interpersonal and cultural gaps, as well as general anxiety can all be buffered by the application of humor. The practitioner also needs to be receptive of the patient-attempted humor as sometimes this can veil or highlight the true questions and concerns. Humor, not unlike beauty, seems to lie in the eye of the beholder. In their article "Use of Humor in Primary Care: Different Perceptions Among Patients and Physicians," Granek-Catarivas et al. demonstrated a significant difference between the patient's perception and the physician's attempt at humor [6]. The unique frames of reference possessed by both the physician and the patient change their ability to identify attempts at humor. While not completely analogous, the difference in knowledge and power between the physician and patient also exists between instructor and student. It seems reasonable then that the instructor's attempted humor might not be received and interpreted equally by the student.

Humor has been shown to improve the interactions within the members of a group, even in a serious or stressful setting. In Burchiel and King's article "Incorporating Fun into the Business of Serious Work: The Use of Humor in Group Process," they were able to show that through the use of humor and playful interaction, the members of a group were able to improve communication, creativity, problem solving, and team building [7]. All of these qualities are important not only in a good simulation but also in the real-life situations for which the students are being prepared.

In the end it can be argued that technique is only as effective as its results. Has there ever been a time where the use of humor did anything more than make a class or a lecture seem a little less boring? In the 1988 article "Teaching and Learning with Humor: Experiment and Replication," in *The Journal of Experimental Education*, Avner Ziv demonstrated on multiple occasions students of a one-semester statistics course scored significantly higher on their final examinations when the class was taught with humor relevant to the subject when compared with a similar group of students who were taught without such embellishment [8]. He then goes on to speculate as to several reasons this might be so. While this may not be directly comparable to medical simulation, the ability of humor to affect retention and comprehension is still intriguing.

Why Humor in Simulation?

With so many factors involved in creating a good simulation, one might ask themselves "Why even bother trying to make this situation funny?" We all have to deal with limited budgets, limited time, and limited participant interest. It's difficult enough trying to juggle these and other things, why should I throw another ball in the air and worry about the students enjoying themselves? We can all learn a lesson from good old-fashioned drive-in B movies and late-night cable sci-fi. They have to deal with many of the same problems we have so they have to rely on creativity and novelty to keep your attention. While no one is really convinced by the actor in the latex mask and foam rubber suit, the overly dramatic screams of the damsel in distress as the camera pans in on her mid-swoon is enough to make us chuckle and keep us watching. The same can be said of someone participating in the simulation. Just like sherbet served between the courses of the fine meal, a little laugh interjected now and again can help to refocus both the participant and the instructor and allow them both to participate more fully in the scenario.

Willing suspension of disbelief is a key component of any good simulation. Anyone who's ever played a role-playing game understands that the more deeply you immerse yourself in the experience, the more you're able to take out of it. The same is true with simulation. A participant who is able to let go of their inhibitions and truly participate in the construct almost certainly benefits more than someone who is simply going through the motions. High-fidelity mannequins, access to nearly unlimited resources, and a dozen supporting cast members mean almost nothing if the message of the simulation is lost on its target. Despite all of our hard work, occasionally it's difficult for the student to share our excitement in the project. Sometimes it's disinterest, sometimes it's stress, and sometimes it's just embarrassment. Any number of factors can hinder the student's participation.

Humor is a great equalizer and can be the answer to these and many other roadblocks. Perhaps this is best understood by temporarily changing roles with the student. You find yourself placed in a room, sometimes alone and sometimes with a group of equally disoriented peers. You're not quite sure what to expect, but you're fairly confident that it's not going to be simple or predictable. You find yourself searching your memory in the hopes you can remember what you're going to be tested on. Rather than reacting to the scenario presented to you, you find yourself trying to anticipate the next horror your instructor has prepared for you. You're worried that you may screw up and make a fool of yourself. In the midst of this anxiety and mounting mental exhaustion, it's no wonder there's limited mental resources available to actually take part in the situation. Enter humor. A well-timed laugh can help you not only relax your mind but also your inhibitions. You see a little of the instructor's humanity, feel a little safer, hopefully share their enthusiasm, and you find yourself slowly but steadily drawn into the simulation. We often try to make our simulations "hyperbolic" (e.g., the unbelievably unreasonable surgeon, the naïve intern saboteur) so the participants realize that we're in a safe place, a fun place, and still an educational place. The little giggle during the arrest doesn't take the participant out of the scenario by the acknowledgement of the artificiality of the simulation, it adds to the theater and allows them to immerse themselves in it, play the role, and hopefully get something out of the experience.

Humor as Component of Multimedia Simulation

Anyone who has ever found themselves in the lounge of a crowded coffee shop, on an elevator at rush hour, or peering through the window of the car next to them at a stoplight can attest to the fact that the age of multimedia information is upon us. It's almost impossible to imagine a student who doesn't have a smart phone, tablet, laptop computer, or any combination thereof. Couple that with the almost ubiquitous presence of high-speed Internet access and today's student has information at their fingertips which once would have been the envy of even the most prestigious academic university. Education is being pulled out of the classroom and becoming a completely immersive experience. This being the case, it seems logical that simulation in healthcare should follow the current trend. In an environment of seemingly limitless information and waning attention spans, how do you hold the student's interest? The answer: give them something they want to watch. A survey of the most frequently viewed items on almost any file sharing service shows an abundance of funny videos. Interjecting some degree of humor into your presentation may make the difference between capturing the student's attention and losing them to the next piece of eye candy.

The purpose of this chapter isn't to be a how-to manual on how to be funny. That should be a function of your unique abilities and perspective. A framework on which to hang your ideas, however, is a nice place to start. A video placed on a website or file server has the potential to reach far more people than could ever fit in a single classroom. The potential audience for such a project is tremendous and exciting. Inside jokes or allusion to little-known people quickly loses its meaning. The humor should be more broad-spectrum yet still relevant to the topic being presented. Today a single person with access to a personal computer and some affordable and readily available software can do things which once would've required the resources of an entire Hollywood studio. If you don't have the skills yet to be the next Stanley Kubrick, an evening with your computer and access to a search engine is usually enough to learn the basics. This is also a good time to go to your favorite video sharing site and see the videos that are trending well. If something is funny enough to get a few million hits, odds are there's something in it you can incorporate into your own simulation.

Myths and Misconceptions About Humor and Simulation

One can easily sit down and think of several reasons why humor has no role in education in any of its various incarnations. We medical folks are generally too serious, anyway. This type of thinking is potentially very limiting as it threatens to steal a potent tool from your repertoire and doesn't necessarily consider the needs of your audience: to learn and to possibly enjoy doing so.

Myth 1: If My Simulation Is Funny It Will Seem Less Professional

In truth, humor in the appropriate amounts can serve to punctuate the most poignant aspects of a scenario. It helps the participants and presenters to relax, focus on the material, and more completely obtain involvement and belief. Humor should be limited and as shown earlier appropriate and relevant to the topic being taught. Why not have your next simulated patient editorialize a bit before going off to sleep? Maybe they keep talking while the mask is on for preoxygenation. Your participants will laugh (our CA1's always do), and they can learn a simple lesson—how to professionally tell a patient to be quiet so they can properly preoxygenate before inducing anesthesia. The groups that don't tell the patient to quiet down and just breathe get a patient that desaturates more quickly and learn the lesson that way. The ones who tell the patient to "shut up" get a well preoxygenated patient but get some debriefing on handling difficult patient encounters properly. You win as an instructor, and they laugh at the ridiculous banter of the patient who just won't be quiet and fall asleep.

Myth 2: I'm Just Not a Funny Person. Dr. X Could Pull This Off but Not Me

Rarely is it ever a good idea to try to be something you're not, be that instructor, healthcare provider, or anything else. That being said, almost everyone has the potential for humor in some capacity. Integrating humor, just like everything in simulation, is about recognizing and utilizing your own talents to their fullest. Bruce Lee suggested the same thing about his martial art Jeet Kune Do: it is about you cultivating your own body as a martial art instrument and then expressing that instrument with the highest degree of efficiency and effectiveness and with total freedom. The more you integrate humor into your presentations the easier it becomes. Your own style emerges as your comfort grows.

Some of our educators are a bit unsure when they are first starting with groups of participants. When they act out certain parts, we dress them up. That is, a wig, some glasses, and a white coat and you've got a nutty professor. The educator usually can't help but embrace the role. The participants realize how ridiculous they look and then the scenario plays out in a friendly way.

Myth 3: What If I Say the Wrong Thing? How Will I Recover?

It's completely understandable to be concerned about spoiling an otherwise well-polished and effective presentation. Ultimately simulation is about flexibility. The mannequin doesn't do what we wanted, hours of setup and preparation laid to waste as the student instantly figures out in seconds what we hoped would take all afternoon or a forgotten misspoken line: these things are familiar to all of us. In the end we have to remember that this is, after all, a simulation. Just as the participants forgive us for our other mistakes, they'll also let us slide on the occasional dud. It happens to the best of us and we all just move on. We usually just tell them to pay no attention to the man behind the curtain as we reboot and start from scratch.

Myth (or Here, Idea) 4: Potential Pitfalls of Humor in Simulation

Just like any powerful tool, humor has the potential to do harm as well as good. When designing a simulation, it's important to remember that lightheartedness and folly might not always be appropriate. As Simon demonstrated in the article "Humor Techniques for Oncology Nurses" [9], a serious or depressing situation doesn't necessarily preclude the use of humor. On the contrary, a gentle and sympathetic comment can be both welcomed and therapeutic in a difficult situation. This has to be balanced against the danger of making light of the patient's suffering. The same holds true for the serious simulation. If the intent is to portray either a very stressful or somber situation, attempts at being funny can be distracting and undermine rather than fortify the simulation's design. Humor is a very valuable tool that helps to pull the student into the situation rather than distract them. For instance, if the goal is to teach a student how to break bad news to a patient or the family, it hardly seems appropriate to do this while waiting for a chuckle. Also, if the intent is to create a confusing and disorienting situation such as a multiple trauma, a coding patient, or significant crisis management, the humorous undertone can serve to dissolve the very tension you're trying to create. In brief, common sense usually dictates where, when, and how much "funny" we inject into a scenario. An 8-h day of laughs is hard to pull off but an 8-h day of misery is easy and, well, miserable.

Self-deprecation in limited amounts can add a sense of humanity and familiarity to a simulation depending upon the relationship the student shares with the instructor. That being said, certain things should be considered completely off-limits. It goes without saying that insulting the student or making comments centered on gender, ethnicity, religion, or disability is completely unacceptable. Anything that might be considered hurtful or offensive not only compromises a relationship with the student it also endangers the integrity and professionalism of the program. Very quickly what was once a warm, relaxing, and safe environment can feel cold, frightening, hostile, and even dangerous. Again, common sense.

As we've already mentioned before, simulation can be fun and it's possible to lose yourself in the roles you've created. It's important to remain cognizant, however, of the fact that the simulation takes place in what is essentially a classroom. The rules of acceptable behavior still hold fast. That being said, aggressive profanity, dirty jokes, and significantly offensive material should best be avoided. It does no good if all the student remembers at the end of the simulation is how uncomfortable they felt while they participated in it.

As the instructor, it's extremely rewarding when you watch a participant become more and more involved in your creation. As Shakespeare wrote in *As You Like It*, "All the world's a stage, and all the men and women merely players." Anyone who teaches in the simulator has to have a little of the acting bug in them, and usually more is better. In general, to hold the attention of the student, our performances have to be grandiose and larger-than-life. A good sense of humor benefits not only the student but also the teacher. Alternatively we want every simulation to be a spectacular educational experience. We want the student to get as much out of it as possible. Few things are more rewarding on both a professional or personal level than watching a group of students become more and more immersed in one of your creations. Humor is nearly always a part of that equation.

Conclusion

We've looked at how you might wedge a little humor into your simulation experience. And we've done this from a few different angles:

- Should you include humor? Yes, just rein it in a little, you budding stand-ups. Use your common sense.
- Should you study humor? Yes, we study everything else! Pay attention to funny people, funny movies—and incorporate it like you would a clinical situation.
- Do you need to justify use of humor? Naah. It has its place. There's a whole book abutting this chapter with tons of evidence about everything else.
- Does the literature back up humor? Sure, though, let's be honest, not with any kind of rigorous science because the NIH doesn't fund comedy. Sad, I know.

So what should you, the budding simulationologist-person, do about weaving some humor into your simulation experience? (This will be tough, but bear with.)

1. Plunk down in front of your TV and watch some Comedy Central while drinking beer and eating nachos. (I told you this would be hard.)
2. Go to YouTube, in the Search place, look up the following:
   Channel, Dr. Gallagher's Neighborhood
   Alternatively, just enter this web address
   http://www.youtube.com/user/DrCGallagher?feature=mhee
   You can see how I have used humor in putting together a ton of simulation videos.
3. Get a hold of *Stand-Up Comedy: The Book*, by Judy Carter (Delta, 1989, there may be newer versions). Even if you don't become a stand-up, you'll learn a thing or two about spicing up your sessions.
4. Go to a local comedy club, keep the receipt! Maybe you'll be able to write it off as a business expense.
5. Attend the IMSH (International Meeting for Simulation in Healthcare) and hang with other simulator people. The "funniness" will rub off on you.

That's it from Simulation Humorville. I hope this little chapter helps breathe a little fun into your educational plans. Now, I wonder what *did* happen when those three mannequins walked into a bar?

References

1. Harvey LC. Humor for healing: a therapeutic approach. Salt Lake City: Academic; 1999.
2. Bennet HJ. The best of medical humor. Philadelphia: Hanley and Belfus; 1997.
3. Bennett H. Humor in medicine. South Med J. 2003;96(12):1257–61.
4. Ziegler JB. Humour in medical teaching. Med J Aust. 1999;171:579–80.
5. Wender RC. Humor in medicine. Prim Care. 1996;23(1):141–54.
6. Granek-Catarivas M. Use of humour in primary care: different perceptions among patients and physicians. Postgrad Med J. 2005;81(952):126–30.
7. Burchiel RN, King CA. Incorporating fun into the business of serious work: the use of humor in group process. Semin Perioper Nurs. 1999;8(2):60–70.
8. Ziv A. Teaching and learning with humor: experiment and replication. J Exp Educ. 1988;57(1):5–15.
9. Simon JM. Humor techniques for oncology nurses. Oncol Nurs Forum. 1989;16(5):667–70.

The Use of Stress to Enrich the Simulated Environment

5

Samuel DeMaria Jr. and Adam I. Levine

Introduction

Although it is considered "safe" since no real patient can be harmed, learning in the simulated environment is inherently stressful. Standing at the head of a mannequin, performing in front of onlookers, and caring for a patient in an environment, where everyone around you seems to be making things worse and help has yet to arrive, are anything but easy. Follow this scenario with a debriefing session where you have to talk about mistakes, feelings, and decisions that played a part in your patient's (simulated) demise, and one has to wonder why anybody would ever want to learn this way.

Experiential learning is widely discussed and accepted as the subtext of the argument for and the utility of simulation-based education (Chap. 3). We learn by doing, we demonstrate our knowledge and skills by performing, and we ultimately want to believe that what we learn in simulation will help us function better in the actual clinical environment. Operating under this premise, the role of stress is rarely discussed in modern simulation-based educational exercises. If stress during simulation is discussed, it is usually framed in a context that includes ways to ameliorate rather than exploit it (Chap. 4). This is in spite of the fact that stress can make a simulation scenario more experiential than the mannequins or equipment being utilized.

Simulation is often presented as a way of augmenting education in the era of work hour restrictions and limited patient exposure for trainees. However, simulation resources are themselves expensive and limited and must be made more efficient vehicles of knowledge delivery; exploiting the stress inherent to simulation or even deliberately ramping up the stress of a scenario may make this possible. In this chapter we present some essential working definitions of stress and learning, a brief overview of stress and its interaction with learning and performance, as well as a practical approach to "dosing" stress so that educators can optimize the learning environment and learners can get the most out of their simulation-based teaching.

S. DeMaria Jr., MD (✉)
Department of Anesthesiology, Icahn School of Medicine at Mount Sinai, New York, NY, USA
e-mail: samuel.demariajr@mountsinai.org

A.I. Levine, MD
Departments of Anesthesiology, Otolaryngology, and Structural and Chemical Biology, Icahn School of Medicine at Mount Sinai, New York, NY, USA

What Is Stress?

Although we have all experienced stress and its meaning is largely self-evident, delving into whether or not stress has a place in simulation requires that certain terms and conditions be defined beforehand. McEwen describes stress as a homeostasis-threatening situation of any kind [1]. Stress can be described in numerous ways, but simply stated: stress is a (usually) negative subjective experience (real or imagined) that impacts one's well-being. It is categorized by physical, mental, and/or emotional strain or tension experienced when a person perceives that expectations and demands exceed available personal or social resources. However, stress has also been characterized as driving performance in a positive way, up to a point (Fig. 5.1). Anxiety, which is closely tied to stress, is a state characterized by somatic, emotional, cognitive, and/or behavioral components. Anxiety can lead to stress and stress can cause one to experience anxiety [2]. However one chooses to define these conditions, they are non-homeostatic, occur interchangeably, and therefore lead to certain physiological measures designed to restore this balance.

The Anatomy and Physiology of Stress

The two pathways activated by stress are the hypothalamic-pituitary-adrenal (HPA) axis and the autonomic nervous system (ANS, especially the sympathetic limb) (Fig. 5.2).

A.I. Levine et al. (eds.), *The Comprehensive Textbook of Healthcare Simulation*,
DOI 10.1007/978-1-4614-5993-4_5, © Springer Science+Business Media New York 2013

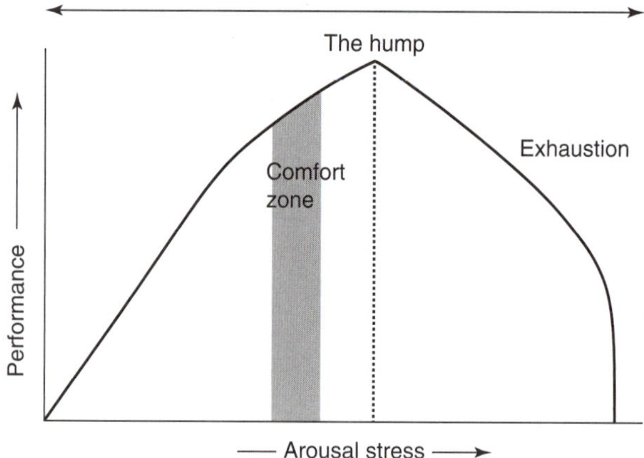

Fig. 5.1 Relationship of human performance and stress. The classic inverted U curve relating stress to performance. In general, certain levels of stress improve performance of specific tasks up to a point where they become detrimental to performance

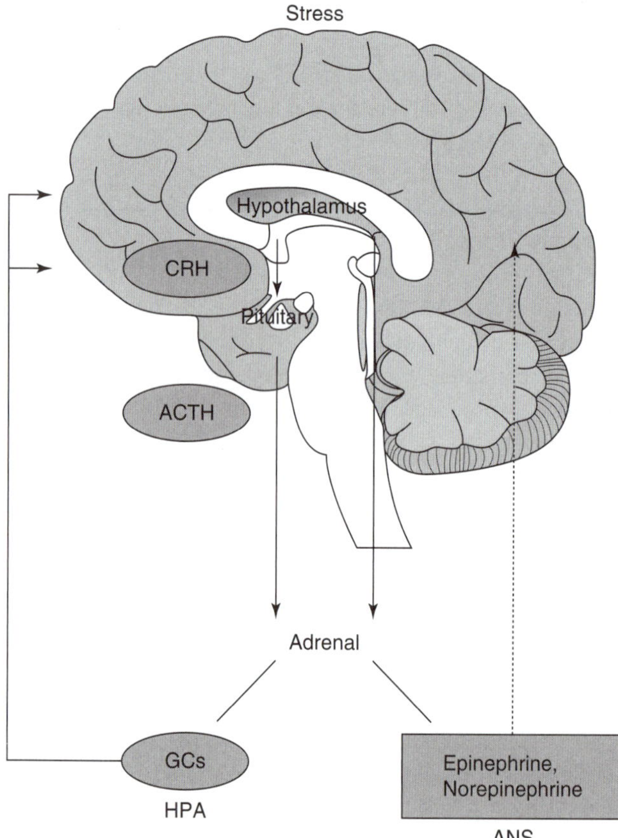

Fig. 5.2 Anatomy of stress. *CRH* corticotropin-releasing hormone, *ACTH* adrenocorticotropic hormone, *GC* glucocorticoid

Stressful events activate the amygdala and a network of associated brain regions. When stress is perceived, a rapid release of norepinephrine from the ANS stimulates alertness, vigilance, and focused attention. The amygdala initially activates the ANS by stimulating the hypothalamus, which in turn causes the release of norepinephrine throughout the body. This release occurs within the first 30 min after exposure to a stressor. The presence of norepinephrine also stimulates the adrenal medulla to release epinephrine.

A slower response simultaneously occurs as corticotrophin-releasing hormone (CRH) is released from the hypothalamus. CRH stimulates the pituitary to secrete endorphins and adrenocorticotropic hormone (ACTH), which induces the release of cortisol (and other glucocorticoids) from the adrenal cortex. The kinetic properties of corticosteroid exposure are slower than those of noradrenaline; peak corticosteroid levels in the brain are not reached earlier than 20 min after stress onset, and normalization takes place after roughly 1–2 h [3]. Cortisol binds with glucocorticoid receptors in the brain and, along with a cascade of neurotransmitter release, leads not only to an enhanced ability to act (i.e., fight or flight) but a mechanism by which the organism is prepared to face similar challenging situations in the future (essentially, a primitive form of learning; usually the memory of a stressful situation as one to avoid in the future).

What Is Learning?

While undeniably linked, learning and memory are slightly different entities. Learning is the acquisition or modification of a subject's knowledge, behaviors, skills, values, or preferences and may involve synthesizing different types of information. Memory is a process by which information is encoded, stored, and retrieved. Therefore, it is possible to remember something, without actually learning from the memory. A complete review of the neurobiology of learning is beyond the scope of this chapter, but certain key concepts are important for the reader and are discussed below (for a review of learning theory, see Chap. 3). Learning occurs through phases of the memory process. From an information-processing perspective, there are three main stages in the creation of a memory [4]:

1. Encoding or registration (receiving, processing, and combining received information)
2. Consolidation or storage (creation of a permanent record of the encoded information)
3. Retrieval, recall, or recollection (calling back the stored information in response to some cue for use in a process or activity; often used as proof that *learning* has occurred)

The pathways encoding memory are complex and modulated by mediators of stress (e.g., cortisol). These mediators can influence memory quality and quantity, and memories can be made more or less extinguishable or accessible by the experience of stress. The amygdala is central in this process as it encodes memories more resistant to extinction than commonly used (i.e., nonstress related) memory pathways.

Stress and Learning

For nearly five decades it has been understood that stress hormones are closely tied to memory. Both memory quantity [5] and quality [6] are affected by stress and stress can variably affect the three phases of memory and therefore potentially affect learning.

Studying the effects of stress on *encoding* alone is difficult because encoding precedes consolidation and retrieval. Therefore, any effect on encoding would naturally affect the other two in tandem. While results are conflicted, with some authors reporting enhanced encoding when learning under stress [7] and others reporting impairment [8], the critical factor appears to be the emotionality of the material being presented for memory [9, 10]. The intensity of the stress also appears to play a role with stress "doses" that are too high or too low leading to poor encoding (roughly reflecting an inverted U, Fig. 5.1) [11].

Remembering stressful experiences or the context surrounding them (i.e., *consolidation* of memory) is an important adaptation for survival; this is avoidance of danger at its most basic level. Considerable evidence suggests that adrenal hormones play a key role in enabling the significance of a stressful experience to impact the strength of a memory [12]. The stress-induced enhancement of memory is directly related to elevated cortisol levels, and this effect is most pronounced for emotionally arousing material [13], likely because the accompanying norepinephrine release interacts with glucocorticoid receptor sensitivity in the brain, priming the brain for improved storage of a stressful event [14]. The effects of stress on memory *retrieval* are overall opposite to those related to memory consolidation, with stress generally impairing retrieval of memories.

In addition to the above quantitative memory effects, it has been hypothesized that stress might also modulate the contribution of multiple memory systems and thus affect how we learn (i.e., the quality of the memory).

Figure 5.3 illustrates the timing of the rise of stress hormones in the basolateral amygdala (BLA), an area central to "emotional" learning [15]. It is important to note that the rise of stress hormones that prime the brain for encoding of memory and, therefore, learning correlates to the general time frame wherein debriefing is usually performed (i.e., post-stress

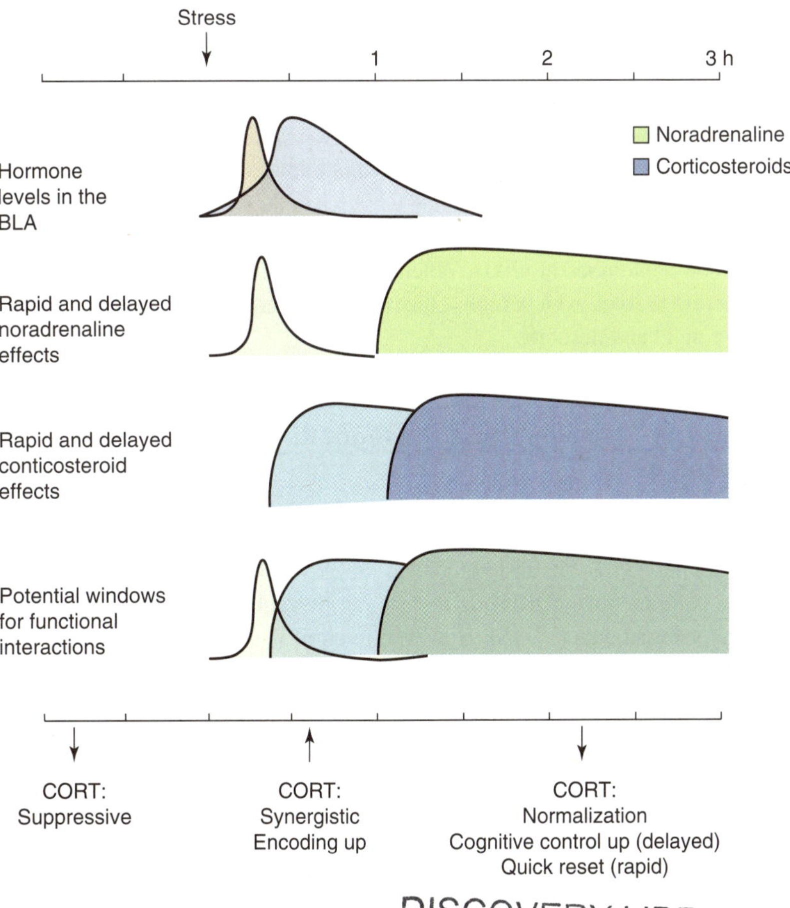

Fig. 5.3 Time line of the rise of stress hormones in the basolateral amygdala. Shortly after stress, noradrenaline levels (*yellow*) in the BLA are transiently elevated. Corticosteroids (*blue*) reach the same area somewhat later and remain elevated for approximately 1–2 h. For a restricted period of time, BLA neurons are exposed to high levels of both hormones (*upper panel*). Noradrenaline primarily works through a rapid G-protein-coupled pathway (*pale yellow*), but secondary genomic effects requiring gene transcription might develop (*bright yellow*). By contrast, effects of corticosteroid hormones are mostly accomplished via nuclear receptors that mediate slow and persistent actions (*bright blue*), although rapid nongenomic actions have also been described in the BLA (*pale blue*). The *lower panel* reflects the windows in time during which the two hormones might functionally interact (*green*). Shortly after stress, corticosteroids are thought to promote effects of noradrenaline (*upward arrow*) enabling encoding of information. Later on, corticosteroid hormones normalize BLA activity (delayed effect via GR), a phase in which higher cognitive controls seem to be restored. *Arrows* are showing the rising or falling levels of cortisol (Reprinted from Joëls et al. [15], Copyright (2011), with permission from Elsevier)

[the simulation]). This, we think, is not an accidental explanation as to why and how simulation and debriefing work in tandem.

At a neurobiological level, stress can be said to enhance learning, but a key factor in this process, which is relevant to simulation-based education, is the learning context. Memory is facilitated when stress and stress hormones are experienced within the context of the learning episode [16] and around the time of the event that needs to be remembered. However, if the hormonal mediators of stress exert their action out of the learning context (e.g., when they are presented during memory retrieval or have no natural relation to the material presented), they are mainly detrimental to memory performance. An example would be eliciting pain or other unpleasant physical phenomena to cause stress and then studying the effects of this stress on learning (this is often done during experiments on the phases of learning in animal models or psychological literature, but does not make practical or ethical sense for medical educators). Fortunately, stress caused by a simulation scenario is nearly always contextual and temporally related to events occurring in a representative clinical environment. In this fashion, appropriately applied and dosed stress will enhance educational benefit derived from a simulation experience by priming the brain for learning during the debriefing process.

Stress, memory, and situation awareness have been demonstrated on a large cultural scale. Stress and extreme emotional content "bookmark" our lives. For the last generation everyone could recall precisely where they were and what they were doing the moment they became aware of President Kennedy's assignation. This social experiment was reproduced during this generation. Everyone knows exactly what they were doing and where they were when they heard that the World Trade Center Buildings were hit by commercial jets on September 11, 2001. When asked, few can recall details from 9/10 or even 9/12, but the recall of details about 9/11 are vivid and durable.

Is Learning Through Stress the *Right* Kind of Learning?

The learning that occurs in a stressful environment is generally characterized as "habit-based," and on the surface, this may be contrary to the rich cognitive thinking required of medical professionals [17, 18]. However, in clinical environments where stressful situations are encountered, interference, ambiguity, and distraction have to be reduced. Fast reactions are required and extensive cognitive reflections cause hesitations that might endanger clarity of thought and action. Thus, the potential "bad" experience of stress (i.e., participant anxiety) is part of a fundamentally adaptive mechanism that allows one to focus on coping with stress in order to form a lasting, easily accessible memory of it for future situations. Simulation-based educators can exploit this adaptive behavior if stress is metered properly.

Although habit-based learning may be the result of stress-induced memory enhancement, it would be naïve to think that learning only takes place during and immediately after a simulation scenario. The emotional impact on the student is a very strong motivator to avoid such negative outcomes and feelings in the future. It could be hypothesized that this triggers significant efforts toward self-reflection, identification of knowledge and performance gaps, and further study to fill identified deficits. These are not such novel concepts; we all learn very early to avoid electric outlets after a gentle pat on the hand, the frustration of poor performance on an exam prompts us to study more in the future, and knowing our clinical material "cold" after experiencing a case that was way over our head or a bad patient outcome are common situations for all clinicians.

While studies are ongoing, limited evidence demonstrating the beneficial effects of inserting deliberate stressors into the simulated environment is available at present. Our group tested the hypothesis that a deliberately stressful simulation scenario (confrontational family member, failed intravenous access, and patient demise) followed by a thorough debriefing would lead to improved long-term retention of ACLS knowledge and skills in a cohort of medical students. While the stressed and unstressed groups had equivalent knowledge retention 6 months after their simulation experience, the stressed group showed improved performance over the unstressed group during a simulated code management scenario and appeared more calm and capable than their counterparts [19].

A similar study using a surgical laparoscopy simulator found that stressed participants had improved skills over an unstressed group of trainees when retested in the simulated environment [20]. Perhaps the stressed cohorts experienced stronger habit-based learning during their training and this translated into better performance some time later? Perhaps they studied more after they experienced stress they may have perceived as attributable to their own knowledge or skill deficits?

Could it be that a stressful simulation leads to an appropriately timed release of mediators (e.g., cortisol) that prime the learner to optimally benefit from the debriefing period? This would make sense at least for our study where the debriefing occurred approximately 30 min after the onset of the stressor and coincided with the classically described cortisol release outlined above. Indeed, several studies have demonstrated rises in biomarkers for stress following simulation experiences, yet little was done to correlate these rises with measurable outcomes related to knowledge and skill acquisition [21–25].

In line with the evidence presented above, severe levels of stress in the simulated environment (just as in the real environment) may lead to poor memory retrieval (measured as impaired performance), and this has been shown in studies of code management simulations [26, 27]. It is likely, however, that poor performance in the simulated environment is of little concern, as long as debriefing occurs after a scenario, capturing the optimal period for learning to occur. For this reason, we do not believe that evidence of poor performance during high levels of stress is an argument against using stressful scenarios. On the contrary, this stress, while it may impair retrieval of knowledge during a scenario, peaks the physiologic readiness to lay down lasting memory during debriefing and the social need to do better next time (perhaps leading to self-reflection and study). This supports the well-accepted and oft reported fact that debriefing is the most important part of any simulation scenario. We do believe, however, that the stress must always be contextual; participants who experience stress due to medical error, lack of knowledge, or poor judgment will derive benefit, while those that merely feel embarrassment or shame are unlikely to be positively affected by the experience.

Stress "Inoculation" and Performance

Although the relationship between stress, memory, and learning is well established and may be beneficial to the educational mission of most simulation groups, its use is still controversial and there is much debate whether to use or avoid its affects. Still an important question should be whether or not the introduction of stress leads to improved actual clinical performance. This is not yet fully elucidated, and perhaps recall and memory enhancement is not the only benefit of introducing stress into the simulated environment. One potential benefit, and one most educators who themselves are involved in actual clinical practice could appreciate, is the use of stress to precondition or "inoculate" students in order to prepare them to manage actual stress during clinical practice. This paradigm has been used in many other arenas: sports, industry, aviation, and the military. As the term inoculation implies, stress inoculation is designed to impart skills to enhance resistance to stress. In brief, the concept is that subjects will be more resistant to the negative effects of stress if they either learn stress-coping strategies ahead of time or if they experience similar contextual stress beforehand.

Stress inoculation training is an approach that has been discussed in systems and industrial psychology for several decades, although it was originally designed as a clinical treatment program to teach patients to cope with physical pain, anger, and phobias [28]. Spettell and Liebert noted that the high stress posed by nuclear power and aviation emergencies warrants psychological training techniques [such as] stress inoculation to avoid or neutralize threats to performance [29]. Although evidence suggests efficacy for stress inoculation training, the overall effectiveness of this approach has not been definitively established in medicine or elsewhere. The theoretical construct, however, should be appealing to simulation educators hoping to train practitioners to be ready and prepared to effectively and decisively manage any fast-paced critical event.

We outlined earlier in this chapter how simulation can induce stress, and several authors have demonstrated this to be true [21–25]. What is perhaps more interesting and clinically relevant is whether this stress leads to clinicians who are more calm and able to provide excellent clinical care in the real environment. Leblanc suggests that since stress can degrade performance, training individuals in stress-coping strategies might improve their ability to handle stress and perform more optimally [30]. Indeed, acute work stressors take a major toll on clinicians, particularly when patients suffer severe injury or death, and may lead to practitioner mental illness and the provision of poor care [31]. Unfortunately, support systems are not universally available and the complexity of the often-litigious medical workplace makes support hard to find.

While simulation will likely not be a panacea for the deeper personal trauma that can result from these scenarios, it can perhaps be used to train clinicians to function at a lower level of stress when similar events are encountered during clinical practice. This is particularly true after a stressful simulation. Here debriefing can be incredibly powerful and the opportunity to illicit the emotional state of the participants should not be overlooked. The classic debriefing "icebreaker" "how did that make you feel?" has even more impact and meaning. Discussing the experience of stress and ways to cope after a scenario is a potent motivator for self-reflection and improvement and certainly a potential area for improvement in the general debriefing process at most centers.

Stress Inoculation: The Evidence

Stressors imposed on the learner *during* simulation-based training may help support the acquisition of stress management skills that are necessary in the applied clinical setting as well. In an early study, a stress inoculation program, in which nursing students were exposed to a stressful situation similar to their clinical experience, was used to help students develop coping skills. It was found that the students experienced less stress and performed better in their clinical rotations after this intervention [32]. In a study of intensivists who underwent a 1-day simulation training course, stress levels as measured by salivary amylase were decreased when subjects encountered a follow-up simulation scenario some time later [23], but performance did not differ. In a similar study of 182 pediatric critical care providers, simulation-based education was found to decrease anxiety in participants, perhaps improving their ability to calmly handle actual clinical events [33]. Harvey et al. [34] suggest training for high-acuity events should include interventions targeting stress management skills as they found that subjects who appraised scenarios as challenges rather than as threats experienced lower stress and better performance in the simulated environment. Perhaps this same paradigm can be translated to the clinical environment if we train participants in a stressful simulation; might they then see the actual situation as a challenge to attack rather than an anxiety-provoking threat to avoid?

The Art: How to Enrich Simulation with Stress

Carefully crafted scenarios are potent mediators of emotionality and stress.

Time pressure; unhelpful, unprofessional, or obstructionist confederates; diagnostic dilemmas; errors; bad outcomes; challenging intraoperative events; difficult patients and family encounters; and failing devices are all individual components of a potentially stressful scenario (Table 5.1). Used individually or together, these can raise and/or lower the emotional impact of a scenario. Supercharged scenarios have the greatest impact on participant recall in our center. In a recent internal survey, we found that our residents recalled scenarios they encountered 2–3 years prior when either the patient did poorly or the scenario was so stressful that it was "seared" into their minds. Scenarios that end in patient demise and those where the resident was the only one who "saved the patient" also appear to be remembered more vividly, as many respondents reported remembering difficult scenarios where they "figured it out at the last minute."

It is our contention that the simulated environment is perfect for the development of stress through error and outcome; first it is the only place in medicine where these can be allowed to occur without true repercussions and second, due to the fact that it is after all a simulator, we believe the stress "dose" is idealized and tempered by the natural ceiling effect created by the trainee's knowledge that no real patient can or will be harmed—participants know this subconsciously and this likely limits how emotional they can truly become over the "piece of plastic."

While we commonly enrich the simulated environment by adding a degree of stress, this is not to say that the environment needs to be an unpleasant, unsuccessful place where participants go to fail and harm patients albeit simulated. What we have recognized is that although stress from failure is a potent and reliable way of activating emotionality in participants, the exhilaration felt by successfully diagnosing an event when others could not or managing a challenging environment with great success has an equally lasting impact on memory retention. When participants succeed after the emotional charge of an exceedingly challenging scenario, this can be particularly empowering. There is no reason for the stress to be delivered in a negative context, and it is as yet unclear whether success or failure is superior in this respect. For this reason (and to avoid all of our scenarios ending poorly—in fact, most do not), we use stressful situations with positive patient outcomes quite often.

Table 5.1 Examples of stressors used deliberately in simulation

Intrinsic to all immersive simulation
• Public demonstration of performance
• Managing rare events
• Managing life-threatening events
• Publicly justifying actions and performance shortcomings
• Simulated scenarios are naturally time compressed and therefore time pressured
• Treating the simulator/simulation as if it were real is embarrassing
• Using equipment that is unfamiliar
• Watching and listening to one's self on video
• Inadequate and unrealistic physical cues to base management decisions
Participants
• Complexity of case out of proportion to participant level of training
• Taking a leadership role
• Taking a team membership role
• Relying on people during a critical event who you never worked with before
• Errors and mistakes
• Failures
Confederates
• Less than helpful support staff
• Dismissive colleagues
• Confrontation with patient, family, other practitioners, and senior faculty
• Anxious, nervous, screaming confederates (patient, family, other healthcare providers)
• Supervising uncooperative, poorly performing, or generally obstructive and unhelpful subordinates
Events
• Rapidly deteriorating vital signs
• Being rushed
• Bad outcome, patient injury or demise
• Ineffective therapeutic interventions
• Unanticipated difficulties
• Diagnostic dilemmas
• Failing devices
• Backup devices unavailable
• Multitasking, triaging, and managing multiple patients simultaneously

The relative emotional impact of each of these is unknown

Incorporating the "inoculation theory" into scenario development is also important at our center where we train anesthesiologists. Figure 5.4 shows the theoretical design of a stress inoculation program.

The first phase of training is educational. The goal of this phase is to understand the experience of stress. This might involve, for our purposes, simply acknowledging that a scenario was stressful during the debriefing. The second phase focuses on skills acquisition and rehearsal; participants learn how to cope with stress. This might involve discussion of crisis resource management skills and the importance of calling for help. During the application phase, these skills are

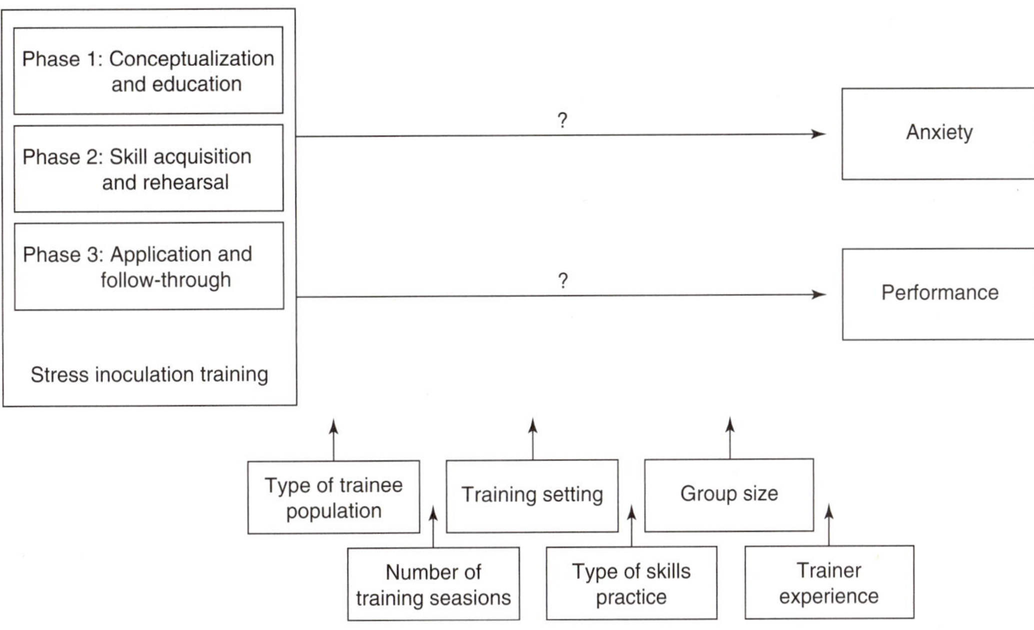

Fig. 5.4 Model of the effects of stress inoculation training on anxiety and performance (From Saunders et al. [35], Copyright 1996 by the Educational Publishing Foundation. Used courtesy of the American Psychological Association)

further developed using deliberate practice throughout multiple simulation scenarios. Based on the effectiveness of the training, the student moves toward varying degrees of anxiety or performance where the balance between these two is critical to training outcome (and ultimately the success of the task needing to be performed under stress).

We derive most of our scenarios from real clinical practice and from trainee feedback. One thing anesthesiology trainees find particularly stressful is contending with a difficult (dismissive, confrontational, judgmental, condescending, or pushy) attending surgeon when the anesthesiology attending is out of the room. For this reason, we expose residents to confederate surgeons who can be at times difficult, at times dangerous, and teach the residents skills to deal with these scenarios professionally and safely. Our residents report that these experiences help to empower them in the actual OR and indeed "inoculate" them to the real environment. Although this example was specific toward anesthesiology training, few healthcare providers work in a vacuum and interdisciplinary care is common place for practically every provider. These difficult interpersonal and professionalism issues can easily be tailored to each individual educator's needs depending on the specialist participating in the simulations.

In addition, stressful respiratory or cardiac arrest ("code") scenarios are used to drive home the point that the "code" environment can be chaotic, disorganized, and rushed. We use these scenarios as an opportunity to teach trainees stress management and crisis resource management and to emphasize professional yet forceful communication when running an arrest scenario. Again, our residents report these scenarios as helpful not only for the knowledge imparted but more importantly for the skills of anticipating and successfully managing these environments professionally and expertly.

Conclusion

Stress is an important and manipulable construct associated with memory formation and should be wielded properly by simulation educators. We know that events with high emotional content are fixed in human memory via a pathway that involves the amygdala [36, 37]. Emotional arousal may enhance one or more of several memory stages, but our common experience tells us that emotional events tend to be well remembered. Extensive scientific evidence confirms anecdotal observations that emotional arousal and stress can strengthen memory.

Over the past decade, there is growing evidence from human and animal subject studies regarding the neurobiology of stress-enhanced memory. Human studies are consistent with the results of animal experiments showing that emotional responses influence memory through the amygdala (at least partially) by modulating long-term memory storage [38]. During and immediately following emotionally charged arousing or stressful situations, several physiological systems are activated, including the release of various hormones [39]. An educator knowledgeable of these responses can employ stress in their simulations to improve learning and perhaps even inoculate trainees to future stress.

References

1. McEwen BS. Definitions and concepts of stress. In: Fink G, editor. Encyclopedia of stress. San Diego: Academic; 2000.
2. Seligman MEP, Walker EF, Rosenhan DL. Abnormal psychology. 4th ed. New York: W.W. Norton & Company, Inc.; 2001.

3. Droste SK et al. Corticosterone levels in the brain show a distinct ultradian rhythm but a delayed response to forced swim stress. Endocrinology. 2008;149:3244–53.
4. Roozendaal B. Stress and memory: opposing effects of glucocorticoids on memory consolidation and memory retrieval. Neurobiol Learn Mem. 2002;78:578–95.
5. Joels M, Pu Z, Wiegert O, Oitzl MS, Krugers HJ. Learning under stress: how does it work? Trends Cogn Sci. 2006;10:152–8.
6. Schwabe L, Oitzl MS, Philippsen C, Richter S, Bohringer A, Wippich W, et al. Stress modulates the use of spatial and stimulus–response learning strategies in humans. Learn Mem. 2007;14: 109–16.
7. Nater UM, Moor C, Okere U, Stallkamp R, Martin M, Ehlert U, et al. Performance on a declarative memory task is better in high than low cortisol responders to psychosocial stress. Psychoneuroendocrinology. 2007;32:758–63.
8. Elzinga BM, Bakker A, Bremner JD. Stress-induced cortisol elevations are associated with impaired delayed, but not immediate recall. Psychiatry Res. 2005;134:211–23.
9. Tops M, van der Pompe GA, Baas D, Mulder LJ, den Boer JAFMT, Korf J. Acute cortisol effects on immediate free recall and recognition of nouns depend on stimulus-valence. Psychophysiology. 2003;40:167–73.
10. Payne JD, Jackson ED, Ryan L, Hoscheidt S, Jacobs WJ, Nadel L. The impact of stress on neutral and emotional aspects of episodic memory. Memory. 2006;14:1–16.
11. Abercrombie HC, Kalin NH, Thurow ME, Rosenkranz MA, Davidson RJ. Cortisol variation in humans affects memory for emotionally laden and neutral information. Behav Neurosci. 2003; 117:505–16.
12. McGaugh JL. Memory—a century of consolidation. Science. 2000;287:248–51.
13. Cahill L, Gorski L, Le K. Enhanced human memory consolidation with postlearning stress: interaction with the degree of arousal at encoding. Learn Mem. 2003;10:270–4.
14. Roozendaal B. Glucocorticoids and the regulation of memory consolidation. Psychoneuroendocrinology. 2000;25:213–38.
15. Joëls M, Fernandez G, Roozendaal B. Stress and emotional memory: a matter of timing. Trends Cogn Sci. 2011;15(6):280–8.
16. Schwabe L, Wolf OT. The context counts: congruent learning and testing environments prevent memory retrieval impairment following stress. Cogn Affect Behav Neurosci. 2009;9(3):229–36.
17. Schwabe L, Wolf OT, Oitzl MS. Memory formation under stress: quantity and quality. Neurosci Biobehav Rev. 2010;34:584–91.
18. Packard MG, Goodman J. Emotional arousal and multiple memory systems in the mammalian brain. Front Behav Neurosci. 2012;6:14.
19. Demaria Jr S, Bryson EO, Mooney TJ, Silverstein JH, Reich DL, Bodian C, et al. Adding emotional stressors to training in simulated cardiopulmonary arrest enhances participant performance. Med Educ. 2010;44(10):1006–15.
20. Andreatta PB, Hillard M, Krain LP. The impact of stress factors in simulation-based laparoscopic training. Surgery. 2010;147(5): 631–9.
21. Girzadas Jr DV, Delis S, Bose S, Hall J, Rzechula K, Kulstad EB. Measures of stress and learning seem to be equally affected among all roles in a simulation scenario. Simul Healthc. 2009;4(3):149–54.
22. Finan E, Bismilla Z, Whyte HE, Leblanc V, McNamara PJ. High-fidelity simulator technology may not be superior to traditional low-fidelity equipment for neonatal resuscitation training. J Perinatol. 2012;32(4):287–92.
23. Müller MP, Hänsel M, Fichtner A, Hardt F, Weber S, Kirschbaum C, et al. Excellence in performance and stress reduction during two different full scale simulator training courses: a pilot study. Resuscitation. 2009;80(8):919–24.
24. Bong CL, Lightdale JR, Fredette ME, Weinstock P. Effects of simulation versus traditional tutorial-based training on physiologic stress levels among clinicians: a pilot study. Simul Healthc. 2010; 5(5):272–8.
25. Keitel A, Ringleb M, Schwartges I, Weik U, Picker O, Stockhorst U, et al. Endocrine and psychological stress responses in a simulated emergency situation. Psychoneuroendocrinology. 2011;36(1):98–108.
26. Hunziker S, Laschinger L, Portmann-Schwarz S, Semmer NK, Tschan F, Marsch S. Perceived stress and team performance during a simulated resuscitation. Intensive Care Med. 2011;37(9):1473–9.
27. Hunziker S, Semmer NK, Tschan F, Schuetz P, Mueller B, Marsch S. Dynamics and association of different acute stress markers with performance during a simulated resuscitation. Resuscitation. 2012;83(5):572–8.
28. Meichenbaum D, Deffenbacher JL. Stress inoculation training. The Counseling Psychologist. 1988;16:69–90.
29. Spettell CM, Liebert RM. Training for safety in automated person-machine systems. Am Psychol. 1986;41:545–50.
30. LeBlanc VR. The effects of acute stress on performance: implications for health professions education. Acad Med. 2009;84(10 Suppl):S25–33.
31. Gazoni FM, Amato PE, Malik ZM, Durieux ME. The impact of perioperative catastrophes on anesthesiologists: results of a national survey. Anesth Analg. 2012;114(3):596–603.
32. Admi H. Stress intervention. A model of stress inoculation training. J Psychosoc Nurs Ment Health Serv. 1997;35(8):37–41.
33. Allan CK, Thiagarajan RR, Beke D, Imprescia A, Kappus LJ, Garden A, et al. Simulation-based training delivered directly to the pediatric cardiac intensive care unit engenders preparedness, comfort, and decreased anxiety among multidisciplinary resuscitation teams. J Thorac Cardiovasc Surg. 2010;140(3):646–52.
34. Harvey A, Nathens AB, Bandiera G, Leblanc VR. Threat and challenge: cognitive appraisal and stress responses in simulated trauma resuscitations. Med Educ. 2010;44(6):587–94.
35. Saunders T, Driskell JE, Johnston JH, Salas E. The effect of stress inoculation training on anxiety and performance. J Occup Health Psychol. 1996;1(2):170–86.
36. Cahill L, Haier RJ, Fallon J, Alkire MT, Tang C, Keator D, et al. Amygdala activity at encoding correlated with long-term, free recall of emotional information. Proc Natl Acad Sci USA. 1996;93:8016–21.
37. Sandi C, Pinelo-Nava MT. Stress and memory: behavioral effects and neurobiological mechanisms. Neural Plast. 2007;2007:78970.
38. Bianchin M, Mello e Souza T, Medina JH, Izquierdo I. The amygdale is involved in the modulation of long-term memory, but not in working or short-term memory. Neurobiol Learn Mem. 1999; 71:127–31.
39. Roozendaal B, Quirarte GL, McGaugh JL. Stress-activated hormonal systems and the regulation of memory storage. Ann NY Acad Sci. 1999;821:247–58.

Debriefing Using a Structured and Supported Approach

6

Paul E. Phrampus and John M. O'Donnell

Introduction

Debriefing is often cited as one of the most important parts of healthcare simulation. It has been described as a best practice in simulation education and is often referred to anecdotally as the point in the session "where the learning transfer takes place." How much participants learn and later incorporate into their practice depends in part on the effectiveness of the debriefing [1–3]. The purpose of a debriefing is to create a meaningful dialogue that helps the participants of the simulation gain a clear understanding of their performance during the session. Key features include obtaining valid feedback from the facilitator, verbalizing their own impressions, reviewing actions, and sharing perceptions of the experience. A skilled debriefing facilitator will be able to use "semi-structured cue questions" that serve to guide the participant through reflective self-discovery [4]. This process is critical in assisting positive change that will help participants to improve future simulation performances and ultimately improve their ability to care for patients.

P.E. Phrampus, MD (✉)
Department of Anesthesiology, Peter M. Winter Institute for Simulation, Education and Research (WISER), Pittsburgh, PA, USA

Department of Emergency Medicine, UPMC Center for Quality Improvement and Innovation, University of Pittsburgh, 230 McKee Place Suite 300, Pittsburgh, PA 15213, USA
e-mail: phrampuspe@upmc.edu

J.M. O'Donnell, RN, CRNA, MSN, DrPH
Nurse Anesthesia Program, University of Pittsburgh School of Nursing, Pittsburgh, PA, USA

Department of Anesthesiology, Peter M. Winter Institute for Simulation, Education and Research (WISER), 360A Victoria Building, 3500 Victoria St., Pittsburgh, PA 15261, USA

Department of Acute/Tertiary Care, University of Pittsburgh School of Nursing, Pittsburgh, PA, USA
e-mail: jod01@pitt.edu

Simulation educational methods are heterogeneous with deployment ranging from partial task training of entry-level students through complicated, interdisciplinary team training scenarios involving practicing professionals. Debriefing has a similar wide and varied development history and evolutionary pathway. Equipment and environmental, student, and personnel resources can greatly influence the selection of a debriefing method. Various techniques and methods have emerged over the last decade based on such factors as the level of the learner, the domain and mix of the learner(s), the amount of time allotted for the simulation exercise, equipment capability, and the physical facilities that are available including audiovisual (AV) equipment, observation areas, and debriefing rooms. Understanding personnel capability and course logistics is crucial to effective debriefing. The level of expertise of the facilitator(s) who will be conducting debriefings, the number of facilitators available, as well as their ability to effectively use the available equipment and technology all play a role in how debriefings are planned and conducted. Other factors that play a role in the design of the debriefing process tie back to the intent and goals of the simulation and how the simulation was conducted. For example, the debriefing style and method of a single stand-alone scenario may be significantly different than the debriefing of a simulation scenario that is part of a continuum of scenarios or learning activities organized into a course.

Development of the Structured and Supported Debriefing Model and the GAS Tool

The Winter Institute for Simulation Education and Research (WISER, Pittsburgh, PA) at the University of Pittsburgh, is a high-volume multidisciplinary simulation center dedicated to the mission that simulation educational methods can improve patient care. Also well recognized for instructor training, the center philosophy acknowledges that training in

A.I. Levine et al. (eds.), *The Comprehensive Textbook of Healthcare Simulation*,
DOI 10.1007/978-1-4614-5993-4_6, © Springer Science+Business Media New York 2013

debriefing is a critical element for the success of any simulation program.

In 2009, WISER collaborated with the American Heart Association to develop the structured and supported debriefing model for debriefing of advanced cardiac life support and pediatric advanced life support scenarios [3]. It was quickly realized that the structured and supported model was scalable and could be easily expanded to meet the debriefing needs of a variety of situations and simulation events. The model derives its name from providing *structured* elements included three specific debriefing phases with related goals, actions, and time allocation estimates. *Supported* elements include both interpersonal support (including development of a safe environment) and objects or media such as the use of protocols, algorithms, and available best evidence to support the debriefing process.

The debriefing *tool* uses the structural framework GAS (gather, analyze, and summarize) as an operational acronym [3]. The final goal was to develop a highly structured approach, which could be adapted to *any* debriefing situation. Another important component was that the model would be easy to teach to a wide variety of instructional faculty with varying levels of expertise in simulation debriefing and facilitation. Structured and supported debriefing is a learner-centered process that can be rapidly assimilated, is scalable, and is designed to standardize the debriefing interaction that follows a simulation scenario. It promotes learner self-reflection in thinking about *what* they did, *when* they did it, *how* they did it, *why* they did it, and *how* they can improve as well as ascertaining if the participants were able to make cause-and-effect relationships within the flow of the scenario. The approach emphasizes both self-discovery and self-reflection and draws upon the learner's own professional experience and motivation to enhance learning. Integration of the educational objectives for each scenario into the analysis phase of the debriefing ensures that the original goals of the educational session are achieved. Further, instructor training in the use of the model emphasizes close observation and identification of gaps in learner knowledge and performance which also are discussed during the analysis phase.

The Theoretical Foundation of the Structured and Supported Debriefing Model

The initial steps in the development of the structured and supported debriefing model were to review debriefing methods and practices currently being used at WISER and determine common elements of effective debriefing by experienced faculty. The simulation and educational literature was reviewed, and the core principles of a variety of learning theories helped to provide a comprehensive, theoretical foundation for the structured and supported model.

The Science of Debriefing

Feedback through debriefing is considered by many to be one of the most important components contributing to the effectiveness of simulation-based learning [1–7]. Participants who receive and assimilate valid information from feedback are thought to be more likely to have enhanced learning and improved future performance from simulation-based activities. Indeed the topic is considered so relevant; two chapters have been devoted to debriefing and feedback in this book (this chapter and Chap. 7). In traditional simulation-based education, debriefing is acknowledged as a best practice and is lauded as the point in the educational process when the dots are connected and "aha" moments occur. While debriefing is only one form of feedback incorporated into experiential learning methods, it is viewed as critical because it helps participants reflect, fill in gaps in performance, and make connections to the real world. The origins of debriefing lie in military exercises and war games in which lessons learned are reviewed after the exercise [8]. Lederman stated that debriefing "incorporates the processing of that experience from which learners are to draw the lessons learned" [9]. Attempts to have the participant engage in self-reflection and facilitated moments of self-discovery are often included in the debriefing session by skilled facilitators.

In simulation education, the experiential learning continuum ranges from technical skills to complex problem-solving situations. Because simulation education occurs across a wide range of activities and with students of many levels of experience, it is logical for educators to attempt to match the debriefing approach with the training level of the learner, the specific scenario objectives, the level of scenario complexity, and the skills and training of the simulation faculty. Additionally, the operational constraints of the simulation exercise must be considered as some debriefing methods are more time-consuming than others. While evidence is mounting with respect to individual, programmatic, clinical, and even system impact from simulation educational approaches, there is little concrete evidence that supports superiority of a particular approach, style, or method of debriefing. In this section we present the pertinent and seminal works that have provided the "science" behind the "art" of simulation-inspired debriefing.

Fanning and Gaba reviewed debriefing from the perspective of simulation education, industry, psychology, and military debriefing perspectives. This seminal paper provides food for thought in the area and poses many questions which still have yet to be answered. The setting, models, facilitation approaches, use of video and other available technology, alternative methods, quality control initiatives, effective evaluation, time frames, and actual need for debriefing are considered. They note that "there are surprisingly few papers in the peer-reviewed literature to illustrate how to debrief, how to teach or learn to debrief, what methods of debriefing exist and how effective they are at achieving learning objectives and goals" [6]. The publication of this paper has had substantial impact on perceptions of debriefing in the simulation educational community and can be viewed as a benchmark of progress and understanding in this area. Following is a review of additional prominent papers that have been published in the subsequent 5-year interval which emphasize methods, new approaches, and the beginnings of theory development in healthcare simulation debriefing. These papers also highlight the gaps in our collective knowledge base:

- Decker focused on use of structured, guided reflection during simulated learning encounters. Decker's work in this chapter drew on a variety of theories and approaches including the work of Schön. Decker adds reflection to the work of Johns, which identifies four "ways of knowing": empirical, aesthetic, personal, and ethical. These ways of knowing are then integrated within a debriefing tool for facilitators [10].
- Cantrell described the use of debriefing with undergraduate pediatric nursing scenarios in a qualitative research study. In this study, Cantrell focused on the importance of guided reflection and used a structured approach including standardized questions and a 10-min time limit. Findings emphasized the importance of three critical elements: student preparation, faculty demeanor, and debriefing immediately after the simulation session [1].
- Kuiper et al. described a structured debriefing approach termed the "Outcome-Present State-Test" (OPT) model. Constructivist and situated learning theories are embedded in the model which has been validated for debriefing of actual clinical events. The authors chose a purposive sample of students who underwent a simulation experience and then completed worksheets in the OPT model. Key to the model is a review of nursing diagnoses, reflection on events, and creation of realistic simulations that mimic clinical events. Worksheets completed by participants were reviewed and compared with actual clinical event worksheets. The authors concluded that this form of structured debriefing showed promise for use in future events [11].
- Salas et al. describe 12 evidence-based best practices for debriefing medical teams in the clinical setting. These authors provide tips for debriefing that arise from review of aviation, military, industrial, and simulation education literature. The 12 best practices are supported by empirical evidence, theoretical constructs, and debriefing models. While the target audiences are educators and administrators working with medical teams in the hospital setting, the principles are readily applicable to the simulation environment [12].
- Dieckmann et al. explored varying debriefing approaches among faculty within a simulation facility focused on medical training. The variances reported were related to differences among individual faculty and in course content focus (medical management vs. crisis management). The faculty role "mix" was also explored, and a discrepancy was noted between what the center director and other faculty thought was the correct mix of various roles within the simulation educational environment [13].
- Dreifuerst conducted a concept analysis in the area of simulation debriefing. Using the framework described by Walker and Avant in 2005, Dreifuerst identified concepts that were defining attributes of simulation debriefing, those concepts that could be analyzed prior to or independently of construction and those concepts to be used for testing of a debriefing theory. Dreifuerst proposes that development of conceptual definitions leading to a debriefing theory is a key step toward clearer understanding of debriefing effectiveness, development of research approaches, and in development of faculty interested in conducting debriefings [14].
- Morgan et al. studied physician anesthetists who experienced high-fidelity scenarios with critical complications. Participants were randomized to simulation debriefing, home study, or no intervention (control). Performance checklists and global rating scales were used to evaluate performance in the original simulation and in a delayed posttest performance (9 months). All three groups improved in the global rating scale (GRS) of performance from their baseline, but there was no difference on the GRS between groups based on debriefing method. A significant improvement was found in the simulation debriefing group on the performance *checklist* at the 9-month evaluation point [15].
- Welke et al. compared facilitated oral debriefing with a standardized multimedia debriefing (which demonstrated ideal behaviors) for nontechnical skills. The

subjects were 30 anesthesia residents who were exposed to resuscitation scenarios. Each resident underwent a resuscitation simulation and was then randomized to a debriefing method. Following the first debriefing, residents completed a second scenario with debriefing and then a delayed posttest 5 weeks later. While all participants improved, there was no difference between groups indicating no difference in effectiveness between multimedia instruction and facilitator-led debriefing [16]. The implications for allocation of resources and management of personnel in simulation education if multimedia debriefing can be leveraged are emphasized by this paper.

- Arafeh et al. described aspects of debriefing in simulation-based learning including pre-briefing, feedback during sessions, and the need for effective facilitation skills. These authors acknowledge the heterogeneity of debriefing situations and describe three specific simulation activities and associated debriefing approaches which were matched based on the objectives, level of simulation, and learning group characteristics. They also emphasized the need for facilitator preparation and the use of quality improvement approaches in maintaining an effective program [5].
- Van Heukelom et al. compared immediate post-simulation debriefing with in-simulation debriefing among 161 third year medical students. Prior to completing a simulation session focused on resuscitation, medical students were randomly assigned to one of the two methods. The participants reported that the post-simulation debriefings were more effective in helping to learn the material and understand correct and incorrect actions. They also gave the post-simulation debriefings a higher rating. The in-simulation debriefing included pause and reflect periods. While not viewed by participants as being equally effective, the pausing that occurred was not seen as having altered the realism of the scenario by the participants [17]. This is important as some educators are reluctant to embrace a pause and reflect approach due to concern of loss of scenario integrity.
- Raemer et al. evaluated debriefing research evidence as a topical area during the Society of Simulation in Healthcare International Consensus Conference meeting in February 2011. These authors reviewed selected literature and proposed a definition of debriefing, identified a scarcity of quality research demonstrating outcomes tied to debriefing method, and proposed a format for reporting data on debriefing. Areas of debriefing research identified as having obvious gaps included comparison of methods, impact of faculty training, length of debriefing, and ideal environmental conditions for debriefing. Models for study design and for presenting research findings were proposed by this review team [18].
- Boet et al. examined face-to-face instructor debriefing vs. participant self-debriefing for 50 anesthesia residents in the area of anesthetist nontechnical skill scale (ANTS). All participants improved significantly from baseline in ANTS performance. There was no difference in outcomes between the two debriefing methods suggesting that alternative debriefing methods including well-designed self-debriefing approaches can be effectively employed [19].
- Mariani et al. used a mixed methods design to evaluate a structured debriefing method called Debriefing for Meaningful Learning (DML)©. DML was compared with unstructured debriefing methods. The unstructured debriefing was at the discretion of the faculty, but the authors noted it typically included a review of what went right, what did not go right, and what needed to be improved for the next time. The DBL approach while highly structured was also more complicated and included five areas: engage, evaluate, explore, explain, and elaborate. The authors reported that the model was based on the work of Dreifuerst. A total of 86 junior-level baccalaureate nursing students were enrolled in the study, and each student was asked to participate in two medical-surgical nursing scenarios. The Lasater Clinical Judgment Rubric was used to measure changes in clinical judgment, and student-focused group interviews elicited qualitative data. No difference was found between the groups in the area of judgment; however, student perceptions regarding learning and skill attainment were better for the structured model [20].

In the 5-year interim since Fanning and Gaba noted that the evidence was sparse regarding debriefing and that our understanding regarding key components is incomplete, there has been some progress but few clear answers. Alternatives to conventional face-to-face debriefing are being explored, theories and methods are being trialed, and several principles have become well accepted regardless of the method. These include maintaining a focus on the student; assuring a positive, safe environment; encouraging reflection; and facilitating self-discovery moments. However, the fundamental questions of who, what, when, where, and how have not been fully answered through rigorous research methodology. It is likely that a "one size fits all" debriefing model will not be identified when one considers the many variables associated with healthcare simulation. The heterogeneity of participants, learning objectives, simulation devices, scenarios, environments, operational realities, and faculty talents require a broad range of approaches guided by specific educational objectives and assessment outcomes.

In this chapter and Chap. 7, two well-established approaches to debriefing are described. Both of these approaches have been taught to hundreds if not thousands of faculty members both nationally and internationally. Both are built upon sound educational theory and have proven track records of success. Both methods have been developed by large and well-established simulation programs with senior simulation leaders involved. Termed "debriefing with good judgment" and "structured and supported debriefing," the contrast and similarities between these two approaches will serve to demonstrate the varied nature of the art and the evolving science of debriefing in simulation education. What should also be apparent is that it may be unimportant how we debrief, but that we debrief at all.

References

1. Cantrell MA. The importance of debriefing in clinical simulations. Clin Simul Nurs. 2008;4(2):e19–e23.
2. McDonnell LK, Jobe KK, Dismukes RK. Facilitating LOS debriefings: a training manual. NASA technical memorandum 112192. Ames Research Center: North American Space Administration; 1997.
3. McGaghie WC, Issenberg SB, Petrusa ER, Scalese RJ. A critical review of simulation-based medical education research: 2003–2009. Med Educ. 2010;44(1):50–63.
4. O'Donnell J, Rodgers D, Lee W, Farquhar J. Structured and supported debriefing using the GAS model. Paper presented at: 2nd annual WISER symposium for nursing simulation, Pittsburgh. 4 Dec 2008; 2008.
5. Arafeh JM, Hansen SS, Nichols A. Debriefing in simulated-based learning: facilitating a reflective discussion. J Perinat Neonatal Nurs. 2010;24(4):302–9.
6. Fanning RM, Gaba DM. The role of debriefing in simulation-based learning. Simul Healthc. 2007;2(2):115–25.
7. Issenberg SB, McGaghie WC. Features and uses of high-fidelity medical simulations that can lead to effective learning: a BEME systematic review. JAMA. 2005;27(1):1–36.
8. Pearson M, Smith D. Debriefing in experience-based learning. Simul/Games Learn. 1986;16(4):155–72.
9. Lederman L. Debriefing: toward a systematic assessment of theory and practice. Simul Gaming. 1992:145–60.
10. Decker S. Integrating guided reflection into simulated learning experiences. In: Jeffries PR, editors. Simulation in nursing education from conceptualization to evaluation. New York: National League for Nursing; 2007.
11. Kuiper R, Heinrich C, Matthias A, et al. Debriefing with the OPT model of clinical reasoning during high fidelity patient simulation. Int J Nurs Educ Scholarsh. 2008;5:Article17.
12. Salas E, Klein C, King H, et al. Debriefing medical teams: 12 evidence-based best practices and tips. Jt Comm J Qual Patient Saf. 2008;34(9):518–27.
13. Dieckmann P, Gaba D, Rall M. Deepening the Theoretical Foundations of Patient Simulation as Social Practice. Simul Healthc. 2007;2(3):183–93.
14. Dreifuerst K. The essentials of debriefing in simulation learning: a concept analysis. Nurs Educ Perspect. 2009;30(2): 109–14.
15. Morgan PJ, Tarshis J, LeBlanc V, et al. Efficacy of high-fidelity simulation debriefing on the performance of practicing anaesthetists in simulated scenarios. Br J Anaesth. 2009; 103(4):531–7.
16. Welke TM, LeBlanc VR, Savoldelli GL, et al. Personalized oral debriefing versus standardized multimedia instruction after patient crisis simulation. Anesth Analg. 2009;109(1): 183–9.
17. Van Heukelom JN, Begaz T, Treat R. Comparison of postsimulation debriefing versus in-simulation debriefing in medical simulation. Simul Healthc. 2010;5(2):91–7.
18. Raemer D, Anderson M, Cheng A, Fanning R, Nadkarni V, Savoldelli G. Research regarding debriefing as part of the learning process. Simul Healthc. 2011;6 Suppl:S52–7.
19. Boet S, Bould MD, Bruppacher HR, Desjardins F, Chandra DB, Naik VN. Looking in the mirror: self-debriefing versus instructor debriefing for simulated crises. Crit Care Med. 2011;39(6): 1377–81.
20. Mariani B, Cantrell MA, Meakim C, Prieto P, Dreifuerst KT. Structured debriefing and students' clinical judgment abilities in simulation. Clin Simul Nurs. 2013;9(5):e147–55.

Theories or educational models which were selected emphasized the need for a student-centric approach; recognized that students are equal partners in the teaching-learning environment; emphasized the environmental, social, and contextual nature of learning; acknowledged the need for concurrent and later reflection; and acknowledged the need for deliberate practice in performance improvement (Table 6.1).

These theories support multiple aspects of the structured and supported model for debriefing. Simulation is a form of experiential learning with curriculum designers focused on creating an environment similar enough to a clinical event or situation for learning and skill acquisition to occur. The goal is to afford participants with the learning tools to allow participant performance in actual clinical care to improve.

In order for a simulated experience to be effective, the objectives for the experience must be conveyed to the participants who are being asked to contribute to the learning environment. This involvement of participants in a truly "democratic" sense was first advocated by Dewey in 1916. Dewey also recognized the power of reflection and experiential learning [5].

Lewin described the importance of experience in his "action research" work, and Kolb extended this work in developing his Experiential Learning Theory [8, 9]. Kolb describes the importance of experience in promoting learning

Table 6.1 Educational and practice theorists and key concepts related to debriefing in simulation

Theorist	Supporting concept for debriefing
Dewey [5]	Experiential learning, reflection, democratization of education
Goffman [6]	Preexisting frameworks of reference based on prior experience (knowledge, attitude, skill) influence current actions
Bandura [7]	Social learning theory. Learning through observation, imitation, and modeling. Self-efficacy critical to learning and performance
Lewin [8] and Kolb [9]	Experiential learning theory. Learning is enhanced by realistic experience. Learning increases when there is a connection between the learning situation and the environment (synergy)
Schön [10]	"Reflective practicum" where faculty act as coach and mentor. Reflection is important both during and after simulation sessions
Lave and Wenger [11]	Situated learning theory. Learning is situated within context and activity. Accidental (unplanned) learning is common
Ericsson [12–15]	Deliberate practice leading to expertise. Performance improvement is tied to repetition and feedback

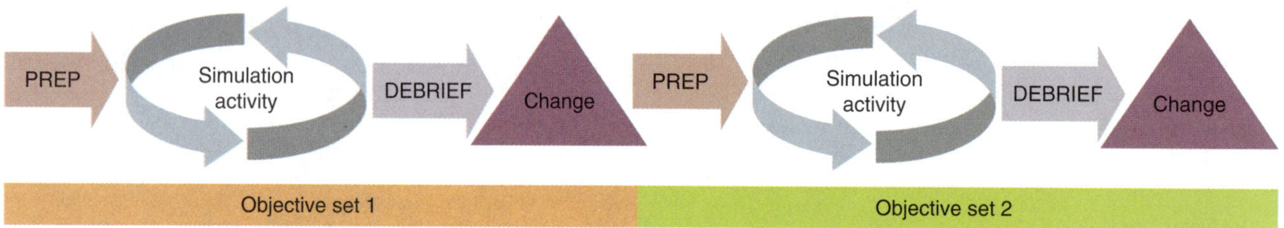

Fig. 6.1 The Ericsson cycle of deliberate practice applied to simulation sessions and incorporating debriefing and planned change

and describes the synergistic impact of environmental realism. Kolb developed a cyclical four-stage learning cycle "Do, Observe, Think, Plan" that describes how experience and action are linked. Kolb's work also emphasizes the need for reflection and analysis [9].

Goffman reported that humans have frames of reference that include knowledge, attitude, skill, and experience elements. Individuals attempt to make sense of new experiences by fitting their actions and understanding to their preexisting frameworks [6]. This is especially important in developing an understanding of "gaps" in participant performance.

Bandura developed the Social Learning Theory. This theory suggests that learning is a socially embedded phenomenon which occurs through observation, imitation, and modeling. Bandura et al. also emphasize that individual self-efficacy is crucial to learning and performance [7]. These constructs are useful in debriefing, as a group debriefing is a fairly complex social environment, and the outcome of a poorly facilitated debriefing session may be a decreased sense of self-efficacy.

Schön described the characteristics of professionals and how they develop their practice. He suggested that one key aspect of professional practice is a capacity to self-reflect on one's own actions. By doing so, the individual engages in a process of continuous self-learning and improvement. Schön suggests that there are two points in time critical to the reflection process. Reflection during an event (reflection in action) and reflection after the event is over (reflection on action) [10]. The facilitator's ability to stimulate participants to reflect on their performance is key during the debriefing process.

Lave and Wenger developed the "situated learning theory," which states in part that learning is deeply contextual and associated with activity. Further, these authors note that transfer of information from one person to another has social and environmental aspects as well as specific context. These authors also indicated that learning is associated with visualization, imitation, and hands-on experience. Accidental (and thus unscripted) learning commonly occurs and learners legitimately gain from observation of performance [11].

Ericsson describes the concept of "deliberate practice" as the route for development of new skills (up to the expert level). In this seminal work, Ericsson points out that the trainee needs to experience multiple repetitions interspersed with meaningful review and learning toward development of expertise [12–15] (Fig. 6.1).

This concept has important implications in simulation development, deployment, and debriefing and is now recognized as a best practice in simulation education [16, 17]. Other literature has emerged and should be used to inform approaches to debriefing. The following are points and best practices regarding debriefing which have been modified from the original paper by Salas which focused on team debriefing in the hospital setting [1, 3, 4, 16–24]:

- Participants want and expect debriefing to occur.
- The gap between performance and debriefing should be kept as short as possible.
- Debriefing can help with stress reduction and closure.
- Performance and perception gaps should be identified and addressed.

- Debriefing enhances learning.
- Environmental conditions are important.
- A "social" aspect must be considered and steps taken to ensure "comfort."
- Participant self-reflection is necessary for learning.
- Instructor debriefing and facilitation skills are necessary.
- Structured video/screen-based "debriefing" also works.
- Lessons can be learned from other fields (but the analogy is not perfect).
- Not everything can be debriefed at once (must be targeted or goal directed).
- Some structure is necessary to meet debriefing objectives.

Based on the theoretical perspectives and the above best practices, faculty are encouraged to ensure that they consistently incorporate several key elements within sessions in order to enhance effectiveness of debriefing:

1. Establish and maintain an engaging, challenging, yet supportive context for learning.
2. Structure the debriefing to enhance discussion and allow reflection on the performance.
3. Promote discussion and reflection during debriefing sessions.
4. Identify and explore performance gaps in order to accelerate the deliberate practice-skill acquisition cycle.
5. Help participants achieve and sustain good performance.

Although the specific structure used in debriefings may vary, the beginning of the debriefing, or the gather phase, is generally used for gauging reaction to the simulated experience, clarifying facts, describing what happened, and creating an environment for reflective learning. It also gives the facilitator an opportunity to begin to identify performance and perception gaps, meaning the differences that may exist between the perception of the participants and the perception of the facilitator.

The most extensive (and typically longest) part of the debriefing is the middle, or analysis phase, which involves an in-depth discussion of observed performance or perception gaps [2]. Performance gaps are defined as the gap between desired and actual performance, while perception gap is the dissonance between the trainee's perception of their performance and actual performance as defined by objective measures. These two concepts must be considered separately as performance and the ability to perceive and accurately self-assess performance are separate functions [25–29]. Since an individual or team may perform actions for which the rationale is not immediately apparent or at first glance seems wrong, an effective debriefing should ideally include an explicit discussion around the drivers that formed the basis for performance/perception gaps. While actions are observable, these drivers (thoughts, feelings, beliefs, assumptions, knowledge base, situational awareness) are often invisible to the debriefer without skillful questioning [6, 19–21]. Inexperienced facilitators often conclude that observed performance gaps are related only to knowledge deficits and launch into a lecture intended to remediate them. By exploring the basis for performance and perception gaps, a debriefer can better diagnose an individual or team learning need and then close these gaps through discussion and/or focused teaching.

Finally, a debriefing concludes with a summary phase in which the learners articulate key learning points, take-home messages, and needed performance improvements, as well as leading them to an accurate understanding of their overall performance on the scenario.

Developing Debriefing Skills

Faculty participating in debriefing must develop observational and interviewing skills that will help participants to reflect on their actions. As in any skill attainment, deliberate practice and instructor self-reflection will assist with skill refinement. New facilitators are often challenged in initiating the debriefing process and find it useful to utilize a cognitive aid such as the GAS debriefing tool (Table 6.2). The use of open-ended questions during debriefings will encourage dialogue and lead to extended participant responses. While it is important to ask open-ended questions, it is equally important for the facilitator to establish clear parameters in order to meet the session objectives. For example, the question "Can you tell us what happened?" may be excessively broad and nondirectional. Alternatively, "Can you tell us what happened between the time when you came in the room and up until when the patient stopped responding?" remains open ended but asks the participant to focus on relevant events as they occurred on a timeline [2, 30].

Some simulation educators suggest that close-ended question (questions that limit participant responses to one or two words) be avoided entirely. However, they are often useful in gaining information about key knowledge or skill areas if phrased appropriately, especially in acute-care scenarios. For example, "Did you know the dose of labetalol?" will provoke a yes or no response and may not provide valuable information for facilitator follow-up or stimulate participant reflection. Alternatively, "What is the dose of labetalol and how much did you give?" provides a more fertile environment for follow-up discussion.

Several communication techniques can be used which promote open dialogue. Active listening is an approach in which the facilitator signals to the participants (both verbally and nonverbally) that their views, feelings, and opinions are important. Key facilitator behaviors include use of nonverbal clues such as appropriate eye contact, nodding, and acknowledging comments ("go ahead," "I understand"). Restating trainee comments (in your own words) and summarizing

Table 6.2 Structured and supported debriefing model. The model consists of three phases with corresponding goals, actions, sample questions, and time frames

Phase	Goal	Actions	Sample questions	Time frame
Gather	Listen to participants to understand what they think and how they feel about session	Request narrative from team leader Request clarifying or supplemental information from team	All: How do you feel? Team Leader: Can you tell us what happened when….? Team members: Can you add to the account?	25%
Analyze	Facilitate participants' reflection on and analysis of their actions	Review of accurate record of events Report observations (correct and incorrect steps) Ask a series of question to reveal participants' thinking processes Assist participants to reflect on their performance Direct/redirect participants to assure continuous focus on session objectives	I noticed… Tell me more about… How did you feel about… What were you thinking when… I understand, however, tell me about the "X" aspect of the scenario… Conflict resolution: Let's refocus—"what's important is not who is right but what is right for the patient…"	50%
Summarize	Facilitate identification and review of lessons learned	Participants identify positive aspects of team or individual behaviors and behaviors that require change Summary of comments or statements	List two actions or events that you felt were effective or well done Describe two areas that you think you/team need to work on…	25%

their comments to achieve clarity are also effective forms of active listening [2, 31].

A second effective debriefing technique is the use of probing questions. This is a questioning approach designed to reveal thinking processes and elicit a deeper level of information about participant actions, responses, and behaviors during the scenario. Many question types can be selected during use of probing questions. These include questions designed to clarify, amplify, assess accuracy, reveal purposes, identify relevance, request examples, request additional information, or elicit feelings [2, 30].

A third technique is to normalize the simulation situation to something familiar to the participants. For example, the facilitator can acknowledge what occurred during the session and then ask the participants "Have you ever encountered something similar in your clinical experience?" This grounds the simulation contextually and allows the participant to connect the simulation event with real-life experience which has the benefit of enhancing transfer of learning.

Another key skill in maintaining a coherent debriefing is redirection. The facilitator needs to employ this skill when the discussion strays from the objectives of the session or when conflict arises. Participants sometimes are distracted by technological glitches or the lack of fidelity of a particular simulation tool. The facilitator task is to restore the flow of discussion to relevant and meaningful pathways in order to assure that planned session objectives are addressed.

Structured and Supported Debriefing Model: Operationally Described

The operational acronym for the structured and supported debriefing model is GAS. GAS stands for gather, analyze, and summarize and provides a framework to help the operational flow of the debriefing, as well as assisting the facilitator in an organized approach to conducting the debriefing (Table 6.2). While there is no ideal time ratio for simulation time to debriefing time, or ideal time for total debriefing, operational realities usually dictate the length of time that can be allocated on the debriefing phase of a simulation course. Using the GAS acronym also provides the facilitator with a rough framework for the amount of time spent in each phase. The gather phrase is allocated approximately 25% of the total debriefing time, the analyze phase is given 50%, and finally the summarize phase is allotted approximately 25%.

Gather (G)

The first phase of the structured and supported model is the gather phase. The goals of this phase are to allow the facilitator to gather information that will help structure and guide the analysis and summary phases. It is time to evoke a reaction to the simulation from participants with the purpose of creating an environment of reflective learning. It is important

Table 6.3 Perception gap conditions

		Student perceptions	
		Performed well	**Performed poorly**
Facilitator perceptions	**Performed well**	Narrow	Wide
	Performed poorly	Wide	Narrow

to listen carefully to the participants to understand what they think and how they feel about the session. Critical listening and probing questions will allow the facilitator to begin to analyze the amount of perception gap that may exist. The perception gap is the difference of the overall opinion of the performance as judged by the participants themselves vs. the opinion of the facilitator. Essentially four conditions can exist, two of which have wide perception gaps in which there is significant discordance between perceptions of the participant and facilitator and two that have narrow perception gaps (Table 6.3). This awareness of the perception gap is a critical element of helping to frame the remainder of the debriefing.

To facilitate the gather phase, the instructor embarks in a series of action to stimulate and facilitate the conversation. For example, the debriefing may begin by simply asking the participants how they feel after the simulation. Alternatively if it is a team-based scenario, facilitators may begin by asking the team leader to provide a synopsis of what occurred during the simulation and perhaps inquire if the participants have insight into the purpose of the simulation. The facilitator may then ask other team members for supporting information or clarifying information, the goal being to determine each of the participant's general perception of the simulation. During the gathering phase open-ended questions are helpful to try to elicit participant thoughts or stream of consciousness so that the facilitator can gain a clear understanding of the participant perceptions. During this phase it is often useful to develop an understanding of whether there is general agreement within the participant group or if there are significant disagreements, high emotions, or discord among the group.

The gather phase should take approximately 25% of the total debriefing time. Once the gather phase is completed, and the facilitator feels that they have elicited sufficient information to proceed, there is a segue into the analyze phase.

Analyze (A)

The analyze phase is designed to facilitate participants reflection *on* and analysis *of* their actions and how individual and team actions may have influenced the outcome of the scenario, or perhaps changes that may have occurred to the patient during the scenario.

During the analyze phase, participants will often be exposed to review of an accurate record of events, decisions, or critical changes in the patient in a way that allows them to understand how the decisions that they made affected the outcomes of the scenario. Simulator log files, videos, and other objective records of events (when available) can often be helpful as tools of reference for this purpose.

Probing questions are used by the facilitator in an attempt to reveal the participants thinking processes. Cueing questions should be couched in a manner that stimulates further reflection on the scenario and promotes self-discovery into the cause-and-effect relationships between decisions and the scenario outcome. For example, a question such as "Why do you think the hypotension persisted?" may allow the participants to realize they forgot to give a necessary fluid bolus.

It is crucial that the facilitator be mindful of the purpose of the session and that the questions selected direct the conversation toward accomplishing the learning objectives (Fig. 6.2). During a simulation scenario, there are many things that occur that *can* be talked about, but it is important to remember that for a variety of reasons, it usually isn't possible to debrief everything. It is the learning objectives that should help to create the screening process that determines what *should* be talked about. Skilled facilitators must continuously direct and redirect participants to assure continuous focus on session objectives, and not let the debriefing conversation stray off-topic.

The skilled facilitator must also continuously be aware of the need for assisting in conflict resolution during the analyze phase. It is important for participants to not focus on who was right and who was wrong but rather encourage an environment of consideration for what would've been right for the comparable actual clinical situation.

The analyze phase is also an ideal time to incorporate the use of cognitive aides or support materials during the discussion. Practice algorithms, professional standards, Joint Commission guidelines, and hospital policies are examples of materials that can be used. These tools allow participants to compare their performance record with the objective-supporting materials and can assist in developing understanding, in providing rationale, and in narrowing the perception gap. It also serves to begin the process of helping learners in calibrating the accuracy of their perception and gaining a true understanding of their overall performance. Importantly, these "objective materials" allow the instructor to defuse participant defensiveness and reduce the tension that can build during a debriefing of a suboptimal performance. Having the participant use these tools to self-evaluate can be useful. Additionally, depending on the design of the scenario and supporting materials, it may be prudent to review completed assessment tools, rating scales, or checklists with the participant team.

Because the analyze phase is designed to provide more in-depth understanding of the participants mindset, insights,

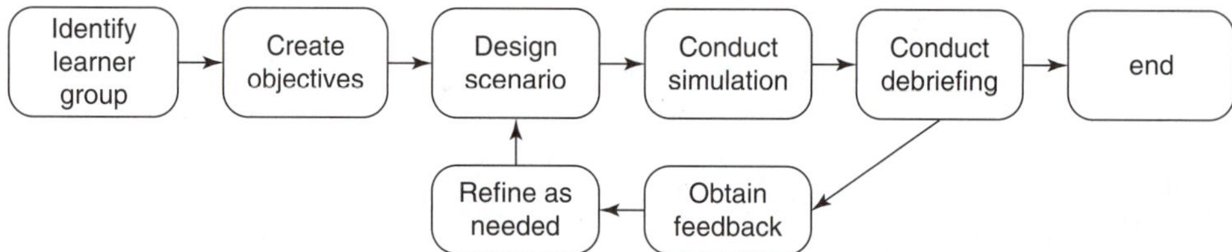

Fig. 6.2 Connection between simulation session objectives and debriefing session (With permission ©Aimee Smith PA-C, MS, WISER)

and reflection of the performance, it is allocated 50% of the total debriefing time. As the goals of the analyze phase are achieved, the facilitator will then transition to the summarize phase.

Summarize (S)

The summarize phase is designed to facilitate identification and review of lessons learned and provide participants with a clear understanding of the most important take-home messages. It continues to employ techniques that encourage learners to reflect over the performance of the simulation. It is designed to succinctly and clearly allow learners to understand their overall performance as well as to reinforce the aspects of the simulation that were performed correctly or effectively, as well as to identify the areas needing improvement for future similar situations.

It is important that the summarize phase be compartmentalized so that the takeaway messages are clearly delivered. Often in the analyze phase, the discussion will cover many topics with varying levels of depth and continuity which can sometimes leave the learners unaware of the big picture of the overall performance. Thus, it is recommended that transition into the summarize phase be stated clearly such as the facilitator making the statement "Ok, now let's talk about what we are going to take away from this simulation."

Incorporating structure into the summarize phase is critical. Without structure, it is possible that the key take-home messages which are tied to the simulation session objectives will be missed. In the structured and supported model, a mini plus-delta technique is used to frame the summarize phase [22]. Plus-delta is a simple model focused on effective behaviors or actions (+) and behaviors or actions which if changed would positively impact performance (Δ). An example of using the plus-delta technique would be asking each team member to relate two positive aspects of their performance, followed by asking each team member to list two things that they would change in order to improve for the next simulation session (Fig. 6.1). This forcing function tied to the plus (positives) and delta (need to improve) elements allows students to clarify, quantify, and reiterate the takeaway messages. At the very end of the summarize phase, the facilitator has the option to explicitly provide input to the participants as to their overall performance rating relative to the scenario if deemed appropriate. This will vary in accordance to the design of the scenario and the assessment tools that are used, or if the assessment is designed to be more qualitative, it may just be a summary provided by the facilitator.

Variability in Debriefing Style and Content

The structured and supported debriefing model provides a framework around which to guide the debriefing process. Entry-level facilitators as well as those who are very experienced are able to use it successfully. There are many factors that determine how long the actual debriefing will take and what will be covered in the debriefing. While there is attention to best practices in debriefing, operational realities often determine how the debriefing session for a given simulation takes place.

The learning objectives for the scenario serve as the initial basis for determining what the actual content of the debriefing should contain. As mentioned previously it is rarely possible to debrief everything that occurs in a given simulation. This is for two principal reasons, the first being the practicality of time and how long participants and faculty member have available to dedicate to the simulation activity. The second is learner saturation level, which is to say there is a finite amount of feedback and reflection possible in a given amount of time.

Other considerations are the structure of the simulation activity. If the simulation is a "stand-alone" or once and done, which is often the case when working with practicing professionals, then debriefing is usually more in-depth and may cover areas including technical as well as nontechnical components. The debriefing may be split into multiple focal areas that allow concentration on particular practice areas or skills (communication, procedural skills, and safety behaviors) for a given point in time.

Phased-domain debriefing is sometimes employed for interprofessional simulation. In phased-domain debriefing, the team is debriefed on common tasks (communications, teamwork, leadership, and other nontechnical skills) followed by a period of time afterward in which team members adjourn and reconvene in their separate clinical domain areas to allow for a more domain-specific discussion (Fig. 6.3).

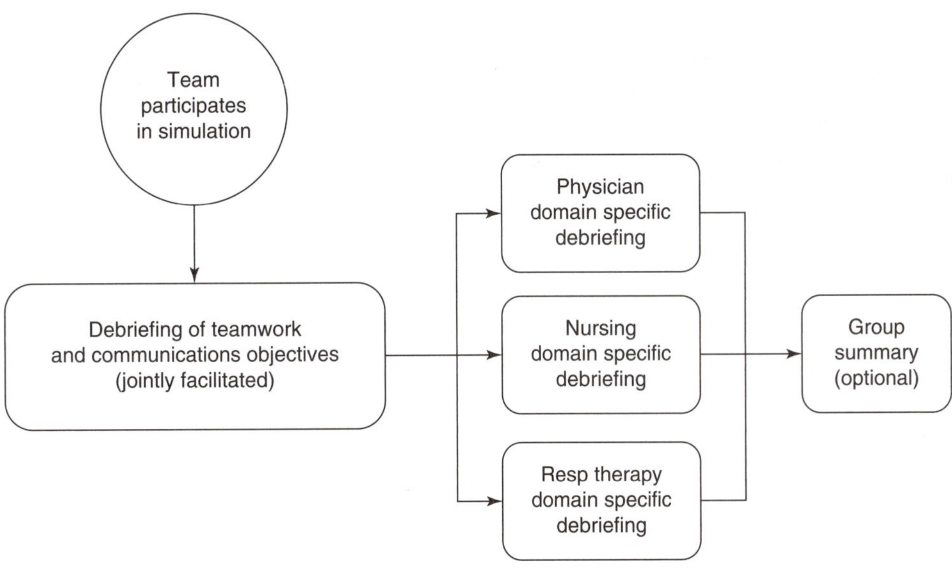

Fig. 6.3 Phased-domain debriefing in simulation. The original group composed of physicians, nurses, and respiratory therapists conducted a team simulation scenario. Debriefing can be divided by clinical domain and separated into group versus domain phases

The structured and supported debriefing model has been successfully deployed in this environment as well.

Simulation scenarios that are part of a course that may include many different learning activities including several simulations are handled somewhat differently. In this example it is very important that the facilitator be aware of the global course learning objectives as well as the individualized objectives for the scenario they are presiding over. This affords the facilitator the ability to limit the discussion of the debriefing for a given scenario to accomplish the goals specific to that scenario, knowing that other objectives will be covered during other educational and simulation activities during the course. This "allocation of objectives" concept is necessary to satisfy the operational realities of the course, which are often time-based and require rotations throughout a given period of time.

Technical resource availability is another consideration in the variability of debriefing. Technical resources such as the availability of selected element video and audio review, simulator log files, projection equipment, access to the Internet and other media, and supporting objects vary considerably from one simulated environment to the next.

The level of the participants and the group dynamics of the participants can factor into the adaptation of best-practice debriefing. Competing operational pressures will often create some limitations on the final debriefing product. For example, when teams of practicing professionals are brought together for team training exercises, they are often being pulled away from other clinical duties. Thus, the pressure is higher to use the time very efficiently and effectively. This is in contrast to student-level simulations, where the limiting factor can be the sheer volume of students that must participate in a given set of simulation exercises.

Challenges in Debriefing

There are a number of challenges associated with debriefing. Some of them involve self-awareness on the part of the facilitator, the skill of the facilitator, as well as resource limitations mentioned earlier. One of most difficult challenges is the need for the facilitator to be engaged in continuous assessment in order to maintain a safe learning environment for the participants.

Controlling the individual passion focus is an important consideration for facilitators and requires self-awareness in order to avoid bias during debriefing. As clinical educators from a variety of backgrounds, it is normal for a facilitator to have a specific passion point around one or more areas of treatment. This can lead the facilitator to subconsciously pay closer attention to that particular area of treatment during the simulation and subsequently focus on it during the debriefing. It is particularly important to maintain focus on the simulation exercise learning objectives when they are not designed in alignment with the passion focus of the facilitator. The facilitator must resist the urge to espouse upon their favorite clinical area during the debriefing. Otherwise the learning objectives for the scenario may not be successfully accomplished.

At times during simulation exercises, egregious errors may occur that need to be addressed regardless of whether they were part of the learning objectives or not. Typically these errors involve behaviors that would jeopardize patient safety in the clinical setting. If the topic surrounding the error is not part of the focal learning objectives for the simulation scenario, it is best to make mention of it, have the participants understand what the error was, describe an appropriate safe response, and then quickly move on. Let the participants know that the area or topic in which the error occurred is not the focus of the simulation, but emphasize that it is important that everyone be aware of safety issues.

The maintenance of a safe learning environment is another aspect of facilitator skill development. For example, difficult participants are sometimes encountered, emotionally charged simulations or debriefings occur and students may fail to "buy in" to the educational method. All of these situations are under the purview of the facilitator to assist in the process that allows self-discovery and allow freedom on the part of the participants to express their thoughts, concerns, and in particular their decision-making thought processes. The facilitator must always be ready to intervene in a way that attempts to depersonalize the discussion to provide a focus on the best practices that would've led to the best care for the patient.

Other factors of maintaining a safe learning environment are typically covered in the orientation to the simulation exercises. Informing participants ahead of time of grading processes, confidentiality factors, and the final disposition of any video and audio recordings that may occur during a simulation will go a long way toward the participant buy-in and comfort level with the simulation process.

Conclusion

The structured and supported model of debriefing was designed as a flexible, learner-centric debriefing model supported by multiple learning theories. The model can be used for almost every type of debriefing ranging from partial task training to interprofessional team sessions. The operational acronym GAS, standing for the phases of the method, gather, analyze, and summarize, is helpful for keeping the debriefing organized and effectively utilized. It is a scalable, deployable tool that can be used by debriefers with skills ranging from novice to expert.

References

1. Cantrell MA. The importance of debriefing in clinical simulations. Clin Simul Nursing. 2008;4(2):e19–23.
2. McDonnell LK, Jobe KK, Dismukes RK. Facilitating LOS debriefings: a training manual. NASA technical memorandum 112192. Ames Research Center: North American Space Administration; 1997.
3. O'Donnell JM, Rodgers D, Lee W, et al. Structured and supported debriefing (interactive multimedia program). Dallas: American Heart Association (AHA); 2009.
4. Decker S. Integrating guided reflection into simulated learning experiences. In: Jeffries PR, editor. Simulation in nursing education from conceptualization to evaluation. New York: National League for Nursing; 2007.
5. Dewey J. Democracy and education: an introduction to the philosophy of education. New York: The Macmillan Company; 1916.
6. Goffman E. Frame analysis: an essay on the organization of experience. New York: Harper & Row; 1974.
7. Bandura A, Adams NE, Beyer J. Cognitive processes mediating behavioral change. J Pers Soc Psychol. 1977;35(3):125–39.
8. Lewin K. Field theory and learning. In: Cartwright D, editor. Field theory in social science: selected theoretical papers. London: Social Science Paperbacks; 1951.
9. Kolb D. Experiential learning: experience as the source of learning and development. Upper Saddle River: Prentice-Hall; 1984.
10. Schön DA. Educating the reflective practitioner: toward a new design for teaching and learning in the professions. 1st ed. San Francisco: Jossey-Bass; 1987.
11. Lave J, Wenger E. Situated learning: legitimate peripheral participation. Cambridge/New York: Cambridge University Press; 1991.
12. Ericsson KA. Deliberate practice and the acquisition and maintenance of expert performance in medicine and related domains. Acad Med. 2004;79(10 Suppl):S70–81.
13. Ericsson KA. Deliberate practice and acquisition of expert performance: a general overview. Acad Emerg Med. 2008;15(11):988–94.
14. Ericsson KA, Krampe RT, Heizmann S. Can we create gifted people? Ciba Found Symp. 1993;178:222–31; discussion 232–49.
15. Ericsson KA, Lehmann AC. Expert and exceptional performance: evidence of maximal adaptation to task constraints. Annu Rev Psychol. 1996;47:273–305.
16. Issenberg SB, McGaghie WC. Features and uses of high-fidelity medical simulations that can lead to effective learning: a BEME systematic review. JAMA. 2005;27(1):1–36.
17. McGaghie WC, Issenberg SB, Petrusa ER, Scalese RJ. A critical review of simulation-based medical education research: 2003-2009. Med Educ. 2010;44(1):50–63.
18. Salas E, Klein C, King H, et al. Debriefing medical teams: 12 evidence-based best practices and tips. Jt Comm J Qual Patient Saf. 2008;34(9):518–27.
19. Rudolph JW, Simon R, Dufresne RL, Raemer DB. There's no such thing as "nonjudgmental" debriefing: a theory and method for debriefing with good judgment. Simul Healthc. 2006;1(1):49–55.
20. Rudolph JW, Simon R, Raemer DB, Eppich WJ. Debriefing as formative assessment: closing performance gaps in medical education. Acad Emerg Med. 2008;15(11):1010–6.
21. Rudolph JW, Simon R, Rivard P, et al. Debriefing with good judgment: combining rigorous feedback with genuine inquiry. Anesthesiol Clin. 2007;25(2):361–76.
22. Fanning RM, Gaba DM. The role of debriefing in simulation-based learning. Simul Healthc. 2007;2(2):115–25.
23. Raemer D, Anderson M, Cheng A, Fanning R, Nadkarni V, Savoldelli G. Research regarding debriefing as part of the learning process. Simul Healthc. 2011;6(Suppl):S52–7.
24. Savoldelli GL, Naik VN, Park J, Joo HS, Chow R, Hamstra SJ. Value of debriefing during simulated crisis management: oral versus video-assisted oral feedback. Anesthesiology. 2006;105(2):279–85.
25. Hodges B, Regehr G, Martin D. Difficulties in recognizing one's own incompetence: novice physicians who are unskilled and unaware of it. Acad Med. 2001;76(10 Suppl):S87–9.
26. Kruger J, Dunning D. Unskilled and unaware of it: how difficulties in recognizing one's own incompetence lead to inflated self-assessments. J Pers Soc Psychol. 1999;77(6):1121–34.
27. Albanese M, Dottl S, Mejicano G, et al. Distorted perceptions of competence and incompetence are more than regression effects. Adv Health Sci Educ Theory Pract. 2006;11(3):267–78.
28. Byrnes PD, Crawford M, Wong B. Are they safe in there? – patient safety and trainees in the practice. Aust Fam Physician. 2012;41(1–2):26–9.
29. Higginson I, Hicks A. Unconscious incompetence and the foundation years. Emerg Med J. 2006;23(11):887.
30. Straker D. Techniques for changing minds: questioning. 2002. http://changingminds.org/techniques/questioning/. Accessed 18 May 2012.
31. Brophy JL. Active listening: techniques to promote conversation. SCI Nurs. 2007;24(2):3.

7 Debriefing with Good Judgment

Demian Szyld and Jenny W. Rudolph

Introduction

Debriefing is the learning conversation between instructors and trainees that follows a simulation [1–3]. Like our patients and other biological organisms, debriefing is composed of both structure and function. Debriefing instructors need to understand the *anatomy* of a debriefing session (structural elements), the *physiology* (what works and how) and *pathophysiology* (what can go wrong), and the *management* options and for these condition (what instructors can do to improve outcomes). Given that structure and function are closely linked, we go back and forth in these two domains hoping to render a full picture for the simulation instructor poised to lead a debriefing.

Typically, debriefings last one to three times as long as the length of the simulation. A simulation session is composed of the scenario and the debriefing that follows. To meet its objectives, a simulation-based course may comprise one or more simulation sessions. A rigorous review of the literature on simulation based medical education lists feedback as one of the most important features [4]. While there might be learning *in action* when learners participate in a simulation, action and experience alone often are not sufficient for significant and sustained change [5]. The debriefing period presents the major opportunity for reflection, feedback, and behavior change; learning *from* action requires external feedback and guided reflection [6, 7]. The instructor's role in providing feedback and guiding reflection is critical, as they must help learners recover from the intense, frequently stressful experience of the simulation and at the same time ensure that reflecting on said experience yields learning and growth in accordance with the stated educational goals of the session [6]. Therefore, the major factors in debriefing are the following: the learning objectives, the simulation that occurred, the learners or participants, and the instructor or debriefer (see Table 7.1).

The role of simulation instructor is broader than the discussion of debriefing. In addition to debriefing, simulation instructors identify or create simulation sessions, prepare for and enact simulations, and evaluate learners and programs. This chapter focuses on the four principles that can enable instructors to effectively prepare and debrief a simulation session in order to achieve their curricular goals (Table 7.2). In this context we will describe the debriefing philosophy of "Debriefing with Good Judgment" [13, 14], an evidence-based and theory-driven structure of formative feedback, reflection, and behavior change that drives the educational process. This approach was developed and tested at the Center for Medical Simulation in Cambridge, Massachusetts, in over 6,000 debriefings and has been taught to more than 1,500 instructors through the Institute for Medical Simulation.

Debriefing with Good Judgment

Learning Objectives Are Clearly Defined Prior to Simulation Session

Clear objectives are requisite for trainees to reliably accomplish curricular goals and for faculty to help them get there. Just as we assess and manage patients with particular goals of hemodynamic stability or other measures of wellness, when learning objectives are clarified in advance, we give ourselves

D. Szyld, MD, EdM (✉)
New York Simulation Center for the Health Sciences, New York, NY, USA

Department of Emergency Medicine, New York University School of Medicine, New York, NY, USA
e-mail: demian.szyld@nyumc.org

J.W. Rudolph, PhD
Center for Medical Simulation, Boston, MA, USA

Department of Anesthesia, Critical Care and Pain Medicine, Massachusetts General Hospital, Boston, MA, USA
e-mail: jwrudolph@partners.org

A.I. Levine et al. (eds.), *The Comprehensive Textbook of Healthcare Simulation*,
DOI 10.1007/978-1-4614-5993-4_7, © Springer Science+Business Media New York 2013

Table 7.1 Definitions

	Definition	Examples
Learning objectives	Two to three observable accomplishments of learners following a simulation session	Treat the reversible causes of PEA arrest Utilize the SPIKES protocol for giving bad news [8] Value and consistently utilize closed loop communication during crisis situations
Simulation	The encounter of individual or group experiences during a simulation session and is discussed during the debriefing	ED patient in shock or cardiac arrest Fire in the labor floor or in the operating room [9, 10] Family meeting to discuss discharger planning [11] or disclose an error [12]
Learners	The participant or participants in a simulation course. Not all learners in a debriefing must participate in each simulation	6 labor floor nurses A complete trauma team (ED nurse, anesthesiologist, EM physician, trauma surgeon, respiratory therapist) Medical and nursing students
Debriefer	The instructor who leads the learners through the debriefing. This person is prepared to discuss the learning objectives and has the ability to give feedback and help learners reflect on their performance as well as prepare for future encounters	A faculty member in the same field as the learners A trained instructor with credentials and expertise in another specialty (clinical or otherwise)

PEA Pulseless Electrical Activity, *ED* Emergency Department

Table 7.2 Four key principles of "Debriefing with Good Judgment"

1. Learning objectives are clearly defined prior to simulation session.
2. Set expectations clearly for the debriefing session.
3. Be curious, give feedback, but do not try to "fix" your learners.
4. Organize the debriefing session into three phases: Reactions, Analysis, and Summary.

and our learners goals to reach by the end of a session. For example, if we want the team members to collaborate on executing the appropriate maneuvers to manage a shoulder dystocia, we know that by the end of the simulation and the debriefing, we want the learners to appreciate what knowledge, skills, or attitudes (KSAs) helped or hindered them in the course of the simulation. We also want them to appreciate which of the effective KSA's to retain and how to modify or change the ineffective ones. Clearly defined learning objectives serve as anchors for both trainees and faculty to focus their attention and discussion. One of the common pitfalls is that realistic, engaging simulations usually represent complex and rich experiences that could yield a myriad of teaching and learning opportunities (much like any interesting clinical experience). Instructors need to be prepared to lead discussions on the chosen topics, even though these represent a very small subset of all the possible thought-provoking conversations. Therefore, in order for faculty to engage deeply in the material, they must have clear understanding of both the details of the case as well as the desired learning outcomes.

Learning objectives, once elucidated and defined, serve a number of critical purposes. They define that considered germane which should be covered during the debriefing and aide the instructor in deciding what topics to steer away from. They allow instructors to develop short didactic "lecturettes" to efficiently describe the current evidence-based or best practices related to a given objective when knowledge gaps exist (usually less than 5 min). Finally, they provide the desired performance level or standard against which observed trainee performance is compared. The ideal learning objective is learner centered, measurable or observable, and specific. For example, when a learning objective reads "Intubate a 4-year-old trauma patient within 15 min of arrival while maintaining cervical stabilization and preventing desaturation," the performance standard is clear and easy to assess.

Whether to reveal the learning objectives at the beginning of the simulation sessions remains controversial. Many believe they should be stated explicitly at the beginning of a course or session; however, there is tension between openly sharing learning objectives with trainees (this helps them focus on how to perform and what to learn) and revealing them only after the trainee had an opportunity to discover them either in action (simulation) or reflection (debriefing). Alternatively, a broader set of goals and objectives can be shared with the students without "ruining" the experiential learning process through discovery. For example, the learning outcome might state: "At the end of the session trainees will deliver medications safely by confirming the right patient, the right medication, the right route of administration, and the right time." Instructors may choose to introduce the session simply by saying that the goal of the session is to practice safety in medication administration. Stating a broader goal can focus learners to the topic and keep them oriented to the activity without prescribing a definite course of action. Instructors can take comfort while sharing specific, observable, measurable learning objectives because as we have repeatedly experienced, knowing what to do is necessary butw not sufficient for expert performance. A complex scenario will challenge many well-prepared learners. The following case studies illustrate the advantages of defining and sharing objectives for both teachers and learners (Table 7.3).

Table 7.3 Case studies for clearly defined learning objectives

Case study	Anatomy	Physiology	Pathophysiology	Management
Instructor utilizes shoulder dystocia case provided by simulation center. No specific learning objectives available	Learners manage the case without a learning goal. Although it is not stated, they are aware that shoulder dystocia and teamwork are taught with simulation The instructor has a general viewpoint for anchoring observations about team performance	During the debriefing learners wonder why they were asked to manage this patient. The instructor gives general commentary about team communication and performance	Learners do not gain new insights about their performance, as they are not provided with specific feedback. They are unable to reflect specifically on areas to improve or correct. Learners regard general comments as undeserved or false praise	Without having specific learning, instructors can teach generic concepts. Instructors can also appeal to the learners as a source of knowledge. Gaining credibility is difficult, as the instructor is not availed of the concepts or evidence
Instructor has clearly outlined learning objectives for the case: "Declare presence of shoulder dystocia in order to avoid injury to the infant's brachial plexus." The objective is *not* shared prior to the scenario	Learners manage the case without a learning goal. Although it is not stated, they are aware that shoulder dystocia and teamwork are taught with simulation. The instructor observes the team performance, focusing communication primarily	During the debriefing learners wonder why they were asked to manage this patient. The instructor gives specific feedback about communication and in particular on the need to declare the condition (shoulder dystocia)	Learners begin the reflection process feeling good about successfully managing the patient. The instructor helps learners reflect on communication and notes that they did not explicitly declare the emergency. Learners no longer feel good about their performance and state that they thought the goal of the scenario was to perform the requisite maneuvers	The instructor validates the learner's performance vis-à-vis the clinical management in an effort to restore positive feeling and attempts to give weight to the communication goal
Instructor has clearly outlined learning objectives: "Declare presence of shoulder dystocia in order to avoid injury to the infant's brachial plexus". The objective *is* shared prior to the scenario	Learners manage the patient and are aware that improving communication during shoulder dystocia is the learning objective	During the debriefing learners reflect on the management of shoulder dystocia including the importance of explicitly stating the diagnosis. The instructor gives feedback about communication and in particular on the need to declare the condition and helps the learners reflect on the challenges of consistently stating their diagnostic thought process	Although the team successfully managed the patient, performed the maneuvers, and delivered the infant after declaring the presence of shoulder dystocia, a rich conversation ensues about the value and tension when being explicit about thought process, since it may benefits the team but could scare the patient and family, some worry that it could increase the risk of litigation	The instructor validates the learners and helps them engage around the stated goals, exploring enablers and barriers to expert performance

In this example a labor floor team gathers for weekly *in situ* simulation. The participants include the anesthesiologist, midwife, labor nurse, and on-call obstetrician. During the case the physical and pharmacologic maneuvers are instituted and the infant is delivered in a timely fashion

Set Expectations Clearly for the Debriefing Session

Benjamin Franklin said, "An ounce of prevention is worth a pound of cure." Although he was referring to fire fighting, the same applies to the beginning of a debriefing session. One of the most common problems debriefers face is the participant that becomes defensive during a debriefing. Setting expectations clearly is the preventive strategy that mitigates this problem. Participants become defensive when they perceive a mismatch between their expectations and their experience. This dissonance is identified by trainees as negative and threatening. Investing time and energy early in the course and in the debriefing to orient learners pays off for instructors [15, 16].

In general, faculty should introduce themselves including their credentials, relevant experience, and any biases or potential conflicts of interests and encourage all participants to follow suit [17]. It can be helpful if faculty put forth a personal goal such as a desire to learn from the experience or improve their abilities. If faculty foster a climate of learning and encourage respectful dialogue from the outset, trainees will aim to maintain and sustain it through the simulation and debriefing periods. A psychologically safe environment allows people to reflect and share their feelings, assumptions, and opinions as well as to speak up and discuss difficulty topics [18].

The *us versus them* dynamic can also contribute to a threatening environment that participants may experience during debriefing. Being on the defensive is triggered when the participant's professional identity is at risk. In the eyes of the participants, the simulation environment is used *by* the instructors *for* the trainees to make mistakes. Participants direct their emotion towards the faculty as they are perceived as both the source of criticism and the causal agent.

Faculty can minimize the effect by showing sympathy during the introduction for example by stating up front that learning with simulation can be confusing or disorienting. Similarly, it is advised that instructors avoid "over selling" the level of realism achieved by a simulation [19]. Although many ask trainees to "suspend their disbelief," an alternative is for educator and student to develop a "contract" collaboratively on rules of engagement within the simulated environment as best as possible given the limitations [20]. The latter strategy is a "virtual contract" where instructors agree to play fair and do their best to set up simulations that are realistic and designed to help trainees learn (not look bad or fail) and trainees agree to engage in the simulation to the best of their ability, treating the simulated patients respectfully and approaching the scenarios professionally.

Many trainees find learning with simulation anxiety-provoking because of its public nature; it uses audio and video recordings for documentation and debriefing, and the potential for assessment and reporting. Setting expectations about confidentiality and the nature of the assessment (formative vs. summative/high stakes) also contributes to a safe learning environment (Table 7.4). Presenting these important limits early in a simulation course can supersede unpleasant surprises for both faculty and learners alike.

Be Curious, Give Feedback, but Do Not Try to "Fix" Your Learners

Judgmental Versus Nonjudgmental Approach

The mindset of the faculty can influence the teaching and learning process in debriefings. An instructor can use inquiry and curiosity to offer performance critique without being overtly critical of the person. One strategy faculty can adopt in order to foster a psychologically safe environment is to assume that the trainee was operating under the best intentions, treating mistakes as puzzles to be solved rather than behaviors to be punished. Debriefers may be ambivalent about judging their trainees' performance and giving direct feedback. They may worry that being critical or negative can jeopardize the teacher-learner relationship. Giving the trainees the benefit of the doubt helps debriefers connect with the student in order to foster self-reflection. The ideal debriefer combines curiosity about and respect for the trainee with judgment about their performance [4]. When trainees feel an alliance with their instructor, trainees may openly share thought processes and assumptions that drove their behavior during the simulation. A healthy dose of curiosity about the learner can transform the tone, body language, timing, framing, delivery, and impact of a simple question such as *what were you thinking when you saw that the patient doing poorly?*

Frames, Actions, and Results

When an instructor witnesses a subpar performance, they could attempt to teach or "fix" the learner by coaching them on their actions. While this may sometimes be effective, often it is not [8]. In the reflective practice model, "frames" (invisible thought processes) lead to "actions" (observable), which in turn lead to "results" (also observable). Coaching at the level of the actions observed may not yield generalizable lessons [5, 6, 13, 14]. For example, the trainee might hold a frame (*ventilating a patient during procedural sedation leads to stomach insufflation, gastric distention, and aspiration of gastric contents – which must be avoided*), which leads to an action (*wait for apnea to resolve rather than ventilate patient with low oxygen saturation*), which in turn leads to a clinical result (*patient suffers anoxic brain injury*). Debriefers hoping for sustainable behavior change should be curious to uncover a trainee's frame as well as the actions these frames might promote. Trainees that can move towards a new (and

Table 7.4 Case studies for set expectations clearly for the debriefing session

Case study	Anatomy	Physiology	Pathophysiology	Management
Welcome and introduction	The simulation instructor states her clinical background/expertise and shares her own desire to improve her ability to perform in critical resuscitations	Trainees respect the instructor because of her critical care experience (7 years as a night nurse) and are interested in her questions as when she leads the debriefing she serves as a fallibility model – she does not have all the answers [21]	Rather than gaining the trust of her trainees, when instructors rely on positional authority, learners can be skeptical, mistrustful, or resentful	Try to ally yourself in the teaching and learning process. Join your learners in the journey. Grant added psychological safety by stating that it is very likely that they will not behave exactly as they would in "real life"
Orientation to the simulation environment. This can be accomplished in writing, via web page or video, or in person	Participants understand or experience the "rules" – how to order and give medications, call consultants, and acquire information from the medical record. They also may have a chance to see the space prior to being in it	Participants lower their defenses, as they know more of what to expect. During the scenario they experience less confusion. If they are surprised, it is because of scenario design, not an artifact of being in a simulation. If they feel defensive, they are unlikely to focus on issues of realism	In the absence of a fair orientation, learners are frequently defensive – this gets in the way of reflection and hinders learning. Signs and symptoms of defensiveness include: quiet participants, statements of low physical or conceptual realism, not forgiving of technological limitations	Do not oversell or undersell the capabilities or realism or the technology [12] Avoid a mismatch between learners' expectations and experience
Set forth the expectation of active participation and agree on the fiction contract [20][a]	Encourage participants to engage in the simulator as well as in the debriefing	Participants will be activated and fully immersed in the care of the patient. They might feel as if they have stopped acting or state that the situation was realistic even though the technology has limitations	Participants do not display expected speed or seriousness for the topic or acuity of the case presented. They do not participate or are not willing to reflect on or discuss difficult topics	Encourage participation by exposing your perspective and goals. Maintain instructor end of the fiction contract – work hard to simulate and situations authentic

The simulation instructor orients the learners to the simulation session including the simulation environment and the debriefing session at the beginning of a course on crisis management

[a]Peter Dieckmann, PhD, introduced the notion of the fiction contract to the healthcare simulation community

improved) frame can improve their performance in future situations as their actions are now the consequence of their improved frame [10–14].

Exploring trainees' frames and examining their actions is not the only purpose of debriefing. The debriefer's role is to help trainees see problems in their frames and understand and appreciate alternatives [15]. Debriefers should avoid attempting to be nonjudgmental since such a position has two major drawbacks – one obvious and one subtle. When withholding judgment, the debriefer is ineffective in giving feedback to the learner as the nonjudgmental approach makes it difficult to share information with the trainee about their performance (usually in the hopes of saving face or keeping within social norms where criticism is construed as malicious). But the more problematic side of this approach is that it is virtually impossible to hide such judgment. Trainees pick up on subtle nonverbal cues projected by the debriefer (mostly subconsciously) when they differ in opinion. This is frequently transparent to the learner and can trigger anxiety or shame and lead to distance. Trainees pick up on this and may become defensive or close minded as they reject the dissonance between what they hear and what they perceive [13, 22].

"Good Judgment" Approach

Given that the judgmental and the nonjudgmental approaches have their limitations (for both learners and faculty), an alternative approach that fosters psychological safety and an effective learning climate for instructors is known as the "good judgment" approach [14]. Faculty aim to be direct about their observations, to share their point of view with the goal of inquiring about the trainees' frames, in the hope to work together towards understanding rather than fixing their behaviors. The combination of an observational assertion or statement with a question (advocacy + inquiry) exposes both the debriefer's observation and judgment. This approach allows instructors to efficiently provide direct feedback to the learner and to explore the trainees' frames during debriefing. Returning to the example of managing a shoulder dystocia, the instructor could say: "I saw the midwife and obstetrician applying suprapubic pressure and doing the McRobert's maneuver to free the baby; however, I did not notice anyone informing the anesthesiologist that they may be needed to prepare for an emergency C-section" (behavioral feedback). This omission could lead to a delay and expose the child to prolonged hypoxia (feedback on the clinical consequences). I am curious to know how you interpreted this (starting the process of eliciting the learner's frames about the situation)? (See Table 7.5.)

This generic approach can be used in any debriefing: (1) observe a result relevant to the learning objective, (2) observe what actions appeared to lead to the result, and (3) use advocacy and inquiry to discover the frames that produced the results. This approach in earnest encompasses this competency for the debriefer.

Organize the Debriefing Session into Three Phases: Reactions, Analysis, and Summary

Debriefing sessions should allow participants in a simulation session time to (1) processes their initial reactions and feelings, (2) describe the events and actions, (3) review omissions and challenges, (4) analyze what happened and how to improve, generalize and apply this new view to other situations, and (5) summarize those lessons learned. This approach is supported by the healthcare debriefing literature and has yielded several debriefing styles or structures [1, 7, 22].

The Reactions Phase

The Reactions Phase is meant to allow trainees to share their emotions and initial reactions – to "blow-off steam" as they transition from the highly activated state of the simulated clinical encounter to the calmer, lower intensity setting of the debriefing room. Trainees open up in this short but important phase to the questions "how did that feel?" or "what are your initial thoughts?" Faculty can validate these initial reactions by active listening techniques and at the same time collect learner-generated goals for the debriefing [23]. It can be difficult for trainees to analyze their actions without this process [24]. Additionally, in the reactions phase trainees should review the main facts of the case (clinical and teamwork challenges alike) so that at the outset all of the participants share an understanding of the key features of the simulation. Faculty sometimes need to fill in some of the clinical or social facts that they may have missed. In summary, the reactions phase is composed of both *feelings* and *facts*.

The Analysis Phase

In the analysis phase, the instructor helps trainees identify major performance gaps with regard to the predefined learning objectives. Trainees and faculty work together to analyze the performance and find ways to fill the performance gap. There are four steps to follow in this process [14]:

1. Observe the gap between desired and actual performance.
2. Provide feedback about the performance gap.
3. Investigate basis for performance gap.
4. Help close the gap through discussion and didactics.

Performance Gaps

Implicit in the third step is that the basis for the performance gap is not uniform among learners. Therefore, generous exploration is required to discover the trainees' assumptions related to the learning objectives. Helping a trainee close the performance gap through discussion and teaching is much easier once they have shared their reasoning and thinking. Although we cannot "fix" or "change" the learner unilaterally, by fostering reflection, supplying new knowledge, encouraging different attitudes, and developing skills and perspectives, debriefers can help trainees close the performance gap.

Table 7.5 Case studies for the nonjudgmental, judgmental, and good judgment debriefing

Case study	Anatomy (debriefer's words to the obstetrician)	Physiology (effect on and response of the learner)	Pathophysiology (learner's thoughts)	Management (intention and thought process of the debriefer)
Nonjudgmental debriefing	"While you performed suprapubic pressure and McRobert's effectively, was there anything you could have done better in terms of communicating with the anesthesiologist?"	Quiet Tentative Guarded	Wonders and tries to guess what the debriefer thinks about their performance Infers that a mistake was made since the debriefer has brought up the topic	Get the trainee to change If I share my judgment, they will be too hurt to be able to learn The best way to learn is if they come to it on their own
Judgmental debriefing	"While you performed suprapubic pressure and McRobert's effectively, you delayed the anesthesiologist and the C-section by not helping them anticipate"	Avoidant Defensive Confrontational	Knows what the debriefer thinks Wants to correct the behavior Does not examine his/her thought process	Get the trainee to change If I share my judgment, they will learn A strong statement cements the learning objective
Good judgment debriefing	"I saw the midwife and obstetrician applying suprapubic pressure and doing the McRobert's maneuver to free the baby but not telling the anesthesiologist that they needed to prepare for an emergency C-section. I worried it could lead to a delay starting the delivery and expose the child to prolonged hypoxia. I am curious to know how you see this?"	Engaged Interested Reflective	Knows what the debriefer thinks Wants to correct the behavior Examines the thought process leading to the behavior	I will create a context in which learners can examine their thoughts and change If I share my judgment, they will know where I am coming from, get clear feedback, and begin to reflect and learn Clear feedback regarding my observation, the clinical consequence and my judgment paired with a short inquiry can help expose trainee's frames. Once these are evident (to them and me) I can help guide them better

An obstetrics team including obstetrician, anesthesiologist, staff nurse, midwife, and charge nurse encounters a shoulder dystocia delivering a child requiring an emergency cesarean section

A brief but important note should be made regarding the nature of performance gaps. They can be small or large, positive or negative. Positive performance gaps are noted when trainees surpass expectations for the case and for their level of training. These positive variances must be explored in order to help trainees and their peers sustain the behavior in future performances. Many debriefers are much more comfortable and effective at giving feedback on negative performance gaps. It is important to help learners and teams understand the range of their performance when they have performed below, at, or above what is expected for the task, topic, and level of training and experience.

Each learning objective treated should yield generalizable lessons that trainees can apply to new clinical settings and different cases. Faculty can facilitate this by making them explicit. For example, what was learned in treating hypoglycemia while searching for other causes of a change in mental status should be generalized to other situations: empiric therapy for a common condition should not preclude nor be delayed by investigation of other causes – treat dehydration in febrile children despite the possibility of sepsis.

The Summary Phase

The summary phase is the final phase of debriefing. Here, instructors should allow trainees to share new insights with each other as they reflect on their past and future performance, process new knowledge, and prepare to transfer gains to future clinical situations. Faculty should signal that the debriefing session is coming to a close and invite trainees to share their current view of what went well and what they hope to sustain as well as what they hope to change or improve in the future. In general, instructors should avoid summarizing at this stage unless the predefined learning objectives were not met nor discussed by the trainees. Another option is to ask participants to share their main "take-home points" from the session and the discussion. Frequently, there is significant diversity from the trainees at this stage that is rewarding for students and teachers alike.

Conclusion

Transparency in learning goals, understanding and use of simulation education and debriefing, mindset towards learning, and the structure of the debriefing can help orient, focus, relax, and prepare trainees for learning during debriefing. Good judgment can help faculty to give direct feedback, share their point of view, and understand their trainees' frames in order to help them sustain and improve their performance.

In this chapter we have shared four key tenets for debriefers. This approach to debriefing favors preparation of goals and specific knowledge of the subject matter including the performance standard so that trainees receive clear feedback. Feedback with good judgment is critical for reflection, and reflection on one's thoughts and actions is the basis of change and learning. As such, the debriefer is a cognitive diagnostician searching for the trainee's frames hoping to diagnose and treat appropriately. In its current state, simulation is confusing enough as it is. Learners benefit from being pointed away from distractions and towards the important lessons by the faculty. Clear, specific, explicit learning objectives can greatly facilitate this process. Following a three-phase debriefing helps trainees as the method is predictable and form and function are aligned. The reactions phase deactivates learners and clarifies what happened in the simulation including many clinical details. In the analysis phase instructors give feedback and help trainees identify and close performance gaps. Learners reach new understandings, in particular about their thoughts, assumptions, beliefs, and experience. During the summary phase trainees prepare to transfer these gains of *new* knowledge, skills, and attitudes to their current and future clinical environments. Central in the educational process of learning with simulation is the debriefing. It is our hope that reading this chapter deepened your understanding and helps you reflect on your practice.

References

1. Darling M, Parry C, Moore J. Learning in the thick of it. Harv Bus Rev. 2005;83(7):84–92.
2. Dismukes RK, McDonnell LK, Jobe KK. Facilitating LOFT debriefings: instructor techniques and crew participation. Int J Aviat Psychol. 2000;10:35–57.
3. Fanning RM, Gaba DM. The role of debriefing in simulation-based learning. Simul Healthc. 2007;2(2):115–25.
4. Issenberg SB, McGaghie WC, Petrusa ER, Lee Gordon D, Scalese RJ. Features and uses of high-fidelity medical simulations that lead to effective learning: a BEME systematic review. Med Teach. 2005;27(1):10–28. doi:10.1080/01421590500046924.
5. Schön D. The reflective practitioner. New York: Basic Books; 1983.
6. Schön D. Educating the reflective practitioner: toward a new design for teaching and learning in the professions. San Francisco: Jossey-Bass; 1987.
7. Kolb DA. Experiential learning: experience as the source of learning and development. Englewood Cliffs: Prentice-Hall; 1984.
8. Baile WF, Buckman R, Lenzi R, Glober G, Beale EA, Kudelka AP. SPIKES-A six-step protocol for delivering bad news: application to the patient with cancer. Oncologist. 2000;5(4):302–11. Retrieved from http://www.ncbi.nlm.nih.gov/pubmed/10964998.
9. Berendzen JA, van Nes JB, Howard BC, Zite NB. Fire in labor and delivery: simulation case scenario. Simul Healthc. 2011;6(1):55–61. doi:10.1097/SIH.0b013e318201351b.
10. Corvetto MA, Hobbs GW, Taekman JM. Fire in the operating room. Simul Healthc. 2011;6(6):356–9. doi:10.1097/SIH.0b013e31820dff18.
11. van Soeren M, Devlin-Cop S, Macmillan K, Baker L, Egan-Lee E, Reeves S. Simulated interprofessional education: an analysis of teaching and learning processes. J Interprof Care. 2011;25(6): 434–40. doi:10.3109/13561820.2011.592229.
12. Wayman KI, Yaeger KA, Paul J, Trotter S, Wise L, Flora IA, et al. Simulation- based medical error disclosure training for pediatric healthcare professionals. J Healthc Qual. 2007;29:12–9.

13. Rudolph JW, Simon R, Dufresne RL, Raemer DB. There's no such thing as a "non-judgmental" debriefing: a theory and method for debriefing with good judgment. Simul Healthc. 2006;1:49–55.
14. Rudolph JW, Simon R, Raemer DB, Eppich WJ. Debriefing as formative assessment: closing performance gaps in medical education. Acad Emerg Med. 2008;15:1010–6.
15. McDonnell LK, Jobe KK, Dismukes RK. Facilitating LOS debriefings: a training manual: NASA; 1997. DOT/FAA/AR-97/6.
16. Simon R, Raemer DB, Rudolph JW. Debriefing assessment for simulation in healthcare© – rater version. Cambridge: Center for Medical Simulation; 2009.
17. Dismukes RK, Smith GM. Facilitation and debriefing in aviation training and operations. Aldershot: Ashgate; 2001.
18. Edmondson A. Psychological safety and learning behavior in work teams. Adm Sci Q. 1999;44:350–83.
19. Rudolph JW, Simon R, Raemer DB. Which reality matters? Questions on the path to high engagement in healthcare simulation. Simul Healthc. 2007;2(3):161–3. doi:10.1097/SIH.0b013e31813d1035.
20. Dieckman P, Gaba DM, Rall M. Deepening the theoretical foundations of patient simulation as social practice. Simul Healthc. 2007;2:183–93.
21. Pisano G. Speeding up team learning. Harv Bus Rev. 2001;79:125–34.
22. Lederman LC. Debriefing: toward a systematic assessment of theory and practice. Simul Gaming. 1992;23:145–60.
23. Merriam SB. Androgogy and self-directed learning: pillars of adult learning theory. New Dir Adult Contin Educ. 2001;89:3–14.
24. Raphael B, Wilson JP. Psychological debriefing. Cambridge: Cambridge University Press; 2000.

Crisis Resource Management

8

Ruth M. Fanning, Sara N. Goldhaber-Fiebert, Ankeet D. Undani, and David M. Gaba

Introduction

Crisis Resource Management (CRM) in health care, a term devised in the 1990s, can be summarized as the articulation of the principles of individual and crew behavior in ordinary and crisis situations that focuses on the skills of dynamic decision-making, interpersonal behavior, and team management [1, 2].

It is a system that makes optimum use of all available resources—equipment, procedures, and people—to promote patient safety. It is a concept that sits within a larger organizational framework of education, training, appraisal, and refinement of processes at both a team and individual level.

Since its earliest iterations, Crisis Resource Management has grown in health-care education and in the provision of health care across multiple domains. The concept has spread from individual disciplines and institutions to entire health-care systems [3–5]. Simulation-based CRM curricula complement traditional educational activities and can be used for other purposes such as the introduction of new staff to unfamiliar work practices and environments or for "fine-tuning" existing interdisciplinary teams.

Increasingly, mandates for CRM-based simulation experiences for both training and certification are issued by professional societies or educational oversight bodies who accredit or endorse simulation programs for these purposes [6]. In some cases medical malpractice insurers encourage CRM curricula for their clinicians, often by offering reduced premiums for those who have undergone training [7]. Nationally and internationally, CRM courses have been created to improve the training and practice of many health-care professionals with the ultimate aim of better and safer patient care. In this chapter we will review the concept of CRM in-depth from its historic, nonmedical origins to its application in health care. We will provide the reader with a detailed working knowledge of CRM in terms of vocabulary, courses, principals, training, and outcomes.

The Origins of CRM

To fully understand CRM in health care, it is useful to explore its origins in parallels drawn from aviation and other high-hazard industries. Exploring where CRM came from and where it is heading in other arenas gives insights into its theoretical underpinnings and also its likely future health-care applications. "Crisis" Resource Management grew out of a number of concepts but was largely modeled on "Cockpit" Resource Management from US commercial aviation, later termed Crew Resource Management. CRM in aviation had its origins in the 1970s and 1980s. Commercial aviation had grown rapidly between the World Wars and dramatically after WWII. Safety within aviation improved remarkably with the advent of the jet engine, which revolutionized aircraft reliability and allowed routine flight above many weather systems. These factors combined with an integrated radar-based air traffic control system spurred a drop in accident rates. However, well into the 1970s and 1980s, aviation accidents still occurred.

R.M. Fanning, MB, MRCPI, FFARCSI (✉)
Department of Anesthesia, Stanford University School of Medicine, Stanford, CA, USA
e-mail: rfanning@stanford.edu

S.N. Goldhaber-Fiebert, MD
Department of Anesthesia, Stanford University School of Medicine, Stanford, CA, USA
e-mail: saragf@stanford.edu

A.D. Undani, MD
Department of Anesthesia, Stanford University School of Medicine, Stanford, CA, USA
e-mail: audani@stanford.edu

D.M. Gaba, MD
Department of Immersive and Simulation-Based Learning, Stanford University, Stanford, CA, USA

Department of Anesthesia, Simulation Center, VA Palo Alto Health Care System, Anesthesia Service,
Palo Alto, CA 1871, USA
e-mail: gaba@stanford.edu

A.I. Levine et al. (eds.), *The Comprehensive Textbook of Healthcare Simulation*,
DOI 10.1007/978-1-4614-5993-4_8, © Springer Science+Business Media New York 2013

Aviation traditionally (especially since WWII) applied human factors engineering principles to cockpit design and pilot selection. In the 1940s human factors principles concentrated mainly on the operator-equipment interface and its role in improving the safety and reliability of flying [8, 9]. The human factors research from the 1940s to 1950s, although fundamental for the more encompassing human factors discipline of recent years, did little to address aviation safety in the era of improved aircraft reliability and design. It was determined that a more holistic approach to the investigation and amelioration of aviation incidents was necessary.

The National Transportation Safety Board and independent airlines' investigations of accidents found that between 1960 and 1980, somewhere between 60 and 80% of accidents in corporate, military, and general aviation were related to human error, initially called "pilot error," referring not so much to the "stick and rudder" skills of flying the plane but to "poor management of resources available in the cockpit"—essentially suboptimal team performance and coordination [8].

Investigators at the NASA-Ames Research Center used structured interviews to gather first-hand information from pilots regarding "pilot error," in addition to analyzing the details of incidents reported to NASA's Aviation Safety Reporting System [8, 10, 11]. From this research they concluded that the majority of "errors" were related to deficiencies in communication, workload management, delegation of tasks, situational awareness, leadership, and the appropriate use of resources. In Europe at this time, the SHEL model of human factors in system design was created. This examined *software* (the documents governing operations), *hardware* (physical resources), *environment* (the external influences and later the role of hierarchy and command in aviation incidents), and *liveware* (the crew) [8, 12, 13].

From many of these threads came the notion of a new form of training, developed to incorporate these concepts into the psyche of pilots and, in later iterations of "Crew" Resource Management, to all crew members. There was a reluctance to use a "band-aid" approach to address the issues but instead a true desire to explore the core elements that would lead to safer aviation practices. In 1979 NASA sponsored the first workshop on the topic providing a forum for interested parties to discuss and share their research and training programs. That same year, United Airlines, in collaboration with Scientific Methods Inc. set about creating "a multifaceted and all encompassing training program that would lead to improved problem solving while creating an atmosphere of openness within its cockpits that would ensure more efficient and safe operations" [10].

This program drew from a number of sources including aviation experience, psychology, human factors, and business managerial models [8, 14]. It combined CRM principles with LOFT (Line Oriented Flight Training), a form of simulation-based training replicating airline flights from start to finish followed by debriefing sessions using videos of the scenarios. This type of training combined the conduct of CRM behaviors with the technical skills of flying the plane. The program was integrated with existing educational programs, reinforced and repeated. By the 1986 workshop on Cockpit Resource Management Training, similar programs had been developed by airlines and military bodies worldwide [10].

CRM and Health Care

During this period of widespread adoption of CRM throughout the airline industry, David Gaba, an anesthesiologist at Veterans Affairs Palo Alto Health Care System (VAPAHCS) and Stanford University, and his colleagues were interested in exploring the behavior of anesthesiologists of varying levels of training and expertise in crisis situations. They were examining patterns of behavior and gaps in knowledge, skills, and performance, akin to the initial exploration of pilot and crew behaviors in the investigations that led to the development of Crew Resource Management in aviation a decade earlier (a detailed history of Gaba's team's work before and during the evolution of ACRM is covered in his personal memoir in Chap. 2 of this book as well as in the paper "A Decade of Experience" [15]).

Beginning in 1986, Gaba and others created a simulated operating room setting where multiple medical events were triggered in or around a patient simulator (CASE 1.2–1.3) in a standardized multi-event scenario [16, 17]. It became apparent from analysis of videotapes from these early experiments that the training of anesthesiologists contained gaps concerning several critical aspects of decision-making and crisis management. As in aviation, the majority of errors were related to human factors including fixation errors rather than equipment failure or use. Although the level of experience played a role in managing critical incidents, human factors were a concern at every level of training and experience, as illustrated in studies including attending anesthesiologists [17–19]. Just like the early days of aviation training, which relied heavily on "stick and rudder" skill training, training in anesthesia (and other fields of medicine) had focused heavily on the medical and technical aspects of patient management but not on the behavioral aspects of crisis management skills that seemed equally important for achieving good patient outcomes in anesthesia and similar fields.

It was time for a paradigm shift, to create a new way of learning the critical skills that were needed to manage challenging situations in anesthesia. Gaba, Howard, and colleagues explored other disciplines to best study and improve the teaching of such elusive skills, in particular the concepts surrounding decision-making in both static and dynamic environments [20–22]. Decision-making in the operating room qualified as a "complex dynamic world" referred to in the "naturalistic decision-making" literature, a world where problems are ill structured, goals are ill defined, time pressure is high, and the environment is full of uncertainty [22].

Creating a training program that addressed skills such as dynamic decision-making in teams, while incorporating a "medically" appropriate set of "Crew Resource Management" principles, required a move away from the traditional didactic classroom setting. Gaba, Howard, and colleagues were training adults—residents and experienced clinicians—with the aim of changing behavior. Adult learning theory and experience suggested that adults preferred learning to be problem centered and meaningful to their life situation, to be actively engaging, and to allow immediate application of what they have learned [23–25]. Thus, to meet these needs the first multimodal "Anesthesia Crisis Resource Management (ACRM)" immersive course was developed in 1989–1990 (first run, September, 1990, with a group of senior anesthesia residents in their last year of training) [26].

At the time of the initial ACRM offering in the 1990s, there was a growing recognition that the practice of medicine was becoming increasingly team orientated, and the skills needed to work as an effective team needed to be addressed. There was an explosion in research exploring teams, how they function, and how to train and assess them, first in the military and then in the business environment. For example, Glickman, Morgan, and Salas looked at the phases of development that characterize team performance, those associated with technical aspects of the task (task work) and those associated with team aspects of the work (teamwork) [27, 28]. Most importantly, it was found that teamwork skills that were consistent across tasks impacted a team's effectiveness [29].

High-risk, high-acuity areas of medicine were the first to incorporate CRM training (e.g., anesthesiology, emergency medicine, critical care, surgery, obstetrics, neonatal units) because of the clear cognitive parallels with aviation and the requirements in these areas to conduct dynamic decision-making and team management. However, the principles are also applicable to less dynamic settings that have less "lethality per meter squared" but a much higher throughput of patients per day. Such arenas include almost all medical disciplines but especially fields like nursing, dentistry, pharmacy, and multiple allied health professions.

Today, CRM is ubiquitous. Since the early days of ACRM, we, like multiple centers across the world, have expanded our Crisis Resource Management courses beyond anesthesiology to cover multiple disciplines (e.g., neonatology, ICU, ED, code teams, rapid response teams) to be run either *in situ* or in dedicated simulation centers, across learner populations from novice to expert, and conducted as single-discipline courses or with multidisciplinary and interprofessional teams [30–35]. CRM courses and CRM instructor courses are now available at numerous centers internationally. They have evolved over time to best suit the learning objectives and cultural needs of the populations they serve as well as the philosophy and pedagogical preferences of the local instructors.

Variations of CRM

Many variants and hybrids of ACRM training have been developed and deployed over multiple health-care domains, disciplines, and institutions; some were connected directly to the VAPAHCS/Stanford work, while others were developed independently.

In the early 1990s, a collaborative project between Robert L. Helmreich of the University of Texas, a pioneer in the aviation side of CRM, and (the now deceased) Hans G. Schaefer, M.D., of the University of Basel created *Team-Orientated Medical Simulation* [36–38]. In this high-fidelity, mannequin-based simulation program, a complete operating room involving all members of the surgical team, including physicians, nurses, and orderlies was designed to teach skills to mixed teams. It focused heavily on the team structure of the learning environment. The course consisted of a briefing, a simulation, and a debriefing, often a laparoscopic case with an event such as a "pneumothorax" to "draw" in all the team members. The courses tended to be shorter than traditional ACRM-styled courses.

At roughly the same time as these interventions came about started, other programs addressing teamwork or CRM in health care were started, mostly using didactic and seminar-style teaching without simulation. Indeed the earliest iterations of CRM in aviation, prior to the introduction of LOFT, relied heavily on similar teaching methods, and in fact, many of the early non-simulation CRM programs in health care grew out of commercial efforts by purveyors of aviation CRM to expand into new markets in health care. Thus, as of the writing of this chapter, one can find courses billed as CRM or CRM-oriented in health care provided by a number of different groups, each with different teaching philosophies. As these programs have developed, there has been an increasing tendency to use multimodal educational techniques—often including simulation—to achieve the desired learning objectives. We will quote a few examples, but there are many others.

In the late 1990s, Dynamics Research Corporation noted a number of similarities between the practice of emergency medicine and aviation, which led to the creation of *MedTeams*. This curriculum was based on a program to train US army helicopter crews in specific behavioral skills which was then tailored to meet the needs of emergency medicine personnel [39–41]. It has since been expanded to labor and delivery, operating room, and intensive care settings. This program was designed to reduce medical errors through the use of interdisciplinary teamwork, an emphasis on error reduction similar to the fifth iteration of CRM in aviation described by Helmreich et al. as the "threat and error management" concept [42]. The program contains three major phases: *site assessment*, *implementation*, and *sustainment* [43]. The *site assessment phase* is conducted both by self-assessment and an on-site facilitator. The *implementation phase* involves classroom didactic or web-based skill-building exercises for participants, plus a "train-the-trainer" instructor program to allow for dissemination of the program throughout the department or institution. MedTeams focuses on generic teamwork skills, targeting disparate teams of three to ten health-care providers, using classroom instruction, videos, and feedback from a facilitator [39]. The *sustainment phase*, seen as the cornerstone of the MedTeams program, involves formal and informal coaching strategies and ongoing evaluation and training. The original MedTeams curriculum did not use simulation.

Medical Team Management is a CRM-based program developed by the US Air Force, styled on the fighter pilot training program, and was created to address deficiencies in the Air Force Hospital system. It uses a variety of training strategies including didactics, web-based seminars, modeling, and case-based scenarios [39]. The program uses established learning theories, founded on well-constructed human factors principles. Participants are expected to perform tasks in the workplace based on their training and discuss their progress at subsequent training sessions. Medical Team Management focuses on reinforcing and sustaining the human factors concepts taught in the program, with periodic drills, team meetings, and follow-up progress reports [39, 44–46].

Dynamic Outcomes Management, now Lifewings, is a CRM-based course developed by Crew Training International [39, 47]. This is a multidisciplinary team-based training, staged, with an educational phase and a number of follow-up phases. The program highly values the use of challenge and response checklists. Participants are encouraged to create and implement their own checklist-based protocols to effect change in their working environment.

In the 2000s, the US Department of Veterans Affairs developed their *Medical Team Training program* [48]. The MTT model was designed, in addition to training CRM principles, to improve patient outcomes and enhance job satisfaction among health care professionals. This program has an application and planning phase, followed by interactive learning and a follow-up evaluative phase. Multimodal video teaching modules for this course were created in collaboration with the Simulation Center of the Palo Alto, CA, VAMC, and the Boston VA Health Care System. As of March 2009, 124 VAMCs participated in the program, representing various clinical units such as operating rooms, intensive care units, medical-surgical units, ambulatory clinics, long-term care units, and emergency departments.

Team Strategies and Tools to Enhance Performance and Patient Safety (TeamSTEPPS™) was developed by the US Department of Defense and the Agency for Healthcare Research and Quality (AHRQ) [49]. It was designed with the aim of integrating teamwork into clinical practice and, in doing so, improving patient safety and the quality and effectiveness of patient care. TeamSTEPPS™ was publicly released in 2006 and materials for TeamSTEPPS™ are freely available through the AHRQ.

The program contains three major phases, starting with a "needs assessment" designed to determine both the requirements of the host institution and their preparedness to take the TeamSTEPPS™ initiative on board. The second phase is one of planning, training, and implementation. Organizations can tailor the program to their specific needs, in a timed manner, referred to as a "dosing" strategy. The third phase of sustainment stresses the need to sustain and spread the concepts within the institution at large.

The educational materials are multimodal, combining didactics with webinars, powerpoints, video vignettes, and other formats selected to best suit the needs of each host institution. TeamSTEPPS™ emphasizes practical techniques and mnemonics to help clinicians execute effective team behaviors (e.g., the highly popular "SBAR" mnemonic for communicating a patient's status). Additional materials and modalities are being continuously added to supplement the "Core TeamSTEPPS™" including leadership skills, TeamsSTEPPS™ for rapid response teams, and most recently various hybrid TeamSTEPPS™ that utilize mannequin-based simulation.

Core Principles of CRM

Despite the evolving nature of CRM in health care—which now comes in various flavors and varieties—as well as advances in health-care practices, the core set of nontechnical skills for health-care teams seems to us to be surprisingly consistent. We present the VA Palo Alto/Stanford formulation of the key points of Crisis Resource Management. Other varieties have substantial similarities to these, but each formulation has its own points of emphasis.

In all our CRM-styled simulation courses, we explicitly teach the "language" of Crisis Resource Management. We explore the concepts of CRM with our course participants using concrete examples drawn initially from non-health-care settings, to impartial health-care settings, before moving on to their own performance. We discuss in detail the "key points" of CRM, their origins and applications. We display them around our debriefing room and give participants pocket-sized aids to refer to throughout the course. Creating this "shared language" sets the scene for rich objective discussion during debriefing sessions. In our CRM instructor

Call for help early
Anticipate and plan
Know the environment
Use all available information
Allocate attention wisely
Mobilize resources
Use cognitive aids
Communicate effectively
Distribute the workload
Establish role clarity
Designate leadership
CRM Key points

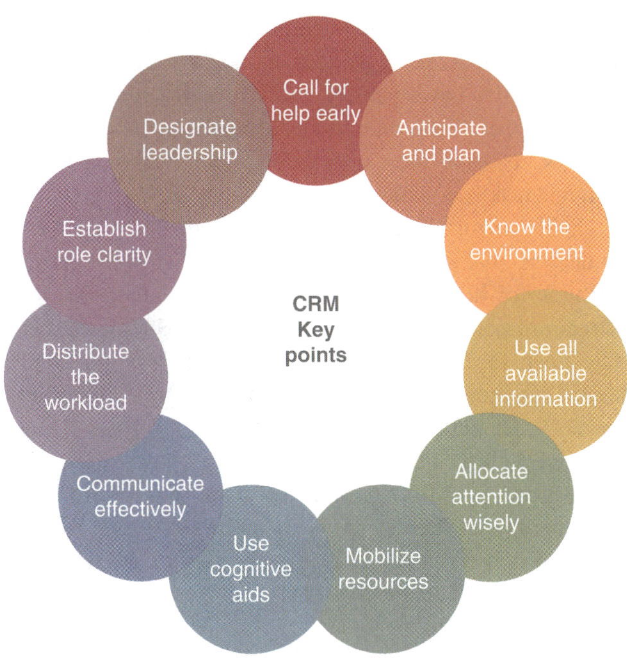

Fig. 8.1 Crisis Resource Management key points (Diagram courtesy of S. Goldhaber-Fiebert, K. McCowan, K. Harrison, R. Fanning, S. Howard, D. Gaba [50])

courses, we emphasize ways of improving discourse around the "key points." As we favor participant-led discussion over facilitator instruction, we illustrate ways to explore the key points using statements, open-ended questions, and other discursive techniques. As we describe the key points below, we will include examples of these techniques.

Conceptually, the key points can be organized into a number of broad categories: Team Management, Resource Allocation, Awareness of Environment, and Dynamic Decision-Making. There are interactions and overlaps among the principles below, as represented in Fig. 8.1.

Team Management

Leadership/Followership

Leadership means to conduct, to oversee, or to direct towards a common goal. In Crisis Resource Management, the "oversight" role of leadership is emphasized (meaning the ability to "see the big picture") to decide what needs to be done and then prioritize and distribute tasks. Questions for this key point include: Who can be or should be the leader? How is the leadership role assigned—hierarchically or by skill set? What happens if there are multiple leaders or the leadership position changes over time? How can we recognize a leader? What are the elements of good leadership? What techniques does the leader employ to ensure that common goals are met?

Any discussion of leadership ultimately broadens to a conversation involving "followership" and questions such as: What are the functions or responsibilities of the "followers" in a team? How can followers aid the leader? Can a follower become a leader? If so, what mechanisms if any, allow this transition to occur effectively?

Role Clarity

Team roles need to be clearly understood and enacted. If the leader is the "head" or director of the team, what roles do the other team members have? How are these roles assigned and recognized? Are these explicit, such as by verbal declarations, by wearing designated hats, vests, or role-specific badge? Or are roles recognized implicitly, such as by where people stand or the tasks they perform? Do roles change over time or in different circumstances, and if so, how are role changes communicated?

Workload Distribution

In complex crisis situations, a multitude of tasks must be performed almost simultaneously. When possible the leader stands back and designates work to appropriate team members. Leaders who immerse themselves in "hands-on" tasks may lose their ability to manage the "larger picture." In situations where the leader is the only person skilled in a particular technique, they may need to temporarily delegate all or part of the leadership responsibility to another team member. Distribution of tasks and leadership roles in a dynamic setting are not intuitive and are best explicitly taught and practiced.

Requesting Timely Help

Generally, it has been found that individuals or teams in crisis situations hesitate to call for help, and when they eventually do so, it may be too late. Thus, we now urge participants to err on the side of calling for help even if they themselves and their colleagues might be able to manage without it. We acknowledge that there are practical limits to how often one can call for help without creating the "boy who cried wolf" phenomenon. When to call for help, and indeed how early is early enough, varies depending on the locale and its resources, time of day, experience and expertise of the clinicians, and complexity of the patient care situation. Simulations often trigger rich discussion about these issues.

Effective Communication

Faulty communication has long been cited as a major contributing factor in the investigation of high profile accidents in high-hazard industries [51, 52]. In medicine, poor communication has been identified as a root cause of medical error in a myriad of health-care settings. Although the diagnosis of "communication failure" can be a "catch-all" assessment that risks masking deeper systems failures, there is no question that communication is of vital importance in crisis management. Improving communication in such settings involves more than simply ensuring the accurate transfer of information. In-depth consideration of how social, relational, and organizational structures contribute to communication failures is also required [53].

Communication skills in dynamic acute patient care arenas—particularly those involving multifaceted teams that are temporary and transitory in nature—require a particular skill set for both followers and leaders. To support the establishment of role clarity and leadership, formal but brief introductions may be used, for example, in the popular "universal protocol" used to prevent wrong site, wrong procedure, and wrong patient surgery [54]. As part of the protocol, a "time out" is performed just prior to incision where team members identify themselves and their roles. In some settings such as a trauma bay in an emergency department, individuals with specific roles may be assigned to stand in certain spots around the patient to provide a nonverbal indication of their roles.

Usually, verbal communication is at the heart of interaction. Ordinarily it should be clear, directed, and calm. When necessary, the leader may need to be more assertive, to quiet team members, or to draw attention to pressing concerns. In these instances, it may be necessary to raise one's voice or sound a whistle to achieve order. Followers may also need to display assertiveness if the goal of "best patient care" is to be achieved. The concept of "Stop the line," a reference to assembly line practice whereby any worker can shut down production if a hazard if found, is increasingly being employed in health-care settings to halt unsafe practices by any member of the team.

Many communications are in the form of orders, requests, or queries. There may be a tendency to utter commands or requests "into thin air" (e.g., "we need a chest tube") without clear direction at a recipient. Such messages are often missed; actions are much more likely to be completed if a recipient is specifically identified. "Closed loop communication" is an effective method to ensure critical steps are completed. The concept originates from "control system theory," where a closed loop system has, in addition to an input and output pathway, a feedback loop to ensure the process has been completed [55]. "Read-back" of orders is a classic everyday example. In commercial aviation, pilots are required by federal regulations to read-back "clearances" and any order having to do with an active runway to air traffic control. Good communication and task coordination requires team members to inform the leader when an assigned task is completed.

Highly performing teams try to establish a "shared mental model" so that everyone is "on the same page." Practical methods for achieving this coordination include out loud "stream of consciousness" commentary by the leader, periodic open recap and reevaluation of the situation by the leader, reminders by whomever is acting as the "recorder," formal "time-outs" before procedures, or a formal patient-centered daily "care plan" in a ward or outpatient setting. The goal is for the team to be aware of the "big picture," with everyone feeling free to speak up and make suggestions in the best interest of the patient if best practices are not being employed or effectively delivered.

Resource Allocation and Environmental Awareness

Know Your Environment

Crisis avoidance or management requires detailed knowledge of the particular clinical environment. Thorough familiarity with the operation of key equipment is vital in many high-tech environments such as the operating room, emergency department, and intensive care unit. Often even very small technical issues can make or break the clinical outcome for the patient. Other aspects of the environment include where equipment, medications, and supplies are located; who is available; and how to access resources when needed. Even familiar settings may take on a different character on the weekend or when different team members are present.

Anticipate and Plan

Effective crisis management "anticipates and plans" for all eventualities, as modified by the specific characteristics of one's environment and the situation. Unlike in a hospital setting, managing a "code" in an outpatient center or nursing home setting may necessitate stabilizing and transferring a patient to another facility, which might require numerous personnel, and extensive planning. Anticipating and planning for a potential transfer early in the patient's treatment can be lifesaving. Such preemptive thinking and action is dynamic as an event unfolds—it is useful to anticipate the worst case of what might transpire and take reasonable steps to get the situation fails to improve ready in case.

Resource Allocation and Mobilization

In the earliest investigations of airline accidents, inadequate utilization of cockpit and out-of-cockpit resources was cited as a leading concern [10]. The concept of "resource" has broadened to include not only equipment but also personnel and cognitive skills. Resources vary from setting to setting and team to team. It is imperative that teams are aware of resources available to them, for example, how to access extra staff, equipment, knowledge and how to mobilize resources early enough to make a difference. Some resources have a particularly long "lead time" so an early decision to put them on alert or to get them mobilized can be critical.

Dynamic Decision-Making

Decision-making, particularly in crisis situations, can be extremely challenging, especially in conditions of dynamic evolution and uncertainty. A number of concepts explored below are integral to the decision-making process in rapidly changing, highly complex environments.

Situation Awareness

The concept of situation awareness has featured heavily in the realms of human factors research. In essence, it has been described as the operator's ability to perceive relevant information, integrate the data with task goals, and predict future events based on this understanding [56, 57]. Situation awareness is an adaptive concept requiring recurrent assessments, tempered by environmental conditions [58, 59].

Gaba and Howard describe three key elements to help enhance situation awareness in health-care settings: (1) sensitivity to subtle cues, (2) dynamic processing as the situation changes, and (3) cognizance of the higher-order goals or special characteristics that will change the otherwise typical response to a situation [60]. Dynamic decision-making in medicine often utilizes matched patterns and precompiled responses to deal with crises, but when the crisis falls outside "usual practice," such recognition-primed decision-making may be insufficient [61].

In a crisis situation, it is easy to become immersed in tasks or to become fixated on a single issue. Human attention is very limited and multitasking is difficult and often unsuccessful. Attention must be allocated where it is needed most. This is a dynamic process and priorities change over the course of the crisis [62]. Distraction and interruption are known vulnerabilities of human beings particularly for "prospective memory"—remembering to do something in the future [63, 64]. When an interruption occurs, it can derail the planned sequence of actions.

Use all Available Information

Multiple information sources including clinical history, monitored data (e.g., blood pressure or oxygen saturation), physical findings, laboratory data, or radiological readings are critical for managing a patient in crisis. Many of these findings change rapidly and require constant vigilance. Some items are measured redundantly, allowing rapid cross-checking of information, which can be prone to artifact, transients, or errors. Electronic health records provide a wealth of clinical information and may incorporate alerts such as drug incompatibilities to aid patient care and safety. The internet provides a secondary source of information, but as in all other sources of information, it requires judicious prioritization.

Fixation Error

A fixation error is the persistent failure to revise a diagnosis or plan in the face of readily available evidence, suggesting that a revision is necessary [62, 65, 66]. Fixation errors are typically of three types. One type of fixation error is called *this and only this*—often referred to as "cognitive tunnel vision." Attention is focused on one diagnosis or treatment plan, and the operator or team is "blind" to other possibilities. Another is *everything but this*, a persistent inability to hone in on the key problem despite considering many possibilities. This may occur for diagnoses that are the most "frightening" possibility or perhaps where treatment for the problem is outside the experience or skill set of the individual. One of the most ominous types of fixation error is the persistent claim that *everything is OK*, in which all information is attributed to artifact or norms and possible signs of a catastrophic situation are dismissed. This type of error often results in a failure to even recognize that a serious problem is present and a failure to escalate to "emergency mode" or to "call for additional help or resources" when time is of the essence.

Individuals and teams who are aware of the potential for fixation error can build "resilience" into their diagnostic and treatment plans by "seeking second opinions" and reevaluating progress. The "10-seconds-for-10-minutes principle" posits that if a team can slow its activities down just a little, it can gain more than enough benefit in rational decision-making and planning to offset the delay [62]. A 10-s pause and recap may reveal information and aid decision-making, preventing diagnostic errors and missteps which effectively "buy extra time" in a crisis situation.

Cognitive Aids

Cognitive aids are tools to help practitioners to remember and act upon important information and plans that experience shows are often "inert" or difficult to use unaided in stressful conditions. Although the term cognitive aid includes "checklists," the concept also includes written protocols guidelines, visual or auditory cues, and alert and safety systems.

Aviation, among other high-hazard industries, has long been successful in using checklists for routine conditions and other written emergency procedures for unanticipated events such as engine failure for many years. Pilots' simulation training reinforces the use of their "Quick Reference Handbooks" for training and handling of real emergency events. Cognitive aids should not be considered a replacement for more detailed understanding of the material. Their use is not a reflection of inadequate or inept personnel. They are however extremely valuable during a crisis because human beings have innate difficulty with recall and cognition at these times. There is value in putting knowledge "in the world" rather than just in people's heads [67].

A common misconception in the past about crisis management in health care was that because immediate lifesaving actions must be performed almost instantaneously, there is little role for cognitive aids. In fact, cognitive aids can be of great value especially, during such time-sensitive critical events, though they must be designed, trained, and used appropriately to make them effective rather than distracting. A vivid example from aviation was the emergency landing of US Airways flight 1549 on the Hudson River, during which the copilot actively read aloud and completed appropriate actions from the "Dual Engine Failure" section of their "Quick Reference Handbook" while the pilot flew the plane and communicated with air traffic control personnel [68].

In health care, we have several challenges to address before practitioners can effectively and efficiently use cognitive aids during an emergency. Though no small task, only when these kinds of aids are familiar, accessible, and culturally accepted will they be used effectively to improve patient care.

The success of the WHO Safe Surgery Checklist (among others) has speeded the tide of change in viewing cognitive aids as important tools enhancing patient care rather than as "crutches" or "cheat sheets." Studies have shown that practitioners often miss critical steps or prioritize ineffectively when managing emergencies, and a growing nascent body of literature is showing that use of cognitive aids can improve performance [69, 70]. Cognitive aid design is a complex endeavor; cognizance of the environment in which the cognitive aid will be used and the user populations are crucial. Attention to layout, formatting and typography in addition to the organization and flow of information is vital. Content can be improved by the utilization of prepublished guidelines and standards of care, employing expert panels. The relevant individual cognitive aids should likely be grouped into easily usable, familiar, and accessible emergency manuals that are available in the appropriate clinical context. Iterative testing of prototypes during simulated emergencies can improve the aids significantly.

Both real-life and simulation-based studies have shown that simply placing the relevant information at the fingertips of practitioners without training them in their use is insufficient [69, 71, 72]. Health-care teams must be familiarized and trained in the use of cognitive aids, with a combination of simulated emergencies and their use in real clinical situations. Gaba, Fish, and Howard in their 1994 book *Crisis Management in Anesthesiology* developed the first useful index of operating room critical events in addition to detailing CRM behaviors [73]. For many years, however, the only commonly available widely promulgated *point of care* cognitive aids for emergency health-care events have been the AHA ACLS guidelines book/cards and the Malignant Hyperthermia poster/wallet card made by MHAUS. The AHA materials are likely the most widely used, contain extremely useful information, and have the necessary benefit of being familiar to most practitioners. However, their font is too small to easily read during a "code,". In addition only ACLS events are covered. Recently, many institutions have adopted a separate "local anesthetic toxicity treatment cart" with the ASRA local anesthetic toxicity treatment guidelines.

The Veterans Health Administration was the first group to employ cognitive aids for both cardiac arrest- and anesthesia-related intraoperative events across multiple centers, finding that although they were deemed useful by a significant number of practitioners, lack of familiarity with the aids resulted in less than optimal uptake [71, 72]. As iteratively improved content and graphics for medical cognitive aids are developed, simulated health-care environments provide an ideal setting for testing and redesign [74]. As Nanji and Cooper point out in a recent editorial, simulation courses also provide a needed opportunity to train practitioners how to appropriately utilize cognitive aids or checklists during emergencies [75]. Burden et al., in their study of the management of operating room crises, illustrated the added value of a reader, working in conjunction with the team leader, in improving patient management in a simulated setting, at least in rarer scenarios such as malignant hyperthermia and obstetric codes [76].

Cognitive aids also have a role in the retention of learning and care delivery. A small randomized control trial showed that cognitive aid use helped to sustain improvement from simulation training that was otherwise lost at 6 months. McEvoy et al. trained anesthesia resident teams with either an AHA cognitive aid or their local MUSC (South Carolina) version [77]. Training improved test scores in both groups, but performance dropped significantly for both groups at 6 months post-training. However, providing the initial cognitive aid at the 6-month follow-up testing returned participant performance to a level comparable to their post test performance immediately after training. Checklists and cognitive aids may also have a role to play in improving the safety culture by changing clinicians' attitudes regarding patient safety [78].

By Example: A Typical CRM Course

Admittedly there are no hard and fast rules regarding how a CRM course should be conducted, but to illustrate the concepts, we offer a description of a typical simulation-based CRM course for anesthesiologists as conducted at our center. The course is multimodal, typically involving initial didactic elements and analysis of prerecorded "trigger videos" (a trigger video is made or selected to trigger discussion by the viewers), with the majority of time spent in a number of mannequin-based simulations and debriefings. In novice CRM courses, we first introduce the participants to the concepts of CRM and familiarize them with the vocabulary in an interactive fashion. We use both health-care and non-health-care videos to introduce the participants to the practice of analyzing performance with the CRM concepts in mind, always stressing that the critique is of the "performance not the performer." This gives participants practice analyzing performance as a group before they do so individually. We follow with a series of simulation scenarios developed with particular learning objectives in mind.

Across scenarios participants rotate roles which are: (a) primary anesthesiologist; (b) first-responder "helping" anesthesiologist who can be called to help but arrives to the crisis unaware of what has transpired; (c) scrub tech, who watches the scenario unfold from the perspective of the surgical team; and (d) the "observer" who watches the scenario in real time via the audio and video links to the simulation room. Each scenario lasts 20–40 min and is followed by an instructor-facilitated group debriefing of similar length, involving all the participants with their unique perspectives. Although substantial learning occurs in the scenarios themselves, the ability to engage in facilitated reflection is considered a critical element of this kind of CRM training [23] (See Chaps. 6 and 7 on debriefing).

Although developed intuitively by the VAPAHCS/Stanford group, its theoretical underpinning fits best with Kolb's theory of experiential learning [79, 80] (See Chap. 3). Our simulation-based CRM courses have an active concrete component, the simulation, along with an integrated reflective observation and abstract conceptualization component—the "making sense of the event"—which takes place during the debriefing process (Figs. 8.2a, 8.2b, 8.2c, and 8.2d). Debriefing in our courses is seen as the central core of the learning process, being highly focused on CRM and systems thinking. We foster discussion rather than direct questions and answers and favor participant discourse over facilitator instruction. Our goal is to encourage the participant-focused learning goals in addition to our own curricular agenda. Each course is part of the 3-year Anesthesiology CRM curriculum (imaginatively named ACRM1, ACRM2, ACRM3) which grows in complexity with the increasing experience of the participants.

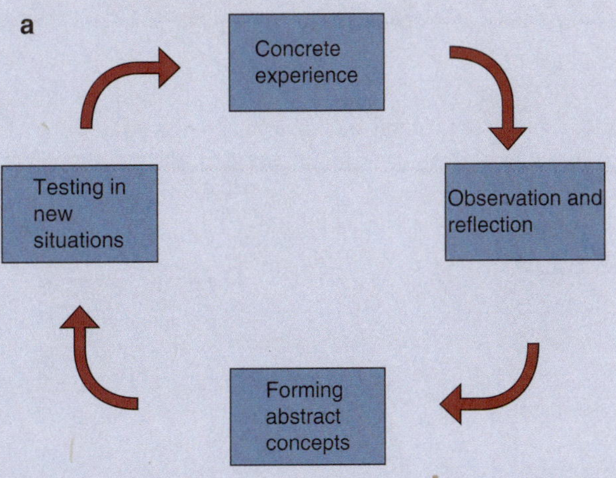

Fig. 8.2a Kolb's model of experiential learning—adaptation to simulation (© 2010 David M. Gaba, MD)

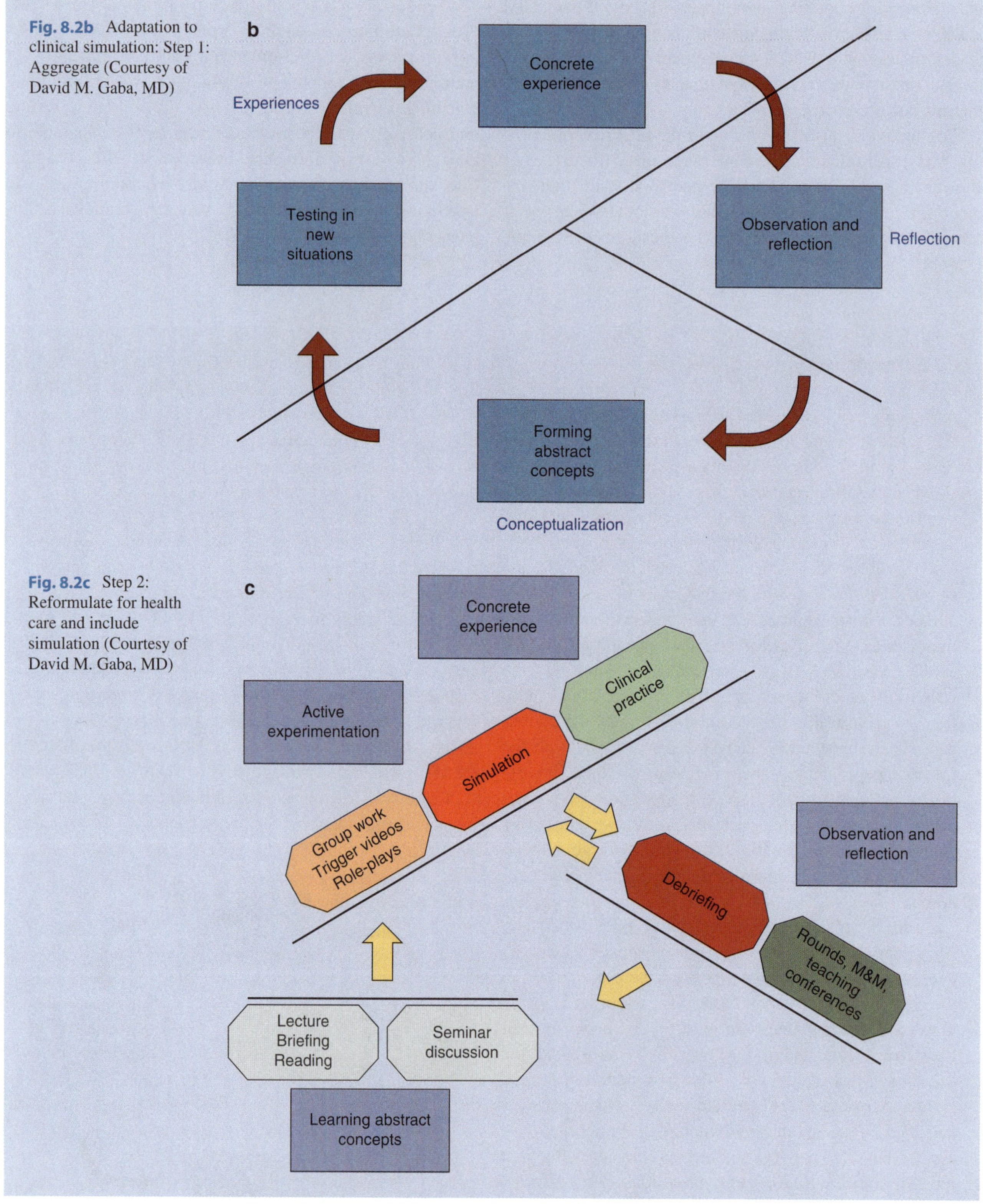

Fig. 8.2b Adaptation to clinical simulation: Step 1: Aggregate (Courtesy of David M. Gaba, MD)

Fig. 8.2c Step 2: Reformulate for health care and include simulation (Courtesy of David M. Gaba, MD)

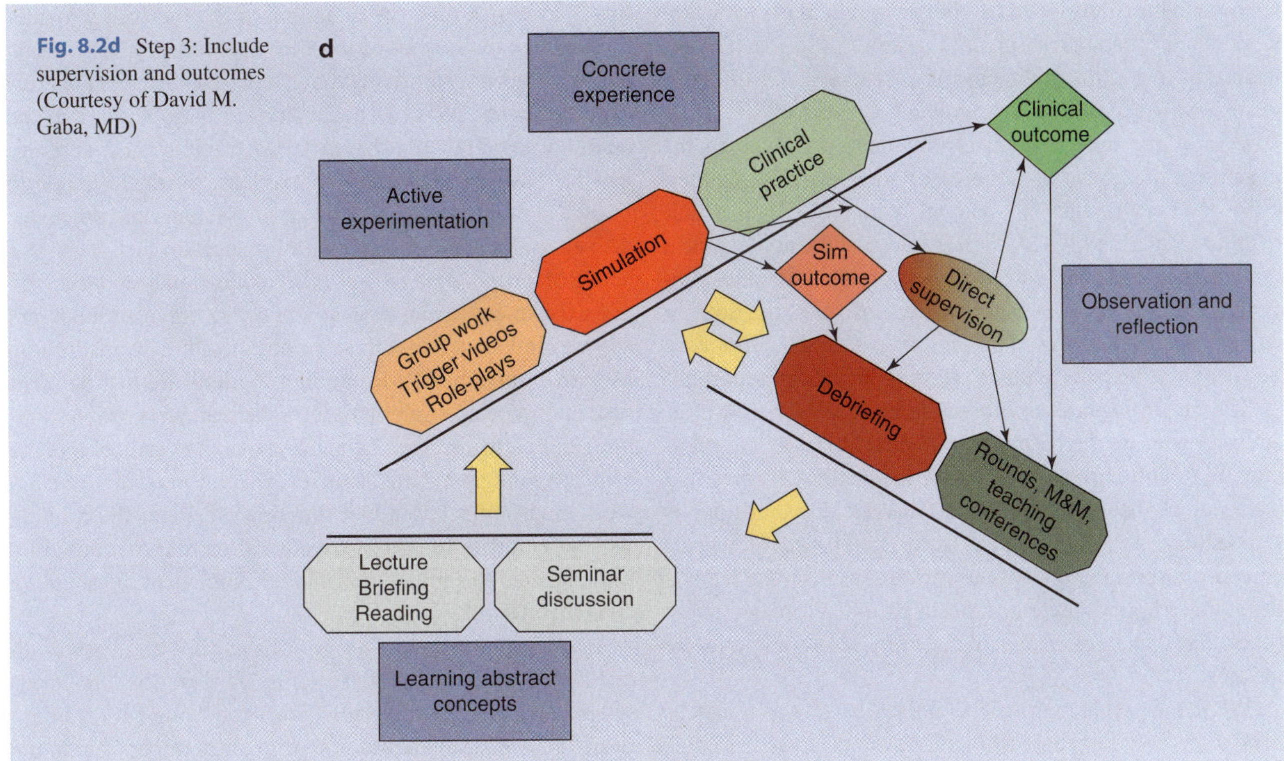

Fig. 8.2d Step 3: Include supervision and outcomes (Courtesy of David M. Gaba, MD)

CRM Training and Assessment

The skills of CRM, although often considered "common sense," have not historically been taught to health-care professionals. A few individuals lucky enough to have absorbed the skills, probably from exposure to role models who are good crisis managers. In general, everyone can improve his or her CRM skills. Thus, as in aviation (and other fields), specific efforts are warranted to teach these skills and to provide opportunities for their controlled practice in a coherent structured fashion.

Crisis Resource Management principles are inherently subjective and do not lend themselves to objective examination systems such as multiple choice tests, checklists of appropriate clinical actions, metrics of psychomotor skill, or time to completion of manual tasks. Nonetheless, simulation provides a unique environment in which to perform assessment of crisis management behaviors. It provides a controlled setting to explore known challenging cases in real time with audio-video recordings, which in themselves allow structured post hoc analyses.

A number of scoring systems have been developed to examine nontechnical or behavioral skills, the core elements of Crisis Resource Management. Perhaps the most well known of these is the ANTS systems (Anesthesia Non-technical Skills) [81]. ANTS was triggered by the so-called NO-TECHS assessment of nontechnical skills in European airline pilots developed by the team of psychologists at the University of Aberdeen (Scotland) led by Rhona Flin [82]. From NO-TECHS, Flin and her student Fletcher joined with anesthesiologists Glavin and Maran to perform in-depth analysis of real-life cases, incident reports, as well as a series of questionnaires to create ANTS. They identified two major categories (i) cognitive and mental skills—including decision-making, planning, and situation awareness and (ii) social and interpersonal skills, including aspects of team working, communication, and leadership. The ANTS system sets out to score skills that can be identified unambiguously through observable behavior, increasing its reliability. It does not, by design, include ratings for "communication" (assuming that this skill is embedded in all the other nontechnical skills).

NOTSS, a nontechnical skills rating system for surgeons, was developed by Yule, Flin and colleagues. An ICU version was created by the same group [83, 84]. OTAS, an observational assessment of surgical teamwork, was conceived by Undre and colleagues in Imperial College, London [85]. This rating is composed of two parts: a task checklist and also a behavioral assessment component largely built around Dickinson and McIntyre's model of teamwork [86]. The behavioral ratings comprised five groups: shared monitoring, communication, cooperation, coordination, and shared leadership. The validity and reliability of the tool has been assessed by Hull and colleagues [87]. Thomas, Sexton, and

Helmreich have developed five behavioral markers for teamwork in neonatal resuscitation teams [88], MedTeams identifies five critical dimensions necessary for effective teamwork linked with 48 observable behaviors [39].

One of the more recent developments involved in the construction and use of subjective nontechnical skills metrics is the Performance Assessment Team concept for a multicenter study (the MOCA AHRQ study) of the nontechnical (and technical) performance of board-certified anesthesiologists undergoing the Maintenance of Certification in Anesthesia (MOCA) Simulation Course in the United States. Several existing paradigms for scoring have been reported.

The Performance Assessment Team in the MOCA project has reviewed the literature on nontechnical scoring systems in health care (including some powerful studies that have not yet been published) and has decided that none is satisfactory enough to adopt as is. Instead, based on the perceived strongest features of the various systems, the team is developing a new integrated set of technical, nontechnical (behavioral anchored subjective scores), and holistic rating metrics.

While the psychometric data on the measures of nontechnical skills and the readiness of such systems to assess clinician performance remains controversial, there is a growing consensus that even imperfect instruments can make a significant contribution to the current systems of measuring clinician performance that have been inadequate to identify and categorize poor clinical ability.

Crisis Resource Management: Legacy and Impact

Creating a CRM-based curriculum and deploying it in a department or even at an institutional level does not guarantee improved efficacy and patient safety. Salas and colleagues, review in 2006 looked at the impact of CRM programs across a number of domains including health care. They illustrated positive reactions among participants, improved learning in general, but variable results with regards to outcomes [89].

Subsequently, a number of studies have shown positive results after the implementation of team-orientated and CRM-type programs [90–93], although a meta-analysis of the evidence basis of "aviation-derived teamwork training in medicine" published in 2010 by Zeltser and Nash did not show a definitive outcome benefit in Healthcare [94]. Gaba pointed out in 2011, in an editorial extending Weinger's analysis of the "pharmacological analogy" for simulation (i.e., considering simulation interventions as if they were a medication) that almost all studies to date of simulation, and especially of CRM-like curricula, have been very small, short in duration, using limited one-time CRM training, without coupling to performance assessment, and without strong reinforcement of CRM principles in actual patient care settings [95, 96]. Under these circumstances the ability to adequately test the impact of the CRM approach is very weak, and it is thus not surprising that a meta-analysis cannot (yet) show a benefit. What is necessary are large studies of the adoption of simulation-based CRM training on a comprehensive basis in health-care institutions, over a long period of time combined with key changes in systems and practices. As yet, no funders have emerged for such studies!

CRM programs like any other educational endeavor do not exist in a vacuum but are subject to organizational and cultural influences that exist in any health-care institution. Moreover, ideally CRM training programs are just one part of a multifaceted strategy to improve teamwork, safety culture, and patient safety. As noted above, it is critical that the principles taught in CRM courses are reinforced in the actual work environment. Without this reinforcement the training will be vitiated. To date, we know of no site that has fully implemented this integration and reinforcement. It remains a challenge for all.

In aviation, the relationship of the pilot and crew with the larger organizational structure is described in terms of an "organizational shell" with the "outer" organizational and cultural elements significantly impacting on the "inner" crew elements. Airlines have much stronger organizational and operational control over the training and work of their air crews than is present in health care [97, 98]. Moreover, the actual practices of flying are strongly regulated by national governments. In the USA, there is *no* federal agency that regulates the practice of health care (the federal government regulates drugs and devices and the payment schemes for elderly and indigent patients, but it does not directly regulate what clinicians actually do or actual health-care practices) [99]. Although "patients are not airplanes," there is still much to be learned from aviation and other industries of high intrinsic hazard concerning the implementation of organizational safety theory—and specific programs such as CRM training—to improve quality and safety outcomes.

Conclusion

In the quest to ensure improvement in patient safety and the quality of patient care, Crisis Resource Management is just one cog in the wheel. To achieve high quality patient care in a safe, reliable setting, where efficiency and cost effectiveness are overarching concerns, a comprehensive program of training, audit, and assessment is necessary. We, in health care, have learned much from our colleagues in aviation, business, psychology, and anthropology. Cross-pollination and adoption of ideas from other disciplines has strengthened the practice of medicine in the past and, in this technological there are vast opportunities to continue this into the future.

References

1. Gaba DM. Crisis resource management and teamwork training in anaesthesia. Br J Anaesth. 2010;105(1):3–6.
2. Helmreich RL, Foushee HC. Why crew resource management? Empirical and theoretical bases of human factors training in aviation. In: Weiner EL, Kanki BG, Helmreich RL, editors. Cockpit resource management. San Diego: Academic; 1993. p. 3–46.
3. The Kaiser Permanente National Healthcare Simulation Collaborative. http://kp.simmedical.com/. Accessed Dec 2011.
4. http://www.simlearn.va.gov/. Accessed Dec 2011.
5. http://www.bannerhealth.com/About+Us/Innovations/Simulation+Education/About+Us/_About+Simulation+Education.htm. Accessed Dec 2011.
6. ACGME. Simulation: new revision to program requirements. http://www.acgme.org/acWebsite/RRC_040_news/Anesthesiology_Newsletter_Mar11.pdf. Accessed Apr 2011.
7. McCarthy J, Cooper JB. Malpractice insurance carrier provides premium incentive for simulation- based training and believes it has made a difference. APSF Newsl. 2007;22(1):17.
8. Helmreich RL, Fousbee CH. Why crew resource management? Empirical and theoretical bases of human factors training in aviation. In: Wiener EL, Kanki BG, Helmreich RL, editors. Cockpit resource management. San Diego: Academic Press Inc; 1993. p. 1–41.
9. Fitts PM Jones RE. Analysis of 270 "pilot error" experiences in reading and interpreting aircraft instruments. Report TSEAA-694-12A. Wright Patterson Air Force Base: Aeromedical Laboratory; 1947.
10. Carroll JE, Taggart WR. Cockpit Resource Management: a tool for improved flight safety (United airlines CRM training). In: Cockpit Resource Management training, proceedings of the NASA/MAC workshop. San Francisco; 1986. p. 40–6.
11. Cooper GE, White MD, Lauber JK. Resource management on the flightdeck: proceedings of a NASA/industry workshop. NASA CP-2120, Moffett Field; 1980.
12. Edwards E. Man and machine: systems for safety. In: Proceedings of British airline pilots' association technical symposium. London: British Airline Pilots Associations; 1972. p. 21–36.
13. Edwards E. Stress and the airline pilot. British Airline Pilots Association medical symposium. London; 1975.
14. Blake RR, Mouton JS. The managerial grid. Houston: Gulf Press; 1964.
15. Gaba DM, Howard SK, Fish KJ, et al. Simulation-based training in anesthesia crisis resource management (ACRM) – a decade of experience. Simul Gaming. 2001;32(2):175–93.
16. Gaba DM, DeAnda A. A comprehensive anesthesia simulation environment: re-creating the operating room for research and training. Anesthesiology. 1988;69(3):387–94.
17. Gaba DM, DeAnda A. The response of anesthesia trainees to simulated critical incidents. Anesth Analg. 1989;68(4):444–51.
18. DeAnda A, Gaba DM. Unplanned incidents during comprehensive anesthesia simulation. Anesth Analg. 1990;71(1):77–82.
19. DeAnda A, Gaba DM. Role of experience in the response to simulated critical incidents. Anesth Analg. 1991;72(3):308–15.
20. Groen GJ, Patel VL. Medical problem-solving: some questionable assumptions. Med Educ. 1985;19(2):95–100.
21. Patel VL, Groen GJ, Arocha JF. Medical expertise as a function of task difficulty. Mem Cognit. 1990;18(4):394–406.
22. Orasanu J, Connolly T, Klein G, et al. The reinvention of decision making. Norwood: Ablex; 1993.
23. Fanning RM, Gaba DM. The role of debriefing in simulation-based learning. Simul Heathc. 2007;2(2):115–25.
24. Knowles M. The modern practice of adult education: from pedagogy to andragogy. San Francisco: Jossey-Bass; 1980. p. 44–5.
25. Seaman DF, Fellenz RA. Effective strategies for teaching adults. Columbus: Merrill; 1989.
26. Howard S, Gaba D, Fish K, et al. Anesthesia crisis resource management training: teaching anesthesiologists to handle critical incidents. Aviat Space Environ Med. 1992;63(9):763–70.
27. Morgan BB, Glickman AS, Woodward EA et al. Measurement of team behaviors in a Navy training environment. Report No TR-86-0140. Norfolk: Old Dominion University, Center for Applied Psychological Studies; 1986.
28. Glickman AS, Zimmer S, Montero RC et al. The evolution of teamwork skills: an empirical assessment with implications for training. Report No TR87-016. Orlando: Naval Training Systems Center; 1987.
29. McIntyre RM, Salas E. Measuring and managing for team performance: emerging principles from complex environments. In: Guzzo R, Salas E, editors. Team effectiveness and decision making in organizations. San Francisco: Jossey-Bass; 1995. p. 149–203.
30. Carne B, Kennedy M, Gray T. Crisis resource management in emergency medicine. Emerg Med Australas. 2012;24(1):7–13.
31. Reznek M, Smith-Coggins R, Howard S, et al. Emergency medicine crisis resource management (EMCRM): pilot study of a simulation- based crisis management course for emergency medicine. Acad Emerg Med. 2003;10(4):386–9.
32. Volk MS, Ward J, Irias N, et al. Using medical simulation to teach crisis resource management and decision-making skills to otolaryngology house staff. Otolaryngol Head Neck Surg. 2011;145(1):35–42.
33. Cheng A, Donoghue A, Gilfoyle E, et al. Simulation-based crisis resource management training for pediatric critical care medicine: a review for instructors. Pediatr Crit Care Med. 2012;13(2):197–203.
34. Kim J, Neilipovitz D, Cardinal P, et al. A pilot study using high-fidelity simulation to formally evaluate performance in the resuscitation of critically ill patients: The University of Ottawa critical care medicine high-fidelity simulation and crisis resource management I study. Crit Care Med. 2006;34(8):2167–74.
35. Sica GT, Barron DM, Blum R, et al. Computerized realistic simulation: a teaching module for crisis management in radiology. Am J Roentgenol. 1999;172(2):301–4.
36. Schaefer HG, Helmreich RL, Scheidegger D. TOMS-Team Oriented Medical Simulation (safety in the operating theatre-part 1: interpersonal relationships and team performance). Curr Anaesth Crit Care. 1995;6:48–53.
37. Schaefer HG, Helmreich RL, Scheidegger D. Human factors and safety in emergency medicine. Resuscitation. 1994;28(3):221–5.
38. Schaefer HG, Helmreich RL. The importance of human factors in the operating room. Anesthesiology. 1994;80(2):479.
39. Medical Team Training: Medical Teamwork and Patient Safety: The Evidence-based Relation. July 2005. Agency for Healthcare Research and Quality, Rockville, MD. http://www.ahrq.gov/research/findings/final-reports/medteam/chapter4.html.
40. Risser DT, Rice MM, Salisbury ML, et al. The potential for improved teamwork to reduce medical errors in the emergency department. The MedTeams Research Consortium. Ann Emerg Med. 1999;34:373–83.
41. Morey JC, Simon R, Jay GD, et al. A transition from aviation crew resource management to hospital emergency departments: the MedTeams story. In: Jensen RS, editor. Proceedings of the 12th international symposium on aviation psychology. Columbus: Ohio State University; 2003. p. 826–32.
42. Helmreich RL, Merritt AC, Wilhelm JA. The evolution of crew resource management training in commercial aviation. Int J Aviat Psychol. 1999;9(1):19–32.
43. http://teams.drc.com/Medteams/Home/Program. Accessed May 2011.
44. Kohsin BY, Landrum-Tsu C, Merchant PG. Medical team management: patient safety overview. Unpublished training materials. Washington, DC: Bolling Air Force Base; 2002.
45. Kohsin BY, Landrum-Tsu C, Merchant PG. Implementation guidance for Medical Team Management in the MTF (Medical

Treatment Facility). Unpublished manuscript. U.S. Air Force Medical Operations Agency. Washington, DC: Bolling Air Force Base; 2002.

46. Kohsin BY, Landrum-Tsu C, Merchant PG. Medical Team Management agenda, homework, observation/debriefing tool, and lesson plan. Unpublished training materials. U.S. Air Force Medical Operations Agency. Washington, DC: Bolling Air Force Base; 2002.
47. http://www.saferpatients.com/. Accessed Apr 2011.
48. Dunn EJ, Mills PD, Neily J, et al. Medical team-training: applying crew resource management in the Veterans Health Administration. Jt Comm J Qual Patient Saf. 2007;33:317–25.
49. http://teamstepps.ahrq.gov/. Accessed May 2011.
50. Crisis Resource Management Diagram. ©2008 Diagram: S. Goldhaber-Fiebert, K. McCowan, K. Harrison, R. Fanning, S. Howard, D. Gaba
51. Helmreich RL, Merritt AD. Culture at work in aviation and medicine: national, organizational, and professional influences. Aldershot: Ashgate; 1998.
52. Weick KE, Sutcliffe KM. Managing the unexpected: assuring high performance in an age of complexity. San Francisco: Jossey-Bass; 2001.
53. Sutcliffe KM, Lewton E, Rosenthal M. Communication failures: an insidious contributor to medical mishaps. Acad Med. 2004;79(2):186–94.
54. http://www.jointcommission.org/facts_about_the_universal_protocol/. Accessed Sept 2011.
55. Lewis FL. Applied optimal control and estimation. New Jersey: Prentice-Hall; 1992.
56. Endsley MR. Measurement of situation awareness in dynamic systems. Hum Factors. 1995;37:65–84.
57. Beringer DB, Hancock PA. Exploring situational awareness: a review and the effects of stress on rectilinear normalization. In: Proceedings of the fifth international symposium on aviation psychology, vol. 2. Columbus: Ohio State University; 1989. pp. 646–51.
58. Sarter NB, Woods DD. Situation awareness: a critical but ill-defined phenomenon. Int J Aviat Psychol. 1991;1:45–57.
59. Smith K, Hancock PA. The risk space representation of commercial airspace. In: Proceedings of the 8th international symposium on aviation psychology. Columbus; 1995.
60. Gaba DM, Howard SK, Small SD. Situation awareness in anesthesiology. Hum Factors. 1995;37(1):20–31.
61. Klein G. Recognition-primed decisions. In: Rouse WB, editor. Advances in man–machine systems research, vol. 5. Greenwich: JAI Press; 1989. p. 47–92.
62. Rall M, Gaba DM, Howard SK, Dieckmann P. Human performance and patient safety. In: Miller RD, Eriksson LI, Fleisher LA, Wiener-Kronish JP, Young WL, editors. Miller's anesthesia. 7th ed. Philadelphia: Churchill Livingstone, Elsevier; 2009. p. 93–149.
63. Stone M, Dismukes K, Remington R. Prospective memory in dynamic environments: effects of load, delay, and phonological rehearsal. Memory. 2001;9:165.
64. McDaniel MA, Einstein GO. Prospective memory: an overview and synthesis of an emerging field. Thousand Oaks: Sage Publications; 2007.
65. DeKeyser V, Woods DD, Masson M, et al. Fixation errors in dynamic and complex systems: descriptive forms, psychological mechanisms, potential countermeasures. Technical report for NATO Division of Scientific Affairs; 1988.
66. DeKeyser V, Woods DD, Colombo AG, et al. Fixation errors: failures to revise situation assessment in dynamic and risky systems. In: Systems reliability assessment. Dordrecht: Kluwer Academic; 1990. p. 231.
67. Norman DA. The psychology of everyday things. New York: Basic Books; 1988.
68. http://www.ntsb.gov/doclib/reports/2010/AAR1003.pdf. Accessed Sept 2011.
69. Harrison TK, Manser T, Howard SK, et al. Use of cognitive aids in a simulated anesthetic crisis. Anesth Analg. 2006;103(3):551–6.
70. Ziewacz JE, Arriaga AF, Bader AM, et al. Crisis checklists for the operating room: development and pilot testing. J Am Coll Surg. 2011;213(2):212–7.
71. Mills PD, DeRosier JM, Neily J, et al. A cognitive aid for cardiac arrest: you can't use it if you don't know about it. Jt Comm J Qual Saf. 2004;30:488–96.
72. Neily J, DeRosier JM, Mills PD. Awareness and use of a cognitive aid for anesthesiology. Jt Comm J Qual Patient Saf. 2007;33(8):502–11.
73. Gaba DM, Fish KJ, Howard SK. Crisis management in anesthesiology. Philadelphia: Churchill Livingstone; 1993.
74. Chu L, Fuller A, Goldhaber-Fiebert S, Harrison TK. A visual guide to crisis management in anesthesia (point of care essentials). Philadelphia: Lippincott Williams & Wilkins; 2011.
75. Nanji KC, Cooper JB. Is it time to use checklists for anesthesia emergencies: simulation is the vehicle for testing and learning. Reg Anesth Pain Med. 2012;37:1–2.
76. Burden AR, Carr ZJ, Staman GW, et al. Does every code need a "reader?" improvement of rare event management with a cognitive aid "reader" during a simulated emergency. Simul Healthc. 2012;7(1):1–9.
77. http://education.asahq.org/sites/education.asahq.org/files/a360.pdf. Accessed Apr 2011.
78. Haynes AB, Weiser TG, Berry WR, et al. Changes in safety attitude and relationship to decreased postoperative morbidity and mortality following implementation of a checklist-based surgical safety intervention. BMJ Qual Saf. 2011;20(1):102–7.
79. Kolb DA. Experiential learning: experience as the source of learning and development. Englewood Cliffs: Prentice Hall; 1984.
80. Kolb's model of experiential learning adapted for simulation (adapted from Kolb DA. Experiential learning: experience as the source of learning and development. Englewood Cliffs: Prentice Hall; 1984. Figure 8.2–5. Figures used with permission. (c) 2010 David M. Gaba, MD).
81. Fletcher G, Flin R, McGeorge P, et al. Anaesthetists' non-technical skills (ANTS): evaluation of a behavioural marker system. Br J Anaesth. 2003;90:580–8.
82. Flin R, Martin L, Goeters K, et al. Development of the NOTECHS (Non-Technical Skills) system for assessing pilots' CRM skills. Hum Factors Aerosp Saf. 2003;3:95–117.
83. Yule S, Flin R, Paterson-Brown S, et al. Development of a rating system for surgeons' non-technical skills. Med Educ. 2006;40:1098–104.
84. Reader T, Flin R, Lauche K, et al. Non-technical skills in the intensive care unit. Br J Anaesth. 2006;96:551–9.
85. Undre AN, Healey A, Darzi CA, et al. Observational assessment of surgical teamwork: a feasibility study. World J Surg. 2006;30:1774–83.
86. Dickinson TL, McIntyre RM. A conceptual framework for teamwork measurement. In: Brannick MT, Salas E, Prince C, editors. Team performance assessment and measurement theory, methods, and applications. New Jersey: Laurence Erlbaum Associates; 1997.
87. Hull L, Arora S, Kassab E, et al. Observational teamwork assessment for surgery: content validation and tool refinement. J Am Coll Surg. 2011;212(2):234–43.
88. Thomas E, Sexton J, Helmreich R. Translating teamwork behaviours from aviation to healthcare: development of behavioural markers for neonatal resuscitation. Qual Saf Health Care. 2004;13 Suppl 1:i57–64.
89. Salas E, Wilson KA, Burke SC, et al. Does crew resource management training work? An update, an extension and some critical needs. Hum Factors. 2006;48:392.

90. Young-Xu Y, Neily J, Mills PD, et al. Association between implementation of a medical team training program and surgical morbidity. Arch Surg. 2011;146(12):1368–73.
91. Neily J, Mills PD, Young-Xu Y. Association between implementation of a medical team training program and surgical mortality. JAMA. 2010;304(15):1693–700.
92. Amour Forse R, Bramble JD, McQuillan R. Team training can improve operating room performance. Surgery. 2011;150(4):771–8.
93. Morey JC, Simon R, Jay GD. Error reduction and performance improvement in the emergency department through formal teamwork training: evaluation results of the MedTeams project. Health Serv Res. 2002;37(6):1553–81.
94. Zeltser MV, Nash DB. Approaching the evidence basis for aviation-derived teamwork training in medicine. Am J Med Qual. 2010;25:12–23.
95. Gaba DM. The pharmaceutical analogy for simulation: a policy prospective. Simul Healthc. 2010;5(1):5–7.
96. Weinger MB. The pharmacology of simulation: a conceptual framework to inform progress in simulation research. Simul Healthc. 2010;5(1):8–15.
97. Gaba DM. Structural and organizational issues in patient safety: a comparison of health care to other high-hazard industries. Calif Manage Rev. 2001;43:83–102.
98. Gaba DM. Out of this nettle, danger, we pluck this flower, safety: healthcare vs. aviation and other high-hazard industries. Simul Healthc. 2007;2:213–7.
99. Gaba DM. Have we gone too far in translating ideas from aviation to patient safety?—No. BMJ. 2011:342, c7309.

Patient Safety

9

Pramudith V. Sirimanna and Rajesh Aggarwal

Introduction

The issue of patient safety is the most paramount topic in healthcare training. The striking statistic that approximately 10% of all patients admitted to hospital encounter some form of harm has been reproduced by many reports throughout the world [1–5]. In 2006, the Institute of Medicine report, *To Err Is Human: Building a Safer Health System*, reported that medical errors are responsible for up to 98,000 hospital deaths each year in USA [6]. Furthermore, each year at least 1.5 million preventable medication errors occur in the USA, and on average, more than one medication error occurs in a hospitalized patient each day [7]. These facts are only compounded by reports that half of all surgical adverse events are preventable [3].

The current paradigm used in healthcare training is based on a loosely structured mentor-student relationship. Traditionally, this Halstedian apprenticeship model relies on the principle of "see one, do one, teach one" where learning occurs within the clinical environment [8]. The unfortunate consequence of such practice results in care of patients being conducted by inexperienced healthcare professionals, thus exposing patients to the potential harm from medical errors. The path towards expertise in any profession is steep and accompanied by a significant learning curve. While surmounting this learning curve, errors are most likely to occur and, in healthcare, have been associated with higher complication and mortality rates [9]. This, of course, is an unacceptable drawback of training the next generation of healthcare professionals. As such, these facts, along with an increase in public and political expectations, have led to the development of strategies outside of the clinical domain to improve competence, reduce time on the learning curve, and thereby reduce patients' exposure to preventable errors.

One such approach is simulation-based training as it allows trainees to develop, refine, and apply knowledge and skills in a risk-free, but immersive and realistic environment. Any errors made are within a safe setting where, through repetitive practice and objective immediate assessment and feedback, the attainment of proficiency can be achieved [10]. Healthcare professionals have developed a variety of methods to train using simulation. For example, simulated and virtual patients through standardized role-plays of history taking, examination, and communication skills can teach fundamentals of patient interaction and clinical skills [11]. Furthermore, bench models using static or interactive mannequin simulators and computer-based virtual reality (VR) simulator can be used for training and assessment of technical and nontechnical skills [12]. The paradigm shift from the traditional temporal experience-based design of training to one that requires certification of competence and proficiency resulted in the development of proficiency-based simulation training curricula [10]. These curricula account for varying rates of learning and allow trainees to practice until a predefined "expert" benchmarked level of technical proficiency is attained [10]. This competency-based method of training results in a standardized model where confirmation of appropriate skill level is confirmed and has further applications into revalidation of ongoing competence [10].

P.V. Sirimanna, MBBS, BSc (Hons)
Division of Surgery, Department of Surgery and Cancer, Imperial College London, Praed Street, London W2 1NY, UK

St. Mary's Hospital, Imperial College NHS Trust, Praed Street, London, UK
e-mail: pramsirimanna@gmail.com

R. Aggarwal, MD, PhD, MA, FRCS (✉)
Division of Surgery, Department of Surgery and Cancer, Imperial College London, Praed Street, 19104 PA, Philadelphia

Department of Surgery, Perelman School of Medicine, University of Pennsylvania, 3400 Spruce Street, 19104 PA, USA

St. Mary's Hospital, Imperial College NHS Trust, Praed Street, London, UK
e-mail: rajesh.aggarwal@imperial.ac.uk; rajesh.aggarwal@uphs.upenn.edu

A.I. Levine et al. (eds.), *The Comprehensive Textbook of Healthcare Simulation*,
DOI 10.1007/978-1-4614-5993-4_9, © Springer Science+Business Media New York 2013

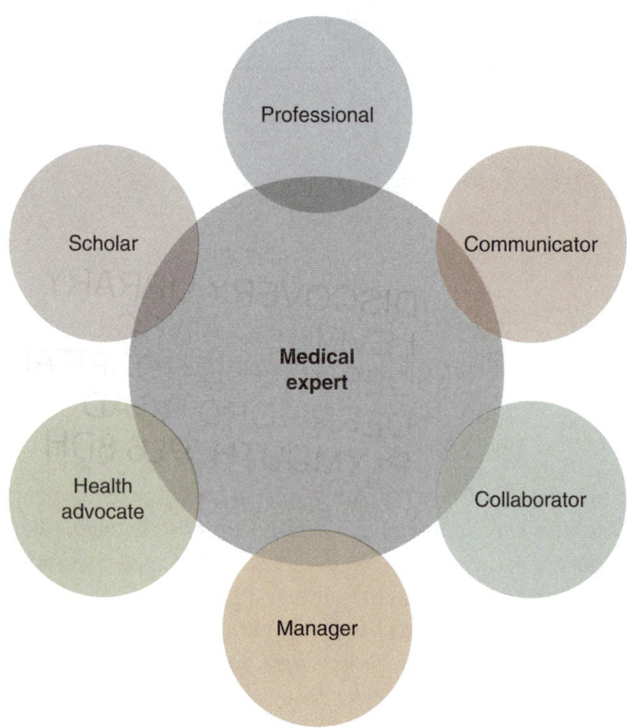

Fig. 9.1 CanMEDs Framework of medical competence from the Royal College of Physicians and Surgeons of Canada highlighting seven key competencies for physicians—medical expert, communicator, collaborator, manager, health advocate, scholar, and professional (Adapted from Ref. [16])

Simulation is also a potent method to allow healthcare professionals to repeatedly practice and safely manage recreated challenging and complex scenarios that are infrequently encountered in clinical practice [13]. Although inexperience is an important factor in medical errors, the majority are systems related [6]. Thus, a further extension of the use of simulation-based training to enhance patient safety is its application in systems and team training [14, 15] (Chaps. 8 and 10).

Healthcare simulation can be used to enhance the broad range of skills that encompass medical competence, which in turn can have an impact on patient safety. Aggarwal et al. suggested the CanMEDs Framework of medical competence from the Royal College of Physicians and Surgeons of Canada [16] as a "viable and tested classification of competency that traverses medical specialties, because it is comprehensive and has been the forerunner of later frameworks" [17]. The CanMED Framework highlights seven key competencies physicians required to provide high-quality care: medical expert, communicator, collaborator, manager, health advocate, scholar, and professional (Fig. 9.1) [16].

Through this chapter we will discuss, in turn, the use of healthcare simulation to improve patient safety through each of the above key competencies that are paramount in developing a healthcare professional capable of providing quality patient care.

The Medical Expert

The idea of the *medical expert* is an umbrella term that can be used to describe a competency that incorporates all aspects of the CanMEDS roles by applying medical knowledge, clinical skills, and professional attitudes to provide patient-centered care [16]. In addition, healthcare practitioners, as *medical experts*, must establish and maintain core clinical knowledge, possess sound diagnostic reasoning and clinical judgment, and acquire procedural skill proficiency [16].

As mentioned previously, a variety of simulation-based training techniques have been used in healthcare education. These techniques provide learners with a risk-free environment to allow deliberate practice, where mistakes can be made and learned from without compromising patient safety. The use of surgical simulators by trainees has been shown to allow surgeons to improve psychomotor skills such as speed, error, and economy of movement as well as procedural knowledge, which contribute to improved performance and confidence in the operating theater [12]. However, simulation-based training comes in a range of varieties.

Box Trainers and Simple Mannequin Simulators

Low-fidelity, inexpensive simulators of procedural skills exist, such as laparoscopic surgery box trainers and mannequins to simulate venipuncture, intravenous cannulation, central venous catheterization, and airway intubation, where learners can develop, practice, and refine skills using real instruments on simulated models. Barsuk et al. reported that residents who underwent training using the Simulan's CentralLineMan central venous catheter (CVC) insertion simulation model displayed decreased complications in the form of fewer needle passes, arterial punctures, and catheter adjustments and had higher success rates during CVC insertion in actual patients compared to residents who trained using traditional methods [18]. In addition, Draycott et al. retrospectively compared the management of shoulder dystocia and the associated neonatal injury before and after introduction of a simulation-based training course using the prototype shoulder dystocia training mannequin (PROMPT Birthing Trainer, Limbs and Things Ltd, Bristol, United Kingdom) [19]. The results of the study concluded that, after training, there was improvement in management of shoulder dystocia and a reduction in neonatal injury [19]. In 2004, the Society of American Gastrointestinal and Endoscopic Surgeons (SAGES) developed the Fundamentals of Laparoscopic Surgery (FLS) program [20]. FLS comprised of a box trainer in which laparoscopic skills can be practiced by performing various abstract tasks and has been previously validated numerously in literature [21, 22]. Subsequently, following endorsement by the American College of Surgeons, the FLS simulator training program has been adopted by the American Board of

Surgery as a requirement for completion of general surgical training [22]. Sroka and colleagues conducted a randomized controlled trial to assess if training to proficiency with the FLS simulator would result in improved operating room performance [23]. It was reported that, after proficiency training on the FLS simulator, surgical residents' performance scores during laparoscopic cholecystectomy were higher than the control group [23]. Furthermore, completion of a proficiency-based FLS simulator training curriculum and subsequent interval training on the FLS simulator was found to be associated with a very high level of skill retention after 2 years [24].

Cadaveric and Animal Tissue Simulators

Human cadaveric and animal tissue has also been used in healthcare simulation training of procedural tasks. In addition to anatomical dissection of human cadavers for medical students and surgical trainees, human cadavers have been used to practice many procedures including laparoscopy and saphenous vein cutdown [25, 26]. Animal models involve the use of either live anesthetized animals or *ex vivo* animal tissues. Such models have been incorporated in many surgical skills courses, for example, the Intercollegiate Basic Surgical Skills course by the Royal College of Surgeons England. Despite a lack of incorporation into discrete proficiency-based training curricula, various studies have used animal models for medical training and assessment of transferability of skills developed from simulation-based training [27–29].

Virtual Reality and Computer-Based Simulation

Virtual reality (VR) simulation has been extensively studied for its ability to provide a safe, high-fidelity, and risk-free environment for healthcare training and assessment [12]. The validity of VR simulation in surgery has been, hitherto, widely demonstrated [12]. Unlike the subjective traditional methods of technical skill assessment, VR simulators provide a valid, objective, and unbiased assessment of trainees, using parameters that cannot easily be measured within the operating theater [30, 31]. Much research has focused upon optimizing the delivery of these benefits with development of repetition and time-based curricula [32, 33]. However, the rate at which a trainee learns may vary, and, as such, these models result in surgeons with varying levels of skill at the end of training period. Thus, proficiency-based training, in which expert benchmark levels are used as performance targets, has been suggested as best able to increase surgical performance to a standardized level of competency [12]. Such training curricula have been developed that allow a strategic methodology for training inexperienced surgeons resulting in a shortened learning curve and attainment of benchmarked expert levels of dexterity [34–36].

Over the past decade, numerous studies have illustrated the benefits of VR simulation on patient safety. Seymour et al. conducted one of the principal studies to show that VR training improves operating performance [37]. In this randomized controlled trial, 16 surgical residents were randomized to either VR training or no VR training [37]. The VR-trained group completed training on the MIST-VR laparoscopic surgical simulator until expert criterion levels were attained. Following this, both groups performed a laparoscopic cholecystectomy, which was reviewed and rated by two independent blinded raters [37]. It was reported that the VR-trained group was faster at gallbladder dissection and six times less likely to make errors, and the non-VR-trained group were five times more likely to injure the gallbladder or burn non-target tissues during their first laparoscopic cholecystectomy [37]. Moreover, two studies reported that VR laparoscopic surgical training to proficiency resulted in significantly better performance when performing basic laparoscopic skills and laparoscopic cholecystectomies in the animate operating environment [29–38]. A recent study by Ahlberg et al. investigated the effect of proficiency-based VR laparoscopic training on outcomes during the early part of the learning curve in the clinical environment [39]. The study showed that VR training to proficiency resulted in significantly fewer errors and a reduction in surgical time in comparison to the control group during the residents' first ten laparoscopic cholecystectomies on actual patients [39]. This notable finding illustrated that the hazardous early part of the learning curve can be shortened and flatter after VR training, thus substantiating the role VR simulation in enhancing patient safety [39]. Most notably, a Cochrane review of the effectiveness of VR training in laparoscopic surgery, based on 23 trials involving 622 participants, confirmed that VR training decreased time taken, increased accuracy, and decreased errors in laparoscopic surgery [40].

The benefits of VR simulation training extend beyond the laparoscopic surgical domain. A pilot study by Sedlack and collaborators showed that computer-based colonoscopy simulation training resulted in a shortened learning curve during the initial 30 patient-based colonoscopies conducted by gastroenterology fellows [41]. Simulator-trained fellows were found to be safer, require less senior assistance, able to define endoscopic landmarks better, and reach the cecum independently on more instances than traditionally trained fellows during the initial part of the learning curve [41]. A further study by Sedlack et al. illustrated that computer-based endoscopy simulator training had a direct benefit to patients by improving patient comfort [42]. Additionally, a recent multicenter, blinded randomized controlled trial provided further evidence for the use of VR endoscopy simulation in reducing the learning curve and improving patient safety [43]. In this study, additional VR colonoscopy simulation-based training resulted in significantly higher objective competency rates during first year gastroenterology fellows' first 100 real colonoscopies [43]. Moreover, as little as 1 h of prior training with a VR bronchoscopy simulator was found to improve the performance of inexperienced residents during basic bronchoscopy on patients compared to peers without similar training and produce a skill level similar to that of more experienced residents [44].

Patient Scenario Simulation

The advent of patient scenario simulation initially utilized a programmed patient paradigm, in which, most commonly, a lay individual would be taught to simulate a medical condition [11]. Harden and Gleeson, in developing the Objective Structured Clinical Examination (OSCE), incorporated this structure into a series of clinical stations comprised of actors performing as simulated patients [11]. Students would rotate through these stations in which aptitude in clinical skills such as history taking, clinical examination, procedural skills, and management plans were tested using a standardized objective scoring system [11]. Since its conception, the OSCE has been used by educational institutions as a valid and reliable method of assessment [17].

A further application of patient scenario simulation that has been investigated is within critical care and, particularly, within training responses to emergency scenarios. Needless to say, it is imperative that healthcare professionals are highly skilled and experienced to deal with these high-risk clinical situations that carry great morbidity and mortality. However, such situations occur with relatively low frequency to gain sufficient experience, and, often, junior members of the medical team, who lack such experience, are the first responders [45]. Therefore, simulation-based training is an attractive technique for medical professionals to practice management of these scenarios outside of the clinical environment. One such technique used in emergency situation training is the computer-controlled patient simulator, SimMan (Laerdal Medical Corporation, Wappingers Falls, NY). Mayo et al. utilized patient-based simulation training to investigate interns' competence in emergency airway management. In this randomized controlled trial, participants were given training on the management of respiratory arrest using the SimMan computer-controlled patient simulator. Such training resulted in significant improvement in airway management skills in actual patient airway events [45]. Furthermore, simulation training using a human patient simulator resulted in improved quality of care provided by residents during actual cardiac arrest team responses [46]. This study illustrated that simulator-trained residents responded to actual cardiac arrest events with great adherence to treatment protocols than non-simulator-trained more experienced residents [46]. Importantly, the durability of the Advanced Cardiac Life Support skills acquired through simulation training was demonstrated by Wayne et al., which reported retention of skills at 6 and 14 months post-training [47].

The recognition of the ability of simulation to be used as a potent tool in healthcare education has resulted in its incorporation into various healthcare educational courses. For example, patient simulation has been integrated in many official acute medical event management courses, such as the worldwide Advanced Trauma Life Support (ATLS) course and the Detecting Deterioration, Evaluation, Treatment, Escalation and Communicating in Teams (DETECT) course in Australia [48].

The Communicator

Communication, written or verbal, is a key attribute that all healthcare professionals must excel at in order to optimize safe, holistic patient care. Not only must communication be effective between healthcare professionals and patients, but also to other healthcare professionals as well as the public as a whole. It is a vital skill that is imperative in every element of clinical practice, especially challenging scenarios such as breaking bad news. The CanMEDs 2005 Framework suggested that, as *communicators*, physicians must effectively facilitate the doctor-patient relationships enabling "patient-centered therapeutic communication through shared decision-making and effective dynamic interactions with patients, families, caregivers, other professionals, and other important individuals" [16]. A competent *communicator* must establish rapport and trust as well as elicit and convey relevant and accurate information from patients, families, and other healthcare professionals in order to develop a common understanding with a shared plan of care [16].

An astonishing statistic provided by the Joint Commission on Accreditation of Health Care Organizations demonstrated that poor communication was causative in two-thirds of almost 3,000 serious medical errors [49]. Compounding this, during a review of 444 surgical malpractice claims, 60 cases were identified as involving communication breakdowns directly resulting in harm to patients [50]. Of these cases of communicative errors, the majority involved verbal communications between one transmitter and one receiver, and the most common communication breakdown involved residents failing to notify attending surgeons of critical events and failure of attending-to-attending handovers [50]. This of course is wholly unacceptable.

Several studies have attempted to investigate methods to improve communication within healthcare practice, including the use of simulation. Correct and thorough communication of patient information during staff shift handover is vital in providing high-quality continued care over the increasingly shift-work-based culture in healthcare. Berkenstadt et al. recognized a deficiency existed within this domain and illustrated that a simulation-based teamwork and communication workshop increased the incidence of nurses communicating crucial information during shift handovers [51].

Moreover, studies have investigated the incorporation of training and assessment of communication skills alongside technical skill acquisition. Kneebone and colleagues developed the Integrated Procedure Performance Instrument (IPPI), which combines technical skills training using inanimate models, with communication challenges in a variety of clinical contexts using standardized simulated patients [52]. Each clinical scenario consists of a bench-top model of a procedural skill, such as wound closure, urinary cauterization, endoscopy, or laparoscopic surgery, and a fully briefed standardized patient [52]. Through such practice, skills to deal with difficult situations such as an anxious, confused, or angry patient can be rehearsed and developed in a safe environment with immediate objective feedback [52]. An extension on this innovative research in 2009 demonstrated that the IPPI format resulted in significantly improved communication skills in residents and medical students [53].

The Collaborator

The CanMEDs 2005 Framework highlights that, in order to deliver optimal patient-centered care, physicians must work effectively within a healthcare team [16]. Such professionals should be competent in participating in an interprofessional healthcare team by recognizing roles and responsibilities of other professionals in relation to their own and demonstrate a respectful attitude towards others in order to ensure where appropriate, multi-professional assessment and management is achieved without conflict [16]. A recent review highlighted the close association between teamwork and patient outcomes in terms of satisfaction, risk-adjusted mortality, complications, and adverse events [54]. As such, techniques to develop and improve teamwork have been investigated.

Other high-risk organizations, such as the airline industry, have demonstrated the use of simulation to improve teamwork skills through Crisis Resource Management, and these techniques have been explored in enhancing patient safety (discussed in the previous chapter). Salas et al. conducted a quantitative and qualitative review of team training in healthcare [55]. They described the "power of simulation" as an effective training tool that creates an environment in which trainees can implement and practice the same mental processes and teamwork skills they would utilize in their actual clinical practice [55]. This review included simulation-based training as an integral aspect of their "eight evidence-based principles for effective planning, implementation and evaluation of team training programs specific to healthcare" (Fig. 9.2) [55]. In addition, simulation has been demonstrated as a key aspect of an education package within a framework for team training in medical education [56].

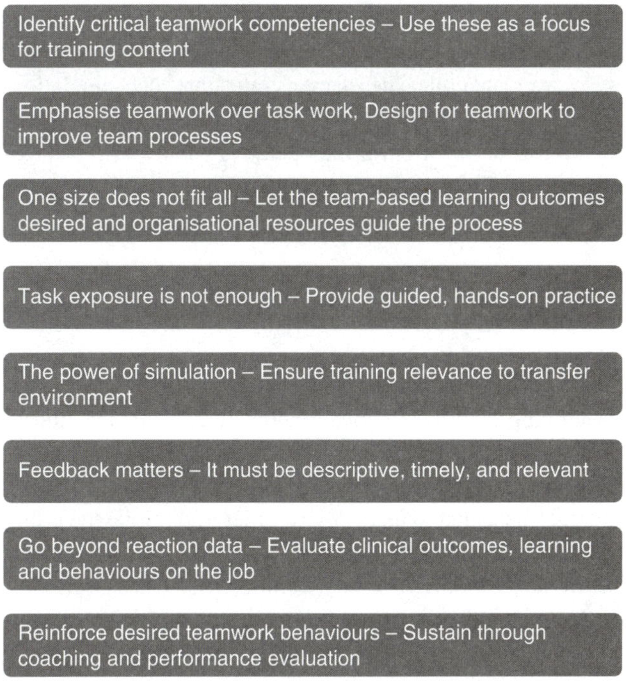

Identify critical teamwork competencies – Use these as a focus for training content

Emphasise teamwork over task work, Design for teamwork to improve team processes

One size does not fit all – Let the team-based learning outcomes desired and organisational resources guide the process

Task exposure is not enough – Provide guided, hands-on practice

The power of simulation – Ensure training relevance to transfer environment

Feedback matters – It must be descriptive, timely, and relevant

Go beyond reaction data – Evaluate clinical outcomes, learning and behaviours on the job

Reinforce desired teamwork behaviours – Sustain through coaching and performance evaluation

Fig. 9.2 Eight principles of team training required for production and implementation of an effective team training program as described by Salas et al. [55]

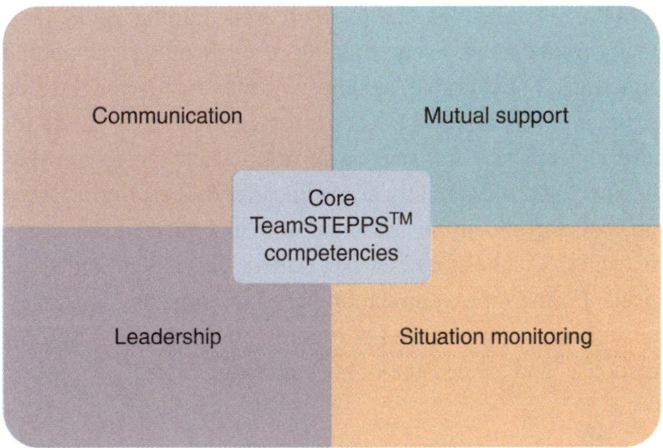

Fig. 9.3 Core TeamSTEPPS™ competencies

Through the collaboration between the Agency for Healthcare Research and Quality and the US Departments of Defense, the TeamSTEPPS™ curriculum was developed. The TeamSTEPPS™ initiative is an evidence-based simulation-based teamwork training system designed to improve patient safety by improving communication and other teamwork skills [57]. The underlying principles of TeamSTEPPS™ comprises of four core competencies that encompass teamwork: leadership, situation monitoring, mutual support, and communication (Fig. 9.3). Emphasis is placed on defining tools and strategies that can be used to gain and enhance proficiency in these competencies [58]. Incorporated within the core curriculum are sessions using patient scenarios, case studies, multimedia, and simulation [58]. Hitherto the TeamSTEPPS™ program has been implemented in multiple regional training centers around the USA as well as in Australia [59]. A recent multi-level evaluation of teamwork training using TeamSTEPPS™ by Weaver and colleagues demonstrated that such simulation-based training significantly increases the degree to which quality teamwork occurred in the operating room [60]. Trainees also reported increased perceptions of patient safety culture and teamwork attitudes [60].

The Manager

An important contributor to optimizing patient safety is by developing a safe, effective healthcare system. Healthcare professionals must play a central role in healthcare organizations and allocate scarce resources appropriately, as well as organize sustainable practices, in order to improve the effectiveness of healthcare [16]. This type of leadership is a key factor in promoting a safety culture, and it has been suggested that, unlike the nursing profession, physicians are yet to develop and utilize skills required for such leadership challenges [61].

As described above, there is evidence to show the positive results of simulation-based training on communication and teamwork of healthcare professionals. However, its use to train management skills has not been illustrated in literature thus far. Despite this, simulation-based training could have many implications in the training of challenging managerial situations. For example, healthcare professionals may be able to practice scenarios where one must apologize to a patient for a serious mistake or manage a situation where a colleague has behaved unprofessionally or unethically. By performing these difficult and uncommon situations in a simulated environment, managerial techniques can be learned, developed, and practiced. Furthermore, simulation-based training has been suggested as a viable method of training error reporting, disaster response, and assessment of hospital surge capacity [62].

The Health Advocate

As health advocates, clinical practitioners have a responsibility to use their expertise and influence to enhance the health of patients, communities, and the population as a whole [16]. Consequently, such advocates highlight inequities, potentially dangerous practices, and health conditions and have attempted to develop strategies to benefit the patient. Examples of the use of simulation in improving health advocacy are scarce. However, simulation-based training has been incorporated into an advocacy training program at Johns Hopkins' Bloomberg School of Public Health in the USA [63]. This program, aimed at graduate students, is designed to develop media advocacy and communication through a multitude of didactic lectures, expert presentations, and practical skills training using a 90-min simulation group exercise [63]. During this exercise, students are divided into groups representing different constituencies, ranging from government to nonprofit organizations, concerned with a local public health issue [62]. Each group is given time to develop a policy position regarding the issues and advocacy strategies to advance its proposed policy improvement [63]. Following this, each participant is placed in a simulated television interview, where challenging questions are asked to help students learn to effectively communicate with advancing a health-policy position [63].

The Scholar

Continual lifelong learning is vital to optimize performance of all healthcare professionals. One must be able to use ongoing learning to maintain and enhance professional activities by reflecting on current practice and critically evaluating literature, in order to make up-to-date evidence-based decisions and make their practice safer [16]. Furthermore, healthcare professionals must facilitate the learning of students, patients, and the wider public as well as be able to contribute to the creation, dissemination, application, and translation of new medical knowledge and practices [16].

Many simulation techniques allow healthcare individuals the opportunity to effectively train delivery of existing knowledge as well as practice the application of new knowledge until proficiency is attained. As an example, during the 1990s, the rapid uptake of laparoscopic surgery was retrospectively described as the "biggest unaudited free for all in the history of surgery" as a result of the unnecessary morbidity and mortality that followed [64]. With the introduction of new technologies, such as robotics or endoluminal surgery, simulation has a unique potential to be used to ensure the learning curve of these techniques does not negatively impact patient safety.

Extending beyond this, an innate aspect of simulation training is reflective practice. Trainees are actively debriefed and given an opportunity to review and critically appraise performance [65]. Moreover, the inherent purpose of simulation is for edification and training and, as such, should be embraced by all healthcare professionals, as *scholars*.

The Professional

Despite the observation that teaching and assessing professionalism is a vital aspect of being a healthcare practitioner with regard to patient safety, unprofessional behaviors are continually reported. As a healthcare *professional*, one should demonstrate a commitment to the health of society and patient safety through ethical practice, integrity, compassion, profession-led regulation, and maintenance of competence [16].

Table 9.1 Seven interactive seminars used in the professionalism curriculum developed by Hochberg

Medical malpractice and the surgeon
Advanced communication skills for surgical practice
Admitting mistakes: ethical and communication issues
Delivering bad news—your chance to become a master surgeon
Interdisciplinary respect—working as a team
Working across language and cultures: the case for informed consent
Self-care and the stress of surgical practice

Adapted from Ref. [68]

Simulation-based training can have an important role in training professionalism. Ginsburg and colleagues conducted a qualitative study utilizing realistic and standardized professional dilemmas in order to aid students' professional development [66]. By using five videotaped reenacted actual scenarios, each depicting a professional dilemma requiring action in response, the reasoning processes of students in response to such circumstances were observed [66]. The simulated professional dilemmas exhibited a variety of typical professionalism issues such as role resistance, communicative violations, accountability, and objectification [66]. It was shown that the students' actions were often motivated by referring to principles, such as honesty, disclosure, and fairness to patient/patient care, as well as obedience or deference to senior figures or loyalty to their team [66]. The study inferred that by using these realistic simulated scenarios of real encounters, it was possible to observe more representative behavioral responses than what would be observed in an examination setting, where students know to "put the patient first" [66].

Hochberg and colleagues at the New York University Medical Center not only displayed that professionalism can be taught through simulation-incorporated methods, but its effects are sustainable in the long term [67, 68]. They tackled the obvious difficulties with teaching professionalism by developing a specially designed Surgical Professionalism in Clinical Education (SPICE) curriculum consisting of seven 1-h interactive sessions where issues of professionalism such as accountability, ethical issues, admitting medical errors, responding to emotion, and interdisciplinary respect were taught using a variety of pedagogic methods (e.g., lectures, video reenactments, role modeling) (Table 9.1) [67]. Surgical residents underwent a six-station OSCE before and after attending the curriculum. This OSCE utilized standardized patients recreating various professionalism scenarios, such as dealing with a colleague showing signs of substance abuse [67]. Surgical residents were scored according to a strict task checklist of criteria and showed a significant improvement in competency of professionalism after completion of the curriculum [67]. Subsequently, this professionalism curriculum was incorporated into surgical resident training at the New York University Medical Center (Fig. 9.4) [68]. Annual evaluation of professionalism skills was conducted subjectively via self-assessments of the residents' professionalism abilities as well as objectively using the same six-station OCSE as previously discussed [68]. In the 3 years post-implementation, aggregate perceived professionalism among surgical residents illustrated a significant positive trend over time with a year-on-year rise [68]. Improvements were observed in all six domains of professionalism: accountability, ethics, altruism, excellence, patient sensitivity, and respect [68]. Furthermore, surgical residents displayed a marked improvement in professionalism as rated by the standardized patients during the annual OSCE [68].

Another challenge in effectively teaching professionalism is the methodology of assessment. Variable rating in evaluation of professionalism by standardized patients, doctors, and lay people has led to the suggestion that multiple assessments by multiple raters at different time intervals are required [69].

Conclusion

Through this chapter we have investigated the effect of simulation on various aspects of healthcare practitioner competence (Fig. 9.4). Strong evidence exists for the use of simulation to teach clinical and procedural skills to develop the *medical expert* as well as teach and assess communication (*communicator*) and teamwork (*collaborator*) skills. Despite this, the routine use of simulation by healthcare professionals to teach these key competencies is few and far between. Simulation has the potential to be used to develop and enhance practitioners as *managers* through the training of management and leadership skills pertinent to patient safety, although further research is required to increase the evidence base. Similarly, the evidence base that simulation enhances healthcare practitioners as *health advocates* and *scholars* remains low, but its use to promote reflective practice provides an important aid to learning. Finally, there is definite evidence to support the application of simulation training practitioners as *professionals* with the advent of curricula incorporating simulated scenarios, ideal for training professionalism. However, further research is required on the best method of assessment of professionalism.

Patient safety is the paramount outcome of importance in the complex process of healthcare delivery. Not only must care be at all times safe, it also must be time efficient and effective in order to be optimal. Several organizations such as hospital departments, national bodies, and international peer-reviewed conferences and journals, in response to the growing awareness and pressures from the public regarding medical errors, have attempted to champion the drive for development and implementation of greater measures to reduce errors. Through identification, assessment, enhancement of practice, and prevention of medical errors, a safer healthcare system can be constructed.

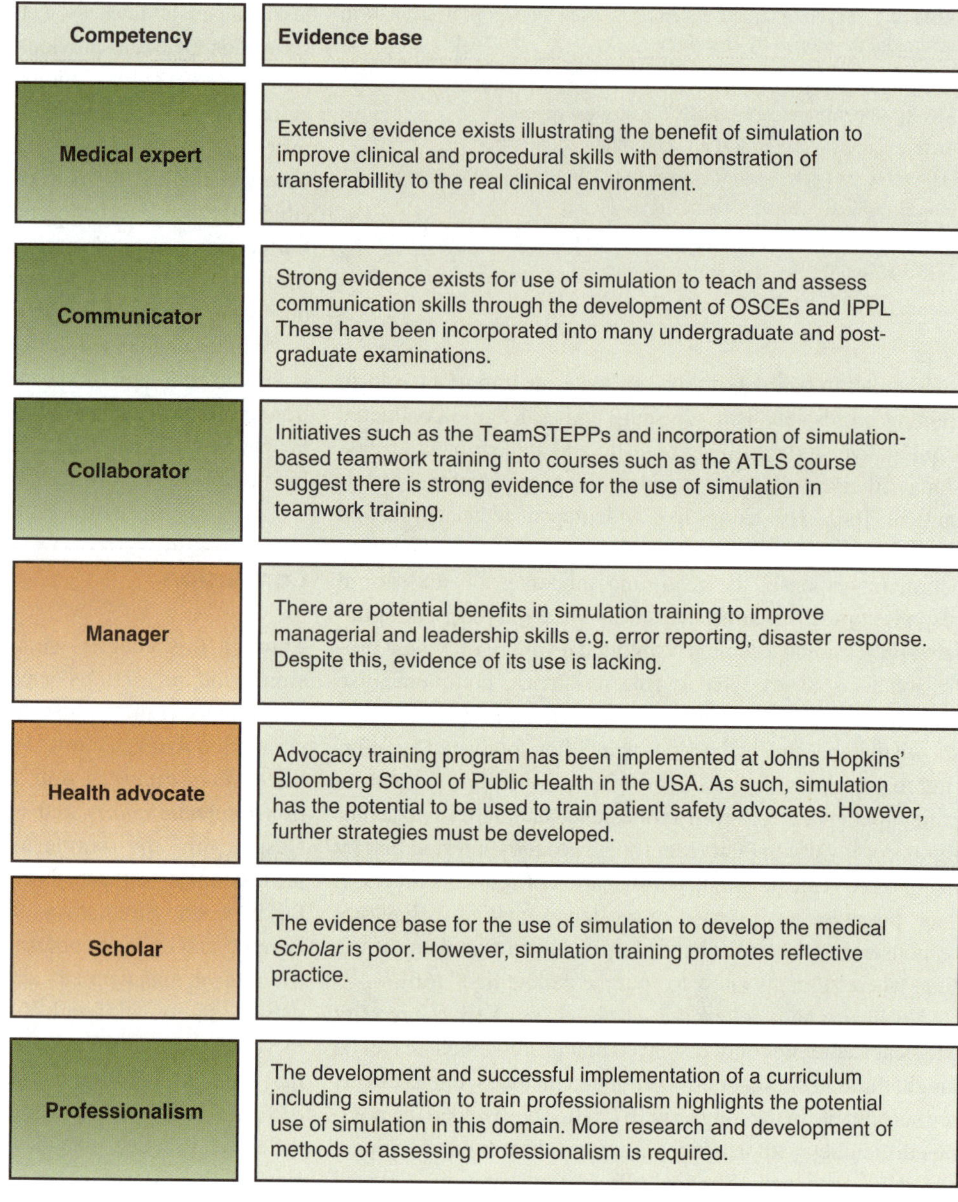

Fig. 9.4 Summary of evidence base for use of simulation in each CanMEDs-defined competency

Healthcare simulation has long been touted as a potential aid to improving patient safety and reducing errors. Since its introduction into healthcare four decades ago with the development of bench-top models and anesthetic scenarios, the advancements in simulation technology and research have been exponential, with its benefits repeatedly demonstrated. Despite this, the relative uptake of simulation-based training in healthcare has been disproportionately low. The mandatory FLS training curriculum has been implemented within the USA, where every surgery resident nationally must demonstrate proficiency in FLS [70]. A further example of an attempt to implement healthcare simulation can be demonstrated at the Israel Center for Medical Simulation [71]. Since its establishment in 2001, this national effort has endeavored to enhance patient safety and promote a culture change in healthcare education within the Israeli medical system. The center contains a vast array of simulation tools ranging from basic mannequin simulators to high-fidelity virtual reality laparoscopic simulators and full-body computerized anesthesia models. These can exist in a multitude of simulated clinical environments, such as virtual intensive care units, emergency rooms, wards, and operating theaters with integrated audiovisual capabilities and one-way mirror control booths for observation and assessment of simulated scenarios. The popularity of this impressive setup with healthcare professionals illustrates its positive impact of patient safety culture [71].

Notwithstanding these exceptions, the difficulties in adoption of simulation-based training stems from a lack of literature pertaining to the effect of simulation on real patient outcomes. Obtaining such data carries obvious difficulties; however, the benefit of simulation on some patient-based outcomes has been investigated, for example, central line infections and stillbirths [17]. Within the UK, the development and collection of patient-reported outcome measures (PROMs) of health-related quality of life after surgery provides a possible direction of future studies to infer the benefit of simulation on patient outcomes.

Unfortunately, despite the obvious benefits of simulation and the need to drive for its further adoption within healthcare, it cannot and should not be viewed upon as a silver bullet to answer all patient safety challenges in the current healthcare climate. It is true that simulation can reduce errors by stemming the early part of the learning curve and instilling a safety culture, but ultimately a system-based approach to promote safe practices and reduce patient harm must also be utilized. With all the benefits of simulation, it is more likely to augment rather than replace extensive real world clinical experience and deliberate practice in the quest to develop expertise, the next challenge to overcome within healthcare education.

In addition, not only should simulation training programs be optimized for learners, trainers must also be appropriately trained by developing dedicated expert clinical facilitators and support staff to ensure teaching is maximal. Similarly, simulation training must be developed to incorporate clinicians of all experience levels, and future research must investigate the use of simulation as tool for credentialing, revalidating, and identifying underperforming healthcare professionals.

There is no doubt that implementation of simulation-based training must gather momentum, where skills can be practiced repeatedly and deliberately in a safe, risk-free environment, and mistakes can be made and learned from. This, in addition to key measures such as guided instruction and judicious "expert" supervision in the real world and further development of a system-based safety culture, will ensure that the challenges of patient safety are overcome.

References

1. Brennan TA, Leape LL, Laird NM, et al. Incidence of adverse events and negligence in hospitalized patients. Results of the Harvard Medical Practice Study I. N Engl J Med. 1991;324:370–6.
2. Wilson RM, Runciman WB, Gibberd RW, et al. The quality in Australian health care study. Med J Aust. 1995;163:458–71.
3. Gawande AA, Thomas EJ, Zinner MJ, et al. The incidence and nature of surgical adverse events in Colorado and Utah in 1992. Surgery. 1999;126:66–75.
4. Vincent C, Neale G, Woloshynowych M. Adverse events in British hospitals: preliminary retrospective record review. BMJ. 2001; 322:517–9.
5. Baker GR, Norton PG, Flintoft V, et al. The Canadian adverse events study: the incidence of adverse events among hospital patients in Canada. Can Med Assoc J. 2004;170:1678–86.
6. Kohn LT, Corrigan JM, Donaldson MS. To err is human: building a safer health system. Washington: National Academy Press; 2000.
7. Bootman JL, Cronenwett LR, Bates DW, et al. Preventing medication errors. Washington: National Academies Press; 2006.
8. Halsted WS. The training of the surgeon. Bull Johns Hopkins Hosp. 1904;15:267–75.
9. A prospective analysis of 1518 laparoscopic cholecystectomies. The Southern Surgeons Club. N Engl J Med. 1991;324:1073–8.
10. Aggarwal R, Darzi A. Technical-skills training in the 21st century. N Engl J Med. 2006;355:2695–6.
11. Harden RM, Gleeson FA. Assessment of clinical competence using an objective structured clinical examination (OSCE). Med Educ. 1979;13:41–54.
12. Aggarwal R, Moorthy K, Darzi A. Laparoscopic skills training and assessment. Br J Surg. 2004;91:1549–58.
13. Agency for Healthcare Research and Quality. Medical errors: the scope of the problem. Rockville: Agency for Healthcare Research and Quality; 2009. Ref Type: Pamphlet.
14. Vincent C, Moorthy K, Sarker SK, et al. Systems approaches to surgical quality and safety: from concept to measurement. Ann Surg. 2004;239:475–82.
15. Salas E, DiazGranados D, Klein C, et al. Does team training improve team performance? A meta-analysis. Hum Factors. 2008; 50:903–33.
16. The CanMEDSs. Better standards. Better physicians. Better care. Ottawa: Royal College of Physicians and Surgeons of Canada; 2005. Ref Type: Report.
17. Aggarwal R, Mytton O, Derbrew M, et al. Training and simulation for patient safety. Qual Saf Health Care. 2010;19 Suppl 2:i34–43.
18. Barsuk JH, McGaghie WC, Cohen ER, et al. Simulation-based mastery learning reduces complications during central venous catheter insertion in a medical intensive care unit. Crit Care Med. 2009; 37:2697–701.
19. Draycott TJ, Crofts JF, Ash JP, et al. Improving neonatal outcome through practical shoulder dystocia training. Obstet Gynecol. 2008;112:14–20.
20. [FLS website] Fundamentals of laparoscopic surgery. Available at: www.flsprogram.org/. Accessed on 15 Mar 2010.
21. Peters JH, Fried GM, Swanstrom LL, Soper NJ, Sillin LF, Schirmer B, et al. Development and validation of a comprehensive program of education and assessment of the basic fundamentals of laparoscopic surgery. Surgery. 2004;135:21–7.
22. Okrainec A, Soper NJ. Trends and results of the first 5 years of Fundamentals of Laparoscopic Surgery (FLS) certification testing. Surg Endosc. 2011;25:1192–8.
23. Sroka G, Feldman LS, Vassiliou MC, Kaneva PA, Fayez R, Fried GM. Fundamentals of laparoscopic surgery simulator training to proficiency improves laparoscopic performance in the operating room-a randomized controlled trial. Am J Surg. 2010;199: 115–20.
24. Mashaud LB, Castellvi AO, Hollett LA, Hogg DC, Tesfay ST, Scott DJ. Two-year skill retention and certification exam performance after fundamentals of laparoscopic skills training and proficiency maintenance. Surgery. 2010;148:194–201.
25. Levine RL, Kives S, Cathey G, Blinchevsky A, Acland R, Thompson C, et al. The use of lightly embalmed (fresh tissue) cadavers for resident laparoscopic training. J Minim Invasive Gynecol. 2006; 13(5):451–6.
26. Wong K, Stewart F. Competency-based training of basic surgical trainees using human cadavers. ANZ J Surg. 2004;74:639–42.
27. Korndorffer Jr JR, Dunne JB, Sierra R, Stefanidis D, Touchard CL, Scott DJ. Simulator training for laparoscopic suturing using performance goals translates to the operating room. J Am Coll Surg. 2005;201(1):23–9.
28. Van Sickle KR, Ritter EM, Smith CD. The pretrained novice: using simulation-based training to improve learning in the operating room. Surg Innov. 2006;13(3):198–204.
29. Aggarwal R, Ward J, Balasundaram I, et al. Proving the effectiveness of virtual reality simulation for laparoscopic surgical training. Ann Surg. 2007;246:771–9.

30. Gallagher AG, Richie K, McClure N, McGuigan J. Objective psychomotor skills assessment of experienced, junior, and novice laparoscopists with virtual reality. World J Surg. 2001;25(11):1478–83.
31. Haque S, Srinivasan S. A meta-analysis of the training effectiveness of virtual reality surgical simulators. IEEE Trans Inf Technol Biomed. 2006;10(1):51–8.
32. Grantcharov TP, Kristiansen VB, Bendix J, Bardram L, Rosenberg J, Funch-Jensen P. Randomized clinical trial of virtual reality simulation for laparoscopic skills training. Br J Surg. 2004;91(2):146–50.
33. Ahlberg G. Does training in a virtual reality simulator improve surgical performance? Surg Endosc. 2002;16(1):126 [Online].
34. Aggarwal R, Grantcharov T, Moorthy K, Hance J, Darzi A. A competency-based virtual reality training curriculum for the acquisition of laparoscopic psychomotor skill. Am J Surg. 2006;191(1):128–33.
35. Aggarwal R, Grantcharov TP, Eriksen JR, Blirup D, Kristiansen VB, Funch-Jensen P, et al. An evidence-based virtual reality training program for novice laparoscopic surgeons. Ann Surg. 2006;244(2):310–4.
36. Aggarwal R, Crochet P, Dias A, Misra A, Ziprin P, Darzi A. Development of a virtual reality training curriculum for laparoscopic cholecystectomy. Br J Surg. 2009;96:1086–93.
37. Seymour NE, Gallagher AG, Roman SA, et al. Virtual reality training improves operating room performance: results of a randomized, double-blinded study. Ann Surg. 2002;236:458–63.
38. Andreatta PB, Woodrum DT, Birkmeyer JD, et al. Laparoscopic skills are improved with LapMentor training: results of a randomized, double-blinded study. Ann Surg. 2006;243:854–60.
39. Ahlberg G, Enochsson L, Gallagher AG, et al. Proficiency-based virtual reality training significantly reduces the error rate for residents during their first 10 laparoscopic cholecystectomies. Am J Surg. 2007;193:797–804.
40. Gurusamy K, Aggarwal R, Palanivelu L, Davidson BR. Systematic review of randomized controlled trials on the effectiveness of virtual reality training for laparoscopic surgery. Br J Surg. 2008;95(9):1088–97.
41. Sedlack RE, Kolars JC. Computer simulator training enhances the competency of gastroenterology fellows at colonoscopy: results of a pilot study. Am J Gastroenterol. 2004;99:33–7.
42. Sedlack RE, Kolars JC, Alexander JA. Computer simulation training enhances patient comfort during endoscopy. Clin Gastroenterol Hepatol. 2004;2:348–52.
43. Cohen J, Cohen SA, Vora KC, et al. Multicenter, randomized, controlled trial of virtual-reality simulator training in acquisition of competency in colonoscopy. Gastrointest Endosc. 2006;64:361–8.
44. Blum MG, Powers TW, Sundaresan S. Bronchoscopy simulator effectively prepares junior residents to competently perform basic clinical bronchoscopy. Ann Thorac Surg. 2004;78:287–91.
45. Mayo PH, Hackney JE, Mueck JT, et al. Achieving house staff competence in emergency airway management: Results of a teaching program using a computerized patient simulator. Crit Care Med. 2004;32:2422–7.
46. Wayne DB, Didwania A, Feinglass J, et al. Simulation-based education improves quality of care during cardiac arrest team responses at an academic teaching hospital: a case–control study. Chest. 2008;133:56–61.
47. Wayne DB, Siddall VJ, Butter J, et al. A longitudinal study of internal medicine residents' retention of advanced cardiac life support skills. Acad Med. 2006;81(10 Suppl):S9–12.
48. DETECT course. Australian Institute of Medical Simulation and Innovation. Available at: http://www.aimsi.org.au/site/detect+msc18_20.php. Accessibility verified 20 Apr 2012.
49. Joint Commission International Center for Patient Safety. Communication: a critical component in delivering quality care. Oakbrook Terrace: Joint Commission on Accreditation of Healthcare Organisations; 2009. Ref Type: Report.
50. Greenberg CC, Regenbogen SE, Studdert DM, et al. Patterns of communication breakdowns resulting in injury to surgical patients. J Am Coll Surg. 2007;204:533–40.
51. Berkenstadt H, Haviv Y, Tuval A, et al. Improving handoff communications in critical care: utilizing simulation-based training toward process improvement in managing patient risk. Chest. 2008;134:158–62.
52. Kneebone R, Nestel D, Yadollahi F, et al. Assessing procedural skills in context: exploring the feasibility of an Integrated Procedural Performance Instrument (IPPI). Med Educ. 2006;40:1105–14.
53. Moulton CA, Tabak D, Kneebone R, et al. Teaching communication skills using the integrated procedural performance instrument (IPPI): a randomized controlled trial. Am J Surg. 2009;197:113–8.
54. Sorbero ME, Farley DO, Mattke S, Lovejoy S. Out- come measures for effective teamwork in inpatient care. RAND technical report TR-462-AHRQ. Arlington: RAND Corporation; 2008.
55. Salas E, DiazGranados D, Weaver SJ, et al. Does team training work? Principles for health care. Acad Emerg Med. 2008;15:1002–9.
56. Ostergaard HT, Ostergaard D, Lippert A. Implementation of team training in medical education in Denmark. Postgrad Med J. 2008; 84:507–11.
57. Clancy CM, Tornberg DN. TeamSTEPPS: assuring optimal teamwork in clinical settings. Am J Med Qual. 2007;22:214–7.
58. King H, Battles J, Baker D, et al. Team strategies and tools to enhance performance and patient safety. Advances in patient safety: new directions and alternative approaches, Performance and tools, vol. 3. Rockville: Agency for Healthcare Research and Quality (US); 2008.
59. TeamSTEPPSTM. Agency for healthcare research and quality. Available at: http://teamstepps.ahrq.gov/. Accessibility verified 20 Apr 2012.
60. Weaver SJ, Rosen MA, DiazGranados D. Does teamwork improve performance in the operating room? A multilevel evaluation. Jt Comm J Qual Patient Saf. 2010;36(3):133–42.
61. Ham C. Improving the performance of health services: the role of clinical leadership. Lancet. 2003;361:1978–80.
62. Kaji AH, Bair A, Okuda Y, et al. Defining systems expertise: effective simulation at the organizational level – implications for patient safety, disaster surge capacity, and facilitating the systems interface. Acad Emerg Med. 2008;15:1098–103.
63. Hearne S. Practice-based teaching for health policy action and advocacy. Public Health Rep. 2008;123(2 Suppl):65–70. Ref Type: Report.
64. Cuschieri A. Whither minimal access surgery: tribulations and expectations. Am J Surg. 1995;169:9–19.
65. Salas E, Klein C, King H, et al. Debriefing medical teams: 12 evidence-based best practices and tips. Jt Comm J Qual Patient Saf. 2008;34:518–27.
66. Ginsburg S, Regehr G, Lingard L. The disavowed curriculum: understanding student's reasoning in professionally challenging situations. J Gen Intern Med. 2003;18:1015–22.
67. Hochberg MS, Kalet A, Zabar S, et al. Can professionalism be taught? Encouraging evidence. Am J Surg. 2010;199:86–93.
68. Hochberg MS, Berman RS, Kalet AL, et al. The professionalism curriculum as a cultural change agent in surgical residency education. Am J Surg. 2012;203:14–20.
69. Mazor KM, Zanetti ML, Alper EJ, et al. Assessing professionalism in the context of an objective structured clinical examination: an in-depth study of the rating process. Med Educ. 2007;41:331–40.
70. Swanstrom LL, Fried GM, Hoffman KI, et al. Beta test results of a new system assessing competence in laparoscopic surgery. J Am Coll Surg. 2006;202:62–9.
71. Ziv A, Erez D, Munz Y, et al. The Israel Center for Medical Simulation: a paradigm for cultural change in medical education. Acad Med. 2006;81:1091–7.

Systems Integration

10

William Dunn, Ellen Deutsch, Juli Maxworthy, Kathleen Gallo, Yue Dong, Jennifer Manos, Tiffany Pendergrass, and Victoria Brazil

Introduction

Are American health-care providers really responsible for 98,000 deaths per year, as described in the Institute of Medicine (IOM) landmark report "To Err is Human" [1]? If so, can simulation play a roll, as a new (and transformational) tool, to improve the quality of health care, both in the USA and globally? Throughout this book, there are examples of ways simulation is used to improve a range of technical, psychomotor, cognitive, and decision-making medical skills, including error prevention and error recovery. Methods and examples of improving crisis resource management (team leadership and team support), safety behaviors, procedural training, and demonstration of proficiency are also described. As such, simulation is a potent tool in several domains including education, assessment, and research, offering opportunities at the operational level of most institutions. The fourth domain of simulation application, "systems integration," is conceptually at a higher plane that is proactively orchestrated and organizationally planned in order to create lasting institutional impact.

Simulation applications within the systems integration construct promote the optimized function of a "complex adaptive system" [2]. This idealized function can only be sustainable within an organization if positive changes are thoughtfully engineered. Health-care leaders have called for the building of a better health-care delivery system that requires "a new engineering and health-care partnership" [3]. The goals of such a system are intrinsically patient centric where the transformed system, according to IOM, is described as safe, effective, timely, efficient, and equitable (Table 10.1) [4].

Simulation will not be the panacea for all deficiencies of health systems. However it can be a viable tool for organizational leadership to solve identified safety, effectiveness, efficiency, and equity problems toward patient-centric optimized care. Simulation is but one of many tools (e.g., informatics technologies, root cause analyses, risk management, community services, biomonitoring) available to improve patient care experiences and outcomes. Identifying how simulation adds value to the reformation of health care is an important task for health-care leaders in partnership with simulation professionals.

"You've got to be very careful if you don't know where you're going because you might not get there."—Yogi Berra

W. Dunn, MD, FCCP, FCCM (✉)
Division of Pulmonary and Critical Care Medicine, Mayo Clinic Multidisciplinary Simulation Center, Mayo Clinic, 200 1st St., SW, Gonda 18, Rochester, MN 55905, USA
e-mail: dunn.william@mayo.edu

E. Deutsch, MD, FACS, FAAP
Department of Anesthesia and Critical Care, Center for Simulation, Advanced Education, and Innovation, The Children's Hospital of Philadelphia, Room 8NW100, 3400 Civic Center Blvd, Philadelphia, PA, USA
e-mail: deutsches@email.chop.edu

J. Maxworthy, DNP, MSN, MBA, RN, CNL, CPHQ, CPPS
School of Nursing and Health Professions, University of San Francisco, San Francisco, CA, USA

WithMax Consulting, 70 Ardilla Rd, 94563 Orinda, CA, USA
e-mail: withmax@comcast.net

K. Gallo, PhD, MBA, RN, FAAN
Center for Learning and Innovation/Patient Safety Institute, Hofstra North Shore-LIJ School of Medicine, North Shore-LIJ Health System, 1979 Marcus Avenue, Suite 101, Lake Success, NY 11042, USA
e-mail: kgallo@nshs.edu

Y. Dong, MD
Division of Pulmonary and Critical Care Medicine, Department of Internal Medicine, Multidisciplinary Simulation Center, Mayo Clinic, 200 First Street SW, Rochester, MN 55905, USA
e-mail: dong.yue@mayo.edu

J. Manos, RS, BSN
Cincinnati Children's Hospital Medical Center, Cincinnati, OH, USA
e-mail: manos@ssih.org

T. Pendergrass, BSN, RN, CPN
Division of Heart Institute, Cincinnati Children's Hospital Medical Center, Cincinnati, OH, USA

V. Brazil, MBBS, FACEM, MBA
School of Medicine, Bond University, Gold Coast, QLD, Australia

Department of Emergency Medicine, Royal Brisbane and Women's Hospital, 21 Jaloon St, Ashgrove, 4060 Qld, Brisbane, QLD, Australia
e-mail: victoria.brazil@gmail.com

A.I. Levine et al. (eds.), *The Comprehensive Textbook of Healthcare Simulation*,
DOI 10.1007/978-1-4614-5993-4_10, © Springer Science+Business Media New York 2013

Table 10.1 Six quality aims for the twenty-first-century health-care system [3]

The committee proposes six aims for improvement to address key dimensions in which today's health care system functions at far lower levels than it can and should. Healthcare should be:
1. Safe—avoiding injuries to patients from the care that is intended to help them.
2. Effective—providing services based on scientific knowledge to all who could benefit and refraining from providing services to those not likely to benefit (avoiding underuse and overuse, respectively).
3. Patient-centered—providing care that is respectful of and responsive to individual patient preferences, needs, and values and ensuring that patient values guide all clinical decisions.
4. Timely—reducing waits and sometimes harmful delays for both those who receive and those who give care.
5. Efficient—avoiding waste, including waste of equipment, supplies, ideas, and energy.
6. Equitable—providing care that does not vary in quality because of personal characteristics such as gender, ethnicity, geographic location, and socioeconomic status.

Reprinted with permission from Ref. [3]

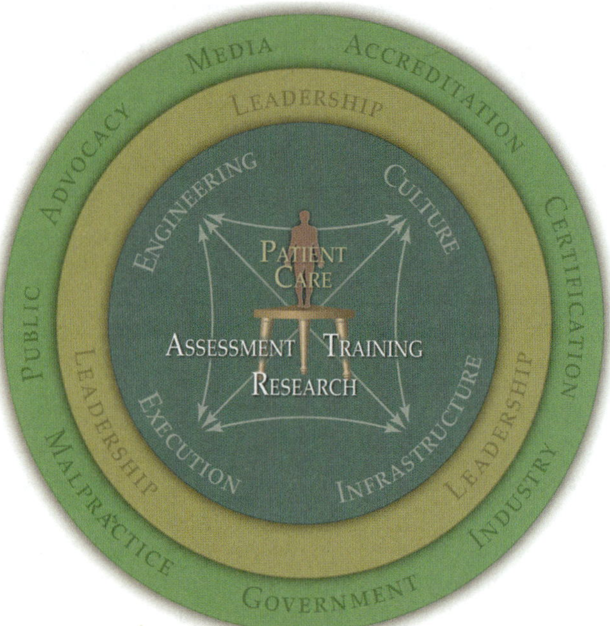

Fig. 10.2 Integration of simulation into organizational complexity (internal and external)

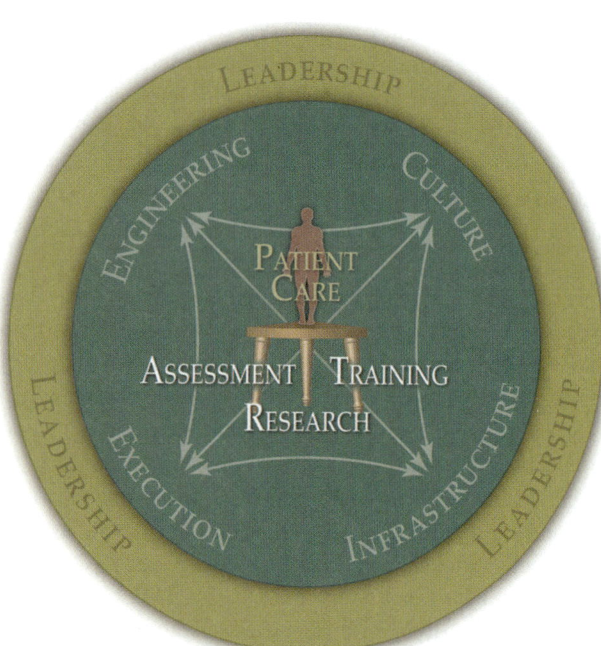

Fig. 10.1 Integration of simulation into organizational complexity

Facilitating value-driven health care at the bedside, health-care organizations utilizing simulation may serve the "common good" by providing education, assessment, quality, safety, and research. Figure 10.1 highlights the relationship between each component of an organization. From a systems standpoint, *delivering* competent, professional patient care is central and the immediate need. The mission of an organization therefore addresses how these system components achieve and highlight the centrality of the safety-focused patient experience. It is the seamless relationship of education (training), assessment, research, and care infrastructures that serves patient needs optimally, within an interdisciplinary framework. Organizations do not function independently however and also have relationships and oversight from external entities including the government, industry, media, accreditation bodies, and other agencies (Fig. 10.2).

Although systems differ, we agree with the IOM that patient centricity must be central to any health-care delivery model. We further assert that simulation affords a needed and transformative set of system improvement tools and opportunities for certain reengineering needs that is unavailable (or suboptimal) via other means; this facilitates integration of process components within our (consistently complex) organizations (i.e., systems). In this chapter, we address the current and potential roll of simulation in improving the quality and safety of patient care delivered at the bedside by discussing simulation's impact at the complex macro-institutional level in a "top-down" rather than a "bottom-up" manner.

Systems Integration from the Perspective of a Simulation Program

Systems integration is defined by the Society for Simulation in Healthcare (SSH) as "those simulation programs which demonstrate consistent, planned, collaborative, integrated and iterative application of simulation-based assessment and teaching activities with systems engineering and risk-management principles to achieve excellent bedside clinical care, enhanced patient safety, and improved metrics across the healthcare system" [5].

Systems integration is a new concept to health care and therefore requires a new and thoughtful approach to meeting these standards. Adopting solutions from other disciplines and industries may offer an innovative "toolkit" that is applicable to the (IOM-driven) transformations essential for health care today.

Systems engineering tools have been used in a wide variety of applications to achieve major improvements in the quality, efficiency, safety, and/or customer centeredness of processes, products, and services in a wide range of manufacturing and services industries [3]. The addition of medical simulation to this evidence-based toolkit is not only complimentary but can enhance the associated transformative effects. Simulation techniques offer opportunities to enhance the accountability of health-care-providers' skills acquisition through formative and summative training, which offer consistency, objectivity, and demonstrated proficiency in the management of clinically realistic and relevant problems.

Health Care as a Complex Adaptive System

Contemporary clinical medicine not only includes the obvious provider-patient interaction but also includes many complex "system" dimensions in the patient care setting. These include health-care provider performance characteristics; organizational factors including physician, nursing, allied health staff availability, environmental considerations, patient, and family member preferences; and the interactions between these components of the complex system [6]. Within organizations, each component is interconnected and interdependent with other system components. The impact of interactions between system components is difficult to predict since they are often remote in time and space. Inadequacy in such system components can negatively affect care delivery. System-related components (patient flow, work environment, information systems, human factors) contribute to delays and errors in care. The World Health Organization (WHO) has suggested that the (1) lack of communication, (2) inadequate coordination, and (3) presence of latent organization failures are important priorities for improving patient safety in developed and developing countries alike [7].

Outside the conceptual "walls" of an organization, complexity remains. Health care is often not delivered within a single "island-like" independent facility. Often, care delivery occurs within a large enterprise or system of systems of health-care delivery. Care across such system components is rarely seamless. Beyond the (larger) enterprise walls exist environmental forces (see Fig. 10.2) including external regulatory agencies, the press, public perception and other market forces, malpractice, and medicolegal concerns.

Health-care delivery systems continue to increase in complexity because of many factors including improvements in technology, advanced diagnostic technology, complex disease processes, increasing accountability and transparency of internal processes, an aging population, workforce shortages, generational differences, social networking, and mobile technology. These factors will transform both patient-provider and provider-provider interactions. Health-care's increased complexity and sophistication comes at a price- increased risk of error and poor patient outcome. Sir Cyril Chantler stated, "Medicine used to be simple, ineffective and relatively safe. Now it is complex, effective and potentially dangerous" [8].

A "Systems Approach" to Improving Health-Care Delivery

Although concepts of systems and engineering applications applied to health care may seem novel, large successful organizations have used systems engineering principles for many years. Dr. Henry Plummer, a Mayo Clinic internist from 1901 to 1936, creatively engineered many aspects of the world's first integrated academic group practice of medicine and surgery and remains a recognized pioneer in conceptually embedding engineering philosophy into the practice of medicine [9]. Plummer's innovations included an integrated inpatient and outpatient medical record, a "master sheet" clinical diagnoses list for research and practice improvement activities, a pneumatic tube system to distribute records and laboratory specimens across multiple geographic sites, and a color-coded lighting system to support central booking and the patient visitation process. All of these inventions remain in use today. In fact, Plummer's novel applications served as the origins of the Division of Systems and Procedures at Mayo Clinic in 1947. Dick Cleeremans (Section Head 1966–1982) stated: "The decision by the Mayo Medical Center to hire *industrial engineers* in those early years was in keeping with the Mayo commitment to the patient, physician/patient relationship and Dr. Plummer's expectation that the system and the organization of the clinical practice were important and a worthy management activity."

More recently, Avedis Donabedian popularized the structure-process-outcome framework with which to assess quality-improvement efforts [10]. Donabedian also described the Systems Engineering Initiative to Patient Safety (SEIPS) framework, designed to improve health-care delivery in complex health-care systems (Fig. 10.3) [10, 11].

System approaches focus on the working environment rather than on the errors of individual providers, as the likelihood of specific errors increases with unfavorable environmental conditions. The effective system intervention is to design, test, and enhance the system's components so it can prevent human error and identify a variety of vulnerabilities such as distraction, fatigue, and other latent factors [12].

The "Systems Approach" Meets "Modeling and Simulation"

Systems-based modeling and simulation (M&S) has several advantages for clinical decision support, systems analysis, and experimentation for multivariate system components

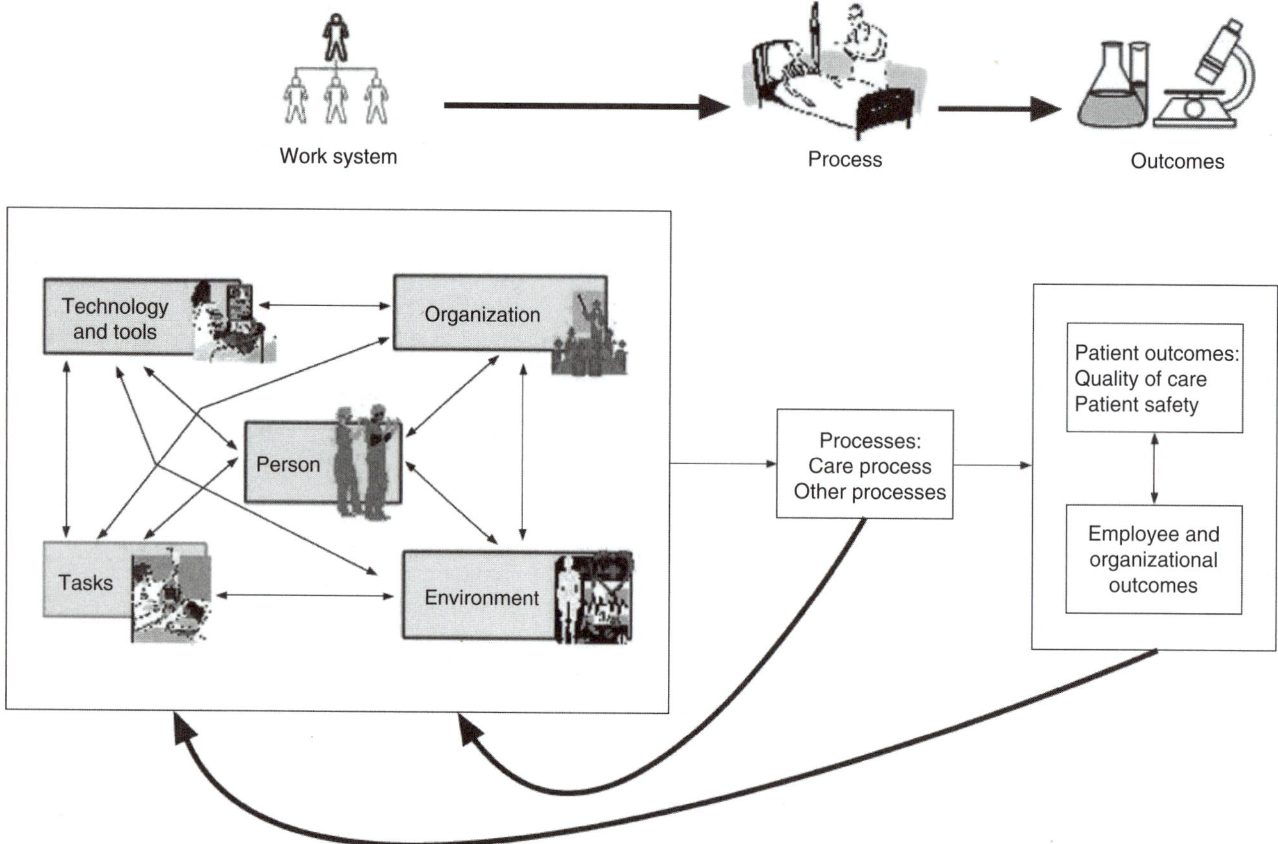

Fig. 10.3 From Carayon et al. work system design for patient safety: The SEIPS model [11] (Used with permission)

that cannot be achieved by traditional quality-improvement processes. Computer modeling can simulate processes of health-care delivery by engineering techniques such as discrete-event simulation. In discrete-event simulation, the operation of a system is represented as a chronological sequence of events; events occur at a particular instant in time, thus defining a change of state in the system [13]. Because discrete-event simulation is time oriented (as clinical patient outcomes often are based on timeliness of delivered care), this form of computer-based simulation lends itself well to systems engineering analyses of contemporary complex health-care systems.

Coupling computer modeling techniques (such as discrete-event simulation) to realistic contemporary simulation programs can provide a synergy of process improvement design and analysis offering exceptionally strong opportunities in transformational process improvement. For instance, novel process optimization mechanisms through integration of engineering principles for health-care system analysis, simulation-based drills, and workflow redesigns for testing proposed interventions (virtual clinical trials or quality improvement) before clinical deployment may reduce the potential for preventable harm to patients.

Consider a patient entering an emergency department with acute abdominal pain, possibly due to a surgical emergency, as the beginning of a "process." Computer models (e.g., a process flow diagram) can readily demonstrate patient time-dependent flow *for a population of such patients*, between the time of emergency room entry to the definitive surgery. Because many process components must occur (history and physical, laboratory analyses, radiographic imaging, consultations) in both series and in parallel, equations describing such patient "traffic" can be defined, which, if accurate enough, can be descriptors of both current and future performance. Such computer-based models are excellent adjuncts for process improvement via immersive experiential simulation such as drills and in situ simulations.

A stepwise M&S approach follows that illustrates the potential for improved health-care delivery process:

Step one, system monitoring: Graphically define a current practice pattern of individual patient flow within a distinct process of delivered care describing the (in series or in parallel) decisions and patient care activities in branching fashion (e.g., trauma assessment and care delivery within an emergency department).

Step two, system modeling: Develop the individual equations defining the time-dependent parameters of the work process flow diagram. The model must replicate reality within reasonable limits, for realistic patient flow care simulations.

Step three, hypothesis generation and system redesign: Practical aspects of delivered care efficiency are optimized (in a hypothetical basis) by altering components of the flow diagram.

Step four, simulation applications to enhance system performance: In center or in situ realistic simulation is utilized to improve individual or team performance.

Step five, feedback loops sustain process improvement: Data monitoring verifies absence of regression to baseline inefficiencies. Simulation "ping" exercises (see example 8 later in the chapter) or drills are used to assess system performance on a perpetual basis.

The National Academy of Engineering and Institute of Medicine of the National Academies directed attention to the issue of systems engineering and integration with their joint report in 2005, *Building a Better Delivery System: A New Engineering/Health Care Partnership* [3]. The proposed collaboration between clinicians, engineers, researchers, educators, and experts from medical informatics and management will provide a clinically relevant, systematic approach and a comprehensive solution to many of the challenging problems in clinical medicine.

System Engineering

The overall goal of systems engineering is to produce a system that meets the needs of all users or stakeholders within the constraints that govern the system's operation. Systems engineering requires a variety of quantitative and qualitative tools for analyzing and interpreting system models (Table 10.2). Tools from psychology, computer science, operations research, management and economics, and mathematics are commonly utilized in systems engineering across a wide array of industries. Quantitative tools include optimization methods, control theory, stochastic modeling and simulation, statistics, utility theory, decision analysis, and economics. Mathematical techniques have the capability of solving large-scale, complex problems optimally using computerized algorithms [14].

Many of the systems engineering tools are found within different quality-improvement strategies, including Six Sigma, Toyota Production System, and Lean. But within these methodologies, examples of system engineering tools that have been utilized in health care include [3]:

- Statistical process control
- Process flowcharting
- Queuing theory
- Quality function deployment
- Failure-modes effect analysis
- Optimization
- Modeling and simulation
- Human-factors engineering

Process Engineering

Process engineering is a subset of systems engineering and represents a system *process* component, essentially a "building block" of a complex adaptive system (Table 10.3). A process is a set of interrelated tasks or steps that together transform inputs into a common output (i.e., workflow) toward a goal, (such as in the assessment steps involved within the "acute abdominal pain" patient group presenting to an emergency department described earlier). The tasks can be executed by people or technology utilizing available resources. Thus, within the processes of (complex adaptive) systems improvement, a focus within individual processes is a natural phenomenon, while recognizing the interrelated

Table 10.2 System analysis tools

Tool/research area	Patient	Team	Organization	Environment
Modeling and simulation				
Queuing methods		X	X	X
Discrete-event simulation		X	X	
Enterprise-management tools				
Supply-chain management		X	X	X
Game theory and contracts		X	X	X
Systems-dynamics models		X	X	X
Productivity measuring and monitoring		X	X	X
Financial engineering and risk analysis tools				
Stochastic analysis and value at risk		X	X	X
Optimization tools for individual decision making			X	X
Distributed decision making (market models and agency theory)			X	X
Knowledge discovery in databases				
Data mining		X	X	X
Predictive modeling		X	X	X
Neural networks			X	X

Reprinted with permission from Ref. [3], Tables 10.3 and 10.4

Table 10.3 Systems engineering versus process engineering

Focus	Systems engineering	Process engineering
Purpose	High-level subsystems or systems	Low-level tasks or steps and the resources/tools required to execute the tasks/steps
Focus	Relationships of interrelated subsystems	Sequence or workflow of interrelated tasks or steps and associated resources/tools
Methodology	Design, analysis, control of relationships between subsystems	Establish workflow or sequence of tasks and required resources/tools
Example of project types	Optimizing patient care processes in a children's hospital using six Sigma methodology	Reducing inpatient turnaround time using a value analysis approach
	Comprehensive perinatal safety initiative to reduce adverse obstetric events	Improving computed tomography scan throughput
	Improving handoff communication	Reducing length of stay for congestive heart failure patients using six Sigma methodology

Modified from Ref. [3]

nature of system (process) component parts. The introduction of new processes, such as technology (and support) associated with the introduction of an electronic medical record (EMR), requires business process redesign *before such processes* are implemented. When, in an effort to meet project management deadlines, engineering processes are rushed or completely ignored, system havoc may ensue.

What Systems Integration Is

In terms of simulation, systems integration (SI) is the recognition of a variety of key principles as one better understands the role and capacity of simulation within the complex adaptive health-care system. This is intended to achieve a functional, highly efficient organization of dynamic teams and processes, interfacing to collectively and artfully optimize patient care. Therefore a simulation program's impact on an organization's intrinsic function includes the following principles as they apply to projects that facilitate seamless and optimal effective heath system process integration.

SI projects are:

- Leadership and mission driven toward safety and quality goals, facilitating optimized care delivery
- Monitored, as appropriate, to assure impact in perpetuity via appropriate metrics
- Described by systems engineering principles and tools
- Interdisciplinary

Simulation can also be used strategically by the health-care organization to achieve business goals. When building new facilities, simulation can be used alone or within Six Sigma or Lean concepts [15, 16], systems engineering tools, to ensure that a facility develops efficient and effective workflows with input from the staff. The new facility can then be tested in simulation to identify and address any process or human factor issues before opening.

Organizational leaders, including clinicians, risk managers, and/or quality/safety process managers, may approach the simulation program with specific safety initiative. Below are a series of eight case studies highlighting the use of simulation for SI purposes.

Example 1

As per organizational policy, the simulation program is contacted by the Chair of Perinatal Services and Risk Management to address a sentinel event that has occurred. An intense review was performed on sentinel events using the following systems and process engineering tools: process flowcharting, quality function deployment, root cause analysis, and statistical process control. A collaborative process among the clinical service, risk management, and the simulation program took place. A comprehensive perinatal safety initiative was developed. It was comprised of the following components: evidenced-based protocols, formalized team training with emphasis on communication, documented competence of electronic fetal monitoring, high-risk obstetrical emergency simulation program, and dissemination of an integrated educational program among all health-care providers. A 2-year study was conducted and demonstrated that this comprehensive program significantly reduced adverse obstetric outcomes, thereby enhancing patient safety, staff, and patient satisfaction.

Example 2

Following an analysis of sentinel event data, an organization concludes that the largest source of preventable mortality for the organization is within the context of patients deteriorating in hospital on the wards, without prompt enough transfer to a higher level of care ("deteriorating patient syndrome"). Root cause analyses, supplemented by survey data, reveal that the primary source of the preventable deaths rests within the cultural aspects (false assumptions, misperceptions, and inadequate communication) of nursing and (on-call) house staff at the time of house staff evaluation. Armed with this conclusion, organizational leadership engages the simulation program to devise and pilot a simulation-based experiential exercise (course) targeting the newly defined deficiencies within the learning goals. Following data analysis, the course is adopted system wide, in a phased approach, with ongoing assessment of both preventable death and cultural survey data.

Example 3

A large organization consists of 15 disparate hospitals within a five-state region. Based on review of the evolving literature, one hospital devises a simulation-based Central Line Workshop, created in an effort to improve consistency of training and reduce line-related complications, including site complications and bacteremia. Following implementation, institutional data demonstrate a reduction in catheter-related bacteremias. Based on this data, organizational leadership decides to:

1. Require simulation-based mandatory standards of training across the organization.
2. Endorse the standardization of all credentialing for central line placement across the organization.
3. Track metrics associated with line-related complications, responding to predefined data metric goals as appropriate.

Example 4

A 77-year-old male with a previously stable and asymptomatic umbilical hernia presents to an emergency department with acute abdominal pain localized to the hernia, associated with evolving abdominal distention. He is otherwise healthy, with the exception of being on therapeutic anticoagulation (warfarin) for a previous aortic valve repair. The patient, the emergency department triage nurse, and the emergency room physician quickly recognize the presence of an incarceration. Due to a series of system inefficiencies, time delays occur, eventuating in a 13-h delay in arrival to the operating room. Dead gut is found, and a primary anastomosis is performed. Five days later, the patient develops repeated bouts of bloody stools associated with breakdown of the anastomosis and dies 12 h later without being seen by a physician.

Following sentinel event review, a process map depicting the steps associated with the evaluation and management of patients having the working diagnosis of umbilical hernia incarceration is created. A computer model is created, depicting the observed process, with discrete-event simulation utilized to computer simulate the actual time delays for a small population of similar patients studied retrospectively. The organization requests the simulation program to develop a realistic simulation process improvement plan, building on the prior work accomplished, to improve the process of incarcerated umbilical hernia patients. Following institution of realistic simulation quality assurance program (involving standardized patients presenting to the emergency department replicating past patients), data demonstrates a 50% reduction in time-to-operating theater, in ten patients within a 2-year period, compared to baseline.

Example 5

Over the past 10 years, a large health-care organization has acquired an array of 20 hospitals, formerly in competition with each other, under a new, semiautonomous organizational structure designed to maintain and capture market share of referrals to the parent academic enterprise. The "hub" of this "hub-and-spoke" organizational model is a well-established and respected organization with well honed, safety-conscious policies and a track record in crisis intervention of perinatal emergencies. A small series of preventable deaths have occurred across the satellite facilities as high-risk, low-frequency events within the small systems. Clinicians within the existing simulation program at the parent organization, seeing examples of referred infants with preventable harm, institute an outreach neonatal resuscitation simulation program. They visit 3 of the 20 satellite facilities and garner positive initial feedback and relationships, albeit in a non-sustainable model of in situ neonatal resuscitation team training.

Leadership at the parent organization learn of a series of malpractice claims associated with financial losses, impacting the institution due to the preventable harm. A cohesive plan is presented to senior leadership by a team represented by the director of the simulation center, the chief legal counsel, safety and quality leadership, and the neonatologists performing the in situ program. After clinical case and financial analyses, a leadership level decision is made to craft an ongoing, dedicate, mandatory, in situ regional program, with ongoing monitoring of learner feedback and clinical outcomes.

Example 6

During an internal quality assessment review, at a regional hospital's emergency department, it was found that mean "door-to-balloon" time for patients with ST elevation myocardial infarction (STEMI) was below locally acceptable standards and norms set by the American Heart Association. In an effort to improve "door-to-balloon" times, the hospital's Quality Council (which includes the director of the simulation center) determined that an in situ simulation of patient journeys would be utilized in an effort to improve system response.

Prehospital providers and multidisciplinary teams from emergency (medical, nursing, patient support) and cardiology (medical, nursing, imaging) participated in a series of in situ simulations of the STEMI patient journey. Simulated (mannequins and monitor emulators) and standardized patients (actors trained to perform as patients with STEMI) were used. "Patients" arrived in the emergency department with a paramedic. Participants were required to identify possible candidates for percutaneous coronary intervention (PCI), provide immediate assessment and management, communicate effectively between teams, and coordinate physical transfer and urgent intervention in the cardiac catheterization suite. After each patient care episode, teams participated in a facilitated debrief to discuss process, teamwork, and communication issues, with a focus on areas for improvement.

Data was collected on the performance against time-based targets and quality-of-care key performance indicators in the simulations. Door-to-balloon times for real STEMI patients presenting to the facility before and after the intervention were collected and analyzed.

Data was collected on participant perceptions of the experience, including the simulation and debrief, and their reflections of how the STEMI patient journey could be improved. Median door-to-balloon times at the facility were 85 min in the 6 months prior to the intervention, and 62 min in the 6 months immediately after the simulation ($p<.05$), and with a change in the "door-to-lab" time of 65 min to 31 min in the corresponding time periods ($p<.01$).

Example 7

During routine competency assessments, the simulation center staff notices a trend in the inability of frontline nursing staff to properly program an infusion pump that was rolled out 3 months earlier at one of the hospitals that utilizes the simulation center. The next week the manager of the simulation center contacts the risk manager of that particular facility. The simulation manager explains in detail the programming challenges that she has witnessed.

The risk manager, utilizing the information provided by the simulation manager, reviews recent incident reports in the electronic incident reporting system. She notices that since the implementation of the new pumps, the number of rapid response team (RRT) calls and code blues outside the ICU has increased by 40%, which raises concern that this increase could be due to improper programming of the pumps. The risk manager shares the information with nursing leadership. Reeducation via experiential exercises within the simulation facility is planned immediately and occurs for frontline nursing staff within the next 2 days. The nursing supervisors, who attend every RRT and code blue, are asked to identify whether the pump programming was a potential cause of the patient decline. Within a week, the number of RRTs and code blues outside the ICU decreases to the levels they had been before the implementation of the pumps and is maintained at this level for a period of over 6 months. To decrease the possibility of similar future issues, the operations director of the simulation program is placed on the equipment purchasing committee such that simulation-based assessments, when deemed appropriate, are performed when new equipment is under evaluation for potential purchase. The challenges and changes to processes and the subsequent outcomes are shared with the performance improvement committee and the board of directors of the hospital.

Example 8 ("Ping" Exercise)

Similar to a submarine's sonar "ping" emitted into surrounding waters in search of an enemy vessel, a simulation exercise (typically in situ) can be utilized to "ping" a clinical environment, searching for latent, or real, failures. The following is an example:

A 300-bed teaching hospital facility's quality team hypothesized that traditionally trained resident physicians perceived to be proficient enough to place central venous catheters (CVCs) alone or under supervision would consistently pass an endorsed, simulation-based, Central Line Workshop (CLW) CVC proficiency examination that incorporates endorsed institutional practice standards.

Resident physicians engaged in performance of CVCs were mandated to enroll in a standardized CLW training program, focusing on training of CVC to demonstrated proficiency standards using ultrasound, universal precautions, and an anatomy-based patient safety curriculum. Experiential training is followed by a "Certification Station" (CS) proficiency assessment. Senior residents and those believed to be adequately proficient (by both program director and self-assessment) in CVC skills were offered the opportunity to "test out" via CS after performing the online course only (no experiential component).

Fifteen (50%) residents "testing out" of simulation-based experiential training performed CS (without completing the standard entire training module). Seven (23%) failed on the first attempt. As a process improvement tool, simulation-based techniques offer the opportunity of assessing the performance of existing systems. In this example, a previously validated system of performance assessment in CVC placement demonstrated imperfect performance by practitioners perceived to be proficient enough to place CVCs alone or under supervision. This exercise demonstrated the weakness of informal CVC placement training exercises and supported the need for standardized experiential training and testing for all residents at the institution placing CVCs. This process (CLW) was therefore incorporated into standard training practice, on an ongoing basis.

Systems Integration Is Not...

Systems integration is not present when a simulation program is developing courses that are not aligned with the strategic plan of the health-care organization or when the primary purpose of a simulation project is for traditional simulation-based training, assessment, and/or research goals. Organizational leadership will typically have very little awareness of most simulation projects occurring within a simulation program. Most courses or programs are naturally developed in relative isolation from organizational leadership and serve defined purposes within a defined process of education, assessment, care delivery, or research. Most programs that are offered specifically for teaching, assessment, or research while valuable are naturally linked to patient safety or quality concept goals, but may not satisfy the rigor of integrating system components, with proactive (engineered) metric assessments of impact. Similarly, a simulation project may have an inadequate feedback loop to the health-care organization and thus not fulfill integrated systems engineering requisites. An example may be found in the following case: The simulation program offers all American Heart Association programs annually—BLS, ACLS, and PALS. No data on resuscitation outcomes from the health service provider is shared with the simulation program. These certifications are a requirement for some hospital personnel and a revenue generator for the program, but the program does not meet the requirements for systems integration.

Systems Integration as a Disruptive Innovation

Disruptive innovation is described by Clayton Christensen as "a process by which a product or service takes root initially in simple applications at the bottom of a market and then relentlessly moves 'up market', eventually displacing established competitors" [17].

Christensen examined the differences between *radical innovation*, which destroys the value of existing knowledge and *incremental innovation* which builds on existing knowledge and creates a "new and improved version." The classic example of a *radical innovation* is the electric light bulb that replaced the candle. Christensen notes that *disruptive innovative* has the destroying value of *radical innovation* but works through industry more slowly. Typically, a disruptive innovation begins unnoticed in an industry as it holds value to only a distinct segment of the market. Its power lies in its ability to meet the needs of this niche that is unaddressed by the current products or services and usually to do so at lower cost. As these disruptive innovations improve their services, they move up the value chain and ultimately become a threat to the market leaders [18, 19].

Certainly simulation, as applied to health care, satisfies all requirements and definitions of being disruptive innovation. Beyond this, however, will simulation-based systems integration (SBSI) move up the value chain in health care and threaten the market leader—*the utilization of a non-systems approach to advance the six IOM Quality Aims?* If there is agreement that the health-care sector is a complex adaptive system, then we must agree that a systems approach to improve health-care delivery is essential. SBSI brings together the components or subsystems of the whole. This is a novel approach and is aligned with Christensen's framework for disruptive innovation: It holds value to a niche segment of the market as it moves through the industry slowly. This niche segment is an important driver behind the rapid growth of an international multidisciplinary organization (based on transformative patient-centric principles including the underlying assumption that simulation represents a "disruptive technology" opportunity), like SSH (Fig. 10.4) [1].

Systems Integration Accreditation via SSH: Raising the Bar

Rationale for the Development of Systems Integration Accreditation

For many health-care facilities with access to simulation, there is a disconnect between what is actually happening within the facility and what is being taught in the simulation program. However, when there is collaboration between

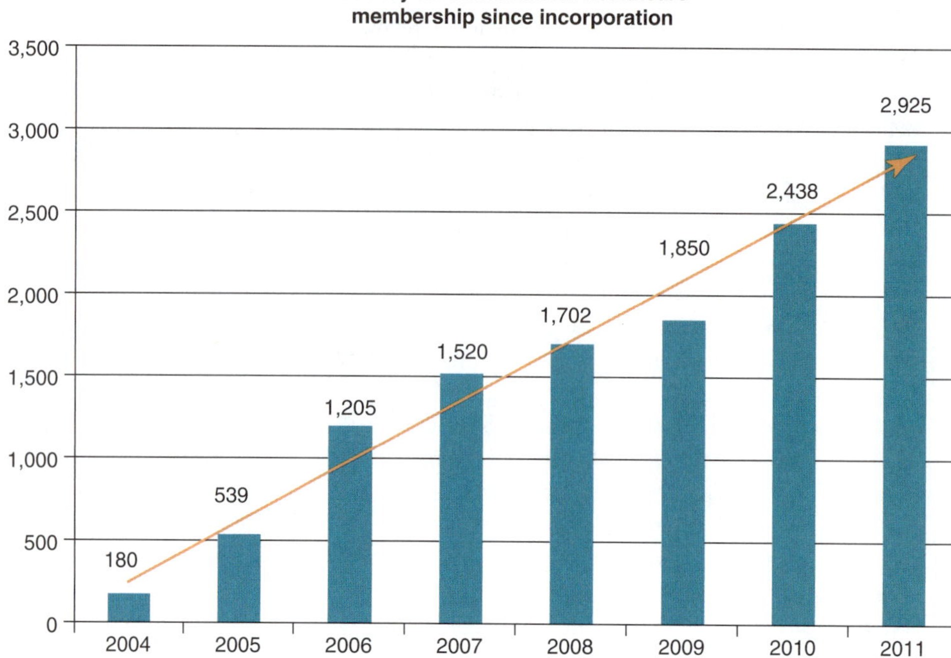

Fig. 10.4 SSIH membership

these entities in the pursuit of decreasing patient harm, the results can be significant. It was identified by the Accreditation Leadership group at SSH that a key aspect of a simulation center of excellence would be the "integration" function.

The Standards in Evolution

A systems integration element was added by the Accreditation Leadership group of SSH to acknowledge a program's high level of organizational integration of simulation consistent with the transformation of health care as espoused by the Institute of Medicine (IOM) principles. A facility must apply for and receive accreditation in at least two other areas (teaching, assessment, research) in order to be accredited in systems integration.

As with all accreditation standards, these will evolve over time, in line with the continually changing health-care landscape. As of January 2012, the standards related to systems integration have completed another iteration to ensure that they are consistent with current practice. Newly endorsed standards, effective January 2012, are provided in Appendix.

Systems integration accreditation by SSH is meant to be challenging, consistent with the transformative goals of the IOM. However, by obtaining compliance with the standards, an institution can be demonstrated to be actively utilizing the simulation program as an effective systems engineering tool, embedded within the organizational safety and quality "toolbox."

"Simulation and Activism: Engineering the Future of Health Care"

Health Workforce Reform: Performance Standardization Credentialing and Accreditation

Certification and accreditation standards provide information about desirable and achievable training, resources, and processes for individuals participating in simulation and for simulation centers, respectively. Articulating these standards provides a mechanism for simulation providers and simulation centers to benchmark their own resources and activities. Workforce standardization is a real and tangible opportunity for organizations. Such a workforce standardization motivator was key in the justification of a major Australian simulation initiative, the Australian Simulation Education and Technical Training program (AusSETT), funded by Health Workforce Australia [20]. The AusSETT project is the result of cooperation across four states, Queensland, South Australia, Victoria, and Western Australia, and represents system integration at a national level.

Educators and professional bodies who certify clinician competence are accountable not only to organizations but also to the larger community. The use of "zero-risk" simulated learning environments for training has led to the use of these same environments for testing and assessment of individuals and teams. Validation of these assessment processes has allowed them to be used for credentialing and recertification of individuals working in a variety of health-care contexts [21–24].

Although many challenges remain before there is widespread adoption [25–27], simulation-based applications continue to evolve in high-stakes testing.

The development of simulation-based assessment should drive collaboration to develop consensus definitions of such standards by professional bodies and health-care regulators. Simulation applications in assessment, research training, and systems integration revolve around the fundamental concept of patient *safety*.

Although admittedly imperfect and not necessarily indicative of mature clinical *competence*, one could conceive of future "skills assessments," based on a set of national standards that can be realistically demonstrated within a simulation environment. Improved health care (and sustainable health) would be the natural and realistic outcome expectation for the global community, based on such system integration principles.

Health Workforce Reform: Risk Management and Malpractice Industry Engagement

Improvements in patient safety (clinical outcomes) have been well demonstrated in the training for, and performance of, a variety of clinical procedures, including central venous catheterization [26], catheter-related bloodstream infections [27], thoracentesis [28], laparoscopic surgery [29], colonoscopy [30], and laparoscopic inguinal hernia repair [31] among others. Due to the rapid demonstration of efficacy of simulation across a large range of procedures and specialties, a recent meta-analysis concluded: "In comparison with no intervention, technology-enhanced simulation training in health professions education is consistently associated with large effects for outcomes of knowledge, skills, and behaviors and moderate effects for patient related outcomes" [32].

Simulation can play a large role in facilitating safest practices through demonstrated proficiency (assessment) and education within a health-care organization. Because of such demonstrable impact, simulation as a quality and safety resource has both great promise and demonstrated efficacy in organizational approaches to risk reduction. Within the Harvard-affiliated system, Gardner et al. demonstrated that a simulation-based team-training course for obstetric clinicians was both well accepted and was justified (internally) in the reduction of annual obstetric malpractice premiums by 10% [33]. This developed as a central component of the CRICO/RMF's (Controlled Risk Insurance Company, Risk Management Foundation) obstetric risk-management incentive program. As such the Harvard medical institutions simulation-based CRM training serves as a strategy for mitigating adverse perinatal events and is a high-profile model for future malpractice industry endeavors, integrating simulation as an organizational risk-management tool into the organizational culture.

Such an organizational loss prevention program is a clear example of integrating simulation within an organizational framework. The intrinsic accountability and feedback architecture, as described above, provides internal ongoing data to the organization, justifying, or modifying as appropriate, the optimal use of simulation in serving patient needs. Beyond obstetrics, risk-management drivers have been utilized within the CRICO/RMF loss prevention "reengineering" system in anesthesiology (with mandatory internal utilization) and laparoscopic surgery [34]. The steps utilized within this process are shown in Table 10.4.

Table 10.4 Organizational steps in the creation of a loss prevention program

Step
Step 1: Analyze malpractice cases
Step 2: Create context
Step 3: Identify and confirm ongoing risk
Step 4: Engineer solutions to risk vulnerability
Step 5: Aggressively train, investing saved "indemnity dollars"
Step 6: Measure impact

Modified from Hanscom [34]

Conclusion

It is exciting to reflect on the dynamic opportunities now afforded to health-related organizations via simulation integration. Using simulation as a tool to define and apply the science of health-care delivery translates into improved patient outcomes. The application of systems thinking and simulation testing/applications of health-care organizational performance may have profound implications for future delivery models. Early experience suggests that future practitioners may be utilized differently for maximum efficiency, value, and affordable care, as traditional duties are disrupted by newer, safer methods of simulation-based training and performance assessment, fully integrated into safety-intense systems of value-driven care. It is critically important that the transformative concepts of the IOM, coupled with the (positive) disruptive potentials of simulation (at "systems" levels), be thoughtfully and carefully applied in new arenas where opportunities for improved, safe, effective, patient-centric, timely, efficient, and equitable health-care delivery exist. Reform in this area could be hampered by the traditional silos of health-care practice and workplace culture that evolved from past eras of health-care reform [35].

Early health-care simulation endeavors promised patient safety through improved *individual and team performance* leading to improved patient care. This chapter has demonstrated how simulation modalities can be used to test and improve health-care *systems* and more profoundly affect patient outcomes and health-care processes. Further progress requires continued collaboration between simulation experts, health-care providers, systems engineers, and policy makers.

Appendix: Council for Accreditation of Healthcare Simulation Programs

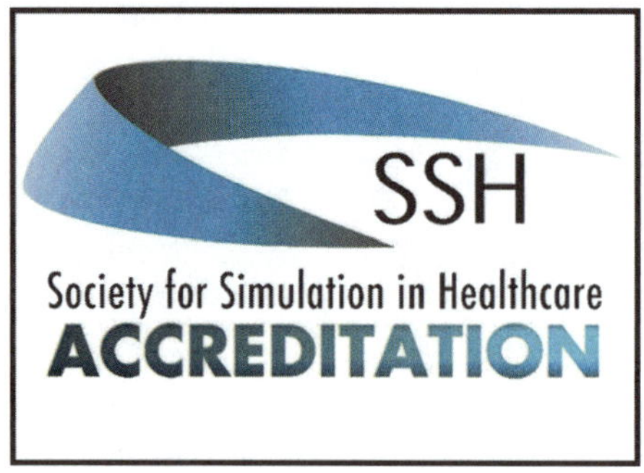

Accreditation Standards and Measurement Criteria

Suggested Revisions as endorsed by Systems Integration Subcommittee of SSH Accreditation Council, amended and authorized by vote of SSH Accreditation Council January 29, 2012

Systems integration: facilitating patient safety outcomes
Application for accreditation in the area of Systems Integration: Facilitating Patient Safety Outcomes will be available to those Programs who demonstrate consistent, planned, collaborative, integrated, and iterative application of simulation-based assessment; quality& safety; and teaching activities with systems engineering and risk management principles to achieve excellent bedside clinical care, enhanced patient safety, and improved outcome metrics across a healthcare system.
Standards specific for accreditation in the area of systems integration & patient safety outcomes
BOLD: Required Criteria
1. MISSION AND SCOPE: *The program functions as an integrated institutional safety, quality, and risk management resource that uses systems engineering principles and engages in bi-directional feedback to achieve enterprise-level goals and improve quality of care.* Provide a brief summary of how the Simulation Program addresses the Mission and Scope requirements described below (not more than 250 words) (a) Systems integration and patient safety activities are clearly driven by the strategic needs of the complex healthcare system(s). (i) There is a documented process in place to link the systems integration and patient safety activities to the strategic plan(s) of the healthcare system(s) Provide a description of the process, including the roles of those responsible for executing the plan to impact systems integration (ii) Provide a Copy of the Mission statement(s) with required elements including Impacting integrated system improvement within a complex healthcare environment Enhancement of the performance of individuals, teams, and organizations Creating a safer patient environment and improving outcomes (iii) Provide evidence from the past two (2) years documenting the simulation program being utilized as a resource by risk management and/or quality/patient safety with bi-directional feedback (iv) Provide a letter (2 pages maximum) from organizational Risk Management, Safety and/or Quality-Improvement leadership supporting the Program's role in achieving organizational risk, quality and/or safety goals (b) There is clear demonstration of impact of the program in improving organizational integrated processes and/or systems, thereby positively (and measurably) impacting patient care environments and/or outcomes, utilizing principles of process engineering for sustained impact (i) The program provides specific documentation of three (3) examples of Simulation used in an integrated fashion to facilitate Patient Safety, Risk Management and/or Quality Outcomes projects/activities. Supporting documentation for each project/activity will include: Documentation of a systems engineering approach used to solve enterprise-defined patient safety concern(s), including design algorithm and bi-directional accountability structure(s) for the activity/project Key project improvement document(s) (e.g. charter, A3, process improvement map, root cause analysis, cycles of improvement, etc.) Documentation of simulation contributing to the achievement of enterprise-level goals and improved quality of care Description of Interprofessional engagement and impact Metric outcomes demonstrating system improvements Report of findings to organizational leadership, including minutes demonstrating review and feedback (ii) Provide evidence that demonstrates sustained (minimum 6 months), positive outcomes achieved by activities in which simulation was used, spanning multiple disciplines (iii) Provide evidence that demonstrates organizational leadership's ongoing assessment of outcome metrics

2. INTEGRATION WITH QUALITY & SAFETY ACTIVITIES: *The Program has an established and committed role in institutional quality assessment and safety processes.*

Provide a brief summary of how the Simulation Program addresses the Integration with quality and Safety Activities requirements described below (not more than 250 words)

(a) There is clear evidence of participation by simulation leadership in the design and process of transformational improvement activities at the organizational level

(i) Provide performance improvement committee rosters and minutes from at least two (2) meetings during the past 2 years to verify contributions of simulation personnel

(ii) Demonstration of accezss to appropriate qualified human factors, psychometric, and/or systems engineering support or resources

References

1. Institute of Medicine (IOM) Committee on Quality of Health Care in America Institute of Medicine. To err is human: building a safer health system. Report no.: 9780309068376, The National Academies Press; 2000.
2. Nielsen AL, Hilwig H, Kissoon N, Teelucksingh S. Discrete event simulation as a tool in optimization of a professional complex adaptive system. Stud Health Technol Inform. 2008;136:247–52.
3. National Academy of Engineering and Institute of Medicine. Building a better delivery system: a new engineering/health care partnership. Washington: National Academies Press; 2005.
4. Institute of Medicine (IOM) Committee on Quality of Health Care in America, Institute of Medicine. Crossing the quality chasm: a new health system for the 21st century. Report no.: 9780309072809, The National Academies Press; 2001.
5. Deutsch ES, Mancini MB, Dunn WF, et al. Informational guide for the accreditation process. https://ssih.org/uploads/committees/2012_SSH%20Accreditation%20Informational%20Guide.pdf. Accessed 24 Jan 2012.
6. Shortell SM, Singer SJ. Improving patient safety by taking systems seriously. JAMA. 2008;299:445–7.
7. Bates DW, Larizgoitia I, Prasopa-Plaizier N, Jha AK. Global priorities for patient safety research. BMJ. 2009;338:1242–4.
8. Chantler C. The role and education of doctors in the delivery of health care. Lancet. 1999;353:1178–81.
9. Kamath JR, Osborn JB, Roger VL, Rohleder TR. Highlights from the third annual Mayo Clinic conference on systems engineering and operations research in health care. Mayo Clin Proc. 2011;86:781–6.
10. Donabedian A. Evaluating the quality of medical care. Milbank Mem Fund Quart. 1966;44:166–206.
11. Carayon P, Schoofs Hundt A, Karsh BT, et al. Work system design for patient safety: the SEIPS model. Qual Saf Health Care. 2006;15:i50–8.
12. Nolan TW. System changes to improve patient safety. Br Med J. 2000;320:771–3.
13. Robinson S. Simulation: the practice of model development and use. New York: Wiley; 2004.
14. Rouse WB, Cortese DA. Engineering the system of healthcare delivery 1st ed. Washington, DC: IOS Press; 2012.
15. Kobayashi L, Shapiro MJ, Sucov A, et al. Portable advanced medical simulation for new emergency department testing and orientation. Acad Emerg Med. 2006;13:691–5.
16. Rodriguez-Paz JM, Mark LJ, Herzer KR, et al. A novel process for introducing a new intraoperative program: a multidisciplinary paradigm for mitigating hazards and improving patient safety. Anesth Analg. 2009;108:202–10.
17. Christensen C. Disruptive innovation. http://www.claytonchristensen.com/key-concepts/. Accessed 27 Mar 2013.
18. Christensen CM. The innovator's dilemma: the revolutionary book that will change the way you do business. New York: Harper Collins; 2000.
19. Smith R. Technology disruption in the simulation industry. J Defense Model Simul. 2006;3:3–10.
20. Bearman M, Brooks PM, Campher D, et al. AusSETT program. http://www.aussett.edu.au/. Accessed 12 Dec 2011.
21. Holmboe E, Rizzolo MA, Sachdeva AK, Rosenberg M, Ziv A. Simulation-based assessment and the regulation of healthcare professionals. Simul Healthc. 2011;6(Suppl):S58–62.
22. Ben-Menachem E, Ezri T, Ziv A, Sidi A, Brill S, Berkenstadt H. Objective structured clinical examination-based assessment of regional anesthesia skills: the Israeli National Board Examination in anesthesiology experience. Anesth Analg. 2011;112:242–5.
23. van Zanten M, Boulet JR, McKinley D. Using standardized patients to assess the interpersonal skills of physicians: six years' experience with a high-stakes certification examination. Health Commun. 2007;22:195–205.
24. Cregan P, Watterson L. High stakes assessment using simulation – an Australian experience. Stud Health Technol Inform. 2005;111:99–104.
25. Amin Z, Boulet JR, Cook DA, Ellaway R, Fahal A, Kneebone R, Maley M, Ostergaard D, Ponnamperuma G, Wearn A, Ziv A. Technology-enabled assessment of health professions education: consensus statement and recommendations from the Ottawa 2010 conference. 2010; Miami; 2010.
26. Barsuk JH, McGaghie WC, Cohen ER, O'Leary KJ, Wayne DB. Simulation-based mastery learning reduces complications during central venous catheter insertion in a medical intensive care unit. Crit Care Med. 2009;37:2697–701.
27. Barsuk JH, Cohen ER, Feinglass J, McGaghie WC, Wayne DB. Use of simulation-based education to reduce catheter-related bloodstream infections. Arch Intern Med. 2009;169:1420–3.
28. Duncan DR, Morgenthaler TI, Ryu JH, Daniels CE. Reducing iatrogenic risk in thoracentesis: establishing best practice via experiential training in a zero-risk environment. Chest. 2009;135: 1315–20.
29. Fried GM, Feldman LS, Vassiliou MC, et al. Proving the value of simulation in laparoscopic surgery. Ann Surg. 2004;240:518–25; discussion 25–8.
30. Sedlack RE, Kolars JC. Computer simulator training enhances the competency of gastroenterology fellows at colonoscopy: results of a pilot study. Am J Gastroenterol. 2004;99:33–7.
31. Zendejas B, Cook DA, Bingener J, et al. Simulation-based mastery learning improves patient outcomes in laparoscopic inguinal hernia repair: a randomized controlled trial. Ann Surg. 2011;254:502–9; discussion 9–11.
32. Cook DA, Hatala R, Brydges R, et al. Technology-enhanced simulation for health professions education: a systematic review and meta-analysis. JAMA. 2011;306:978–88.
33. Gardner R, Walzer TB, Simon R, Raemer DB. Obstetric simulation as a risk control strategy: course design and evaluation. Simul Healthc. 2008;3:119–27.
34. Hanscom R. Medical simulation from an insurer's perspective. Acad Emerg Med. 2008;15:984–7.
35. Ludmerer KM. Time to heal: American medical education from the turn of the century to the era of managed care. Oxford: Oxford University Press; 2005.

Competency Assessment

11

Ross J. Scalese and Rose Hatala

Introduction

Writing this chapter on a topic as broad as "competency assessment" posed a somewhat daunting challenge. There are so many facets of assessment (about each of which whole chapters and indeed whole textbooks could be/have been written). We don't claim to be "the world's leading authorities" on any one aspect of assessment, but over the years we have both gained significant research [1–3] and practical [4, 5] experience with assessment methodologies, in particular as they relate to using simulations for evaluative purposes. Because simulation enthusiasts sometimes think that these modalities constitute a universe unto themselves, where fundamental principles of education don't apply, we will start each discussion in generic terms and then explore the relevance of simulations to each topic. Accordingly, our goal in this chapter is to provide a fairly comprehensive introduction to assessment, including important terms and concepts, as well as a broad framework for thinking first about the evaluation of competence in general and then, more specifically, about the application of simulation methods in the assessment context.

Historical Perspective

In the 1960s, Stephen Abrahamson conducted pioneering work employing simulations in medical education—first with Howard Barrows using "programmed patients" (what we now call simulated or standardized patients [SPs]) [6] and later with Denson and Wolf describing the first computer-enhanced mannequin, "Sim One" [7]. Interestingly, whereas Sim One was used mainly for training (of anesthesiology residents), SPs were initially developed specifically for assessment (of neurology clerkship students), as a proposed solution to some of the methodological challenges with traditional testing of clinical skills in actual patient care settings. Barrows and Abrahamson first reported this foundational work nearly 50 years ago, but the opening paragraph of that article offers a definition of assessment and description of its purposes, as well as a rationale for using simulation in this context, which are still extremely relevant today: "As in all phases of medical education, measurement of student performance is necessary to determine the effectiveness of teaching methods, to recognize individual student difficulties so that assistance may be offered and, lastly, to provide the basis for a reasonably satisfactory appraisal of student performance. However, the evaluative procedure must be consistent with the goals of the particular educational experience. Difficulties occur in clinical clerkships because adequate testing in clinical teaching is beset by innumerable problems" [6].

We will return to this quotation several times throughout this chapter, as we explore different facets of assessment in general, as well as the specific applications of simulation methods for evaluative purposes.

Definition of Terms

A quick online search using a dictionary application yields the following definition of *assessment*: "the evaluation or estimation of the nature, quality, or ability of someone or something" [8]. This broad but useful definition includes the closely related term *evaluation*, which to a certain extent connotes more of a quantitative estimation of a given characteristic of someone or something. In the educational context, some authors draw a distinction between these terms, reserving "assessment" for methods of obtaining information used

R.J. Scalese, MD, FACP (✉)
Division of Research and Technology, Gordon Center for Research in Medical Education, University of Miami Miller School of Medicine, 016960 (D-41), Miami, FL 33101, USA
e-mail: rscalese@med.miami.edu

R. Hatala, MD, MSc
Department of Medicine, University of British Columbia, Suite 5907, Burrard Bldg., Vancouver, BC V6Z 1Y6, Canada

Department of Medicine, St. Paul's Hospital, 1081 Burrard St., Vancouver, BC, V6Z 1Y6, Canada

A.I. Levine et al. (eds.), *The Comprehensive Textbook of Healthcare Simulation*, DOI 10.1007/978-1-4614-5993-4_11,

to draw inferences about *people* and "evaluation" for similar systematic approaches used to determine characteristics about some instructional unit or educational *program*. (Note that the quotation above from Barrows and Abrahamson refers to both reasons why "measurement of student performance is necessary" [6]). For the purposes of discussion in this chapter, we will use these terms almost interchangeably, although generally our considerations will focus on the assessment of learning, skill acquisition, or other educational achievement by people, namely, healthcare professionals in training or in practice.

Similarly, the discussion to follow will employ two other closely related terms: in general, we will refer broadly to medical "simulations," meaning any approximation of an actual clinical situation—thus including computer-based virtual patients, standardized patients, and so on—that attempts to present assessment problems realistically. On the other hand, we define "simulators" more narrowly to mean medical simulation *devices* designed to imitate real patients, anatomic regions, or clinical tasks; these run the gamut of technologies that encompasses part task trainers, computer-enhanced mannequins, and virtual reality (VR) simulators. Various simulation modalities will be described in greater detail in chapters that follow in the next section of this textbook, but, again, the focus here will be on the use of simulations for assessment purposes. In this context, those undergoing evaluation will see cues and consequences very much like those in actual clinical environments, and they must act as they would under real-world conditions. Of course, for various reasons—engineering limitations, cost and time constraints, psychometric requirements, and so on—a simulation will never be completely identical to "the real thing" [9].

As is unavoidable in any discussion on simulation, this brings us to another important term: "fidelity." We will use this in a very general way to describe aspects of the likeness of the simulation to the real-life circumstances it aims to mirror. This authenticity of duplication can refer not only to the appearance of the simulation ("physical" or "engineering fidelity") but also to the behaviors required within the simulated environment ("functional" or "psychological fidelity") [10]. Because of these different facets of fidelity, much inconsistency in defining and using the term exists in the simulation literature; to compound this problem, "high fidelity" has also come to imply "high tech" because advanced technology components (e.g., some of the full-body computer-enhanced mannequins or virtual reality devices) may contribute to the increasing realism of simulations available today. We will explore the idea of fidelity in greater depth later in the chapter (see section "Validity").

Throughout the chapter, we will follow common usage with general terms like "tools," "techniques," and "modalities." Whenever possible, however, we will use two other terms more specifically, drawing a distinction between assessment *methods* and rating *instruments*. We can think of a transportation analogy: "Methods" would refer to travel by air, ground, or sea, and the correlate would be assessment by written exam, performance-based tests, or clinical observation. Within these categories are further subclassifications: ground travel can be via car, bus, or motorcycle, just as performance-based tests can be conducted as a long case or as a simulation. Rating "instruments," on the other hand, are used in conjunction with almost all of the assessment methods to measure or judge examinee performance and assign some type of score. These most commonly include things like checklists and global rating scales, and detailed discussion of such instruments is beyond the scope of this chapter.

One final note as something of a disclaimer: we (the authors) naturally draw on our personal educational and clinical experiences to inform the discussion that follows. Therefore, we will frequently cite examples within the contexts of physician education and the North American systems with which we are most familiar. This is not to discount invaluable contributions and lessons learned from experiences in nursing and other healthcare professions or in other countries; rather, our intention is simply to illustrate points that we feel are broadly applicable to simulation-based education across the health professions worldwide.

Outcomes-Based Education

So why is it important for us to talk about assessment? For most of the last century, discussion in the health professions education literature focused chiefly on the teaching/learning *process*; for example, issues of curriculum design (traditional separation of the basic and clinical sciences vs. a more vertically and horizontally integrated approach) and content delivery (the more common large-group, instructor-led lecture format vs. small-group, problem-based and student-centered learning) dominated the debate among educationists. Earlier chapters in this textbook similarly addressed educational process questions, this time in the context of simulation-based teaching environments; for example, (how) should we use humor or stress to enhance the learning experience or what are different/preferred methods of debriefing.

Somewhere along the line, however, amid all the discourse about various ways of teaching and optimal processes to promote student learning, our focus wavered and we lost sight of the final *product*: at the end of the day, what is a graduating medical or nursing student supposed to look like? What competencies does a resident or fellow need to have at the completion of postgraduate training? What knowledge, skills, and attitudes does a practicing clinician need to possess in order to provide safe and effective patient-centered care? Glaring examples [11, 12] of what a healthcare professional is *not* supposed to look like (or do) brought things sharply back into focus; over the last decade or so, the issue of public accountability, perhaps more than any other influence, has driven a paradigm shift toward *outcomes-* or *competency-based education* [13, 14]. In response to public demand for assurance that doctors and other healthcare providers are competent, academic institutions and professional organizations worldwide have increased self-regulation and set quality standards that their graduates or practitioners must meet. Of course, it is not sufficient merely to list various competencies or expected outcomes of the educational process: implicit in the competency-based model is the need to demonstrate that required outcomes have actually been achieved. It is this essential requirement that assessment fulfills.

Global Core Competency Frameworks

In keeping with the evolution to this outcomes-based educational model, then, many different organizations and accrediting bodies have enumerated core competencies that describe the various knowledge, skills, and attitudes that healthcare professionals should possess at various stages in their training and, most importantly, when they are entering or actually in practice. Examples include the Institute for International Medical Education's definition of the "global minimum essential requirements" of *undergraduate* medical programs, which are grouped within seven broad educational outcome-competence domains: (1) professional values, attitudes, behavior, and ethics; (2) scientific foundation of medicine; (3) clinical skills; (4) communication skills; (5) population health and health systems; (6) management of information; and (7) critical thinking and research [15]. These "essentials" are meant to represent only the core around which different countries could customize medical curricula according to their unique requirements and resources. Accordingly, focusing on what the graduating medical student should look like, in the UK, the General Medical Council (GMC) describes "Tomorrow's Doctors" with knowledge, skills, and behaviors very broadly grouped under three outcomes [16], whereas the five schools in Scotland organize their scheme based on three slightly different essential elements and then within these further elaborate 12 domains encompassing the learning outcomes that "The Scottish Doctor" should be able to demonstrate upon graduation [17].

By contrast, in North America, the most commonly used competency-based frameworks focus on outcomes for *graduate* medical education programs; in Canada, the Royal College of Physicians and Surgeons (RCPSC) outlines in the CanMEDS framework seven roles that all physicians need to integrate to be better doctors [18], and in the United States, the Accreditation Council for Graduate Medical Education (ACGME) describes desired outcomes of physician training categorized under six general competencies [19]. The GMC in the UK, in their guidance about what constitutes "Good Medical Practice" [20], outlines desired attributes for doctors not only in postgraduate training but also in clinical practice in that country. Although the number and definition of essential outcomes vary somewhat among different frameworks, the fundamental description of what a physician should look like at the end of medical school, upon completion of postgraduate training, and on into professional practice is strikingly similar across these and other schemes. In like fashion, nursing, physician assistants, veterinary medicine, and other health professions all enumerate the core competencies required of trainees and practitioners in those fields [21–24].

Criteria for Good Assessment

Before we can discuss various methods to assess any of the outcomes described in these competency frameworks, we should first establish criteria for judging the quality of different evaluation tools. Such appraisal has traditionally focused on the psychometric properties of a given test, particularly its reliability and validity, but more recently assessment experts have proposed additional factors to consider when weighing the advantages and disadvantages of various modalities and deciding which to use for a specific purpose [25, 26].

Reliability

In its simplest conception, reliability means consistency of performance. In the context of educational testing, reliability is a property of *data* produced by an assessment method and refers to the reproducibility of scores obtained from an exam across multiple administrations under similar conditions. An analogy to archery is sometimes drawn to illustrate this concept: imagine two archers (representing two different assessments) taking aim at a target where different rings are assigned different point values. Each archer has several tries, and one hits the bull's-eye every time, while the other hits the same spot in the outer ring every time. Both archers would receive the same score on each trial, and, in this sense, they would be considered equally reliable.

We refer to this as *test-retest reliability* when, as in the archery example, the same individuals undergo the exact same assessment but at different times. Another aspect of reliability is *equivalence*: this is the degree to which scores are replicable if either (1) the same test is administered to different groups (sharing essential characteristics, such as level of training) or (2) the same examinees take two different forms of the exam (matched for number, structure, level of difficulty, and content of questions). Yet another facet of reliability is *internal consistency*: this concept is related to that of equivalence, in that correlations are calculated to gauge reproducibility of scores obtained by two different measures, this time using different questions (e.g., all the odd- vs. even-numbered items) within the same exam. The chief advantage of this so-called split-half method is practicality because reliability coefficients can be calculated from a single test administration [27, pp. 57–66; 28, pp. 15–17; 29, pp. 307–308].

Thus far we have been speaking about assessment instruments that produce data that can be objectively scored (e.g., answers to multiple-choice questions are either right or wrong). Scoring for other evaluation methods, however, often entails some subjectivity on the part of human raters, thereby introducing measurement variance that will potentially limit the reliability of resulting data. In these cases, attention must be paid to other types of reliability. *Inter-rater reliability* refers to the agreement of scores given to the same candidate by two or more independent examiners. Even in situations where there is only one person marking a given assessment, *intra-rater reliability* is important, as it represents the consistency with which an individual assessor applies a scoring rubric and generates data that are replicable over time, either across multiple examinees on a given day or upon rescoring (e.g., by videotape review) of the same performances at a later date [27, pp. 66–70; 28, pp. 16–17; 29, pp. 308–309].

Reliability of Simulation-Based Assessments

Assessments of clinical competence, however, are somewhat different than other evaluation settings (e.g., intelligence testing), in which there are ordinarily just two main sources of variance in measurement: (1) "exam" factors and (2) "examinee" factors. By addressing the reliability problems discussed above, we attempt to control for those "exam" variables—issues related to the assessment instrument itself or the raters using the tool—such that the construct of interest (in this case, differing intelligence among examinees) accounts for most of the observed variation in scores. Almost by definition, though, the assessment equation in the context of health professions education contains a third variable representing "patient" factors (or disease process or clinical task). Indeed, Barrows and Abrahamson were referring chiefly to reliability issues when they said "…adequate testing in clinical [settings] is beset by innumerable problems" [6, p. 802]. Their solution, novel at the time, was to employ simulations, whose programmability confers a generally high degree of reliability: SPs can be trained to present history and physical exam findings in a consistent manner, and simulators can be programmed to respond in a reproducible way to various maneuvers and even invasive procedures. In this way, simulations eliminate the risk of harm to real patients and minimize the variability inherent in actual clinical encounters. The ability to present assessment problems accurately and repeatedly in the same manner to any number of examinees is one of the key strengths of simulations for evaluation purposes. This reproducibility becomes particularly important when high-stakes decisions (e.g., licensure and specialty board certification) hinge on these assessments, as is discussed in greater detail in Chap. 12.

Validity

Tightly interconnected with reliability, the concept of validity is perhaps more nuanced and, consequently, often misunderstood. One definition of validity is the degree to which a test measures what it was intended to measure. Back to the archery analogy: both archers—one who hit the bull's-eye every time and one who hit the same spot in the outer ring every time—are equally reliable. If these archers represent two different assessments, both of whose aim is to measure some outcome represented by the bull's-eye, then clearly the first archer's shots would be considered more valid. Thus, whereas reliability relates to consistency, validity refers to accuracy. In other words, validity reflects the degree to which we are "on target" with our assessments.

This simplified notion of validity, however, belies a significant evolution over the past 40–50 years in our understanding of the concept. As an associate editor (RH) and external reviewers (both authors) for health professions journals, we often receive submitted manuscripts that describe study methods in terms such as "Using the *previously validated* 'XYZ Checklist'…." The implication is that validity is an attribute of particular rating instruments or evaluation methods per se—in our example above, that the shots themselves are valid or not—but we feel this is a misconception. Whereas reliability is a property of the data collected in an assessment, validity is a characteristic of the *interpretations* of this data. Validity is not intrinsic to a given assessment method or the scores derived from a particular test; rather, it is the *inferences* we draw and *decisions* we make based on those scores that are valid (or not). If both archers' aim is to measure the same construct (say, distance to the bull's-eye determined by the length of a string attached to the arrow), then the first archer's shots would lead to more valid conclusions about what the "true" distance is to the bull's-eye.

The Validity Argument

Consequently, establishing validity is not as straightforward as conducting one study of an assessment and calculating some "validity coefficient." Instead, the validation process involves making a structured and coherent argument, based on theoretical rationales and the accumulation of empiric evidence, to support (or refute) intended interpretations of assessment results [30, pp. 21–24; 31]. The concept of validity is critically dependent on first specifying the purpose of an assessment and then considering other factors related to the particular context in which it takes place: "There is no such thing as a *valid test*! The score from any given test could be used to make a variety of decisions in different contexts and with different examinee populations; evidence to support the validity of one type of interpretation in one context with one population may or may not support the validity of a different interpretation in a different context with a different population" [28, p. 10]. Hence, if the purpose of our archery contest had been to measure the distance, not to the bull's-eye but to the outer ring of the target, then the second archer's shots would lead to more valid decisions based on the length of string attached to those arrows. If the aim, however, was to evaluate a completely different construct (for instance, the distance to something that was located in the opposite direction behind the archers' backs), then no valid or meaningful interpretation could be made based on results of either assessment, despite their both yielding highly reliable results.

These last two examples illustrate the point that inferences or decisions based on scores may not be valid despite having reliable data for consideration. The contrary proposition, however, is not true: without reliable data, meaningful interpretation is impossible. Thus, as mentioned at the very beginning of this section, reliability and validity are inextricably bound in the context of assessment, with reliability of measurement being a necessary (but insufficient) prerequisite for valid interpretation and decision-making based on evaluation results. In fact, assumptions and assertions about reliability issues constitute just one step in a whole series of inferences we make whenever we draw conclusions from a given assessment.

Kane's Validity Framework

Michael Kane proposed an approach to validity that systematically accumulates evidence to build an overall argument in support of a given decision based on test results. This argument is structured according to four main links in the "chain of inferences" that extends from exam administration to final interpretation:

1. *Scoring*—inferences here chiefly concern collecting data/making observations. Evidence for/against these inferences examines whether the test was administered under standardized conditions, examinee performance/responses were captured accurately, scoring rubrics and conversion/scaling procedures were applied consistently and correctly, and appropriate security protocols were in place.
2. *Generalization*—inferences here mainly pertain to generalizing specific observations from one assessment to the "universe" of possible test observations. Evidence for/against these inferences chiefly addresses whether appropriate procedures were used for test construction and sampling from among possible test items and reliability issues were addressed, including identification of sources of variance in observed scores or sources of measurement error and checks for internal consistency.
3. *Extrapolation*—inferences here principally involve extrapolating from observations in the testing environment to performance in actual professional practice. Evidence for/against these inferences analyzes the degree to which scores on the exam correspond to other variables/outcomes of interest or predict real-world performance.
4. *Decision*—inferences here form the basis for the final interpretation or actions based on scores. Evidence for/against this component explores whether procedures for determination of cut scores were appropriately established and implemented; decision rules follow a theoretical framework that is sound and applicable to the given context; decisions are credible to examinees, the professional community, and other stakeholders, including the public; and consideration was given to the consequences of such decisions when developing the assessment [28, pp. 12–22; 32].

Characteristics of different assessment methods influence which components of the validity argument are typically strongest and which usually represent "the weakest link." Threats to the validity of any of the assumptions weaken the overall argument in support of a given interpretation. For example, with written assessments such as MCQ exams used for board certification, scoring and generalization components of the validity argument are generally strong: exam conditions and security are tightly controlled and grading of examinee responses is objective, and because such exams typically feature a large number of items, there is ample research evidence demonstrating robust measurement properties and high reliability. On the other hand, the greatest threats to the validity of decisions based on written exam scores come in the form of arguments concerning the extrapolation of results. Although they directly measure knowledge and, to a certain extent, problem-solving skills requiring application of this knowledge, by their nature, written assessments can provide only indirect information about actual examinee behaviors in real clinical settings. Empirical evidence demonstrating a relationship between scores on standardized written exams and some other performance-based assessment would strengthen the validity of inferences in this extrapolation component, as well as the overall argument in favor of using scores on such an exam to make, say, selection decisions for further training [33, 34].

Validity Argument for Simulation-Based Assessments

In similar fashion, we can use Kane's argument-based approach to consider validity issues as they relate to simulation-based assessments. For instance, during our discussion about reliability, we highlighted the programmability of simulations as one of their strengths for evaluation purposes. We assume, therefore, that all examinees receive test stimuli presented in a reproducible and standardized manner, but threats to the validity of this assumption are not difficult to imagine: simulators might malfunction or SPs might deviate from the script and decide to "ad lib." The argument to support assumptions made in the *scoring* component, then, could include evidence that mannequins are periodically tested to ensure proper operation, that SPs receive extensive training regarding their roles, and that quality control checks for internal consistency are made by observing SP performances.

Concerning inferences about the generalizability of test observations from one "snapshot" in time, the relatively small number of items on most simulation-based assessments is problematic. For example, the leap from a single evaluation of a surgical resident's performance on a virtual reality (VR) laparoscopy trainer to what the same resident's performance might be over many different observations of related surgical skills (with the same simulator or even different forms of simulation) is a potentially risky inference. This problem of case or content specificity (also called "construct underrepresentation" in the validity literature [30]) constitutes one of the major threats to validity across many assessment modalities, particularly those based on observational methods, whether in simulated environments or in real clinical settings. The only effective way to reinforce this "weak link" in the *generalization* component of the validity argument is by increasing the number of cases in an assessment. One of the advantages of simulations is that more cases can be developed and implemented as needed (within the constraint of available resources), unlike assessments based on observation of actual clinical encounters, which are generally restricted to the patients, conditions, or procedures available in the hospital or clinic on a given day [28, pp. 18–19; 33]. Development of multi-station examination formats—with many, brief, and varied simulations rather than one long testing scenario, such as in Objective Structured Clinical Examinations (OSCEs)—was another attempt to solve just such problems with the generalizability of results from clinical assessments.

The next component of the validity argument—*extrapolation*—also requires evidence to substantiate assumptions that examinee performance under test conditions is likely to be representative of future performance, this time in actual clinical situations, rather than just under similar testing conditions. Such evidence could be drawn from empiric correlation of assessment data with real-world variables of interest, such as level of experience or patient care outcomes. For example, the argument that performance on a VR endoscopy simulator is predictive of competence performing real endoscopies would be strengthened if (1) attending gastroenterologists with many years of endoscopy experience score higher on a test utilizing the simulator than postgraduate trainees with limited real-life experience, who in turn score higher than novices with no endoscopy experience, and/or (2) those scoring higher on the simulation-based test have lower rates of complications when performing endoscopies on real patients than those with lower test scores and vice versa. Experiments to gather evidence in support of the first hypothesis are frequently conducted because prospective studies designed to test the second would raise significant ethical, and possibly legal, questions!

In contradistinction to written tests, where the extrapolation component of the validity argument is often the weakest link (because they simply cannot replicate psychomotor and other elements of real-world clinical tasks), the high degree of realism of VR and other modern simulators seems prima facie to strengthen the "predictive validity" of assessment methods using these technologies. It is here that the idea of fidelity becomes important, as it is often cited to support the extrapolation phase of the validity argument: the assumption is that the more authentic the simulation (as with some high-tech simulators currently available), the more likely it is that performance in the assessment will predict real-world behaviors. Of course, we have already stated that a simulation, by its very nature, is never completely identical to "the real thing." Indeed, the more we manipulate aspects of a scenario (e.g., to improve standardization or include rare clinical content), the more artificiality we introduce. Consequently, steps to strengthen the scoring and generalization components of our validity argument may come at the cost of weakening the extrapolation link to real-world clinical practice [33].

Moreover, as mentioned very early in this chapter, the concept of fidelity has many facets, and we should take care to differentiate among them. Engineering fidelity refers to the degree to which the simulation device or environment reproduces the physical appearance of the real system (in this case, actual clinical encounters), whereas psychological fidelity refers to the degree to which the simulation duplicates the skills and behaviors required in real-life patient care situations [10]. At this point, we should recall our basic definition of validity—the degree to which a test measures what it was intended to measure—from which it becomes clear that high-level psychological fidelity is much more important than engineering fidelity, because real-world behaviors, not just appearances, are the ultimate "target" of our assessments. After all, "appearances can be deceiving." For instance, while it may seem that we are assessing cardiopulmonary resuscitation (CPR) skills using a "high-fidelity" human patient simulator, outcome measures may correlate better with examinees' prior exposure/practice with that particular mannequin than with actual level of proficiency in performing CPR, or returning to the earlier example of a VR endoscopy simulator, scores may turn out to correlate better with users' experience playing video games than with actual procedural experience. In such cases, factors other than the competency of interest influence scores, introducing a major threat to validity known as "construct-irrelevant variance" [28, pp. 20–21; 30]. Data obtained from the assessment may still be highly reliable, because this source of measurement error is not random but systematic, making it sometimes difficult to detect. Especially with assessments employing high-tech simulators, therefore, description of orientation sessions for all examinees to control for the confounding variable of familiarity with the "hardware" could strengthen the extrapolation phase of the validity argument. Beyond components of the simulation itself, a related threat to validity can arise due to the manner in which rating instruments are constructed and used: if scores are derived, say, from a checklist of action items, examinees might learn to "game the system" by stating or performing numerous steps that they might not actually do in real life in order to maximize points on the test. To argue against this potential threat to validity, evidence could be presented about procedures used to minimize effects of such a "shotgun approach," including differential weighting of checklist items and penalties for extraneous or incorrect actions [28].

As with most testing methodologies, especially when high-stakes determinations rest on assessment results, the final interpretation or *decision* phase of the validity argument for simulation-based methods should offer evidence that cut scores or pass/fail judgments were established using defensible standards [35, 36]. Moreover, the assessment process and resulting final decisions must be credible to various stakeholders: even if ample evidence supports the scoring, generalization, and extrapolation portions of the validity argument, final interpretations of test scores are only valid if parties to whom resulting decisions are important believe they are meaningful. For example, the public places trust in the process of board certification to guarantee that practitioners are competent and duly qualified in a given specialty. If numerous "bad apples" (who ultimately commit malpractice) were found to have cleared all the requisite evaluation hurdles and still somehow slipped through the system, then the validity of such certification decisions would be called into question.

Educational Impact

Samuel Messick was a psychologist and assessment expert who articulated the view that consideration of the consequences of testing is an important component of the validation process [37]. This shifted the discussion in the education community from one focused mostly on the scientific or psychometric evaluation of test data to a broader discourse on the secondary effects of assessment implementation and decisions. "Assessment drives learning." As is captured in this often repeated expression, one clear consequence of testing is the influence it can have on what teachers choose to teach and what students choose to study. Lambert Schuwirth and Cees van der Vleuten are two thought leaders (from Maastricht University in the Netherlands) who have carried Messick's view into the realm of health professional education and spoken eloquently about the need to look beyond reliability and validity as the sole indicators of assessment quality and also consider the educational impact, both positive and negative, of testing programs. Moreover, they argue that it is not enough to simply acknowledge that learners will be motivated to study in different ways by both the content and form of required examinations; we should actually capitalize on this phenomenon by purposely designing assessment systems in such a way as to steer learners' educational efforts in a desirable direction [38].

Educational Impact of Simulation-Based Assessments

One of the most notable examples of the way simulation-based assessment has driven learning can be seen with the introduction of the Step 2 Clinical Skills component (Step 2 CS) of the United States Medical Licensing Examination (USMLE) [39]. Developed by the National Board of Medical Examiners (NBME), this multistep examination is required for physician licensure in the United States. The Step 2 CS component was added to assess hands-on performance of history-taking and physical examination skills as well as attributes of professionalism. Simulations are central to this exam, in that examinees interact with and evaluate a series of SPs, who are trained not only to provide the history and mimic certain physical exam findings but also to score candidates' performance of these clinical tasks using standardized checklists. The impact of introducing this additional step to the USMLE was felt even before full implementation: as soon as the final decision to add the new exam component was announced, medical schools altered curricula to increase emphasis on teaching and learning these clinical skills, including development of "mock board" exams at local institutions to give their students practice with this testing format. In fact, special simulation labs and clinical skills centers sprang up with astounding rapidity, such that now—only 8 years after introduction of the Step 2 CS exam—nearly every medical school in the USA has a well-established program utilizing SPs for teaching and assessing these clinical skills.

To the extent that history-taking and physical exam skills are considered fundamental competencies for any physician to practice safely and effectively, increased emphasis on teaching and learning these skills would appear to be a beneficial effect of the assessment program. Sometimes, however, the impact on educational and other learner attributes can be unexpected and negative and due not so much to examination content as testing format. What has been observed at the examination is that some students take a "shotgun" approach, aiming to "tick all the boxes" by asking numerous irrelevant questions in the history and performing many examination maneuvers, with little attention to those elements that will be of highest yield in a patient with certain signs and symptoms. In addition, many students perform history taking in a robotic manner, seeking only factual information rather than developing a more humanistic and patient-centered approach. If, as mentioned in the previous section, examinees are trying to "game the system" in this way, then this represents a threat to the predictive validity of the assessment process. If, on the other hand, we are to infer that such student behaviors can be extrapolated to performance in actual patient care settings, then clearly the impact of the assessment process will have been negative. In response to this observed effect, the NBME announced that the scoring rubric for interpersonal communication elements in the Step 2 CS would change in 2012 [40]. There is no doubt that this, in turn, will impact the way communication skills are taught, learned, and assessed in the future; questions about the magnitude, direction, and ultimate benefit (or harm) of this continuing evolution remain.

Catalytic Effect

Recently a panel of health professions educational experts elaborated a consensus statement and recommendations concerning seven "criteria for good assessment" [26]. We have already discussed most of these factors to be weighed in judging the quality of assessment programs, including (using their terminology) (1) validity or coherence, (2) reproducibility or consistency, (3) equivalence, (4) acceptability, and (5) educational effect. In their treatment of the last element, however, they draw a distinction between the impact that testing has on individual learners—"the assessment motivates those who take it to prepare in a fashion that has educational benefit" [26]—and what they call *catalytic effect*: "the assessment provides results and feedback in a fashion that creates, enhances, and supports education; it drives future learning forward" [26]. The working group emphasized this as a (sixth) separate criterion against which to judge assessments, viewing it as both important and desirable. This kind of catalytic effect can influence medical school curricula, provide impetus to reform initiatives, and set national priorities in medical education, such as we described as a result of the simulation-based assessments in the USMLE Step 2 CS exam.

Purposes of Assessment

The overarching reasons for conducting an assessment have a clear relationship to the educational impact it is likely to make. Just as the purpose of an assessment was of fundamental importance to the process of validation, so, too, this context must be considered in order to anticipate the probable consequences of implementing a new evaluation scheme. On one hand, testing carried out primarily to determine whether (and to what degree) learners achieve educational objectives is said to be for *summative* purposes. This usually occurs at the end of a unit of instruction (e.g., exams at the end of a course, year, or program) and typically involves assignment of a specific grade or categorization as "pass or fail." Not infrequently summative assessments involve high-stakes decisions, such as advancement to the next educational level or qualification for a particular scope of practice, and, therefore, these are the types of assessments most likely to have a catalytic educational effect. We have already mentioned some of the ways (both positive and negative) that such high-stakes exams can influence not only the study patterns and behaviors of individual learners but also local institutions' curricula and even national educational agendas. On the other hand, assessments undertaken chiefly to identify particular areas of weakness in order to direct continued learning toward the goal of eventual improvement are said to serve a *formative* purpose. Although often thought of as distinct components of an educational system, this is the area where teaching and testing become intertwined. While it might seem that formative assessments, by definition, will have a positive educational impact, care must be exercised in how the formative feedback is given, lest it have unanticipated negative effects. This can be especially true with simulation-based methods: because of the high level of interactivity, and depending on the degree of psychological fidelity, learners can suspend disbelief and become significantly invested in the outcomes of a given situation. Imagine then the possible negative consequences of designing a testing scenario—even if intended to teach lessons about dealing with bad outcomes or difficult emotional issues—wherein the patient always dies. Occasionally individuals will instead learn detrimental coping strategies or adopt avoidance behaviors if confronted with similar clinical circumstances in the future. Awareness of the fact that our choice of evaluation methods, whether for summative or formative purposes, will have some educational impact, and attempts to anticipate what these effects might be can lead to better assessment systems and improved learning outcomes.

Feasibility

Finally, all of the discourse about reliability and validity issues and educational impact would be strictly academic if an assessment program cannot be implemented for practical reasons. Feasibility is the remaining (seventh) criterion to consider for good evaluation systems, according to the expert group's consensus statement: "The assessment [should be] practical, realistic, and sensible, given the circumstances and context" [26]. Here again we see the importance of context, with local resources being a limiting factor in whether an assessment can be developed and actualized. The first consideration regarding resources is usually financial, but other "costs" including manpower needs and technical expertise must be tallied when deciding whether, for example, a school can mount a new OSCE examination as a summative assessment to decide who will graduate. In addition, too much attention is often paid to start-up costs and not enough consideration is given to resources that will be required to sustain a program. Ultimately, analysis about the feasibility of an assessment should ask not only whether we *can* afford the new system but also whether we *should* expend available resources on initiation, development, maintenance, and refinement of the assessment.

Feasibility of Simulation-Based Assessments

When a needs analysis indicates that simulation-based methods would be the best solution for an evaluation problem on theoretical and educational grounds, costs are usually the first challenge to realization for practical reasons. If simulators, especially newer computer-enhanced mannequins and virtual reality devices, are to be employed, their purchase costs may be prohibitive. The upfront expenses are obvious, but ongoing costs must also be calculated, including those for storage, operation, repair, and updating of the devices over time. For example, beyond the initial costs for high-tech simulators, which sometimes exceed six figures, maintenance and extended service contracts for these devices can easily cost thousands of additional dollars per year. These equipment costs can be considerable, but personnel costs may be more so, especially because they are recurring and are often overlooked in the initial budget calculation: simulation center employees usually include technical personnel who perform upkeep of simulators, administrative staff for scheduling and other day-to-day operational issues, and, if the simulations are undertaken for formative purposes, instructors who may or may not need to have professional expertise in the area of interest. The reckoning must also include indirect costs in time and manpower, which can be substantial, for simulation scenario development, pilot testing, and so on.

Costs for relatively low-tech simulations, likewise, often receive less attention than they deserve: for instance, examinations using SPs for assessment of clinical skills are quite expensive to develop and implement [41]. There are costs related to recruiting and training the SPs, as well as supervision and evaluation of their performance in the assessment role. If the program is designed for widespread (e.g., national) implementation, then this can become a full-time job for the SPs. In addition, testing centers must be built, equipped, and maintained. If raters other than SPs score examinee performances in real time, their employment and training represent yet additional expenses, especially if the assessment requires health professionals with technical expertise as raters, with opportunity costs owing to the time away from their regular clinical duties. For an assessment program like this to be feasible, there must be funding to cover these costs, which oftentimes are passed on to examinees in the form of fees. Practical issues such as these were among the principal reasons why implementation of the USMLE Step 2 CS exam was delayed for many years after the decision was made to incorporate this additional step in the licensure process, and one of the ongoing criticisms about this exam pertains to the additional financial burden it imposes on medical students who are already heavily in debt.

Weighing Assessment Criteria

In judging how good an assessment may be in terms of the criteria described above, different stakeholders will value and prioritize different characteristics. Decisions based on results of testing matter to numerous parties, including individual learners, teachers and their respective programs, professional and regulatory bodies, and, ultimately, the patients on whom the health professionals undergoing these assessments might practice. Obviously not all criteria will or can receive equal emphasis in designing evaluation programs, so various factors must be balanced according to the purpose and context of the assessment. For example, a high-stakes summative exam (e.g., for licensure or board certification) must fulfill criteria related to the need for accountability to regulators and patients, as well as fairness and credibility for examinees and other health professionals. Therefore, validity and reliability considerations may trump educational impact. By contrast, for formative assessments, educational effect is a more desirable attribute than, say, exact reproducibility or equivalence of different exams. As just stated, no matter the purpose of the assessment, feasibility issues will be important because they determine whether a planned testing program will actually come to fruition; clearly though, the practicality issues will vary considerably depending on the purpose, scale, stakes, and other contextual features of an exam [26]. For assessment planners using simulation-based methods, the trade-offs and differential weighting of different quality criteria will be the same as for various other evaluation methods.

Assessment Methods

In consideration of these criteria, as well as the outcomes framework operational in a given setting, numerous assessment modalities exist for evaluating relevant competencies. As George Miller stated: "It seems important to start with the forthright acknowledgement that no single assessment method can provide all the data required for judgment of anything so complex as the delivery of professional services by a successful physician" [42]. Moreover, it is beyond this chapter's scope to describe all the available assessment methodologies in great detail; as we stated at the outset, entire chapters and textbooks have been written about these topics, and we refer the reader to several excellent sources for more in-depth discussion—including detailed descriptions with examples of different testing formats, treatment of technical and psychometric issues, analysis of research evidence to support decisions to use a number of modalities, and consideration of advantages, limitations, and practical matters involved with implementation of various assessment methods [43–47]. Instead, we will provide a brief overview of the general types of assessment modalities, with limited examples, and emphasize the importance of choosing evaluation methods that are aligned with the competencies being tested as well as other assessment dimensions.

To organize our thinking about so many different methodologies, it is helpful to group them into a few broadly defined categories. Based on several similar classification schemes [48, pp. 5–9; 49, pp. 7–8; 50], we will consider the following as they apply to the evaluation of health professionals: (1) written and oral assessments, (2) performance-based assessments, (3) clinical observation or work-based assessments, and (4) miscellaneous assessments (for methods that defy easy classification or span more than one category) (see Table 11.1).

Table 11.1 General categories and examples of assessment methods

Category	Examples
Written and oral assessments	Multiple-choice questions (MCQ)
	Matching and extended matching items
	True-false and multiple true-false items
	Fill-in-the-blank items
	Long and short essay questions
	Oral exams/vivas
Performance-based assessments	Long and short cases
	Objective Structured Clinical Examinations (OSCE)
	Simulation-based assessments
Clinical observation or work-based assessments	Mini-Clinical Evaluation Exercise (mini-CEX)
	Direct Observation of Procedural Skills (DOPS)
	360° evaluations/multisource feedback
Miscellaneous assessments	Patient surveys
	Peer assessments
	Self-assessments
	Medical record audits
	Chart-stimulated recall
	Logbooks
	Portfolios

Written and Oral Assessments

Written Assessments

Written tests have been in widespread use for nearly a century across all fields and stages of training; indeed, scores on written examinations often carry significant weight in selection decisions for entry into health professional training programs, and, as such, written tests can constitute high-stakes assessments. Written exams—whether in paper-and-pencil or computer-based formats—are the most common means used to assess cognitive or knowledge domains, and these generally consist of either *selected-response*/"closed question" (e.g., multiple-choice questions [MCQs] and various matching or true-false formats) or *constructed-response*/"open-ended question" (e.g., fill-in-the-blank and essay question) item formats. MCQs, in particular, have become the mainstay of most formal assessment programs in health professions education because they offer several advantages over other testing methods: MCQs can sample a very broad content range in a relatively short time; when contextualized with case vignettes, they permit assessment of both basic science and clinical knowledge acquisition and application; they are relatively easy and inexpensive to administer and can be machine scanned, allowing efficient and objective scoring; and a large body of research has demonstrated that these types of written tests have very strong measurement characteristics (i.e., scores are highly reliable and contribute to ample validity evidence) [46, pp. 30–49; 51–54].

Oral Assessments

Like written tests, oral examinations employ a stimulus–response format and chiefly assess acquisition and application of knowledge. The difference, obviously, is the form of the stimulus and response: As opposed to pencil-and-paper or computer test administration, in oral exams, the candidate verbally responds to questions posed by one or more examiners face to face (hence the alternate term "vivas," so-called from the Latin *viva voce*, meaning "with the live voice"). In traditional oral exams, the clinical substrate is typically the (unobserved) interview and examination of an actual patient, after which the examinee verbally reports his or her findings and then a back-and-forth exchange of questions and answers ensues. Examiners ordinarily ask open-ended questions: Analogous to written constructed-response-type items, then, the aim is to assess more than just retention of facts but also ability to solve problems, make a logical argument in support of clinical decisions, and "think on one's feet." An advantage of oral exams over, say, essay questions is the possibility of dynamic interaction between examiner(s) and candidate, whereby additional queries can explore why an examinee answered earlier questions in a certain way. The flip side of that coin, however, is the possibility that biases can substantially affect ratings: Because the exam occurs face to face and is based on oral communication, factors such as examinee appearance and language fluency may impact scores. Oral exams face additional psychometric challenges in terms of (usually) limited case sampling/content specificity and, due to differences in examiner leniency/stringency, subjectivity in scoring. These issues pose threats to the reliability of scores and validity of judgments derived from oral assessment methods [46, pp. 27–29; 55, pp. 269–272; 56, p. 324; 57, pp. 673–674].

Performance-Based Assessments

Long Cases

Performance-based tests, in very general terms, all involve formal demonstration of what trainees can actually do, not just what they know. Traditional examples include the "long case," whereby an examiner takes a student or candidate to the bedside of a real patient and requires that he or she shows how to take a history, perform a physical examination, and perhaps carry out some procedure or laboratory testing at the bedside. Because examinees usually answer questions about patient evaluation and discuss further diagnostic work-up and management, long cases also incorporate knowledge assessment (as in oral exams), but at least some of the evaluation includes rating the candidate's performance of clinical skills at the bedside, not just the cognitive domains. Long (and/or several short) cases became the classic prototype for clinical examination largely because this type of patient encounter was viewed as highly authentic, but—because patients (and thus the conditions to be evaluated) are usually chosen from among those that happen to be available in the hospital or clinic on the day of the exam and because examiners with different areas of interest or expertise tend to ask examinees different types of questions—this methodology again suffers from serious limitations in terms of content specificity and lack of standardization [46, pp. 53–57; 55, pp. 269–281; 56, p. 324; 57, pp. 673–674].

Objective Structured Clinical Examination (OSCE)

Developed to avoid some of these psychometric problems, the Objective Structured Clinical Examination (OSCE) represents another type of performance-based assessment [58]: OSCEs most commonly consist of a "round-robin" of multiple short testing stations, in each of which examinees must demonstrate defined skills (optimally determined according to a blueprint that samples widely across a range of different content areas), while examiners rate their performance according to predetermined criteria using a standardized marking scheme. When interactions with a "patient" comprise the task(s) in a given station, this role may be portrayed by actual patients (but outside the real clinical context) or others (actors, health professionals, etc.) trained to play the part of a patient (simulated or standardized patients [SPs]; "programmed patients," as originally described by Barrows and Abrahamson [6]). Whereas assessment programs in North America tend to use predominantly SPs, real patients are more commonly employed in Europe and elsewhere. One concern about the OSCE method has been its separation of clinical tasks into component parts: Typically examinees will perform a focused physical exam in one station, interpret a chest radiograph in the next, deliver the bad news of a cancer diagnosis in the following station, and so forth. A multiplicity of stations can increase the breadth of sampling (thereby improving generalizability), but this deconstruction of what, in reality, are complex clinical situations into simpler constituents appears artificial; although potentially appropriate for assessment of novice learners, this lack of authenticity threatens the validity of the OSCE method when evaluating the performance of experts, whom we expect to be able to deal with the complexity and nuance of real-life clinical encounters. An additional challenge is that OSCEs can be resource intensive to develop and implement. Nonetheless, especially with careful attention to exam design (including adequate number and duration of stations), rating instrument development, and examiner training, research has confirmed that the OSCE format circumvents many of the obstacles to reliable and valid measurement encountered with traditional methods such as the long case [46, pp. 58–64; 57, 59].

Simulation-Based Assessments

Besides their use in OSCEs, SPs and other medical simulators, such as task trainers and computer-enhanced mannequins, often represent the patient or clinical context in other performance-based tests [60, pp. 245–268; 61, pp. 179–200]. Rather than the multi-station format featuring brief simulated encounters, longer scenarios employing various simulations can form the basis for assessment of how individuals (or teams) behave during, say, an intraoperative emergency or mass casualty incident. We will elaborate more on these methods in later sections of this chapter, and specialty-specific chapters in the next section of the book will provide further details about uses of simulations for assessment in particular disciplines.

Clinical Observation or Work-Based Assessments

Clinical observational methods or work-based assessments have in common that the evaluations are conducted under real-world conditions in the places where health professionals ordinarily practice, that is, on the ambulance, in the emergency department or operating room or clinic exam room, on the hospital ward, etc. Provider interactions are with actual patients, rather than with SPs, and in authentic clinical environments. The idea here is to assess routine behaviors in the workplace ("in vivo," if you will) as accurately as possible, rather than observing performance in artificial ("in vitro") exam settings, such as the stations of an OSCE or even during long cases. Consequently, such observations must be conducted as unobtrusively as possible, lest healthcare providers (or even the patients themselves) behave differently because of the presence of the observer/rater. Work-based evaluation methods have only recently received increasing attention, largely due to growing calls from the public for better accountability of health professionals already in practice, some of whom have been found to be incompetent despite having "passed" other traditional assessment methods during their training [49, p. 8].

Mini-Clinical Evaluation Exercise (Mini-CEX)

Examples of work-based assessment methods include the Mini-Clinical Evaluation Exercise (mini-CEX), which features direct observation (usually by an attending physician, other supervisor, or faculty member) during an actual encounter of certain aspects of clinical skills (e.g., a focused history or physical exam), which are scored using behaviorally anchored rating scales. Because the assessment is brief (generally 15 minutes or so; hence the term "mini"), it can relatively easily be accomplished in the course of routine work (e.g., during daily ward rounds) without significant disruption or need for special scheduling; also, because this method permits impromptu evaluation that is not "staged," the clinical encounter is likely to be more authentic and, without the opportunity to rehearse, trainees are more likely to behave as they would if not being observed. The idea is that multiple observations over time permit adequate sampling of a range of different clinical skills, and use of a standardized marking scheme by trained raters allows measurements to be fairly reliable across many observers [46, pp. 67–70; 62, pp. 196–199; 63, p. 339].

Direct Observation of Procedural Skills (DOPS)

Direct Observation of Procedural Skills (DOPS) is another method similar to the mini-CEX, this time with the domains of interest focused on practical procedures. Thus DOPS can assess aspects such as knowledge of indications for a given procedure, informed consent, and aseptic technique, in addition to technical ability to perform the procedure itself. Again, the observations are made during actual procedures carried out on real patients, with different competencies scored using a standardized instrument generally consisting of global rating scales. For this and most other work-based methods based on brief observations, strong measurement properties only accrue over time with multiple samples across a broad range of skills. One challenge, however, is that evaluation of such technical competencies usually requires that expert raters conduct the assessments [46, pp. 71–74].

360° Evaluations

By contrast, not all methods require that supervisory or other experienced staff carry out the observations. In fact, alternative and valuable perspectives can be gained by collecting data from others with whom a trainee interacts at work on a daily basis. Thus, peers, subordinate personnel (including students), nursing and ancillary healthcare providers, and even patients can provide evaluations of performance that are likely more accurate assessments of an individual's true abilities and attitudes. A formal process of accumulating and triangulating observations by multiple persons in the trainee's/practitioner's sphere of influence comprises what is known as a 360° evaluation (also termed multisource feedback). Despite the fact that formal training seldom occurs on how to mark the rating instruments in these assessments, research has demonstrated acceptable reliability of data obtained via 360° evaluations, and, although aggregation of observations from multiple sources can be time and labor intensive, this process significantly decreases the likelihood that individual biases will impact ratings in a systematic way [46, pp. 82–85; 62, p. 199; 64].

Miscellaneous Assessments

Patient, Peer, and Self-Assessments

This "miscellaneous" category includes a variety of evaluation methods that don't fit neatly under any one of the previous headings. In some cases, this is an issue of semantics related to how we define certain groupings. For example, we include in the classification of clinical observation or work-based assessments only those methodologies whereby data is collected on behaviors directly observed at the time of actual performance. On the other hand, if an assessment method yields information—albeit concerning real-world behaviors in the workplace—that is gathered indirectly or retrospectively, we list it here among other miscellaneous modalities. Therefore, as an example, patient satisfaction questionnaires completed immediately following a given clinic appointment that inquire about behaviors or attitudes the practitioner demonstrated during that visit would be included among clinical observation methods, such as part of 360° evaluations, whereas patient surveys conducted by phone or mail two weeks after a hospital admission—necessarily subject to recall and other potential biases—and based on impressions rather than observations would be grouped in the miscellaneous category. Similarly, peer assessments could be classified under more than one heading in our scheme. Self-assessments of performance, while they may have some utility for quality improvement purposes, are seldom used as a basis for making high-stakes decisions. Such ratings are extremely subjective: Personality traits such as self-confidence may influence evaluation of one's own abilities, and research has demonstrated very poor correlation between self-assessments and judgments based on more objective measurements [63, pp. 338–339].

Medical Record Audits and Chart-Stimulated Recall

Chart audit as the basis for assessing what a clinician does in practice is another method of evaluation that we could classify in different ways: Clearly this is an indirect type of work-based assessment, whereby notes and other documentation in the written or electronic medical record provide evidence of what practitioners actually do in caring for their patients, but this can also represent a form of peer or self-assessment, depending on who conducts the audit. In any case, a significant challenge arises in choosing appropriate criteria to evaluate. Medical record review is also a relatively time- and labor-intensive assessment method, whose measurement properties are ultimately dependent on the quality (including completeness, legibility, and accuracy) of the original documentation [62, p. 197, 63, pp. 337–338; 65, pp. 60–67; 69–74].

Chart-stimulated recall is a related assessment method based on review of medical records, which was pioneered by the American Board of Emergency Medicine as part of its certification exams and later adopted by other organizations as a process for maintenance of certification. In this case, the charts of patients cared for by the candidate become the substrate for questioning during oral examination. Interviews focus retrospectively on a practitioner's clinical judgment and decision-making, as reflected by the documentation in actual medical records, rather than by behaviors during a live patient encounter (as in traditional vivas or long cases). Chart-stimulated recall using just three to six medical records has demonstrated adequate measurement properties to be used in high-stakes testing, but this exam format is nonetheless expensive and time consuming to implement [55, p. 274, 65, pp. 67–74; 66, pp. 899, 905].

Logbooks and Portfolios

Logbooks represent another form of written record, usually employed to document number and types of patients/conditions seen or procedures performed by health professionals in the course of their training and/or practice. Historically, "quota" systems relied on documentation in logs—formerly paper booklets and nowadays frequently electronic files—of achievement of a defined target (for instance, number of central lines to be placed) to certify competence in a given area. These quotas were determined more often arbitrarily than based on evidence, and although some research suggests that quality of care is associated with higher practice volume [63, p. 337], other studies clearly show that experience alone (or "time in grade") does not necessarily equate with expertise [67]. Additional challenges exist in terms of the accuracy of information recorded, irrespective of whether logbooks are self-maintained or externally administered. As a result, few high-stakes assessment systems rely on data derived from logbooks per se; instead, they are ordinarily used to monitor learners' achievement of milestones and progression through a program and to evaluate the equivalence of educational experiences across multiple training sites [46, pp. 86–87; 63, p. 338].

The definition of portfolios as a method of assessment varies somewhat according to different sources: Whether the term is used in the sense of "a compilation of 'best' work" or "a purposeful collection of materials to demonstrate competence," other professions (such as the fine arts) have employed this evaluation method far longer than the health professions [68, p. 86]. A distinguishing feature of portfolios versus other assessment modalities is the involvement of the evaluee in the choice of items to include; this affords a unique opportunity for self-assessment and reflection, as the individual typically provides a commentary on the significance and reasons for inclusion of various components of the portfolio. Many of the individual methods previously mentioned can become constituents of a portfolio. An advantage of this method, perhaps more than any other single "snapshot" assessment, is that it provides a record of progression over time. Although portfolio evaluations don't readily lend themselves to traditional psychometric analysis, the accumulation of evidence and triangulation of data from multiple sources, although laborious in terms of time and effort, tend to minimize limitations of any one of the included assessment modalities. Nonetheless, significant challenges exist, including choice of content, outcomes to assess, and methods for scoring the portfolio overall [46, pp. 88–89; 68, 69, pp. 346–353; 70].

Rating Instruments and Scoring

We stated early on that this chapter's scope would not encompass detailed discussion of various rating instruments, which can be used with practically all of the methods described above to measure or judge examinee performances during an assessment. Reports of the development and use of different checklists and rating scales abound, representing a veritable "alphabet soup" of instruments known by clever acronyms such as RIME (Reporter-Interpreter-Manager-Educator) [71], ANTS (Anesthetists' Non-Technical Skills) [72], NOTSS (Non-Technical Skills for Surgeons) [72], SPLINTS (Scrub Practitioners' List of Intraoperative Non-Technical Skills) [72], and others too numerous to count. Because development of such rating instruments should follow fairly rigorous procedures [73, 74], which can be time and labor intensive, we realize that many readers would like a resource that would enable them to locate quickly and use various previously reported checklists or rating forms. Such a listing, however, would quickly become outdated. Moreover, once again we caution against using rating instruments "off the shelf" with the claim that they have been "previously validated": although the competency of interest may generally be the same, the process of validation is so critically dependent on context that the argument in support of decisions based on data derived from the same instrument must be repeated each time it is used under new/different circumstances (e.g., slightly different learner level, different number of raters, and different method of tallying points from the instrument). That said, the rigor with which validation needs to be carried out depends on the stakes of resulting assessment decisions, and tips are available for adapting existing rating instruments to maximize the strength of the validity argument [62, pp. 195–201]. Finally, it should be noted that we use rating instruments themselves only to capture observations and produce data; the manner in which we combine and utilize these data to derive scores and set standards, which we interpret to reach a final decision based on the assessment, is another subject beyond the scope of this chapter, but we refer the interested reader to several sources of information on this and related topics [75–77].

Multidimensional Framework for Assessment

In further developing a model for thinking about assessment and choosing among various methods, we suggest consideration of several dimensions of an evaluation system: (1) the outcomes that need to be assessed, (2) the levels of assessment that are most appropriate, (3) the developmental stage of those undergoing assessment, and (4) the overall context, especially the purpose(s), of the assessment (see Fig. 11.1). We will explore each of these in turn.

Outcomes for Assessment

In keeping with the outcomes-based educational paradigm that we discussed earlier, we must first delineate what competencies need to be assessed. We (the authors) are most familiar with the outcomes frameworks used in medical education in our home countries (the USA and Canada), and we

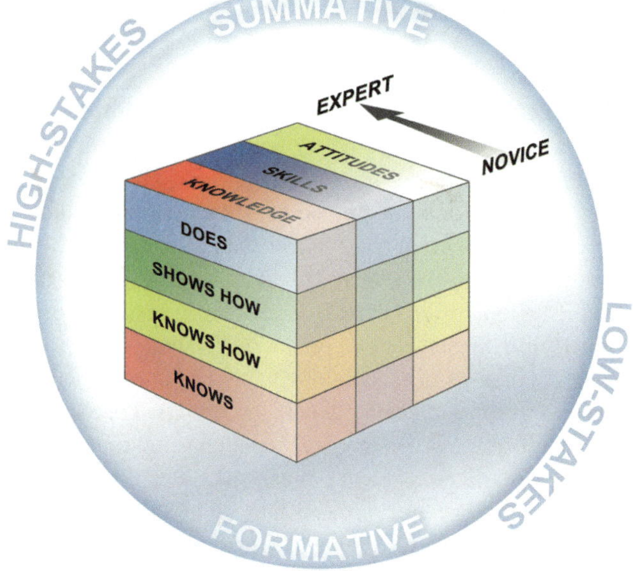

Fig. 11.1 Multidimensional framework for assessment

Table 11.2 ACGME competencies and suggested best methods for assessment

Competency	Required skills	Suggested assessment methods[a]
Patient care and procedural skills	Caring and respectful behaviors	*SPs*, patient surveys (1)
	Interviewing	OSCE (1)
	Informed decision-making	Chart-stimulated recall (1), oral exams (2)
	Develop/carry out patient management plans	Chart-stimulated recall (1), *simulations* (2)
	Preventive health services	Medical record audits (1), logbooks (2)
	Performance of routine physical exam	*SPs*, OSCE (1)
	Performance of medical procedures	*Simulations* (1)
	Work within a team	360° evaluations (1)
Medical knowledge	Investigatory and analytic thinking	Chart-stimulated recall, oral exams (1), *simulations* (2)
	Knowledge and application of basic sciences	MCQ written tests (1), *simulations* (2)
Practice-based learning and improvement	Analyze own practice for needed improvements	Portfolios (1), *simulations* (3)
	Use of evidence from scientific studies	Medical record audits, MCQ/oral exams (1)
	Use of information technology	360° evaluations (1)
Interpersonal and communication skills	Creation of therapeutic relationship with patients	*SPs*, OSCE, patient surveys (1)
	Listening skills	*SPs*, OSCE, patient surveys (1)
Professionalism	Respectful, altruistic	Patient surveys (1)
	Ethically sound practice	360° evaluations (1), *simulations* (2)
Systems-based practice	Knowledge of practice and delivery systems	MCQ written tests (1)
	Practice cost-effective care	360° evaluations (1)

[a]Based on ACGME Toolbox of Assessment Methods [78]
1 the most desirable, *2* the next best method, *3* a potentially applicable method

will draw on these as examples for the discussion to follow. As previously mentioned, the ACGME outlines six general competencies: (1) patient care and procedural skills, (2) medical knowledge, (3) practice-based learning and improvement, (4) interpersonal and communication skills, (5) professionalism, and (6) systems-based practice [19]. While differing slightly in number, there is significant overlap between the six ACGME competencies and the outcomes expected of specialist physicians, which the CanMEDS framework describes in terms of seven roles that doctors must integrate: the central role is that of (1) medical expert, but physicians must also draw on the competencies included in the roles of (2) communicator, (3) collaborator, (4) manager, (5) health advocate, (6) scholar, and (7) professional to provide effective patient-centered care [18].

Accordingly, one way to choose among assessment modalities is to align various methods with the outcomes to be assessed. For example, when they elaborated the six general competencies (and a further number of "required skills" within each of these domains), the ACGME also provided a "Toolbox of Assessment Methods" with "suggested best methods for evaluation" of various outcomes [78]. This document lists thirteen methodologies—all of which were described in the corresponding section of this chapter (see Box)—and details strengths and limitations of each assessment technique. The metaphor of a "toolbox" is apt: a carpenter often has more than one tool at his disposal, but some are better suited than others for the task at hand. For example, he might be able to drive a nail into a piece of wood by striking it enough times with the handle of a screwdriver or the end of a heavy wrench, but this would likely require more time and energy than if he had used the purpose-built hammer. Similarly, while 360° evaluations are "a potentially applicable method" to evaluate "knowledge and application of basic sciences" (under the general competency of "medical knowledge"), it is fairly intuitive that MCQs and other written test formats are "the most desirable" to assess this outcomes area, owing to greater efficiency, robust measurement properties, etc. Table 11.2 provides an excerpt from the ACGME Toolbox showing suggested methods to evaluate various competencies, including some of the newer domains ("practice-based learning and improvement" and "systems-based practice") that are not straightforward to understand conceptually and, therefore, have proven difficult to assess [79] (see Table 11.2).

In similar fashion, when the Royal College of Physicians and Surgeons of Canada described several "key" as well as other "enabling" competencies within each of the CanMEDS roles, they provided an "Assessment Tools Handbook," which lists important methods for assessing these competencies [80]. Just like the ACGME Toolbox, this document describes strengths and limitations of contemporary assessment techniques and ranks various tools according to how many of the outcomes within a given CanMEDS role they are appropriate to evaluate. For example, within this framework, written tests are deemed "well suited to assessing many of the [medical expert] role's key competencies" but only "suited to assessing very specific competencies within the [communicator] role." We could situate any of these sets of outcomes along one axis in our assessment model, but for illustrative purposes, we have distilled various core competencies into three categories that encompass all cognitive ("knowledge"), psychomotor ("skills"), and affective ("attitudes") domains (see Fig. 11.1).

Levels of Assessment

The next dimension we should consider is the level of assessment within any of the specified areas of competence. George Miller offered an extremely useful model for thinking about the assessment of learners at four different levels:

1. *Knows*—recall of basic facts, principles, and theories.
2. *Knows how*—ability to apply knowledge to solve problems, make decisions, or describe procedures.
3. *Shows how*—demonstration of skills or hands-on performance of procedures in a controlled or supervised setting.
4. *Does*—actual behavior in clinical practice [42].

This framework is now very widely cited, likely because the description of and distinction between levels are highly intuitive and consistent with most healthcare educators' experience: we all know trainees who "can talk the talk but can't walk the walk." Conceptualized as a pyramid, Miller's model depicts knowledge as the base or foundation upon which more complex learning builds and without which all higher achievement is unattainable; for example, a doctor will be ill equipped to "know how" to make clinical decisions without a solid knowledge base. The same is true moving further up the levels of the pyramid: students cannot possibly "show how" if they don't first "know how", and so on. Conversely, factual knowledge is necessary but not sufficient to function as a competent clinician; ability to apply this knowledge to solve problems, for example, is also required. Similarly, it's one thing to describe ("know how") one would, say, differentiate among systolic murmurs, but it's another thing altogether to actually perform a cardiac examination including various maneuvers ("show how") to make the correct diagnosis based on detection and proper identification of auscultatory findings. Of course, we always wonder if our trainees perform their physical exams using textbook technique or carry out procedures observing scrupulous sterile precautions (as they usually do when we're standing there with a clipboard and rating form in hand) when they're on their own in the middle of the night, with no one looking over their shoulder. This—what a health professional "does" in actual practice, under real-life circumstances (not during a scenario in the simulation lab)—is the pinnacle of the pyramid, what we're most interested to capture accurately with our assessments.

Although termed "Miller's pyramid," his original construct was in fact a (two-dimensional) triangle, which we have adapted to our multidimensional framework by depicting the levels of assessment along an axis perpendicular to the outcomes being assessed (see Fig. 11.1). Each (vertical) "slice" representing various areas of competence graphically intersects the four (horizontal) levels. Thus, we can envision a case example that focuses on the "skills" domain, wherein assessment is possible at any of Miller's levels:

1. *Knows*—a resident can identify relevant anatomic landmarks of the head and neck (written test with matching items), can list the contents of a central line kit (written test with MCQ items or fill in the blanks), and can explain the principles of physics underlying ultrasonography (written test with essay questions).
2. *Knows how*—a resident can describe the detailed steps for ultrasound-guided central venous catheter (CVC) insertion into the internal jugular (IJ) vein (oral exam).
3. *Shows how*—a resident can perform ultrasound-guided CVC insertion into the IJ on a mannequin (checklist marked by a trained rater observing the procedure in the simulation lab).
4. *Does*—a resident performs unsupervised CVC insertion when on call in the intensive care unit (medical record audit, logbook review, or 360° evaluation including feedback from attendings, fellow residents, and nursing staff in the ICU).

Choice of the most appropriate evaluation methods (as in this example) should aim to achieve the closest possible alignment with the level of assessment required. It is no accident, therefore, that the various categories of assessment methods we presented earlier generally correspond to the different levels of Miller's pyramid [46, pp. 22–24; 48, pp. 2–5]: written and oral assessments can efficiently measure outcomes at the "knows" and "knows how" levels, while performance-based assessments are most appropriate at the "shows how" level, and clinical observation or work-based and other miscellaneous assessment methods are best suited to evaluating what a clinician "does" in actual practice (see Table 11.3). Of course, because of the hierarchical nature of Miller's scheme, methods that work for assessment at the upper levels can also be utilized to evaluate more fundamental competencies; for instance, 360° evaluations (directly) and chart-stimulated recall (indirectly) assess real-world behaviors, but they are also effective (albeit, perhaps, less efficient) methods to gauge acquisition and application of knowledge. In addition, the interaction between these two dimensions—outcomes of interest and levels of assessment—describes a smaller set of evaluation tools that are best suited to the task. For this reason, although multiple techniques might have applications for assessment of a given ACGME competency, the Toolbox suggests relatively few as "the most desirable" methods of choice [78].

Stages of Development

As any doctor who has been educated in North America—where the period of training between finishing high school

Table 11.3 Levels of assessment and corresponding assessment methods

Level of assessment[a]	Assessment category	Example(s)
Does	Clinical observation or work-based assessments	Mini-Clinical Evaluation Exercise (mini-CEX) Direct Observation of Procedural Skills (DOPS) 360° evaluations (multisource feedback)
	Miscellaneous assessments	Patient surveys, peer and self-assessments Medical record audits and chart-stimulated recall Logbooks and portfolios
Shows how	Performance-based assessments	Long and short cases Objective Structured Clinical Examinations (OSCE) Simulation-based assessments
Knows how	Written and oral assessments	Fill-in-the-blank items Long and short essay questions Oral exams/vivas
Knows	Written and oral assessments	Multiple-choice questions (MCQ) Matching and extended matching items True-false and multiple true-false items Oral exams/vivas

[a]Based on Miller's pyramid framework [42]

and beginning independent clinical practice is, at minimum, seven years and, much more commonly, eleven to fourteen years—can attest, acquisition of the knowledge, skills, and attitudes required to become a competent (much less an expert) health professional is not accomplished overnight! The notion of "*lifelong* learning" has almost become trite, yet it has significant implications for the entire educational process, including any assessment system: just as styles of learning (and, therefore, of teaching) should evolve across the continuum of educational levels, so, too, methods of assessment must change according to an individual's developmental stage [49, pp. 5–6].

One way to describe the formational steps to becoming a health professional is simply in terms of training phases: using physician education as an example, one progresses from medical student to resident to practicing doctor. We can even subdivide these periods of training: within undergraduate curricula, there is generally an early/preclinical phase followed by a later/clinical phase, and in graduate medical education programs, there is internship, then residency, followed by fellowship. Expectations for what competencies should be achieved at particular training levels differ, and methods to assess these outcomes should vary accordingly. For instance, we would expect a first-year medical student (MS-1) who has just completed one month of the gross anatomy and pathology courses to be able to identify the gall bladder and relevant structures in the right upper quadrant of the abdomen, but not to be able to perform surgery to remove them. Therefore, it would be appropriate to test MS-1 students using a written exam requiring them to match photos of anatomic specimens with a corresponding list of names or a laboratory practical exam requiring them to identify (either in writing or orally) tagged structures in their dissections. On the other hand, we would expect a fourth postgraduate year (PGY-4) general surgery resident to be able not only to master the competencies (and "ace" the exams) mentioned above but also to be able to perform laparoscopic cholecystectomy, as assessed either on a virtual reality simulator or by direct observation in the operating room. Of course, there is an assumption that merely spending a certain amount of time in training will result in the acquisition of certain knowledge, skills, and attitudes, when, in fact, as previously mentioned, we often find this not to be true [67]. Such a notion, based as it is on educational *process* variables (phase of training or "time in grade"), runs completely countercurrent to the whole *outcomes*-based model.

Other templates for describing stages of development of health professions trainees have been proposed. For example, the "RIME" scheme [81] originated to evaluate medical students and residents during internal medicine training in the USA but has since been used more broadly across medical specialties. This framework assesses trainees with a focus on their achievement of developmental milestones as defined by observable behaviors: *Reporter*—reliably gathers information from patients and communicates with faculty (can answer the "what" questions). *Interpreter*—demonstrates selectivity and prioritization in reporting, which implies analysis, and develops reasonable differential diagnosis (can answer the "why" questions). *Manager*—actively participates in diagnostic and treatment decisions for patients (can answer the "how" questions). *Educator*—demonstrates self-reflection and self-education to acquire greater expertise, which is shared with patients and colleagues toward common goal of continuous improvement [71]. Using a different model, the Royal College of Obstetricians and Gynecologists (RCOG) in the UK assesses trainees' achievement of competency "targets" as they progress through different stages based on the degree of supervision required: level 1—*observes*; Level 2—*assists*; Level 3—*direct supervision*; Level 4—*indirect supervision*; and Level 5—*independent* [82].

An alternative model of skill acquisition that is generally applicable to the developmental progress of any learners, not just health professionals, was proposed by the Dreyfus brothers in terms of five stages with corresponding mental frames:

1. *Novice*—the learner shows "rigid adherence to taught rules or plans" but does not exercise "discretionary judgment."
2. *Advanced beginner*—the learner begins to show limited "situational perception" but treats all aspects of work separately and with equal importance.
3. *Competent*—the learner can "cope with crowdedness" (multiple tasks and accumulation of information), shows some perception of actions in relation to longer-term goals and plans deliberately to achieve them, and formulates routines.
4. *Proficient*—the learner develops holistic view of situation and prioritizes importance of aspects, "perceives deviations from the normal pattern," and employs maxims for guidance with meanings that adapt to the situation at hand.
5. *Expert*—transcends reliance on rules, guidelines, and maxims; shows "intuitive grasp of situations based on deep, tacit understanding"; and returns to "analytical approaches" only in new situations or when unanticipated problems arise [83].

Again according to this model, individuals at each stage learn in different ways. Curriculum planning, therefore, should attempt to accommodate these various learning styles by including different instructional methods at distinct stages of training; the corollary of this proposition is that assessment methodologies should change in corresponding fashion [49, pp. 5–6]. Thus, there is a progression according to developmental stage (graphically illustrated as a color gradient) within a given competency as well as within a given assessment level, adding another dimension to our evaluation system framework (see Fig. 11.1).

Assessment Context

Other sources have suggested a three-dimensional model such as forms the core of our assessment framework thus far [49, pp. 3–6]. We feel, however, that additional dimensions merit close attention. In particular, as we have emphasized when discussing the concepts of validity and feasibility, consideration of the larger setting in which an assessment takes place is of vital importance, including interrelated factors such as the outcomes framework employed, geographic location, and availability (or paucity) of resources. As stated earlier, perhaps the most crucial contextual element is the purpose of the test. The possible reasons for conducting any assessment are manifold. Most important in the outcomes-based model is determination of whether prespecified learning objectives have been accomplished. Moreover, such measurement of educational outcomes not only identifies individuals whose achievements overall meet (or do not meet) minimum standards of acceptable performance (summative assessment) but also elucidates particular areas of weakness with an eye toward remediation and quality improvement (formative assessment). Note once more that Barrows and Abrahamson referred to each of these different purposes of assessment strategies: in addition to curriculum or program evaluation ("…to determine the effectiveness of teaching methods…")—not our particular focus here—they also allude to both formative assessment ("…to recognize individual student difficulties so that assistance may be offered…") and summative assessment ("…to provide the basis for a reasonably satisfactory appraisal of student performance") [6]. Although they were speaking about evaluation of competency in the context of an undergraduate medical clerkship, such discussion applies broadly across the continuum of educational levels and multiple health professions. Unlike some of the other parameters we have discussed in our assessment framework, however, there is no clear demarcation between what constitutes a summative versus a formative assessment: even high-stakes examinations conducted mainly for summative purposes, such as for professional licensure or board certification, provide some feedback to examinees (such as subsection scores) that can be used to improve future performance, and, therefore, serve a formative purpose as well. Although often described as opposing forces in assessment, the distinction between summative and formative evaluations is somewhat arbitrary. In fact, more recently the terminology has evolved and the literature refers to "assessment *of* learning" (rather than summative assessment) and "assessment *for* learning" (meaning formative assessment), with a keen awareness that the two purposes are inextricably intertwined.

Similarly, there is no absolute definition of what constitutes a high-stakes assessment versus medium or low stakes: to the extent that performance in a single simulation scenario (generally considered low stakes) might ultimately steer a student toward specialization in a particular area, the ramifications to future patients for whom that individual cares may be very important. Because there is no clear dividing line between such "poles"—the boundaries are blurred, as opposed to more linear demarcations within the three other core dimensions of our model as constructed thus far—we have chosen to depict this fourth dimension of our assessment framework as a sphere (or concentric spheres), which graphically represents the contextual layers that surround any assessment (see Fig. 11.1).

Simulation-Based Assessment in Context

Now where does simulation-based assessment fit into all of this? The discussion heretofore has elaborated a broad framework for thinking generally about the evaluation of clinical competence and for choosing the best assessment methods for a given purpose, but we have said relatively little about specific applications of simulation in this setting. In preceding sections, we emphasized the importance of examining contextual relationships, of situating a given idea, concept, or method against the wider backdrop. This is, ultimately, a book about simulation, so why did the editors choose to conclude the introduction and overview section with two chapters devoted to the topic of assessment? In that context, the final part of this chapter will explore (1) how trends in the use of simulation for assessment purposes follow the overall movement toward simulation-based education in the health professions and (2) the particular role of simulation-based methods for the evaluation of competence within our outcomes-based model.

Drivers of Change Toward Simulation-Based Education

As already mentioned, seminal publications about healthcare simulation date as far back as the 1960s, but it is only in the last decade or two that health professions educators worldwide have embraced simulation methods and dramatically increased their use not only for teaching but also for assessment. This represents a fundamental paradigm shift from the traditional focus on real patients for training as well as testing. Earlier chapters of this book trace the history of healthcare simulation and describe some of the drivers behind these recent trends, especially the uses of simulation for *teaching and learning*, but many of the same forces have shaped the evolution of simulation-based *assessment* over the same period.

Changes in Healthcare Delivery and Academic Medicine

For example, managed care has led to higher volumes but shorter appointment times for outpatient visits (including patients with conditions for which inpatient treatment was previously the norm) and higher acuity of illnesses but shorter hospital stays for patients who are admitted. Together with recent restrictions on trainee work hours, pressures on faculty to increase clinical service and research productivity have negatively impacted the time they have available to spend with their students [84, 85]. In the aggregate, these changes have dramatically altered the educational landscape at academic medical centers, but what is most often discussed is the resulting reduction in learning opportunities with actual patients; less often considered is how such changes also limit occasions for assessment of trainees' or practitioners' skills, especially their behaviors in the real-world setting (i.e., at the "shows how" and "does" levels in Miller's scheme). Thus, in addition to their psychometric shortcomings, traditional assessment methods featuring live patient encounters (such as the long case) nowadays face the extra challenge of decreased patient availability as the substrate for clinical examinations.

Such limitations likewise impact more recently developed assessment methods: undoubtedly, many of us know the experience of arriving with a trainee to conduct a mini-CEX, only to find the patient that was intended for examination out of the room to undergo some diagnostic test or treatment. At other times, patients may be too ill, become embarrassed or fatigued, or otherwise behave too unpredictably to be suitable for testing situations, especially if multiple examinees are involved or if very high reliability is required. These problems underscore how opportunistic the educational and assessment process becomes when dependent on finding real patients with specific conditions of interest. Simulations, by contrast, can be readily available at any time and can reproduce a wide variety of clinical conditions and situations on demand and with great consistency across many examinees, thereby providing standardized assessments for all [86].

Technological Developments

Advances in technology, especially computers, have transformed the educational environment across all disciplines. Regarding assessment, in particular, the advent of computing technology first facilitated (via optical scanning machines and computerized scoring) the widespread implementation of MCQ exams and, more recently, creation of test items with multimedia content for MCQs and other written formats, which examinees answer directly on the computer rather than taking traditional paper-and-pencil tests. Significant advantages of this method of exam delivery include improved efficiency and security, faster grading and reporting of scores, and easier application of psychometrics for test item analysis. Additionally, artificial intelligence programs permit natural language processing—to analyze and score exams with constructed-response item formats—as well as adaptive testing, whereby sequential questions posed to a particular examinee are chosen based on how that individual answered previous items, probing and focusing on potential gaps in knowledge rather than on content the examinee has evidently mastered. Such adaptive testing makes estimation of examinee proficiency more precise and more efficient. Computerized testing also allows use of interactive item formats to assess clinical judgment and decision-making skills: examinees are presented patient cases and asked to gather data and formulate diagnostic and treatment plans; the computer cases unfold dynamically and provide programmed responses to requested information, on which examinees must base ongoing decisions; and these scenarios can also incorporate the element of time passing. Thus, some types of computer-based cases are simulations in the broadest sense and reproduce (more realistically than traditional paper-and-pencil patient management problems) tasks requiring the kinds of judgments and decisions that clinicians must make in actual practice [87].

Other advances in engineering and computer technology—including increased processor speeds and memory capacity, decreased size, improved graphics, and 3-D rendering—have led to development of virtual reality (VR) simulators with highly realistic sound and visual stimuli; incorporation of haptic (i.e., touch and pressure feedback) technologies has improved the tactile experience as well, creating devices especially well suited to simulating (and to assessing) the skills required to use some of the newer diagnostic and treatment modalities, particularly endoscopic, endovascular, and other minimally invasive procedures.

Patient Safety and Other Considerations

The chapters preceding this one discuss the topic of simulation-based training of healthcare practitioners to manage rare/critical incidents and to work effectively in teams [88], and they also highlight important related issues concerning patient safety [89, 90]. Such analysis inevitably leads to comparisons with other professions operating in high-risk performance environments [91–93], especially commercial aviation. No argument in favor of simulation-based training in crisis resource management is more compelling than images of US Airways Flight 1549 floating in the Hudson River [94]! When that dramatic tale is recounted—often crediting Captain Chesley B. "Sully" Sullenberger's quick thinking and calm handling of the situation to his pilot training—reports usually emphasize the use of simulations to *teach* aircrew how to handle emergencies like the bird strike that disabled both engines on that aircraft. Far less often mentioned, however, is the fact that simulation-based *assessment* is also a fundamental component of aviation training programs: pilots do not earn their qualifications to fly an airplane until they "pass" numerous tests of their competence to do so. Interestingly, even the terminology used—to be "*rated* in the 767 and 777" means to be deemed competent to fly those particular types of aircraft—indicates how central the evaluation or assessment process is to aviation training.

Yet, obviously, aeronautics instructors cannot stop to teach proper protocols during an actual in-flight emergency nor can they wait for a real catastrophic engine failure to occur to evaluate crew skills in responding to such an incident. There are no "time-outs" during a plane crash! Simulations, on the other hand, allow instructors to take advantage of "teachable moments" *and* afford opportunities to assess the competence of trainees, all without risk of harm. The situation is completely analogous in the health professions: even if we could predict when it would happen, we usually wouldn't pause to pull out clipboards and rating forms to evaluate nurse/physician team skills in the middle of a real "code blue." Simulations, on the other hand, permit assessment in a safe, controlled environment, where the experience becomes appropriately learner centered, instead of focused on the well-being of the patient, as is required in actual clinical settings.

Closely related to these safety issues are important ethical concerns about "using" real patients (even SPs) for teaching or testing purposes, with the debate focused especially on settings that involve sensitive tasks (e.g., male and female genital examination) or the potential for harm (e.g., invasive procedures). For instance, although it would be most realistic to assess intubation skills of medical students or anesthesiology interns during live cases in the operating room, is it ethical to allow novices to perform such procedures on real patients—whether for training or assessment purposes—when mistakes could jeopardize patients' health? Using cadavers or animals as substitutes for live humans raises other ethical questions, with animal welfare issues in particular receiving much public scrutiny, and these also lack a certain degree of authenticity. Alternatively, employing simulators—such as some of the computer-enhanced mannequins that have highly realistic airway anatomy as well as programmable physiologic responses—to assess invasive procedural skills circumvents many of these obstacles.

Curriculum Integration and Alignment

Therefore, in healthcare, just as in aviation, simulation-based assessment should become every bit as important as simulation-based teaching and learning. These facets of simulation are inextricably bound in the training environment, such that everyone involved in flying expects not only that they will learn and practice in flight simulators or other simulation scenarios, but also that they will undergo regular skills testing, not just during their initial training and certification but also during periodic reassessments that are routine and ongoing throughout one's career. It is in this way that aviation has developed a safety-oriented culture and maintained its remarkable record of safe flying over many decades. Pointing to this example and striving to achieve similar results in our provision of healthcare, specialties such as anesthesiology, critical care, and emergency medicine have led the patient safety movement, making it one of the most important factors influencing the increased use of simulations for health professional education over the past few decades.

Along similar lines, as the chapter immediately preceding this one emphasized, we in the health professions need to integrate simulation within our systems of education *and* practice. Research has shown that, in order to maximize their educational effect, simulation activities shouldn't be optional or "just for fun"; systematic reviews have identified integration of simulation within the curriculum as one of the features most frequently reported in studies that demonstrate positive learning outcomes from simulation-based education [1–3]. Such curricular integration is best accomplished when a master plan or "blueprint" identifies and aligns desired learning outcomes with instructional and assessment methods. Notice once again that the specification of expected outcomes is the first step in the curriculum planning process! Especially when it comes to simulation-based methods, all too often the process begins with the available technology: "We bought this simulator (because we had 'use it or lose it funds'), now let's see what we can teach/test with it." This proverbial "cart before the horse" mentality often leads to misalignment between purpose and methods and, in the area of assessment, to major threats to the validity of decisions based on evaluation results.

Simulation-Based Methods Within the Assessment Framework

As suggested when we introduced our assessment framework, the choice of best methods from among the numerous tools available for a given evaluation can be guided by aligning different testing modalities (see Table 11.1) along multiple dimensions of an assessment system (see Fig. 11.1).

Outcomes for Assessment

Therefore, starting with the competencies to be assessed, simulations—taken in the broadest sense, running the gamut from written patient management problems and computerized clinical case simulations to SPs, and from task trainers and mannequins to virtual reality devices—can be employed to evaluate almost any outcomes. Among these various domains, however, simulations seem best suited to assess a wide range of "skills" and "attitudes," although certainly they also have applications in the evaluation of "knowledge." For example, in the course of testing a resident's ability to perform chest compressions (a psychomotor skill) on a mannequin and to work as part of a team (a nontechnical skill) during a simulated cardiac arrest, we can also glean information about knowledge of current basic life support algorithms, proper number and depth of chest compressions, etc.; requiring that the resident also delivers bad news to a confederate SP in the scenario—"despite attempted resuscitation, your loved one has died"—facilitates assessment of additional skills (interpersonal communication) as well as aspects of professionalism (respectful attitudes). According to the ACGME Toolbox of Assessment Methods, a consensus of evaluation experts rated simulations "the most desirable" modalities to assess those of the six general competencies that primarily encompass clinical skills domains ("patient care and procedural skills" and "interpersonal and communication skills"), whereas simulations were "the next best method" to gauge "professionalism" and only "a potentially applicable" technique to evaluate areas of "practice-based learning and improvement" [78] (see Table 11.2).

Looking alternatively at the assessment of competencies delineated in the CanMEDS framework, simulations earned the highest rating ("well suited to assessing *many* of the role's key competencies") for the "medical expert" and "collaborator" roles and were thought to be "well suited to assessing *some* of the role's key competencies" for the "manager" and "professional" roles [80]. For instance, use of high-fidelity human patient simulators to evaluate anesthesiology residents' crisis resource management (CRM) skills affords opportunities to test aspects not only of the central "medical expert" role, but also of the "manager," "communicator," and "professional" roles [95]. Again, although it is clear in this example that various cognitive domains could also be evaluated by means of simulation, technical skills and affective attributes seem most amenable to measurement using these techniques. In other words, simulation-based methods are often the best tools for "nailing" assessments of psychomotor as well as nontechnical clinical skills. Extending the metaphor, however, provides a cautionary reminder in the expression: "Give a kid a hammer…" Lest everything start to look like a nail, advocates of simulation strategies must remain mindful of the fact that they are not the optimal solution for every assessment problem!

Levels of Assessment

We can also approach the choice of testing methods from the perspective of assessment levels by matching different modalities with corresponding tiers in Miller's scheme (see Table 11.3). Inspection of Table 11.3 reveals that simulation methods are among the performance-based assessment tools most appropriate for evaluation at the "shows how" level within any of the outcomes domains. Again, because the construct of the Miller model is such that one level necessarily builds upon those below, methods well suited for testing competencies at this performance level often yield information about more basic levels as well; thus, in addition to assessing ability to demonstrate a focused physical (say, pulmonary) exam, simulations (such as SPs or pulmonary task trainers) can be employed to gauge fund of knowledge (about lung anatomy) and clinical reasoning (using exam findings to narrow the differential diagnosis for a complaint of dyspnea). On the other hand, simulation methods may not be as efficient or possess as strong psychometric properties across a wider range of content at the "knows" and "knows how" levels as, for example, written tests consisting of numerous MCQs and matching items. Furthermore, the converse proposition is rarely true: although written and oral assessments are the preferred methods to evaluate what someone knows, they are not appropriate for formal demonstration of what individuals can actually do. Thus, it makes little sense (despite long-standing custom) to assess the capability to perform a procedure by *talking* about it (as in oral board exams for certification in some surgical specialties).

The brief examination stations of an OSCE form one of the most common settings in which we find simulations employed for performance-based evaluations; in various stations, examinees must demonstrate their ability to carry out defined tasks via interaction with SPs, task trainers, or mannequins. Obviously, use of simulations in this context ordinarily restricts the level of assessment (to the "shows how" or lower tiers) in Miller's model—since examinees are aware that the clinical encounter is a simulation, they might behave differently than they would under real-world conditions—but creative work using other forms of simulation, such as "incognito SPs," can also allow us to assess what a health professional "does" in actual practice [96–98]. Akin to using "secret shoppers" to evaluate the customer service skills of retail employees, incognito or "stealth" SPs present, for example, in the clinic or emergency department to providers who are unaware that the encounter is, in fact, a simulation, thereby affording rare opportunities for assessment at the highest level of multiple competencies, including authentic behaviors and attitudes that are otherwise very difficult to evaluate.

In trying to choose the best evaluation methods for a given purpose, we have thus far considered different dimensions of our framework separately; that is, we have tried to match various assessment tools with either the outcomes being assessed *or* the level of assessment. It stands to reason, however, that the optimal method(s) will be found where these constructs intersect. A Venn diagram, as a two-dimensional representation of this exercise in logic, would indicate that the best uses of simulation-based methods are for assessment of psychomotor (i.e., clinical or procedural) skills and non-technical (i.e., affective or attitude) competencies at the "shows" how level.

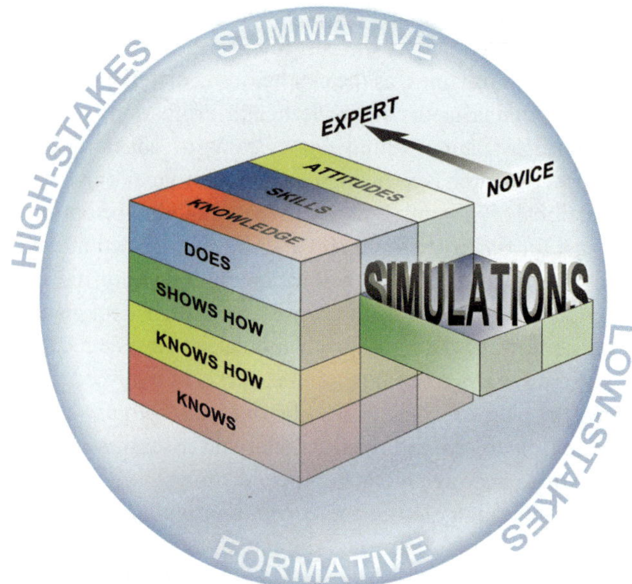

Fig. 11.2 Use of simulation-based methods within a multidimensional framework for assessment

Stages of Development

Alternatively, we can depict this graphically using our multidimensional framework and revisit the toolbox metaphor once again: numerous evaluation methods are the tools contained in different compartments of the toolbox, which are organized in columns according to outcomes and in rows corresponding to assessment levels. Having already determined the best place to keep simulation methods (see Fig. 11.2), we must still decide which tools among several available in those "drawers" are best suited to assess learners at different developmental stages.

For example, simulations with varying degrees of fidelity are more or less appropriate for novices versus experts. Breaking down complex skills into component parts makes it easier for beginning learners to focus on one task at a time and master sequential elements. Simulations with low to medium physical and psychological fidelity (such as an intubation task trainer consisting only of a head, neck, and inflatable lungs) present manageable levels of cognitive load for novices, whereas this group may become overwhelmed by trying to learn the task of endotracheal intubation during a full-blown scenario consisting of a multifunctional human patient simulator in a realistic operating room (OR) setting with numerous participants including SPs playing the role of various OR staff. Choosing the right rating instruments to use in simulation-based assessments should also involve consideration of level of training. To be confident that beginners have learned the systematic process needed to perform certain procedures, we typically use checklists of action items that are important to demonstrate.

By contrast, advanced trainees or experienced practitioners develop a more holistic approach to clinical problem solving and learn which steps they can skip while still reliably arriving at the correct conclusion. Thus, they sometimes score lower than beginners on checklist-based assessments [99]. Global ratings using behaviorally anchored scales are probably more appropriate instruments to use when evaluating this group. In addition, the artificiality of lower fidelity simulations weakens the extrapolation component of the argument and may threaten the validity of decisions based on such assessment of performance by experts. High-fidelity simulations, on the other hand, such as hybrids combining SPs with task trainers [100] more realistically imitate actual clinical encounters, where healthcare providers must bring to bear multiple competencies simultaneously (e.g., performing a procedure while communicating with the patient and demonstrating professional and respectful attitudes), so interpretations of results from such assessments are likely to be more valid.

Assessment Context

Continuing this last example, moving the location of the hybrid simulation-based evaluation from a dedicated testing center or simulation lab to the actual clinical setting in which a trainee or practitioner works (so-called "in situ" simulation) can also enhance the authenticity of the scenario [101], thus greatly strengthening inferences that performances in the assessment are likely to be predictive of behaviors in real-world practice. Similarly, the simulation testing environment should be reflective of the local context, including elements that typically would (or would not) be found in particular hospitals or in certain countries or geographic regions, depending on availability of resources. Testing scenarios should be designed with sensitivity to religious, social, or cultural mores, such as appropriate interactions between genders or between superiors and subordinates. Finally, and very importantly, the purpose of the assessment will influence the choice of simulation-based methods: for instance, a station testing physical exam skills during a summative exam for licensure—where criteria related to reliability are paramount—might employ a mannequin simulator because of its programmability and high level of reproducibility of exam findings. By contrast, an impromptu formative assessment of a student's history-taking skills during a medical school clerkship—where educational effect is an important characteristic—might use a nursing assistant who happened to be working in the clinic that day (rather than a well-trained SP) to portray the patient.

Conclusion

Consideration of the different dimensions in the assessment framework we have proposed can guide not only choice of assessment strategies in general (i.e., whether to use a performance-based vs. other test) and selection of particular methods within a given category (e.g., simulation-based exam vs. a long case) but also decisions to use a specific form of simulation among the possible modalities available. Clearly these multiple dimensions are interrelated, and thinking about areas of interaction will help identify strengths to capitalize on and potential challenges to try to mitigate. Specification of the outcomes to be assessed is the first step in the current competency-based educational paradigm. These must then be considered in the context of desired assessment level, examinee stage of training or experience, and overall purpose of the assessment. Alignment of these various elements will improve chances that more quality criteria will be met from the perspective of multiple stakeholders, including those undergoing the assessment, teachers and schools, accreditation organizations, and, ultimately, the public whom we as healthcare professionals all serve.

References

1. Issenberg SB, McGaghie WC, Petrusa ER, Lee Gordon D, Scalese RJ. Features and uses of high-fidelity medical simulations that lead to effective learning: a BEME systematic review. Med Teach. 2005;27(1):10–28.
2. McGaghie WC, Issenberg SB, Petrusa ER, Scalese RJ. A critical review of simulation-based medical education research: 2003–2009. Med Educ. 2010;44(1):50–63.
3. Cook DA, Hatala R, Brydges R, et al. Technology-enhanced simulation for health professions education: a systematic review and meta-analysis. JAMA. 2011;306(9):978–88.
4. Hatala R, Kassen BO, Nishikawa J, Cole G, Issenberg SB. Incorporating simulation technology in a Canadian internal medicine specialty examination: a descriptive report. Acad Med. 2005;80(6):554–6.
5. Hatala R, Scalese RJ, Cole G, Bacchus M, Kassen B, Issenberg SB. Development and validation of a cardiac findings checklist for use with simulator-based assessments of cardiac physical examination competence. Simul Healthc. 2009;4(1):17–21.
6. Barrows HS, Abahamson S. The programmed patient: a technique for appraising student performance in clinical neurology. J Med Educ. 1964;39:802–5.
7. Abrahamson S, Denson JS, Wolf RM. Effectiveness of a simulator in training anesthesiology residents. J Med Educ. 1969;44(6):515–9.
8. Stevenson A, Lindberg CA, editors. New Oxford American Dictionary. 3rd ed. New York: Oxford University Press; 2010.
9. McGaghie WC. Simulation in professional competence assessment: basic considerations. In: Tekian A, McGuire CH, McGaghie WC, editors. Innovative simulations for assessing professional competence. Chicago: Department of Medical Education, University of Illinois at Chicago; 1999. p. 7–22.
10. Maran NJ, Glavin RJ. Low- to high-fidelity simulation – a continuum of medical education? Med Educ. 2003;37 Suppl 1:22–8.
11. Quirey Jr WO, Adams J. National Practitioner Data Bank revisited – the lessons of Michael Swango, M.D. Virginia State Bar Web site. http://www.vsb.org/sections/hl/bank.pdf. Accessed 30 Aug 2012.
12. The Shipman Inquiry. Second report: The police investigation of March 1998. Official Documents Web site. http://www.official-documents.gov.uk/document/cm58/5853/5853.pdf. Published 2003. Accessed 30 Aug 2012.
13. Harden RM, Crosby JR, Davis M. An introduction to outcome-based education. Med Teach. 1999;21(1):7–14.
14. Harden RM, Crosby JR, Davis MH, Friedman M. AMEE guide no. 14: outcome-based education: part 5. From competency to meta-competency: a model for the specification of learning outcomes. Med Teach. 1999;21(6):546–52.
15. Schwarz MR, Wojtczak A. Global minimum essential requirements: a road towards competence-oriented medical education. Med Teach. 2002;24(2):125–9.
16. General Medical Council. Tomorrow's Doctors – outcomes and standards for undergraduate medical education. 2nd ed. London: General Medical Council; 2009.

17. Scottish Deans' Medical Curriculum Group. The Scottish Doctor – learning outcomes for the medical undergraduate in Scotland: a foundation for competent and reflective practitioners. 3rd ed. Dundee: Association for Medical Education in Europe; 2007.
18. Frank JR, editor. The CanMEDS 2005 physician competency framework. Better standards. Better physicians. Better care. Ottawa: The Royal College of Physicians and Surgeons of Canada; 2005.
19. Accreditation Council for Graduate Medical Education. Core program requirements categorization. ACGME 2012 Standards – Categorization of Common Program Requirements Web site. http://www.acgme-nas.org/assets/pdf/CPR-Categorization-TCC.pdf. Published 7 Feb 2012. Updated 2012. Accessed 24 June 2012.
20. General Medical Council. Good medical practice. 3rd ed. London: General Medical Council; 2009.
21. American Association of Colleges of Nursing. The essentials of baccalaureate education for professional nursing practice. Washington, D.C.: American Association of Colleges of Nursing; 2008.
22. Core competencies for nurse practitioners. National Organization of Nurse Practitioner Faculties (NONPF) Web site. http://nonpf.com/displaycommon.cfm?an=1&subarticlenbr=14. Updated 2012. Accessed 30 Aug 2012.
23. Competencies for the physician assistant profession. National Commission on Certification of Physician Assistants Web site. http://www.nccpa.net/pdfs/Definition%20of%20PA%20Competencies%203.5%20for%20Publication.pdf. Published 2006. Accessed 30 Aug 2012.
24. Core competencies. Association of American Veterinary Medical Colleges Web site. http://www.aavmc.org/data/files/navmec/navmec-corecompetencies.pdf. Published 2012. Accessed 30 Aug 2012.
25. Van Der Vleuten CPM, Schuwirth LWT. Assessing professional competence: from methods to programmes. Med Educ. 2005;39(3):309–17.
26. Norcini J, Anderson B, Bollela V, et al. Criteria for good assessment: consensus statement and recommendations from the Ottawa 2010 conference. Med Teach. 2011;33(3):206–14.
27. Axelson RD, Kreiter CD. Reliability. In: Downing SM, Yudkowsky R, editors. Assessment in health professions education. New York: Routledge; 2009. p. 57–74.
28. Clauser BE, Margolis MJ, Swanson DB. Issues of validity and reliability for assessments in medical education. In: Holmboe ES, Hawkins RE, editors. Practical guide to the evaluation of clinical competence. Philadelphia: Mosby/Elsevier; 2008. p. 10–23.
29. McAleer S. Choosing assessment instruments. In: Dent JA, Harden RM, editors. A practical guide for medical teachers. 2nd ed. Edinburgh: Elsevier/Churchill Livingstone; 2005. p. 302–10.
30. Downing SM, Haladyna TM. Validity and its threats. In: Downing SM, Yudkowsky R, editors. Assessment in health professions education. New York: Routledge; 2009. p. 21–56.
31. Downing SM. Validity: on the meaningful interpretation of assessment data. Med Educ. 2003;37(9):830–7.
32. Kane MT. An argument-based approach to validity. Psych Bull. 1992;112(3):527–35.
33. Kane MT. The assessment of professional competence. Eval Health Prof. 1992;15(2):163–82.
34. McGaghie WC, Cohen ER, Wayne DB. Are United States Medical Licensing Exam Step 1 and 2 scores valid measures for postgraduate medical residency selection decisions? Acad Med. 2011;86(1):48–52.
35. Wayne DB, Fudala MJ, Butter J, et al. Comparison of two standard-setting methods for advanced cardiac life support training. Acad Med. 2005;80(10 Suppl):S63–6.
36. Wayne DB, Butter J, Cohen ER, McGaghie WC. Setting defensible standards for cardiac auscultation skills in medical students. Acad Med. 2009;84(10 Suppl):S94–6.
37. Messick S. Validity. In: Linn R, editor. Educational measurement. 3rd ed. New York: American Council on Education/Macmillan; 1989. p. 13–103.
38. Schuwirth LW, van der Vleuten CP. Changing education, changing assessment, changing research? Med Educ. 2004;38(8):805–12.
39. Federation of State Medical Boards of the United States/National Board of Medical Examiners. 2012 Bulletin of Information. Philadelphia: United States Medical Licensing Examination.
40. Bulletin: Examination content. United States Medical Licensing Examination (USMLE) Web site. http://www.usmle.org/bulletin/exam-content/#step2cs. Published 2011. Accessed Aug 2012.
41. Hodges B, Regehr G, Hanson M, McNaughton N. An objective structured clinical examination for evaluating psychiatric clinical clerks. Acad Med. 1997;72(8):715–21.
42. Miller GE. The assessment of clinical skills/competence/performance. Acad Med. 1990;65(9 Suppl):S63–7.
43. Downing SM, Yudkowsky R, editors. Assessment in health professions education. New York: Routledge; 2009.
44. Holmboe ES, Hawkins RE, editors. Practical guide to the evaluation of clinical competence. Philadelphia: Mosby/Elsevier; 2008.
45. Dent JA, Harden RM, editors. A practical guide for medical teachers. 2nd ed. Edinburgh: Elsevier/Churchill Livingstone; 2005.
46. Amin Z, Seng CY, Eng KH. Practical guide to medical student assessment. Singapore: World Scientific; 2006.
47. Norman GR, van der Vleuten CPM, Newble DI, editors. International handbook of research in medical education. Dordrecht: Kluwer Academic; 2002.
48. Downing SM, Yudkowsky R. Introduction to assessment in the health professions. In: Downing SM, Yudkowsky R, editors. Assessment in health professions education. New York: Routledge; 2009. p. 1–20.
49. Norcini J, Holmboe ES, Hawkins RE. Evaluation challenges in the era of outcome-based education. In: Holmboe ES, Hawkins RE, editors. Practical guide to the evaluation of clinical competence. Philadelphia: Mosby/Elsevier; 2008. p. 1–9.
50. Newble D. Assessment: Introduction. In: Norman GR, van der Vleuten CPM, Newble DI, editors. International handbook of research in medical education, vol. 2. Dordrecht: Kluwer Academic; 2002. p. 645–6.
51. Downing SM. Written tests: constructed-response and selected-response formats. In: Downing SM, Yudkowsky R, editors. Assessment in health professions education. New York: Routledge; 2009. p. 149–84.
52. Hawkins RE, Swanson DB. Using written examinations to assess medical knowledge and its application. In: Holmboe ES, Hawkins RE, editors. Practical guide to the evaluation of clinical competence. Philadelphia: Mosby/Elsevier; 2008. p. 42–59.
53. Downing SM. Assessment of knowledge with written test forms. In: Norman GR, van der Vleuten CPM, Newble DI, editors. International handbook of research in medical education, vol. 2. Dordrecht: Kluwer Academic; 2002. p. 647–72.
54. Schuwirth LWT, van der Vleuten CPM. Written assessments. In: Dent JA, Harden RM, editors. A practical guide for medical teachers. 2nd ed. Edinburgh: Elsevier/Churchill Livingstone; 2005. p. 311–22.
55. Tekian A, Yudkowsky R. Oral examinations. In: Downing SM, Yudkowsky R, editors. Assessment in health professions education. New York: Routledge; 2009. p. 269–86.
56. Marks M, Humphrey-Murto S. Performance assessment. In: Dent JA, Harden RM, editors. A practical guide for medical teachers. 2nd ed. Edinburgh: Elsevier/Churchill Livingstone; 2005. p. 323–35.
57. Petrusa ER. Clinical performance assessments. In: Norman GR, van der Vleuten CPM, Newble DI, editors. International handbook of research in medical education, vol. 2. Dordrecht: Kluwer Academic; 2002. p. 673–710.
58. Harden RM, Gleeson FA. Assessment of clinical competence using an objective structured clinical examination (OSCE). Med Educ. 1979;13:41–54.
59. Yudkowsky R. Performance tests. In: Downing SM, Yudkowsky R, editors. Assessment in health professions education. New York: Routledge; 2009. p. 217–43.
60. McGaghie WC, Issenberg SB. Simulations in assessment. In: Downing SM, Yudkowsky R, editors. Assessment in health professions education. New York: Routledge; 2009. p. 245–68.

61. Scalese RJ, Issenberg SB. Simulation-based assessment. In: Holmboe ES, Hawkins RE, editors. Practical guide to the evaluation of clinical competence. Philadelphia: Mosby/Elsevier; 2008. p. 179–200.
62. McGaghie WC, Butter J, Kaye M. Observational assessment. In: Downing SM, Yudkowsky R, editors. Assessment in health professions education. New York: Routledge; 2009. p. 185–216.
63. Davis MH, Ponnamperuma GG. Work-based assessment. In: Dent JA, Harden RM, editors. A practical guide for medical teachers. 2nd ed. Edinburgh: Elsevier/Churchill Livingstone; 2005. p. 336–45.
64. Lockyer JM, Clyman SG. Multisource feedback (360-degree evaluation). In: Holmboe ES, Hawkins RE, editors. Practical guide to the evaluation of clinical competence. Philadelphia: Mosby/Elsevier; 2008. p. 75–85.
65. Holmboe ES. Practice audit, medical record review, and chart-stimulated recall. In: Holmboe ES, Hawkins RE, editors. Practical guide to the evaluation of clinical competence. Philadelphia: Mosby/Elsevier; 2008. p. 60–74.
66. Cunnington J, Southgate L. Relicensure, recertification, and practice-based assessment. In: Norman GR, van der Vleuten CPM, Newble DI, editors. International handbook of research in medical education, vol. 2. Dordrecht: Kluwer Academic; 2002. p. 883–912.
67. Vukanovic-Criley JM, Criley S, Warde CM, et al. Competency in cardiac examination skills in medical students, trainees, physicians, and faculty: a multicenter study. Arch Intern Med. 2006;166(6):610–6.
68. Holmboe ES, Davis MH, Carraccio C. Portfolios. In: Holmboe ES, Hawkins RE, editors. Practical guide to the evaluation of clinical competence. Philadelphia: Mosby/Elsevier; 2008. p. 86–101.
69. Davis MH, Ponnamperuma GG. Portfolios, projects and dissertations. In: Dent JA, Harden RM, editors. A practical guide for medical teachers. 2nd ed. Edinburgh: Elsevier/Churchill Livingstone; 2005. p. 346–56.
70. Tekian A, Yudkowsky R. Assessment portfolios. In: Downing SM, Yudkowsky R, editors. Assessment in health professions education. New York: Routledge; 2009. p. 287–304.
71. Pangaro L, Holmboe ES. Evaluation forms and global rating scales. In: Holmboe ES, Hawkins RE, editors. Practical guide to the evaluation of clinical competence. Philadelphia: Mosby/Elsevier; 2008. p. 24–41.
72. Flin R, Patey R. Non-technical skills for anaesthetists: developing and applying ANTS. Best Pract Res Clin Anaesthesiol. 2011;25(2):215–27.
73. Stufflebeam DL. Guidelines for developing evaluation checklists: The checklists development checklist (CDC). Western Michigan University: The Evaluation Center Web site. http://www.wmich.edu/evalctr/archive_checklists/guidelines_cdc.pdf. Published 2010. Accessed 31 Aug 2012.
74. Bichelmeyer BA. Checklist for formatting checklists. Western Michigan University: The Evaluation Center Web site. http://www.wmich.edu/evalctr/archive_checklists/cfc.pdf. Published 2003. Accessed 31 Aug 2012.
75. Yudkowsky R, Downing SM, Tekian A. Standard setting. In: Downing SM, Yudkowsky R, editors. Assessment in health professions education. New York: Routledge; 2009. p. 119–48.
76. Norcini J, Guille R. Combining tests and setting standards. In: Norman GR, van der Vleuten CPM, Newble DI, editors. International handbook of research in medical education, vol. 2. Dordrecht: Kluwer Academic; 2002. p. 811–34.
77. Norcini J. Standard setting. In: Dent JA, Harden RM, editors. A practical guide for medical teachers. 2nd ed. Edinburgh: Elsevier/Churchill Livingstone; 2005. p. 293–301.
78. Accreditation Council for Graduate Medical Education/American Board of Medical Specialties. Toolbox of assessment methods. http://www.partners.org/Assets/Documents/Graduate-Medical-Education/ToolTable.pdf. Updated 2000. Accessed 27 June 2012.
79. Duffy FD, Holmboe ES. Competence in improving systems of care through practice-based learning and improvement. In: Holmboe ES, Hawkins RE, editors. Practical guide to the evaluation of clinical competence. Philadelphia: Mosby/Elsevier; 2008. p. 149–78.
80. Bandiera G, Sherbino J, Frank JR, editors. The CanMEDS assessment tools handbook. An introductory guide to assessment methods for the CanMEDS competencies. Ottawa: The Royal College of Physicians and Surgeons of Canada; 2006.
81. Pangaro L. A new vocabulary and other innovations for improving descriptive in-training evaluations. Acad Med. 1999;74(11): 1203–7.
82. Introduction to the basic log book. Royal College of Obstetricians and Gynaecologists Web site. http://www.rcog.org.uk/files/rcog-corp/uploaded-files/ED-Basic-logbook.pdf. Published 2006. Accessed 31 Aug 2012.
83. 'Staged' models of skills acquisition. University of Medicine and Dentistry of New Jersey Web site. http://www.umdnj.edu/idsweb/idst5340/models_skills_acquisition.htm. Accessed 31 Aug 2012.
84. Issenberg SB, McGaghie WC, Hart IR, et al. Simulation technology for health care professional skills training and assessment. JAMA. 1999;282(9):861–6.
85. Fincher RE, Lewis LA. Simulations used to teach clinical skills. In: Norman GR, van der Vleuten CPM, Newble DI, editors. International Handbook of Research in Medical Education, vol. 1. Dordrecht: Kluwer Academic; 2002. p. 499–535.
86. Collins JP, Harden RM. AMEE education guide no. 13: Real patients, simulated patients and simulators in clinical examinations. Med Teach. 1998;20:508–21.
87. Clauser BE, Schuwirth LWT. The use of computers in assessment. In: Norman GR, van der Vleuten CPM, Newble DI, editors. International handbook of research in medical education, vol. 2. Dordrecht: Kluwer Academic; 2002. p. 757–92.
88. Gaba DM. Crisis resource management and teamwork training in anaesthesia. Br J Anaesth. 2010;105(1):3–6.
89. Institute of Medicine. To err is human: building a safer health system. Washington, D.C.: National Academy Press; 2000.
90. Department of Health. An organisation with a memory: report of an expert group on learning from adverse events in the NHS. London: The Stationery Office; 2000.
91. Goodman W. The world of civil simulators. Flight Int Mag. 1978;18:435.
92. Wachtel J, Walton DG. The future of nuclear power plant simulation in the United States. In: Simulation for nuclear reactor technology. Cambridge: Cambridge University Press; 1985.
93. Ressler EK, Armstrong JE, Forsythe G. Military mission rehearsal: from sandtable to virtual reality. In: Tekian A, McGuire CH, McGaghie WC, editors. Innovative simulations for assessing professional competence. Chicago: Department of Medical Education, University of Illinois at Chicago; 1999. p. 157–74.
94. N.Y. jet crash called 'miracle on the Hudson'. msnbc.com Web site. http://www.msnbc.msn.com/id/28678669/ns/us_news-life/t/ny-jet-crash-called-miracle-hudson/. Published 15 Jan 2009. Updated 2009. Accessed 10 June 2012.
95. Berkenstadt H, Ziv A, Gafni N, Sidi A. Incorporating simulation-based objective structured clinical examination into the Israeli National Board Examination in Anesthesiology. Anesth Analg. 2006;102(3):853–8.
96. Borrell-Carrio F, Poveda BF, Seco EM, Castillejo JA, Gonzalez MP, Rodriguez EP. Family physicians' ability to detect a physical sign (hepatomegaly) from an unannounced standardized patient (incognito SP). Eur J Gen Pract. 2011;17(2):95–102.
97. Maiburg BH, Rethans JJ, van Erk IM, Mathus-Vliegen LM, van Ree JW. Fielding incognito standardised patients as 'known' patients in a controlled trial in general practice. Med Educ. 2004;38(12):1229–35.

98. Gorter SL, Rethans JJ, Scherpbier AJ, et al. How to introduce incognito standardized patients into outpatient clinics of specialists in rheumatology. Med Teach. 2001;23(2):138–44.
99. Hodges B, Regehr G, McNaughton N, Tiberius R, Hanson M. OSCE checklists do not capture increasing levels of expertise. Acad Med. 1999;74(10):1129–34.
100. Kneebone R, Kidd J, Nestel D, Asvall S, Paraskeva P, Darzi A. An innovative model for teaching and learning clinical procedures. Med Educ. 2002;36(7):628–34.
101. Kneebone RL, Kidd J, Nestel D, et al. Blurring the boundaries: scenario-based simulation in a clinical setting. Med Educ. 2005;39(6):580–7.

Simulation for Licensure and Certification

12

Amitai Ziv, Haim Berkenstadt, and Orit Eisenberg

Introduction

Throughout their careers, health professionals are subjected to a wide array of assessment processes. These processes are aimed at evaluating various professional skills including knowledge, physical exam and communication skills, and clinical decision-making. While some of these assessments are used for formative evaluation, others are employed for summative evaluation in order to establish readiness and competence for certification purposes. Unfortunately, the traditional emphasis of medical education has been on the "easy to measure" (i.e., cognitive skills and knowledge) and not necessarily on what is "important to measure," ignoring in many ways the sound assessment of "higher order skills" considered to be crucial for the safe delivery of quality care, such as safety skills (e.g., handover, adherence to guidelines, error recovery, calling for help, documentation skills), teamwork skills (e.g., leadership, followership, communication, counseling, interprofessional skills), and personal traits (e.g., integrity, motivation, capacity, humility, risk-taking traits). These skills are crucial to ensuring that a licensed and certified physician is capable of delivering quality care.

In the past two decades, there has been a growing interest in simulation-based assessment (SBA) as demonstrated by the fact that SBA has been incorporated in a number of high-stakes certification and licensure examinations [1]. The driving forces for this change mostly stem from the patient safety movement and the recognition of the medical community and the general public that medical education and its traditional assessment paradigm has a share in the suboptimal patient safety that surfaced in the American Institute of Medicine's "To Err is Human" report in 1999. Furthermore, the recognized link between safety and simulation and the understanding that SBA has the power to serve as a vehicle for cultural change towards safer and more ethical medical education has led education and accreditation bodies to search for means to become more accountable for the health professional "products" they produce. The need to develop and adapt competency-based assessment for certification and recertification policies has emerged as a part of this accountability. Other contributing factors driving SBA forward are the global migration of healthcare professionals and the increased need for proficiency gatekeeping on behalf of healthcare systems that absorb health professionals who were trained in foreign educational systems that might not have rigorous enough proficiency training in their curriculum. Finally, SBA is also driven by the rapidly developing simulation industry which provides more modern simulators including some built-in proficiency metrics.

Compared with other traditional assessment methods (i.e., written tests, oral tests, and "on the job" assessments), SBA has several advantages: the ability to measure actual performance in a context and environment similar to those in the actual clinical field; the ability to assess multidimensional professional competencies including knowledge, technical skills, clinical skills, communication, and decision-making as well as higher order competencies such as safety skills and teamwork skills; the ability to test predefined sets of medical scenarios

A. Ziv, MD, MHA (✉)
Medical Education, Sackler School of Medicine, Tel Aviv University, Tel Aviv, Israel

Patient Safety and Risk Management, Israel Center for Medical Simulation (MSR), Chaim Sheba Medical Center, Tel Hashomer 52621, Israel
e-mail: zamitai@post.tau.ac.il

H. Berkenstadt, MD
Department of Anesthesiology and Intensive Care, Sackler Faculty of Medicine, Tel Aviv University, Tel Aviv, 69978, Israel

Department of Anesthesiology, Sheba Medical Center, Ramat Gan, Israel
e-mail: haim.berkenstadt@sheba.health.gov.il

O. Eisenberg, PhD
MAROM—Assessment and Admissions Centers, National Institute for Testing and Evaluation, P.O. Box 26015, Jerusalem 91260, Israel

Assessment Unit, The Israel Center for Medical Simulation, Tel Hashomer, Israel
e-mail: orit@nite.org.il

A.I. Levine et al. (eds.), *The Comprehensive Textbook of Healthcare Simulation*,
DOI 10.1007/978-1-4614-5993-4_12,

according to a test blueprint, including the presentation of rare and challenging clinical scenarios; the ability to present standard, reliable, and fair testing conditions to all examinees; and the fact that SBA entails no risk to patients [2, 3].

This chapter deals with the role SBA can and should play in regulatory-driven assessment programs for healthcare students and providers seeking licensure and certification. Regulatory programs are defined as processes required by external entities as a condition to maintain some form of credentials, including certification within a discipline, licensure, and privileges within an institution and/or health systems [4]. We will also describe the Israeli experience in SBA at MSR—the Israel Center for Medical Simulation [5]—and highlight our insights from over 10 years of experience in conducting regulatory-driven SBA programs with focus on the barriers, challenges, and keys to success.

Brief History and Review of Current Use of Simulation-Based Licensure and Certification

The foundation for SBA as a regulatory requirement began in the 1960s and 1970s when basic and advanced life support courses—partially based on simple mannequins/simulators—were introduced and endorsed as a standard requirement by medical and licensure associations [6]. Another important aspect that contributed to the foundation of SBA was the introduction of simulated/standardized patients (SPs) and the objective structured clinical examination (OSCE) approach in the 1970s. The OSCE methodology matured in the 1990s and throughout the twenty-first century, especially by being employed more and more by regulatory boards around the world as the tool of choice to assess medical school graduates' clinical skills, as part of a certification process. Inspired by the work done by the Medical Council of Canada (MCC) which launched an OSCE-based licensure for all its local and foreign graduates (titled Qualifying Examination Part II (MCCQE Part II)) [7], the Educational Commission for Foreign Medical Graduates (ECFMG) [8] launched its CSA (Clinical Skills Assessment) in 1998 for US foreign graduates. This exam was subsequently (2004) modified and endorsed by the National Board of Medical Examiners (NBME) to become the United States Medical Licensing Examination Step 2 Clinical Skills (USMLE Step II CS) required for US graduates as well [9]. More recently, the American Board of Surgery has begun to require a successful completion of the Fundamentals of Laparoscopic Surgery (FLS) course for initial certification of residents in surgery [10, 11]. These are just a few examples of the late-twentieth–early-twenty-first-centuries' paradigm shift to include simulation-based exams as a well-established and well-recognized high-stakes assessment tool worldwide for healthcare professional certification [1, 12–15].

SBA endorsement is increasing in other healthcare professions, although less published academically. In nursing, for example, OSCEs are being used in Quebec, Canada, as part of the registered nurse licensure examination [16] and for licensure of nurse practitioners in British Columbia and Quebec. An assessment that includes OSCEs is required for all foreign-educated nurses desiring to become registered in any Canadian province [17]. In the last decade, SBA utilizing SPs is increasingly used also for the admission and screening of candidates to medical schools' interpersonal/noncognitive attributes [18–21].

Simulation-Based Licensure and Certification: Challenges and Keys for Success

SBA requires multi-professional collaboration. To achieve an effective test for any high-stakes context, the involvement of experts from three different fields—content experts, simulation experts, and measurement experts (i.e., psychometricians)—is mandatory. In the following section, we will try to highlight some of the main concerns or challenges that are inherent to SBA and suggest how the triple professional collaboration assists in facing these challenges and ensuring a successful measurement in SBA.

Does SBA Really Simulate Reality?

The rapid development of medical simulation technology, including advanced computerized full-body mannequin simulators and task trainers, greatly expands the horizons of possible clinical skills that could be assessed using simulation [1]. However, recognizing the limitations of current simulation technology, for example, the inability of existing mannequin simulators to sweat or change skin color makes SBA incomplete in its ability to authentically simulate certain clinical conditions [22]. In addition, some of the important job characteristics (e.g., team management) are also difficult to simulate in a standard measurable way that is required for high-stakes assessment. These limitations can be partially overcome by providing (by the simulator operator—verbally or in a written form) examinees those missing features which are not presented by the simulator and/or through utilizing a hybrid (SP and a simulator) model and/or through using a standard mock team member for team management evaluation. Regardless of the strategy, the limitations of the simulator being utilized must be recognized and furnished to the participants.

SBA developers should be well aware of these limitations. After content experts define test goals and test blueprints (i.e., a list of content domains and clinical skills to be measured) with the assistance of psychometricians, the simulation experts should suggest their perspective on the appropriate simulation module(s) to be used. With the acknowledgment that not everything can be simulated, one should keep in mind that SBA should not be the automatic replacement of other assessment methods. Rather, it should be viewed as a complementary tool and used only when it can serve a sound measurement and when it has a real added value to the overall assessment of the health professional.

Can SBA Really Measure What We Want It to Measure?

SBA Scoring Strategies

If SBA is used in a high-stakes licensure/certification context, it is essential that scores be reliable and valid. Two main factors contribute to measurement accuracy in SBA: the metrics (measurement method) and the raters. Developing assessment rubrics is certainly one of the main challenges in SBA, and it requires the cooperation between content experts and psychometricians. The first decision in this process should be what type of measurement method (analytic/checklist or holistic) is suitable for each simulation model or scenario [1]. For a typical clinical skills simulation scenario, checklists can be constructed to tap explicit processes such as history taking, physical examination, and clinical treatment steps. Although checklists have worked reasonably well and have provided modestly reproducible scores depending on the number of simulated scenarios [1], they have been criticized for a number of reasons. First, checklists, while objective in terms of scoring, can be subjective in terms of construction [23]. While specific practice guidelines may exist for some conditions, there can still be considerable debate as to which actions are important or necessary in other conditions. Without expert consensus, one could question the validity of the scenario scores. Second, the use of checklists, if known by those taking the assessment, may promote rote behaviors such as employing rapid-fire questioning techniques. To accrue more "points," examinees may ask as many questions as they can and/or perform as many physical examination maneuvers as are possible within the allotted time frame. Once again, this could call into questioning the validity of the scores. Third, and likely most relevant for SBA of advanced professionals (i.e., licensure and certification context), checklists are not conducive to scoring some aspects of professional case handling such as timing or sequencing of tasks, communication with patients and team members, and decision-making [1]. For these reasons, it is unlikely that checklist-based scoring alone will adequately satisfy.

Holistic scoring (or global scoring), where the entire performance is rated as a whole or when several generally defined performance parameters are rated, is also often used in SBA [1]. Rating scales can effectively measure certain constructs, especially those that are complex and multidimensional, such as communication and teamwork skills [24, 25], and they allow raters to take into account egregious actions and/or unnecessary patient management strategies [26]. Psychometric properties of global rating scales have yielded reliable measurement [26, 27] and, for advanced practitioners seeking licensure, have a major role in assessment.

SBA Raters, Importance, Development, and Maintenance

The other main factor that affects measurement quality in SBA is the raters. After choosing the preferred scoring method and investing in its development using relevant expertise, one has to make sure that qualified raters are employed for the actual measurement. Recruiting good raters and assuring their ongoing commitment for a regulatory re-accruing certification or licensure project is a challenge. Often, when a new SBA project is presented, there is good enthusiastic spirit among senior professionals in the profession that is being tested. It is easy to recruit these professionals for the rater position in the first few testing cycles. However, as the time goes by and the test becomes more routine, recruitment and ongoing maintenance of raters becomes more difficult. Therefore, it is essential to come up with ways to raise raters' commitment to the SBA project. For example, one may consider reimbursing raters for their participation in the test, awarding academic credit, or providing them with other promotional benefit. Furthermore, efforts should be made to ensure that the raters' role in the test group is highly regarded as a prestigious position with good reputation. In addition, it is highly crucial to generate the support of the regulators of the national, regional, or relevant local medical systems who must define the SBA project as high on their priorities' order.

In addition to recruiting good and collaborative raters, the most important component of SBA regarding the raters is their training [4]. While the raters in SBA are almost always senior experts in the profession being tested, they are not experts in measurement. "Train the rater" workshops are a crucial element of the SBA development and implementation, which contain two components: presentation of the test format and scoring methodology coupled with multiple scoring exercises with emphasis on raters' calibration. The calibration process should be based on preprepared scoring exercises (i.e., video clips) in which raters score examinees' performance individually and afterwards discuss their ratings with special attention allotted to outlier ratings.

Can Examinees in SBA Show Their Real Ability?

Although current simulation methodology can mimic the real medical environment to a great degree, it might still be questionable whether examinees' performance in the testing environment really represents their true ability. Test anxiety might increase in an unfamiliar testing environment; difficulty to handle unfamiliar technology (i.e., monitor, defibrillator, or other devices that may be different than the ones used in the examinee's specific clinical environment) or even the need to "act as if" in an artificial scenario (i.e., talking to a simulator, examining a "patient" knowing he/she is an actor) might all compromise examinees' performance.

The best solution to the main issues raised above is the orientation of examinees to the simulated environment. Examinees must be oriented to the test environment and receive elaborated instructions regarding the local technology and the main principles of SBA-required behavior. It is also of great value that examinees get the chance to practice in the relevant simulation methodology. In addition, raters and testers should be instructed to support examinees who have difficulty to "get into the role-playing" by reminding them throughout the test to behave "as if they are in the actual clinical setting."

Is SBA Worth the Investment?

SBA is an expensive venture! As mentioned before, the development stage requires involvement of diverse and costly human resources (psychometric, simulation, and content experts). Raters' hours are also costly (senior content experts that leave their routine clinical work for several days per year are not inexpensive), and the challenging logistical preparation and operation during testing days also requires a substantial human and infrastructural investment. In addition, unlike written tests, the number of examinees per testing day is limited by the size of the simulation facility and the availability of simulators and raters. This fact makes it necessary to develop more testing forms (to avoid leak of confidential test information), which also increases test costs and complicates validity.

In order to justify the huge investment in financial, human, and technological resources, the SBA professionals must supply proof for the psychometric qualities and added value of a test over other less costly approaches. Boulet [1] reviewed the issues of reliability and validity evidence in SBA. He described some studies that showed evidence for internal consistency within and across scenarios, studies that deal with inter-rater reliability and generalizability (G), and studies that were conducted to specifically delimit the relative magnitude of various error sources and their associated interactions. Boulet also emphasized the importance of using multiple independent observations for each examinee to achieve good enough test reliability.

The validity of a simulation-based assessment relates to the inferences that we want to make based on the examination scores [28]. There are several potential ways to assess the validity of test scores. For SBA, especially for tests used for certification and licensure, content validity and construct validity have been reported extensively [1, 29–33]. However, predictive validity, which is the most crucial validity aspect for this type of test, is also the most complicated one to prove, and much research effort is still needed to establish this aspect of SBA [1, 34, 35].

To conclude, in high-stakes licensure and certification SBA, the purpose of the evaluations is, most often, to assure the public that the individual who passes the examination is fit to practice, either independently or under supervision. Therefore, the score-based decisions must be validated and demonstrated to be reliable using a variety of standard techniques, and SBA professionals should preplan reliability and validity studies as integral parts of the development and implementation of the tests.

The Israeli Experience: The Israeli Center for Medical Simulation (MSR)

Since its establishment in 2001, one of the main strategic goals of MSR, the Israel Center for Medical Simulation [36] (Fig. 12.1), was to promote simulation-based certification and accreditation in a wide range of medical professions on a national level. This goal was set because of the deep recognition of the important influence that traditional healthcare education and assessment had in the current suboptimal reality of patient safety and healthcare quality. The traditional deficiency and almost absence of high-stakes clinical skills assessment of health professionals throughout their career has contributed to the lack of competency standards for healthcare professionals as they advance from one stage to the next in their professional path, as well as when they are expected to demonstrate maintenance of competency (MOC) to safely serve their patients. Thus, with the establishment of MSR, 2 years after the release of the "To Err is Human" report, it was clear that setting new competency standards on a national level via simulation-based high-stakes assessment could convey an important message regarding the accountability of the healthcare licensure system to ensure patient safety through improving health professionals' readiness and preparedness to fulfill their professional roles in high-quality and safety standards.

From its outset, a strategic alliance and close collaboration was established between MSR and the National Institute for Testing and Evaluation (NITE) in Israel, an institute that specializes in measurement and provides psychometric services to all Israeli universities and higher-education colleges [37]. Expert psychometricians from NITE work routinely at MSR and together with the regulatory professional bodies who assign content experts for their exams, and MSR's

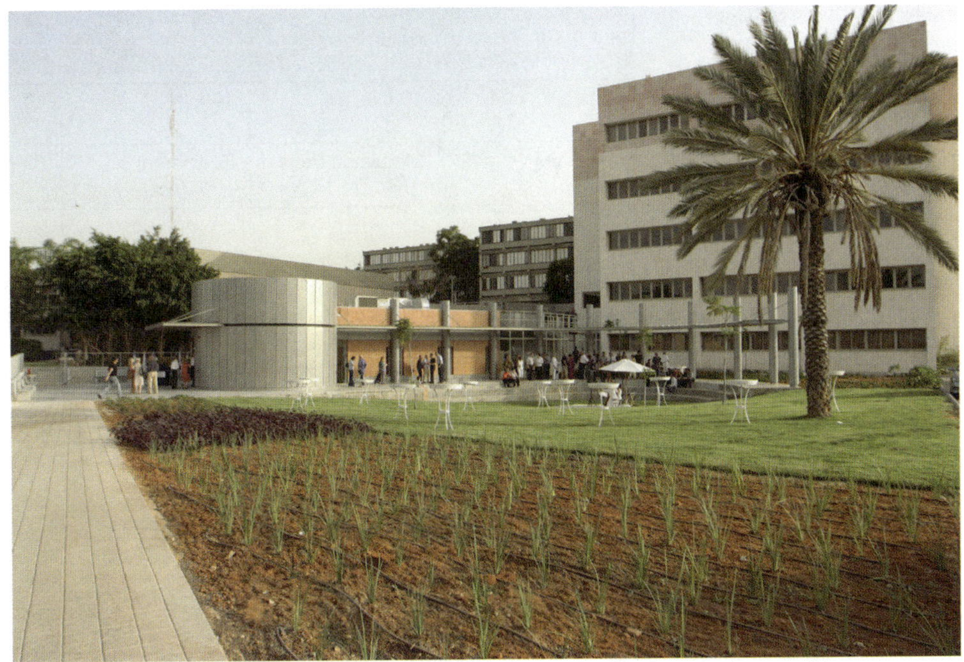

Fig. 12.1 MSR, the Israel Center for Medical Simulation

professional staff—with its simulation expertise—a team with all three domains of expertise, was formed. This team collaboratively develops and implements various simulation-based testing programs at MSR—to serve the needs identified by Israel's healthcare system regulators.

In the following section of this chapter, we will describe the evolution of MSR's national SBA programs conducted in collaboration with NITE and with Israel's health professional regulatory bodies. We will also highlight the lessons learned and special insights which surfaced during the course of the development and implementation of these SBA programs.

The Israeli Board Examination in Anesthesiology

As in other medical professions, Israeli anesthesiology residents are subjected to a written mid-residency board examination and an oral board exam at the end of their five and a half years of residency training. Acknowledging the possible benefits of SBA and the lack of a structured performance evaluation component, the Israeli Board of Anesthesiology Examination Committee decided in 2002 to explore the potential of adding an OSCE component to the board examination process. The initial decision was that the SBA would be complementary to the existing board examination process and that SBA would be a task-driven test where relevant tasks are incorporated into realistic and relevant simulated clinical scenarios.

Being the first high-stakes test to be developed at MSR, this test evolved gradually since its first initiation demonstrating a dynamic development and ongoing attempts to improve various aspects of the SBA. Following are a few examples that reflect this dynamic approach on behalf of the test development committee: realism of scenarios improved by presenting a "standardized nurse" to the stations and by using more advanced simulation technology; scoring method was upgraded throughout the years (e.g., critical "red flag" items that examinee had to perform in order to pass were removed, checklist format was modified to improve raters' ability to score examinees' performance), a two-stage scenario model was developed and adopted to include a simulation-based scenario which is followed by a "debriefing" or an oral examination used to assess the examinee's understanding of the previously performed scenario, and his ability to interpret laboratory results and tests; and finally, in terms of the SBA role in certification, passing the simulation-based test has become a prerequisite for applying to the oral board examination although recently due to logistic reasons the SBA stations are part of the oral board exams.

Major components of the SBA include an orientation day for examinees held at MSR a few weeks before the examination. During this day, the examinees familiarize themselves with the test format and the technological environment (simulators, OR equipment, etc.). Another major component is the examiners' orientation and retraining ("refresher") before each test. Table 12.1 describes the actual examination format, and Table 12.2 presents an example of a checklist used during the examination.

Nineteen examination cycles were held since 2002, and the number of examinees in each cycle was 25–35. The board examination in anesthesiology achieved good psychometric characteristic with satisfying inter-rater agreement, good

Table 12.1 Anesthesiology board examination format

Examination stations	Regional anesthesia	Anesthesia equipment	Trauma management	Resuscitation
Time allotment	18 min	18 min	18 min	18 min
Simulator	Simulated Patient (SP)	Equipment	SimMan	SimMan
No. of examiners	2	2	2	2
Other personnel needed			Technician & Nurse/Paramedic	Technician & Nurse/Paramedic

Table 12.2 An example of an evaluation checklist for the assessment of axillary block performance (only part of the checklist is presented)

The examiner requests the examinee to start performing the block according to the following steps: patient positioning, anatomical description, insertion point and direction of needle advancement and specification of type and volume of local anesthetic injected.				
Examinee's expected action			Done	Not done
1	Patient positioning	Arm abduction		
		Elbow at 90°		
		Axillary artery		
		Pectoralis major		
		Coracobrachialis		
2	Direction of needle insertion	45° angle		
The examiner stops the examinee and says, "Now that you have demonstrated the performance of the block, I would like to ask a number of questions".				
3	The examiner presents a nerve detector and a model of the arm to the examinee, and asks him/her to demonstrate and describe its use	Correct connection between the stimulator and model		
		Output set at 0.8–1.0 mA		
		Frequency set at 1–2 Hz		
		Expected response of the hand		
		Injection when twitches are present at 0.1–0.4 mA		
4	The examiner asks, "After advancing the needle 2 cm, a bony structure is encountered. What is this structure and what will you do?"	Humerus		
		The needle has to be re-angled superiorly or inferiorly		
5	During injection the SP complains of pain radiating to the hand. The examiner asks, "What is the reason for this complaint, and what should be done?"	Intraneural needle placement		
		Immediate cessation of injection		

intra-case reliability, as well as good structure validity and face validity [30, 38, 39]. In addition to the satisfactory psychometric qualities, the process of incorporating SBA into the board examination paradigm has had several important implications. Analysis of frequent errors in the test yielded important and precious feedback to the training programs aiming at highlighting areas of skills deficiencies (e.g., identifying and managing technical faults in the anesthesia machine) [40], with the hope that it would drive educational improvements in residency. The effort to keep high psychometric standards in the SBA inspired the test committee to aspire to the same standards in the oral exam. Hence, a more structured oral exam was developed, and an obligatory "train the rater" workshop was conducted to improve raters' oral examination skills.

Paramedics Certification Exam

Paramedics training in Israel includes a 1-year course followed by an accreditation process that includes evaluation by the training program supervisor, a written examination, and a simulation-based exam at MSR. The SBA includes four stations with scenarios in four major professional areas: trauma management,

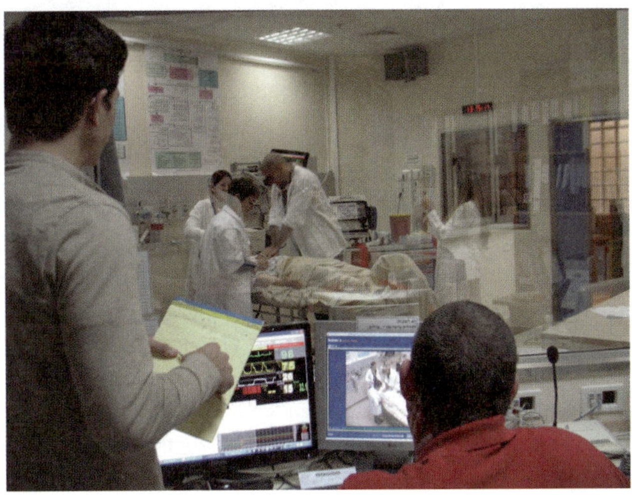

Fig. 12.2 Team Management Training at MSR, the Israel Center for Medical Simulation

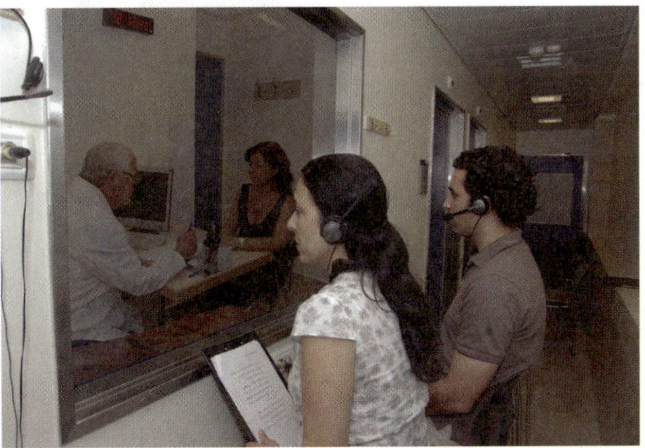

Fig. 12.3 OSCE for Advanced Nursing Accreditation at MSR, the Israel Center for Medical Simulation

cardiology, pediatrics, and respiratory emergencies. Various relevant simulators are used, and two of the test stations include an actor (SP) in a hybrid format that combines communication with the SP and clinical performance on a mannequin simulator. Since one of the core characteristics of the paramedics' profession is team management, this had to become an integral part of the assessment in the simulation-based test (Fig. 12.2). Therefore, examinees perform as team leaders in all station and are assisted by two other more junior paramedics who are still in the paramedic course—and therefore are not test subjects (in fact, this experience serves also as part of the junior paramedics' orientation for their future certification exam). The score in each station is composed of yes/no checklist items (70%) (20–30 items per station), holistic parameters (20%) assessed on a 1–6 scale (time management, team leadership, etc.), and one general holistic assessment (10%) on a 1–10 scale. The SPs in the two hybrid stations also score examinees' performance. The final score per station is a weighted average of the SP score (10%) and the professional rater score (90%).

The paramedics certification test takes place 4–5 times a year with about 25 examinees per day. A month before each test, an orientation takes place in which examinees practice at MSR on scenarios similar to the ones used in the actual test and receive feedback based on a "test like" scoring form. The raters (two raters per station) also participate in a mandatory "train the rater" workshop. Several psychometric features of this test are routinely measured, inter-rater agreement varies from 75 to 95%, and face validity, as reflected in participants' feedbacks, is also very high.

National Registration Exam for Nurse Specialists

In Israel, to become a certified nurse specialist in any of the 16 defined nursing professions (intensive care, pediatric intensive care, psychiatry, oncology, etc.), one must undertake a yearlong specialty course. In 2008, recognizing the need of performance measures to the registration process, the nursing authority in Israel's ministry of health decided to collaborate with MSR and NITE and develop a simulation-based test to replace the written multiple choice certification test. Currently, 16 different tests are developed annually for the various nursing specialties, requiring teams of nurse specialists to work closely with the simulation experts and psychometricians on the test content in each profession.

All exams have a common format that includes 11 stations with various combinations of the following station types:

(a) High-fidelity simulation—measuring clinical competence in a scenario using high-fidelity mannequin simulators.
(b) SP stations—measuring clinical competence, including communication with patients (Fig. 12.3).
(c) Debrief stations—following the SP station, the examinee is debriefed on the scenario and his/her performance and decision-making using questions such as what was your diagnosis? what facts regarding the patient led you to that diagnosis? and why did you choose a specific treatment?
(d) Video-/PPT-based case analysis stations—written open-ended items all relating to a specific case, presented either in video or in Power Point Presentation.
(e) Short computerized multiple choice test.

The raters in this examination are nurse specialists in the respective fields. All raters participate in an obligatory train the rater workshop before each test. The National Registration Exam for Nurse Specialists has been running for 3 years with 650–1,000 examinees per year in 13–16 different nursing professions. Unfortunately, the small numbers of examinees in each profession make it difficult to compute the psychometric parameters. However, in three professions, the number of examinees is relatively high: intensive care (about 160 examinees per year), midwifery (60–80 per year), and primary care in the community (40–50 per year). In these professions, internal consistency ranged from 0.6 to 0.8. In addition, inter-rater disagreement rate in all tests was less than 5% (unpublished data), indicating satisfactory reliability. At the moment, long-term predictive validity research is being conducted to measure the correlation between test scores and supervisor and peer evaluations in the workplace.

The "MOR" Assessment Center: Selection of Candidates to Medical Schools

Medical school admissions traditionally rely heavily on cognitive variables, with noncognitive measures assessed through interviews only. In recognition of the unsatisfactory reliability and validity of traditional interviews, medical schools are increasingly exploring alternative approaches that can provide improved measures of candidates' personal and interpersonal qualities.

In 2004, the Tel Aviv University Sackler School of Medicine appointed MSR and NITE to join forces with its admission committee in order to develop and implement an original assessment system for the selection of its candidates, focused exclusively on their noncognitive attributes.

The MOR assessment center that was developed included three main assessment tools:

1. A biographical questionnaire
2. An ethical judgment and decision-making questionnaire
3. A set of OSCE-like behavioral stations

For a full description of the questionnaires and the original behavioral stations structure, see Ziv et al. [18].

The raters of candidates' attributes in the behavioral stations are faculty members (doctors, nurses, psychologists, social workers) as well as SPs. They score candidates' behaviors on a standard structured scoring form that includes four general parameters (each divided into 2–6 scored items): interpersonal communication skills, ability to handle stress, initiative and responsibility, and maturity and self-awareness. All raters are trained in 1-day mandatory train the rater workshops.

The MOR assessment center has greatly evolved throughout the years. First, other Israeli faculties joined the project, including the medical faculty at the Technion, the dental school at Tel Aviv University, and recently, the new medical school at the Bar-Ilan University. Second, the number of behavioral stations increased (from 8 to 9), and different types of stations were added. Currently, the system includes 3 SP stations (a challenging encounter with an actor that does not require any medical knowledge), 2 debrief stations, 3 structured mini interviews, one group dynamic station, and one team station with an SP.

Ninety-six candidates are tested at MSR per testing day. In each testing day, about 40 raters are occupied in two testing shifts. A total of over 1,000 examinees are tested per year.

The MOR assessment center has good internal reliability, good test-retest reliability, satisfactory inter-rater reliability, and high face validity [18, 41]. However, the main challenge of establishing predictive validity has not yet been met. We hope to overcome some political and economic obstacles to achieve this goal in the near future.

Simulation-Based Licensure and Certification: The Authors' Vision

Following 10 years of promoting SBA in Israel, we are proud to recognize a high degree of vertical (among different seniority levels) and horizontal (among different medical professions) penetration of SBA into the healthcare system. For example, over 50% of the anesthesiologists in the country experienced SBA as examiners and/or as examinees. Similarly, SBA was a central professional experience to most Israeli paramedics, the full cohort of the incoming generation of the advanced specialty nurses and over 80% of Israel's current generation of medical students who were screened via an SBA screening process conducted at MSR. Thus, in addition to the wide exposure of trained faculty from all the above professions who served as raters for those SBA programs, Israel has now a substantial group of change agents who convey the moral message, inherent in SBA, as a means to set new proficiency standards for readiness and certification in health care.

We strongly believe that the widespread penetration of SBA within Israel's healthcare system has contributed in many ways to expedite important educational processes. First, in the spirit of the "assessment drives education" concept, the fact that SBA has been widely endorsed by leading healthcare regulators has motivated a growing interest in simulation-based medical education. In many medical institutions and healthcare professional schools who became more aware of the need to focus on the provision of sound training to their students/health providers, this has led to broad use of simulation modalities. Second, SBA has helped to identify deficiencies in the skill sets of examinees and thus served as an important feedback mechanism to training and educational programs which triggered changes in the focus of training and curricular programs accordingly. Finally, as the collaborative teams of simulation, content, and measurement experts gained more and more experience in this rather demanding and resource-consuming field of SBA, important psychometric/logistical/administrative processes have been developed and substantially improved, thus enabling improved cost-effectiveness of the SBA program as a whole.

Lessons Learned

As we strongly believe that SBA is a reflection of a very important and rapidly growing safety and accountability movement in health care, we would like to summarize this chapter with some of the important lessons we learned during the course of developing and conducting national SBA programs at MSR. First, and perhaps the most important lesson, is that the process of incorporating SBA requires courageous leadership and strong belief in the cause on behalf of the professional and regulatory boards. High-stakes competency assessment needs to be an explicit goal and a strategic decision of professional boards. Thus, together with simulation experts and psychometric backup, these bodies should launch the process with readiness to fight for the cause and defend the movement to SBA in the profession. A second important lesson is not to wait for the completion of the development of the ultimate SBA exam as a launching condition, as this could never be completed. Rather, "dive into the SBA water" and apply the SBA as complementary to the traditional assessment tools, with the understanding that the process is an ongoing "work in progress." Thus, SBA should be continuously improved in small increments following feedback from examiners and examinees as well as thorough research and evaluation of the process. Finally, SBA must be accompanied by ongoing research aiming at improving processes of test development and rater training as well as research regarding the impact of the incorporation of SBA into a given profession. These studies should attempt to explore the impact of the SBA on the educational processes in the given field and ultimately on the quality and safety of healthcare delivery provided by those who met the SBA standards in that given field.

Conclusion

The challenges surrounding SBA as it develops in the years to come are many. That said, incorporation of SBA into licensure and certification processes is feasible. The integration of "higher-order skills" into the assessment paradigm, the measurement of the "difficult to measure" yet "important to measure" skills (like professionalism, safety, and teamwork skills), should serve as a road map for medical educators who strive to set new standards for healthcare providers' readiness to serve the public with safe and high-quality medicine. As medicine advances on this never-ending quality improvement and safety journey, simulation-based assessment should be viewed as one of the most powerful modalities in ensuring quality care.

References

1. Boulet JR. Summative assessment in medicine: the promise of simulation for high-stakes evaluation. Acad Emerg Med. 2008;15:1017–124.
2. Gaba DM. Do as we say, not as you do: using simulation to investigate clinical behavior in action. Simul Healthc. 2009;4:67–9.
3. Scalese RJ, Issenberg SB. Simulation-based assessment. In: Holmboe ES, Hawkins RE, editors. A practical approach to the evaluation of clinical competence. Philadelphia: Mosby/Elsevier; 2008.
4. Holmboe E, Rizzolo MA, Sachdeva A, Rosenberg M, Ziv A. Simulation based assessment and the regulation of healthcare professionals. Simul Healthc. 2011;6:s58–62.
5. MSR Israel Center for Medical Simulation. Available at: http://www.msr.org.il/. Accessed Oct 2006.
6. Issenberg SB, McGaghie WC, Petrusa ER, Lee Gordon D, Scalese RJ. Features and uses of high-fidelity medical simulations that lead to effective learning: a BEME systematic review. Med Teach. 2005;27:10–28.
7. Medical Council of Canada. Medical Council of Canada qualifying Examination Part II (MCCQE Part II). 2008. Medical Council of Canada.
8. Whelan G. High–Stakes medical performance testing: the Clinical Skills Assessment Program. JAMA. 2000;283:1748.
9. Federation of State Medical Board, Inc. and National Board of Medical Examiners. United States Medical Licensing Examination: Step 2 clinical skills (cs) content description and general information. 2008. Federation of State Medical Board, Inc. and National Board of Medical Examiners.
10. American Board of Surgery. ABS to Require ACLS, ATLS and FLS for General Surgery Certification. Available at: http://home.absurgery.org/default.jsp?news_newreqs. Accessed 27 May 2011.
11. Soper NJ, Fried GM. The fundamentals of laparoscopic surgery: its time has come. Bulletin of the American College of Surgeons. 2008. Available at: http://www.flsprogram.org/wp-content/uploads/2010/10/FLSprogramSoperFried.pdf. Accessed 7 Mar 2011.
12. Petrusa ER. Clinical performance assessment. In: Norman GR, van der Vleuten CPM, Newble DI, editors. International Handbook of Research in Medical Education. Dordrecht: Kluwer Academic Publications; 2002.
13. Tombeson P, Fox RA, Dacre JA. Defining the content for the objective structured clinical examination component of the Professional and Linguistic Assessment Board examination: development of a blueprint. Med Educ. 2000;34:566–72.
14. Boyd MA, Gerrow JD, Duquette P. Rethinking the OSCE as a tool for national competency evaluation. Eur J Dent Educ. 2004; 8:95.
15. Boulet JR, Smee SM, Dillon GF, Gimplr JR. The use of standardized patient assessments for certification and licensure decisions. Simul Healthc. 2009;4:35–42.
16. Ordre des Infirmieres et Infirmiers Quebec. Available at: http://www.oiiq.org/. Accessed 7 Mar 2011.
17. College and Association of Registered Nurses of Alberta. Available at:http://www.nurses.ab.ca/carna/index.aspx?WebStructureID_3422. Accessed 7 Mar 2011.
18. Ziv A, Rubin O, Moshinsky A, et al. MOR: a simulation-based assessment centre for evaluating the personal and interpersonal qualities of medical school candidates. Med Educ. 2008;42: 991–8.
19. Harris S, Owen C. Discerning quality: using the multiple mini-interview in student selection for the Australian National University Medical School. Med Educ. 2007;41(3):234–41.
20. O'Brien A, Harvey J, Shannon M, Lewis K, Valencia O. A comparison of multiple mini-interviews and structured interviews in a UK setting. Med Teach. 2011;33(5):397–402.
21. Eva KW, Rosenfeld J, Reiter HI. Norman GR An admissions OSCE: the multiple mini-interview. Med Educ. 2004;38(3):314–26.
22. Issenberg SB, Scalese RJ. Simulation in health care education. Perspect Biol Med. 2008;51:31–46.
23. Boulet JR, van Zanten M, de Champlain A, Hawkins RE, Peitzman SJ. Checklist content on a standardized patient assessment: an ex post facto review. Adv Health Sci Educ. 2008;13:59–69.
24. Baker DP, Salas E, King H, Battles J, Barach P. The role of teamwork in the professional education of physicians: current status and assessment recommendations. Jt Comm J Qual Patient Saf. 2005;31:185–202.
25. van Zanten M, Boulet JR, McKinley DW, de Champlain A, Jobe AC. Assessing the communication and interpersonal skills of graduates of international medical schools as part of the United States Medical Licensing Exam (USMLE) Step 2 Clinical Skills (CS) Exam. Acad Med. 2007;82(10 Suppl l):S65–8.

26. Weller JM, Bloch M, Young S, et al. Evaluation of high fidelity patient simulator in assessment of performance of anesthetists. Br J Anaesth. 2003;90:43–7.
27. Morgan PJ, Cleave-Hogg D, Guest CB. A comparison of global ratings and checklist scores from an undergraduate assessment using anesthesia simulator. Acad Med. 2001;76:1053–5.
28. Downing SM. Validity: on the meaningful interpretation of assessment data. Med Educ. 2003;37:830–7.
29. Newble D. Techniques for measuring clinical competence: objective structured clinical examinations. Med Educ. 2004;38:199–203.
30. Berkenstadt H, Ziv A, Gafni N, Sidi A. The validation process of incorporating simulation-based accreditation into the anesthesiology Israeli national board exams. Isr Med Assoc J. 2006;8: 728–33.
31. Murray DJ, Boulet JR, Avidan M, et al. Performance of residents and anesthesiologists in a simulation based skill assessment. Anesthesiology. 2007;107:705–13.
32. Girzadas Jr DV, Clay L, Caris J, Rzechula K, Harwood R. High fidelity simulation can discriminate between novice and experienced residents when assessing competency in patient care. Med Teach. 2007;29:452–6.
33. Rosenthal R, Gantert WA, Hamel C, et al. Assessment of construct validity of a virtual reality laparoscopy simulator. J Laparoendosc Adv Surg Tech A. 2007;7:407–13.
34. Tamblyn R, Abrahamowicz M, Dauphinee D, et al. Physician scores on a national clinical skills examination as predictors of complaints to medical regulatory authorities. JAMA. 2007;298:993–1001.
35. Hatala R, Issenberg SB, Kassen B, Cole G, Bacchus CM, Scalese RJ. Assessing cardiac physical examination skills using simulation technology and real patients: a comparison study. Med Educ. 2008;42:628–36.
36. Ziv A, Erez D, Munz Y, Vardi A, Barsuk D, Levine I, et al. The Israel Center for Medical Simulation: a paradigm for cultural change in medical education. Acad Med. 2006;81(12):1091–7.
37. National Institute for Testing and Evaluation. Available at: http://www.nite.org.il/. Accessed Oct 2006.
38. Berkenstadt H, Ziv A, Gafni N, Sidi A. Incorporating simulation-based objective structured clinical examination into the Israeli National Board Examination in Anesthesiology. Anesth Analg. 2006;102(3):853–8.
39. Ziv A, Rubin O, Sidi A, Berkenstadt H. Credentialing and certifying with simulation. Anesthesiol Clin. 2007;25(2):261–9.
40. Ben-Menachem E, Ezri T, Ziv A, Sidi A, Berkenstadt H. Identifying and managing technical faults in the anesthesia machine: lessons learned from the Israeli Board of Anesthesiologists. Anesth Analg. 2011;112(4):864–6. Epub 2011 Feb 2.
41. Gafni N, Moshinsky A, Eisenberg O, Zeigler D, Ziv A. Reliability estimates: behavioural stations and questionnaires in medical school admissions. Med Educ. 2012;46(3):277–88.

Part II

Simulation Modalities and Technologies

13 Standardized Patients

Lisa D. Howley

Introduction

Standardized patients (SPs) are individuals who have been carefully selected and trained to portray a patient in order to teach and/or evaluate the clinical skills of a healthcare provider. Originally conceived and developed by Dr. Howard Barrows [1] in 1964, the SP has become increasingly popular in healthcare and is considered the method of choice for evaluating three of the six common competencies [2] now recognized across the continuum of medicine.

The standardized patient, originally called a "programmed patient," has evolved over 50 years from an informal tool to a ubiquitous, highly sound modality for teaching and evaluating a broad array of competencies for diverse groups of trainees within and outside of healthcare. Barrows and Abrahamson [1] developed the technique of the standardized patient in the early 1960s as a tool for clinical skill instruction and assessment. During a consensus conference devoted to the use of standardized patients in medical education, Barrows [3] described the development of this unique modality. He was responsible for acquiring patients for the Board Examinations in Neurology and Psychiatry and soon realized that the use of real patients was not only physically straining but also detrimental to the nature of the examination. Patients would tire and alter their responses depending upon the examiner, time of day, and other situational factors.

Barrows also recognized the need for a more feasible teaching and assessment tool while instructing his medical students. In order to aid in the assessment of his neurology clerks, he coached a woman model from the art department to simulate paraplegia, bilateral positive Babinski signs, dissociated sensory loss, and a blind eye. She was also coached to portray the emotional tone of an actual patient displaying these troubling symptoms. Following each encounter with a clerk, she would report on his/her performance. Although initially controversial and slow to gain acceptance, this unique standardized format eventually caught the attention of clinical faculty and became a common tool in the instruction and assessment of clinical skills across all disciplines of healthcare.

This chapter will present a historical overview of the standardized patient, prevalence, current uses, and challenges for using SPs to teach and assess clinical competence. A framework for initiating, developing, executing, and appraising SP encounters will be provided to guide the process of integrating SP encounters within medical and healthcare professionals' education curricula.

Common Terminology and Uses

The title "SP" is used, often interchangeably, to refer to several different roles. Originally, Dr. Barrows referred to his SPs as "programmed" or "simulated patients." Simulated patients refer to those SPs trained to portray a role so accurately that they cannot be distinguished from the actual patient. The term "standardized patient" was first introduced almost two decades later by psychometrician, Dr. Geoff Norman and colleagues [4], to iterate the high degree of reproducibility and standardization of the simulation required to offer a large number of trainees a consistent experience. Accurate simulation is necessary but not sufficient for a standardized patient. Today, the term "SP" is used interchangeably to refer to simulated or standardized patient or participant. Refer to Appendix for a description of the common SP roles and assessment formats.

The use of standardized patients has increased dramatically, particularly over the past three decades. A recent census by the Liaison Committee on Medical Education [5] reported that 96% of US Medical Schools have integrated OSCEs/standardized patients for teaching and assessment

L.D. Howley, MEd, PhD
Department of Medical Education,
Carolinas HealthCare System,
Charlotte, NC, USA
e-mail: lisa.howley@carolinashealthcare.org

A.I. Levine et al. (eds.), *The Comprehensive Textbook of Healthcare Simulation*,
DOI 10.1007/978-1-4614-5993-4_13, © Springer Science+Business Media New York 2013

within their curricula. Today, ironically, the internal medicine clerkships (85%) are more likely, and the neurology clerkships (28%) are least likely to incorporate SPs into their curricula for the assessment of clinical knowledge and skills. Approximately 50% or more of the clerkships in internal medicine, OBGYN, family medicine, psychiatry, and surgery use SP exams/OSCEs to determine part of their students' grades. In addition, many medical licensing and specialty boards in the United States and Canada are using standardized patients to certify physician competencies [6, 7]. Notable examples include (a) the National Board of Medical Examiners, (b) the Medical Council of Canada, (c) the Royal College of Physicians and Surgeons of Canada, and (d) the Corporation of Medical Professionals of Quebec. Numerous other healthcare education programs are also using SPs for instruction and assessment [8].

As SP methodologies expanded and became more sophisticated, professionals working in the field became more specialized, and a new role of educator was born – the "SP educator." An international association of SP educators (ASPE) was created in 1991 to develop professionals, advance the field, and establish standards of practice for training SPs, designing, and evaluating encounters. Its diverse members include SP educators from allopathic medicine, as well as osteopathy, dentistry, pharmacy, veterinary medicine, allied health, and others [9]. This association is currently collaborating with the Society for Simulation in Healthcare to develop certification standards for professional SP educators [10].

Standardized patients can be used in a variety of ways to teach, reinforce, and/or assess competencies of healthcare professionals. In the early decades of SP use, their primary role was formative and instructional. Although still widely used for the teaching and reinforcement of clinical skills, as the practice has matured and evidence has mounted, SPs have been integrated into certification and licensure examinations in the United States, Canada, and increasing numbers of other countries.

Table 13.1 Advantages and challenges of using SPs

Advantages
Feasibility: Available any time and can be used in any location
Flexibility: Able to simulate a broad array of clinical presentations; faculty able to direct learning objectives and assessment goals
Fidelity: Highly authentic to actual patient and family dynamics
Formative: Able to provide immediate constructive feedback to trainees; provide unique patient perspective on competencies
Fend: Protect real patients from repeated exposure to novice skills of trainees; able to simulate highly sensitive and/or emotional content repeatedly without risk to real patient; protect trainees from anxiety of learning skills on real patients
Facsimile: Encounters are reproduced allowing numerous trainees to be taught and assessed in a standard environment
Fair: SP encounters are standardized and controlled allowing for reduction of bias, equitable treatment of trainees, and equal opportunity to learn the content
Challenges
Fiscal: Lay person working as SPs require payment for time spent training and portraying their roles
Fidelity: Certain physical conditions and signs cannot be simulated with SPs (can be overcome with hybrid simulation)
Facility: Requires expertise to recruit and train SPs, develop related materials, and evaluate appropriately

Advantages and Challenges

There are several advantages to using SPs to train and evaluate healthcare professionals. Table 13.1 includes a summary of the advantages and challenges of using SPs in teaching and assessment. The most notable advantages include increased opportunity for direct observation of trainees in clinical practice, protection of real patients from trainees' novice skills and repeated encounters, standard and flexible case presentation, and ability to provide feedback and evaluation data on multiple common competencies.

Historically, prior to the 1960s, clinical teaching and evaluation methods consisted primarily of classroom lecture, gross anatomy labs, bedside rounds of real patients, informal faculty observations, oral examinations, and multiple-choice tests. Prior to the introduction of the SP, there was no objective method for assessing the clinical skills of trainees. This early simulation opened doors to what is today a recommended educational practice for training and certification of healthcare professionals across geographic and discipline boundaries.

An SP can be trained to consistently reproduce the history, emotional tone, communicative style, and physical signs of an actual patient without placing stress upon a real patient. Standardized patients also provide faculty with a standard assessment format. Learners are assessed interacting with the same patient portraying the same history, physical signs, and emotional content. Unlike actual patients, SPs are more flexible in types of cases presented and can be available at any time during the day and for extended periods of time. SPs can be trained to accurately and consistently record student performance and provide constructive feedback to the student, greatly reducing the amount of time needed by clinical faculty members to directly observe trainees in practice.

SPs can also be trained to perform certain basic clinical procedures and, in turn, aid in the instruction of trainees. When SPs are integrated within high-fidelity simulation experiences (hybrid simulations), they enhance the authenticity of the experience and provide increased opportunities to teach and assess additional competencies, namely, interpersonal communication skills and professionalism.

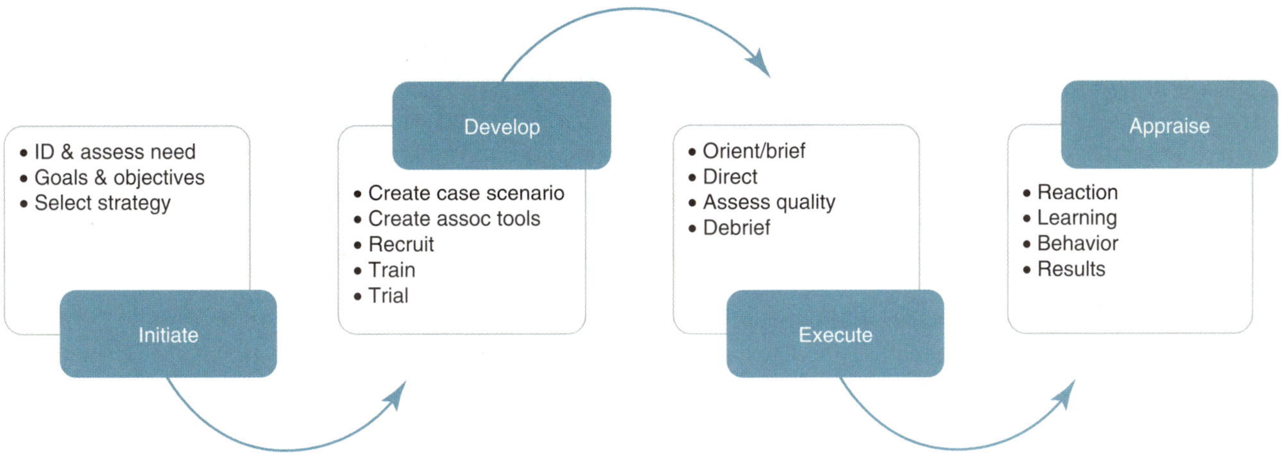

Fig. 13.1 The IDEA Framework: a stepwise process for preparing and using SPs in healthcare education

Framework for SP Encounters

Effective SP encounters require a systematic approach to development. Figure 13.1 displays a stepwise approach for preparing and using SPs in healthcare education. The IDEA framework is intended to serve as a guide to developing SP encounters, particularly for SP assessments (OSCE, CPX). Each of the four steps (Initiate, Develop, Execute, and Appraise) is described throughout this chapter with increased emphasis on the first two. This framework does not generally apply to a single large-group SP demonstration and assumes that the SP encounters are repeated to teach and/or evaluate multiple trainees.

Initiate: Initial Considerations for Using SPs in Healthcare

When initiating an SP encounter, it is important to clarify the purpose of the exercise. Encounters are intended to reinforce, instruct, and/or assess competencies. When designing an encounter to assess, the intent should be clarified as formative (to monitor progress during instruction) or summative (to determine performance at end of instruction). Due to the increased stakes, summative assessments generally require more rigor during the development process. However, all assessments require some evidence to support the credibility of the encounters and the performance data they derive. It is recommended that the developer consider at the earliest stage how she/he will determine whether the encounter performed as it was intended. How will you appraise the quality of the SP encounter? Attention paid to the content, construction of data gathering tools, training of SPs, and methods for setting performance standards throughout the process will result in more defensible SP encounters.

Goals and Objectives

Next, it is important to consider the competencies and performance outcomes that the encounter is intended to address. SP encounters are best suited for teaching and assessing patient care as well as the affective competencies, interpersonal and communication skills, and professionalism. If the specific competencies and objectives have been predefined by a course or curriculum, it is simply a matter of determining which are most appropriate to address via the SP encounter. Alternatively, there are several methods to determine the aggregate needs of trainees, including the research literature, association and society recommendations, accreditation standards, direct observations of performance, questionnaires, formal interviews, focus group, performance/test data, and sentinel events. This data will help the developers understand the current as well as the ideal state of performance and/or approach to the problem. For detailed information on assessing the needs of trainees, see Kern et al. [11].

Writing specific and measurable objectives for an SP encounter and overall SP activity is an important task in directing the process and determining what specific strategies are most effective. Details on writing educational goals and objectives can be found in Amin and Eng [12]. Sample trainee objectives for a single SP encounter include: (1) to obtain an appropriate history (over the telephone) from a mother regarding her 15-month old child suffering from symptoms of an acute febrile illness, (2) differentiate relatively mild conditions from emergent medical conditions requiring expeditious care, and (3) formulate an appropriate differential diagnosis based on the information gathered from the mother and on the physical exam findings provided to the learner. This encounter which focused on gathering history and formulating a differential diagnosis was included within an extended performance assessment with the overall objective to provide a standard and objective measure of medical students' clinical skills at the end of the third year of undergraduate medical education [13].

It is strongly recommended, particularly when multiple encounters are planned, that a blueprint be initiated to guide and direct the process. The blueprint specifies the competencies and objectives to be addressed by each encounter and how they align to the curricula [14]. This ensures that there is a link to what is being taught, reinforced, or assessed to the broader curriculum. The content of the blueprint will vary according to the nature of the encounter. If developers plan an SP assessment, then this document may be supplemented by a table of specifications, which is a more detailed description of the design.

Questions to consider at this stage in the development process include: What is the need? What do trainees need to improve upon? What external mandates require or support the use of the educational encounter? What is currently being done to address the need? What is the ideal or suggested approach for addressing the need? What data support the need for the educational encounter? What is the current performance level of trainees? What will the trainees be able to do as a result of the educational encounter?

Strategies

SPs can be used in a variety of ways, and the strategy should derive from the answers to the above questions. In general, these strategies fall within two areas: instruction or assessment. Several sample strategies for each of these broad areas will be described below.

Instruction

Although SPs are used to enhance a large group or didactic lecture to demonstrate a procedure, counseling technique, or steps in physical examination, their greatest instructional benefit is found in small group or individualized sessions where experiential learning can take place. For example, an SP meets with a small group of trainees and a facilitator. He or she is interviewed and/or physically examined by the facilitator as a demonstration, and then the trainees are provided the opportunity to perform while others observe. One variation to the small group encounter is the "time-in/time-out" technique, originally developed by Barrows et al. [15]. During this session, the interview or physical exam is stopped at various points in order for the group to engage in discussion, question the thoughts and ideas of the trainee, and provide immediate feedback on his/her performance. During the "time-out," the SP acts as though he or she is no longer present and suspends the simulation while remaining silent and passive. When "time-in" is called, the SP continues as if nothing had happened and is unaware of the discussions which just occurred. This format allows for flexible deliberate practice, reinforcement of critical behaviors, peer engagement, and delivery of immediate feedback on performance.

Another example of an effective individual or small group teaching encounter is a hybrid [16] or combination SP with high-fidelity technical simulators. During these encounters, technical simulators are integrated with the SP to provide the opportunity for trainees to learn and/or demonstrate skills that would be otherwise impossible or impractical to simulate during an SP encounter (i.e., lung sounds, cardiac arrest, labor, and childbirth). For example, Siassakos et al. [17] used a hybrid simulation to teach medical students the delivery skills of a baby with shoulder dystocia as well as effective communication strategies with the patient. In this simulation encounter, the SP was integrated with a pelvic model task trainer and draped to appear as though the model were her own body. The SP simulated the high-risk labor and delivery and subsequently provided feedback to the students on their communication skills. This hybrid encounter was found to improve the communication skills of these randomly assigned students compared to those of their control group.

Another example which highlights the importance of creating patient-focused encounters is by Yudkowsky and colleagues [18]. They compared the performance of medical students suturing a bench model (suture skin training model including simulated skin, fat, and muscular tissue) with and without SP integration. When the model was attached to the SP and draped as though his/her actual arm, student performance in technical suturing as well as communication was significantly weaker compared to performance under non-patient conditions. This research negates the assumption that novice trainees can translate newly acquired skills directly to a patient encounter and reminds us of the importance of context and fidelity in performance assessment [19]. The authors concluded that the hybrid encounter provided a necessary, intermediate, safe opportunity to further hone skills prior to real patient exposure.

Most SP encounters are single sessions, where the trainee interacts with the SP one time and not over a series of encounters. However, the use of SPs in longitudinal encounters has been shown to be very effective, particularly for teaching the complexities of disease progression and the family dynamics of healthcare. In order to address family-centered care objectives, Pugnaire et al. [20] developed the concept of the standardized family at the University of Massachusetts Medical School. Initially termed the "McQ Standardized Family Curriculum," these longitudinal instructional SP encounters involved multiple participants portraying different family members. Medical students participated in several encounters over the course of their clerkship. More recently, Lewis et al. [21] incorporated SPs into a series of three encounters to teach residents how to diagnose, treat, and manage a progressive disease (viz., Alzheimer's) over the 10-year course of the "patient's" illness. The sessions took place over three consecutive days, but the time was lapsed over these years to simulate the progressive illness. These sessions provided opportunities for deliberate practice and reinforced continuity of care.

Over 40 years ago, Barrows [22] described the use of SPs in a clinical "laboratory in living anatomy" where lay persons were examined by medical students as a supplement to major sections of the gross anatomy cadaver lab. This early experiential use of SPs led to the more formal role of the Patient Instructor and the Gynecological Teaching Associate (GTA), developed by Stillman et al. [23] and Kretzschmar [24], respectively.

SPs are used to teach physical examination skills. The patient instructor is a lay person with or without physical findings who has been carefully trained to undergo a physical examination by a trainee and then provide feedback and instruction on the performance using a detailed checklist designed by a physician [23]. At the University of Geneva [25], faculty used PIs with rheumatoid arthritis to train 3rd year medical students to interview and perform a focused musculoskeletal exam. The carefully trained PIs were able to provide instruction on examination and communication skills during a 60-min encounter. As a result, students' medical knowledge, focused history taking, and musculoskeletal exam skills improved significantly from pre- to post session. The authors concluded that "grasping the psychological, emotional, social, professional and family aspects of the disease may largely be due to the direct contact with real patients, and being able to vividly report their illness and feelings. It suggests that the intervention of patient-instructors really adds another dimension to traditional teaching." Henriksen and Ringsted [26] found that PIs fostered patient-centered educational relationships among allied health students and their PIs. When compared to traditional, faculty-led teaching encounters, a class delivered by PIs with rheumatism trained to teach basic joint examination skills and "respectful patient contact" was perceived by the learners as a safer environment for learning basic skills.

The GTA has evolved over the years, and the majority of medical schools now use these specialized SPs to help teach novice trainees how to perform the gynecologic, pelvic, and breast examinations and how to communicate effectively with their patient as they do so. Kretzschmar described the qualities the GTA bring to the instructional session as including "sensitivity as a woman, educational skill in pelvic examination instruction, knowledge of female pelvic anatomy and physiology, and, most important, sophisticated interpersonal skills to help medical students learn in a non-threatening environment." Today, the vast majority of medical schools now use GTAs to teach students these invasive examinations (typically during year 2). Male urological teaching associates (UTAs) have also been used to teach trainees how to perform the male urogenital exam and effective communication strategies when doing so. UTAs have been shown to significantly reduce the anxiety experienced by second year medical students when performing their first male urogenital examination, particularly with regard to female students [27].

Assessment

There is a vast amount of research which supports the use of SP assessment as a method for gathering clinical performance data on trainees [28]. A detailed review of this literature is beyond the scope of this chapter. However, defensible performance assessments depend on ensuring quality throughout the development as well as execution phases and should be considered early as an initial step in the process for preparing and using SPs in assessment. Norcini et al. [29] outline several criteria for good assessment which should be followed when initiating, developing, executing, and appraising SP assessments. These include validity or coherence, reproducibility or consistency, equivalence, feasibility, educational effect, catalytic effect, and acceptability.

One related consideration is "content specificity": Performance on a single encounter does not transfer to subsequent encounters [30]. This phenomenon has theoretical as well as practical implications on the design, administration, and evaluation of performance assessments. Namely, decisions based on a single encounter are indefensible because they cannot be generalized. When making summative decisions about trainee performance, the most defensible approach is to use multiple methods across multiple settings and aggregate the information to make an informed decision about trainee competence. According to Van der Vleuten and Schuwirth, "one measure is no measure," and multiple SP encounters are warranted for making evidence-based decisions on trainee performance [31].

There are several additional practical decisions which need to be made at this stage in the process. Resources, including costs, time, staff, and space, may limit the choices and are important considerations at this stage in the process. Questions include: Does the encounter align to the goals and objectives of the training program? Is the purpose of the encounter to measure or certify performance or to inform and instruct trainees? Formative or summative? Limited or extended? Do the goals and objectives warrant hybrid simulation or unannounced SP encounters? What is the optimal and practical number of encounters needed to meet the goals and objectives of the exercise? What is the anticipated length of the encounters? How many individual SPs will be needed to portray a single role? Is it possible to collaborate in order to share or adapt existing resources?

SP assessments commonly take one of the following two formats: (a) objective-structured clinical examination (OSCE) or the (b) clinical practice examination (CPX). The OSCE is a limited performance assessment consisting of several brief (5–10-min) stations where the student performs a very focused task, such as a knee examination, fundoscopic examination, or EKG reading [32, 33]. Conversely, the CPX is an extended performance assessment consisting of several long (15–50-min) stations where the student interacts with patients in an unstructured environment [15]. Unlike the OSCE format, trainees are not given specific instructions in a CPX. Consequently, the CPX is more realistic to the clinical environment and provides information about trainees' abilities to interact with a patient, initiate a session, and incorporate skills of history taking, physical examination, and patient education.

As in any written test, the format of the performance assessment should be driven by its purpose. If, for example, faculty are interested in knowing how novice trainees are performing specific fragmented tasks such as physical examination or radiology interpretation, then the OSCE format would be suitable. If, however, the faculty are interested in knowing how they are performing more complex and integrated clinical skills such as patient education, data gathering, and management, then the CPX or unannounced SP formats would be an ideal choice. As stated earlier, the primary advantages of using SP encounters to assess performance include the ability to provide highly authentic and standard test conditions for all trainees and focus the measurement on the specific learning objectives of the curriculum. SP assessments are ideally suited to provide performance information on the third and fourth levels of Miller's [34] hierarchy: Does the trainee "show how" he is able to perform and does that performance transfer to what he actually "does" in the workplace?

The current USMLE Step 2CS [35] is an extended clinical practice exam of twelve 15-min SP encounters. Each encounter is followed by a 10-min post encounter where the student completes an electronic patient note. The total testing time is 8 h. The examination is administered at five testing facilities across the United States where students are expected to gather data during the SP encounters and document their findings in a post-encounter exercise. SPs evaluate the data gathering performance, including history taking, physical examination, and communication/interpersonal skills. Synthetic models, mannequins, and/or simulators may be incorporated within encounters to assess invasive physical examination skills.

Another less common but highly authentic method for the assessment of healthcare providers is the unannounced SP encounter. During these incognito sessions, SPs are embedded into the regular patient schedule of the practitioner, who is blinded to the real versus simulated patient. Numerous studies have shown that these SPs can go undetected by the physicians in both ambulatory and inpatient settings [36]. The general purpose of these encounters is to evaluate actual performance in practice: Miller's [34] ubiquitous fourth and highest ("does") level of clinical competence. For example, Ozuah and Reznik [37] used unannounced SPs to evaluate the effect of an educational intervention to train pediatric residents' skills at classifying the severity of their asthmatic patients. Six individual SPs were trained to simulate patients with four unique severities of asthma and were then embedded within the regular ambulatory clinics of the residents. Their identities were unknown to the trainee and the preceptor, and those residents who received the education were significantly better able to appropriately classify their patients' conditions in the true clinical environment.

Develop: Considerations and Steps for Designing SP Encounters

The development of SP encounters will vary depending on the purpose, objectives and format of the exercise. This section will describe several important aspects of developing SP encounters including case development, recruitment, hiring, and training. Table 13.2 lists several questions to consider at this stage of SP encounter development.

Table 13.2 Questions for evaluating SP assessments

Questions to consider when designing a summative SP assessment include: 1. Is the context of the encounter realistic in that it presents a situation similar to one that would be encountered in real life? 2. Does the encounter measure competencies that are necessary and important? 3. Does it motivate trainees to prepare using educationally sound practices? Does participation motivate trainees to enhance their performance? 4. Is the encounter an appropriate measure of the competencies in question? Are there alternative more suitable methods? 5. Does the encounter provide a fair and acceptable assessment of performance? 6. Are the results consistent between and among raters? 7. Do existing methods measuring the same or similar construct reveal congruent results? 8. Does the assessment provide evidence of future performance? 9. Does the assessment differentiate between novice and expert performance? 10. Do other assessments that measure the same or similar constructs reveal convergent results? 11. Do other assessments that measure irrelevant factors or constructs reveal divergent results? 12. Is the assessment feasible given available resources?
A formative assessment will require increased attention to the feedback process. In addition to questions 1–4 above, the following should be considered when designing formative assessments: 1. How will the individual trainee's performance be captured, reviewed, interpreted, and reported back to the learner? 2. How will the impact of the feedback be evaluated?

Nature of Encounter

If the nature of the encounter is instructional and the SP is expected to provide direct instruction to the trainee, a guide describing this process should also be developed. The guide will vary greatly depending on several factors, including the duration, nature, and objectives of the encounter. Sample contents include a summary of the encounter and its relationship to the curriculum; PI qualifications and training requirements; schedules; policies; relevant teaching aids or models and instructions for their use during sessions; instructional resources including texts, chapters, or videotaped demonstrations; and models for teaching focused procedures or examinations. For a sample training manual for PIs to teach behavioral counseling skills, see Crandall et al. [38].

An encounter incorporated within a high-stakes assessment intended to determine promotion or grades will require evidence to support the validity, reliability, and acceptability of the scores. In this case, the individual encounter would be considered in relation to the broader context of the overall assessment as well as the evaluation system within which it is placed. For principles of "good assessment," see the consensus statement of the 2010 Ottawa Conference [29] which is an international biennial forum on assessment of competence in healthcare education.

Case Development

Although not all encounters require the SP to simulate a patient experience, the majority requires a case scenario be developed which describes in varying detail his/her role, affect, demographics, and medical and social history. The degree of detail will vary according to the purpose of the encounter. For those which are lower stakes or those that do not require standardization, the case scenario will be less detailed and may simply outline the expectations and provide a brief summary of his character. Conversely, a high-stakes encounter which includes simulation and physical examination will require a fully detailed scenario and guidelines for simulating the role and the physical findings. Typically, a standardized encounter would require a case scenario which includes a summary, a description of the patient's presentation and emotional tone, his current and past medical history, lifestyle preferences and habits, and family and social history. If the SP is expected to assess performance, the scenario will also include a tool for recording the performance and a guide to carefully describe its use. If the SP is expected to provide verbal or written feedback to the trainee, a guide describing this process should also be included.

Although issues related to psychometrics are beyond the scope of this chapter, the text below will describe a standard process for developing a single SP encounter intended for use in one of multiple stations included in a performance assessment. For a comprehensive description of psychometric matters, see the *Practice Guide to the Evaluation of Clinical Competence* [39] and the *Standards for Educational and Psychological Testing* [40].

In order to facilitate the case selection and development processes, physician educators should be engaged as clinical case consultants. Often if encounters are designed to assess trainee performance, multiple physician educators will be surveyed to determine what they believe to be the most important topics or challenges to include, the key factors which are critical to performance, and how much weight should be placed upon these factors.

Once the topic or presenting complaint for the case has been selected, this information should be added to the blueprint described above. The next step is to gather pertinent details from the physician educator. Ideally, the case scenario will be based on an actual patient with all identifying information removed prior to use. This will make the encounter more authentic and ease the development process. Additionally, Nestel and Kneebone [41] recommend a method for "authenticating SP roles" which integrates actual patients into all phases of the process, including case development, training, and delivery. They argue that SP assessments may reflect professional but not real patient judgments and by involving actual patients into the process, a more authentic encounter will result. This recommendation is further supported by a recent consensus statement [29] which calls for the incorporation of the perspectives of patients and the public within assessment criteria. One effective strategy for increasing the realism of a case is to videotape actual patient interviews about their experiences. The affect, language, and oral history expressed by the actual patients can then be used to develop the case and train the SPs.

A common guide to case development is based on the works of Scott, Brannaman, Struijk, and Ambrozy (see Table 13.3). The 15 items listed in Table 13.3 have been adapted from the *Standardized Patient Case Development Workbook* [42]. Once these questions are addressed, typically the SP educator will transpose the information and draft training materials, the SP rating scale/checklist, and a guide for its use. See Wallace [43] Appendix A for samples of each of the above for a single case. This draft will then be reviewed by a group of experts. One method for gathering content-related evidence to support the validity of the encounter is to survey physician experts regarding several aspects of the encounter. This information would then be used to further refine the materials. Sample content evaluation questions include: (1) Does the encounter reinforce or measure competencies that are necessary for a (level) trainee? (2) Does the encounter reinforce or measure competencies that are aligned to curricular objectives? (3) How often would you expect a (level) trainee to perform such tasks during his/her training? (4) Does the encounter require tasks or skills infrequently encountered in practice that may result in high patient risk if performed poorly? (5) Is the context of the encounter realistic

Table 13.3 SP encounter pertinent details

1. Major purpose of encounter
2. Essential skills and behaviors to be assessed during encounter
3. Expected differential diagnosis (if relevant) or known diagnosis
4. SOAP note from original patient
5. Setting (as relevant): place, time of day, time of year
6. A list of cast members (if relevant) and their roles during the encounter
7. Patient characteristics (as relevant): age, gender, race, vitals at time of encounter, appearance, affect
8. Relevant prior history
9. Expected encounter progression (beginning, middle, end)
10. Contingency plans for how SP responds to certain actions/ comments throughout encounter
11. Information to be made available to the trainee prior to encounter
11. Current symptoms
12. Relevant past medical and family history
13. Relevant currently prescribed and OTC medications
14. Relevant social history
15. SP recruitment information (as relevant): age range, physical condition, gender, race/origin, medical conditions or physical signs which may detract from the case, requirements to undergo physical examination, positive physical exam findings

Reprinted from Scott et al. [42], with permission from Springer

in that it presents a situation similar to one that a provider might encounter in professional practice? (6) Does the encounter represent tasks that have been assessed elsewhere either in writing or on direct observation?

Very little attention has been paid to the development of SP cases and related materials in the published literature. In a comprehensive review of literature over a 32-year period, Gorter et al. [44] found only 12 articles which reported specifically on the development of SP checklists in internal medicine. They encourage the publication and transparency of these processes in order to further develop reliable and valid instruments. Despite the lack of attention in published reports, the design and use of the instruments used by the SP to document and/or rate performance is critical to the quality of the data derived from the encounter. Simple binary (done versus not done) items are frequently used to determine whether a particular question was asked or behavior was performed. Other formats are typically used to gather perspectives on communication and professionalism skills, such as Likert scales and free text response options. Overall global ratings of performance are also effective, and although a combination of formats is most valuable, there is evidence to suggest that these ratings are more reliable than checklist scores alone [45].

SP Recruitment and Hiring

There are several qualities to consider when recruiting individuals to serve as SPs. The minimum qualifications will vary depending upon the nature of the role and the SP encounter. For example, if hired to serve as a PI, then teaching skills and basic anatomical knowledge would be necessary. If recruiting someone to portray a highly emotional case, an individual with acting experience and/or training would be beneficial. In addition to these qualities, it is important to screen potential SPs for any bias against medical professionals. SPs with hidden (even subconscious) agendas may disrupt or detract from the encounters. A screening question to address this issue includes "Tell us about your feelings towards and experiences with physicians and other healthcare professionals." Additionally, it is important to determine if the candidate has had any personal/familial negative experiences with the role she is being recruited to portray. Although we do not have empirical data to support this recommendation, common sense tells us that repeated portrayal of a highly emotive case which happens to resemble a personal experience may be unsettling to the SP. Examples include receiving news that she has breast cancer, portraying a child abuser, or a patient suffering from recent loss of a parent. Identifying potential challenging attitudes and conflicting personal experiences in advance will prevent potential problems in the execution phase.

Identifying quality SPs can be a challenge. Several recruiting resources include: theater groups or centers, volunteer offices, schools, minority groups, and student clubs. Advertisements in newsletters, intranet, and social media will typically generate a large number of applicants, and depending on the need, this may be excessive. The most successful recruiting source is your current pool of SPs. Referrals from existing SPs have been reported as the most successful method for identifying quality applicants [45].

It is ideal if individual SPs are not overexposed to the trainees: Attempts should be made to avoid hiring SPs that have worked with the same trainees in the past. Always arrange a face-to-face meeting with a potential SP before hiring and agree to a trial period if multiple encounters. After the applicant completes an application, there are several topics to address during the interview including those listed in Table 13.4.

The amount of payment SPs receive for their work varies according to the role (Table 13.5), encounter format, expectations, and geography. A survey of US and Canadian SP Programs [46] revealed that the average hourly amount paid to SPs for training was $15 USD, $16 USD for role portrayal, and $48 USD for being examined and teaching invasive physical examination skills. The rates were slightly higher in the western and northeastern US regions.

SP Training

The training of SPs is critical to a successful encounter. Figure 13.2 displays a common training process for SPs for a simulated, standardized, encounter with expectations for assessment of trainees' skills. This process is intended to serve as a model and should be adapted to suit the needs of the encounter and the SPs being trained. Unfortunately, there is a lack of evidence to support specific training SP methods. A comprehensive review of SP research reports [47] found that, although data from SP encounters is frequently used to make decisions about efficacy of the research outcomes, less than 40% of authors made any reference to the methods for training the SPs and/or raters.

For a comprehensive text on training SPs, see *Coaching Standardized Patients for Use in the Assessment of Clinical*

Table 13.4 SP interview questions

Suggested discussion topics and questions for the potential SP include:
Discussion of encounter specifics and general nature of the role
Assess for potential conflicting emotions which may impede performance or impact the SP
Assess comfort with undergoing and/or teaching physical examination
Review training and session schedule
Determine if SP is appropriate for specific case
If relevant, discuss need for health screening and universal precautions training
Common questions to expect during the recruitment process include:
What is an SP? Why are they used in healthcare education?
Isn't being an SP just like being an actor?
What is the encounter format?
How do SPs assess trainees?
Where do the cases come from?
How does this benefit the trainee?
What is required of me?
How will I be trained?
How much time is required?
How much do I get paid?

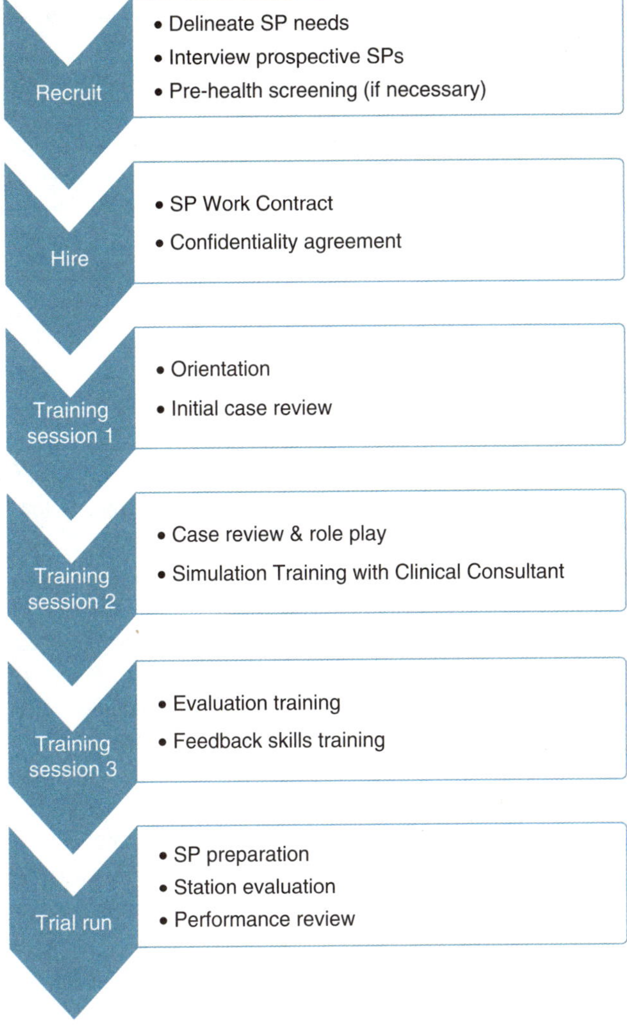

Fig. 13.2 Common training process for SP encounters

Table 13.5 Qualities of standardized patients according to role

	SP		PI/GTA/UTA	
	Assessment?		Assessment?	
	Yes	No	Yes	No
Intelligence	×	×	×	×
Excellent *communication skills*	×	×	×	×
Ability to simultaneously attend to (internal) role and (external) performance of learners	×		×	
Ability to deliver constructive feedback	×		×	×
Ability to accurately recall and record performance	×		×	
Conscientiousness and timeliness	×	×	×	×
Flexibility in schedule	×	×	×	×
Respect for healthcare professionals	×	×	×	×
Acting *skills*	×	×		
Teaching *skills*			×	×
Teamwork *skills*	×	×	×	×
Medical *knowledge*			×	×

Competence [43]. Wallace described six skills critical to an effective simulated standardized performance. The following should be attended to throughout the training process:

1. Realistic portrayal of the patient
2. Appropriate and unerring responses to whatever the student says or does
3. Accurate observation of the medical student's behavior
4. Flawless recall of the student's behavior
5. Accurate completion of the checklist
6. Effective feedback to the student (written or verbal) on how the patient experienced the interaction with the student.

As stated above, the type and duration of training will vary depending upon the expectations and purpose of the encounter. Details regarding training sessions for role portrayal, instruction, evaluation, and feedback will be described below. Training SPs to simulate a standardized role with no further expectations will take 1–2 h during one or two sessions. If you expect them to document and/or rate the performance of the trainees, an additional 2–3-h session will be required. A trial run with all major players and simulated trainees to rehearse the actual encounter is strongly encouraged. This session typically takes an additional 1–3 h and, depending on performances, may lead to additional training. In 2009, Howley et al. [46] surveyed SP Programs throughout the USA and Canada and found that the average amount of time reported to train a new SP before performing his role was 5.5 (SD = 5) and was reported by the majority of respondents as being variable according to the type of encounter. For example, if expected to teach trainees, the amount of preparation will be significantly lowered if the PI has prior training in healthcare delivery.

Regardless of the role that the SP is to being trained to perform, all SPs should be oriented to the use of SPs in healthcare, policies and procedures of the program, and general expectations of the role. It is also beneficial to share the perspectives of trainees and other SPs who participated in similar encounters to highlight the importance of the contribution he/she is about to make to healthcare education.

Role Portrayal

After the initial orientation, the SP reviews the case scenario with the SP educator. If multiple individuals are being hired to portray the same role, the SPs should participate as a group. Standardization should be clearly defined, and its impact on their performance should be made explicit throughout the training. During a second session, the SP reviews the case in greater depth with the SP educator. If available, videotaped samples of the actual or similar case should be shown to demonstrate desired performance. Spontaneous versus elicited information should be carefully differentiated, and the SPs should have the opportunity to role-play as the patient while receiving constructive feedback on their performances. A clinical case consultant also meets with the SPs to review clinical details and if relevant, describe and demonstrate any physical findings. In order to provide the SPs with greater understanding of the encounter, the consultant should also demonstrate the interview and/or physical examination while each SP portrays the role. The final training session should be a trial run with all the major players including simulated trainees to provide the SPs with an authentic preparatory experience. During this trial, the SP educator and the clinical consultant should evaluate the performance of all SPs and provide constructive comments for enhancing their portrayal. See Box 13.1 for an *SP Critique Form* for role portrayal. These questions should be asked multiple times for each SP during the training process and throughout the session for continuous quality improvement. Depending on performance during the trial run, additional training may be required to fully prepare an SP for his role. As a final reminder, prior to the initial SP encounter, several "do's and don'ts" of simulation should be reviewed (see Box 13.2 for sample).

Teaching

Patient instructors, including GTAs and UTAs, will often participate in multiple training methods which typically includes an apprentice approach. After initial recruitment and orientation, she/he would observe sessions led by experienced PIs, then serve as a model and secondary instructor for the exam, and finally as an associate instructor. Depending on the expectations of the PI role, the training may range from 8 to 40 h prior to participation and additional hours to maintain skills. General participation and training requirements for PIs include (1) health screening examination for all new and returning PIs, (2) universal precautions training, (3) independent study of anatomy and focused physical examination, (4) instructional video review of the examination, (5) practice sessions, (6) performance evaluation by physician and fellow PIs, and (7) ongoing performance evaluation for quality assurance and to enhance standardization of instruction across associates.

Evaluation/Rating

There is strong data to support the use of SPs to evaluate history taking, physical examination, and communications skills of (particularly junior) trainees [48, 49]. If an SP is expected to document or evaluate performance, it is imperative that she/he be trained to do so in an accurate and unbiased manner. The goals of this session are to familiarize the SPs with the instrument(s) and to ensure that they are able to recall and document/rate performance according to the predetermined criteria. The instrument(s) used to document or rate performance should be reviewed item-by-item for clarity and intent. A guide or supplement should accompany the evaluation instruments which clearly defines each item in

Box 13.1: SP Critique Form I

Evaluator: _______________ SP: __________________

SP Critique Form: Role Portrayal

1. Is the SP's body language consistent with the case description?
Yes No (If no, describe why)

2. Is the delivery (tone of voice, rate of speech, etc.) consistent with the case description?
Yes No (If no, describe why)

3. Does the SP respond to questions regarding the presenting complaint accurately?
Yes No (If no, describe why)

4. Does the SP respond to questions regarding his/her previous medical history accurately?
Yes No (If no, describe why)

4. Does the SP respond to questions regarding his/her lifestyle accurately?
Yes No (If no, describe why)

5. Does the SP simulate clinical findings accurately?
Yes No (If no, describe why)

6. Does the SP depict his/her case in a realistic manner?
Yes No (If no, describe why)

7. Does the SP refrain from delivering inappropriate information or leading the trainee?
Yes No (If no, describe why)

behavioral terms. The instruments should be completed immediately after each encounter to increase recall and accuracy. A training technique to increase the accuracy of ratings is to review and call attention to errors commonly made by SPs (and raters in general) when completing scales. Sample effects include halo/horn, stereotyping, Hawthorne, rater drift, personal perception, and recency. Several vignettes are developed, each depicting one of these errors, and the SPs are expected to determine which error is being made in each example and discuss its impact on the performance rating.

Another effective method for training SPs to use evaluation tools includes showing a videotaped previous SP encounter and asking the SPs to individually complete the instrument based on the performance observed in the encounter. The instrument may be completed during (or immediately after) the encounter, repeat with another sample

Box 13.2: SP Reminders

Do's and Don'ts of Simulation

Do

…be both accurate and consistent each time you portray the case. Your goal is to present the essence of the patient case, not just the case history, but the body language, physical findings, and emotional and personality characteristics.

Don't

…embellish the case. Don't be creative in the details of the case and stray from the standardized information.

Do

…maintain role throughout the encounter no matter what the trainee may say or do in attempt to distract you from your role.

Don't

…break from your role. Even if the trainee breaks from his/her role, the best thing to do is keep being you, the patient. Generally, trainees will regain the role if you don't miss a beat.

Do

…incorporate aspects of your own life when these details do not detract from the reality of the simulation. Try to feel, think, and react like the patient would. Begin to think about how "you" feel rather than the more distant stance of how the "patient" feels.

Don't

…view the case as a script to be memorized since you will lose some of the reality of portraying a real patient.

Do

…provide constructive feedback in your evaluation checklist as seen from the patient's point of view.

Don't

…simply restate in your feedback what the trainee did or did not do during the encounter.

Do

…self-monitor your comfort level with the role. You must believe in the plausibility of the role in order to assume it. Also be sure that a simulation striking "too close to home" does not impact your ability to portray the role. If this is the case, then this role may not be a good match for you.

Do

…take the role seriously and carefully review the details of the case. Ask questions as you see possible discrepancies in the role and seek clarification when needed.

encounter, and require the SPs to complete the instrument afterwards via recall. Afterwards, collect the instruments and tally the results for visual presentation. The SPs then discuss, as a group, those items about which they disagree. Rating scales can be particularly challenging in forming consensus, but in general, a behaviorally anchored scale will result in greater agreement of ratings. If necessary, replay the videotape to resolve any misunderstood behaviors that arise during the training exercise.

Feedback

One of the greatest benefits of SP encounters is the immediate feedback delivered by the SP to the trainee. Whether provided in writing or orally, training SPs to provide constructive feedback to the trainees is critically important. As in other areas, the training content and duration will vary according to the nature of the role and the purpose of the encounter. There are several resources available for feedback training which can be readily adapted to suit the needs of a particular encounter [50–52].

The primary goal of this training session is to equip the SPs with the knowledge and skills to provide quality constructive feedback to the trainees. Feedback is defined as "information communicated to the learner that is intended to modify the learner's thinking or behavior for the purpose of improved learning" [53]. SPs should be trained to deliver feedback that is descriptive and nonevaluative. The focus of the feedback should be consistent with the intent and expertise of the SP. Unless the SPs are serving as trained instructors, the SP should limit the feedback to how the patient felt during the encounter. In other words, feedback regarding clinical skills should be reserved for those faculty or others who hold this expertise. The SOAP model and DESC script are two effective methods for training SPs to frame and deliver constructive feedback to trainees [51].

Once the parameters and principles of the feedback have been reviewed, training should continue with opportunities for the SPs to put this knowledge into practice. To begin, ask the SPs to view a videotaped encounter and assume the role of the SP in the video. Immediately afterwards, ask the SP to deliver feedback to the "trainee" who in this exercise is simulated by another SP or a staff member. The SP role-plays delivering feedback while an observer critiques the performance. Refer to Box 13.3 for sample questions to guide the critique.

The SPs ability to provide constructive written feedback should not be ignored. Many of the same principles of constructive feedback apply to both oral and written communications. One method for reinforcing the SPs writing skills is to provide a series of feedback statements, some of which are inappropriate. Ask the SPs to review each statement and, when appropriate, rewrite to reflect a more constructive comment.

Trial Run

After SPs have been trained to perform their various roles (simulator, evaluator, and/or instructor), it is important to provide an opportunity to trial the encounter. These dress rehearsals should proceed as the actual event to allow for final preparation and fine-tuning of performance. Depending on the nature of the encounter/s, the objectives of the trial run may include: provide SPs with a better understanding of the format of the encounter, critique the SPs role portrayal, determine the SPs evaluation skills, orient and train staff, and test technical equipment. Simulated trainees should be invited to participate and provide feedback on the encounter, including the SPs portrayal. Although minor revisions to the cases may be made between the trial and the first encounter, it is preferable for the materials to be in final form prior to this session. Videotape review of the encounter/s with feedback provided to the SPs is an excellent method to further enhance SP performance and reinforce training objectives. The SP Critique Forms (Boxes 13.1 and 13.3) described above can be used to provide this feedback.

Execute and Appraise: Steps to Administer and Evaluate SP Encounters

The administration of SP encounters will vary by level of complexity and use of outcomes. This final section will summarize several recommendations for ensuring a well-run encounter. However, the efforts expended earlier to align the encounter to relevant and appropriate objectives; to recruit, hire, and train SPs suited to perform and evaluate trainee performance; and to construct sound training and scoring materials will go a long way to strengthen the encounter and the outcomes it yields.

Major Players

Directing an SP encounter can be a very complex task. Depending on the number of simultaneous encounters, the number of roles, the nature of the cases, and the number of trainees, the production may require dozens of SPs and staff support. See Table 13.6 for a description of major players and their roles in an SP assessment.

Orientation/Briefing

As with any educational offering, the orientation of the trainees to the SP encounter is critical to the overall quality of the experience. Trainees should know the purpose and expectations of the encounter/s; they should be made aware of the quality of the educational experience, how it is aligned to their curricula, instructions on how to progress through the encounter/s, implications of their performance, and how they can provide feedback on the encounter/s for future enhancements. Ideally, trainees should be able to self-prepare for the

Box 13.3: SP Critique Form II

Evaluator: _______________ SP: ___________________

SP Critique Form: Feedback

The SP began by asking the trainee whether he/she would like feedback.
Yes No

The SP began the feedback session by allowing the learner to describe how he/she felt the interaction went.
Yes No (If no, describe why)

The SP provided feedback about a performance strength.
Yes No (If no, describe why)

The SP provided feedback about behaviors that the learner could do something about.
Yes No (If no, describe why)

The SP's feedback was specific.
Yes No (If no, describe why)

The SP's feedback was nonevaluative.
Yes No (If no, describe why)

The SP checked to ensure that the feedback was received.
Yes No (If no, describe why)

The SP provided appropriate feedback within his/her expertise and intent of the encounter.
Yes No (If no, describe why)

The SP provided a sufficient amount of feedback.
Yes No (If no, describe why)

From Howley and McPherson [51]

Table 13.6 OSCE/SP assessment major players and their roles

Role	Responsibilities
Exam director	Oversee the entire production; facilitate the development of the cases, training materials, post-encounter stations, related instruments, and setting of examination standards
Exam steering committee	Address issues ranging from review of exam blueprint to justification and procurement of financial support
Clinical case consultant(s)	Provide guidance on case including evaluation instruments, train SPs on physical findings and assess quality of portrayal, set examination passing standards, define remediation strategies
SP educator(s)	Recruit, hire, and train all SPs; provide ongoing feedback on quality of SP performance; contribute to the development of the cases, training materials, post-encounter stations, and related instruments
SP	Complete all prescreening requirements and training sessions, continually monitor self and peer performances, present case, and evaluate trainees' performance timely, consistently, and accurately throughout the examination
Administrative assistant(s)	Maintain paperwork for all SPs and support staff, create schedules, prepare materials
Proctor(s)	Monitor time schedule throughout examination, proctor trainees during interstation exercises, oversee "smooth" functioning of the examination
Technical assistant	Control video monitoring equipment to ensure proper capture, troubleshoot all technical difficulties as they arise

encounter by reviewing relevant literature, training videos, policies and procedures, etc. These preparation strategies are consistent with Knowles et al.'s [54] assumptions of adult learners, including that they need to know what they are going to experience, how it applies to their daily practice, and how they can self-direct their learning.

When orienting and executing SP encounters, it is important to maintain fidelity by minimizing interactions with the SPs outside of the encounters. Trainees should not see the SPs until they greet them in the simulation. In addition, an individual SP should not engage with the same trainees while portraying different roles. Although this may be impractical, steps should be taken to avoid overexposure to individual SPs. During an encounter, the SP should always maintain his character (with the notable exception of the "time-in, time-out" format). If the trainee breaks role, the SP should not reciprocate.

Quality Assurance

Intra-evaluation methods, such as inter-rater agreement and case portrayal checks, should be implemented to monitor quality. Woehr and Huffcutt [55] found that raters who were trained on the standards and dimensionality for assigning ratings were more accurate and objective in their appraisals of performance. Specific methods include an *SP Critique Form* (Box 13.1), or a similar tool, to audit the accuracy and realism of the role. If multiple encounters are required over an extended period of time, critiques should be done periodically to assess performance. Similarly, the SPs delivery of written and oral feedback should also be monitored to prevent possible performance drift (see Box 13.3). Similar quality assurance measures have been shown to significantly reduce performance errors by SPs [56]. A second approach to assuring quality is to introduce additional raters in the process. A second rater views the encounter (in real or lapsed time) and completes the same rating and checklist instruments of the SP. An assessment of the inter-rater agreement will help determine if the ratings are consistent and if individual SPs need further training or recalibrating.

Debriefing

Although there are clear guidelines for debriefing trainees following simulation encounters [57], there is a paucity of published reports on debriefing SPs. It is important to debrief or de-role the SP following the encounter. This is particularly important for those cases which are physically or emotionally challenging. Methods used to detach the SP from his role include discussions about his orientation and trainee behaviors during the sessions. Casual conversations about future plans and life outside of their SP role will also facilitate the debrief process. The goal of this process is to release tensions, show appreciation for the work, distance the SP from the emotions of the role, and allow the SP to convey his feelings and experiences about his performance [58].

Evaluation

The evaluation of the encounter should be integrated throughout the entire IDEA process. Data to defend the quality of the encounter is gathered initially when multiple stakeholders are involved in identifying the needs of the trainees, in developing the case and associated materials, and in training the SPs. Evaluation of the outcomes is critical to assess the overall value of the offering as well as areas for future enhancement. Appraisal evidences for the validity, reliability, and acceptability of the data resulting from performance assessments were described earlier. This evidence determined the utility of the SP assessment in making formative and summative decisions.

A common 4-step linear model by Kirkpatrick and Kirkpatrick [59] can be used to appraise the encounter/s, particularly instructional strategies. This model includes the following progressive outcomes: (1) *reaction* to the offering (how he felt about the experience), (2) whether *learning* occurred (pre to post differences in performance), (3) whether *behavior* was effected (generalizable to actual behaviors in practice), and (4) whether this produced *results* in improvements in patient care or system enhancements (impactful on his patients or the system in which he practices). The majority of SP encounters have focused on the levels 1 and 2 of this model with participant surveys and pre-posttests of performance and/or knowledge to measure the effect of the encounter on knowledge, comprehension, and/or application. Levels 3 and 4 are relatively difficult to measure; however, if the encounter/s can be attributed to positive changes at these levels, the outcomes are commendable.

Conclusion

Whether the purpose is to certify a level of achievement, provide feedback to trainees about their clinical skills, or provide faculty with information about curriculum effectiveness, standardized patients will continue to play a vital role in the education of our healthcare professionals. Although the development of optimal SP encounters requires time, commitment, and resources, the reward is our ability to instruct and assess trainees in a safe, authentic, and patient-centered environment.

Appendix: Brief Glossary of Common Roles and Encounter Formats

Common roles	
Standardized patient	A lay person trained to portray a medical patient's relevant history, physical findings, and affect. SPs may be used in assessment or instructional encounters. They can also be trained to provide feedback on the performance of trainees. Typically, multiple lay persons are trained to portray the same patient in a *standard* fashion to allow for repeated performance and fair assessment of numerous trainees in a short time period
Simulated patient	A lay person trained to portray a medical patient's relevant history, physical findings, and affect. SPs may be used in assessment or instructional encounters. They can also be trained to provide feedback on the performance of trainees. Typically, educators differentiate simulated from standardized patients based on whether there are single or multiple lay persons trained to simulate the role in a low- or high-stakes encounter, respectively
Simulated participant or confederate	A lay person trained to portray a family member, friend, or nurse of a "patient" during a hybrid simulation encounter. The "patient" in these encounters is a high-fidelity human patient simulator. SPs may be used in assessments or instructional encounters to increase the fidelity and/or evaluate the performance of the individual or team of trainees. They can also be trained to provide feedback on the observed performance
Patient instructor or educator	A lay person trained to provide instruction on the physical examination using his/her own body. This instruction is typically delivered in small group settings where the trainees have the opportunity to view demonstrations of the exam as well as practice these newly acquired skills on the PI. These lay persons are trained on physical exam skills, teaching techniques, and delivering constructive feedback to trainees
Gynecological teaching associate	A female patient instructor specific to the gynecological examination
Urological teaching associate	A patient instructor specific to the male urogenital examination
Formats and methods	
OSCE	An objective-structured clinical examination is a limited performance assessment consisting of several brief (5–10-min) stations where the student performs a very focused task, such as a knee examination, fundoscopic examination, or EKG reading [27]. SPs are often integrated within these examinations to simulate patients, evaluate performance, and provide feedback to trainees
CPX	The clinical practice examination is an extended performance assessment consisting of several (15–50-min) stations where the student interacts with patients in an unstructured environment [15]. Unlike the OSCE format, students are not given specific instructions in a CPX. Consequently, the CPX is realistic to the clinical environment and provides information about a student's abilities to interact with a patient, initiate a session, and incorporate skills of history taking, physical examination, and patient education
Hybrid simulation	A simulation that integrates standardized, simulated patients and/or participants with technologies, such as high-fidelity simulators, task trainers, and/or medium-fidelity mannequins [16]
Patient encounter	A general term for the station or setting where a single simulation takes place
Unannounced standardized patient	An SP who has been covertly integrated into the real clinical practice environment to evaluate the performance of a healthcare professional

References

1. Barrows HS, Abrahamson S. The programmed patient: a technique for appraising student performance in clinical neurology. J Med Educ. 1964;39:802–5.
2. Outcome Project: General Competencies. Accreditation Council for Graduate Medical Education; 1999. Available from http://www.acgme.org/outcome/comp/compmin.asp. Accessed 11 Oct 2011.
3. Barrows HS. An overview of the uses of standardized patients for teaching and evaluating clinical skills. Acad Med. 1993;68(8):443–53.
4. Norman GR, Tugwell P, Feightner JW. A comparison of resident performance on real and simulated patients. J Med Educ. 1892;57:708–15.
5. LCME Annual Questionnaire Part II. 2011. Available from www.aamc.org/curriculumreports. Accessed 15 Nov 2011.
6. Klass DJ. "High-Stakes" testing of medical students using standardized patients. Teach Learn Med. 1994;6(1):28–32.
7. Reznick RK, Blackmore D, Dauphinee WD, Rothman AI, Smee S. Large scale high stakes testing with an OSCE: report from the Medical Council of Canada. Acad Med. 1996;71:S19–21.
8. Coplan B, Essary AC, Lohenry K, Stoehr JD. An update on the utilization of standardized patients in physician assistant education. J Phys Assist Educ. 2008;19(4):14–9.
9. Association of Standardized Patient Educators (ASPE). Available from http://www.aspeducators.org/about-aspe.php. Accessed 15 Nov 2011.
10. Association of Standardized Patient Educators (ASPE). Important certification survey for SP Educators. 14 Sept 2011. Available from: ASPE http://aspeducators.org/view_news.php?id=24. Accessed 15 Nov 2011.
11. Kern DE, Thomas PA, Howard DM, Bass EB. Curriculum development for medical education: a six-step approach. Baltimore: Johns Hopkins University Press; 1998.
12. Amin Z, Eng KH. Basics in medical education. 2nd ed. Hackensack: World Scientific; 2009.
13. Doyle LD. Psychometric properties of the clinical practice and reasoning assessment. Unpublished dissertation, University of Virginia School of Education. 1999.
14. Bashook PG. Best practices for assessing competence and performance of the behavioral health workforce. Adm Policy Ment Health. 2005;32(5–6):563–92.
15. Barrows HS, Williams RG, Moy HM. A comprehensive performance-based assessment of fourth-year students' clinical skills. J Med Educ. 1987;62:805–9.
16. Kneebone RL, Nestel D, Vincent C, Darzi A. Complexity, risk and simulation in learning procedural skills. Med Educ. 2007;41(8):808–14.
17. Siassakos D, Draycott T, O'Brien K, Kenyon C, Bartlett C, Fox R. Exploratory randomized controlled trial of a hybrid obstetric simulation training for undergraduate students. Simul Healthc. 2010;5:193–8.
18. Yudkowsky R, Hurm M, Kiser B, LeDonne C, Milos S. Suturing on a bench model and a standardized-patient hybrid are not equivalent tasks. Poster presented at the AAMC Central Group on Educational Affairs annual meeting, Chicago, 9 Apr 2010.
19. Cumming JJ, Maxwell GS. Contextualising authentic assessment. Assess Educ. 1999;6(2):177–94.
20. Pugnaire MP, Leong SL, Quirk ME, Mazor K, Gray JM. The standardized family: an innovation in primary care education at the University of Massachusetts. Acad Med. 1999;74(1 Suppl):S90–7.
21. Lewis T, Margolin E, Moore I, Warshaw G. Longitudinal encounters with Alzheimers disease standardized patients (LEADS). POGOe – Portal of Geriatric Online Education; 2009. Available from: http://ww.pogoe.org/productid/20246
22. Barrows HS. Simulated patients in medical teaching. Can Med Ass J. 1968;98:674–6.
23. Stillman PL, Ruggill JS, Rutala PJ, Sabers DL. Patient instructors as teachers and evaluators. J Med Educ. 1980;55:186–93.
24. Kretzschmar RM. Evolution of the gynecological teaching associate: an education specialist. Am J Obstet Gyn. 1978;131:367–73.
25. Bideau M, Guerne PA, Bianci MP, Huber P. Benefits of a programme taking advantage of patient-instructors to teach and assess musculoskeletal skills in medical students. Ann Rheum Dis. 2006;65:1626–30.
26. Henriksen AH, Ringsted C. Learning from patients: students perceptions of patient instructors. Med Educ. 2011;45(9):913–9.
27. Howley LD, Dickerson K. Medical students' first male urogenital examination: investigating the effects of instruction and gender anxiety. Med Educ Online [serial online] 2003;8:14. Available from http://www.med-ed-online.org.
28. Howley LD. Performance assessment in medical education: where we've been and where we're going. Eval Health Prof. 2004;27(3):285–303.
29. Norcini J, Anderson B, Bollelea V, Burch V, Costa MJ, Duvuvier R, et al. Criteria for good assessment: consensus statement and recommendations for the Ottawa 2010 Conference. Med Teach. 2011;33(3):206–14.
30. Elstein A, Shulman L, Sprafka S. Medical problem solving: an analysis of clinical reasoning. Cambridge: Harvard University Press; 1978.
31. Van der Vleuten CPM, Schuwirth LWT. Assessment of professional competence: from methods to programmes. Med Educ. 2005;39:309–17.
32. Harden R, Gleeson F. Assessment of clinical competence using an objective structured clinical examination (OSCE). Med Educ. 1979;13:41–54.
33. Harden V, Harden RM. OSCE Annotated Bibliography with Contents Analysis: BEME Guide No 17. 2003 by AMEE. Available at: http://www2.warwick.ac.uk/fac/med/beme/reviews/published/harden/beme_guide_no_17_beme_guide_to_the_osce_2003.pdf
34. Miller GE. The assessment of clinical skills/competence/performance. Acad Med. 1990;65(9):S63–7.
35. Educational Commission for Foreign Medical Graduates (ECFMG®) Clinical Skills Assessment (CSA®) Candidate Orientation Manual. 2002 by the ECFMG. Available at: http://www.usmle.org/pdfs/step-2-cs/content_step2cs.pdf
36. Rethans JJ, Gorter S, Bokken L, Morrison L. Unannounced standardized patients in real practice: a systematic literature review. Med Educ. 2007;41(6):537–49.
37. Ozuah PO, Reznik M. Using unannounced standardized patients to assess residents' competency in asthma severity classification. Ambul Pediatr. 2008;8(2):139–42.
38. Crandall S, Long Foley K, Marion G, Kronner D, Walker K, Vaden K, et al. Training guide for standardized patient instructors to teach medical students culturally competent tobacco cessation counseling. MedEdPORTAL; 2008. Available from: www.mededportal.org/publication/762.
39. Holmboe ES, Hawkins RE. Practical guide to the evaluation of clinical competence. Philadelphia: Mosby Publishing Company; 2008.
40. AERA, APA, & NCME. Standards for educational and psychological testing. Washington, D.C.; 1999.
41. Nestel D, Kneebone R. Authentic patient perspectives in simulations for procedural and surgical skills. Acad Med. 2010;85(5):889–93.
42. Scott CS, Brannaman V, Struijk J, Ambrozy D. Standardized patient case development workbook [book online]. University of Washington School of Medicine; 1999. Available at: www.simportal.umn.edu/training/SPWORKBOOK.RTF. Accessed 11 Nov 2011.

43. Wallace P. Coaching standardized patients for use in the assessment of clinical competence. New York: Springer Publishing Company; 2007. p. 152.
44. Gorter S, Rethans JJ, Scherpbier A, Van der Heijde D, Houben H, Van der Vleuten C, et al. Developing case-specific checklists for standardized-patient-based assessments in internal medicine: a review of the literature. Acad Med. 2000;75(11):1130–7.
45. Hodges B, Regehr G, McNaughton N, Tiberius R, Hanson M. OSCE checklists do not capture increasing levels of expertise. Acad Med. 1999;74:1129–34.
46. Howley LD, Gliva-McConvey G, Thornton J. Standardized patient practices: initial report on the survey of US and Canadian Medical Schools. Med Educ Online. 2009;14:7.
47. Howley LD, Szauter K, Perkowski L, Clifton M, McNaughton N. Quality of standardized patient research reports in the medical education literature: review and recommendations. Med Educ. 2008;42(4):350–8.
48. Stillman PL, Swanson DB, Smee S, et al. Assessing clinical skills of residents with standardized patients. Ann Intern Med. 1986;105(5):762–71.
49. Martin JA, Reznick RK, Rothman A, et al. Who should rate candidates in an objectives structured clinical examination? Acad Med. 1996;71(2):170–5.
50. Howley L. Focusing feedback on interpersonal skills: a workshop for standardized patients. MedEdPORTAL; 2007. Available from: www.mededportal.org/publication/339.
51. Howley L, McPherson V. Delivering constructive formative feedback: a toolkit for medical educators. [Unpublished book] Presented at the annual educational meeting of the Accreditation Council of Graduate Medical Education, Nashville, Mar 2011.
52. May W. WinDix training manual for standardized patient trainers: how to give effective feedback. MedEdPORTAL; 2006. Available from: www.mededportal.org/publication/171.
53. Shute VJ. Focus on formative feedback. Rev Educ Res. 2008;78(1): 153–89.
54. Knowles MS, Holton EF, Swanson RA. The adult learner. Houston: Gulf Publishing; 1998.
55. Woehr DJ, Huffcutt AI. Rater training for performance appraisal: a quantitative review. J Occup Organ Psychol. 1994;67:189–205.
56. Wallace P, Garman K, Heine N, Bartos R. Effect of varying amounts of feedback on standardized patient checklist accuracy in clinical practice examinations. Teach Learn Med. 1999;11(3):148–52.
57. Fanning RM, Gaba DM. The role of debriefing in simulation based learning. Simul Healthc. 2007;2(2):115–25.
58. Cleland JA, Abe K, Rethans JJ. The use of simulated patients in medical education, AMEE Guide 42. Med Teach. 2009;31(6): 477–86.
59. Kirkpatrick DL, Kirkpatrick JD. Evaluating training programs: the four levels. 3rd ed. San Francisco: Berrett-Koehler Publishing Company; 2006.

Computer and Web Based Simulators

14

Kathleen M. Ventre and Howard A. Schwid

Introduction

Acceleration of the patient safety movement over the last decade has brought a heightened level of scrutiny upon the traditional time-based, apprenticeship model of medical education. Throughout the twentieth century, the guiding principle of medical education was that time served in the clinical setting was a reasonable proxy for professional competency and the capacity for independent practice. Historically, physicians have been trained through a largely haphazard process of practicing potentially risky interventions on human patients, and the types of situations physicians gained experience in managing during their training years were determined largely by serendipity. In 2003 and again in 2011, the Accreditation Council for Graduate Medical Education instituted progressive restrictions on the number of hours that American physician trainees can spend in direct patient care or on-site educational activities. These changes were intended to address a growing appreciation of the patient safety threat posed by fatigue-related medical errors. However, they would also limit allowable training time to a degree that created a need for fresh approaches that are capable of bridging a growing "experience gap" for physicians-in-training.

Increasing regulatory pressures have revived interest in using simulation technology to help transform the traditional time-based model of medical education to a criterion-based model. Human patient simulation has undergone a period of considerable growth since 2003, resulting in the establishment of a dedicated professional journal and yearly international meeting whose attendance increased 15-fold between 2003 and 2008 [1]. The majority of simulation taking place in medical education today involves the use of full-scale, computer-driven mannequins that are capable of portraying human physiology and around which a realistic clinical environment can be recreated. In this sense, mannequin simulators are uniquely suited for creating training scenarios capable of satisfying the highest requirements for equipment fidelity, environment fidelity, and psychological fidelity, or the capacity to evoke emotions in trainees that they could expect to experience in actual practice. However, there are significant logistical challenges associated with gathering work-hour limited trainees at sufficiently frequent intervals to foster maintenance of clinical competency using mannequin simulation. Moreover, the high cost of equipping and maintaining a state-of-the-art simulation facility places significant limitations on the ability of mannequin simulation to integrate fully into existing curricula. Although staffing costs are the single most expensive part of mannequin simulation, descriptive reports of academic simulation programs commonly avoid a thorough accounting of instructor salaries, technician salaries, and opportunity costs when defending their cost-effectiveness or sustainability [2–5].

As the medical simulation field matures, there is growing interest in the use of complementary technologies such as computer screen-based simulators, to make simulation more affordable and more accessible to health-care professionals. Screen-based simulators are designed in the image of popular gaming devices that present information on a computer screen, in the form of dynamic graphical images and supplementary text. The operator interacts with the user interface using keyboard, joystick, touchpad, or computer mouse controls. Contemporary screen-based simulators for medical education owe their earliest origins to a prototype from the early 1960s, which Entwisle and colleagues developed to provide instructor-free training in differential diagnosis [6]. This was a desk-sized, LGP-30 digital computer (Royal

K.M. Ventre, MD (✉)
Department of Pediatrics/Critical Care Medicine,
Children's Hospital Colorado/University of Colorado,
13121 E 17th Ave, MS 8414, L28-4128,
Aurora, CO 80045, USA
e-mail: kathleen.ventre@ucdenver.edu

H.A. Schwid, MD
Department of Anesthesiology and Pain Medicine,
University of Washington School of Medicine,
Seattle, WA, USA
e-mail: hschwid@u.washington.edu

A.I. Levine et al. (eds.), *The Comprehensive Textbook of Healthcare Simulation*,
DOI 10.1007/978-1-4614-5993-4_14, © Springer Science+Business Media New York 2013

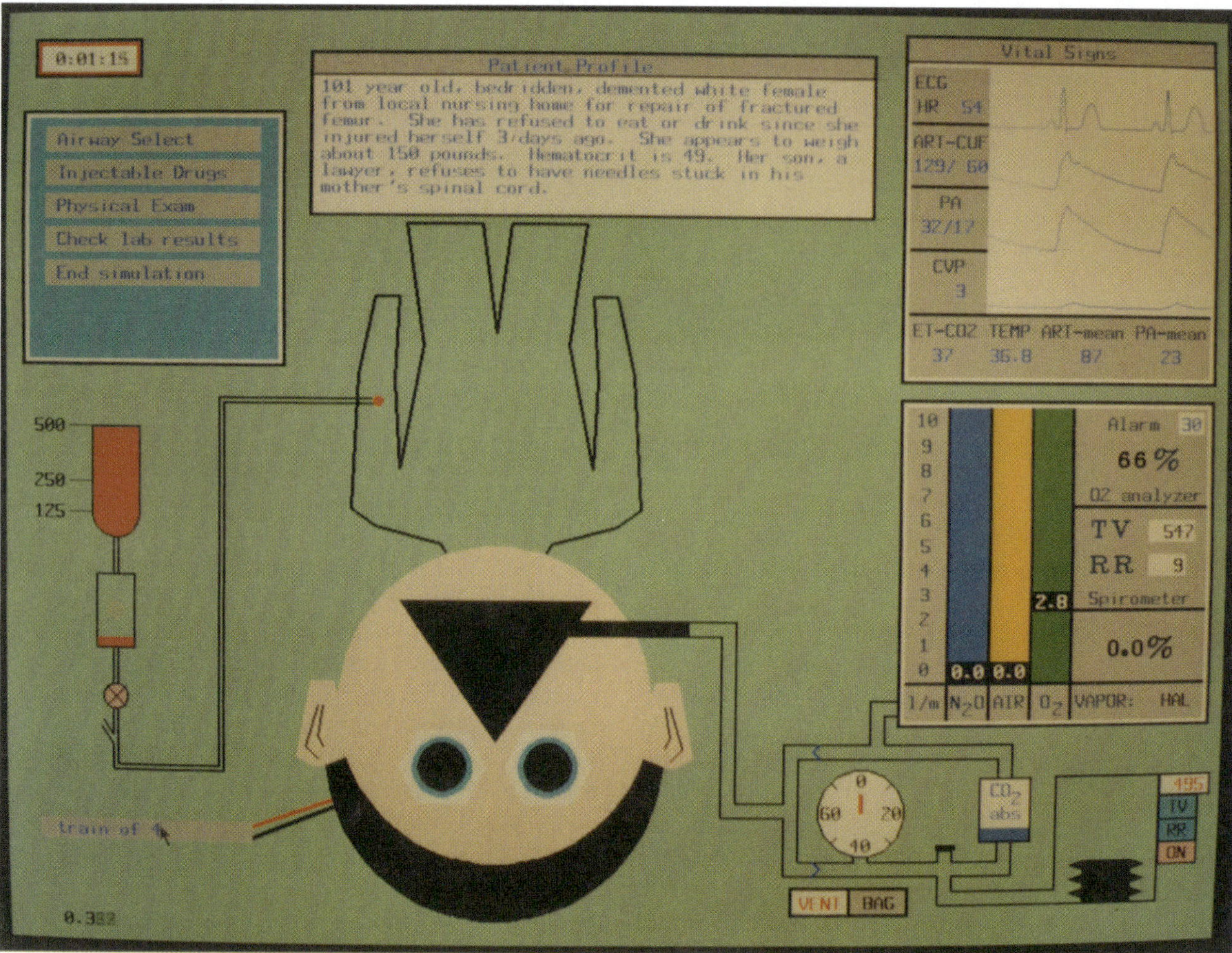

Fig. 14.1 A screen-based simulator for general anesthesia training, ca. 1987. The simulator's mouse-controlled graphics display is shown, depicting a patient, the patient history, and key aspects of the operating room environment (From Schwid [7])

Precision Corporation, Port Chester NY) that was programmed to randomly generate hypothetical patients with one of six possible diagnoses. Each "patient" possessed a unique array of physical findings, as determined from symptom frequency tables that were painstakingly assembled by the investigators and subsequently stored by the computer for each diagnosis. The computer would display the words "yes", "no", or "no information" in response to a student typing individual symptoms from a master list. If the student ultimately arrived at an incorrect diagnosis at the end of this process, the computer would issue a prompt to enter additional queries. It took 4 full minutes for the computer to generate each hypothetical patient and ready itself for student queries, and the entire program operated at the limits of the computer's 4,096-word memory.

By the early 1980s, personal computer (PC) technology had become powerful and inexpensive enough to make widespread availability of more sophisticated screen-based simulators a realistic possibility. Created in the image of flight simulators from the same era, these "second-generation" medical simulators were originally designed as anesthesiology trainers that could mathematically model how pharmaceuticals interact with circulatory, respiratory, renal, and hepatic pathophysiology [7]. The interface to the simulator contained a graphics display that recreated key aspects of the operating room environment, including a patient, an array of airway management options, and a monitor showing ECG, central venous pressure, and systemic and pulmonary arterial waveforms (Fig. 14.1). An anesthesia machine, oxygen analyzer, spirometer, circle system, ventilator, nerve stimulator, and flow-inflating anesthesia bag were also represented on the display. These capabilities supported the portrayal of realistic and dynamic clinical scenarios using an intuitive interface that allowed the operator to interact with the device as he or she would interact with an actual patient. This "Flight Simulator for Anesthesia Training" set the standard for screen-based simulators that were designed for training health-care professionals in the decades that followed.

The Fidelity Spectrum in Screen-Based Simulation

Screen-based simulators for health-care education now encompass a broad spectrum of fidelity, a term that describes the number and authenticity of sensory or environmental "cues" that the simulator provides as part of the context surrounding the clinical scenario it depicts. Occupying the highest end of the environmental and psychological fidelity spectrum are "virtual reality" trainers. These are highly sophisticated screen-based simulators that are capable of representing complex physical spaces in three dimensions while allowing multiple users to interact with virtual objects and animated versions of one another ("avatars") within the virtual environment [8]. Positioned somewhat lower on the fidelity spectrum are "conventional" screen-based simulators, which aspire to represent fewer aspects of the physical environment, yet demonstrate a degree of fidelity sufficient to refine clinical judgment and develop the cognitive structures that are required to execute complex tasks in a reliable manner.

All screen-based simulators, regardless of their fidelity level, address some of the inherent disadvantages of mannequin simulation. First, because screen-based simulations are entirely conducted on a personal computer or within a web browser, they offer unparalleled flexibility of the time and place in which the training exercises occur. Second, every correct or incorrect decision the operator makes during the simulation can be captured and tracked quite easily, rendering screen-based simulation highly suitable for developing or assessing competency in large groups of health-care providers. In the case of virtual reality simulators, even physical movements can be captured and tracked, a feature which renders them capable of driving trainees to higher levels of technical skill performance. Finally, screen-based simulations offer significant cost advantages over mannequin simulation [9]. While screen-based simulations can have high initial development costs, they do not require an instructor to be present while the trainee completes an exercise.

While virtual reality simulators possess a set of attributes that will ultimately allow instructors to extend screen-based simulation objectives beyond the cognitive domain into the technical and affective domains, fulfillment of their potential to truly transform simulation training remains dependent on additional research and development. This chapter will focus on conventional screen-based simulation, an area in which there has been considerable growth over the past several years.

Core Technical Standards for Screen-Based Simulators

There are several key attributes possessed by all screen-based simulators that allow them to operate "intelligently" and provide an effective learning experience without the need for instructor presence (Table 14.1). First, screen-based simulators have a *graphical user interface* that displays the simulator "output." The display includes an image of the patient that changes according to how the simulated scenario unfolds and shows monitored clinical parameters that are appropriate for the type of setting in which the scenario is supposed to be occurring. For example, scenarios that are occurring in an emergency department or hospital ward setting should at least show an ECG tracing sweeping across the cardiac rhythm monitor, and perhaps an oxygen saturation tracing. Scenarios that are occurring in the operating room or an intensive care setting should add dynamic waveform displays for arterial blood pressure, central venous pressure, and end-tidal carbon dioxide, as well as pulmonary arterial catheter waveforms, if applicable. Audible alarms and/or monitor tones can provide realistic environmental cues that deepen the operator's engagement with the simulation. The graphical user interface should operate as intuitively as possible, so that the trainee can provide "input" to the simulator using a computer mouse, touchpad, or simple keyboard controls, as appropriate for the device on which the program is operating. The key to ensuring interface simplicity is to maintain a very clear idea of the training objectives and limit the "scene detail" portrayed in the displays to only those elements that are required to manage the case. Although initial development of an elegant user interface involves considerable effort and expense, individual components such as cardiac rhythm displays, patient images depicting various stages of resuscitation, the defibrillator, and a representation of other medical devices can be reused as part of any number of scenarios, thus reducing the overall development costs [8].

Table 14.1 Key attributes of screen-based simulators

Easy-to-use graphical user interface
Models and states to predict simulated patient responses
Automated help system
Automated debriefing and scoring
Automated case record
Case library
Learning management system compatibility

Screen-based simulators must be developed around a simulation "engine" that governs how the simulated patient responds to the operator's interventions during the case. The engine consists of mathematical *models* of pharmacology as well as cardiovascular and respiratory physiology. The pharmacokinetic model predicts blood and tissue levels as well as elimination for any drug administered to the simulated patient. The pharmacodynamic model predicts the effects of any drug on heart rate, cardiac contractility, vascular resistance, baroreceptor response, respiratory drive, and other physiologic parameters. The cardiovascular model predicts changes in cardiac output and blood pressure in response to these effects, and the respiratory model predicts subsequent alterations in gas exchange which are reflected in the simulated patient's blood gas. Thus, the individual models interact with one another to emulate and portray complex human pathophysiology. What appears to the operator as a dynamic yet coherent case scenario is actually modeled using a finite number of *states*. The case author designs a set of states, each of which describes the physiologic condition of the patient at various points as the simulation unfolds. Each state moves to the next if a set of predetermined transition conditions are met. The physiologic status of the simulated patient, as represented in the simulator as vital sign changes, laboratory values, and other cues, is constantly updated by the combination of model predictions and transitions between states. Discussion of how a finite state machine interacts dynamically with mathematical models to depict a realistic clinical scenario is available in Schwid and O'Donnell's 1992 description of a malignant hyperthermia simulator [10].

Screen-based simulators should also contain a series of embedded feedback devices to provide guidance to the trainee as he or she navigates the case scenario. These include an *automated help system* which provides real-time information about drug dosing and mechanism of action, as well as on-demand suggestions for the trainee about what he or she should do next for the patient [11]. In addition, these simulators should contain an *automated debriefing system* that captures all of the management decisions that were made during the case [12]. This system recognizes when the operator has met all the learning objectives for the scenario and issues feedback that the simulation has ended. However, if the patient does not survive in the scenario, the debriefing system issues feedback suggesting the operator practice the case again. In either situation, when the scenario is over, the debriefing system provides a time-stamped record of decisions the operator made while managing the case. In addition, the *case record* produces a complete log of the user's management decisions and patient responses [13]. It also indicates where the user gained or lost points during the scenario and issues a score for overall performance.

Ideally, the simulator software package would include a set of pre-written, ready-to-use case scenarios, or a *case library* [14, 15]. Each simulation case scenario in the library is represented by a data file that is read and interpreted by the simulator program. There are many possible formats for the data file including simple text or XML (extended markup language) [16, 17]. It is desirable for case authors to share their case scenarios with one another in order to facilitate development of a large library of content. At this time, there is no single standard case format, but the Association of American Medical Colleges supports a web-based, accessible format at its medical education content repository, MedEdPORTAL (https://www.mededportal.org/). See, for example, a case scenario for anaphylaxis which comes complete with learning objectives and debriefing messages [18].

In recent years, many health-care organizations have adopted ways to centralize and automate the administration of training modules to their clinician workforce. These "learning management systems" (LMS) are software applications capable of importing and managing a variety of e-learning materials, provided the learning modules comply with the system's specifications for sharable content (e.g., Sharable Content Object Reference Model or "SCORM"). *LMS compatibility* is rapidly becoming a desirable attribute for screen-based simulators, as they progress from operating as installed applications on individual computer terminals to applications that can operate within web browsers. Integrating screen-based simulation into a learning management system gives administrators the ability to chart health-care professionals' progress through a diverse library of training cases. As standardized scoring rubrics for screen-based simulations are developed and validated, learning management systems will also be able to securely track specific competencies, as assessed using screen-based simulation rather than traditional multiple-choice testing.

Examples of Screen-Based Simulators

Several software companies now market case-based simulations that are designed to operate on personal computers. Mad Scientist Corporation (www.madsci.com) and Anesoft Corporation (www.anesoft.com) have each been in this business for approximately 25 years. Both produce a suite of programs that offer training in the management of adult and pediatric acute and critical care scenarios. Anesoft Corporation has a particularly extensive range of case-based simulators encompassing the domains of adult and pediatric critical care, neonatology, obstetrics, anesthesiology, and bioterrorism (Table 14.2). This chapter will focus its discussion on Anesoft screen-based simulators and a couple of other innovative and promising research prototypes.

Table 14.2 Anesoft case-based medical simulators

Anesoft case-based medical simulators
ACLS Simulator
PALS Simulator
Anesthesia Simulator
Critical Care Simulator
Sedation Simulator
Pediatrics Simulator
Obstetrics Simulator
Neonatal Resuscitation Simulator
Bioterrorism Simulator
Hemodynamics Simulator

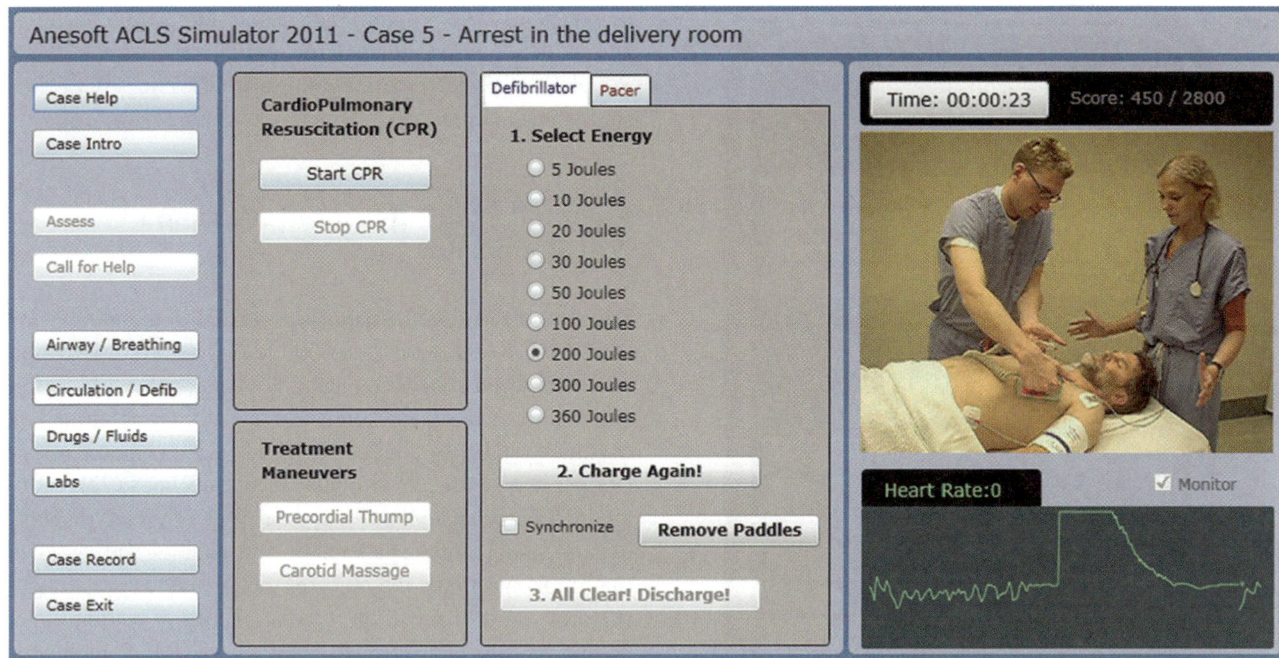

Fig. 14.2 Graphical user interface for the Anesoft ACLS Simulator 2011. Dynamic photographic images show the patient, 2 resuscitators, and the actions the user commands them to perform by using a mouse or touchpad to interact with the interface buttons. Note the dynamic cardiac rhythm waveform in the lower right of the figure, which depicts the upward voltage deflection (and subsequent voltage decay) associated with the countershock. *Note*: *In the Anesoft Simulators, the patient and the resuscitators shown in the photographic images are portrayed by actors*

Anesoft Advanced Cardiac Life Support (ACLS) Simulator

The Anesoft ACLS Simulator was developed almost 20 years ago, to address the observation that knowledge of the American Heart Association guidelines for management of cardiac arrest states decayed quickly following formal classroom training [19–22]. The program was originally designed as an installed application that could run on Windows (Microsoft Corporation, Redmond WA) computers [23]. Two modules are contained within the ACLS Simulator package. The "Rhythm Simulator" is designed to teach and reinforce a structured approach to recognizing common cardiac rhythm disturbances. The second module is the ACLS megacode simulator itself, whose graphical user interface displays dynamic photographic images of the simulated patient and two resuscitators, as well as a cardiac monitor displaying the patient's current rhythm sweeping across the screen (Fig. 14.2). The user controls the actions of the resuscitators by interacting with the interface using a computer mouse and a series of dashboard buttons. The ACLS Simulator contains an automated debriefing system and a built-in, on-demand help system that prompts the user to take the next appropriate action in each scenario. At the conclusion of each case, the simulator produces a detailed, downloadable or printable case record summarizing all of the decisions the trainee made during the scenario and assigns a score for overall performance. The *ACLS Simulator 2011* assesses user performance according to the American Heart Association's 2010 Guidelines for Cardiopulmonary Resuscitation and Emergency Cardiovascular Care [24]. *ACLS Simulator 2011* operates on Windows and Macintosh computers in almost any browser. The simulator contains a case library consisting of 16 cases covering ACLS guidelines for the management of ventricular fibrillation/pulseless ventricular tachycardia, ventricular tachycardia with pulse, pulseless electrical activity, and assorted other tachycardic and bradycardic dysrhythmias. Completion of *ACLS Simulator 2011* cases is not sufficient for provider credentialing through the American Heart Association but does entitle the user to as many as 8 American Medical Association Physician Recognition Award Category 2 Continuing Medical Education credits. A couple of key distinctions between *ACLS 2011* and earlier versions of the simulator are that it operates completely within any web browser and it meets SCORM and Aviation Industry Computer-Based Training Committee ("AICC") standards, which means that the simulator is now compatible with many institutional learning management systems. Most recently, the *ACLS Simulator 2011* has been modified so that it can port to mobile devices. The more streamlined "iPhone and iPad" (Apple Corporation, Cupertino CA) and "Android" (Google, Menlo Park CA) versions of the simulator contain the same drug library as the parent version, but contain only 12 cases. While the mobile version allows defibrillation, it

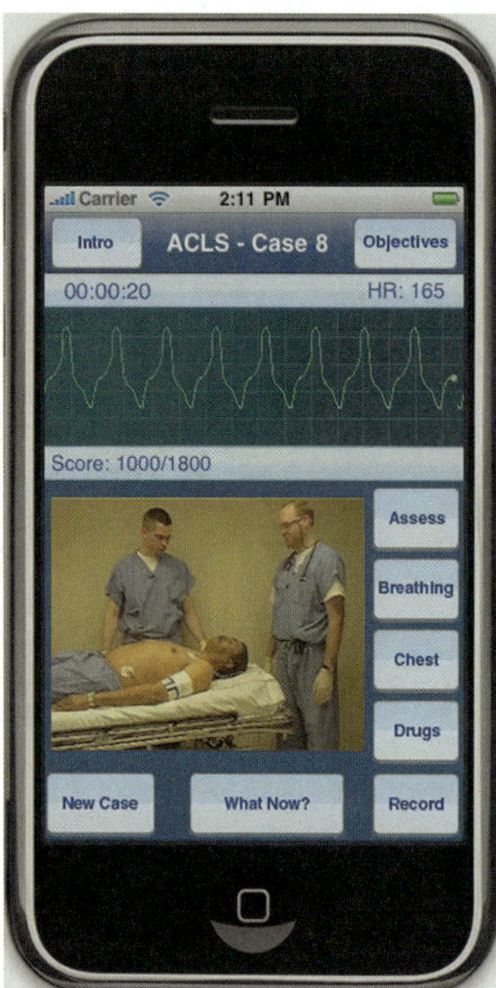

Fig. 14.3 Anesoft ACLS 2011, "iPhone and iPad" version. As compared to the full-scale ACLS Simulator 2011, this user interface is simplified but still shows dynamic photographic images of the patient and resuscitators and shows a dynamic cardiac rhythm waveform. Elapsed scenario time (*upper left*) and the running score tally are also displayed

does not allow transcutaneous pacing, IV fluid management, lab values, caselog downloading/printing, or CME credits (Fig. 14.3). The "Rhythm Simulator" is not included as part of the mobile ACLS Simulator package but is available separately.

Laerdal HeartCode® ACLS Simulator

HeartCode® ACLS (Laerdal Corporation, Stavanger, Norway) has many similarities to the Anesoft ACLS Simulator. It is also a web-based program that enables students to diagnose and treat a number of Advanced Cardiac Life Support scenarios [25]. The package has a total of ten cases with one BLS case, two megacode scenarios, and seven other emergencies. The program includes on-line help (coaching) and automated debriefing. Unlike with the Anesoft ACLS Simulator, the electrocardiogram in HeartCode® ACLS is a static image rather than a dynamic, sweeping waveform.

Anesoft Pediatric Advanced Life Support (PALS) Simulator

The Anesoft PALS Simulator was created in the mold of its adult (ACLS) counterpart in 2006 [26]. The original version was configured to operate on any Windows-compatible computer and was designed to provide robust training in the key cognitive aspects of conducting an advanced pediatric resuscitation in accordance with published guidelines [27]. As in the ACLS Simulator, the graphical user interface displays dynamic images of the patient, the resuscitators, and a cardiac rhythm monitor, and the operator directs the resuscitators to perform various interventions using a series of buttons and a mouse-controlled menu (Fig. 14.4a). The PALS Simulator also contains an automated debriefing system and on-demand help system, and the simulator's drug information library provides dosing guidelines appropriate for pediatric patients.

In 2011, the Anesoft PALS Simulator was modified to operate completely within a web browser [26]. *PALS Simulator 2011* assesses user performance according to the American Heart Association's 2010 Guidelines for Cardiopulmonary Resuscitation and Emergency Cardiovascular Care [27]. It also features improvements to the user interface (Fig. 14.4b) and other modifications that were suggested in a survey of multidisciplinary pediatric health-care professionals who provided feedback on the original version of the PALS Simulator [28]. The simulator's original library of 12 cases was extended to 16 cases for the 2011 version, in response to user feedback. In addition to the original 12 cases representing the 4 major PALS treatment algorithms (supraventricular tachycardia, pulseless electrical activity, ventricular fibrillation/pulseless ventricular tachycardia, and bradycardia), *PALS Simulator 2011* now includes 4 Pediatric Emergency Assessment, Recognition, and Stabilization ("PEARS") cases that emphasize averting cardiac or respiratory arrest through prompt reversal of shock or other forms of cardiopulmonary distress [29]. *PALS Simulator 2011* also contains a basic case scenario that serves as a structured tutorial on how the simulator operates. Users who complete cases on *PALS Simulator 2011* do not automatically receive provider credentialing through the American Heart Association but are entitled to as many as 8 American Medical Association Physician Recognition Award Category 2 Continuing Medical Education credits. *PALS Simulator 2011* is also SCORM and AICC compliant. PALS Simulator for iPhone, iPad, and Android devices is under development.

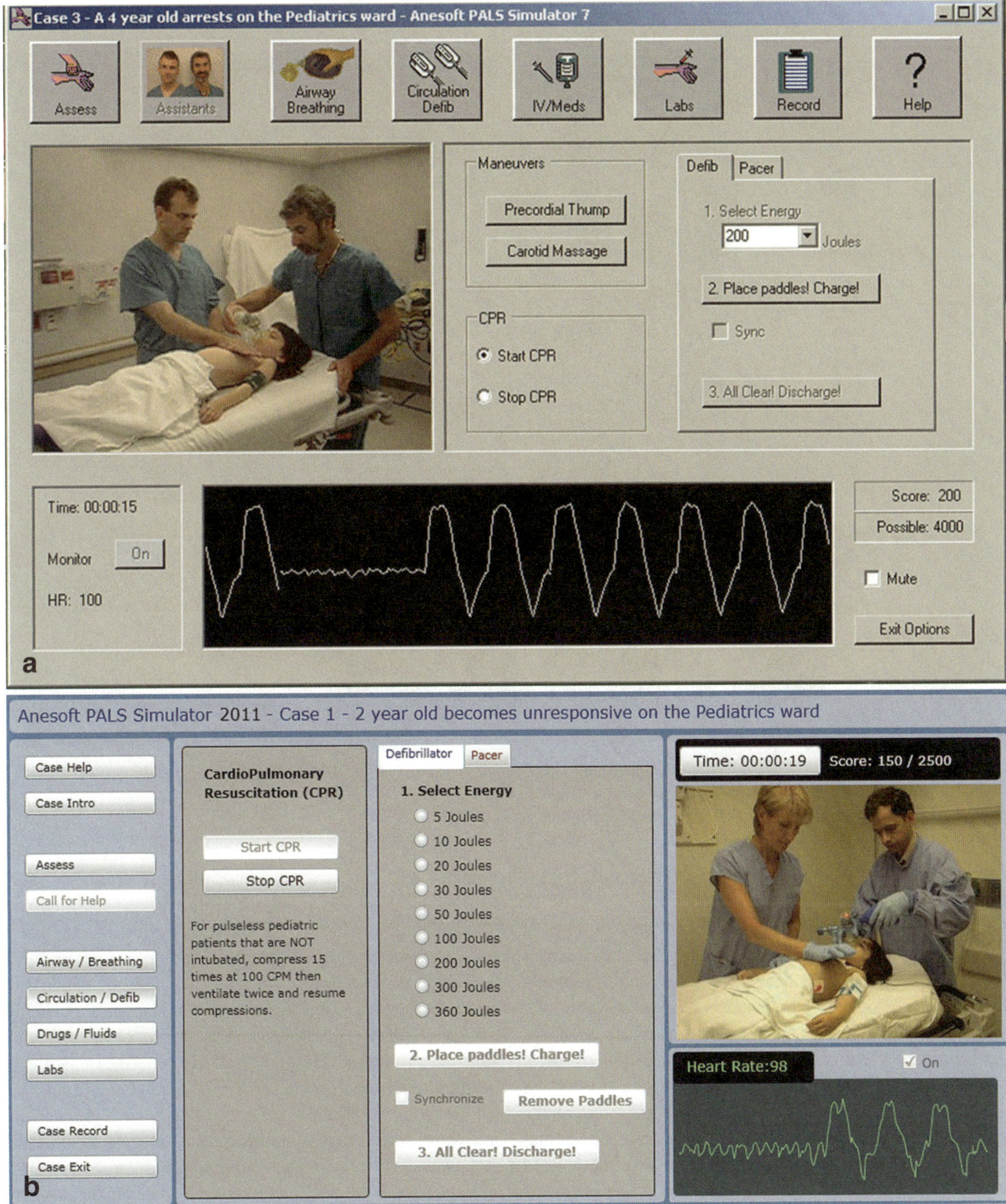

Fig. 14.4 (**a**) Graphical user interface for the Anesoft PALS Simulator 2006. Dynamic photographic images of the patient and 2 resuscitators are shown. The resuscitators execute tasks as commanded by the user using a mouse or touchpad to interact with the interface buttons. A dynamic cardiac rhythm waveform sweeps across the *bottom* of the screen as shown. (**b**) Anesoft PALS Simulator 2011 graphical user interface. Dynamic photographic images depict the patient, the resuscitators, and the actions the user commands the resuscitators to perform. A dynamic cardiac rhythm waveform sweeps across the "monitor screen" at *lower right*; artifact from chest compressions is superimposed over the underlying rhythm

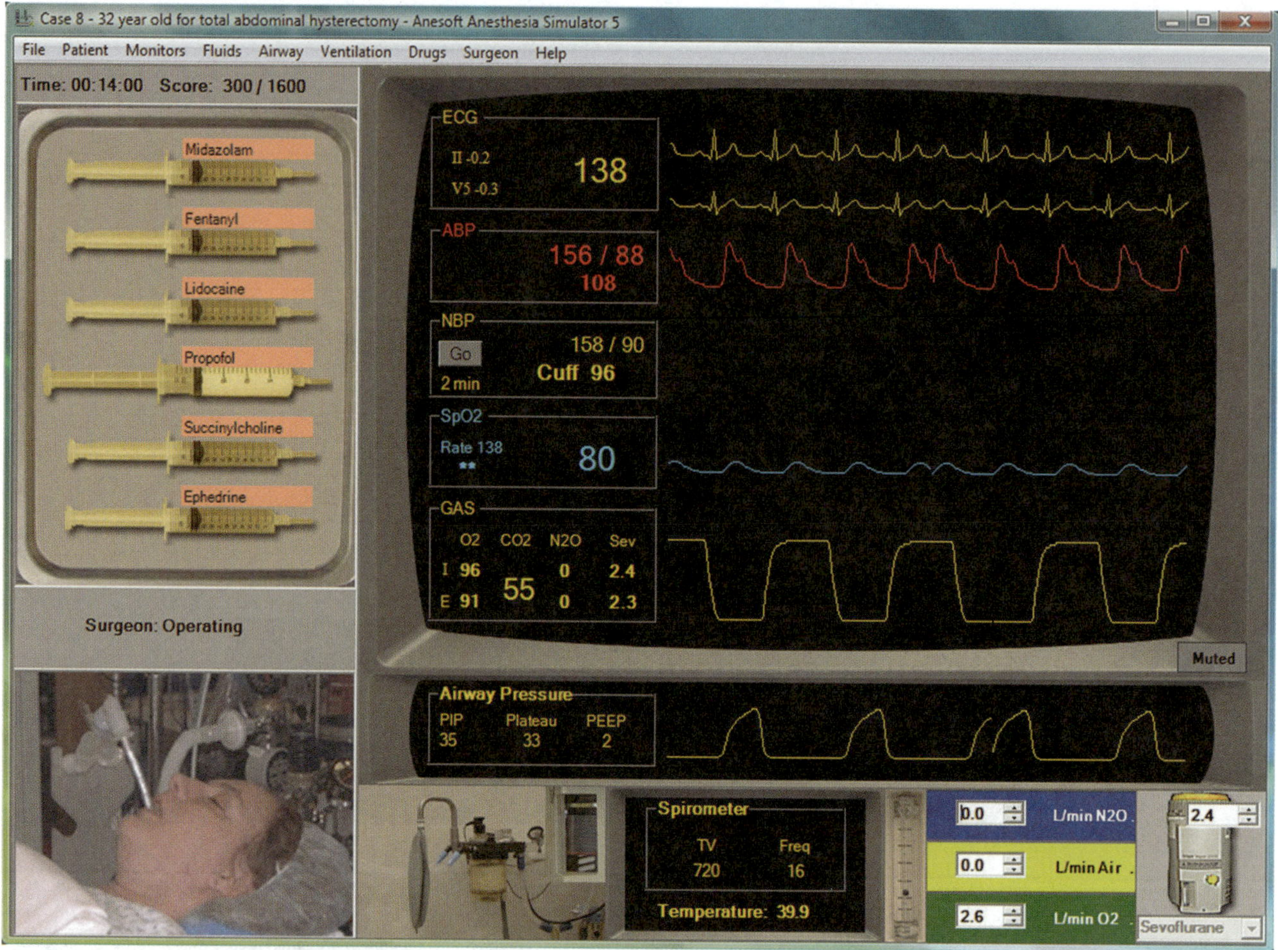

Fig. 14.5 User interface for the Anesoft Anesthesia Simulator. Dynamic cardiac rhythm, hemodynamic, and respiratory waveforms sweep across the monitor screen. An image of the patient is depicted at *lower left*. The surgeon's activities are represented as supplementary text above the patient image

Anesoft Anesthesia and Critical Care Simulators

The Anesoft Anesthesia Simulator has undergone a series of technical improvements and iterative upgrades since it was first introduced more than 20 years ago [13]. The current version is able to operate as an installed application on any Windows computer. The user interface displays an image of the patient, dynamic waveforms for monitored physiologic parameters, audible monitor tones, a representation of the anesthesia machine and spirometer, and a status report on the surgeon's activities during the case (Fig. 14.5). The simulator contains an on-demand help system, an automated debriefing system, and a drug library containing over 100 medications. Mathematical models of pharmacokinetic, pharmacodynamic, cardiovascular, and respiratory interactions predict the simulated patient's response to medications and are capable of representing both normal patients and patients with underlying acute or chronic illness. The simulator contains a library of 34 cases representing a range of anesthesia emergencies as well as scenarios spanning a clinical spectrum from regional anesthesia to specialty-specific domains such as cardiovascular, obstetric, pediatric, and neurosurgical anesthesia. The Anesoft Anesthesia Simulator is used in more than 50 countries worldwide and has been translated into Spanish and Portuguese [30].

The original version of Anesoft's Sedation Simulator was created more than a decade ago, as the product of a collaborative research project between the Department of Radiology at Cincinnati Children's Hospital Medical Center, the Department of Anesthesiology at the University of Washington, and Anesoft Corporation [31]. The project's objectives were to develop an interactive screen-based simulator that could train radiologists in the management of analgesia during painful procedures and in responding to critical incidents such as complications following contrast media administration. The Sedation Simulator has since undergone a series of upgrades and improvements, owing partly to additional contributions from content experts representing gastroenterology and dental surgery. The current version of the simulator operates as an installed application on any Windows computer and contains a library of 32 adult and pediatric case scenarios representing a range of circumstances such as anaphylaxis, agitation, aspiration, apnea, bradycardia,

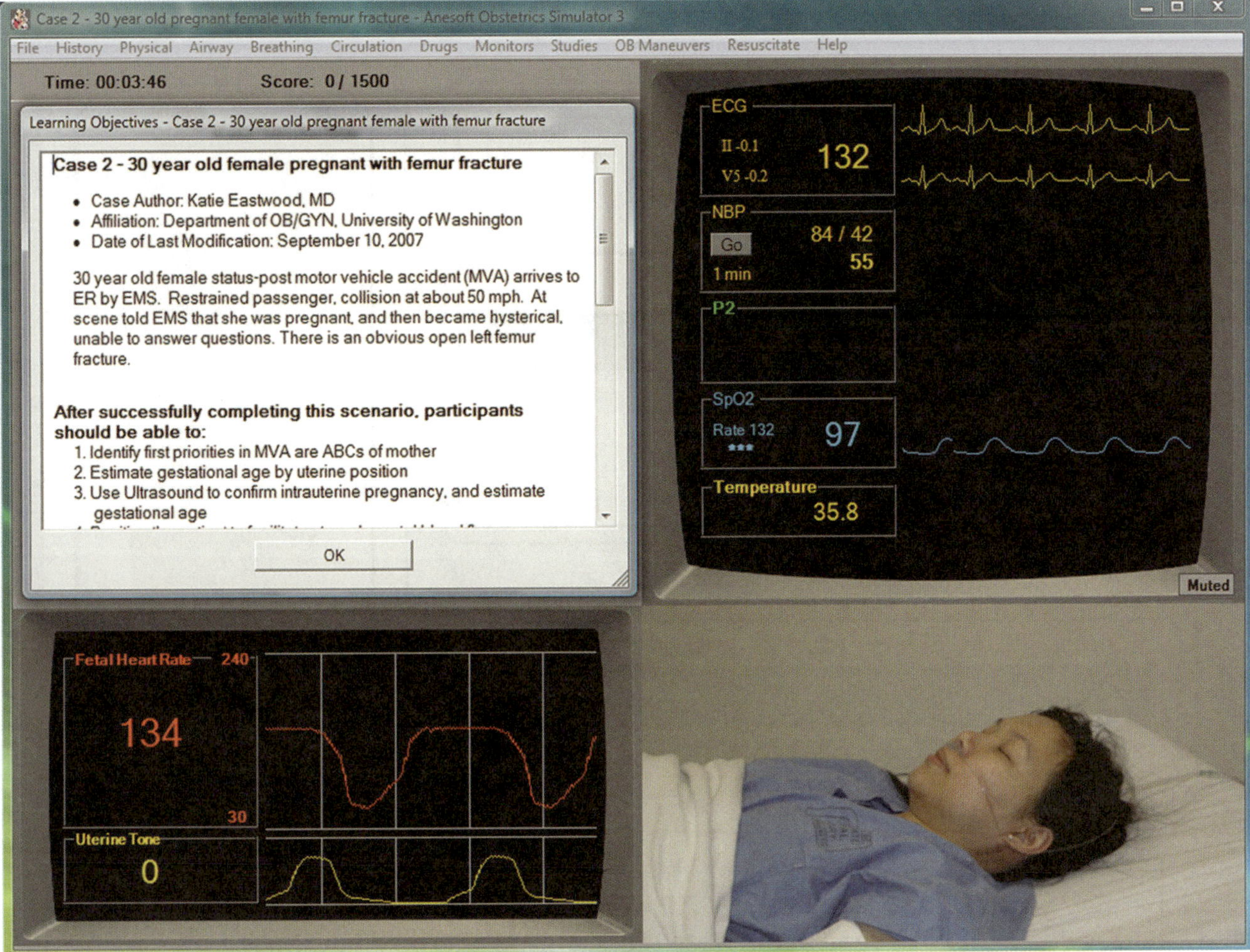

Fig. 14.6 User interface for the Anesoft Obstetrics Simulator. Dynamic cardiac rhythm and respiratory waveforms sweep across the monitor at *upper right*. Dynamic fetal heart and uterine tone tracings sweep across the monitor at *lower left*. An image of the patient is shown at *lower right*

hypotension, and myocardial ischemia. The user interface displays images of the patient as well as dynamic waveforms reflecting desired monitored parameters such as a cardiac rhythm tracing, peripheral oxygen saturation, and end-tidal capnography. Noninvasive blood pressure readings are also displayed. Comments and questions from the "proceduralist" are provided for the sedation provider (i.e., the simulator user) in the form of status updates that are displayed on the screen.

Anesoft's (adult) Critical Care Simulator possesses many of the attributes of the Anesthesia Simulator but is designed to portray clinical scenarios that take place in an emergency department or intensive care unit setting [32]. Accordingly, the user interface displays only those parameters that are routinely monitored in either of those environments. The Critical Care Simulator operates on Windows computers and contains a library of six case scenarios. Anesoft's Pediatrics Simulator is analogous to the Critical Care Simulator. Its user interface displays images of pediatric patients and its case library contains six scenarios representing complex acute and critical illness states [33].

The Anesoft Obstetrics Simulator was developed to train clinicians in the management of obstetric emergency scenarios [34]. The simulator operates on Windows computers, and its user interface displays images of the patient and all dynamic waveforms representing typical monitored parameters including an electrocardiogram tracing, blood pressure, peripheral oxygen saturation, and patient temperature. In addition, uterine tone and a fetal heart tracing are displayed (Fig. 14.6). The case library contains eight scenarios covering a range of obstetric emergencies such as placental abruption, postpartum hemorrhage, ectopic pregnancy, trauma, and cardiac arrest.

The Anesoft Neonatal Simulator also works on Windows computers and is designed to train clinicians in the management of important delivery room emergencies [35]. The user interface displays images of the neonate and any interventions the resuscitators are performing. Monitored physiologic parameters that are displayed on the interface include the infant's cardiac rhythm and peripheral oxygen saturation tracing. The case library contains 12 scenarios, including fetal heart rate decelerations, severe fetal bradycardia, meconium-stained amniotic fluid, and meconium aspiration.

The Bioterrorism Simulator is the final example in this summary of Anesoft's portfolio of interactive case-based

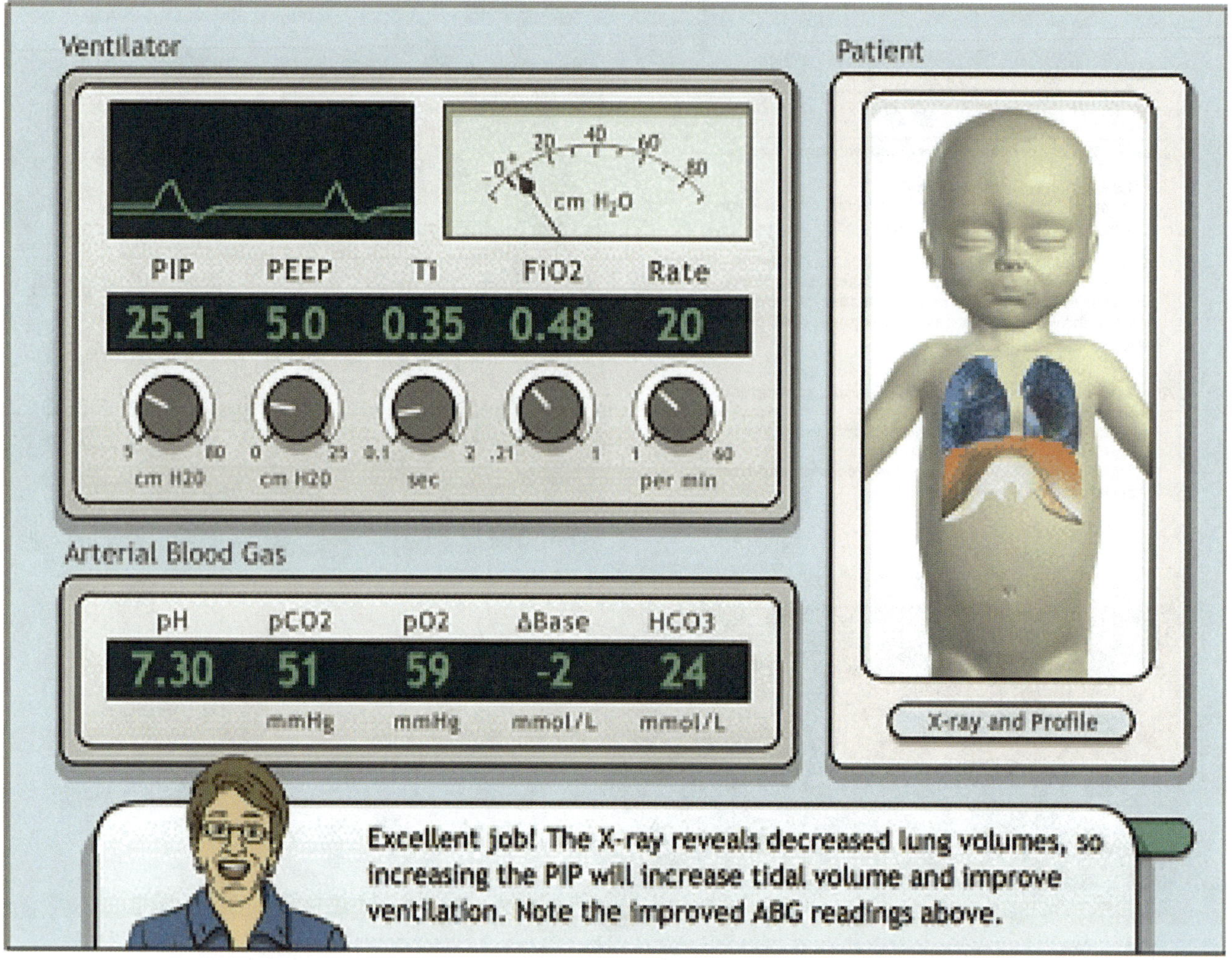

Fig. 14.7 User interface for the Interactive Virtual Ventilator. A representation of the infant is shown, along with the ventilator console and controls, and a blood gas display. A pop-up avatar (shown at the *bottom* of the image) provides feedback on interventions selected by the operator

simulators. The Bioterrorism Simulator was developed in 2002 as a multilateral collaboration involving the Anesoft Corporation, experts from the military, and content experts from the specialties of infectious diseases, public health, critical care, and toxicology [36]. It works in both Windows and Macintosh browsers, and its objective is to train first responders to recognize, diagnose, and treat patients who demonstrate signs and symptoms of possible exposure to biological or chemical agents, while avoiding personal contamination. The user interface displays an image of the patient and dynamic waveform displays of all monitored physiologic parameters. An on-demand help system provides real-time assistance with appropriate case management. The case library contains 24 scenarios reflecting a range of clinical presentations from what content experts believe to be the most likely terrorist threats: anthrax, botulism, ebola virus, plague, tularemia, smallpox, and nerve agent or vesicant exposures. At the conclusion of each scenario, the automated debriefing system produces a detailed record of correct and incorrect decisions made during the case.

New Horizons: The "Virtual NICU," Transparent Reality, and Multiuser Simulation

The unique throughput advantages of screen-based simulation have been incorporated into a national strategy to reengineer neonatal nurse practitioner (NNP) training, in order to better meet the growing demand for a skilled NNP workforce [37]. The "Neonatal Curriculum Consortium" is a group of experienced NNPs whose overall vision is to develop robust, standardized, interactive training modules and host them on an Internet site that is scheduled to be completed in 2012. Interactive training incorporating regular use of these modules would then be integrated into existing NNP training curricula across the United States. In collaboration with the Institute for Interactive Arts and Engineering at the University of Texas at Dallas, the Neonatal Curriculum Consortium has developed an innovative, case-based, web-enabled simulator called the "Interactive Virtual Ventilator" (Fig. 14.7). The user interface displays a representation of a patient, a chest x-ray, blood gas data, and a representation of a ventilator, an airway pressure gauge, and a ventilator waveform. The ventilator console contains inspiratory and expiratory pressure controls, as well as inspiratory time, FiO_2, and ventilator rate controls that the learner can manipulate in order to produce changes in blood gas values. There is a built-in help system in the form of a pop-up avatar of a "coach" who provides feedback on whether the trainee made appropriate or inappropriate ventilator adjustments and offers a brief commentary explaining the rationale for the correct answer. Graduate NNP students at the University of Texas at Arlington pilot tested the Interactive Virtual Ventilator in 2010, and their feedback will be incorporated into future simulator modifications and improvements [38].

Virtual Anesthesia Machine

Well-designed screen-based simulators do not seek to faithfully recreate all aspects of the physical environment, but rather seek only to achieve a level of fidelity that is sufficient to develop a cognitive structure that will foster reliable approaches to patient management. Embedded within these interactive screen-based simulations are sophisticated mathematical models that are predicting the clinical response to the trainee's management decisions and governing the functions of life support equipment such as the anesthesia machine. Importantly, the trainee is guided by the output of these models as reflected in abrupt changes in the patient's condition, but both the physiologic mechanisms determining the patient's clinical changes and the internal workings of key pieces of equipment are completely inaccessible to learners. Thus, the reductive output displays on these simulations may be enough to impart procedural knowledge but are limited in their ability to foster a deeper understanding of human physiology or about how life support equipment actually works. Investigators at the University of Florida developed the "Virtual Anesthesia Machine" (VAM) simulator in 1999 to facilitate construction of a mental model for how an anesthesia machine works [39] because problems with the anesthesia machine have been shown to cause negative outcomes in patients [40]. The VAM uses Adobe Shockwave and Flash Player technology (Adobe Systems Inc., San Jose CA) to allow interactive visualization of all of the machine's internal connections and the effects of manipulating its external controls. In addition, gas flows, gas concentrations, and gas volumes are color coded to make them easier for a student to dynamically track. In 2008, Fischler and colleagues designed a study to determine whether individuals who were trained using this transparent VAM would learn more effectively than those who were trained using a version of the VAM that visually represented an anesthesia machine as a photographic image and showed only bellows movement and standard, externally mounted pressure gauge needles but represented none of the machine's internal mechanisms [41]. The investigators alternately assigned 39 undergraduate students and 35 medical students with no prior knowledge of the anesthesia machine to train using either the transparent or the "opaque" VAM. Detailed manuals were provided to each student in order to help structure the learning experience. Although separate versions of the manual were created to coordinate with each assigned simulator type, both versions provided a thorough orientation to how the anesthesia machine operates. Learning assessments were conducted 1 day after training and consisted of identifying anesthesia machine components, short-answer questions about the machine's internal dynamics, and multiple-choice questions on how to operate the anesthesia machine safely. Subjects assigned to the transparent VAM scored significantly higher on the multiple-choice questions ($P=0.009$) as well as the short-answer questions requiring a functional knowledge of machine functions and internal dynamics ($P=0.003$). These findings have important implications for training anesthesiologists. To the extent that human error during anesthesia machine operation can be averted through training methods that are better able to develop a sound, functioning mental map of the device, a favorable impact on patient outcomes may be achievable through regular use of media such as the transparent VAM (Fig. 14.8). The concept of "transparent reality" simulation may also find future application in teaching health-care professionals to understand the intricate circulatory physiology of patients with complex congenital heart disease. Transparent reality modeling holds enormous promise for making screen-based simulators more robust training devices capable of imparting a deeper understanding of complex biological and mechanical systems.

Up to this point, all the simulators presented have been designed for a single learner at a time. In the current era of multiplayer on-line gaming, there is no reason that screen-based medical simulators should not be developed to support multiple concurrent users. Several efforts are underway to introduce screen-based simulation programs involving multiple health-care professionals that have been designed to improve teamwork and interpersonal communication. The MedBiquitous virtual patient system has been used to enable paramedic students to work together on five different scenarios [42]. Duke University's Human Simulation and Patient Safety Center developed 3DiTeams [43], a three-dimensional simulation environment to practice team coordination skills (Fig. 14.9). While these efforts are still in the early stages of evaluation, the promise for future training of health-care professionals is clear.

Applications I: Training Impact of Screen-Based Simulators

Evidence supporting an important role for screen-based simulation in the training of health-care professionals is weighted toward assessments of learner perceptions about the technology, as well as post-training assessments of clinical skills, which are typically carried out in a mannequin laboratory setting. Learners' reactions to this technology are usually

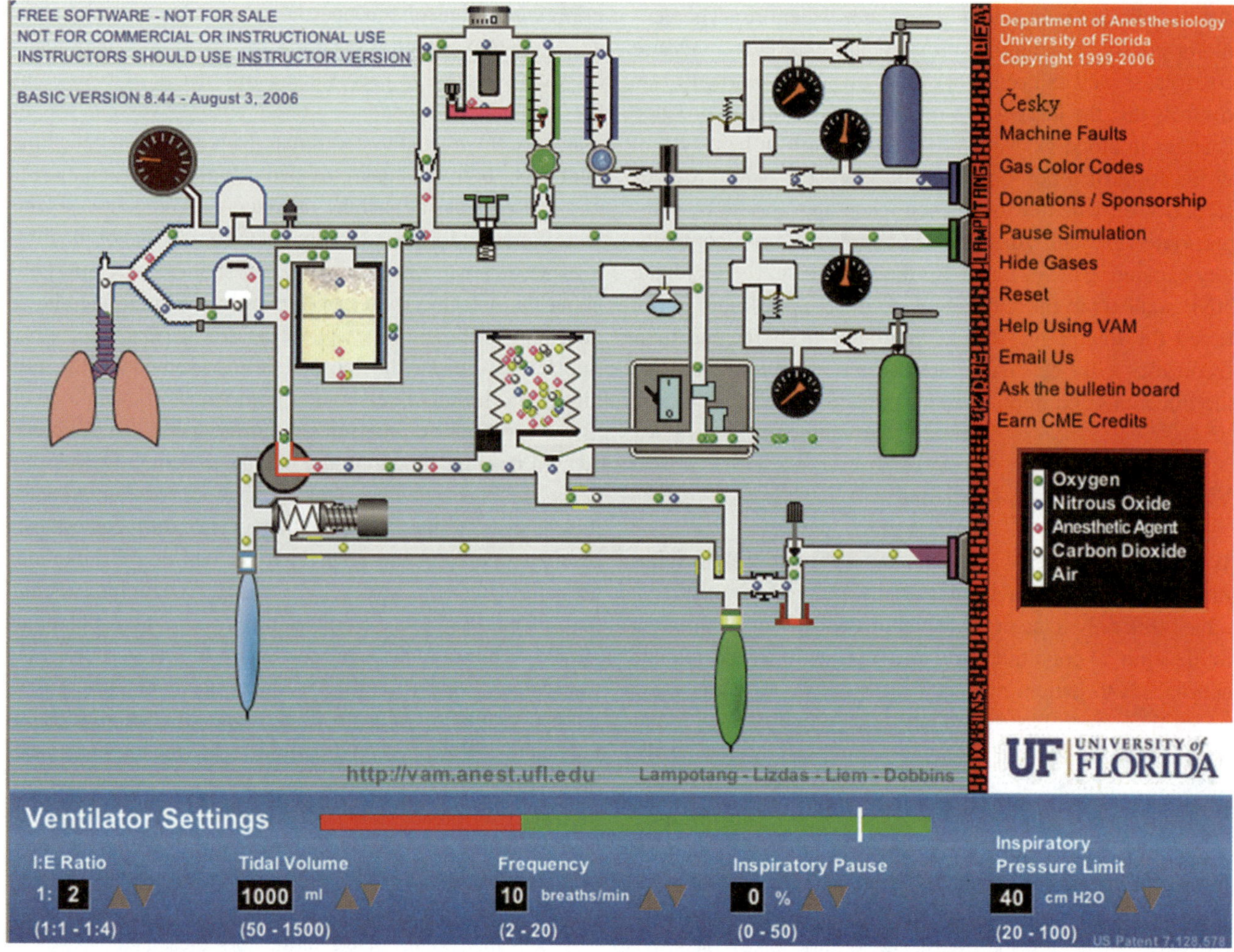

Fig. 14.8 The "Virtual Anesthesia Machine." Color coding is enabled in the exercise depicted here, in order to represent gas flows, gas concentrations, and gas volumes. The color legend is shown at *right*. Ventilator parameters are adjustable and are shown at the *bottom* of the image

highly favorable, regardless of whether they are asked to consider the merits of a particular screen-based simulator in general [13, 28, 44, 45] or in comparison to a lecture presenting the same material [46]. The largest available study on user perceptions collected feedback from 798 multidisciplinary pediatric providers in a university-affiliated children's hospital who had used a newly developed, screen-based Pediatric Advanced Life Support Simulator [28]. Simulator users were asked to indicate their level of agreement that the simulator was an effective training tool or that the simulator filled a gap in their current training regimen, using a 5-point Likert-style scale ranging from "strongly disagree" to "strongly agree." Ninety-five percent of respondents indicated they agreed or strongly agreed that the PALS Simulator is an effective training tool. The strength of the respondents' agreement with this statement was not related to their professional discipline. Eighty-nine percent agreed or strongly agreed that the simulator filled a gap in their training; physicians agreed with this statement more strongly than nurses ($P=0.001$). Respondents cited the simulator's realism, its capacity to facilitate regular practice, and its on-demand help feature as the three attributes they valued most.

There are several published investigations designed as comparative efficacy studies of case-based screen simulators in relation to either "traditional" classroom or paper-based training methods [46–49] or mannequin simulators [50, 51]. Two of these studies evaluated the Laerdal MicroSim case-based cardiac arrest simulator [49, 51] (Laerdal Medical, Stavanger Norway), and four evaluated Anesoft screen-based simulators [46–48, 50]. The evidence can be summarized as indicating that screen-based simulation imparts procedural knowledge better than classroom (lecture) training [46, 49], is *more* efficacious than independent study of standardized preprinted materials, and is as efficacious as mannequin simulation [50, 51] in preparing health-care professionals to manage clinical emergency scenarios on a mannequin simulator [47, 48]. There are three screen-based simulation studies which are notable for having particularly well-controlled

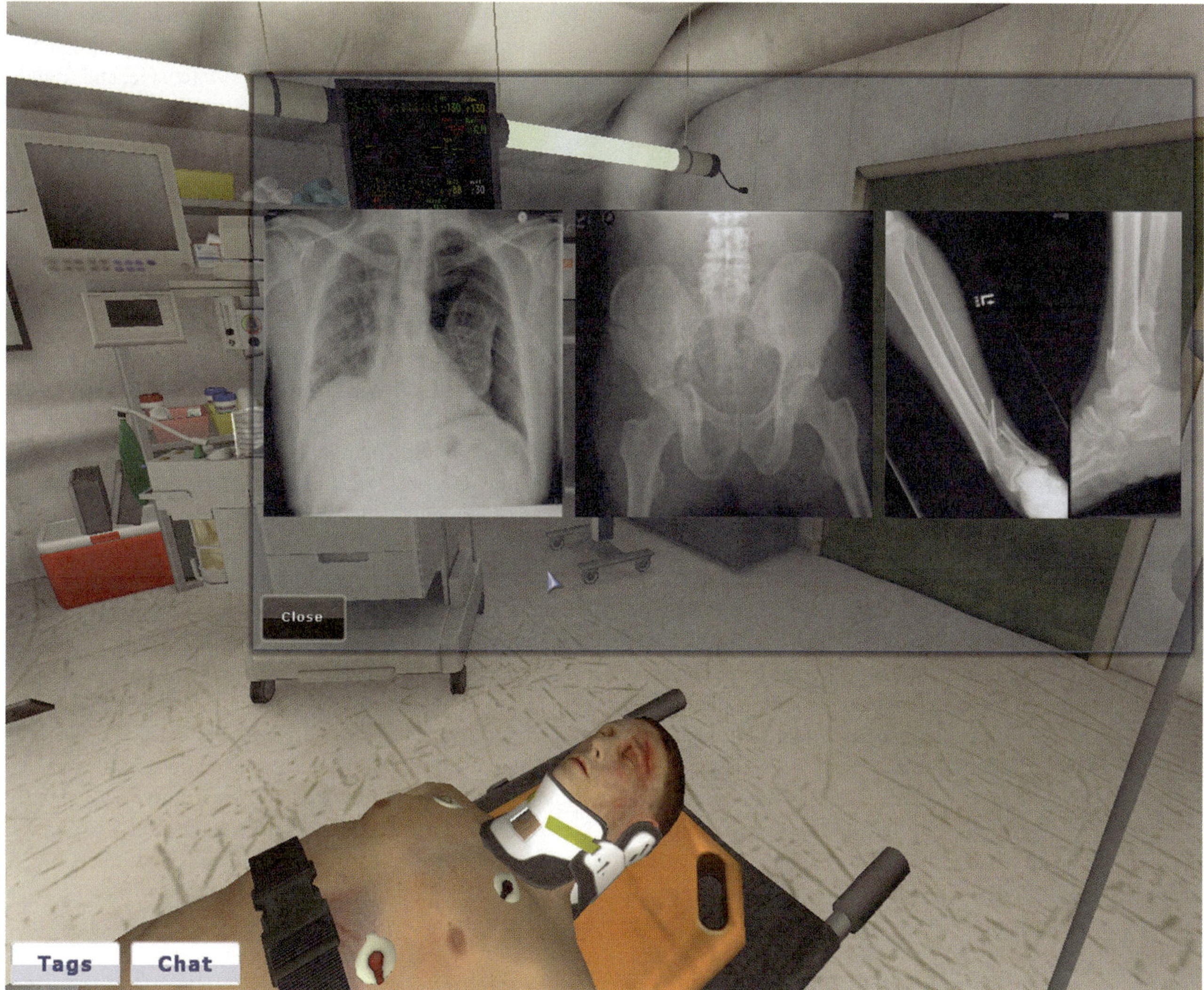

Fig. 14.9 Screen image from the "3DiTeams" Simulator. A representation of the patient and a series of radiographic images are shown in an emergency department setting

protocols [47, 48, 50]; each was conducted in a single center. The first is a prospective trial to determine whether the Anesoft ACLS Simulator imparted knowledge of American Heart Association ACLS guidelines better than a standard textbook review [47]. The investigators randomized 45 ACLS-certified anesthesiology residents, fellows, and faculty to review ALCS guidelines using either printed American Heart Association materials or using the ACLS screen-based simulator, 1–2 months prior to managing a standardized mock resuscitation on a full-scale mannequin simulator. Individual performance during the resuscitation was videotaped and later scored by two blinded observers using a structured checklist. The investigators found that study participants who prepared using the ACLS Simulator performed significantly better during the mock resuscitation than those who prepared using printed materials (mean checklist score 34.9 of 47 possible points [SD 5.0] vs 29.2 points [SD 4.9]; $P<0.001$). Covariate analysis revealed that the performance differences were not related to the time each participant spent studying. The second well-controlled screen-based simulation study is a prospective study to evaluate whether exposure to a screen-based anesthesia simulator with written debriefing prepared anesthesia trainees to manage anesthesia emergencies better than a paper handout [48]. The investigators randomized 31 first-year anesthesiology residents to prepare for a clinical assessment on a mannequin simulator by either managing 10 anesthesia emergencies on an interactive, case-based anesthesia simulator (Anesoft Corporation, Issaquah WA) or by studying a handout that discussed how to manage the same ten emergency scenarios. Handout content was reproduced directly from content stored within the simulator's built-in help function for each case. All participants prepared independently, except those assigned to the simulator group received written feedback from faculty who reviewed the case records that the simulator generated upon completion of each scenario. The clinical assessment that took place on the mannequin simulator consisted of four standardized emergency scenarios that were chosen from the ten scenarios the participants had prepared to manage. Performance during the mannequin scenarios was videotaped and scored by two blinded observers who used a consensus process to rate each participant using a structured checklist. This study found that participants who prepared using the simulator scored significantly better during the mannequin simulation exercise than those who prepared using printed materials (mean score 52.6 ± 9.9 out of 95 possible points vs 43.4 ± 5.9 points; $P = 0.004$). The third reasonably well-controlled study was a prospective study that compared the training efficacy of a screen-based anesthesia simulator (Anesoft Corporation, Issaquah WA) and a mannequin simulator (Eagle Simulation Inc, Binghamton NY) [50]. These investigators divided 40 anesthesia trainees into two groups of roughly equal clinical experience. One group trained using the screen-based simulator, and the other trained using the mannequin simulator. During the training, participants in each group were randomly exposed to either an anaphylaxis scenario or a malignant hyperthermia scenario and were debriefed in a structured fashion following the conclusion of the training exercises. One month after training, participants were tested on anaphylaxis management using the assigned simulator. Performance during both training and testing was evaluated by two blinded observers who marked the time at which each participant announced the correct diagnosis and also completed a structured assessment tool. Regardless of the assigned simulator, participants in either group who saw the same scenario in testing as they saw during training scored better on the test. However, there was no association between the assigned simulator and either the time elapsed before announcing the correct diagnosis during the test or the overall performance score. This observation provides support for the training efficacy of screen-based simulation, despite clear limitations in physical fidelity.

Although varied in their design and in the level of evidence they provide, published studies appear to confirm the training efficacy of screen-based simulators that meet contemporary technical standards with regard to the user interface, simulation engine, and automated systems for providing feedback on case management. What is missing from the available studies is a determination of whether the knowledge gained from screen-based simulators transfers to the actual clinical environment. This follows from the fact that the simulations evaluated in the studies are designed to prepare health-care workers to manage critical (yet treatable) events that occur too rarely for them to master during the course of actual patient-care activities. Thus, the training outcomes must be assessed in a structured laboratory environment, where virtually all aspects of the case presentation can be controlled and the scenario can be restaged as often as necessary to complete the study within a reasonable timeframe. Of course, assessing training outcomes using mannequin simulation is expensive, resource-intensive, and fraught with challenges, including the scarcity of valid and reliable assessment tools and the difficulty of capturing key clinician behaviors in the context of a dynamic and often emotionally charged scenario. These are major barriers to scaling simulation research on a level that would make conducting well-controlled, appropriately powered multicenter trials more practicable.

Applications II: Assessment of Clinical Knowledge

Using screen-based simulation for assessment purposes can potentially overcome many of the challenges associated with evaluating clinician behaviors in either the mannequin laboratory or the actual clinical setting. Although clearly limited in its capacity to evaluate psychomotor skills or whether a clinician knows how to manipulate specific types of medical equipment, screen-based simulation offers an unequalled capacity to record and analyze clinicians' cognitive error patterns in a highly efficient fashion. A couple of studies have described the use of screen-based simulation to prospectively evaluate clinicians' management strategies for critical events. In the first study, investigators used an early version of the Anesoft Anesthesia Simulator (the "Anesthesia Simulator Consultant") to assess how 10 anesthesia residents, 10 anesthesiology faculty, and 10 private practice anesthesiologists managed a variety of critical event scenarios which they encountered on the simulator [52]. The cases were presented to each participant in random fashion, so that no participant was aware of which scenarios he or she would confront. Each participant had to manage at least one cardiac arrest scenario. The investigators encouraged participants to vocalize their thinking process as they managed the cases. Participant vocalizations were recorded manually, and management decisions executed through the user interface were recorded by the simulator software. The investigators identified numerous errors and outright management failures that were committed by members of each participant category. The observed error patterns included *incorrect diagnosis* (e.g., interpreting loss of the end-tidal carbon dioxide trace as bronchospasm), *fixation errors* (e.g., asking for a new monitor but not seeking additional diagnostic information when confronted with loss of the end-tidal carbon dioxide trace), *emergency medication dosing errors*, and *deviation from ACLS management protocols*. In fact, only 30% of participants managed the simulated cardiac arrest according to published ACLS guidelines. The elapsed time since each participant's last formal ACLS training predicted whether the arrest was managed successfully. Seventy-one percent of participants who had ACLS training within 6 months of the study managed the arrest successfully, while only 30% of those who had ACLS training between 6 months and 2 years prior to the study managed it successfully. Of those who last had ACLS training 2 or more years before the study, none managed the arrest successfully. Interestingly, the types of errors observed in this study were similar to those that other investigators had described while studying anesthesiologists' responses to critical incidents that were staged on a full-scale mannequin simulator [53, 54].

In a more recent prospective study, Ventre and colleagues used a modified version of the Anesoft PALS Simulator to evaluate the performance of pediatric health-care providers on four PALS scenarios [55]. This study advanced the case for using screen-based simulation for assessment purposes by involving a diverse group of nationally recognized American Heart Association content experts to develop a valid scoring system for the simulator. With input from this expert panel of three pediatric emergency medicine physicians and three pediatric intensivists, the investigators developed a consensus-based algorithm for scoring the management of four standardized PALS cases: supraventricular tachycardia (SVT), pulseless electrical activity (PEA), ventricular fibrillation (VF), and bradycardia (Brady). The consensus scoring system was then attached to the simulator software. All management decisions executed through the user interface were recorded by the simulator software, and the simulator's automated help system was disabled for the study. One hundred multidisciplinary PALS providers completed the PALS scenarios on the PALS screen-based simulator. Forty percent of participants were recruited immediately after completing a traditional PALS course. The remainder reported last having PALS training between 1 month and 2 years before enrolling in the study. Participants were proctored and were not permitted to use cognitive aids while managing the scenarios. The average time it took for each participant to complete all four scenarios on the simulator was 13.8 min. The investigators found that management of all four simulated scenarios frequently deviated from consensus guidelines. The highest scores were achieved on the SVT scenario, and the lowest scores were achieved on the PEA scenario. Physician status predicted a higher aggregate score as well as higher scores on the SVT, PEA, and Brady scenarios ($P<0.05$ for all comparisons). Participants who completed the scenarios on the same day as they completed PALS training scored higher only on the SVT scenario ($P=0.041$). As in the Anesthesia Simulator assessment study [52], the types and frequencies of errors recorded by the PALS Simulator in this study were similar to those that had been reported in prior studies that used a mannequin simulator to evaluate how pediatric provider teams manage SVT and arrest states [56, 57]. The unparalleled reliability of computerized scoring and the concordance of findings between computer-based assessment studies and mannequin-based assessment studies make a very strong case for using computer-based simulators to efficiently and rigorously evaluate health-care workers against explicit performance criteria.

Applications III: Evaluation of Treatment Guidelines and Novel Monitoring Displays

The experience from large-scale industrial accidents and attacks of bioterrorism offers important lessons for the international health-care community regarding how these incidents can be managed most effectively. For instance, retrospective reviews of the 1984 Union Carbide disaster in India and the 1995 sarin attack on Tokyo subway stations revealed that a lack of clear protocols for how to treat exposed individuals contributed to delays in diagnosis and treatment [58–61]. In both the Tokyo attack and the 1994 sarin attack in Matsumoto Japan, contamination of health-care workers was another major problem [61–63]. Within the USA and worldwide, increased emphasis has recently been placed on enhancing the health-care system's preparedness to respond to a biological or chemical agent of mass destruction. However, the rarity of these kinds of events makes it difficult to prospectively validate triage and treatment protocols in order to verify that they are easy to use, have the proper scope, and result in reliable recognition of likely exposures, contamination risks, completion of initial resuscitation priorities, and timely administration of definitive therapy. Evaluating the performance of triage and treatment guidelines in a real-world setting would require trained observers to determine whether every branch point in the algorithm resulted in a correct decision for any patient in a diverse group of exposed individuals. This would be an expensive and laborious process.

At least one group of investigators has used screen-based simulation to guide the development, pilot testing, and iterative refinement of a novel bioterrorism triage algorithm [63, 64]. Bond and colleagues recently described the development of an algorithm designed to assist health-care workers during their initial encounter with exposed adult or pediatric patients who may have been exposed to several agents and who are manifesting different levels of symptom severity and physiologic stability. The algorithm used the patient's primary symptom complex to guide health-care workers to promptly isolate appropriate patients and address initial resuscitation priorities *before* making a final diagnosis, while still assuring that patients who require a specific antidote receive it in a timely fashion. The investigators tested each draft of the treatment algorithm on the Anesoft Bioterrorism Simulator. The simulator's case library provided a validation cohort of simulated adult and pediatric patients who were exposed to a variety of agents conferring a range of infectious or contamination risks and who exhibited various states of physiologic derangement. The physiologic models in the simulator engine ensured that the simulated patients would respond in appropriate ways to the interventions the algorithm suggested at any point during the case. Through completing the case scenarios, the investigators determined that the scope of the algorithm must encompass situations in which there are potentially conflicting priorities, such as unstable patients with possible nerve agent exposure who require airway support and early antidote administration but who also present a concomitant risk of health-care worker contamination. Managing these types of scenarios led investigators to revise the algorithm to allow definitive treatment before decontamination, yet provided for health-care worker protection, in situations where this approach would offer the optimal chances for survival [64]. Thus, the simulated cases helped expose flaws in the algorithm, which the investigators addressed through iterative cycles of making adjustments to the working draft, then repeating each scenario until the algorithm was able to direct appropriate triage and treatment of all simulated patient scenarios.

Screen-based simulators have also been used to evaluate the impact of novel clinical monitoring displays on physician response times. A group of investigators in Salt Lake City developed an innovative graphic monitoring display that incorporates the many discrete physiologic variable displays that clinicians must factor into clinical decision making in intensive care environments. The new display serves as a visual "metaphor" for representing 30 physiologic parameters as colors and shapes, rather than traditional waveforms and numerals [65]. The investigators compared the new display with traditional monitor displays, using the "Body Simulation" (Advanced Simulation Corporation, San Clemente CA) screen-based anesthesia simulator as the reference display [66]. Ten anesthesiology faculty members were randomly assigned to manage a case scenario on the screen-based simulator using either the traditional monitor waveform displays (control condition) or the new, integrated monitor display (experimental condition). Both groups used observed images of the simulated patient, the anesthesia record, the anesthesia machine, and other physiologic data on supplementary screens contained within the simulator's user interface. All audible alarms were silenced for the study period, so that interventions were made based on visual stimuli only. Four critical events were simulated, during which study participants were asked to vocalize when they perceived a change in the patient's condition, and then vocalize what caused the change. The investigators analyzed recordings of participants' vocalizations to determine the time it took for them to notice a perturbation in the patient's condition and the time it took for them to identify the cause of this change. The study demonstrated that in two of the four critical events those who used the new, integrated display noticed a physiologic change in the simulated patient faster than those who observed the traditional display. The "integrated display" group also correctly identified the critical events significantly faster than the traditional group. In three out of four of the critical events, this difference achieved statistical significance.

Conclusion

There has been tremendous growth in the field of screen-based simulation over the past 20 years, corresponding with advances in computer technology and a need for fresh approaches to the growing problem of how to best develop and maintain a skilled health-care workforce amid concurrent budgetary constraints, duty-hour restrictions, and ongoing scrutiny of the safety and reliability of patient-care practices. While screen-based simulators are designed to recreate only limited aspects of the physical environment, those meeting contemporary technical standards achieve a level of fidelity sufficient to impart procedural knowledge better than traditional textbook or paper-based methods, and possibly as well as mannequin simulation. Moreover, their unparalleled reliability and throughput capacity make them highly promising tools for assessing and tracking cognitive performance for research or administrative purposes. The recent emergence of web-enabled simulators will make screen-based simulations easier for learners to access, easier for institutions to install, and easier to revise through downloadable updates. The Internet also opens up a host of potential new directions for screen-based simulation, including a capacity to support multiple participants who manage a simulated scenario as a team, in a real-time, networked environment. Thus, future generations of screen-based simulators are likely to be able to represent more of the interpersonal and team coordination aspects of professional practice. Going forward, screen-based simulation stands to play a major role in research designed to identify performance deficiencies that can be translated into opportunities for targeted curricular and care process improvement.

References

1. Historical facts, dates, places, numbers. Society for Simulation in Healthcare. 2008. http://www.ssih.org/public/ssh_content. Accessed 30 Apr 2008.
2. Weinstock PH, Kappus LJ, Kleinman ME, Grenier B, Hickey P, Burns JP. Toward a new paradigm in hospital-based pediatric education: the development of an onsite simulator program. Pediatr Crit Care Med. 2005;6:635–41.
3. Nishisaki A, Hales R, Biagas K, et al. A multi-institutional high-fidelity simulation "boot camp" orientation and training program for first year pediatric critical care fellows. Pediatr Crit Care Med. 2009;10:157–62.
4. Weinstock PH, Kappus LJ, Garden A, Burns JP. Simulation at the point of care: reduced-cost, in situ training via a mobile cart. Pediatr Crit Care Med. 2009;10:176–81.

5. Calhoun AW, Boone MC, Peterson EB, Boland KA, Montgomery VL. Integrated in-situ simulation using redirected faculty educational time to minimize costs: a feasibility study. Simul Healthc. 2011;6(6):337–44.
6. Entwisle G, Entwisle DR. The use of a digital computer as a teaching machine. J Med Educ. 1963;38:803–12.
7. Schwid HA. A flight simulator for general anesthesia training. Comput Biomed Res. 1987;20:64–75.
8. Taekman JM, Shelley K. Virtual environments in healthcare: immersion, disruption, and flow. Int Anesthesiol Clin. 2010;48:101–21.
9. Schwid HA, Souter K. Cost-effectiveness of screen-based simulation for anesthesiology residents: 18 year experience. In: American Society of Anesthesiologists annual meeting, New Orleans, 2009.
10. Schwid HA, O'Donnell D. Educational malignant hyperthermia simulator. J Clin Monit. 1992;8:201–8.
11. Schwid HA, O'Donnell D. The anesthesia simulator consultant: simulation plus expert system. Anesthesiol Rev. 1993;20:185–9.
12. Schwid HA. Components of a successful medical simulation program. Simulation Gaming. 2001;32:240–9.
13. Schwid HA, O'Donnell D. The anesthesia simulator-recorder: a device to train and evaluate anesthesiologists' responses to critical incidents. Anesthesiology. 1990;72:191–7.
14. Smothers V, Greene P, Ellaway R, Detmer DE. Sharing innovation: the case for technology standards in health professions education. Med Teach. 2008;30:150–4.
15. Posel N, Fleiszer D, Shore BM. 12 tips: guidelines for authoring virtual patient cases. Med Teach. 2009;31:701–8.
16. Triola MM, Campion N, McGee JB, Albright S, Greene P, Smothers V, Ellaway R. An XML standard for virtual patients: exchanging case-based simulations in medical education. AMIA Annu Symp Proc. 2007:741–5.
17. Schwid HA. Open-source shared case library. Stud Health Technol Inform. 2008;132:442–45.
18. Schwid HA. Anesthesia Simulator-Case 5-Anaphylactic reaction. MedEdPORTAL 2009. Available from www.aamc.org/mededportal. (ID=1711). Accessed on 2 Nov 2011.
19. Stross JK. Maintaining competency in advanced cardiac life support skills. JAMA. 1983;249:3339–41.
20. Curry L, Gass D. Effects of training in cardiopulmonary resuscitation on competence and patient outcome. Can Med Assoc J. 1987; 137:491–6.
21. Gass DA, Curry L. Physicians' and nurses' retention of knowledge and skill after training in cardiopulmonary resuscitation. Can Med Assoc J. 1983;128:550–1.
22. Lowenstein SR, Hansbrough JF, Libby LS, Hill DM, Mountain RD, Scoggin CH. Cardiopulmonary resuscitation by medical and surgical house-officers. Lancet. 1981;2:679–81.
23. Schwid HA, Rooke GA. ACLS Simulator. Issaquah: Copyright Anesoft Corporation; 1992.
24. Field JM, Hazinski MF, Sayre MR, et al. Part 1: executive summary: 2010 American Heart Association Guidelines for Cardiopulmonary Resuscitation and Emergency Cardiovascular Care. Circulation. 2010;122:S640–56.
25. HeartCode® ACLS. Copyright Laerdal Corporation, Stavanger Norway, 2010.
26. Schwid HA, Ventre KM. PALS Simulator. Copyright Anesoft Corporation, Issaquah, 2006, 2011.
27. Kleinman ME, Chameides L, Schexnayder SM, et al. Part 14: pediatric advanced life support: 2010 American Heart Association Guidelines for Cardiopulmonary Resuscitation and Emergency Cardiovascular Care. Circulation. 2010;122:S876–908.
28. Ventre KM, Collingridge DS, DeCarlo D. End-user evaluations of a personal computer-based pediatric advanced life support simulator. Simul Healthc. 2011;6:134–42.
29. Ralston ME, Zaritsky AL. New opportunity to improve pediatric emergency preparedness: pediatric emergency assessment, recognition, and stabilization course. Pediatrics. 2009;123:578–80.
30. Schwid HA. Anesthesia simulators – technology and applications. Isr Med Assoc J. 2000;2:949–53.
31. Medina LS, Racadio JM, Schwid HA. Computers in radiology. The sedation, analgesia, and contrast media computerized simulator: a new approach to train and evaluate radiologists' responses to critical incidents. Pediatr Radiol. 2000;30:299–305.
32. Schwid HA, Gustin A. Critical Care Simulator. Issaquah: Copyright Anesoft Corporation; 2008.
33. Schwid HA, Bennett T. Pediatrics Simulator. Issaquah: Copyright Anesoft Corporation; 2008.
34. Schwid HA, Eastwood K, Schreiber JR. Obstetrics Simulator. Issaquah: Copyright Anesoft Corporation; 2008.
35. Schwid HA, Jackson C, Strandjord TP. Neonatal Simulator. Issaquah: Copyright Anesoft Corporation; 2006.
36. Schwid HA, Duchin JS, Brennan JK, Taneda K, Boedeker BH, Ziv A, et al. Bioterrorism Simulator. Issaquah: Copyright Anesoft Corporation; 2002.
37. LeFlore J, Thomas PE, Zielke MA, Buus-Frank ME, McFadden BE, Sansoucie DA. Educating neonatal nurse practitioners in the 21st century. J Perinat Neonatal Nurs. 2011;25:200–5.
38. LeFlore J, Thomas P, McKenzie L, Zielke M. Can a complex interactive virtual ventilator help to save babies' lives: an educational innovation for neonatal nurse practitioner students [abstract]. Sim Healthc. 2010;5:A106.
39. Lampotang S. Virtual anesthesia machine. Copyright University of Florida. 2000. http://vam.anest.ufl.edu/simulations/configurablevam.php. Accessed on 3 Nov 2011.
40. Caplan RA, Vistica MF, Posner KL, Cheney FW. Adverse anesthetic outcomes arising from gas delivery equipment: a closed claims analysis. Anesthesiology. 1997;87:741–8.
41. Fischler IS, Kaschub CE, Lizdas DE, Lampotang S. Understanding of anesthesia machine function is enhanced with a transparent reality simulation. Simul Healthc. 2008;3:26–32.
42. Conradi E, Kavia S, Burden D, Rice A, Woodham L, Beaumont C, et al. Virtual patients in a virtual world: training paramedic students for practice. Med Teach. 2009;31:713–20.
43. Taekman JM, Segall N, Hobbs G, et al. 3Di Teams: healthcare team training in a virtual environment. Anesthesiology. 2007;107:A2145.
44. Cicarelli DD, Coelho RB, Bensenor FE, Vieira JE. Importance of critical events training for anesthesiology residents: experience with computer simulator. Rev Bras Anestesiol. 2005;55:151–7.
45. Biese KJ, Moro-Sutherland D, Furberg RD, et al. Using screen-based simulation to improve performance during pediatric resuscitation. Acad Emerg Med. 2009;16 Suppl 2:S71–5.
46. Tan GM, Ti LK, Tan K, Lee T. A comparison of screen-based simulation and conventional lectures for undergraduate teaching of crisis management. Anaesth Intensive Care. 2008;36:565–9.
47. Schwid HA, Rooke GA, Ross BK, Sivarajan M. Use of a computerized advanced cardiac life support simulator improves retention of advanced cardiac life support guidelines better than a textbook review. Crit Care Med. 1999;27:821–4.
48. Schwid HA, Rooke GA, Michalowski P, Ross BK. Screen-based anesthesia simulation with debriefing improves performance in a mannequin-based anesthesia simulator. Teach Learn Med. 2001;13:92–6.
49. Bonnetain E, Boucheix JM, Hamet M, Freysz M. Benefits of computer screen-based simulation in learning cardiac arrest procedures. Med Educ. 2010;44:716–22.
50. Nyssen AS, Larbuisson R, Janssens M, Pendeville P, Mayne A. A comparison of the training value of two types of anesthesia simulators: computer screen-based and mannequin-based simulators. Anesth Analg. 2002;94:1560–5.
51. Owen H, Mugford B, Follows V, Plummer JL. Comparison of three simulation-based training methods for management of medical emergencies. Resuscitation. 2006;71:204–11.
52. Schwid HA, O'Donnell D. Anesthesiologists' management of simulated critical incidents. Anesthesiology. 1992;76:495–501.

53. DeAnda A, Gaba DM. Role of experience in the response to simulated critical incidents. Anesth Analg. 1991;72:308–15.
54. Gaba DM, DeAnda A. The response of anesthesia trainees to simulated critical incidents. Anesth Analg. 1989;68:444–51.
55. Ventre KM, Collingridge DS, DeCarlo D, Schwid HA. Performance of a consensus scoring algorithm for assessing pediatric advanced life support competency using a computer screen-based simulator. Pediatr Crit Care Med. 2009;10:623–35.
56. Hunt EA, Walker AR, Shaffner DH, Miller MR, Pronovost PJ. Simulation of in-hospital pediatric medical emergencies and cardiopulmonary arrests: highlighting the importance of the first 5 minutes. Pediatrics. 2008;121:e34–43.
57. Shilkofski NA, Nelson KL, Hunt EA. Recognition and treatment of unstable supraventricular tachycardia by pediatric residents in a simulation scenario. Sim Healthc. 2008;3:4–9.
58. Dhara VR, Dhara R. The Union Carbide disaster in Bhopal: a review of health effects. Arch Environ Health. 2002;57:391–404.
59. Dhara VR, Gassert TH. The Bhopal syndrome: persistent questions about acute toxicity and management of gas victims. Int J Occup Environ Health. 2002;8:380–6.
60. Okumura T, Suzuki K, Fukuda A, et al. The Tokyo subway sarin attack: disaster management, part 1: community emergency response. Acad Emerg Med. 1998;5:613–7.
61. Morita H, Yanagisawa N, Nakajima T, et al. Sarin poisoning in Matsumoto, Japan. Lancet. 1995;346:290–3.
62. Nozaki H, Hori S, Shinozawa Y, et al. Secondary exposure of medical staff to sarin vapor in the emergency room. Intensive Care Med. 1995;21:1032–5.
63. Subbarao I, Johnson C, Bond WF, et al. Symptom-based, algorithmic approach for handling the initial encounter with victims of a potential terrorist attack. Prehosp Disaster Med. 2005;20:301–8.
64. Bond WF, Subbarao I, Schwid HA, Bair AE, Johnson C. Using screen-based computer simulation to develop and test a civilian, symptom-based terrorism triage algorithm. International Trauma Care (ITACCS). 2006;16:19–25.
65. Michels P, Gravenstein D, Westenskow DR. An integrated graphic data display improves detection and identification of critical events during anesthesia. J Clin Monit. 1997;13:249–59.
66. Smith NT, Davidson TM. BODY Simulation. San Clemente: Copyright Advanced Simulation Corporation; 1994.

15 Mannequin Based Simulators

Chad Epps, Marjorie Lee White, and Nancy Tofil

Introduction

The first computer-controlled full-scale mannequin simulator, Sim One®, developed in the 1960s, required a number of computers and operators to function. Today's control systems are much more compact and vary in their use of electronic, computer, pneumatic, and fluid controls. Due to the phenomenal growth of computer hardware and software technology, today's mannequins may be completely tetherless and controlled from a portable device that models highly sophisticated physiologic and pharmacologic principles. These mannequin-based simulators are commonly referred to as full-scale simulators, high-fidelity simulators, or realistic simulators.

Mannequin-based simulators are only one piece of a fully immersive environment (Fig. 15.1). To bring mannequins to life, there must be an operator, or a team of operators, to designate inputs to the mannequin. The mannequin's output such as physical findings, physiologic data, and other verbal cues can create a greater immersive environment that will have an effect on the learner. The learner, through their actions and interventions, also affects the immersive environment. The operator may adjust inputs to both the mannequin and the immersive environment to vary and optimize the experience for the learner.

Mannequin-based simulators should be viewed as part of the spectrum of simulation. For clarity, mannequin-based simulators will be assumed to include simulators that have the ability to display a range of physical attributes and physiologic parameters, are life-sized, and have the ability to have controllable inputs that result in outputs. The mannequin-based simulators in this chapter are controlled by a computer platform (Figs. 15.2 and 15.3) which allows for programmability as well as "on the fly" changes and come in four general sizes: adult, child (5–12 years old), infant (2–18 months old), and neonate (0–2 months old). Mannequin-based part-task trainers will also be considered in this chapter.

Control and Modeling

Broadly speaking, mannequin simulators are either operator-driven or autonomous. Operator-driven mannequins rely on the instructor, rather than modeling, to drive the simulator. Responses to interventions are controlled by the operator since there is typically limited ability of the mannequin to provide intervention feedback. Autonomous simulators utilize mathematical modeling algorithms to prompt changes in status or physiology based on intervention. For example, giving intravenous fluids to an autonomous simulator will correct signs of hypovolemia automatically (i.e., increased blood pressure with a reduction of heart rate), while the same intervention in an operator-driven mannequin requires changing of the appropriate vital signs by the operator. A learner's perspective of the simulated scenario is the same regardless of type, but the operator's ability to control the scenario varies. Operator-driven mannequins are typically less complicated and easy to control but are dependent on the operator to ensure that the physiologic data (e.g., vital signs) are realistic. Realism is less of an issue with autonomous simulators, but the plethora of physiologic parameters that can be manipulated can be overwhelming and generally requires at least a modest understanding of the physiologic mechanisms.

C. Epps, MD (✉)
Departments of Clinical and Diagnostic Services and Anesthesiology, University of Alabama at Birmingham, 1705 University Blvd., SHPB 451, Birmingham, AL 35294-1212, USA
e-mail: cepps@uab.edu

M.L. White, MD, MPPM, MEd
Departments of Pediatrics and Emergency Medicine, Pediatric Simulation Center, University of Alabama at Birmingham, Birmingham, AL, USA
e-mail: mlwhite@peds.uab.edu

N. Tofil, MD, MEd
Department of Pediatrics, Division of Critical Care, Pediatric Simulation Center, University of Alabama at Birmingham, Birmingham, AL, USA
e-mail: ntofil@peds.uab.edu

A.I. Levine et al. (eds.), *The Comprehensive Textbook of Healthcare Simulation*,
DOI 10.1007/978-1-4614-5993-4_15, © Springer Science+Business Media New York 2013

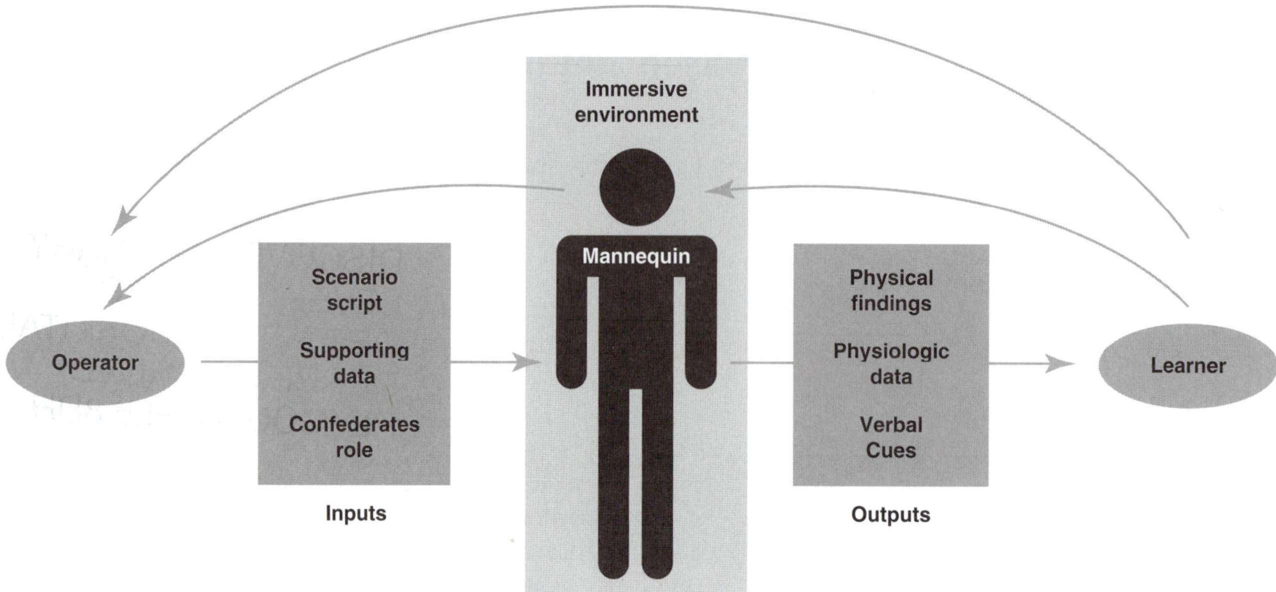

Fig. 15.1 Mannequin-based simulators placed in the larger simulation context which includes an immersive environment, inputs and outputs, and an operator learner pairing

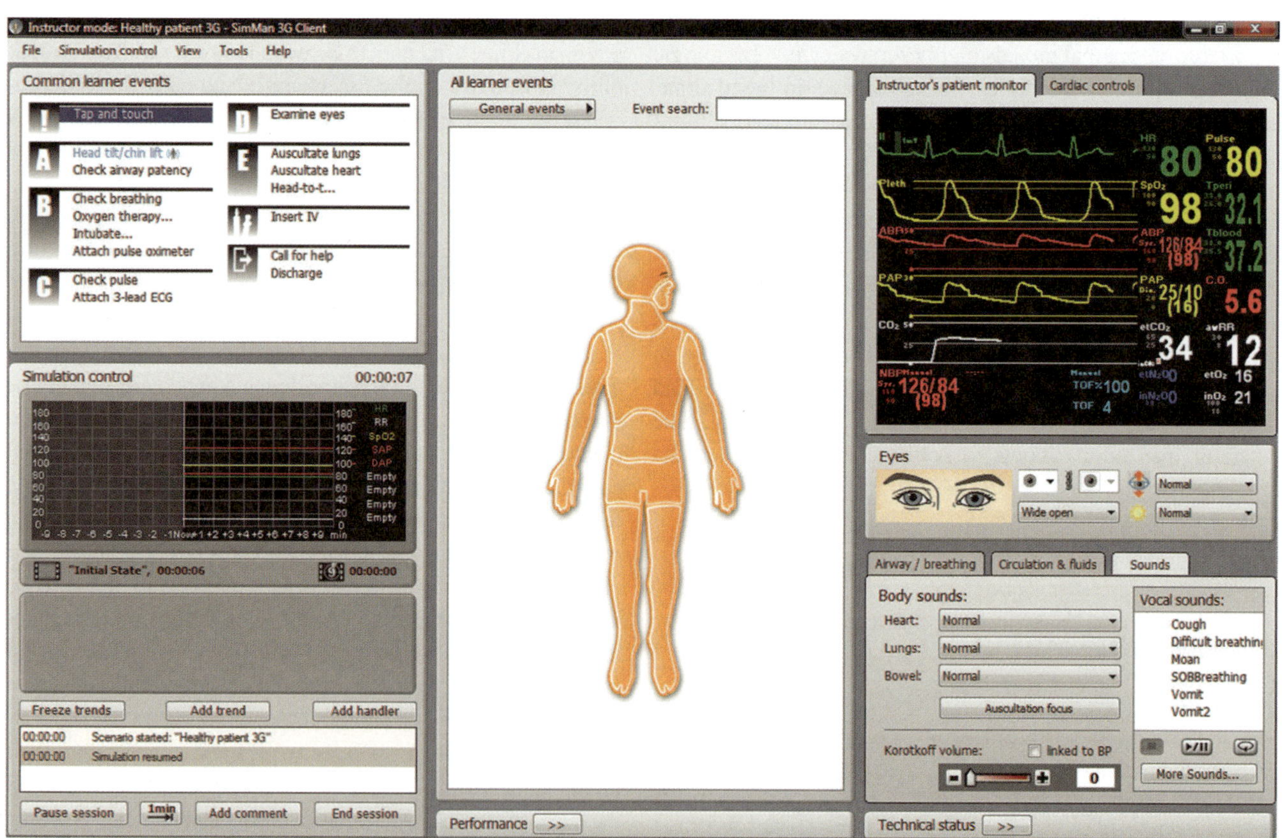

Fig. 15.2 SimMan® 3G user interface (Photo courtesy of Laerdal Medical. All rights reserved)

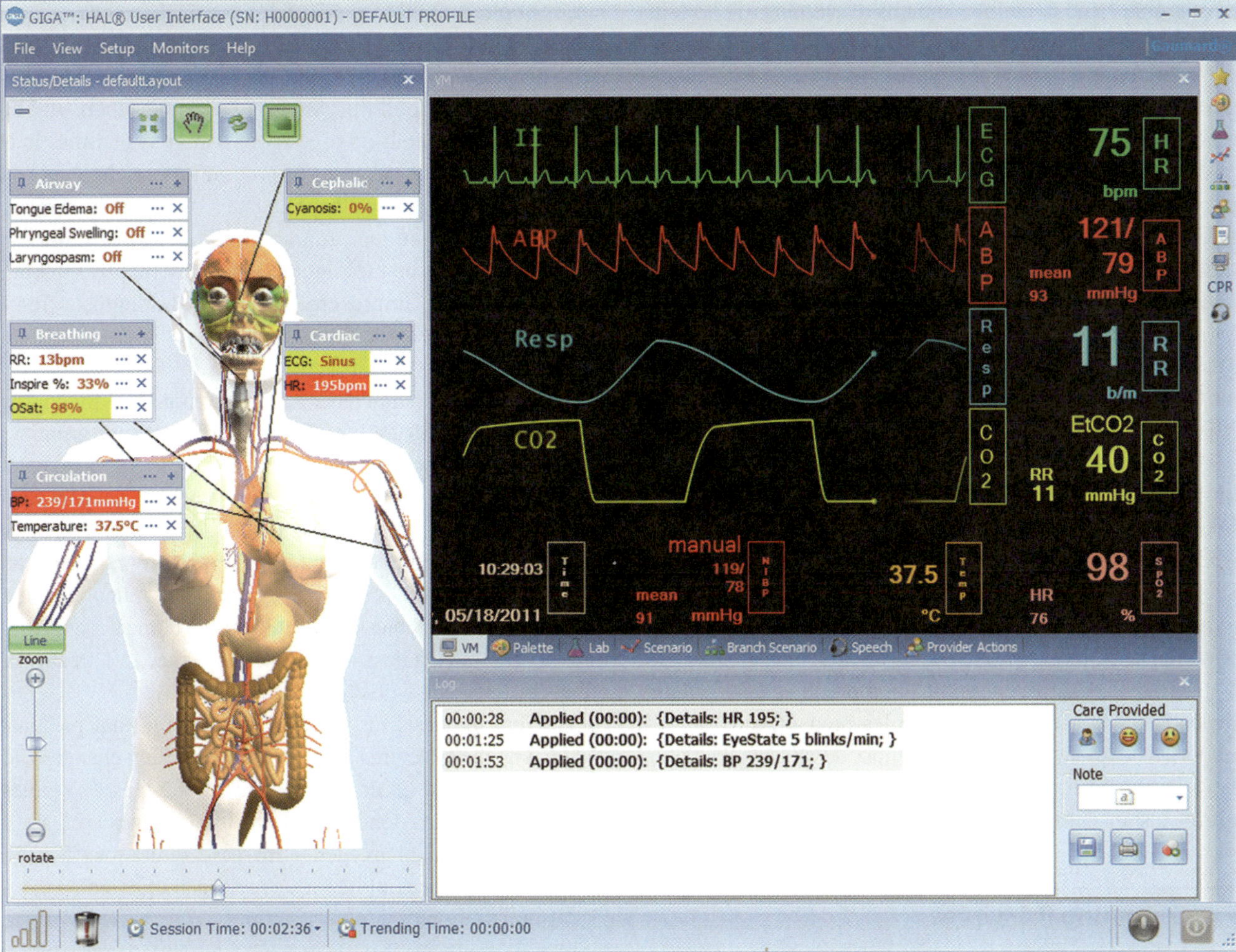

Fig. 15.3 Gaumard's GIGA user interface (Photo courtesy of Gaumard Scientific 2012. All rights reserved)

Even though a simulator may be primarily operator-driven, varying degrees of physiologic modeling may be included that allows for autonomous changes. For example, some operator-driven mannequins may respond to the application of oxygen or use of bag-valve mask by increasing the simulator's oxygen saturation without input from the operator. Additionally, some operator-driven mannequins detect electrical current and can respond to cardioversion, defibrillation, or pacing.

Complex mathematical models are crucial to the development of today's autonomous mannequin simulators to predict physiological and pharmacological responses. These models first appeared in screen-based simulators before being integrated into mannequin simulators. The models use mathematical terms to describe the relationship between two or more physiologic parameters and behave similarly to real-life processes. The model acts as an "engine" for the simulator and is affected by learner intervention as well as events scripted by the operator. By accurately generating physiologic responses to learner actions, these models can reduce, for instance, the need for operators to specify moment-to-moment vital signs, significantly reducing the operator's workload to allow more time for observing learner activity.

Not all patient conditions can be easily modeled. Because of inter-patient variability and the large number of contributing factors, there is no way to predict exactly when, for example, a patient will have a cardiac event. A model can, however, calculate the likelihood of such an event based on the information available.

Fidelity

Fidelity refers to the degree a simulator is able to reproduce a real-world environment. Though levels of fidelity are not formally defined, it is generally accepted that the advanced mannequin-based simulators discussed in this chapter are in the higher-fidelity ranges. These "full-scale" or "high-fidelity" simulators are usually found in high-fidelity environments and designed to interact with healthcare providers on both the psychomotor and cognitive domains of learning [1]. Fidelity ultimately depends on the intended application. A mannequin designed for neurologic surgery would not be considered high fidelity in a simulated labor and delivery setting where the objectives focus on techniques of vaginal delivery.

Mannequin features such as realistic heart sounds, palpable pulses, and the ability to speak add to simulation fidelity. Though these advanced features come at a higher cost [2], there are many studies that indicate training with realistic mannequins improves clinical performance (ACLS [3], detection of murmurs [4]), and improves skills with full-mannequin simulators (airway management [5], medical emergencies [6], PALS [7], ACLS [8], trauma management [9]). Conversely, some studies indicate that learners training with higher-fidelity mannequins have no advantage in skills or knowledge compared to learners training with lower-fidelity modalities [10–12]. There appears to be insufficient evidence to make a final determination on how fidelity correlates with effectiveness or clinical outcomes. It is important to note, however, that learners consistently report greater satisfaction with more realistic high-fidelity mannequins [12, 13]. In some regards, the most appropriate level of fidelity depends on the learners and the learning objectives. It is important to note that even the most advanced simulators have important limitations and none rival the sophistication of, for instance, flight simulators used by pilots.

Programming Principles

Commonly the simulation scenario will last approximately one-third of the allotted time allowing two-thirds of the time for debriefing (Chaps. 6 and 7). Depending on the complexity of the case, the types of learners, and the learning objectives, the simulation scenario may only last a matter of minutes. Due to this relatively short time frame, clinical treatments such as administering a fluid bolus, which may typically occur over 5 min, often occur over 1 min or even instantly in simulation. These time-scaling properties are generally built into the commonly available programming platforms. When programming these treatment effects on the simulator and monitor, it is important that they do not occur too fast to be unrealistic but not too slow that the intensity of the session is lost.

All simulators can be run "on the fly," meaning without a preexisting program. This works very well when very few changes occur or only one change occurs at a time. For example, if a patient develops supraventricular tachycardia (SVT), one can simply change the rhythm from normal sinus rhythm to SVT. This change can be detected on the patient monitor (increase in heart rate and loss of P waves) as well as the simulator (increases in palpable pulse rate and heart sounds). Clinically speaking, however, many changes occur over time and multiple changes may occur simultaneously. For example, a child in shock will have increased heart rate, decreased blood pressure with either a narrowed or widened pulse pressure, increased respiratory rate, and decreased end-tidal carbon dioxide. If this child is given fluids, there will be multiple simultaneous changes over a period of time. It is very difficult for an operator to program these changes "on the fly" and have each of these changes over simultaneously over time. The common programming platforms, however, allow scenarios to be programmed in a way that by clicking one state such as "improvement" or "fluid administration," all of these changes begin at once and occur over a specified time (Fig. 15.4).

Operator-driven simulators can be programmed by adjusting vital signs, simulator voice/sounds (i.e., vomiting, grunting, crying), and physical exam findings. The programmer must have a working knowledge of expected changes caused by various treatments. Either too great, small, fast, or slow decreases the believability of the scenario. If the person programming the scenario has limited clinical experience, it is important that they work with someone more familiar with clinical manifestations to carefully adjust magnitudes and speed of treatment effects by someone with clinical experience.

Trending is a helpful programming feature that prevents sudden unbelievable vital sign changes. Trending changes can be programmed to occur over seconds to minutes. Examples of effective changes done through the use of trends are:

1. Administration of oxygen – Increase saturations 5–10% over 30–60 s depending on scenario pathophysiology.
2. Administration of intravenous fluids – Decrease heart rate by 5–10 beats per minute over 30–60 s and increase blood pressure by 5–10 mmHg over 30–60 s.
3. Administration of neuromuscular blocking agent – Decrease respiratory rate to zero over 5–30 s depending on particular agent administered.
4. Administration of dopamine – Increase blood pressure by 5–10 mmHg and increase heart rate 5–10 beats per minute over 30–60 s.
5. Seizure – Increase heart rate by 25–50 beats per minute, increase blood pressure 20–40 mmHg, over 5–10 s, and increase end-tidal carbon dioxide by 10–30 over 1–2 min.
6. Administration of anticonvulsants to treat seizures – Reverse above changes over a similar time frame.
7. Worsening – This trend can be programmed which the operator can activate when participants enter. This may be preferable to starting the physiologic changes when the scenario is opened. It can be hard to predict the exact entrance of participants.
8. Shock – This can be an excellent example of a worsening change. Heart rate gradually increases, respiratory rate increases, end-tidal carbon dioxide decreases, and blood pressure decreases. Both systolic and diastolic pressure can decrease together or they can widen or narrow depending on the type of shock.

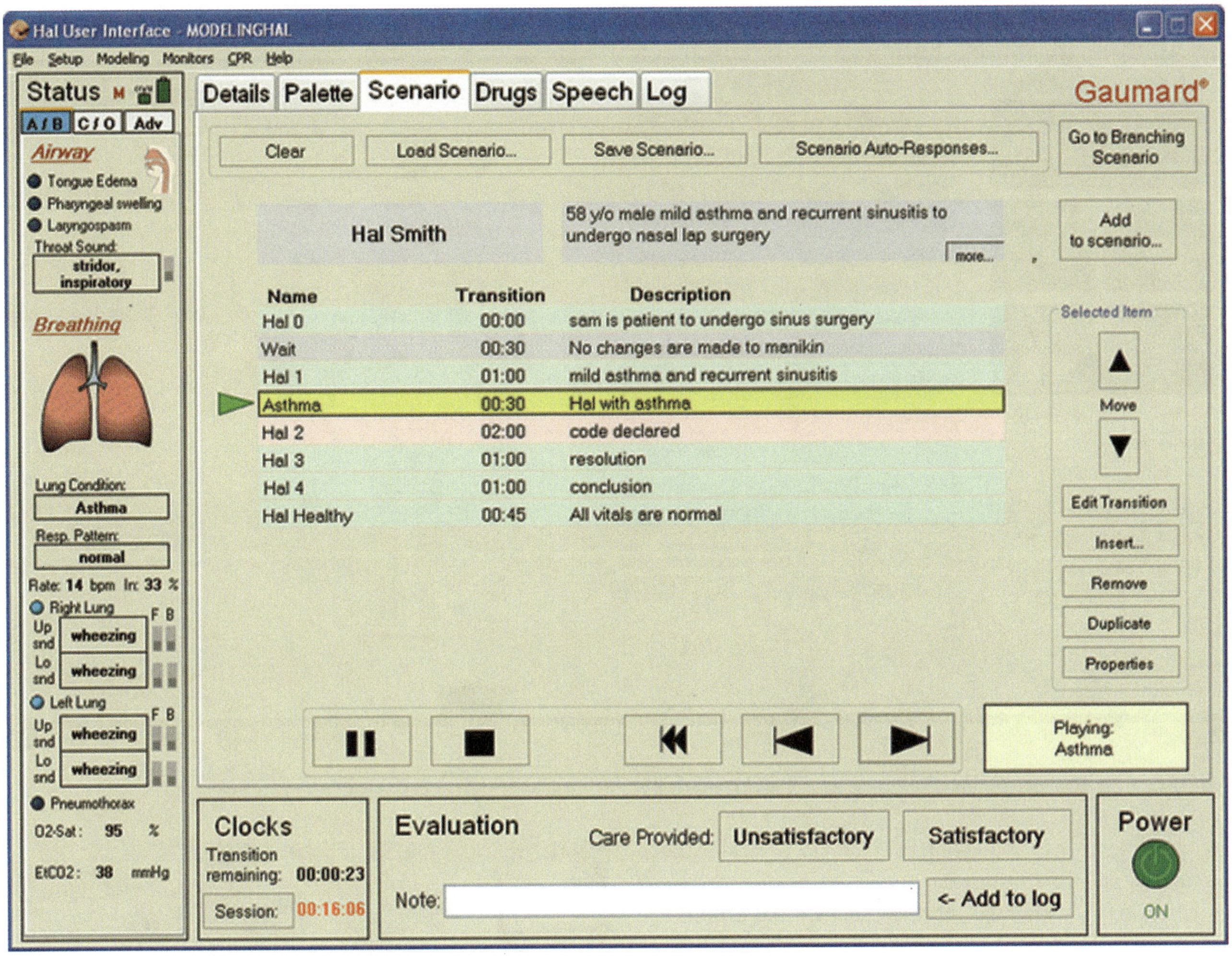

Fig. 15.4 Scenario palette of the HAL® user interface (Photo courtesy of Gaumard Scientific 2012. All rights reserved)

As these trends are created, they can be saved and used again for any other scenario. For example, many cases will have a component of hypoxia which is improved with oxygen. You can insert this trend into any of these cases.

Autonomous simulators are programmed by adjusting simulator physiology or by programming events that result in physiologic changes. For instance, if the operator wants to simulate shock, they may simply program the simulated patient to lose 10% of their blood volume over a desired time frame. Unlike operator-driven simulators that require the operator to actually change the vital signs, autonomous simulators will improve by infusing blood. The physiology of autonomous simulators is complex but sometimes needs to be adjusted slightly to make changes occur at a different rate or degree. Complex trending in autonomous simulators may be replaced by the use of scenarios that contain multiple physiologic changes in each state. In addition, if more than one physiologic change is programmed, these changes may interact and affect each other. It is crucial to test these combined physiology changes to ensure a reasonable degree of believability.

CAE Healthcare (formerly METI) has one programming platform that functions autonomously, HPS, and a newer programming platform that functions more as operator-driven, Müse® (Fig. 15.5). Laerdal and Gaumard (Fig. 15.3) platforms are mostly operator-driven but may still respond autonomously to some interventions. All platforms include the ability to log and time stamp most physiological, pharmacological, and event data. Some platforms also automatically log advanced values such as alveolar and blood gases, cardiac output, and hematocrit values. These logs can aid in the programming of scenarios and events based on past simulations that were, perhaps, initially performed "on the fly."

Nontechnical aspects of scenario programming are important as well. As shown in Fig. 15.1, supporting data such as mock laboratory results, appropriate radiographs improve the fidelity of the scenario. In addition, confederates such as parents, spouses, nurses, doctors, and consultants assist both the reality of the case as well as help move the scenario if learners are frustrated or misinterpret a finding which leads them to a completely different set of differential diagnoses

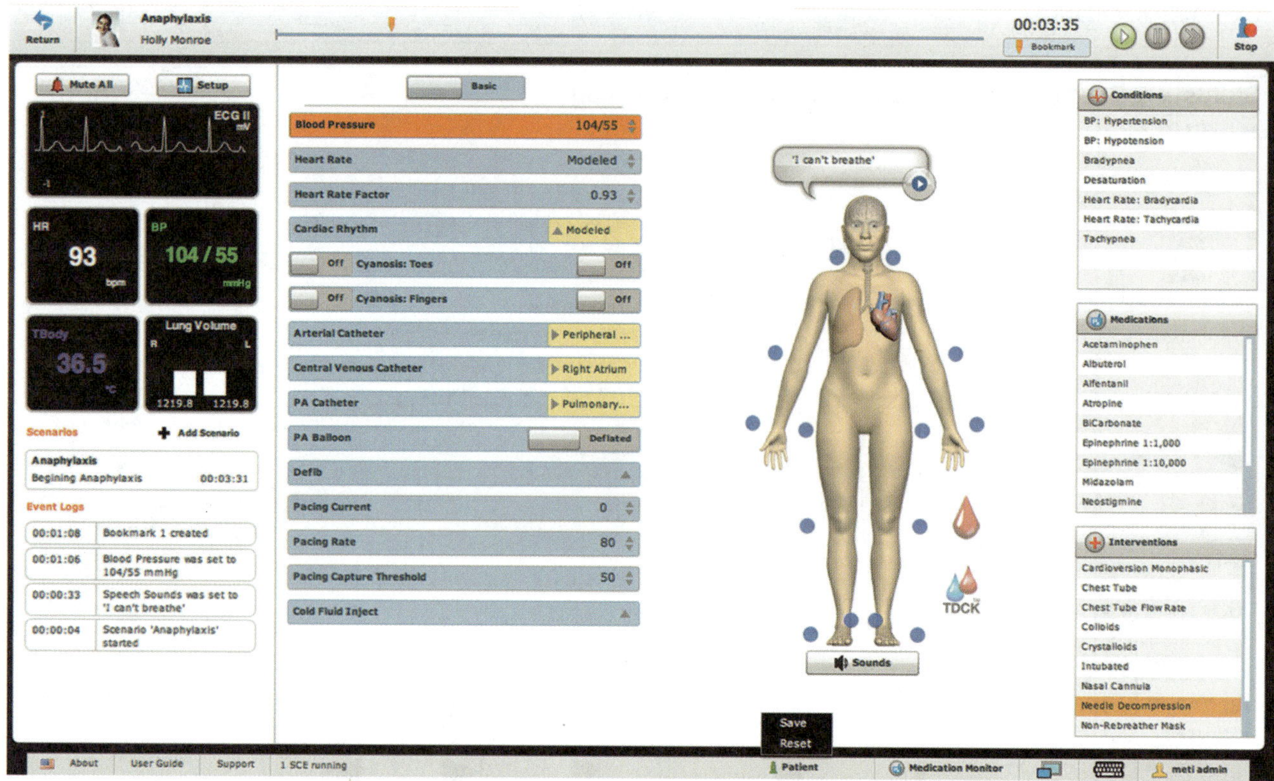

Fig. 15.5 CAE Healthcare's Müse® user interface (Photo courtesy of CAE Healthcare ©2012 CAE Healthcare)

and therapies. An example of this is the use of stridor in the Laerdal infant. This inspiratory sound can be misinterpreted as wheezing. If learning objectives include the differential diagnosis of stridor such as laryngotracheitis and foreign body, this will not be considered if the physical finding misinterpretation finding is not corrected. Confederates can gently redirect learners with statements such as "It sounded more like stridor than wheezing to me" or "I think the noise is occurring during inspiration and not expiration." Their verbal cues as referenced in Fig. 15.1 are often crucial.

Feature Considerations

Respiratory

Most mannequins generate realistic breath sounds while the chest wall moves with respiration. Oxygen sensors are built in some models allowing for detection of changes in inspired oxygen concentration and, according to physiologic models, change the saturation accordingly. In addition, more advanced mannequin modeling considers patient-specific factors such as weight, functional residual capacity, cardiac output, shunt, and dead space. The rate of saturation and desaturation may be adjusted in some mannequins giving the instructor more control over timing of the scenario. Some models include a gas analyzer and may detect anesthetic gases (Fig. 15.6).

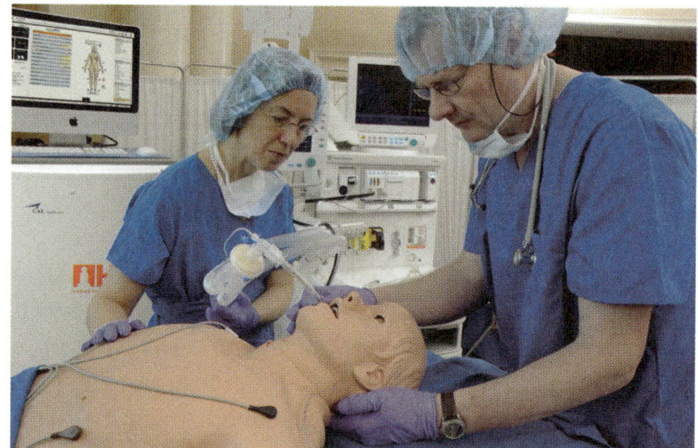

Fig. 15.6 METI HPS® Human Patient Simulator has an optional anesthesia delivery system (Photo courtesy of CAE Healthcare ©2012 CAE Healthcare)

Some mannequins may be attached to an external carbon dioxide source to simulate end-tidal carbon dioxide. Mannequins capable of exhaling carbon dioxide may do so in one of two ways. Some mannequins release an unprecise amount of carbon dioxide intended solely for qualitative assessment (e.g., to produce a positive response with a colorimetric carbon dioxide detector). Other mannequins produce model-driven condition-specific carbon dioxide waveforms capable of generating a capnogram.

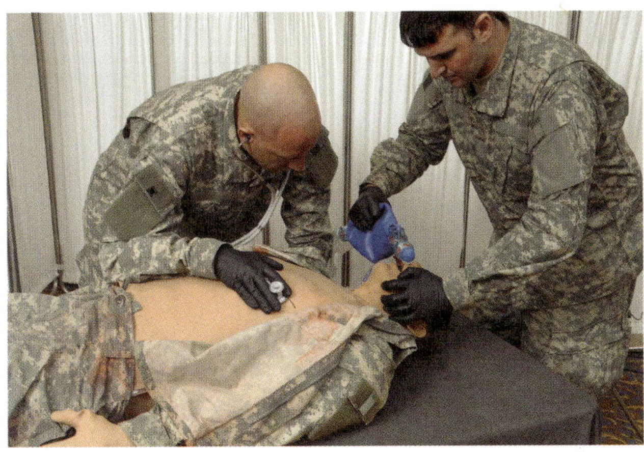

Fig. 15.7 Heart sounds being auscultated on METI iStan® (Photo courtesy of CAE Healthcare ©2012 CAE Healthcare)

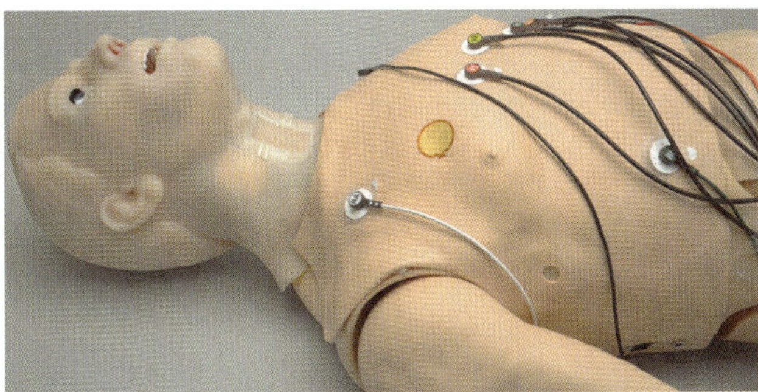

Fig. 15.8 HAL® S3201 connected to real 12-lead ECG (Photo courtesy of Gaumard Scientific 2012. All rights reserved)

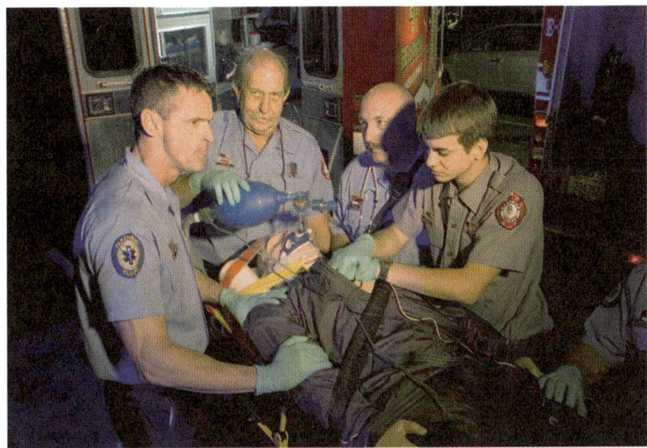

Fig. 15.9 Chest compressions performed on METIman® (Photo courtesy of CAE Healthcare ©2012 CAE Healthcare)

Use of computer-controlled mannequins in the intensive care setting is limited by the capacity to respond physiologically to complex changes in mechanical ventilator modes and settings (PEEP, I-E ratios, pressure control, etc.). More recently simulators have been introduced with dependable dynamic airway and lung compliance, variable respiratory rates, and I-E ratios to accommodate mechanical ventilatory support. Most mannequins do, however, interface well with high-frequency oscillatory ventilation.

Cardiovascular

Pulse volume and strength is typically palpable at multiple anatomic locations and may dissipate with decreasing blood pressure. A range of heart sounds is present and may be auscultated using a standard stethoscope (Fig. 15.7). Most high-fidelity mannequins include a library of rhythms, and some are capable of generating a real electrocardiogram signal when connected to real equipment (Fig. 15.8). Many valvular heart diseases may be simulated and autonomous mannequins demonstrate hemodynamic behavior that reflects valvular lesions automatically. Learners sometimes find it difficult to hear or interpret mannequin heart sounds accurately with the notable exception of Harvey® the cardiopulmonary patient simulator designed for this purpose. Some mannequins simulate realistic jugular venous distension based on cardiac status. Almost all models are capable of full chest compressions and some provide feedback on effectiveness (Fig. 15.9).

Airway

Most mannequin simulators allow for realistic bag-valve-mask intervention as well as endotracheal and nasotracheal intubation. Depth and position of endotracheal tube placement are sensed and respond appropriately in some models. Gastric distension typically results if a tube is placed in the esophagus. Operators may manipulate airway conditions to facilitate cannot ventilate and/or cannot intubate scenarios. This may be achieved through glottic and/or tongue swelling, trismus, laryngospasm, or bronchial occlusion. Cricothyrotomy is possible through replaceable neck skins. Some models are capable of oral secretions to add even more realism to airway manipulation.

In most situations, a dedicated airway trainer is superior to full-body mannequin simulators in terms of airway realism and manipulation. Even so, most model-based mannequins have an airway capable of basic airway interventions including placement of endotracheal tubes and laryngeal mask airways, mask ventilation, jet ventilation, and cricothyrotomy. In most cases, advanced airway techniques such as double-lumen tracheal tube placement and retrograde intubation are also possible. Mannequins with realistic tracheal and bronchial anatomy allow for direct laryngobronchoscopy and even practice of foreign body removal.

Neurologic

Many mannequin simulators have eyes that open, blink, and close depending on the state of consciousness (Fig. 15.10).

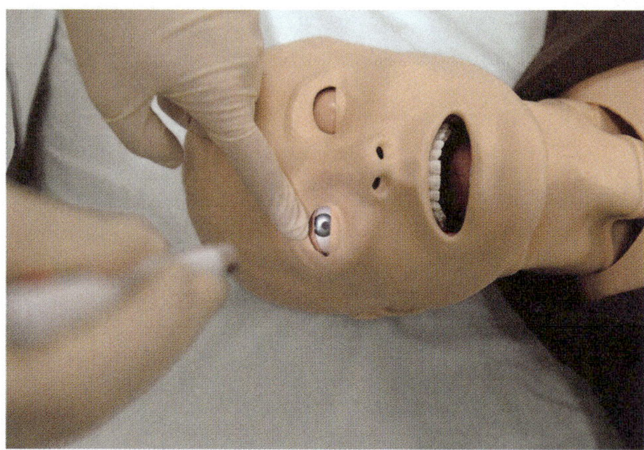

Fig. 15.10 SimMan® 3G eye signs (Photo courtesy of Laerdal Medical. All rights reserved)

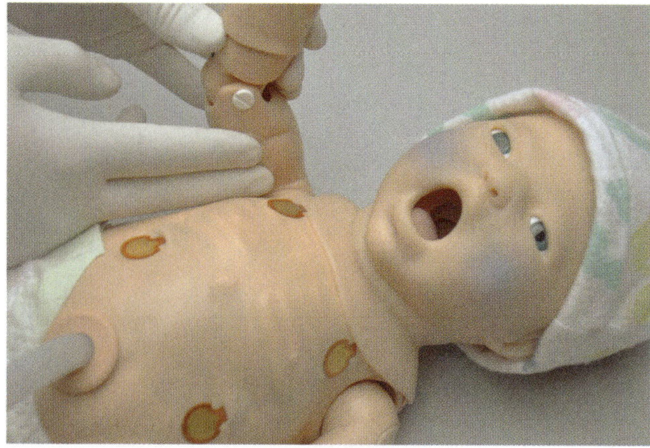

Fig. 15.11 Newborn HAL® S3010 includes cyanosis as a standard feature (Photo courtesy of Gaumard® Scientific 2012. All rights reserved)

Some mannequins feature pupils that change automatically in response to light or programmed states, while other mannequins have eyes that may be manually rotated to select a pupil size. Many full-scale mannequins also include embedded speakers that allow an operator to speak as the patient making the system a virtual standardized patient. The capacity to seize is included in some models though it is generally limited to movement of the head in adults and children or torso in infants. Degree of drug-induced paralysis may be monitored in at least one mannequin model by use of a peripheral nerve stimulator that simulates adductor pollicis muscle twitches. Some infant mannequins allow for assessment of the anterior fontanelle which may be bulging in when intracranial pressure in elevated.

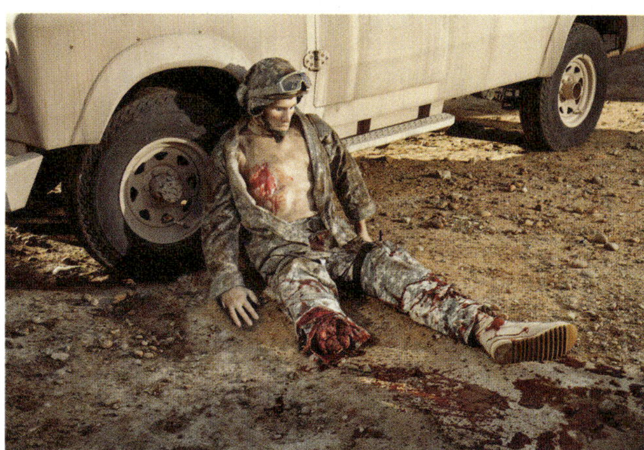

Fig. 15.12 CAE Caesar™ trauma patient simulator is built with modular limbs that may be moulaged for amputation (Photo courtesy of CAE Healthcare ©2012 CAE Healthcare)

Extremities

Generally all mannequin simulators have some degree of articulation though some are more limited than others. Some mannequins are capable of circumoral and/or peripheral cyanosis (Fig. 15.11). Various add-on kits are available to facilitate trauma conditions such as amputations (Fig. 15.12).

Pharmacologic Intervention

Select mannequins include drug recognition systems that identify drug, concentrations, and dosages administered via a bar-coded syringe filled with sterile water (Fig. 15.13) or radiofrequency identification tags (Fig. 15.14). These mannequins have varying degrees of pharmacologic modeling to autonomously initiate a realistic response. Some mannequins may be fitted with anesthesia delivery kits to allow for simulation of various anesthetic gas administrations.

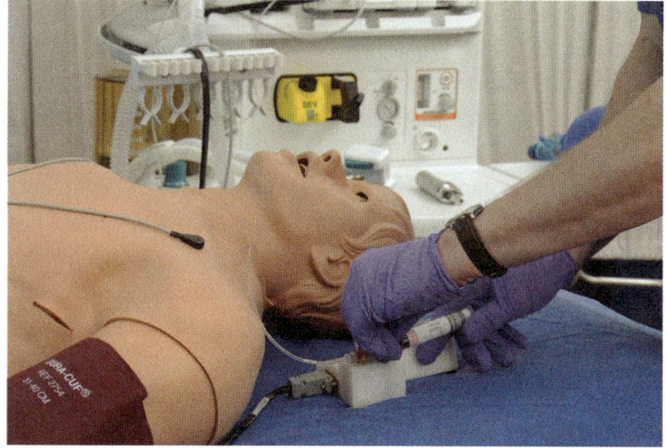

Fig. 15.13 METI HPS® Human Patient Simulator drug recognition system uses barcode technology to accurately identify drug administered, concentration, and dose (Photo courtesy of CAE Healthcare ©2012 CAE Healthcare)

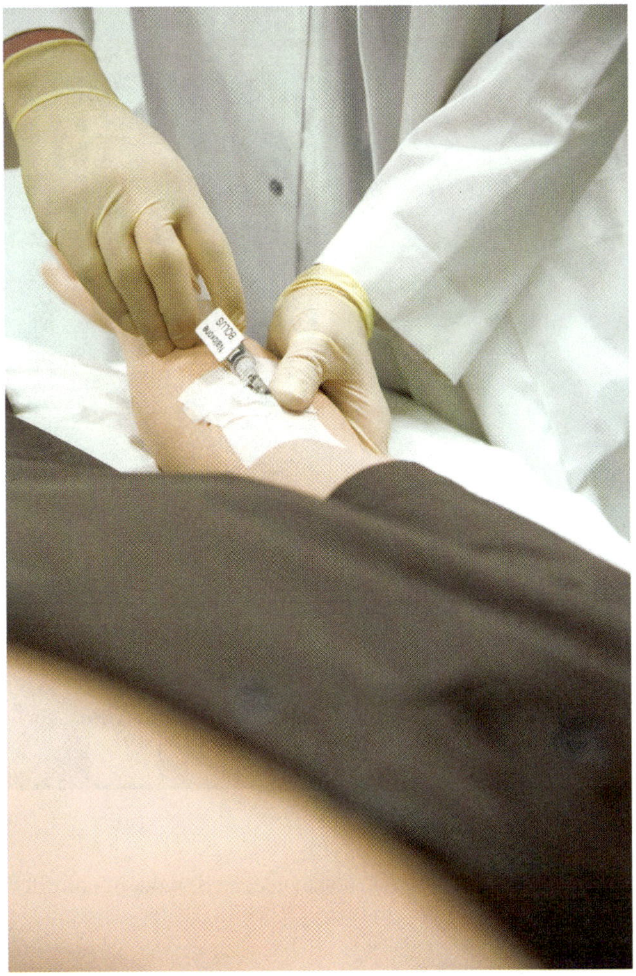

Fig. 15.14 SimMan® 3G advanced drug recognition system uses radiofrequency identification tags (Photo courtesy of Laerdal Medical. All rights reserved)

Procedural Intervention

Mannequins may be used for training invasive procedures such as chest tube insertion, needle thoracotomy, pericardiocentesis, diagnostic peritoneal lavage, urinary catheter placement, surgical cricothyroidotomy, and various other interventions. Intravenous catheter placement and arterial sampling are available on some models and may result in blood "flashback" to assist the learner in verifying placement. Mannequin skin and internal tubing, however, are rarely durable enough to make this a practical procedure during routine simulations. Most pediatric mannequins are capable of intraosseous access and infusion as well.

Interface with Existing Equipment

Vital signs are typically displayed on an accompanying monitor. Some mannequin simulators have the ability to interface with standard patient monitoring equipment, while other simulators require a monitor to be attached to the control computer that generates the clinical data that is displayed. Some manufacturers also include the ability to display clinical images such as chest radiographs (Fig. 15.15) or electrocardiograms.

Portability

Mannequins often are used in a fixed location though more recently developed mannequins are more portable. Institutions utilizing in situ simulations value mannequins that are easily transported. In addition, simulators are sometimes transported outside the facility for training purposes. Mannequin portability has greatly increased in recent years due to availability of tetherless mannequins, rechargeable batteries, and reduced size of associated equipment including cabling, hoses, and compressors necessary to operate the mannequin. Many pediatric simulators and associated equipment can be contained in a portable crib or isolette.

Cost

Although not a "feature" per se, another significant point of comparison for mannequin-based simulators are the costs. In general, cost will rise with the degree of technicality and advanced features. The initial purchase price should be considered as well as costs associated with service contract, upgrades, associated software, and hardware requirement. It is not uncommon for new features to become available that may require an additional investment. Because simulators vary in their ease of operability, another cost consideration is the degree to which varying levels of operators may be trained to use the equipment.

Regardless of features, it should be noted that mannequin simulators today are fairly unreliable compared to comparatively priced devices used on a daily basis. The degree of unreliability seems to increase with the complexity of the mannequin. Busy centers realize the importance of having an experienced simulationist that can quickly address these sudden problems. It is generally advisable to maintain warranty coverage in order to address these expected malfunctions and required repairs.

Examples of Mannequin Simulators

At the writing of this chapter, there are three primary companies that produce programmable mannequin-based simulators in North America: Laerdal (Stavanger, Norway), CAE Healthcare (Sarasota, Florida), and Gaumard (Miami, Florida). All three companies manufacture adult and pediatric simulators.

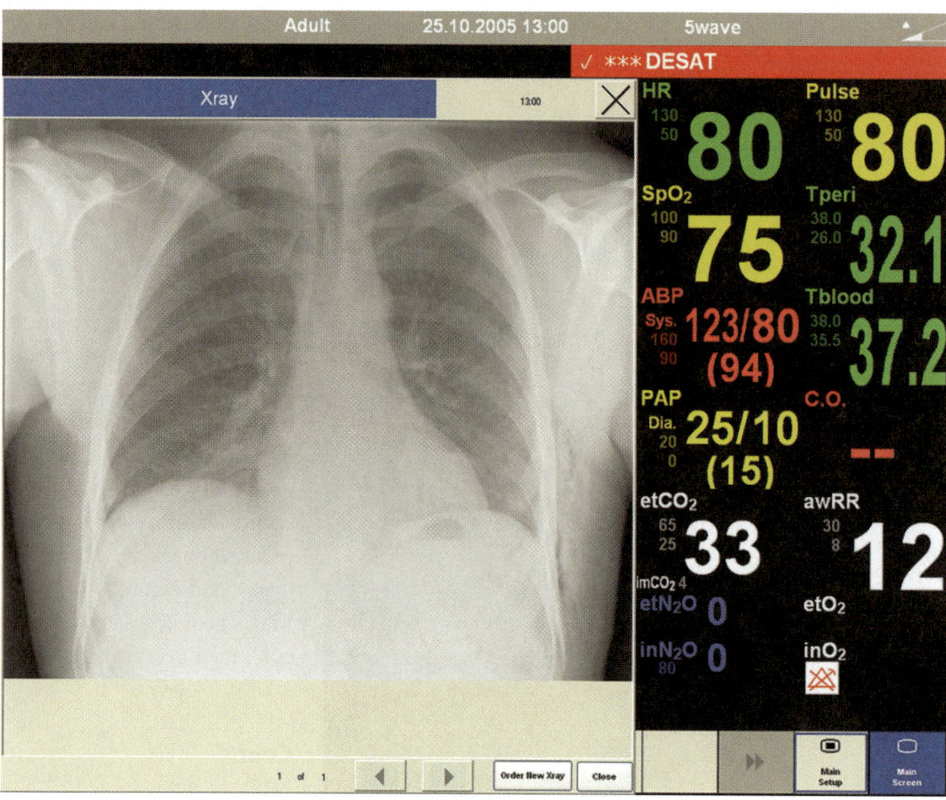

Fig. 15.15 Chest radiography displayed on SimMan patient monitor (Photo courtesy of Laerdal Medical. All rights reserved)

Adult Mannequin Simulators

Though features differ between models and companies, mannequins with similar price points are generally comparable (Table 15.1; Figs. 15.16, 15.17, 15.18, and 15.19). Although prescribing every mannequin in detail is beyond the scope of this chapter, a few adult mannequins with distinguishing characteristics are described below. For completeness the reader is referred to Table 15.1 for side by side comparisons of equipment.

Human Patient Simulator, HPS (CAE Healthcare)

The Human Patient Simulator (HPS), initially commercialized by Loral Data Systems, then Medical Education Technologies (METI) and now CAE Healthcare, is a full-sized mannequin supported by gas analyzer and advanced physiologic and pharmacologic modeling (Fig. 15.20). Though HPS development dates back to the late 1980s, it remains one of the most complex and comprehensive patient simulators available. The HPS was the first patient simulator with the ability to provide respiratory gas exchange, anesthesia delivery, and patient monitoring with real physiological clinical monitors making it ideal for simulations involving anesthesia, critical care, and respiratory care. In addition to commonly available feature, some of the enhanced capabilities include light-responsive pupils, thumb twitch to peripheral nerve stimulator, drug recognition, variable lung compliance and airways resistance, and model-controlled urinary output.

Emergency Care Simulator, ECS (CAE Healthcare)

Although similar in appearance to the HPS, the ECS is more mobile, has autonomous capabilities (i.e., will desaturate spontaneously during apneaic episodes) and therefore is more modestly priced. It lacks the ability to interface with actual physiologic monitors, inhaled anesthetic agent detection, or produce a true capnograph.

Caesar™ (CAE Healthcare)

Caesar was developed by the Center for Integration of Medicine Innovative Technology (CIMIT) in collaboration with the Telemedicine and Advanced Technology Research Center (TATRC) of the US Army Medical Research and Material Command for use by combat medics in the battlefield and other military-based environments (Figs. 15.23 and 15.24). Features such as video-based screen eyes not affected by debris in the field and a rugged, durable, water-resistant design makes Caesar ideal for a variety of terrain, climates, and environmental conditions. Caesar is operated by a tetherless autonomous physiologically modeled interface preloaded with trauma scenarios and is anatomically accurate with complete articulation of joints and spine. Other features include a hemorrhage control system with tourniquet sensors, IV access, and multiple trauma-related procedural

Table 15.1 Comparison of mannequins

Adult mannequin simulator comparison									
	HPS (CAE)	iStan (CAE)	METIman (CAE)	ECS (CAE)	SimMan Essential (Laerdal)	SimMan 3G (Laerdal)	HAL S3000 (Gaumard)	Hal S3201 (Gaumard)	Susie 2000 (Gaumard)
General									
Autonomous	Yes	Yes	Yes	Yes	No	No	No	No	No
Tetherless	No	Yes	Yes	No	Yes	Yes	Yes	Yes	Yes
Real monitors	Yes	No	No	No	No	No	No	Yes	Yes
Airway/respiratory									
Trismus	No	Yes	No	No	Yes	Yes	No	No	No
Articulating mandible	No	Yes	No	No	Yes	Yes	No	Yes	No
Breakaway teeth	Yes	Yes	Yes	Yes	No	No	No	No	No
Nasal intubation	Yes	Yes	Yes[a]	Yes	Yes	Yes	Yes	Yes	No
Bronchial occlusion	Yes	Yes	Yes	Yes	No	Yes	No	Yes	No
Laryngospasm	Yes	Yes	Yes	Yes	Yes	Yes	Yes	Yes	Yes
Airway occlusion	Yes	Yes	Yes	Yes	Yes	Yes	No	Yes	Yes
Airway resistance	Yes	Yes	Yes[a]	Yes	Yes	Yes	No	Yes	No
Oral secretions	Yes	No	Yes[a]	No	No	Yes	No	No	No
Cardiovascular									
CO_2 detection	Yes	Yes	Yes	Yes	Yes	Yes	No	Yes	No
JVD	No	Yes	No	No	No	No	No	No	No
Cyanosis	No	Yes	No	No	No	Yes	Yes	Yes	Yes
Capillary refill	No	Yes	No	No	No	No	No	No	No
Pulse sites	Yes	14	14	14	11[a]	14	10	12	12
ECG detectable	Yes	No	No	Yes	No	No	Yes	Yes	Yes
Neuro									
Reactive pupils	Yes	Yes	Yes	No	No	Yes	Yes	Yes	Yes
Convulsions	No	Yes	Yes	Yes[a]	No	Yes	No	Yes	No
Procedural									
Intraosseous	No	Yes	Yes[a]	Yes	Yes	Yes	No	Yes	No
Intravenous	Yes	No	Yes	Yes	Yes	No	Yes	Yes	Yes
IM injection	Yes	No	Yes	Yes	Yes	Yes	Yes	Yes	Yes
Finger stick glucose	No	No	No	No	No	No	No	No	Yes
Needle thoracostomy	Yes	Yes	Yes[a]	Yes	Yes	Yes	Yes	Yes	No
Chest tube	Yes	Yes	Yes	Yes	Yes	Yes	Yes[a]	Yes	No
Chest tube output	Yes	Yes	Yes	Yes	No	No	No	No	No
Peridcardiocentesis	Yes	No	No	Yes	No	No	No	No	No
Urinary catheterization	Yes	Yes	Yes	Yes	Yes	Yes	No	Yes	Yes
Urinary output	Yes	No	Yes[a]	Yes	No	Yes	No	No	Yes

[a]Availability depends on model and may be an add-on feature

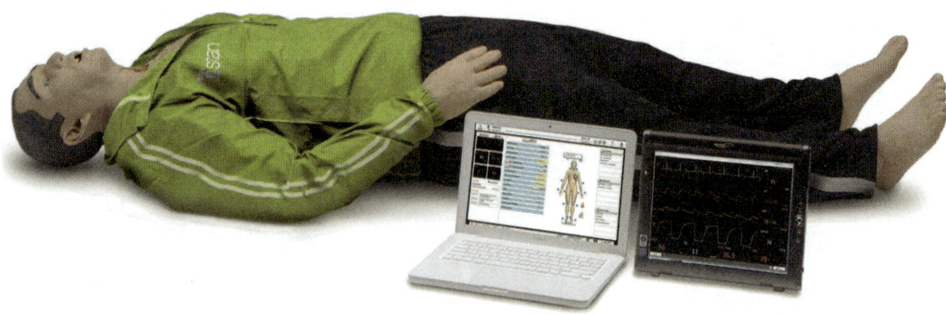

Fig. 15.16 METI iStan® (Photo courtesy of CAE Healthcare ©2012 CAE Healthcare)

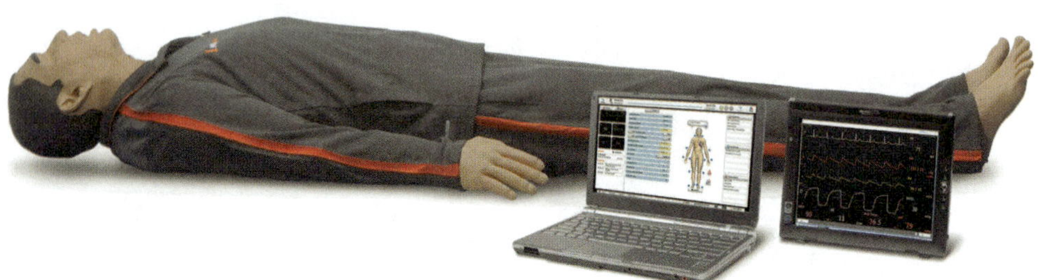

Fig. 15.17 METIman® (Photo courtesy of CAE Healthcare ©2012 CAE Healthcare)

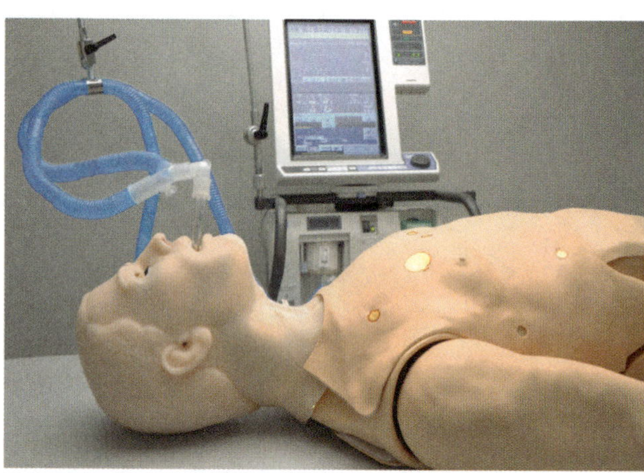

Fig. 15.18 HAL® S3201 (Photo courtesy of Gaumard® Scientific 2012. All rights reserved)

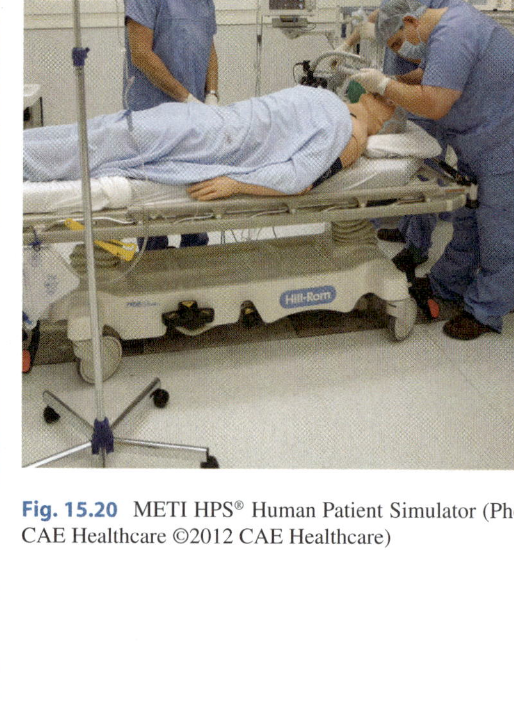

Fig. 15.20 METI HPS® Human Patient Simulator (Photo courtesy of CAE Healthcare ©2012 CAE Healthcare)

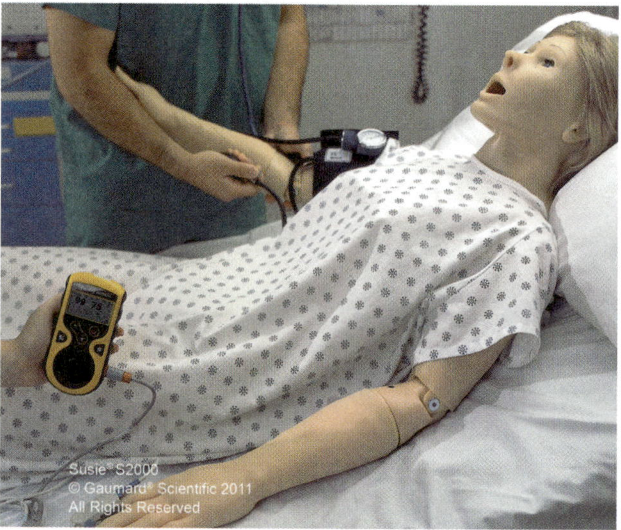

Fig. 15.19 SUSIE® S2000 (Photo courtesy of Gaumard® Scientific 2012. All rights reserved)

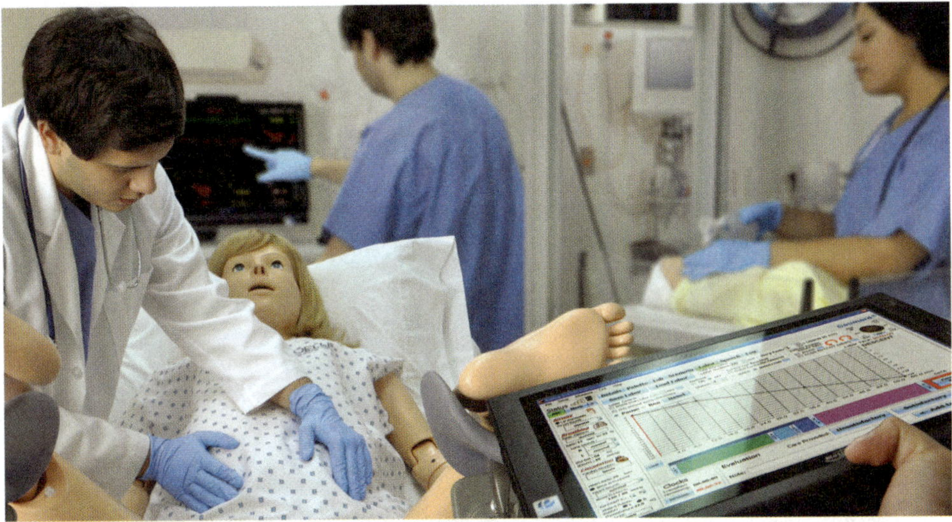

Fig. 15.21 NOELLE® Maternal and Neonatal Simulation System (Photo courtesy of Gaumard® Scientific 2012. All rights reserved)

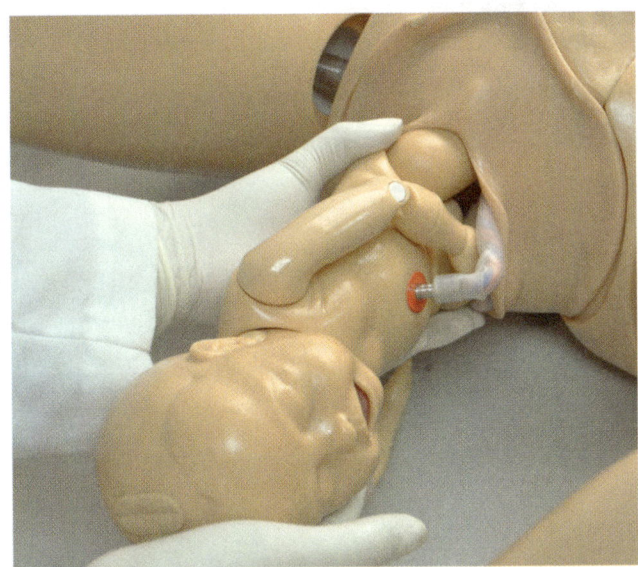

Fig. 15.22 NOELLE® Maternal and Neonatal Simulation System (Photo courtesy of Gaumard® Scientific 2012. All rights reserved)

interventions like needle thoracostomy and airway management.

NOELLE® (Gaumard)

The NOELLE® Maternal and Neonatal Birthing Simulator (Figs. 15.21 and 15.22) provides a complete birthing experience before, during, and after delivery. A variety of birthing scenarios including breech delivery, shoulder dystocia, and postpartum hemorrhage are preprogrammed, and learners may choose normal vaginal or instrumented delivery. In addition to the features expected of any adult mannequin simulator (breath sounds, realistic airway, pulses, etc.), NOELLE is capable of simulating caesarean sections, fundal massage, and episiotomy repairs. NOELLE® may be purchased with an accompanying Newborn HAL® allowing for neonatal resuscitation/monitoring after the simulated birth. The system is equipped with vital sign and perinatal (fetal) monitoring. Recently, a midrange NOELLE was introduced that, while retaining most of the obstetric-related functionality, lacks some of the advanced non-obstetric features such as advanced eye systems and wireless functionality.

SimMan™ (Laerdal)

SimMan™ is a computer-operated total-body mannequin simulator and was one of the first totally mobile computer-controlled mannequins (Fig. 15.25). SimMan™ includes a patented airway system for highly realistic airway manipulation. SimMan™ can be operated on the fly or with user-generated scenarios and, like other Laerdal simulators, is supported by SimStore, a unique online resource for purchasing annual or capital licenses for predeveloped scenarios and simulation content. The newest model, SimMan™ 3G, includes radiofrequency identification technology in chin and arm for drug recognition, an internal air compressor in each leg, internal reservoirs for water and simulated blood to emulate exsanguination and secretions (Fig. 15.26), and intraosseous line placement (Fig. 15.27).

Pediatric Mannequin Simulators

Pediatric mannequin simulators are available in a variety of size and age ranges from premature infants to older children. Many common features of pediatric mannequins are found in Table 15.2 and are summarized below.

PediaSIM (CAE Healthcare)

PediaSIM is a child simulator that is available as a Human Patient Simulator (HPS) or Emergency Care Simulator (ECS)

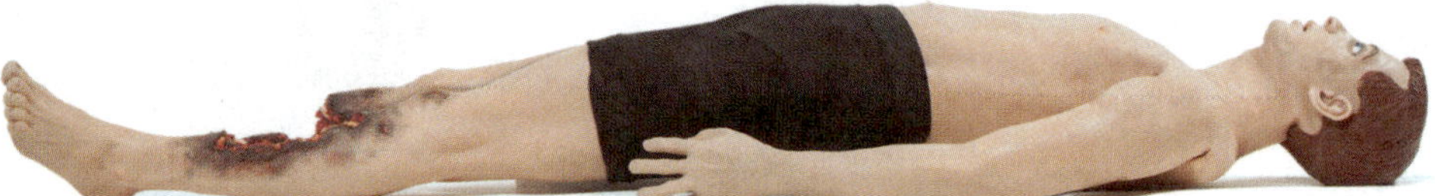

Fig. 15.23 CAE Caesar™ trauma patient simulator (Photo courtesy of CAE Healthcare ©2012 CAE Healthcare)

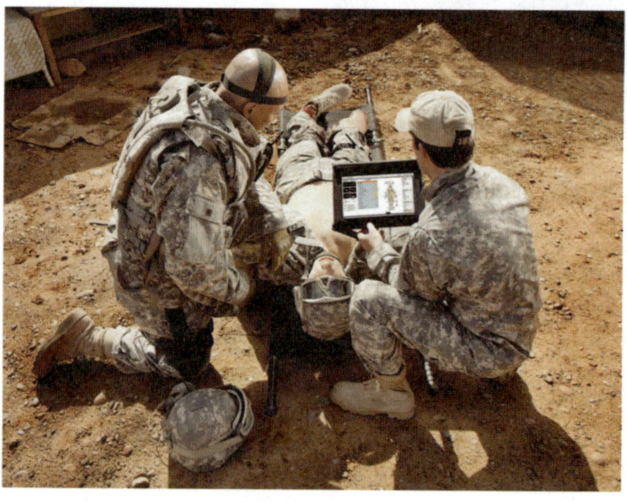

Fig. 15.24 CAE Caesar™ trauma patient simulator (Photo courtesy of CAE Healthcare ©2012 CAE Healthcare)

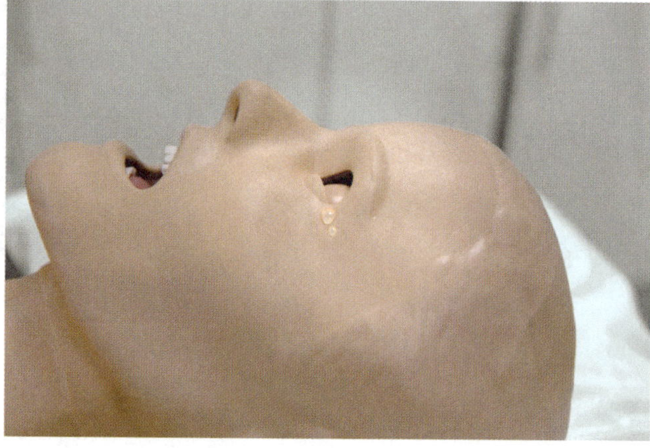

Fig. 15.26 SimMan® 3G eye secretions (Photo courtesy of Laerdal Medical. All rights reserved)

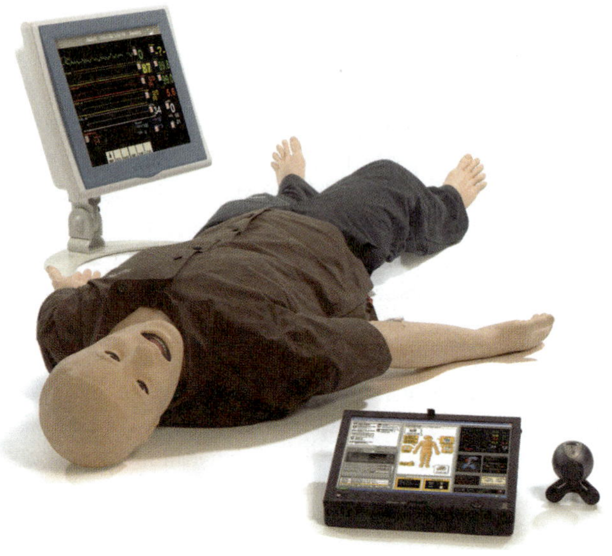

Fig. 15.25 SimMan® 3G (Photo courtesy of Laerdal Medical. All rights reserved)

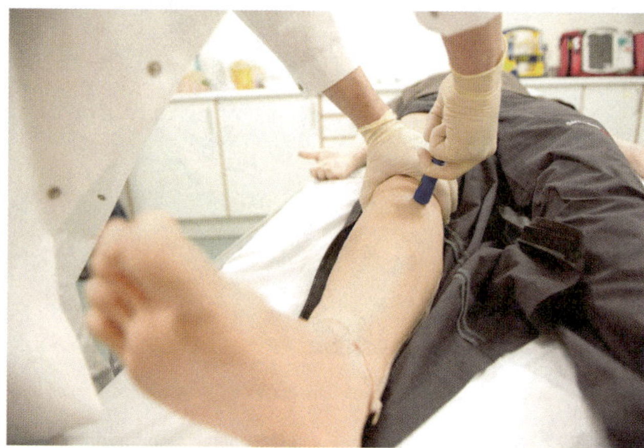

Fig. 15.27 SimMan® 3G intraosseous access (Photo courtesy of Laerdal Medical)

version (Fig. 15.28). Similar to the adult versions the HPS is necessary for use of anesthetic gases. There are also features in this simulator allowing medications with bar codes to be scanned and computer-controlled secretions. Some of the pharmacokinetic modeling, however, may be too fast or slow. The ECS version offers many of the same features as the HPS but they are not as automated. For example, tears can be produced connecting a syringe with sterile water to the tears tubing and pushing slowly. This often can be done very subtly by confederates. This simulators eyes open and close and has a wireless microphone allowing for the controller to talk for the simulator. The voice comes from a speaker mounted in the simulator's head. Both versions come with a full monitor. PediaSIM can be controlled using either the autonomous HPS or operator-driven Müse® platform and can be used to simulation patients approximately 6–10 years old.

Pediatric HAL (Gaumard)

Pediatric HAL comes in 1-year-old and 5-year-old versions which are similar in their functionality, operation, and programming (Fig. 15.29). Both simulators are wireless

Table 15.2 Common features of pediatric mannequins

Pediatric mannequin simulator comparison							
	Child			Infant		Neonate	
	SimJunior (Laerdal)	Pediatric HAL (Gaumard)	PediaSIM (CAE)	SimBaby (Laerdal)	BabySIM (CAE)	SimNewB (Laerdal)	Newborn HAL (Gaumard)
General							
Autonomous	No	No	Yes	No	Yes	No	No
Tetherless	Yes	Yes	Yes	No	Yes	No	Yes
Airway/respiratory							
Laryngospasm	No	No	Yes	Yes	Yes	No	No
Inflatable tongue	Yes	No	Yes	Yes	No	No	No
Airway occlusion	No	No	Yes	Yes	Yes	No	No
Cricothyrotomy	No	No	Yes	No	No	No	No
Nasal intubation	Yes	Yes	Yes	No	Yes	No	Yes
Cardiovascular							
CO_2 detection	No	No	Yes[a]	Yes	Yes	Yes	No
Cyanosis	No	Yes	No	Yes	No	Yes	Yes
Pacing	Yes	No	Yes	Yes	Yes	No	No
Pulse sites	8	8	12	4	4	3	3
ECG detectable	Yes	No	Yes	No	Yes	No	No
Neuro							
Reactive pupils	No	Yes	No	No	No	No	No
Convulsions	Yes	Yes	No	Yes	No	No	Yes
Bulging fontanelle	No	No	No	Yes	Yes	No	No
Procedural							
Intraosseous	Yes	Yes	Yes	Yes	Yes	Yes	Yes[a]
Intravenous	Yes	Yes	Yes	Yes	No	No	Yes[a]
Umbilical cath	No	No	No	No	No	Yes	Yes
Needle thoracostomy	No	No	Yes[a]	Yes	Yes	Yes	Yes
Chest tube	No	No	Yes	Yes	Yes	No	No
Urinary catheterization	No	Yes	Yes	No	Yes	No	Yes
Urinary output	No	No	Yes	No	Yes	No	No

[a]Availability depends on model and may be an add-on feature

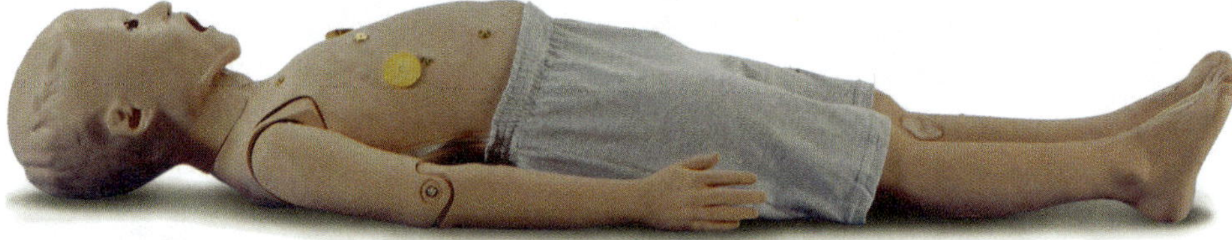

Fig. 15.28 METI PediaSIM® pediatric patient simulator (All rights reserved. Photo courtesy of CAE Healthcare ©2012 CAE Healthcare)

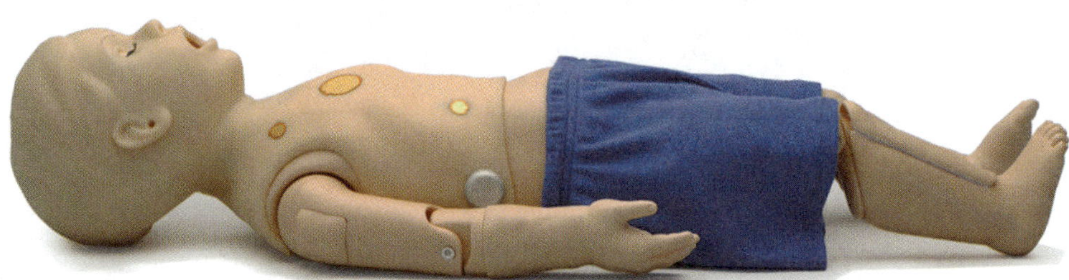

Fig. 15.29 Pediatric HAL® S3005 (Photo courtesy of Gaumard® Scientific 2012. All rights reserved)

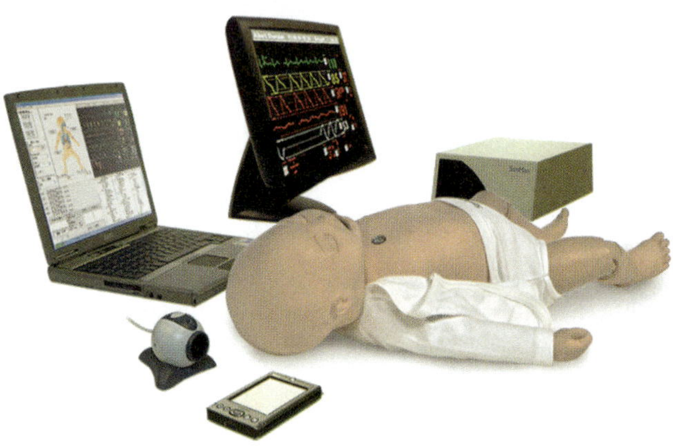

Fig. 15.30 SimBaby™ (Photo courtesy of Laerdal Medical. All rights reserved)

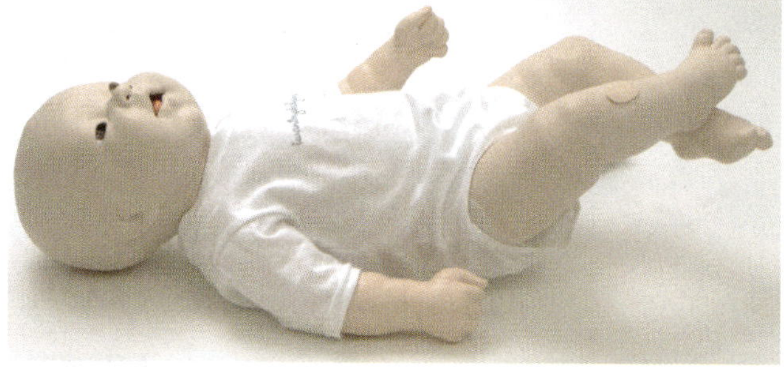

Fig. 15.31 METI BabySIM® (Photo courtesy of CAE Healthcare ©2012 CAE Healthcare)

making them easier to transport to in situ scenarios and non-hospital-based cases. They both function on a tablet computer controlled by a "touch pen." They have eyes which open and close and pupils which can react to light. They both can "speak" via prerecorded age appropriate words and phrases. They can have a tracheostomy tube placed. Monitors are available but not standard. It is the opinion of the authors that the 1-year-old HAL appears more 18 months to 3 years old. The 5-year-old HAL can be used to simulation patients approximately 5–8 years old.

SimBaby (Laerdal)

SimBaby uses the same platform as SimNewB and the original SimMan allowing easy transfer of operating skills (Fig. 15.30). This simulator comes with a full monitor with capabilities to display electrocardiograms and digital radiographs utilizing the touch screen technology. It has six age appropriate verbal sounds. There is an anterior fontanelle which can be sunken, normal, or full. The components necessary to function can be placed in a hospital crib allowing for relatively easy movement for in situ hospital scenarios. SimBaby can be modified to include an umbilical task trainer [14]. This infant simulator can be used to simulate patients approximately 1 week to 18 months old.

BabySIM (CAE Healthcare)

BabySIM has the physiology of a 6-month-old infant (Fig. 15.31). It uses the Müse® operating platform and comes with a touch screen monitor. It has blinking eyes and the pupil size can be changed manually.

PEDI Blue Neonatal Simulator with SmartSkin Technology (Gaumard)

PEDI Blue Neonatal represents a 4 lb newborn allowing simulation of initial care such as suctioning, obtaining umbilical access, and intubation. An optional leg is available for intraosseous access and an optional arm is available for intravenous access and injections. This simulator has the capabilities of peripheral and central cyanosis.

PREMIE Blue Simulator with SmartSkin Technology (Gaumard)

The PREMIE Blue (Fig. 15.32) simulates a 28-week premature infant with variable skin color based on the effectiveness of resuscitation. This simulator includes intraosseous, intravenous, and intramuscular sites as well as heel stick capabilities for capillary blood samples.

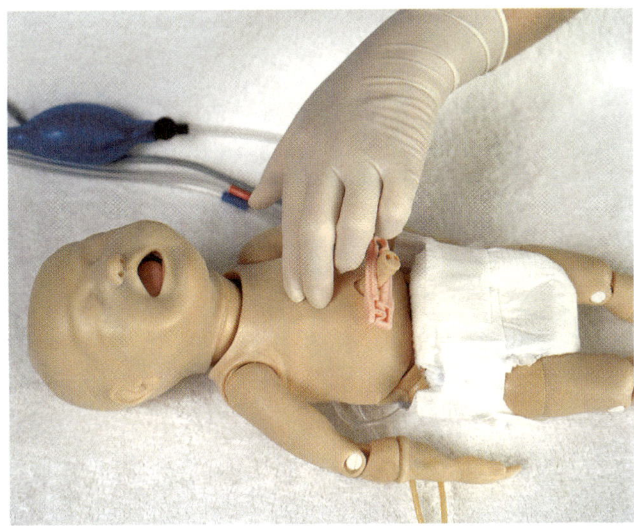

Fig. 15.32 PREMIE™ Blue Simulator with SmartSkin™ Technology (Photo courtesy of Gaumard® Scientific 2012. All rights reserved)

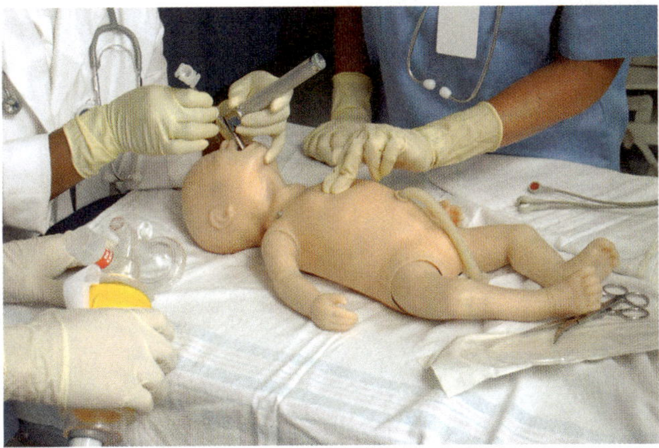

Fig. 15.33 SimNewB® (Photo courtesy of Laerdal Medical. All rights reserved)

SimNewB (Laerdal)

SimNewB represents a 7 lb newborn that is capable of simulating initial tone (limp, normal tone, spontaneous movement, seizures, etc.), cyanosis, and crying (Fig. 15.33). There is an umbilicus with two arteries and one vein all of which can be cannulated. It includes a standard monitor with the same features and properties of the other Laerdal simulators. This simulator can be intubated. There is no fontanelle and a peripheral venous catheter cannot be performed.

Part-Task Trainers

Historically nursing literature documents the use of leg and arm models to learn bandaging in 1874 [15]. Many healthcare practitioners have experienced the use of various foods (oranges to learn injection techniques) or body parts (bones for intraosseous line placement [16]) to learn procedure-specific skills. Modern task trainers, however, generally take plastic form and allow for basic skill acquisition in a safe, risk-free environment. Perhaps the most familiar are compression models used for cardiopulmonary resuscitation training.

Part-task trainers (PTTs) represent a continuum of the mannequin-based simulation spectrum. Cooper and Taqueti define a PTT as one that replicates only a portion of a complete process or system [17]. Most PTTs utilized in healthcare incorporate only the relevant anatomical section pertinent to a particular procedural skill. There is a significant body of scholarly work documenting the effectiveness of PTTs [18]. Part-task trainers are often the most commonly utilized modality for myriad reasons including cost, size, and risk. Part-task trainers can be effectively used to teach novices the basics of psychomotor skills [19] and can allow for maintenance and fine-tuning of expert skills. Many centers find that PTTs minimize wear and tear and hence maintenance costs for high-fidelity mannequins when capabilities are duplicated. Part-task trainers, similar to mannequin-based simulators, also vary in their fidelity and features ranging from PTTs constructed of common household objects to highly evolved PTTs capable of complicated virtual tasks (see Chap. 16). In a 2008 article, Cooper and Taqueti noted over 20 types of PTTs available or in development [20]. At the time of this writing, the list is significantly longer. This section seeks to outline the various major categories and uses of anatomically based PTTs in four categories: (1) airway management, (2) invasive procedures, (3) skills-based teaching, and (4) learning and special situations, primarily surgical.

Airway Management

Airway management skills require considerable practice to acquire competency. There are multiple PTTs that replicate various portions of the anatomic airway with varying degrees of realistic head, neck, and chest anatomy (Figs. 15.34 and 15.35). These trainers allow for skill development in bag-valve masking, placement of nasal airways, oral airways, endotracheal tubes, and supraglottic devices as well as tracheostomy care (Fig. 15.36). Some airway PTTs offer sufficiently correct bronchial anatomy for fiberoptic bronchoscopy and even foreign body removal. At least one study showed that trainees can develop responses to and skill in management of emergency airway situations [21]. In addition, PTTs have been developed for attaining competency in rescue airway skills such as cricothyrotomy and tracheotomy (Fig. 15.37).

Invasive Procedures

Suturing and Knot Tying Trainers

Many healthcare providers have tied their first surgical knots on peg boards using recycled equipment. Specialized knot

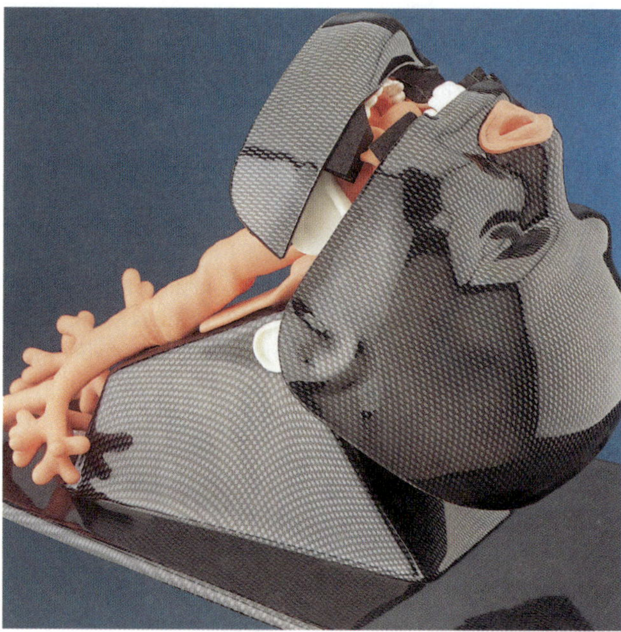

Fig. 15.34 AirSim Bronchi provides anatomically correct detail down to the fourth-generation bronchi (Photo courtesy of Trucorp, Ltd. All rights reserved)

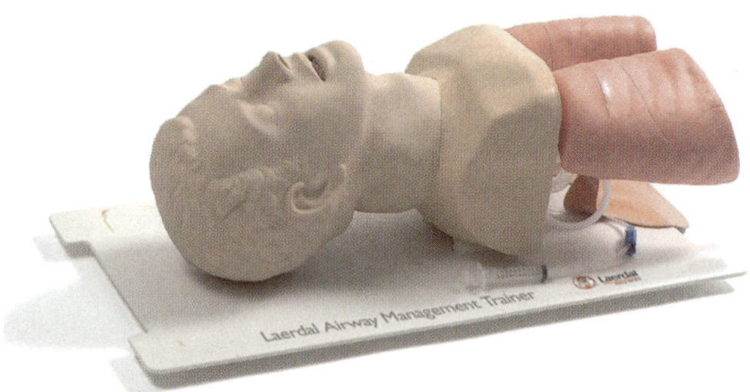

Fig. 15.35 Laerdal® Airway Management Trainer (Photo courtesy of Laerdal Medical. All rights reserved)

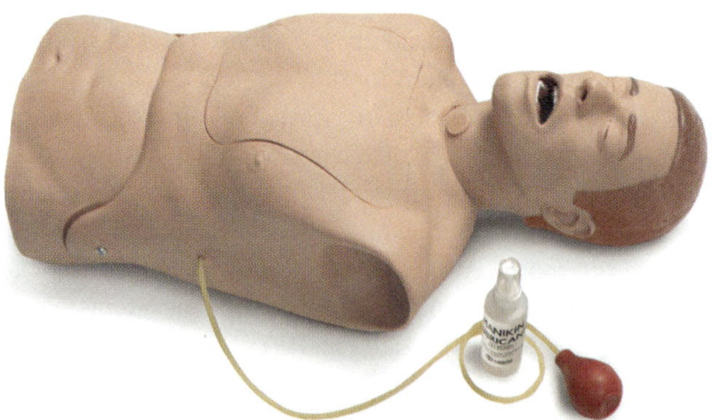

Fig. 15.36 Laerdal NG Tube and Trach Care Trainer (Photo courtesy of Laerdal Medical. All rights reserved)

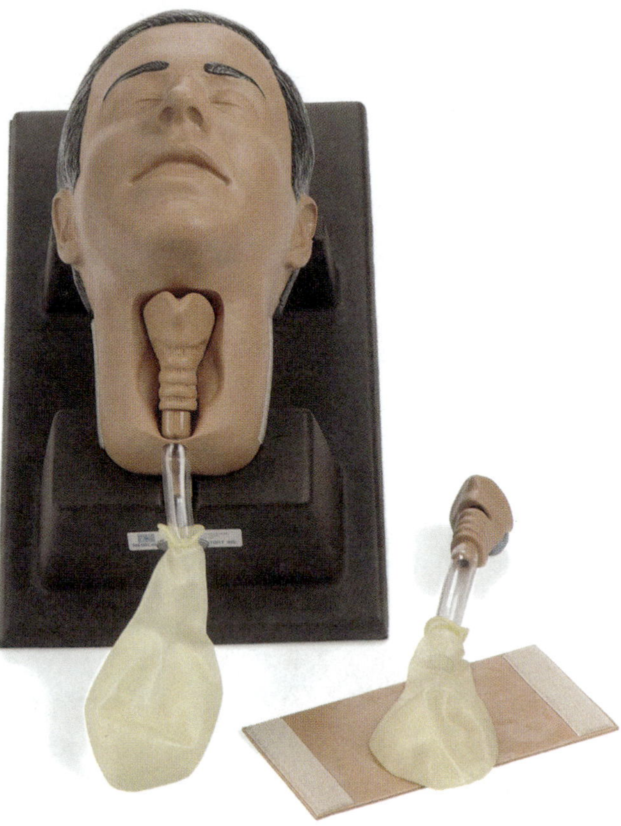

Fig. 15.37 Cricoid Stick Trainer allows practice of surgical cricothyrotomy skills (Photo courtesy of Laerdal Medical. All rights reserved)

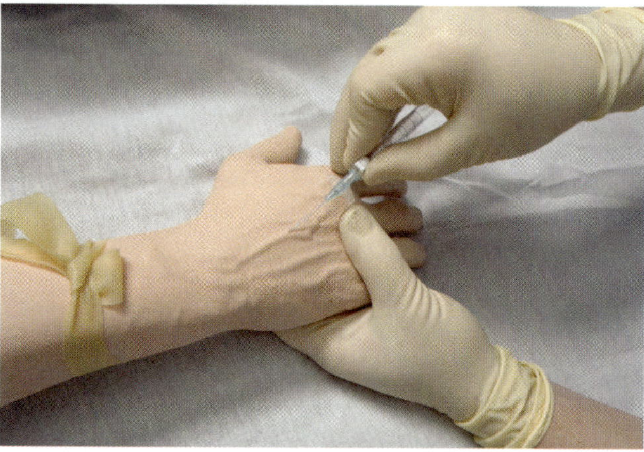

Fig. 15.38 Laerdal IV Training Arm has replaceable skin and veins designed for peripheral intravenous therapy (Photo courtesy of Laerdal Medical. All rights reserved)

tying boards and surgical skills development platforms are also available for this purpose. Suture practice arms and hands made with soft vinyl skin over stitchable foam are useful for cutting and laceration repair. Models have also been developed to teach laparotomy opening and closing with attention to the layers of the abdominal wall.

Intravenous Access

Venipuncture PTTs, often models of arms or hands, are widely used in healthcare training. Intravenous (IV) access arms come with differing sizes and depths of veins (Figs. 15.38 and 15.39). These PTTs allow learners to

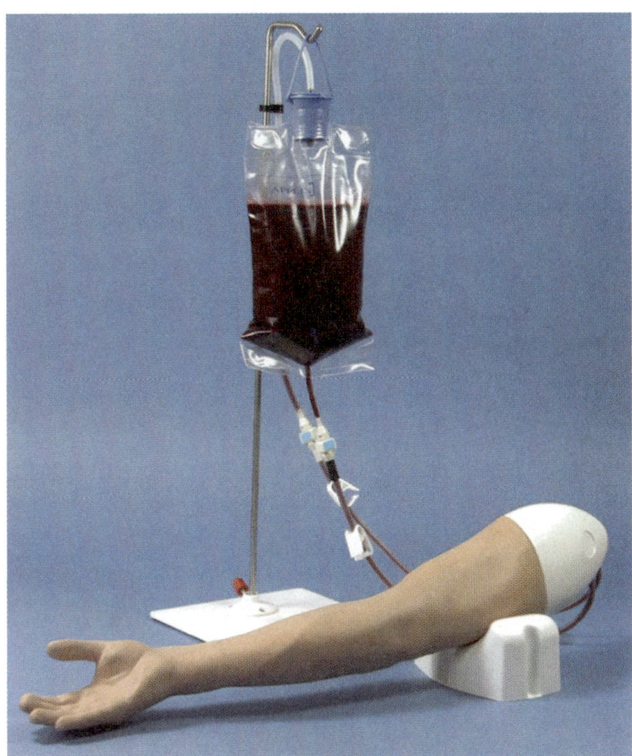

Fig. 15.39 Standard venipuncture arm (Photo courtesy of Limbs & Things ©2012 www.limbsandthings.com)

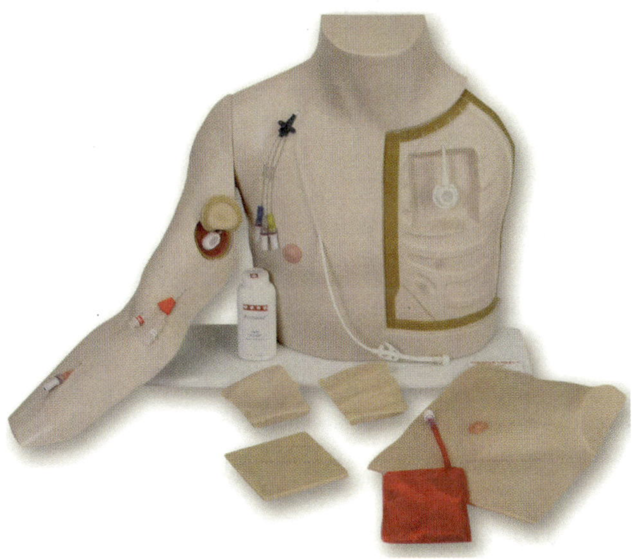

Fig. 15.40 Chester Chest™ (Photo courtesy of Vata, Inc. ©2012 www.vatainc.com)

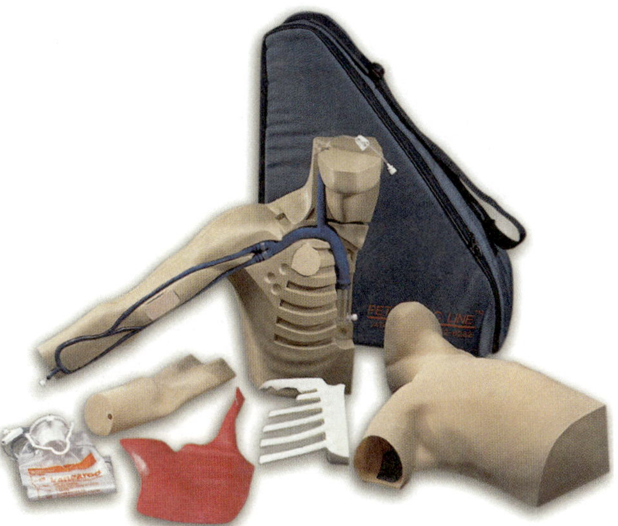

Fig. 15.41 Peter PICC Line™ (Photo courtesy of Vata, Inc. ©2012 www.vatainc.com)

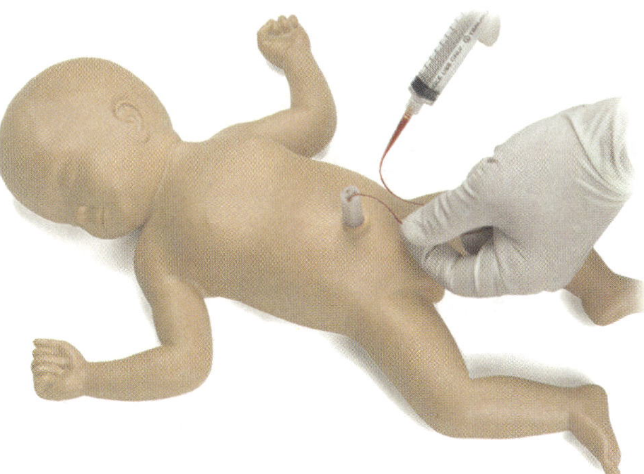

Fig. 15.42 Baby Umbi: female newborn infant reproduction designed for the practice of umbilical catheterization (Photo courtesy of Laerdal Medical. All rights reserved)

become comfortable wearing gloves and using sterile technique. Some models have the ability to demonstrate a realistic "flashback" of simulated blood to confirm proper needle placement and may have veins which "roll." Others allow for injection of fluids and withdrawal of blood.

Central line PTTs are also widely available some of which are adaptable for the use of ultrasound (Figs. 15.40 and 15.41). Currently models are available that allow for central vascular catheterization using the subclavian, supraclavicular, internal jugular, and femoral approach and are available in both adult and pediatric sizes. Infant and neonatal trainers are available for umbilical venous (Fig. 15.42) and arterial line as well as intraosseous line placement (Fig. 15.43). Significant research has documented that important patient safety goals can be met with intentional practice by trainees prior to performing these skills in the clinical setting [22].

Arterial puncture PTTs are available with a variety of features for blood collection and/or catheterization including palpable arterial pulsation and natural flashback of artificial blood.

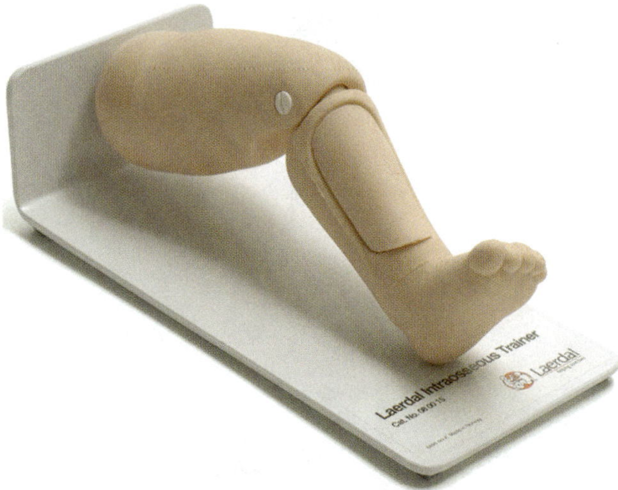

Fig. 15.43 Laerdal intraosseous trainer (Photo courtesy of Laerdal Medical. All rights reserved)

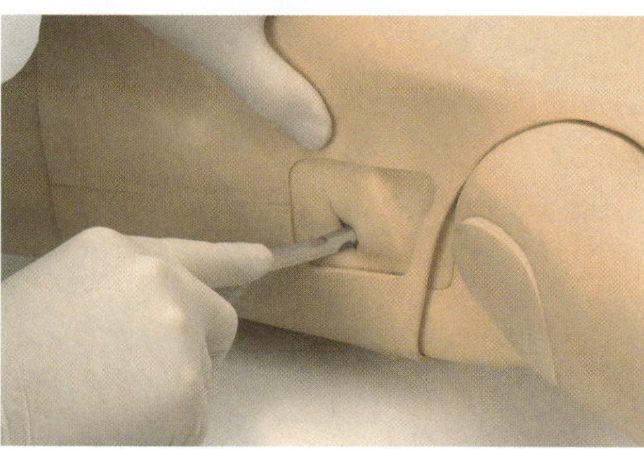

Fig. 15.45 Chest tube placement (Photo courtesy of Laerdal Medical. All rights reserved)

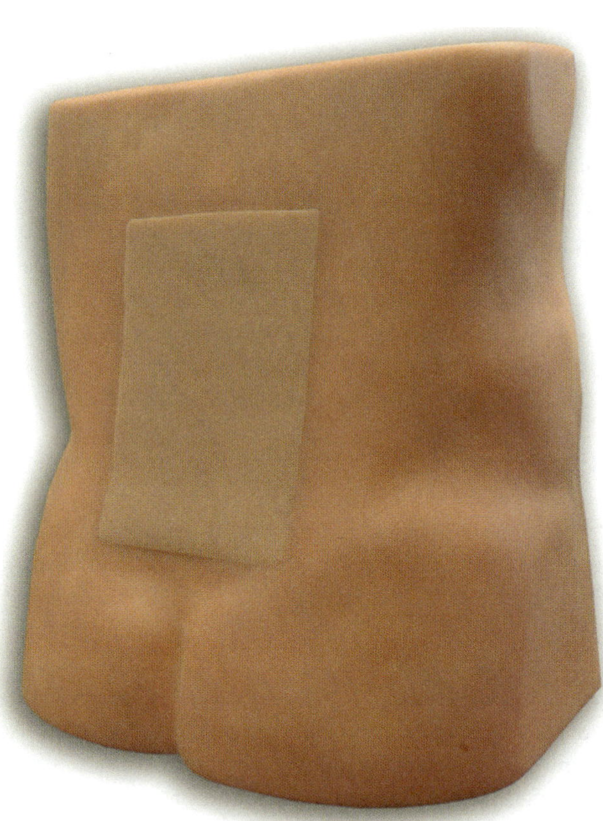

Fig. 15.44 Lumbar puncture/epidural trainer (Photo courtesy of Simulab. All rights reserved)

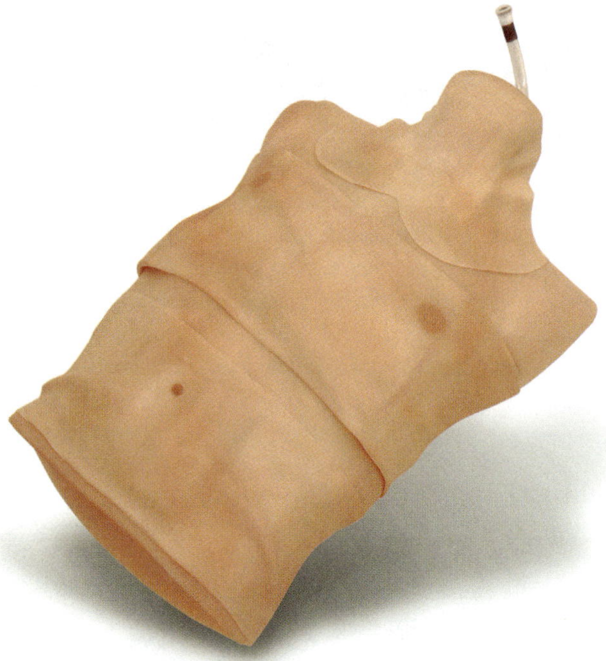

Fig. 15.46 TraumaMan® (Photo courtesy of Simulab. All rights reserved)

Lumbar Puncture and Epidural Trainers

Several lumbar puncture and epidural PTTs are commercially available (Fig. 15.44). Both infant and adult models have been used in educational settings [23]. An area of active research is looking at the transferability to the clinical setting of simulated lumbar puncture training [19].

Thorax Procedures

While many of the full-body mannequins offer the capability for needle thoracostomy, chest tube placement (Fig. 15.45), paracentesis, and pericardiocentesis, many centers find it helpful to utilize procedure-specific PTTs to assist in developing competency for each. Indeed, it is now common for torso-based surgical PTTs such as TraumaMan® (Fig. 15.46) to be used as part of Advanced Trauma Life Support (ATLS) courses [24]. In addition, PTTs are available for teaching the concepts of closed water-seal drainage systems as well as their setup and maintenance.

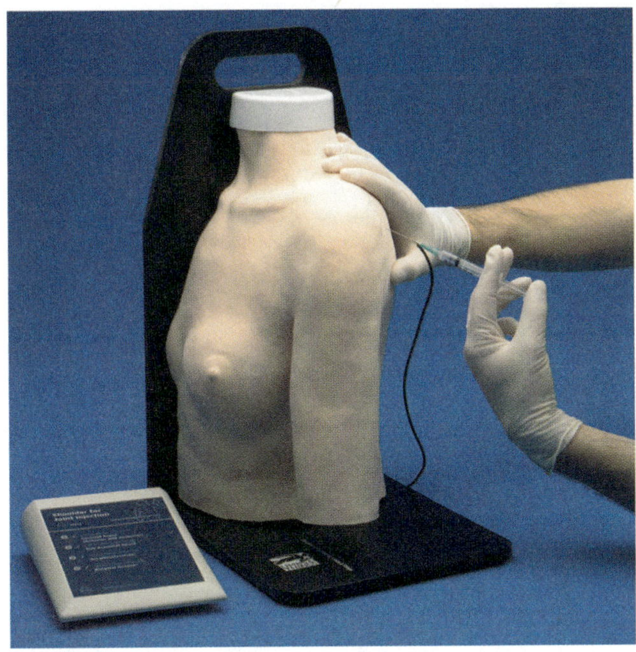

Fig. 15.47 Shoulder for joint injection (Photo courtesy of Limbs & Things ©2012 www.limbsandthings.com)

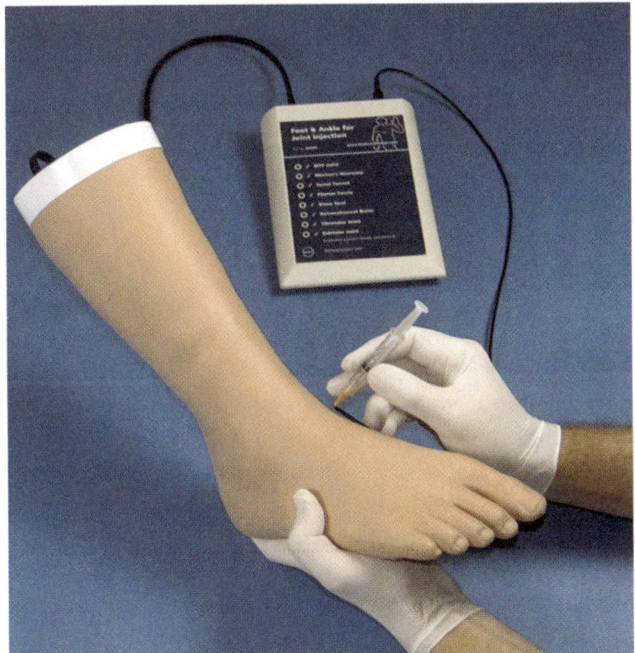

Fig. 15.48 Foot and ankle for joint injection (Photo courtesy of Limbs & Things ©2012 www.limbsandthings.com)

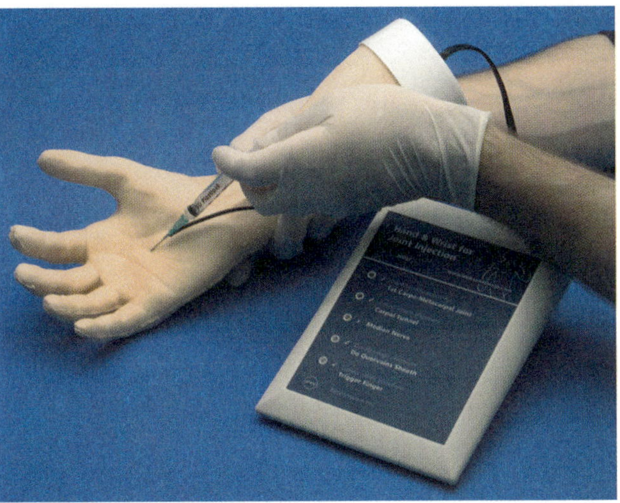

Fig. 15.49 Hand and wrist for joint injection (Photo courtesy of Limbs & Things ©2012 www.limbsandthings.com)

Orthopedic Joint and Anesthetic Block Trainers

Injection models are available for the shoulder, pelvis, lumbosacral spin, elbow, wrist, hip, ankle, and knee (Figs. 15.47, 15.48, and 15.49). Several models give audio feedback when an internal structure is touched with an errant needle. Part-tasks trainers for complex regional and central block techniques are also available.

Other Skills-Based Teaching and Learning

Breast Exam Trainer

Several breast examination PTTs are available for and may include the axillary and/or clavicular regions. Some breast exam PTTs may be worn like a costume and comes with interchangeable inserts to allow for identification of masses of various sizes and consistencies. This model can be used in integrated simulations.

Prostate Exam Simulator/Pelvic Examination Trainers/Urinary Catheter Trainers

Multiple PTTs are available for both anatomic instruction and procedural practice of male and female urinary catheter placement and perineal care (Fig. 15.50). Pathological conditions involving the prostate and colon can be varied in some models. There is a normal feeling of resistance and pressure as a catheter passes through the urethra, and artificial urine flows through the catheter when it enters the bladder. Pelvic simulators are designed to facilitate pelvic examination and tumor detection (Fig. 15.51). Basic simulators allow for palpation and manipulation of bony landmarks and organs, while more advanced simulators are designed for surgical procedures such as pelvic floor reconstruction.

Nasogastric Tube and Tracheostomy Care Trainers

Several PTTs been developed for instruction in the care of patients with tracheostomies and, in many cases, include the ability to place nasogastric tubes and practice gastrointestinal care via nasal and oral routes. In addition to commercially

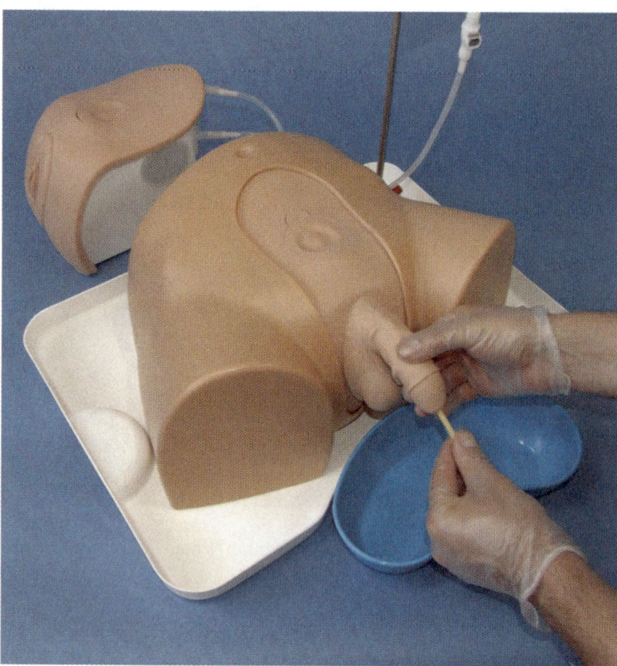

Fig. 15.50 Advanced catheterization trainer (Photo courtesy of Limbs & Things ©2012 www.limbsandthings.com)

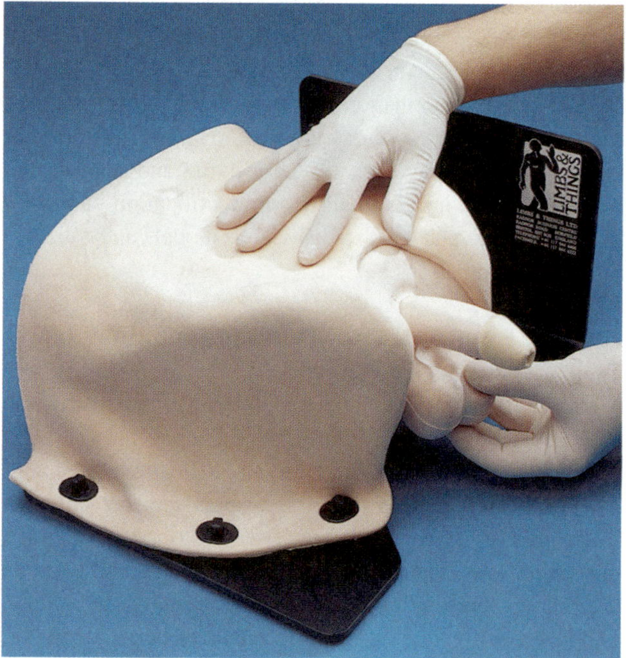

Fig. 15.51 Clinical male pelvic trainer designed for testicular and rectal examination (Photo courtesy of Limbs & Things ©2012 www.limbsandthings.com)

available trainers, low-cost alternatives have been published [25, 26].

Ear and Eye Exam Models

Ear PTTs are available which allows for examination of the tympanic membrane directly with an otoscope and can also be used to practice earwax and foreign body removal. Eye PTTs have also been designed to allow for fundoscopic exam with variable slides, depth, and pupil diameter.

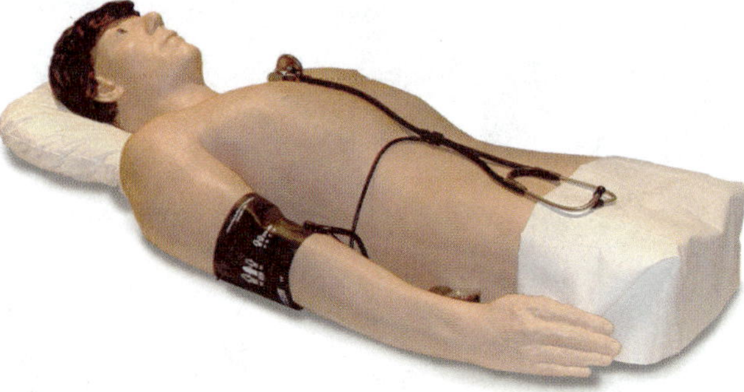

Fig. 15.52 Harvey® the Cardiopulmonary Patient Simulator (Photo courtesy of Laerdal Medical. All rights reserved)

Harvey®

Harvey® was the first cardiopulmonary simulation system introduced in 1968 at the American Heart Association Scientific Sessions (Fig. 15.52). Harvey® can demonstrate almost any cardiac condition by varying blood pressure, heart sounds, pulses, and respirations. Learners can view bilateral jugular venous pulse waveforms and arterial pulses as well as precordial impulses. Harvey® is a proven system to teach transferrable bedside skills and improve learner confidence and diagnostic abilities [27–29]. Harvey® now comes with a computer-based curriculum that allows for user-driven learning as well.

Surgical Simulators

There are multiple forms of surgical simulators currently available: nonanatomic, anatomic, and virtual. Some surgical simulators are not anatomically correct and, in fact, may not resemble anatomy at all because they focus on the handling of instruments used to perform surgery. The number of anatomically based surgical trainers on the market is currently growing and includes the recent release of Surgical Chloe™ by Gaumard (Figs. 15.53 and 15.54), a full-body surgical simulator that incorporates the lifelike use of real surgical instruments. Virtual surgical simulators are the most common and are discussed in Chap. 16.

PTT Development

There is active PTT development ongoing at many simulation centers around the world. In part driven by local factors and most certainly by cost, many innovative models are being developed, exhibited in posters, and published in journals such as the Journal of the Society of Simulation in Healthcare. Many surgical centers are using PTTs in combination with biological tissue to teach thoracic and cardiovascular surgical skills [30, 31]. A middle fidelity model for

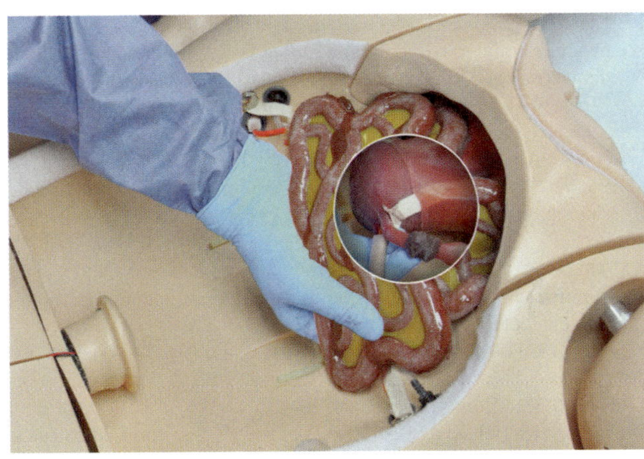

Fig. 15.53 Surgical Chloe™ S2100 (Photo courtesy of Gaumard® Scientific 2012. All rights reserved)

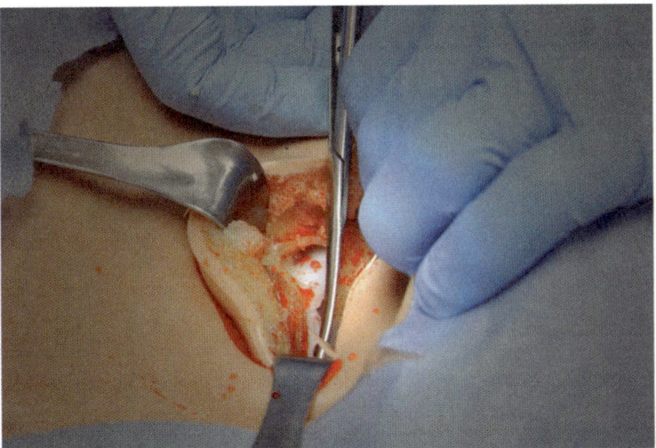

Fig. 15.54 Surgical Chloe™ S2100 (Photo courtesy of Gaumard® Scientific 2012. All rights reserved)

teaching a laparoscopic pyloromyotomy has been demonstrated to have face and content validity [32]. Urologists report the use of boar urinary tract mounted in an acrylic frame [33]. Emergency physicians at Evanston Northwestern Healthcare developed a homemade simulated sheep trachea holder with a skin layer that bleeds to improve their cricothyrotomy training as well as adapted on older airway trainer to simulate epistaxis [34]. Emergency physicians at the University of Alabama at Birmingham have developed an ultrasound-friendly model to measure intraocular pressure. Other emergency physicians have developed a PTT for pericardiocentesis which can be constructed in a home kitchen [35]. Models to teach inguinal anatomy and exploration of common bile duct anatomy are also available in part-task, low-fidelity formats.

The widespread use and value of part-task-trainers cannot be underestimated. However, their ultimate impact on patient care is likely to be magnified when their ability to simulate psychomotor skills can be placed in a critical thinking environment [36]. Unlike many of the full-mannequin simulators which allow for inputs by programmers and interaction or physiologic variability, part-task trainers are primarily designed to be used in a static environment. Improvements in these devices have generally been the development of virtual environments. However, an important trend is the combination of part-task trainers with either standardized patients (live actors) or full-mannequin simulators to allow for task completion in a more fully immersive environment [14, 37].

Conclusion

Mannequin-based simulators have become common place in the education of healthcare providers either as full-body high-fidelity simulators or part-task trainers. High-fidelity mannequin-based simulators are computer-controlled manufacturer-specific platform that may be model-driven (autonomous), operator-driven, or a combination of each. The variety of features currently available allows for realistic interaction and intervention and typically includes some level of automation using a variety of sensors. As technology continues to advance, the hope is that future models will include an even more expanded list of features. The ability of mannequins to move purposefully will greatly enhance the fidelity of simulation scenarios. In addition, though some mannequins can produce sounds that mimic cough and regurgitation, physical cough and regurgitation are also desirable. New technology will likely enhance the ability of mannequin skin to better mimic conditions such as cyanosis, rashes, hives, diaphoresis, and the ability to change temperature. The ability of mannequins to interface with more advanced monitoring modalities (e.g., electroencephalography, bispectral index) will also greatly enhance the simulated experience as well. Many of these desirable features are already available as homemade or third-party add-ons but will hopefully become integrated into future mannequin offerings.

References

1. Bloom BS. Taxonomy of educational objectives; the classification of educational goals. 1st ed. New York: Longmans, Green; 1956.
2. Iglesias-Vazquez JA, Rodriguez-Nunez A, Penas-Penas M, Sanchez-Santos L, Cegarra-Garcia M, Barreiro-Diaz MV. Cost-efficiency assessment of Advanced Life Support (ALS) courses based on the comparison of advanced simulators with conventional manikins. BMC Emerg Med. 2007;7:18.
3. Wayne DB, Didwania A, Feinglass J, Fudala MJ, Barsuk JH, McGaghie WC. Simulation-based education improves quality of care during cardiac arrest team responses at an academic teaching hospital: a case–control study. Chest. 2008;133(1):56–61.
4. Fraser K, Wright B, Girard L, et al. Simulation training improves diagnostic performance on a real patient with similar clinical findings. Chest. 2011;139(2):376–81.
5. Mayo PH, Hackney JE, Mueck JT, Ribaudo V, Schneider RF. Achieving house staff competence in emergency airway management: results of a teaching program using a computerized patient simulator. Crit Care Med. 2004;32(12):2422–7.

6. Owen H, Mugford B, Follows V, Plummer JL. Comparison of three simulation-based training methods for management of medical emergencies. Resuscitation. 2006;71(2):204–11.
7. Donoghue AJ, Durbin DR, Nadel FM, Stryjewski GR, Kost SI, Nadkarni VM. Effect of high fidelity simulation on Pediatric Advanced Life Support training in pediatric house staff: a randomized trial. Pediatr Emerg Care. 2009;25(3):139–44.
8. Rodgers DL, Securro Jr S, Pauley RD. The effect of high fidelity simulation on educational outcomes in an advanced cardiovascular life support course. Simul Healthc. 2009;4(4):200–6.
9. Marshall RL, Smith JS, Gorman PJ, Krummel TM, Haluck RS, Cooney RN. Use of a human patient simulator in the development of resident trauma management skills. J Trauma. 2001;51(1):17–21.
10. Knudson MM, Khaw L, Bullard MK, et al. Trauma training in simulation: translating skills from SIM time to real time. J Trauma. 2008;64(2):255–63; discussion 263–4.
11. Hoadley TA. Learning advanced cardiac life support: a comparison study of the effects of low- and high fidelity simulation. Nurs Educ Perspect. 2009;30(2):91–5.
12. Campbell DM, Barozzino T, Farrugia M, Sgro M. High fidelity simulation in neonatal resuscitation. Paediatr Child Health. 2009;14(1):19–23.
13. Cherry RA, Williams J, George J, Ali J. The effectiveness of a human patient simulator in the ATLS shock skills station. J Surg Res. 2007;139(2):229–35.
14. Sawyer T, Hara K, Thompson MW, Chan DS, Berg B. Modification of the Laerdal SimBaby to include an integrated umbilical cannulation task trainer. Simul Healthc. 2009;4(3):174–8.
15. Lees FS, Acland HW. Handbook for hospital sisters. London: W. Ibister & Co.; 1874.
16. Ota FS, Yee LL, Garcia FJ, Grisham JE, Yamamoto LG. Which IO model best simulates the real thing? Pediatr Emerg Care. 2003;19(6):393–6.
17. Cooper JB, Taqueti VR. A brief history of the development of mannequin simulators for clinical education and training. Qual Saf Health Care. 2004;13 suppl 1:i11–8.
18. Nestel D, Groom J, Eikeland-Husebo S, O'Donnell JM. Simulation for learning and teaching procedural skills: the state of the science. Simul Healthc. 2011;6(Suppl):S10–3.
19. Kessler DO, Auerbach M, Pusic M, Tunik MG, Foltin JC. A randomized trial of simulation-based deliberate practice for infant lumbar puncture skills. Simul Healthc. 2011;6(4):197–203.
20. Cooper JB, Taqueti VR. A brief history of the development of mannequin simulators for clinical education and training. Postgrad Med J. 2008;84(997):563–70.
21. Ellis C, Hughes G. Use of human patient simulation to teach emergency medicine trainees advanced airway skills. J Accid Emerg Med. 1999;16(6):395–9.
22. Britt RC, Novosel TJ, Britt LD, Sullivan M. The impact of central line simulation before the ICU experience. Am J Surg. 2009;197(4):533–6.
23. Uppal V, Kearns RJ, McGrady EM. Evaluation of M43B Lumbar puncture simulator-II as a training tool for identification of the epidural space and lumbar puncture. Anaesthesia. 2011;66(6):493–6.
24. Block EF, Lottenberg L, Flint L, Jakobsen J, Liebnitzky D. Use of a human patient simulator for the advanced trauma life support course. Am Surg. 2002;68(7):648–51.
25. Pothier PK. Create a low-cost tracheotomy model for suctioning simulation. Nurse Educ. 2006;31(5):192–4.
26. Pettineo CM, Vozenilek JA, Wang E, Flaherty J, Kharasch M, Aitchison P. Simulated emergency department procedures with minimal monetary investment: cricothyrotomy simulator. Simul Healthc. 2009;4(1):60–4.
27. Ewy GA, Felner JM, Juul D, Mayer JW, Sajid AW, Waugh RA. Test of a cardiology patient simulator with students in fourth-year electives. J Med Educ. 1987;62(9):738–43.
28. Hatala R, Issenberg SB, Kassen B, Cole G, Bacchus CM, Scalese RJ. Assessing cardiac physical examination skills using simulation technology and real patients: a comparison study. Med Educ. 2008;42(6):628–36.
29. Issenberg SB, McGaghie WC, Gordon DL, et al. Effectiveness of a cardiology review course for internal medicine residents using simulation technology and deliberate practice. Teach Learn Med. 2002;14(4):223–8.
30. Carter YM, Marshall MB. Open lobectomy simulator is an effective tool for teaching thoracic surgical skills. Ann Thorac Surg. 2009;87(5):1546–50; discussion 1551.
31. Lodge D, Grantcharov T. Training and assessment of technical skills and competency in cardiac surgery. Eur J Cardiothorac Surg. 2011;39(3):287–93.
32. Plymale M, Ruzic A, Hoskins J, et al. A middle fidelity model is effective in teaching and retaining skill set needed to perform a laparoscopic pyloromyotomy. J Laparoendosc Adv Surg Tech A. 2010;20(6):569–73.
33. Grimsby GM, Andrews PE, Castle EP, Wolter CE, Patel BM, Humphreys MR. Urologic surgical simulation: an endoscopic bladder model. Simul Healthc. 2011;6(6):352–5.
34. Pettineo CM, Vozenilek JA, Wang E, Flaherty J, Kharasch M, Aitchison P. Simulated emergency department procedures with minimal monetary investment: cricothyrotomy simulator. Simul Healthc. 2009;4(1):60–4. doi:10.1097/SIH.1090b1013e31817b39572.
35. Daniel Girzadas D, Zerth H, Harwood R. An inexpensive, easily constructed, reusable task trainer for simulating ultrasound-guided pericardiocentesis. Acad Emerg Med. 2009;16(s1):S279.
36. Boet S, Borges BC, Naik VN, et al. Complex procedural skills are retained for a minimum of 1 yr after a single high fidelity simulation training session. Br J Anaesth. 2011;107(4):533–9.
37. Girzadas Jr DV, Antonis MS, Zerth H, et al. Hybrid simulation combining a high fidelity scenario with a pelvic ultrasound task trainer enhances the training and evaluation of endovaginal ultrasound skills. Acad Emerg Med. 2009;16(5):429–35.

16

Virtual Reality, Haptic Simulators, and Virtual Environments

Ryan Owens and Jeffrey M. Taekman

A good hockey player plays where the puck is. A great hockey player plays where the puck will be.
—Wayne Gretzky

Introduction

Traditional, ineffective forms of passive education are crumbling under the demands of learners who have grown up digital [1]. Today's learners use technology to communicate, to play, and to learn. In 2000, Charles Friedman wrote that medical education was "stuck in time" but predicted a paradigm shift in pedagogy enabled by new technologies [2]. Although technology-enabled education has been growing in popularity, the pedagogy behind online "lectures" remains the same. Passive lecture-based education is known to be ineffective in changing behaviors [3]. What is needed are interactive forms of online education that take full advantage of modern technology and are better aligned with modern learning theory.

Over the last decade, we have been witness to an explosive growth in the use of simulation in healthcare. As Gaba points out, "simulation is a technique, not technology" [4]. However, many of the tools we use in simulation are technology dependent, and computer capabilities are expanding rapidly. Moore's Law—the law that states computing power doubles every 18 months—shows no signs of slowing [5]. With improvement in computer and communication technology, we can expect incredible advances in learning technology.

R. Owens, MD (✉)
Department of Neurological Surgery,
Duke University Medical Center,
615 Morningside Dr, Durham, NC 28036, USA
e-mail: ryan.owens@duke.edu

J.M. Taekman, MD
Department of Anesthesiology, Duke University
School of Medicine, Durham, NC, USA

Department of Anesthesiology,
Human Simulation and Patient Safety Center,
Duke University Medical Center,
100 Trent Drive, Box 3094, Durham, NC 27710, USA
e-mail: jeffrey.taekman@duke.edu

Virtual reality (VR) is "a term that applies to computer-simulated environments that can replicate physical presence in places in the real world, as well as in imaginary worlds." Those familiar with early phases of virtual reality often conjure up images of head-mounted displays and data suits, but more recently virtual reality can also be used to describe highly visual, 3D environments developed with commercial game technology such as the UnReal Engine from Epic Games.

Today's video game players socialize, collaborate, and relax in shared virtual environments (VEs). As the technology behind video games improves, there has been a growing interest in using the technology for purposes beyond entertainment, the so-called serious games [6]. What constitutes a "game" versus a simulation is an ongoing debate, well beyond the scope of this chapter. We will take a high-level approach using the term games-based learning (GBL) to denote learning activities built upon video game technology. Whether the end product is a "game" or a simulation is immaterial, both are a means to the end—producing competent healthcare workers, able to care for patients safely and effectively in a rapidly changing environment.

This chapter focuses on simulation capabilities enabled by rapidly advancing computer and gaming technologies: virtual reality, haptics, and virtual environments. We will first consider procedural-based simulators and then turn our attention to virtual environments. The domains of procedural-based simulation and virtual environments are on a technological collision course. The end result will be new learning paradigms that empower a revolution in healthcare learning and assessment.

Virtual Reality and Haptic Simulators

With the creation of resident work hour limitations and subsequent decrease in operative training coupled with increased focus on patient safety and medicolegal concerns, surgical

A.I. Levine et al. (eds.), *The Comprehensive Textbook of Healthcare Simulation*,
DOI 10.1007/978-1-4614-5993-4_16, © Springer Science+Business Media New York 2013

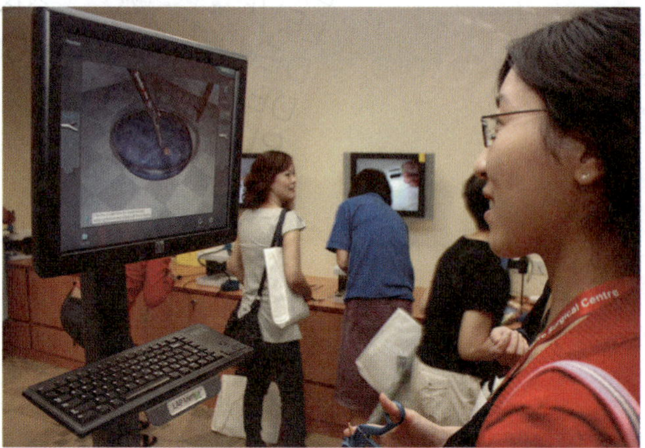

Fig. 16.1 Participants using virtual reality haptic simulators in a conference setting

education via the traditional Halsteadian route of teaching on live patients is becoming increasingly difficult. Currently, cadaveric dissection is the gold standard for such technical training. However, this is expensive, increases risk of disease transmission to the trainee, and cannot sufficiently replicate pathology the surgeon or proceduralist will see intraoperatively during practice—what you see is what you get. Models are another method of surgical training being used. However, most models such as saw bones are cumbersome and unrealistic and again fail to replicate pathology the surgeons might see in the operating room. Many disciplines (as evidenced by the depth and breadth of this book's content)—including general surgery, urology, otolaryngology and gynecology gastroenterology, and pulmonology—are turning to virtual reality haptic simulators to enhance surgical and procedural training away from the actual clinical environment as a solution to the aforementioned obstacles to training (Fig. 16.1).

These devices in general process a physical interface (e.g., laparoscopic instrument, laparoscopic camera, bronchoscope, or colonoscopes) that replicates the actual devices used in clinical practice, with respect to feel, heft, and controllers. The operator interacts with the virtual, computer-generated clinical environment (abdomen, tracheobronchial tree, colon) by engaging the physical device into a "mannequin". Moving the device (advancing, withdrawing, turning left and right) produces accurate movement in the virtual environment. The positioning of the physical device in the virtual environment produces images on the display, optional force feedback (i.e., haptics, see below) and tissue deformity (movement, bleeding, or procedural success). Many of these devices have additional ports where other instruments can be deployed into the virtual environment to replicate interventions (cutting, needling, suturing, irrigation, or lavage). Several even possess performance matrices (procedure time, motion economy, structures visualized) and standardized feedback can be generated and followed over time and used to compare individual performance or to compare individuals to one another. Figure 16.2 demonstrates a typical surgical virtual reality simulator.

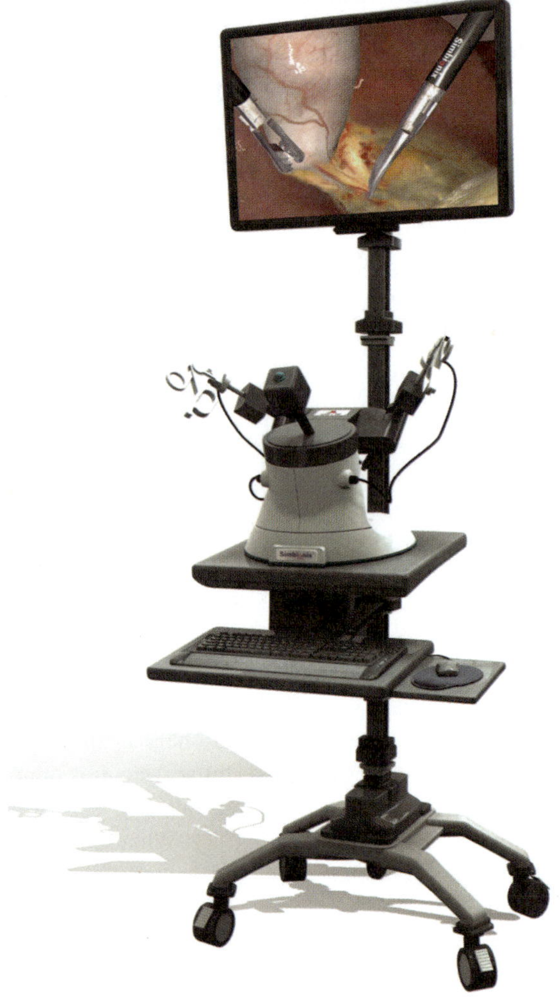

Fig. 16.2 LAP Mentor™ Express is a non-haptic laparoscopic training system provided at a lower cost. Available in either portable or optional tower including touch screen settings

Haptic feedback is defined as the combination of sensory input through the tactile receptors in the skin and the kinesthetic receptors in the muscles, tendons, and joints [7, 8]. Haptic surgical simulators have been created, most notably in laparoscopic surgery, but can now be found in nonlaparoscopic surgical subspecialties such as ear, nose, and throat, orthopedic, and neurological surgery. Surgical simulators in each area are reviewed below as well as pertinent studies evaluating the effectiveness of haptic feedback in enhancing surgical training.

Laparoscopic Surgical Simulators

General Surgery

The need for simulation in general surgery arose mostly for the introduction and popularization of laparoscopic surgery in the 1980s. Despite the small incisions and proposed "minimal access," it became quite clear it carried a higher complication rate and a steep learning curve for surgeons trying to adapt to this new technology [9]. Upon further investigations, it was found these deficiencies stemmed from psychomotor challenges related to the new cumbersome interaction with the videoscopic interface. Thus, a number of laparoscopic simulators were developed including but not limited to GI Mentor, ProMIS, LapSim Simulator, MIST-VR, and XiTact SA.

Within the last decade, the American College of Surgeons Residency Review Committee has mandated that all programs institute a skills laboratory curriculum with laparoscopic box trainers and virtual reality simulators as minimally acceptable equipment [8]. Haptic feedback distinguishes the box trainer from many of the virtual reality-based systems. However, more commonly, efforts are being made to equip the virtual reality simulators with adequate haptic feedback as exemplified by Procedicus, MIST, Lapsim, Reachin, and Virtual Endoscopic Surgery Trainer to create a more realistic feel to the virtual reality simulator.

The development and validation of a comprehensive fundamentals of laparoscopic surgery (FLS) was described by Peters et al. [10]. In this chapter, the importance of testing technical skills in laparoscopy was emphasized as a distinctly separate skill set that must be obtained by the practicing physician, and learning these skills can be accomplished outside of the operating theater [10]. The five tasks designed for evaluation are as follows: peg transfer, pattern cutting, ligating loop, suturing with an intracorporeal knot, and suturing with an extracorporeal knot. Figure 16.3a–g demonstrates the Simbionix Lap Mentor including the device (Fig. 16.3a), the instruments (Fig. 16.3b) and the screenshot portraying classic laparoscopic skills like peg transfers (Fig. 16.3c), and suturing (Fig. 16.3e). Completion is required for all trainees as of 2010 in order to sit for the American Board of Surgery exams.

Box trainers are used by several programs to enhance laparoscopic skills. Typically, these simulators use actual laparoscopic equipment including laparoscope, camera, light source, trocars, and authentic laparoscopic instruments. The instruments are placed into the training area via an opaque covering. The simulators usually require an experienced mentor and the trainee is evaluated on time to completion and number of errors. Studies show both improvement in laparoscopic skills and improved performance in the operative theater [11]. Although these simulators allow for haptic feedback while using authentic laparoscopic tools, the simulators lack the ability to simulate the actual surgery and are limited to fundamental skills.

Virtual reality simulators have risen in popularity secondary to success demonstrated in the aviation community and the demand for higher fidelity simulators capable of more than just simple task-oriented simulation. These simulators entail a virtual environment on a computer screen with three-dimensional graphics taken from actual MRI or CT scans. Instruments are created virtually that track the trainee's movement and updated in real time. Haptic feedback is included in the higher end simulators but with an increased cost and represents varying levels of realism.

Seymour et al. [9] validated the use of virtual reality in improving operating room performance. Sixteen surgical residents at various levels of training were randomized into virtual reality trained group or a non-virtual reality trained group. The virtual reality group was trained on a MIST-VR laparoscopic trainer without haptic feedback. The results of the study showed that residents without virtual reality laparoscopic simulator training were nine times more likely to transiently fail in making progress, five times more likely to injure the gallbladder or burn nontarget tissue, and overall were six times more likely to commit errors.

The importance of haptic feedback in these simulators has been a subject of interest for some time. Panait et al. [8] examined the role of haptic feedback in laparoscopic simulation training by evaluating performance of medical students on two FLS tasks, peg transfer, and pattern cutting, on laparoscopic simulators with and without haptic feedback. In the simpler peg transfer, the study shows haptic feedback has no effect on performance; however, faster completion and a trend toward fewer errors were seen in the more complex pattern cutting task. The study concluded haptic feedback allows superior precision in more advanced surgical tasks.

In order to truly validate the importance of haptic feedback in laparoscopic simulators, it must be shown to enhance training when simulating actual surgical tasks. One study that examined this notion compared traditional box simulators with haptic feedback versus a VR laparoscopic simulator without haptic feedback. The study found participants significantly prefer haptic feedback when simulating an actual complex laparoscopic task [7]. Again, this study reiterates the finding that haptic feedback is preferred when simulating complex surgical tasks.

Alternatively, haptic feedback does not universally prove to be advantageous in the literature. Salkini et al. [12] investigate the role of haptic feedback on the Simbionix LapMentor II while performing three laparoscopic tasks in novice medical students. Similar to previous studies, the students were split into a haptic and a non-haptic group and asked to perform

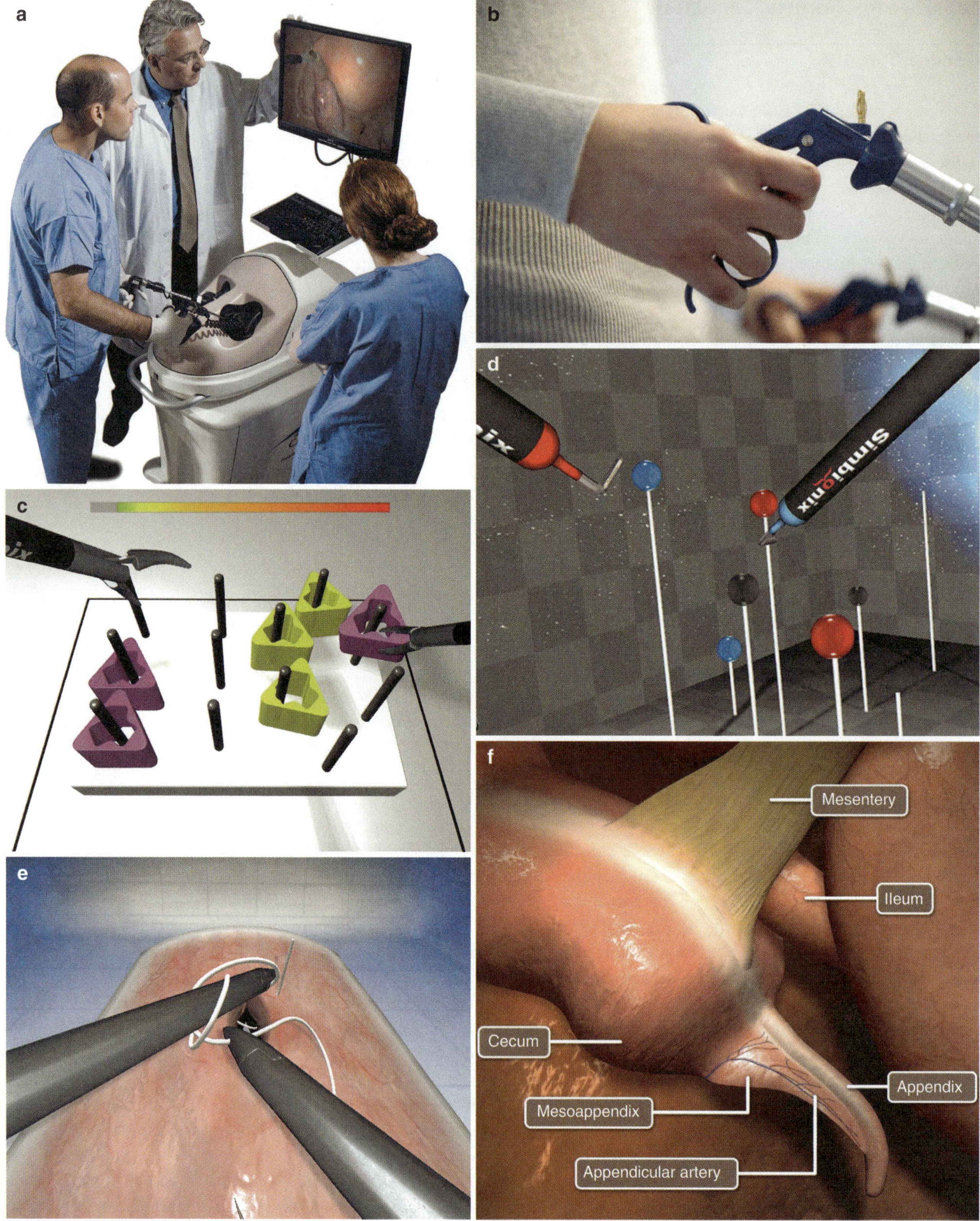

Fig. 16.3 (**a**–**g**) Device, instruments, and screenshots of the Lap Mentor (Photo courtesy of Simbionix)

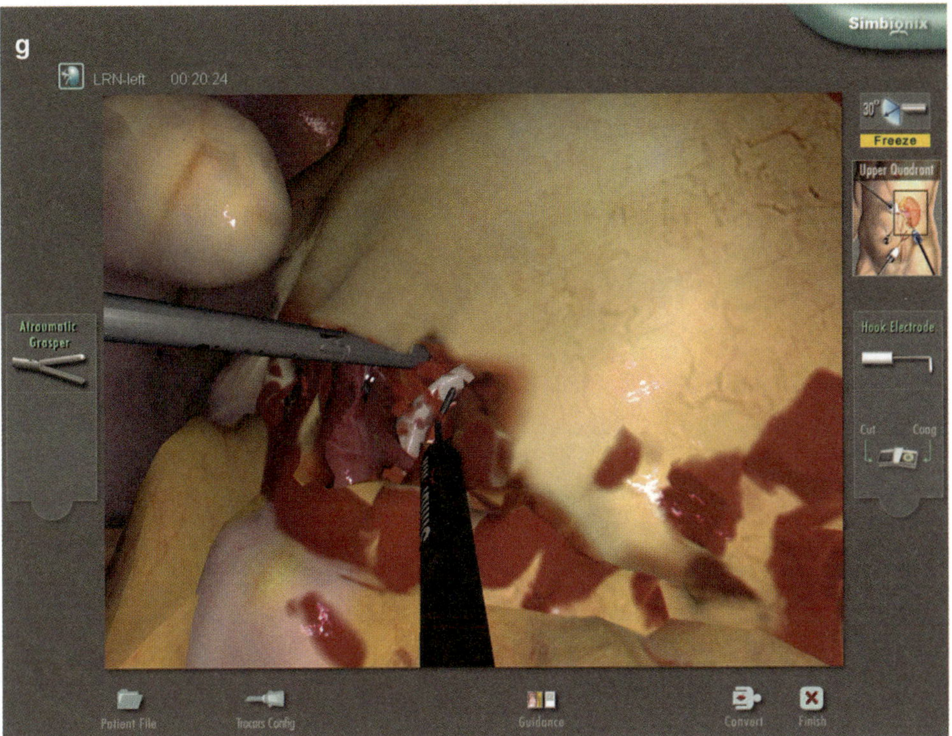

Fig. 16.3 (continued)

these tasks. No differences were noted between in speed, accuracy, or economy of movement between the two groups [12]. However, it should be noted that one of the tasks was clipping a tubular structure which was initially eliminated from FLS secondary to having no discriminatory value [10]. Overall, general surgery has been a pioneer in the creation and integration of haptic surgical simulation into the curriculum of surgical trainees.

Thoracic Surgery

Haptic simulators have also found a place in the training of thoracic surgeons. Solomon et al. [13] have reported the development of a haptic enable virtual reality cognitive simulator for video-assisted thoracoscopic lobectomy (VATS). The simulator was created through adaptation of anatomy explorer models and a previously developed simulation engine. Cognitively, this simulator allows for 13 anatomic identifications and 20 high yield lung cancer learning points. The procedural components to the simulator allow for placement of trocars, manipulation of the thoracoscope for exploration of the pertinent anatomy, stapling, and haptic-enabled gross dissection of the lung tissue to expose underlying hilar structures [13].

Unfortunately, the simulator does not allow haptic feedback for fine motor tasks such as dissecting around the hilar vessels, and validation for this interface is ongoing. Additionally, the significance of the gross haptic feedback currently enabled in the current system has not been evaluated in regard to impact subsequent improvement in the operative theater. Nonetheless, this project represents the progression of haptic simulators to simulate actual procedures as opposed to fundamental training tasks in yet another subspecialty of surgery.

Gynecological Surgery

The use of laparoscopic simulators in gynecological surgery was recently detailed [11]. Training systems using virtual reality for laparoscopic bilateral tubal ligation, hysteroscopic resection of myoma, endometrial ablation, and removal of a tubal ectopic pregnancy have all been described. However, these are at various stages of development and validation. The use of haptic feedback in these simulators is currently unclear. Figure 16.4a–d shows gynecological surgery simulators in use, including the DaVinci robot simulation (Fig. 16.4d).

Non-laparoscopic Surgical Simulators

Otolaryngology

Haptic simulators have also been created for the field of otolaryngology in order to train residents in endonasal techniques as well as temporal bone dissection. Tolsdorff et al. [14]

reported a new virtual reality paranasal sinus surgery simulator. The simulator is a standard PC-based program with haptic feedback that presents a highly realistic environment to learn surgical anatomy and navigation in a complex anatomical space. Further studies are needed on this simulator to validate its usefulness in improving operative performance in residents [14]. Another endonasal simulator, the Endoscopic Sinus Surgical Simulator, has been studied and shown to have a positive effect on early operative performance of trainees [15].

Temporal bone dissection is another area of otolaryngology that has a haptic enable VR simulator currently studied for its use in self-directed learning. The CSIRO/University of Melbourne system is run on a standard desktop PC and utilizes a 3D model that the user interacts with through shutter glasses and haptic devices. This particular system was studied as a part of a randomized blinded control trial evaluating the role of this simulator in self-directed learning [16]. Two groups of medical students were randomly divided. One group received training via temporal bone models and video, whereas the other group underwent training on the VR simulator using self-directed curriculum. Afterward, both groups were given 1 h to complete a temporal bone dissection which was subsequently graded. Results indicated that the VR group showed better performance on all four outcome measures recorded in the study. Studies showing improved operative performance have yet to be performed with this model.

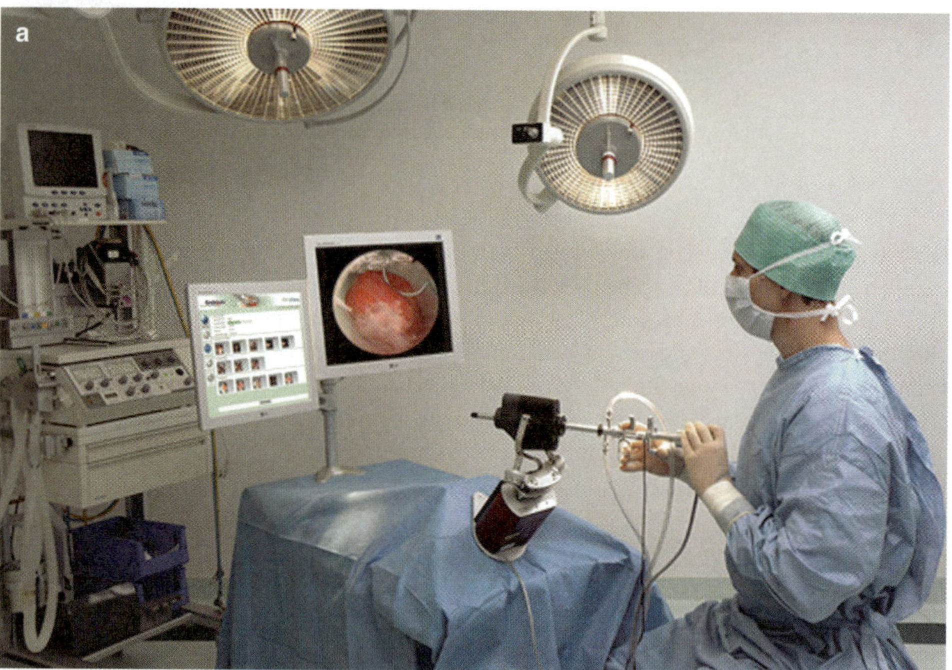

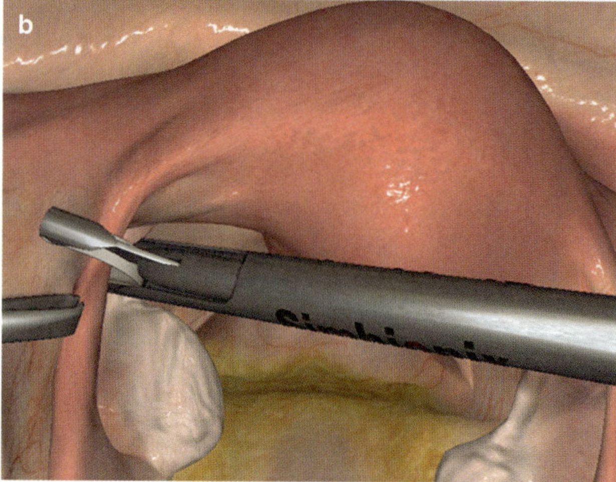

Fig. 16.4 (**a**–**d**) Gynecological surgery VR simulation (VirtaMed HystSim™) (Photo courtesy of Simbionix)

Fig. 16.4 (continued)

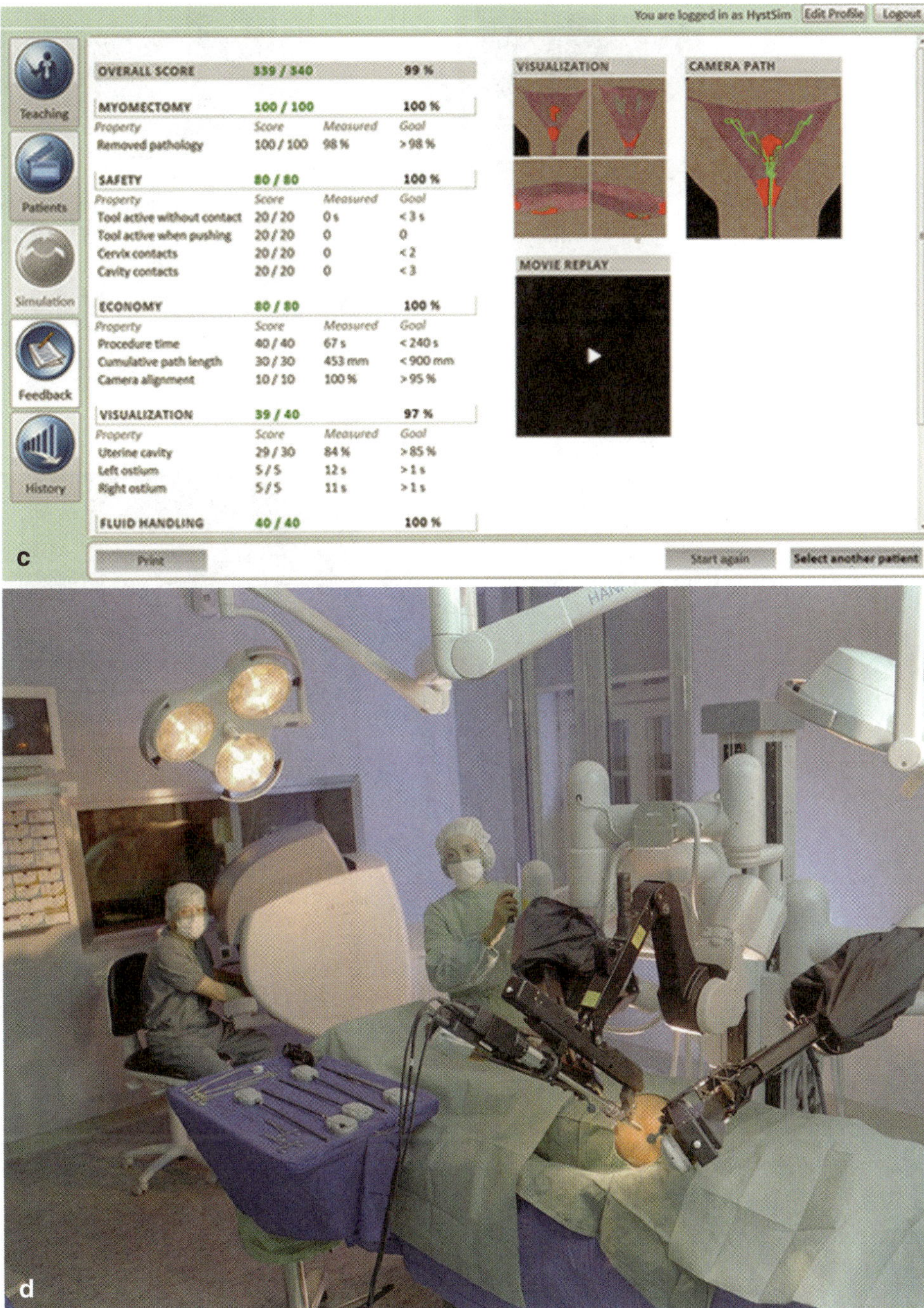

Orthopedics

Simulators have been introduced into orthopedic surgical training in the form of knee and shoulder arthroscopic simulators. A systematic review of knee and shoulder arthroscopy was performed evaluating five studies that investigated knee arthroscopy and four studies for shoulder arthroscopy [17]. These studies were all found to have high levels of internal validity and consistency for computer simulation. In the nine studies evaluated, one study investigated the transfer of knee arthroscopic skills from the simulator to the operative theater [18]. Twenty junior orthopedic trainees were randomized to two groups with one group trained on the simulator with expert supervision while the other group observed diagnostic arthroscopy in the operative theater. Afterward, the participants were graded in the operative theater based on global assessment scale as well at the Orthopedic Competence Assessment Project score. Results show the simulator group outperformed the non-simulator trained group on both, concluding that these skills do in fact translate to performance in

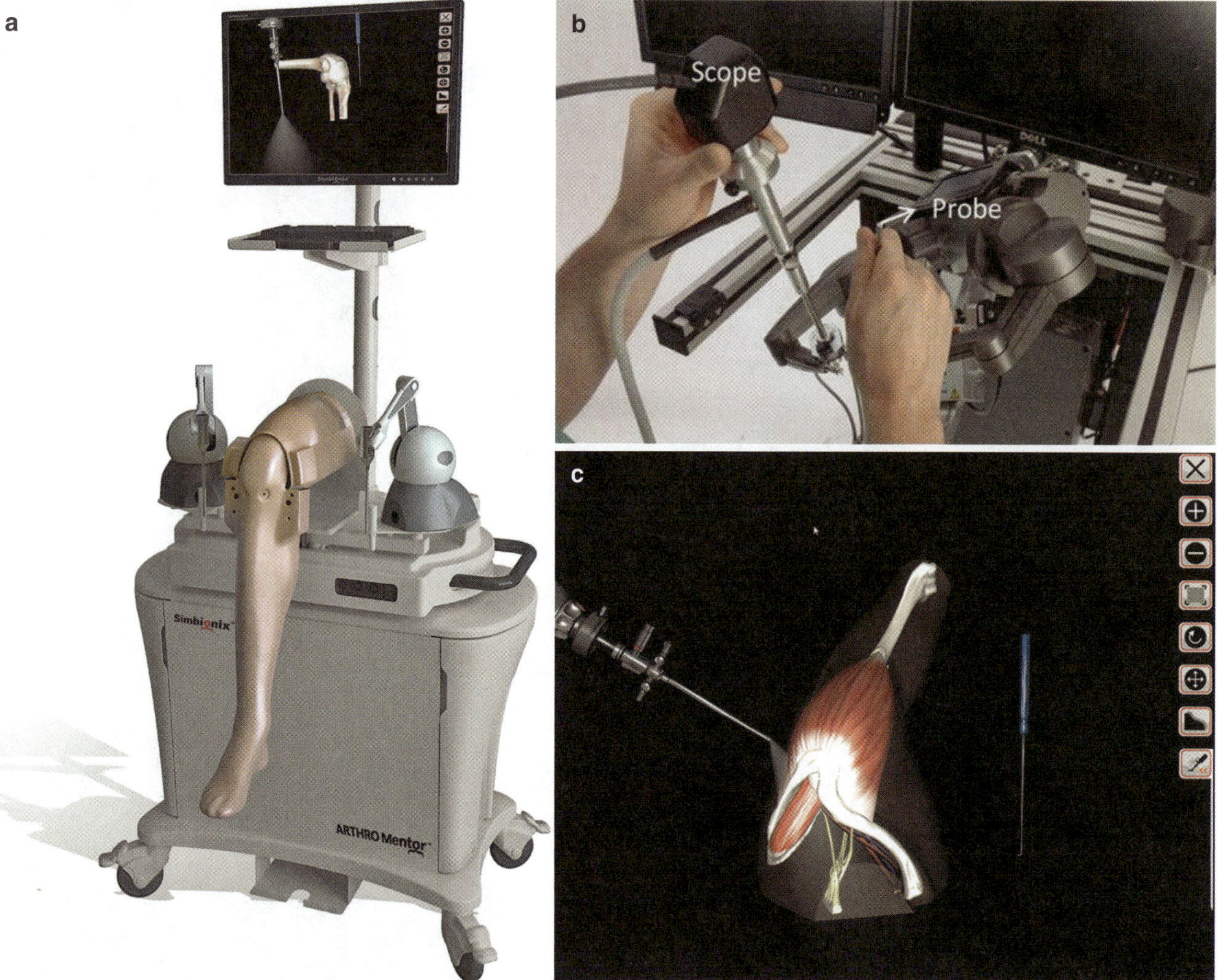

Fig. 16.5 (a–c) Arthro Mentor (Photo courtesy of Simbionix)

the operative theater. The role of haptic feedback was not evaluated in these studies. Figure 16.5a–c shows an orthopedic VR simulator, including the device, the hand controls, and a screenshot.

Neurological Surgery

VR simulators in neurological surgery have been created for the areas of cranial skull base surgery, neuro-oncology, ventriculostomy placement, and placement of spinal hardware. In skull base surgery, Dextroscope was created initially as a tool to create patient-specific volumetric models that can be manipulated in 3D space with the use of handheld controllers. The Dextroscope was originally designed to assist in operative planning and to evaluate 3D anatomy prior to operative intervention [19–21]. Wong et al. [22] created a procedural application for this model that allowed clipping of intracranial aneurysms [22]. To our knowledge, there are no current studies that have looked at enhancement of trainee performance on this simulator. Another simulator that is increasing in popularity in neurological surgery is the ImmersiveTouch. This system improves on the concept of Dextroscope by the addition of electromagnetic head-tracking goggles that allows a user-centered stereoscopic perspective and the addition of haptic feedback [23]. Using this simulator, trainees can perform a virtual ventriculostomy. In addition to this module, ImmersiveTouch also has a spine module that recreates the placement of pedicle screws for spinal fixation. Studies are currently ongoing regarding the transfer of these skills to the operative theater [21].

More recently, a haptic-enabled VR simulator has been created called NeuroTouch. The main components are a stereo vision system and bimanual haptic tool manipulators. The simulation software engine runs three processes for computing graphics, haptic feedback, and mechanics [24]. The goals of this training system are to safely remove the tumor without damaging normal tissue with an ultrasonic aspirator and to maintain hemostasis using bipolar cautery. The prototypes are currently being dispersed throughout training programs in Canada for beta testing and validation.

Procedural-based simulation is advancing rapidly and is on a collision course to intersect with other forms of simulation and visualization enabled by the rapid advancement of technology.

Nonsurgical Procedural Simulators

Endovascular Simulators

Endovascular interventions are another area of medicine where simulation has been utilized. Much of this discipline is becoming more minimally invasive with the creation of endovascular technologies. As we have seen in laparoscopic surgery, these minimally invasive techniques can possess a steep learning curve due to decreased tactile feedback and working in a 2D environment. Currently, several high-fidelity endovascular simulators are commercially available including Procedicus VIST, Angio Mentor, and Sim Suite. These simulators offer haptic, visual, and aural interfaces in order to create a lifelike environment to perform the procedures. In particular, coronary artery stenting and peripheral angioplasty are simulated and appear to be the most studied.

Three studies performed using Procedicus VIST simulator show simulator use improves procedure time, contrast volume used, and fluoroscopy time [25–27]. Furthermore, the simulators were shown to have good construct validity given the ability to consistently distinguish novice from expert as well as show significant improvement with practice in novice users. In peripheral artery angioplasty, similar results were found in similar studies [28, 29]. However, Chaer et al. went one step further and performed the first randomized trial to show translation of endovascular simulation skills to the clinical environment [30]. The study concluded residents trained on the simulator scored higher on a global rating scale for performance than those without training. Thus, it is likely simulation training in vascular surgery will become increasingly integrated into resident training. Figure 16.6 shows VR endovascular simulators in use.

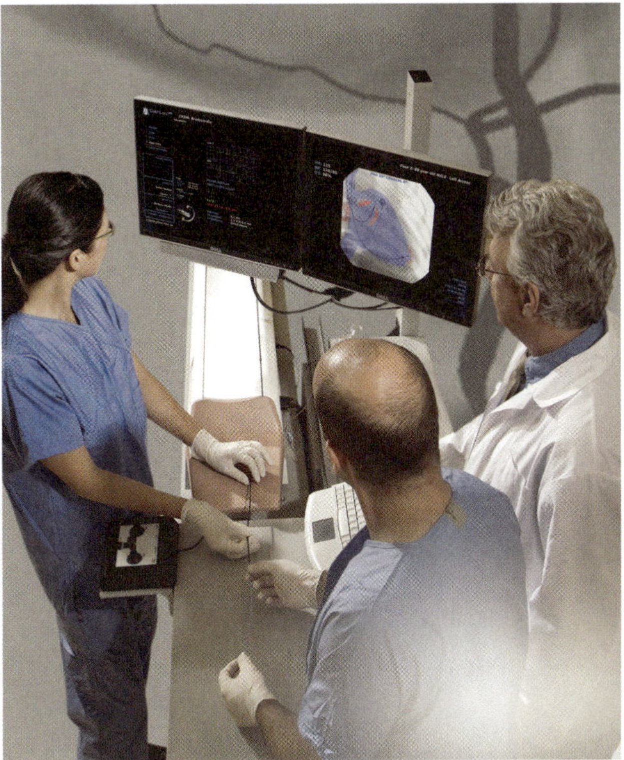

Fig. 16.6 VR endovascular simulation (Photo courtesy of CAE Healthcare ©2012 CAE Healthcare)

Bronchoscopy

Bronchoscopy is performed by anesthesiologist, cardiothoracic and trauma surgeons, critical care physicians, and otolaryngologists. Training on these procedures varies across disciplines and institutions. Proficiency is currently based on a minimum number of procedures to perform at many facilities. Several virtual reality high-fidelity simulators, including Accutouch bronchoscopy simulator (CAE) (Fig. 16.7) and GI Bronch Mentor (Simbionix) (Fig. 16.7a, b), are currently available commercially. Several studies have documented improvement of skills with these simulators; for example, participants trained on the simulator are less likely to experience wall contact, red out, and complete the procedure more efficiently [31].

Endoscopy

Gastroenterologist also utilizes virtual reality simulators in order to train for endoscopic procedures. The bronchoscopy simulators mentioned above also possess endoscopy capabilities. There are two simulators currently on the market for use, Accutouch from CAE and GI Bronch Mentor. Both are virtual reality simulators equipped with haptic feedback (Figs. 16.7, 16.8a–c, and 16.9).

Multiple types of endoscopes are available depending on the procedure being simulated; both upper and lower GI endoscopy can be replicated. These simulators also involve upper and lower endoscopic procedures and are complete with haptic feedback. Comprehensive metrics are also included with these model [32]. Although studies have shown the GI Bronch Mentor to have good construct validity and improve skills when tested on a simulator, there are no

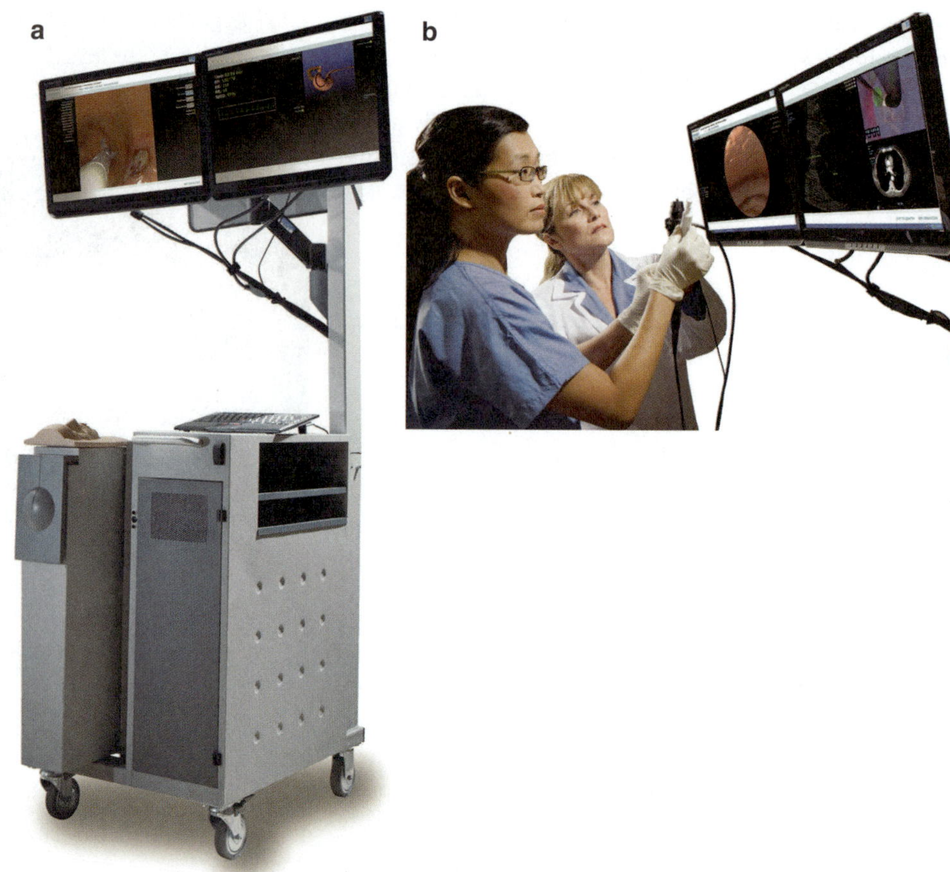

Fig. 16.7 (**a**, **b**) Accutouch endoscopy simulator (Photo courtesy of CAE Healthcare © 2012 CAE Healthcare)

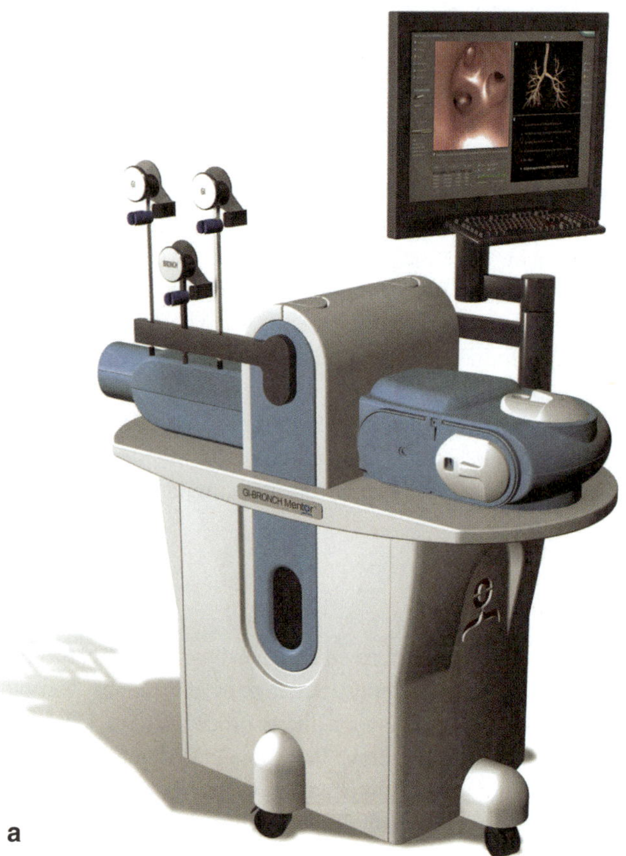

Fig. 16.8 (**a–c**) Use of the GI Bronch Mentor (Photo courtesy of Simbionix)

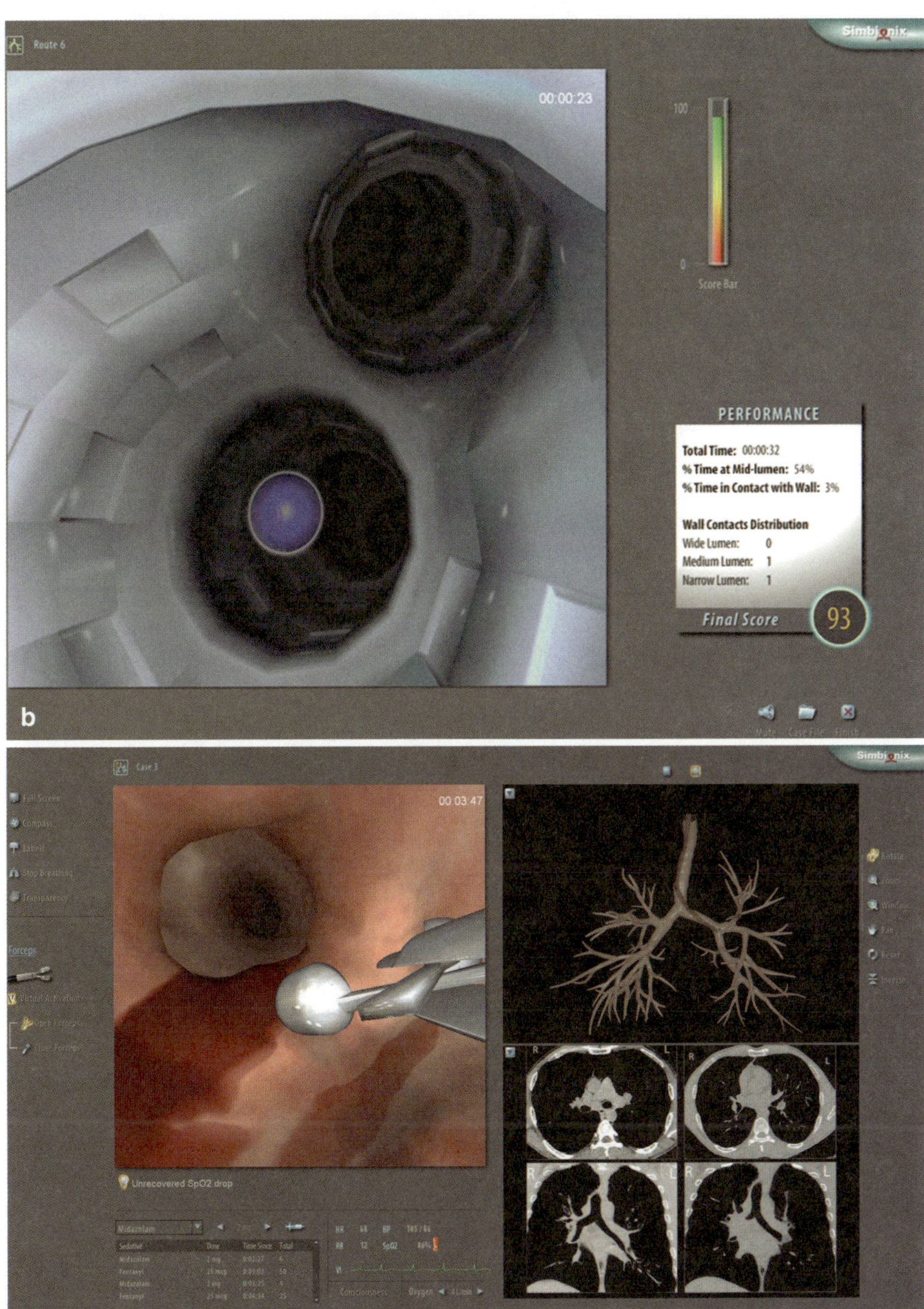

Fig. 16.8 (continued)

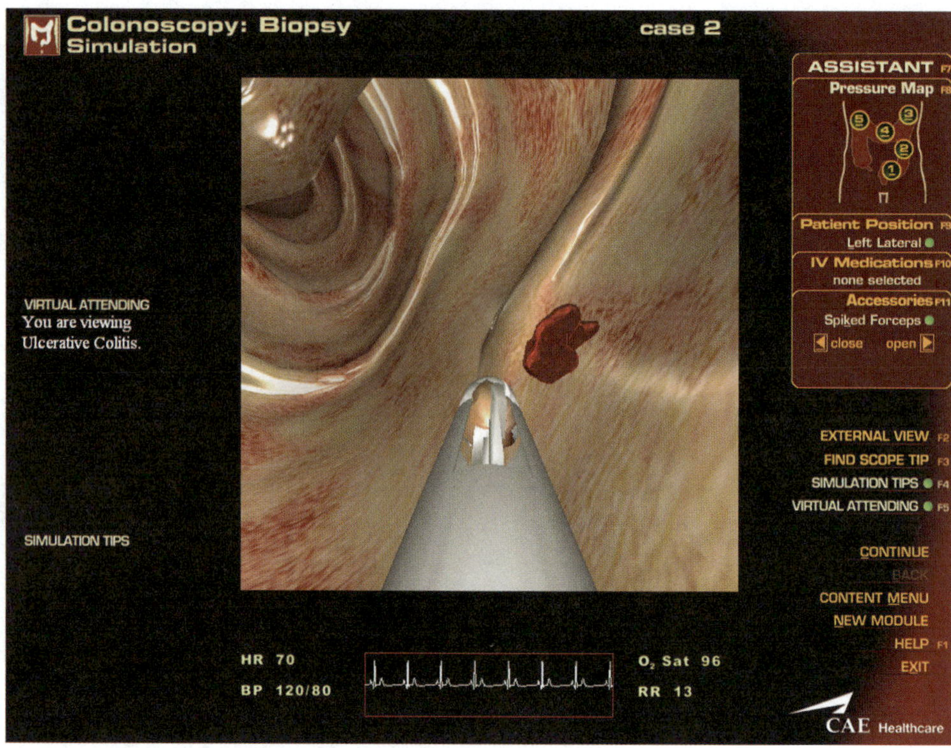

Fig. 16.9 A screenshot of the colonoscopy module from the Accutouch endoscopy simulator (Photo courtesy of CAE Healthcare © 2012 CAE Healthcare)

studies that describe transfer of these skills to a clinical environment.

Virtual Platforms and Environments

Technological advancement is accelerating and so too are changes in healthcare. The purpose of healthcare education is to train workers who can competently care for their patients today while building a foundation for lifelong learning.

The need for lifelong learning in healthcare's rapidly changing environment prompted the American Board of Medical Specialties (ABMS) and its 24 member boards in 2000, to promote Maintenance of Certification (MOC) to "evolve recertification programs towards continuous professional development" [33]. Continuous professional development requires objective proof that the workers' practice is improving. These demands are forcing a shift in healthcare pedagogy toward interactive forms of learning formats capable of changing behavior.

Although the system targets competence for its workforce, many of us aspire to become experts in our field. According to Ericsson et al., the development of expertise requires 10,000 h of deliberate practice [34]. Deliberate practice is *not* time spent in patient care; instead, it requires time rehearsing, practicing, and reflecting on one's actions—striving to improve with each and every repetition.

Deliberate practice is hard work, requiring motivation, endurance, and a grasp of domain-specific nuances of behavior. Unlike other domains where deliberate practice has been studied (e.g., music, chess playing), healthcare professionals cannot easily or ethically "practice" with live patients [35]. Through various forms of simulation, healthcare workers now have tools to aid in their pursuit of expertise.

Unfortunately, today's physical simulators, because of their high cost, limitations on learner throughput, and need for highly trained facilitators, offer limited opportunities for deliberate practice—there simply are not enough simulators or facilitators to handle the sheer number of hours required.

What is needed is a robust, scalable, easily accessible, personal, interactive learning platform that enables learners to practice new skills, make mistakes, receive immediate feedback, and reflect on how they might improve—a scalable platform for deliberate practice. What is needed is the Ultimate Learning Platform.

The Ultimate Learning Platform

What might this Ultimate Learning Platform look like? In science we are often taught to visualize the end product first (e.g., a table or figure) and design our experiment backward from there. If we use the same approach for healthcare learning, the Ultimate Learning Platform would have the following features (Table 16.1).

Table 16.1 Features of the Ultimate Learning Platform: a comparison of mannequin-based learning (MBL), procedural simulation (procedural), single-player games-based learning (GBL single), and multiplayer games-based learning (GBL multi)

Features of the Ultimate Learning Platform	MBL	Procedural	GBL (single)	GBL (multi)
Interactive	×	×	×	×
Participate individually		×	×	
Participate in teams	×			×
Peer instruction	×		×	×
Engages multiple senses	×	×	×	×
Sense of touch	×	×		
Offers immediate feedback	×	×	×	×
Opportunity for reflection	×	×	×	×
Self-paced reflection		×	×	
Chaining		×	×	×
Individual remediation		×	×	
Inexpensive to build				
Inexpensive to maintain			×	×
Accessible 24/7/365			×	×
Accessible from anywhere			×	×
Mobile delivery			×	×
Learning at the point of care	×		×	×
On-demand/just-in-time delivery			×	
Self-directed		×	×	
Facilitator independent		×	×	×
Self-paced learning		×	×	
Scalable			×	×
Distributable			×	×
Personalized			×	
Adaptive			×	×
Adjustable levels of fidelity			×	×
Back-end analytics		×	×	×
Automated assessment		×	×	×
Expandable content	×		×	×
Extensible platform			×	×
Reusable assets	×	×	×	×
Augment reality		×	×	×
Manipulate time	×	×	×	×
Standardize experience		×	×	×
Learners remain anonymous		×	×	×

- Interactive—Interactivity is a key element in engagement and information retention. It is also a key to changing learner behaviors [36]. Unlike current passive learning (e.g., lectures), the Ultimate Learning Platform would offer a high level of interactivity as well as immediate feedback to the learner.
- Participate individually or in teams (especially interprofessional teams)—Healthcare is delivered in teams. There is a national push for interprofessional education with physicians, nurses, and other health professionals learning side by side. The Ultimate Learning Platform would provide profession-specific topics for learners to master individually. Once competence is reached, the learner would participate in a "capstone" exercise with learners from other professions—applying their new knowledge in a realistic interprofessional exercise.
- Social—Peer instruction enhances learning and is far more effective than traditional, passive forms of education [37, 38]. The Ultimate Learning Platform not only would enable learners to interact with one another at a distance but also would offer learning exercises designed to encourage peer-to-peer interaction. Using data fed to a central learning management system,

groups could be automatically (or manually) matched based on performance or other criteria (e.g., disparate learning styles) to optimize group dynamics.

- Engage multiple senses—The more senses engaged in the learning process, the stronger the imprint in our memory. Uni-sensory (reading) or dual-sensory (lectures) learning experiences do not engage multisensory pathways and, thus, likely result in a suboptimal learning [39]. The Ultimate Learning Platform would engage multiple senses throughout the learning process.
- Offers immediate feedback—Immediate feedback, with time for reflection, is crucial for learning, mastery, and engagement [40]. The Ultimate Learning Platform would offer immediate and constant feedback to the learner at every phase of the learning process.
- Allows time for reflection—Individual reflection following feedback is critical in the learning process. Experience, feedback, reflection, and repetition are the cycle required for mastery. The Ultimate Learning Platform would allow adequate time for reflection/deliberate practice.
- Builds on and reinforces previously learned concepts—When learning complex tasks, the most powerful learning exercises offer small, incremental doses of experience that build upon one another. Complex tasks should be broken down to key components, each component sequentially practiced until mastery is achieved. This approach, known as "concurrent chaining," is a more efficient and effective method of learning complex tasks than an attempting to master an entire complex behavior at once [41]. The Ultimate Learning Platform would have a library of complex tasks for the learner to master, one step at a time.
- Allows remediation—Despite numerous barriers, individuals, hospitals, and health systems all learn through failure [42]. When a failure occurs, the learner must reflect and then try alternative pathways to the desired goal. The Ultimate Learning Platform would offer frequent feedback and remediation should the learner not perform a task adequately, allowing them to learn from their failure and repeat the exercise until success is achieved.
- Inexpensive—Lecture-based education has endured for so long partly due to its relatively low cost when compared to other educational methods. Interactive methods such as mannequin-based learning (MBL) or problem-based learning, because of their small learner-to-facilitator ratios, are more labor intensive and thus costly. The Ultimate Learning Platform would be inexpensive—offering interactivity while minimizing the need for numerous (expensive) trained facilitators. Further savings would be realized through the reuse of objects (e.g., art work, animations) that could be reused ad infinitum.
- Accessible 24/7/365, from anywhere—Today's learners have grown up with the world of information at their fingertips [43]. Learners want access to education where ever they may be—at the hospital, at home, or while commuting. The Ultimate Learning Platform would be accessible 24 h a day, 7 days a week, and 365 days a year through a variety of platforms (e.g., computers, iPad, or Smart Phones).
- Mobile delivery inside and outside of the hospital—Healthcare workers are highly mobile. In a single day a physician may work in numerous disparate locations. The Ultimate Learning Platform would be available at all times on a variety of devices, regardless of the user's location.
- Just-in-time delivery—Learning is enhanced when new information can be applied immediately [3]. The Ultimate Learning Platform would contain a broad range of material, allowing the learner to experience disease states, procedures, pieces of equipment, or other critical events just prior to needing the information for patient care.
- Self-directed—Lifelong learning requires a balance between mastering new information, staying current in the areas you are passionate about, and filling educational gaps. Every learner is unique in their learning pace, style, interests, and needs. The Ultimate Learning Platform would accommodate for these differences, offering a balance between what the learner needs and what they desire.
- Self-paced—Most interactive healthcare education occurs in groups, giving each individual little control over the pace of their learning. Within groups, it is likely some members master information more quickly than others, leading to learning disparities between group members. The Ultimate Learning Platform would allow learners to master core concepts at their own pace. Only after mastering core concepts would group activities be opened to the individual. Should they need more time to master a group concept, the platform would search for and recommend supplemental learning experiences.
- Scalable/distributable—Current methods of interactive learning do not scale well to large learning communities (e.g., team training for an entire health system). The Ultimate Learning Platform would be able to scale to accommodate the learning needs of an individual, a small group, or multiple hospitals.
- Personalized—Every learner is different. Each has their own learning strengths, weaknesses, and style.

The Ultimate Learning Platform would personalize education playing on the individual's strengths and minimizing or augmenting their weaknesses.

- Adaptive—Different learners master concepts at different speeds. It may take one learner a week to master concept that another grasps the same material within minutes. The Ultimate Learning Platform would adapt to these differences and offer level-appropriate learning content to the end user.
- Adjustable levels of fidelity—Maran and Glavin suggested that fidelity has two dimensions: psychological (does the task match the behaviors needed to be accomplished in the real world) and engineering (does the simulation "look" real) [44]. Although a great deal of emphasis has been placed on engineering fidelity in healthcare simulation (adding significantly to cost), psychological fidelity is much more important when learning [45]. The Ultimate Learning Platform would allow adjustable levels of psychological and engineering fidelity appropriate to the learner and the learner's task at hand.
- Back-end analytics—The speed and power of computers and communication networks continues to grow. We now have the opportunity to aggregate and analyze huge repositories of data. The Ultimate Learning Platform would collect learning information and feed it into a data warehouse. The aggregated data, when analyzed, could enable a revolution in healthcare learning. Through analyzing large information sets, we would have objective data to guide the development of more efficient and efficacious methods of mastery learning.
- Expandable and extensible—The equipment, process, and procedures in healthcare change rapidly. The Ultimate Learning Platform should be expandable and extensible to meet these needs—new modules and features added individually over time, expanding the overall breadth of content and capabilities of the system.
- Reusable—Elements within a learning platform should be reusable. For instance, a piece of equipment, avatar, or animation needs to be modeled once. It can then be reused infinitely in thousands of new modules with little additional incremental cost. Although the cost of the Ultimate Learning Platform is high initially, the cost falls substantially over time.

Table 16.2 Major developers of virtual environments in healthcare

	Virtual Heroes	SAIC	Breakaway Games	Clinispace
Location	North Carolina	Virginia	Maryland	California
Industry	Defense contractor	Defense contractor	Defense contractor	Education
Core game engine	Unreal/HumanSim	Unity/Olive 3D	Unity/Pulse!	Unity
Physiology	Engine (Body.dll)	Engine (HumMod)	No	Table based
Sample Projects	Zero Hour		Dental Implant Training	BattleCare
	HumanSim preview		Pulse!	
	Moonbase Alpha			

Video game technology, built specifically for education, could meet many of the criteria of the Ultimate Learning Platform (see Table 16.2).

Platforms

When building GBL, there are two alternatives. Develop the games in-house or contract with a vendor. At the time this was written, there are four major vendors focused on healthcare VEs: Clinispace, SAIC, Breakaway Games, and Virtual Heroes. Several universities also have site-based game development studios (e.g., University of Texas, Dallas). The technology behind VEs (and marketplace) is evolving quickly. For an overview of the vendors and their projects, see Table 16.2.

Emerging Trends That Will Influence the Future of Learning

As mentioned, the Ultimate Learning Platform does not yet exist. There are, however, several converging trends that lead us to believe video game technology will ultimately fulfill the need. These trends include: (1) the convergence of increasingly powerful computers and communication technologies, (2) the increase in popularity of online education, (3) the increasing use of simulation, and (4) push for "big data."

Convergence of Computers and Communication Technologies

The last decade has seen incredible growth of computer and networking power. These improvements have led to massive innovations in the capabilities of commercial game technology. With these changes, video games have moved from being an independent activity to highly collaborative, interactive, and engaging form of entertainment.

The lessons learned from video games, including fostering engagement, stoking motivation, and improving cognition, hold the promise of revolutionizing education. We can now build the next generation of interactive learning and assessment technologies—enabling an understanding of learning that heretofore has been unimaginable.

Rise of Online Education

Over the past decade, largely due to the increased power of computers and networking, there has been a massive shift toward online education. In 2010, 31 percent of higher education students took at least one course online [46]. Unfortunately, "online education" today still leaves much to be desired, relying heavily on passive, lecture-based material. Recently, in healthcare, there has been a call for a change in pedagogy, using technology to "flip" the classroom [47].

Our future vision of healthcare education includes an evidence-based, technology-enabled pedagogy that relies heavily on self-directed and peer-to-peer interactive learning. Resource intensive methods of teaching (e.g., MBL) will not be eliminated but instead will be reserved for capstone exercises or times when GBL lacks the proper capabilities (e.g., bag-mask ventilation when learning how to sedate a patient).

Rise of Simulation

The growth of simulation in healthcare has been nothing short of astonishing. We can use publications within a specialty to gauge growth. In a recent review by Ross, simulation manuscripts in the specialty journals of anesthesiology showed a 126% increase in a 3-year moving average between 2001 and 2010. The vast majority of publications in anesthesiology utilized mannequins and were focused primarily on learning (as opposed to other uses such as process improvement) [48]. The majority of simulation was mannequin based. Other specialties, such as surgery, might have different ratios of preferred simulator type, but the trend is clear; simulation use is increasing in healthcare.

"Big Data"

"Big data," the most important trend of all, has little to do with simulators themselves but, instead, has to do with the output, aggregation, and interpretation of data generated by the technology. Big data is defined as "data sets so large and complex they become awkward to work with using on-hand database management tools. Difficulties include capture, storage, search, sharing, analysis, and visualization." Big data holds the promise for us, for the first time in history, to gain significant insight into the pedagogy behind healthcare learning. Data streaming from simulators can be fed into local, national, or international databases. By mining these large data sets, we will be able to (1) build formative and summative assessments of individuals, (2) benchmark individuals to each other (locally, nationally, or internationally), (3) study educational effectiveness and outcomes, (4) use the analysis to redesign systems to maximize engagement and learning efficiency, and (5) understand the local, national, or international impact of discreet educational interventions. Big data from healthcare education will require a whole new breed of scientist focused on "learning analytics." Ultimately, we expect this knowledge to transform healthcare education.

How Many Learners at a Time? Multiplayer Versus Single Player

Through the remainder of the chapter, we will discuss the comparative advantages and disadvantages of GBL when compared to physically based simulators. In order to fully comprehend these arguments, one must understand the different types of GBL.

Single Player

In a single-player GBL exercise, the learning is targeted at a single individual (see Fig. 16.10). We expect single-player GBL to be especially useful in the early phases of learning. Autonomous embedded avatar physiology is a critical component in this vision. In this type of learning, an individual works through the learning module at their own pace, making and reflecting on errors as they occur. In an adaptive learning system, the platform would adjust the difficulty based on the learner's performance. If they make too many mistakes—the challenge becomes easier. If they are making few mistakes, the challenge becomes harder. Only after mastering the core concepts individually will the learner be eligible for multiplayer, collaborative exercises.

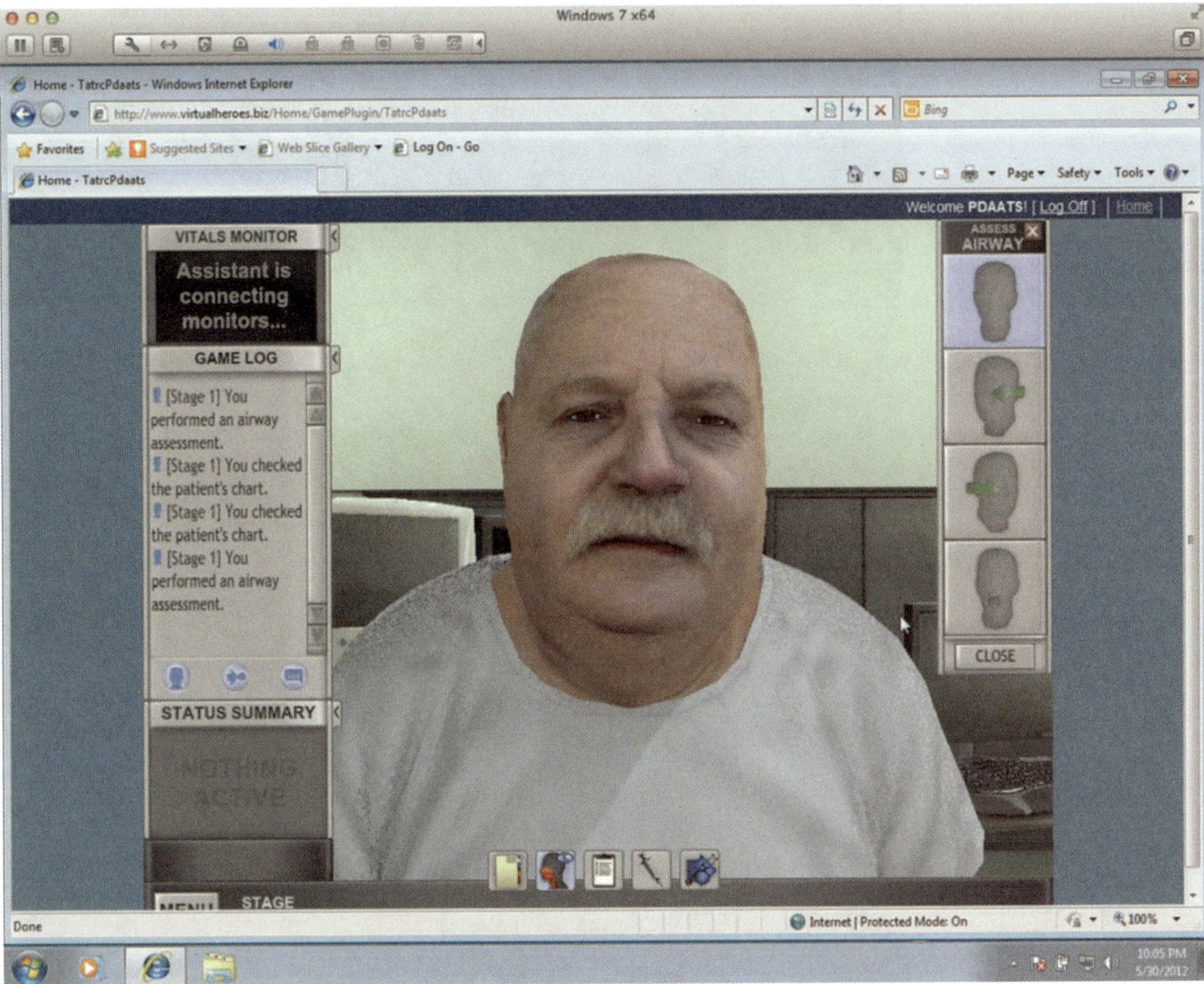

Fig. 16.10 Sample of a single-player games-based learning environment developed for non-anesthesia military personnel to practice the cognitive skills of deep sedation and rapid sequence intubation. The learner must evaluate each of ten patients and develop and execute individual plans. The learner's choices are tracked automatically. Following each case, the learner is compared to an anesthesiologist and can reflect on differences in practice. Each case can be repeated multiple times until mastery. Pre-deployment Anesthesia and Anaphylaxis Training System (PDAATS), currently under development, is funded by the Telemedicine and Advanced Technology Research Center (TATRC) of the US Army Medical Research and Materiel Command (Screenshots courtesy of the Virtual Heroes Division of Applied Research Associates)

Multiplayer

There are two types of multiplayer GBL types: facilitated (see Figs. 16.11 and 16.12) and non-facilitated. Facilitated multiplayer GBL requires a trained facilitator to lead the exercise and the subsequent debrief such as 3DiTeams. The actions of the learners can still be automatically logged, but the facilitator is primarily responsible for driving exercise forward.

Non-facilitated multiplayer allows learners to work together with preprogrammed "non-player characters" (NPC) much like the commercial game World of Warcraft [49]. Feedback in non-facilitated multiplayer experiences is generated primarily by the technology and/or peer-to-peer interactions but also can be given by a trained facilitator.

Any action taken in any virtual environment (single player or multiplayer) can be logged and sent to a learning management system.

Advantages and Disadvantages of Mannequin-Based Learning Compared to Games-Based Learning

Advantages of GBL Versus MBL

Simulation is effective method of learning [50]. MBL will continue to have a role in medical education, but as capabilities of other forms of simulation grow, its role will likely

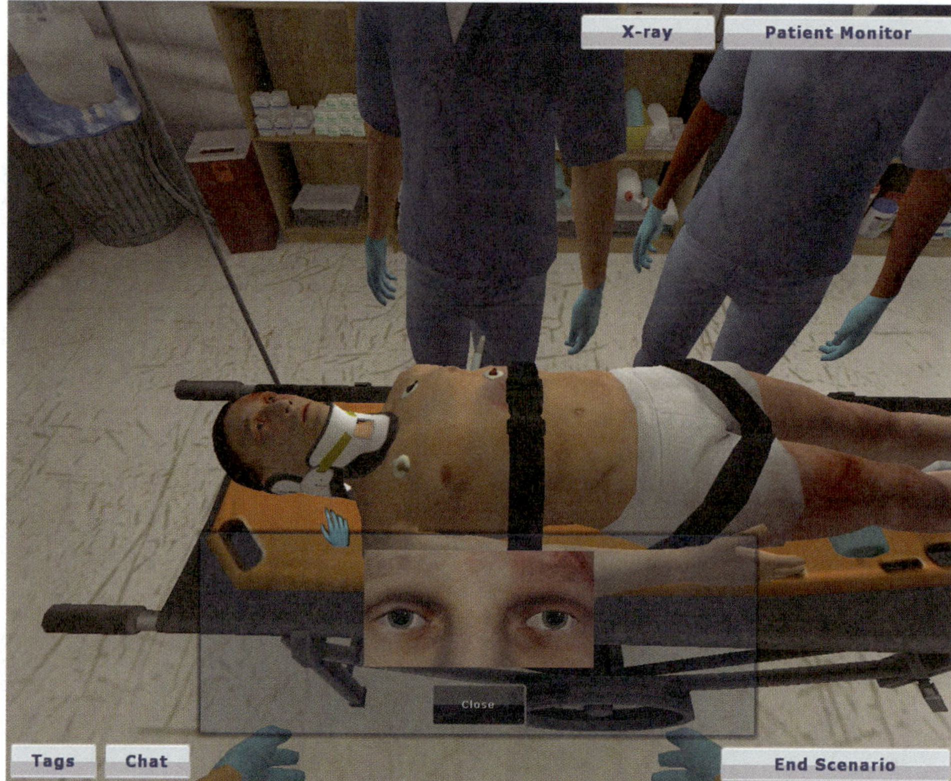

Fig. 16.11 Sample of a facilitator-led multiplayer training environment for team training. In this example the patient (avatar) has his own physiology driven by a physiology engine. Each healthcare worker can connect to the shared virtual environment from anywhere in the world. The facilitator controls unexpected "complications" deciding when (or if) to add them to the scenario. The scenario is "filmed" and may be played back during a debriefing. 3DiTeams (circa 2007) funded by the Telemedicine and Advanced Technology Research Center (TATRC) of the US Army Medical Research and Materiel Command (Screenshots courtesy of the Virtual Heroes Division of Applied Research Associates)

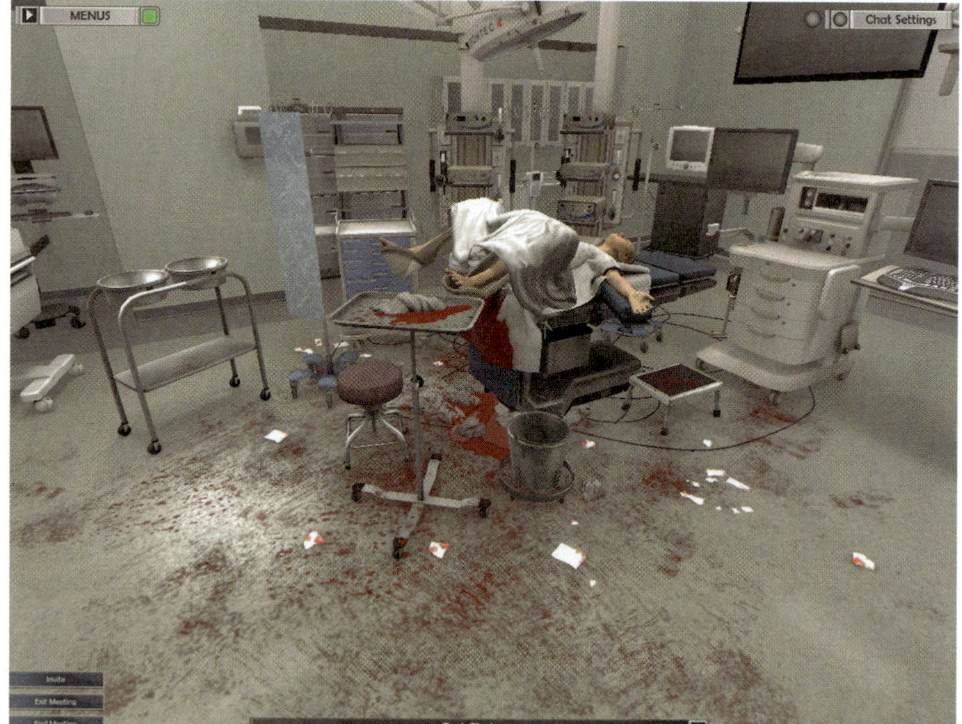

Fig. 16.12 Sample of a more recent facilitator-led multiplayer training environment (currently under development) for team training in the setting of postpartum hemorrhage. 3DiTeams obstetrics is being built on the Immersive Learning Environments @ Duke (ILE@D) Platform and will be used both for team training and massive hemorrhage protocol training. Note the improved visual fidelity compared to the original 3DiTeams. Choices made during the scenario, mouse clicks, and other data are automatically captured by the platform and, in a later version, to automate feedback. The interaction can be "recorded" and played back for a traditional debrief (Funded by Department of Health and Human Services. Screenshots courtesy of the Virtual Heroes Division of Applied Research Associates)

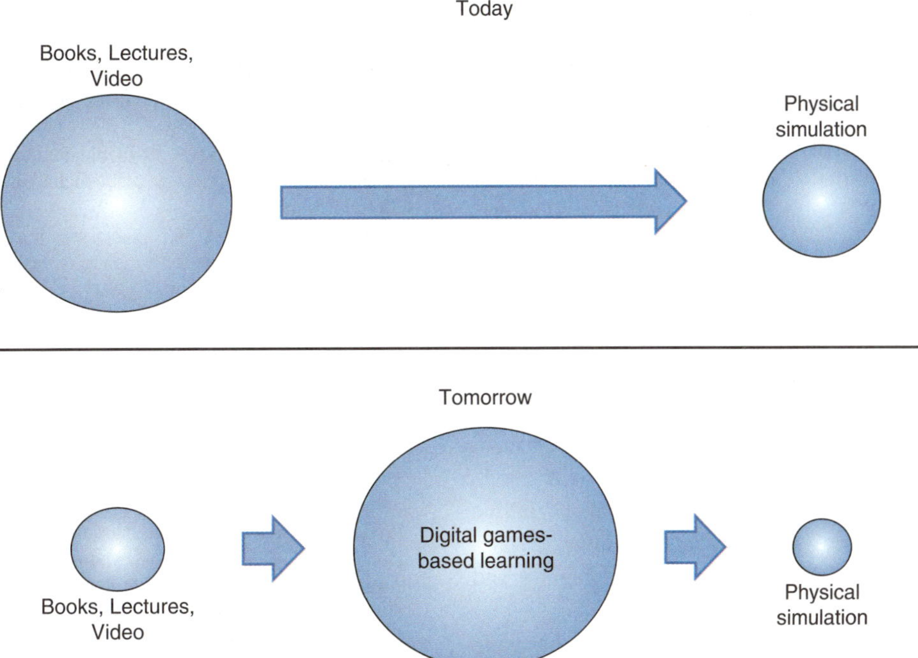

Fig. 16.13 Comparison of simulation learning today and tomorrow (circle size represents relative amount of learning in each format). Today, most learners gain basic knowledge from books, the web, or lectures then attempt to directly apply that knowledge in facilitator-led simulation scenarios. In the future, we believe there will be an additional step between basic information acquisition (from books and lectures) and face-to-face interaction. This intermediate step, games-based learning, will reduce the need for face-to-face interactions and will result in more efficient use of simulation resources when face-to-face learning is required. Overall, through the integration of games-based learning, we expect the efficiency of simulation to improve significantly

change. More convenient, distributable, and less expensive forms of simulation (e.g., GBL) will command an increasing proportion of the market for training. GBL is not perfect, but it possesses many of the features we desire in a learning platform. Technological advantages of GBL over MBL include the following: (1) scalability, (2) distributability, (3) the ability to augment reality, (4) the ability to manipulate and warp time, (5) mobile delivery, (6) the ability to reuse assets, (7) the ability to standardize content (to share curriculum or develop high-stakes assessment), (8) adjustable levels of fidelity, and (9) automated tracking and assessment.

In addition, there are many advantages for the learner using GBL when compared to MBL: (1) convenience, (2) self-paced learning, (3) adaptive to learner making it easier or harder based on grasp of material, (4) social that allows for peer-to-peer interaction with or without facilitator, (5) frequent and immediate feedback, (6) concurrent chaining of complex behaviors, (7) frequent rewards through completion of tasks, (8) easy remediation, and (9) ability to remain anonymous while still working with peers.

Disadvantages of GBL Versus MBL

GBL is not perfect and currently suffers from the following shortcomings when compared to MBL: (1) the stigma that game technology is only for "fun" and cannot be used for serious learning, (2) lack of evidence to support (or refute) GBL as a viable learning option, (3) lack of haptics (sense of touch) in virtual environments, and (4) the need to hard code much of the experience (making spontaneous interaction much more difficult).

From a learner's perspective, GBL may also have the following disadvantages: (1) A learner that is a computer novice or has little computer acumen may not find VEs amenable to learning, (2) a learner with little or no experience in gaming environments may struggle with game mechanics (and lose sight of the learning objectives), and (3) nonverbal communication is poor in VEs (again with an unknown effect on learning outcomes).

Immersive Virtual Environments

ILE@D—Immersive Learning Environments @ Duke

Currently, in our lab in the Duke University Human Simulation and Patient Safety Center, we are trying to position virtual environments as an intermediate step between basic knowledge acquisition and face-to-face interaction (see Fig. 16.13). Central to this vision is the development of ILE@D (Immersive

Learning Environments @ Duke), a shared common virtual environment platform for interprofessional learning—our first step toward the Ultimate Learning Platform. ILE@D is a three-dimensional, collaborative world accessible from any Internet-connected computer that provides an innovative, interactive "front-end" to distance education in the healthcare professions. ILE@D maximizes face-to-face interactions between teachers and students through preparatory self-directed, team-based, and facilitator-led activities in the virtual environment. We are designing a flexible architecture to allow creation of a library of locales, tools, medicines, procedures, patient profiles, events, and avatar responses. Once these libraries are created, they can be shared across a range of scenarios. The ILE@D framework, which supports open standards, and a plug-in architecture will become a hub of virtual healthcare education and research. Current healthcare applications under development in the ILE@D ecosystem include: (1) deep sedation training, (2) handover training, (3) teamwork and communication training, and (4) postpartum hemorrhage training.

We expect the future of healthcare education to be made up of blended or hybrid learning solutions that are heavily dependent on interactive learning delivered via GBL-ILE@D will fulfill this need.

Disruptive Technology

Clay Christensen, in his seminal book, *The Innovator's Dilemma* [51], spoke of disruptive technology. A disruptive technology is a new technological advance that is initially ignored because it only offers a fraction of the features of the state-of-the art legacy product. Ultimately, through cycles of development, the disruptive technology improves until the point where it overtakes the legacy technology—and in its wake, the legacy company withers. We have seen this cycle repeat itself many times including with cameras, movies, desktop computers, and other technology. Initially, GBL will be utilized primarily in blended learning solutions. Ultimately, we believe MBL, a recent disruptor of medical education, will be disrupted itself, increasingly supplanted by the rapidly improving capabilities of GBL. With these changes will come a revolution in our understanding and enjoyment of lifelong learning.

Conclusion

The convergence of computer hardware, communication networks, haptic technology, and consumer electronics/gaming technology will result in the simulation products that are currently unimaginable. We believe this convergence will usher in a new generation of tools and technology for healthcare learning that are efficient, efficacious, and engaging. Ultimately, these tools and the data derived from them will change the very nature of healthcare learning.

References

1. Taekman JM, Shelley K. Virtual environments in healthcare: immersion, disruption, and flow. Int Anesthesiol Clin. 2010;48(3): 101–21.
2. Friedman CP. The marvelous medical education machine or how medical education can be "unstuck" in time. Med Teach. 2000;22(5):496–502.
3. Davis D. Does CME, work? An analysis of the effect of educational activities on physician performance or health care outcomes. Int J Psychiatry Med. 1998;28(1):21–39.
4. Gaba D. The future vision of simulation in health care. Qual Saf Health Care. 2004;13(Suppl 1):i2–10.
5. Lundstrom M. Applied physics. Moore's law forever? Science. 2003;299(5604):210–1.
6. Annetta LA, Minogue J, Holmes SY, Cheng M-T. Investigating the impact of video games on high school students' engagement and learning about genetics. Comput Educ. 2009;53(1):74–85.
7. Botden SM, Torab F, Buzink SN, Jakimowicz JJ. The importance of haptic feedback in laparoscopic suturing training and the additive value of virtual reality simulation. Surg Endosc. 2008;22(5):1214–22.
8. Panait L, Akkary E, Bell RL, Roberts KE, Dudrick SJ, Duffy AJ. The role of haptic feedback in laparoscopic simulation training. J Surg Res. 2009;156(2):312–6.
9. Seymour NE, Gallagher AG, Roman SA, et al. Virtual reality training improves operating room performance: results of a randomized, double-blinded study. Ann Surg. 2002;236(4):458–63;discussion 463–4.
10. Peters JH, Fried GM, Swanstrom LL, et al. Development and validation of a comprehensive program of education and assessment of the basic fundamentals of laparoscopic surgery. Surgery. 2004;135(1):21–7.
11. Chou B, Handa VL. Simulators and virtual reality in surgical education. Obstet Gynecol Clin North Am. 2006;33(2):283–96, viii–ix.
12. Salkini MW, Doarn CR, Kiehl N, Broderick TJ, Donovan JF, Gaitonde K. The role of haptic feedback in laparoscopic training using the LapMentor II. J Endourol. 2010;24(1):99–102.
13. Solomon B, Bizekis C, Dellis SL, et al. Simulating video-assisted thoracoscopic lobectomy: a virtual reality cognitive task simulation. J Thorac Cardiovasc Surg. 2011;141(1):249–55.
14. Tolsdorff B, Pommert A, Hohne KH, et al. Virtual reality: a new paranasal sinus surgery simulator. Laryngoscope. 2010;120(2):420–6.
15. Edmond CVJ. Impact of the endoscopic sinus surgical simulator on operating room performance. Laryngoscope. 2002;112(7 Pt 1):1148–58.
16. Zhao YC, Kennedy G, Yukawa K, Pyman B, O'Leary S. Improving temporal bone dissection using self-directed virtual reality simulation: results of a randomized blinded control trial. Otolaryngol Head Neck Surg. 2011;144(3):357–64.
17. Modi CS, Morris G, Mukherjee R. Computer-simulation training for knee and shoulder arthroscopic surgery. Arthroscopy. 2010;26(6):832–40.
18. Howells NR, Gill HS, Carr AJ, Price AJ, Rees JL. Transferring simulated arthroscopic skills to the operating theatre: a randomised blinded study. J Bone Joint Surg Br. 2008;90(4):494–9.
19. Malone HR, Syed ON, Downes MS, D'Ambrosio AL, Quest DO, Kaiser MG. Simulation in neurosurgery: a review of computer-based simulation environments and their surgical applications. Neurosurgery. 2010;67(4):1105–16.
20. Alaraj A, Lemole MG, Finkle JH, et al. Virtual reality training in neurosurgery: review of current status and future applications. Surg Neurol Int. 2011;2:52.
21. Robison RA, Liu CY, Apuzzo ML. Man, mind, and machine: the past and future of virtual reality simulation in neurologic surgery. World Neurosurg. 2011;76(5):419–30.
22. Wong GK, Zhu CX, Ahuja AT, Poon WS. Craniotomy and clipping of intracranial aneurysm in a stereoscopic virtual reality environment. Neurosurgery. 2007;61(3):564–8; discussion 568–9.

23. Lemole GMJ, Banerjee PP, Luciano C, Neckrysh S, Charbel FT. Virtual reality in neurosurgical education: part-task ventriculostomy simulation with dynamic visual and haptic feedback. Neurosurgery. 2007;61(1):142–8; discussion 148–9.
24. Delorme S, Laroche D, Diraddo R, Del Maestro R. NeuroTouch: a physics-based virtual simulator for cranial microneurosurgery training. Neurosurgery. 2012;71(1 Suppl Operative):32–42.
25. Dayal R, Faries PL, Lin SC, et al. Computer simulation as a component of catheter-based training. J Vasc Surg. 2004;40(6):1112–7.
26. Hsu JH, Younan D, Pandalai S, et al. Use of computer simulation for determining endovascular skill levels in a carotid stenting model. J Vasc Surg. 2004;40(6):1118–25.
27. Patel AD, Gallagher AG, Nicholson WJ, Cates CU. Learning curves and reliability measures for virtual reality simulation in the performance assessment of carotid angiography. J Am Coll Cardiol. 2006;47(9):1796–802.
28. Aggarwal R, Black SA, Hance JR, Darzi A, Cheshire NJ. Virtual reality simulation training can improve inexperienced surgeons' endovascular skills. Eur J Vasc Endovasc Surg. 2006;31(6):588–93.
29. Dawson DL, Meyer J, Lee ES, Pevec WC. Training with simulation improves residents' endovascular procedure skills. J Vasc Surg. 2007;45(1):149–54.
30. Chaer RA, Derubertis BG, Lin SC, et al. Simulation improves resident performance in catheter-based intervention: results of a randomized, controlled study. Ann Surg. 2006;244(3):343–52.
31. Davoudi M, Colt HG. Bronchoscopy simulation: a brief review. Adv Health Sci Educ. 2009;14(2):287–96.
32. Desilets DJ, Banerjee S, Barth BA, et al. Endoscopic simulators. Gastrointest Endosc. 2011;73(5):861–7.
33. ABMS Maintenance of Certification [Internet]. abms.org. Available from http://www.abms.org/Maintenance_of_Certification/ABMS_MOC.aspx. Cited 3 Aug 2012.
34. Ericsson KA, Krampe RT, Teschromer C. The role of deliberate practice in the acquisition of expert performance. Psychol Rev. 1993;100(3):363–406.
35. Ziv A, Wolpe PR, Small SD, Glick S. Simulation-based medical education: an ethical imperative. Simul Healthc. 2006;1(4):252–6.
36. Davis D, O'Brien M, Freemantle N, Wolf F, Mazmanian P, Taylor-Vaisey A. Impact of formal continuing medical education: do conferences, workshops, rounds, and other traditional continuing education activities change physician behavior or health care outcomes? JAMA. 1999;282(9):867–74.
37. Crouch C, Mazur E. Peer instruction: results from a range of classrooms. Phys Teach. 2002;40:206–9.
38. Nicol DJ, Boyle JT. Peer instruction versus class-wide discussion in large classes: a comparison of two interaction methods in the wired classroom. Stud Higher Educ. 2003;28(4):457–73.
39. Shams L, Seitz AR. Benefits of multisensory learning. Trends Cogn Sci (Regul Ed). 2008;12(11):411–7.
40. Csikszentmihalyi M. Flow: the psychology of optimal experience. 1st ed. New York: Harper Perennial Modern Classics; 2008.
41. Mayo M. Video games: a route to large-scale STEM education? Science. 2009;323(5910):79–82.
42. Edmondson AC. Learning from failure in health care: frequent opportunities, pervasive barriers. Qual Saf Health Care. 2004;13 suppl 2:ii3–9.
43. Tapscott D. Grown up digital. McGraw-Hill Professional; US. 2009.
44. Maran NJ, Glavin RJ. Low- to high-fidelity simulation—a continuum of medical education? Med Educ. 2003;37 Suppl 1:22–8.
45. Norman G, Dore K, Grierson L. The minimal relationship between simulation fidelity and transfer of learning. Med Educ. 2012;46(7):636–47.
46. Allen IE, Seaman J. Going the distance: Online education in the United States, 2011. Babson Park: Babson Survey Research Group; 2011. Available from http://sloanconsortium.org/publications/survey/going_distance_2011.
47. Prober CG, Heath C. Lecture halls without lectures—a proposal for medical education. N Engl J Med. 2012;366(18):1657–9.
48. Ross AJ, Kodate N, Anderson JE, Thomas L, Jaye P. Review of simulation studies in anaesthesia journals, 2001–2010: mapping and content analysis. Br J Anaesth. 2012;109(1):99–109.
49. World of Warcraft [Internet]. us.battle.net. Available from http://us.battle.net/wow/en/?. Cited 3 Aug 2012.
50. Cook DA, Hatala R, Brydges R, et al. Technology-enhanced simulation for health professions education: a systematic review and meta-analysis. JAMA. 2011;306(9):978–88.
51. Christensen CM. The innovator's dilemma: the revolutionary national best seller that changed the way we do business. HarperCollins Publishers, NY; 2000.

Part III

Simulation for Healthcare Disciplines

Simulation in Anesthesiology

17

Laurence Torsher and Paula Craigo

Introduction

The specialty of anesthesiology has been at the forefront of healthcare simulation from its development and early applications to pioneering simulation for residency training requirements and maintenance of specialty board status. As such, the specialty of anesthesiology has a rich and mature experience with simulation. In this chapter we will explore the application of simulation to the field of anesthesiology with regard to training, assessment, and maintenance of competence. Given the specialty's extensive experience, much of the chapter will be devoted to the "art" of simulation with a detailed discussion of scenario, course, and curricular development.

The Specialty of Anesthesiology

"Although good clinical care in anesthesia has many components, the ability to diagnose and treat acute, life-threatening perioperative abnormalities is near the top of most anesthesiologists' lists" [1]. David Gaba's statement still rings true, and anesthesiology training aims to ensure competence in all aspects of perioperative care for patients of all ages and conditions. In addition to a broad base of clinical knowledge and judgment, procedural skills must be mastered to a level permitting flexible, creative, and adaptive application. The cognitive abilities necessary for intraoperative vigilance and responses to emergency and critical situations must be developed to a high level and complemented by the communication and leadership skills needed to conduct a coordinated team response. Additionally, graduates must possess skills that foster a commitment to lifelong learning throughout the coming decades of practice, while practicing anesthesiologists require maintenance of skills, and opportunities to acquire new knowledge and skills.

During the last few decades, the scope of practice of anesthesiologists has increased to encompass care outside the surgical suite including clinical environments such as the intensive care units, inpatient and pain medicine clinics, and preoperative clinics. This expanded base of practice requires anesthesiologists to have a broader training program that focuses on cognitive, procedure, and leadership skills to foster patient safety beyond the operating room. Recently, four roles have been used to describe the professional anesthesiologist: the professional artist (providing a safe anesthetic), the good Samaritan (managing patient pain, fear, and anxiety), the servant (serving the hospital by providing optimal care in the OR as well as facilitating the roles of other services in the hospital, e.g., care of critically ill patients), and the coordinator (administrative roles facilitating smooth functioning of the hospital, e.g., OR scheduling, airway management backup, roles in safety and education) [2]. The most comprehensive role is that of the servant, despite its seemingly negative connotation: aiding other providers in caring for the acutely or critically ill patient, thus supporting and facilitating the effectiveness and safety of the entire hospital system. Research in the workplace demonstrates that the performance of individuals with a broader vision of their work is superior to those whose professional understanding is narrow [3]. Though anesthesia residency education may focus primarily on one's individual operative management, particularly in settings in which residents provide most of the intraoperative care, broadening trainee's vision of their professional responsibilities is an important aspect of their education.

L. Torsher, MD (✉) • P. Craigo, MD
Department of Anesthesiology,
College of Medicine, Mayo Clinic,
Charlton 1-145, 200 First Street, SW,
Rochester, MN 55905, USA
e-mail: torsher.laurence@mayo.edu;
craigo.paula@mayo.edu

A.I. Levine et al. (eds.), *The Comprehensive Textbook of Healthcare Simulation*,
DOI 10.1007/978-1-4614-5993-4_17, © Springer Science+Business Media New York 2013

Table 17.1 A summary of graded levels of education evaluation

Kirkpatrick levels [117]	McGaghie [118]: education as translational research	Miller's pyramid [119]
1. Reaction		
2. Learning	T1—learning seen in controlled setting	Knows
3. Behavior	T2—learning used in patient care setting	Knows how/what
		Shows how/what
		Does
4. Results	T3—learning improved patient care	

Graduate medical education has a strong experiential base. Residents learn by taking care of patients under the supervision of faculty, not only through reading, attending lectures, and participating in discussions with faculty and peers. Faculty also model important skills and attitudes and are responsible for assessing learners' readiness for progression and eventual graduation into independent practice. This supervised practice and role modeling bears resemblance to apprenticeship. The modern application of apprenticeship in medical education was championed by Flexner, who integrated structured scientific study, and Osler, who introduced clinical clerkships into American medical education and derided the lecture hall as a "bastard substitute" for bedside teaching by a master physician [4]. The apprenticeship approach to medical education is familiar to many current medical faculty members, because it would resemble their own experiential training. However, changes in graduate medical education in recent years have raised concerns that experiential training may be inadequate to prepare anesthesiologists for decades of practice [4].

Trainee work-hour restrictions have resulted in a decrease in clinical exposure to both total number of cases and case diversity [5]. Public demand for increased safety and accountability has increased supervision of learners and intolerance of trainee error. Failure to learn critical management skills may result not only from lack of opportunity for independent practice but also from a learner's inability to perform the procedure with sufficient safety and facility to permit performance on an actual patient. Trainees worry that they are not ready to take up independent practice after graduation [6].

Identifying the trainee who is competent to perform a clinical procedure under varying levels of supervision (completed milestone) is an important issue and a major focus of the Accreditation Council of Graduate Medical Education (ACGME). Without formal assessment training, faculty members generally use their own, however limited, observations and perception of competency, to assess learners. Competence may be assumed simply because no evidence to the contrary is available to the staff. The learner may simply be required to demonstrate proof of the number of times they have performed a procedure (ACGME case log) and less often queried about their practical or theoretical knowledge prior to patient care. More commonly the trainee is simply asked if he or she can handle the procedure or situation. Trainees may have to bring forward the claim that they are competent or be deprived of practice opportunities.

Some cases are particularly rare during residency training and make sufficient experience unlikely to develop. It is unlikely that a resident in anesthesia will see a case of malignant hyperthermia or undiagnosed pheochromocytoma; general anesthesia for cesarean section may occur only one or two times during a residency, yet the practicing anesthesiologist must be proficient and capable of recognizing and managing rare life-threatening events that may occur in these situations. Several studies have demonstrated wide variation in performance of groups that were presumably similarly trained [7, 8]. This concerning level of variability raises questions over the effectiveness and reliability of the medical education system.

Competence is a necessary prerequisite for independence, but does not in and of itself indicate the ability for independent practice [9]. Even if competent to handle routine cases, independence requires the ability to recognize the nonroutine and predict and manage associated critical events. The resident's ability to recognize and manage rare and critical events may be very difficult for faculty to predict or determine. Competence also depends on the complexity of the procedure and how often it is performed. Behaviors denoting "competence" might be demonstrated a few times and subsequently lost. Early learners would be less able to deal with differences in equipment, staff, or systems support. This is the gap between competency and capacity for professional independence, better delineated by the development of milestones in professional education.

Moving beyond the time-based model of education, in which training is defined primarily in terms of the length, there is the potential to make residency training more efficient [10]. Some learners grasp things more quickly, while others need more hands-on practice and repetition. Even those adept learners may have more difficulty mastering some specific aspects of anesthesia practice. Rather than identifying competence in terms of time in training, proficiency should be identified based on an achieved set of abilities (competencies and milestones). The trainee is then able to move on to more advanced applications or add other types of training to his portfolio.

Advantages of Simulation for Anesthesia Education and Assessment

Though definitive evidence for simulation's superiority to more traditional approaches of evaluation and education is still being sought, its intuitive appeal has led to its acceptance into medical education programs. In the United States, simulation experiences are now a requirement in anesthesia residency training [11] as well as a part of Maintenance of Certification in Anesthesiology for professionals in practice [12]. However, it is worth noting that although written and oral exams have been utilized for many years as a method to determine competency, they have not been definitively shown to reliably differentiate safe from unsafe practitioners.

In addition to learning and rehearsing management of clinical problems, simulation can be useful in developing procedural, communication, teaching, and leadership skills. Simulation allows practice of rare but critical events. For some skills and topics, the experiential learning offered through simulation may produce outcomes superior to that which can be achieved via the clinical setting using more traditional techniques.

Learning while doing requires reflection; debriefing is a structured form of reflection that is at the heart of simulation-based education. Enhanced opportunity for reflection and improvement in a safe and guided setting with repetition and further assessment is an essential part of the simulation experience. Rather than the "fog of war" experienced when managing an actual surgical or anesthetic crisis, simulation affords the opportunity to take a step back; thoughtfully consider actions; incorporate feedback from faculty, peers, and recordings; and develop a plan for improvement. This experiential learning occurs in a safe, learning-focused environment, unlike actual clinical settings in which patients are at risk, the resident/anesthesiologist functions on a public stage, and criticism, legal action, loss of position or public humiliation may result. It is for this reason that it is critical that simulation creates and maintains a safe learning atmosphere.

Once training is complete, it can be difficult for established practitioners to learn new skills in a typical practice setting. Some skills build on foundations from earlier training; other skills present a paradigm shift and are less likely to be learned on the job after board certification. For example, the introduction of ultrasound into anesthesia practice could have been facilitated by use of task trainers outside of clinical practice.

Simulation may also be used for formative and summative assessment. Formative assessment or "feedback" is a key component of learning and improvement in knowledge and skills in medical education. Summative assessment, in which one's knowledge and skills are summarized and reported, is used more for testing. As research accumulates and simulation technology advances, there is a slow progression from formative to summative assessment. Boulet and Murray have recently reviewed the challenges of developing summative assessments [13], including defining the skills to be measured, developing a simulation to assess those skills and the metrics to measure the performance, and building a case for the validity of the simulation task as well as the reliability and usability of the metrics.

Simulation-based assessment may give different results from usual assessment tools. Anesthesia educators know the difficulties of training residents who do well on written tests but are ineffective in the clinical setting. Even residents who do well in one area may not do well in another, because competency is specific to both the content and context in which it is situated. In addition to cognitive errors, learners may have ingrained misunderstandings and habitual thought process errors that require correction before independent practice. In the clinical setting, these faults may never surface unless a particular event or fortuitous question reveals the deficiency. Simulation affords a setting in which the resident can be put in a position of decision-making and independent practice not normally available to them. The scenario is then allowed to play out without faculty interference or intervention, until errors and deficiencies are revealed.

Simulation offers the opportunity to practice and calibrate self-reflection. The American Board of Medical Specialties emphasizes self-directed learning, which assumes an ability to self-assess, as an integral part of maintenance of certification. Davis et al., in a systematic review on physician self-assessment compared to an external standard, determined that the majority of studies showed either a negative, minimal, or no association between self-assessment and external measures [14]. Thus, learners who present the greatest educational challenges are frequently those who fail to recognize their own limitations. As Hodges et al. described it, "those who know less also know less about what they know" [15]. Those who performed less well rated themselves inappropriately highly and, in contrast to high-performing and middle-performing subjects, failed to correct or calibrate their self-assessments toward more accurate estimations after exposure to other's performance and self-assessments [15, 16]. Simulation presents opportunities for guidance by a facilitating faculty, review of videotapes, and other means of correlating self-rating with external standards [17].

Of concern is a study by Wenk et al., demonstrating an increase in confidence in learners after completion of simulation learning that was not associated with an improvement in performance [18]. It is possible that this phenomenon is more likely to occur with medical students, who have less clinical context in which to evaluate and interpret the simulation experience.

There have been limitations on the level and impact of research in the use of stimulation in anesthesia education and evaluation. Much research is limited to Kirkpatrick level 1 ("learners liked it") (see Table 17.1); the highest level (improved patient outcomes) is the hardest to demonstrate but more valuable. Others argue that the question now is not "Why simulation?" but "How best to use simulation?" It is suggested that the role of research now is not to prove that simulation is good or better than other modalities but to clarify the specific areas in which it works best and define the details of how best to use it [19].

Technology and Techniques

Although entire chapters in this textbook are devoted to the discussion of simulation technology, there are a number of particular part-task trainers in addition to the full-scale mannequin simulators that have specific application to the training and assessment of anesthesiologists and anesthesia providers.

Part-Task Trainers

Task trainers are devices designed to teach a specific skill. They may be higher fidelity, simulating a patient or body part in realistic detail, or a more rudimentary model that simply lets the novice master the basic steps of a clinical task. Task trainers currently on the market are often criticized for their lack of fidelity with skeptics saying they offer a crude model at best. In actuality, a more complex trainer might detract from the learning experience by increasing cognitive load.

The role of the task trainer is not to convert a novice into an expert but to allow mastery of the basics of a technique so that when managing an actual patient, the learner can focus on the more sophisticated and subtle aspects of the task while providing a more efficient, safe, and comfortable experience for the patient.

Airway Trainers

Choosing an appropriate airway task trainer requires first establishing clear goals and objectives for the training. For airway skills, bag-and-mask ventilation, direct laryngoscopy, placement of supraglottic devices, fiberoptic intubation, and one-lung ventilation require trainers with differing anatomy and attributes (Fig. 17.1).

Most of the airway trainers on the market allow bag-and-mask ventilation and have sufficient mobility of the head, jaw, and neck to allow practice of proper placement of oral and nasal airways, ventilating mask, and positioning of the head and neck. Many airway trainers can be modified into "homegrown" airway trainers for more advanced skills such as regional anesthesia trainers for illustration of superior laryngeal and recurrent laryngeal nerve blocks (Fig. 17.2).

For training in direct laryngoscopy, appropriate upper airway anatomy, trachea, esophagus, as well as mobility in the jaw and neck to facilitate laryngoscopy will be needed. These attributes permit practice of laryngoscopy of normal anatomy and allow positioning of the head, alignment of the laryngoscope, and passage of the endotracheal tube. Typically limited to head, neck, and upper torso, these trainers are reasonably priced and quite durable, but do not effectively simulate the difficult airway. Still, they can be used to practice the fundamentals of bag-and-mask ventilation, placement of oral and nasal airways, direct laryngoscopy, and inserting rescue devices used in airway management.

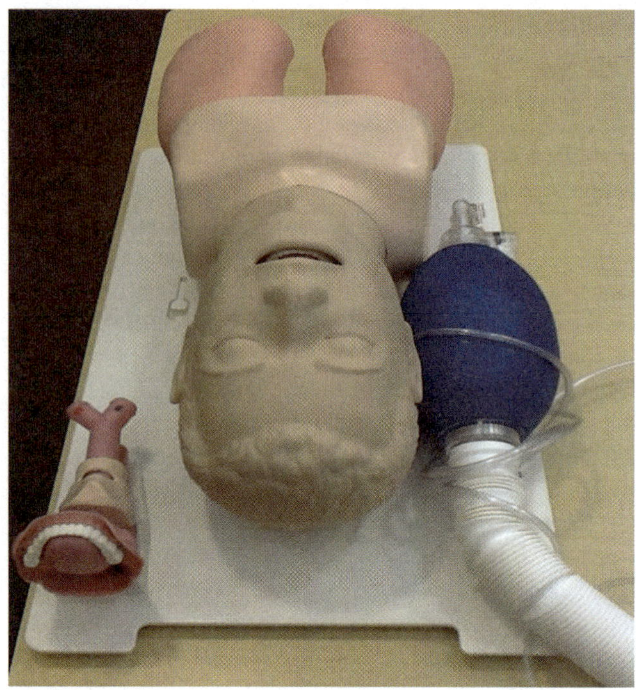

Fig. 17.1 Traditional airway trainer used for teaching basic airway skills with anatomical airway model for illustration of normal anatomy

The next level of sophistication in airway task trainers allows alteration of normal anatomy to mimic the difficult airway. Typically bladders are inflated to mimic a swollen tongue and/or hypopharynx; electrically activated devices decrease mobility of the jaw and/or neck to simulate "can't-intubate/can't-ventilate" situations. The simulated difficult airway may not exactly recreate clinical experience but provides the opportunity to work through the steps of management. Some of these simulators provide an audible tone mimicking a pulse oximeter as the oxygen saturation falls, to add a realistic sense of urgency. Although more expensive than the simple head task trainer, they are still far cheaper than the full-scale mannequin.

At the highest level of sophistication, high-fidelity simulation mannequins have complexly engineered anatomy that allows recreation of both straightforward and complicated airways in addition to modeling the rest of the body. These mannequins are very expensive and prone to breakdown, so to use them simply as an airway trainer may be inefficient and ill advised (Fig. 17.3). They do have the added benefit of showing the systemic effects of prolonged attempts at airway management such as hypoxia, hemodynamic instability, and changes in pulmonary mechanics.

Airway devices may not work as well in a trainer as in a live patient. It can be difficult to get an adequate seal with supraglottic devices such as the laryngeal mask airway, but

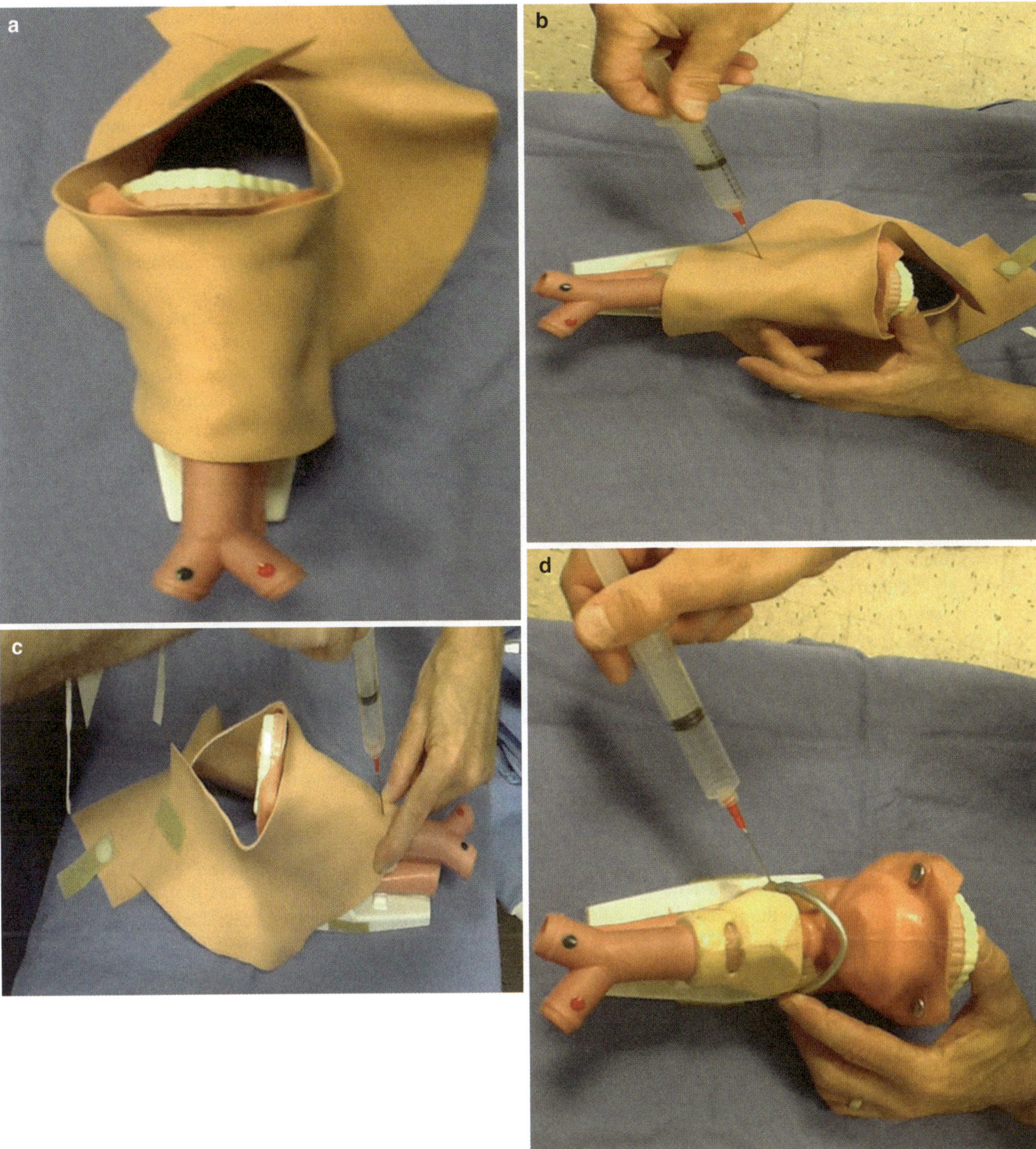

Fig. 17.2 Homegrown airway regional anesthesia trainer showing (**a**) airway anatomic model covered with skin from mannequin simulator. Performance of (**b**) superior laryngeal nerve block and (**c**) transtracheal nerve block. (**d**) With skin off the design of the trainer is shown to involve a stylet for use as a hyoid bone and tape to simulate a cricothyroid membrane

practice in placement is still valuable. Video laryngoscopes work well in most (Fig. 17.3).

Finally, animal models have been used for many decades. Isolated pig tracheas, available from most slaughterhouses, provide a very realistic model for needle and surgical cricothyrotomy.

Bronchoscopy Trainers

Video laryngoscopes have decreased the number of bronchoscopic intubations being done by anesthesia trainees [20], so simulation training for bronchoscopic airway management becomes more important than ever as this skill is practiced less

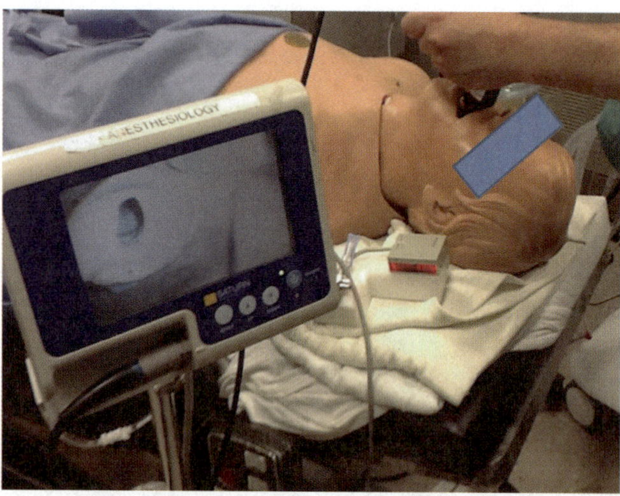

Fig. 17.3 Use of a glidescope to intubate the METI HPS

in the clinical setting. Component skills of bronchoscopy are recognition of the anatomy and manipulation of the scope.

Airway trainers provide a model of the proximal airway; however, most of them are only anatomically accurate to the level of the carina. Homemade models using branching tubes permit the learner to practice "driving" the scope. Although these models are not anatomic, they allow mastery of manipulation and control of an actual bronchoscope. There does not appear to be enhanced skill acquisition with sophisticated bronchoscopic simulators compared with less sophisticated models when the bronchoscopic objective is securing the airway [21, 22].

Screen-based high-fidelity bronchoscopic trainers consist of a controller resembling a bronchoscope and a screen-based system showing simulated images of the anatomy. Advantages include learning to drive the scope as well as detailed anatomy; a tutorial is frequently built in to the system. If the goal is simply to learn bronchoscopic anatomy, a screen-based bronchoscopic anatomy trainer that uses keyboard or mouse controls for bronchoscopic control may suffice. An example is Bronchoscopy Simulator [23], a free Web-based application developed by the University of Toronto. However, the anesthesiology trainee will necessarily need to develop psychomotor skills related to bronchoscopy, and this cannot be accomplished with keyboard controlled screen-based simulators. Scope manipulation as well as anatomic knowledge may be learned using a high-fidelity bronchoscopy model, an anatomic model of the upper airway, larynx, trachea, and bronchi through which the learner must manipulate the scope (Fig. 17.4).

Central Line Placement Trainers

Models for learning central line placement consist of the upper torso and typically provide palpable anatomy (bony landmarks) as well as arterial and venous systems that can be cannulated. Arterial systems with lifelike pulsations add another level of complexity and fidelity (Fig. 17.5). Trainers are also available for cannulation of femoral vessels.

Questions to consider before integrating these simulators include: Will the trainer be used to learn cannulation of the internal jugular or subclavian veins? Does it provide the landmarks needed for the techniques that we emphasize in our center? Does the level of complexity match our needs, recognizing that complexity adds cost as well as increasing the risk of malfunction and cost of maintenance?

If the model will be used to teach ultrasound (US)-guided central venous cannulation, the fidelity of ultrasound images produced should be assessed. Images may be provided not only of the vessels but of surrounding anatomy (trachea, muscles, and nerves); arterial and venous vessels may be distinguishable by the image shape and pulsatile motion. Not all models will have all of these features, so it is up to the buyer to determine which are important for the curriculum that you are developing. Most central line placement task trainers consist of a base and a replaceable component through which the needle is inserted. Cost of the disposables as well as their durability (how many needle punctures they can withstand, how the US image degrades after multiple needle passes, etc.) needs to be integrated into purchase decisions.

Though task trainers are a useful component of education, safely placing a central line requires far more than piercing the correct vessel, that is, setup of the procedure tray, patient preparation and positioning, identification of landmarks, puncture of the vessel, insertion and confirmation of guidewire location, dilation of the tissue path, and finally placement and confirmation of the venous line itself, all while monitoring the patient's status, comfort, and possible cardiac arrhythmias and maintaining sterile technique. The task training exercise needs to include all of these to develop safe trainees, rather than ones who can simply get a needle into a vessel. Limiting the frequency of actual dilation and cannulation in practice sessions can prolong the longevity of disposable portions of the trainer. By emphasizing these basics on the task trainer, bedside teaching with actual patients can focus on more advanced skills such as recognizing variations in anatomy and communicating with the patient. Alternatively, screen-based central line simulators are being developed that serve as a tutorial for the steps of central line placement without the physical mannequin. This allows trainees to rehearse the key steps of line placement without the need for a mannequin. Given that these steps are equally important to the psychomotor aspects of line placement with regard to patient safety, these simulators may prove useful to training programs.

Echocardiography Trainers

Transesophageal echocardiography (TEE) requires manual skills to manipulate the TEE probe to obtain the desired

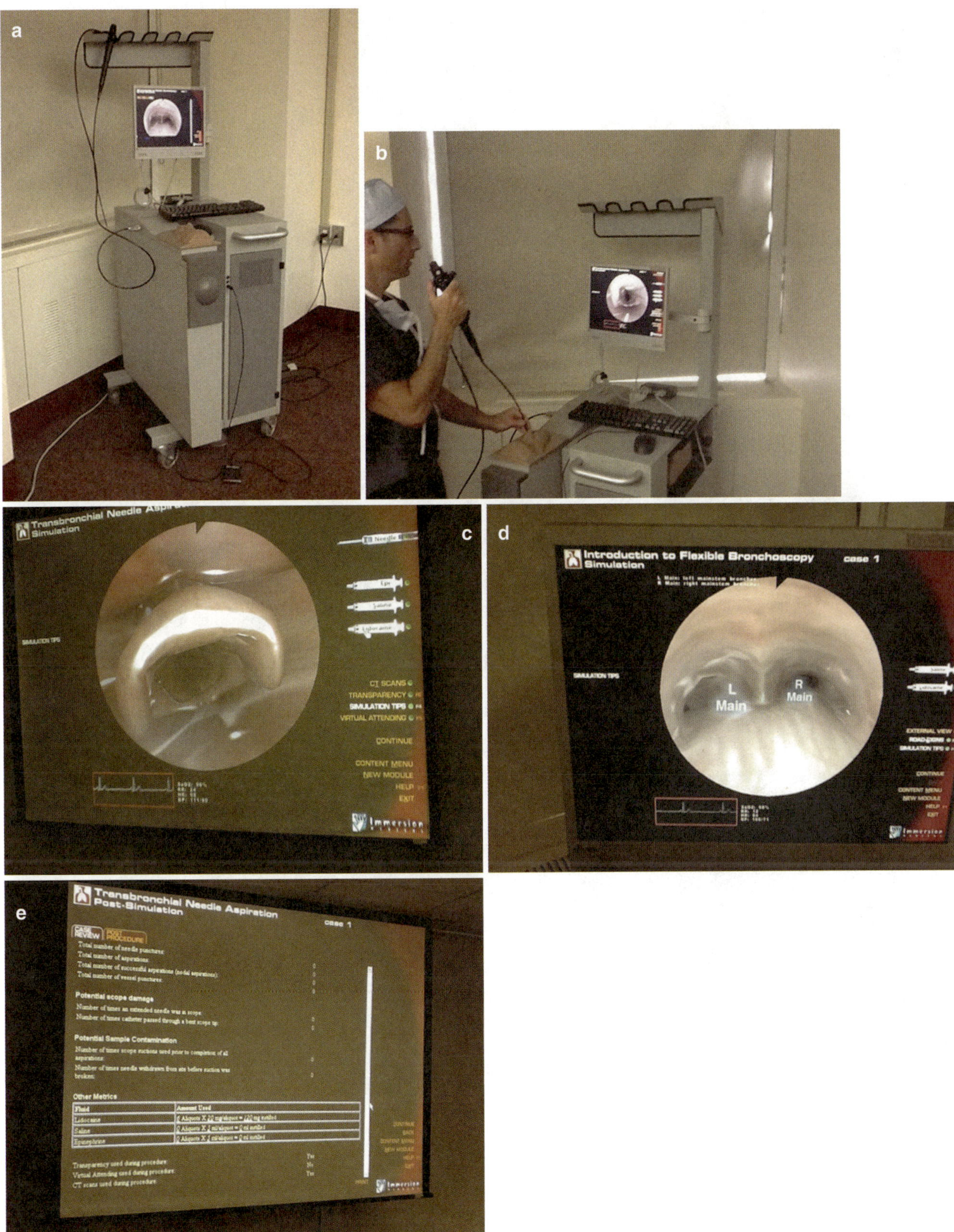

Fig. 17.4 Virtual bronchoscopy simulator. (**a**) Simulator setup. (**b–d**) Simulator use and airway images. (**e**) Performance metrics

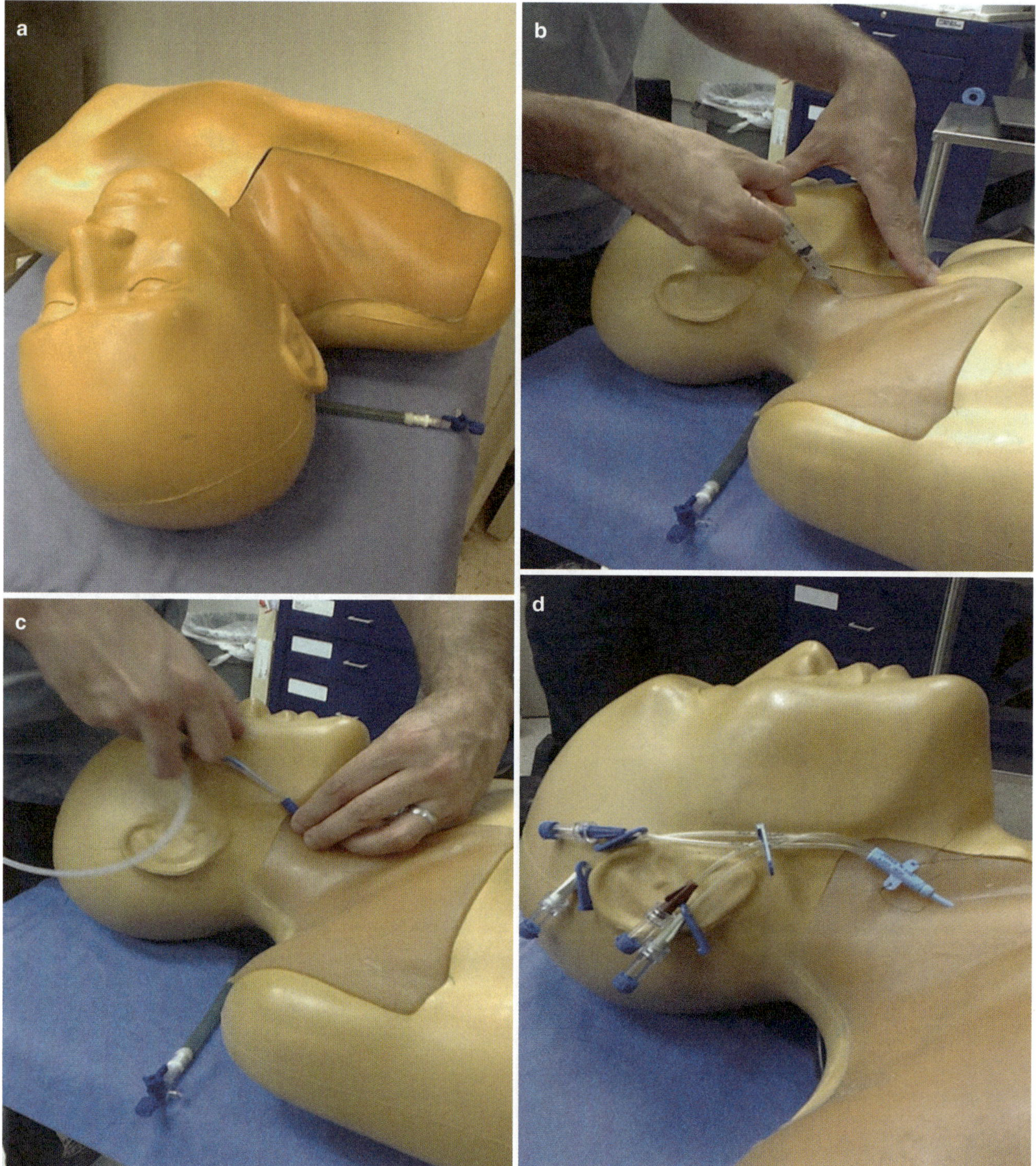

Fig. 17.5 (**a–d**) Central venous cannulation trainer showing participant performing steps of internal jugular vein cannulation

images as well as the knowledge to interpret these images. Many of the TEE trainers on the market focus exclusively on image interpretation; they may be screen- or Web-based and lack a TEE probe. They tend to be modestly priced and are often intended for self-study.

Manipulating the TEE probe in response to suboptimal images, which necessitates a TEE-like probe with which to practice, may challenge novices. Trainers developed to address these needs consist of either a model with an "image-able" static cardiac model within it that the learner evaluates

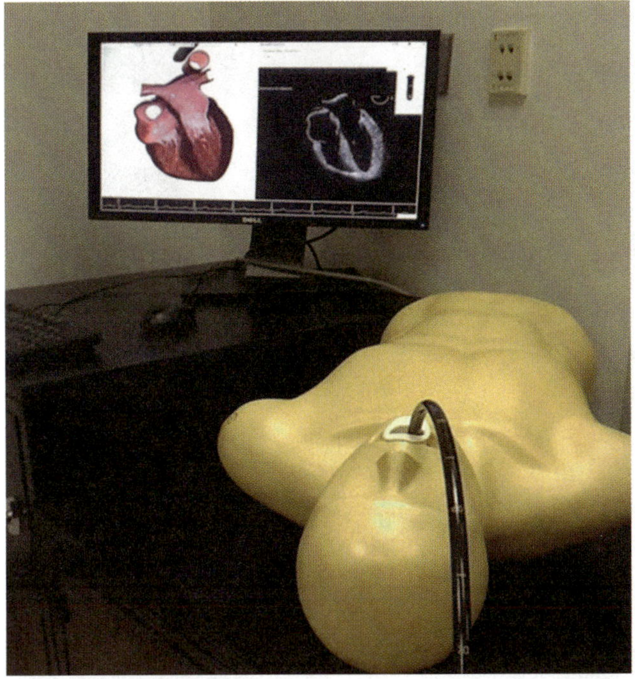

Fig. 17.6 TEE simulator

with a standard echo machine (e.g., the Blue Phantom cardiac model) or alternatively one in which a controller that resembles a TEE probe interacts with a computer model to provide simulated views (e.g., CAE or HeartWorks). A static cardiac model in a mannequin or thorax is appealing because it allows use of the actual TEE equipment in your clinical setting. The disadvantages are that it is a static model, not a beating heart, and it ties up clinical equipment. Computer-simulated systems often include an online tutorial along with the models, simulate a beating heart, and are dedicated teaching systems not tying up clinical equipment. Most trainers that simulate TEE provide transthoracic echo training as well, which may be additionally useful for PACU and ICU settings (Fig. 17.6).

Regional Anesthesia Trainers

Regional anesthesia under US guidance requires a learner to master not only ultrasonography and sonoanatomy but the eye-hand coordination to maneuver the needle in three dimensions in response to the images. Models for ultrasound probe manipulation and needle control must provide a target image within a medium that mimics the feel of directing the needle to reach that target. Commercial products typically consist of a target imbedded in a gel that facilitates imaging. After repeated needle passage, gel-based models tend to show needle tracks on US imaging, image quality is degraded, and hence, their durability is limited. Homemade models may be made by placing targets, for example, olives within cuts of meat. Large nerves, such as the sciatic, as well as sizable cuts of meat can be purchased from an abattoir or a cooperative butcher. Anatomy and sonoanatomy required for successful regional anesthesia practice may be effectively learned from print material or screen-based tutorials as well, though as with central line simulators, there is no psychomotor component.

Epidural and spinal anesthesia simulators typically consist of a torso with an imbedded synthetic spinal column that includes a ligamentum flavum and a spinal cord within a fluid-filled thecal sac (Fig. 17.7). There may be some flexibility in the torso and spine to allow optimal and suboptimal positioning. Not all models can be used in both the upright and lateral decubitus position. These trainers can reasonably recreate the touch, feel, and consistency of a normal human back and the structures involved in neuraxial regional techniques. Their primary utility lies in letting the novice practice all the basic steps of an uncomplicated spinal or epidural technique. Some models allow ultrasound imaging. Homemade models have been described using bananas as targets to recreate the loss of resistance associated with epidural placement [24].

The Science of Simulation Education

What Is Effective Simulation?

The characteristics that make simulation an effective educational tool have been described throughout the literature [25]. Well-defined goals are requisite to being able to determine whether or not the simulation has been successful in meeting educational goals, and there must be a clear way to determine when the goals have been met. Feedback and the opportunity for repetitive practice are important. Simulation should be integrated into the curriculum in a meaningful way and not technology-driven. The level of difficulty should be appropriate for the learners, but there must be the availability of multiple levels of difficulty. Ideally the capacity for individualization through the use of different teaching strategies can also enhance simulation-based education effectiveness. Some representation of clinical variation and how to adapt to it is useful. Finally, simulation should take place in a safe environment for learning.

As already mentioned and covered in great detail throughout this text, debriefing is critical. It is where learning takes place. Different kinds of debriefing can be equally effective, whether guided by a facilitator or self-directed using a written guide [26]. Similarly, although video review is frequently part of debriefing, some have suggested that it may not be necessary for success and need not be used universally [27, 28]. For a more complete description of scenario debriefing including best practices and theory, see Chaps. 6 and 7.

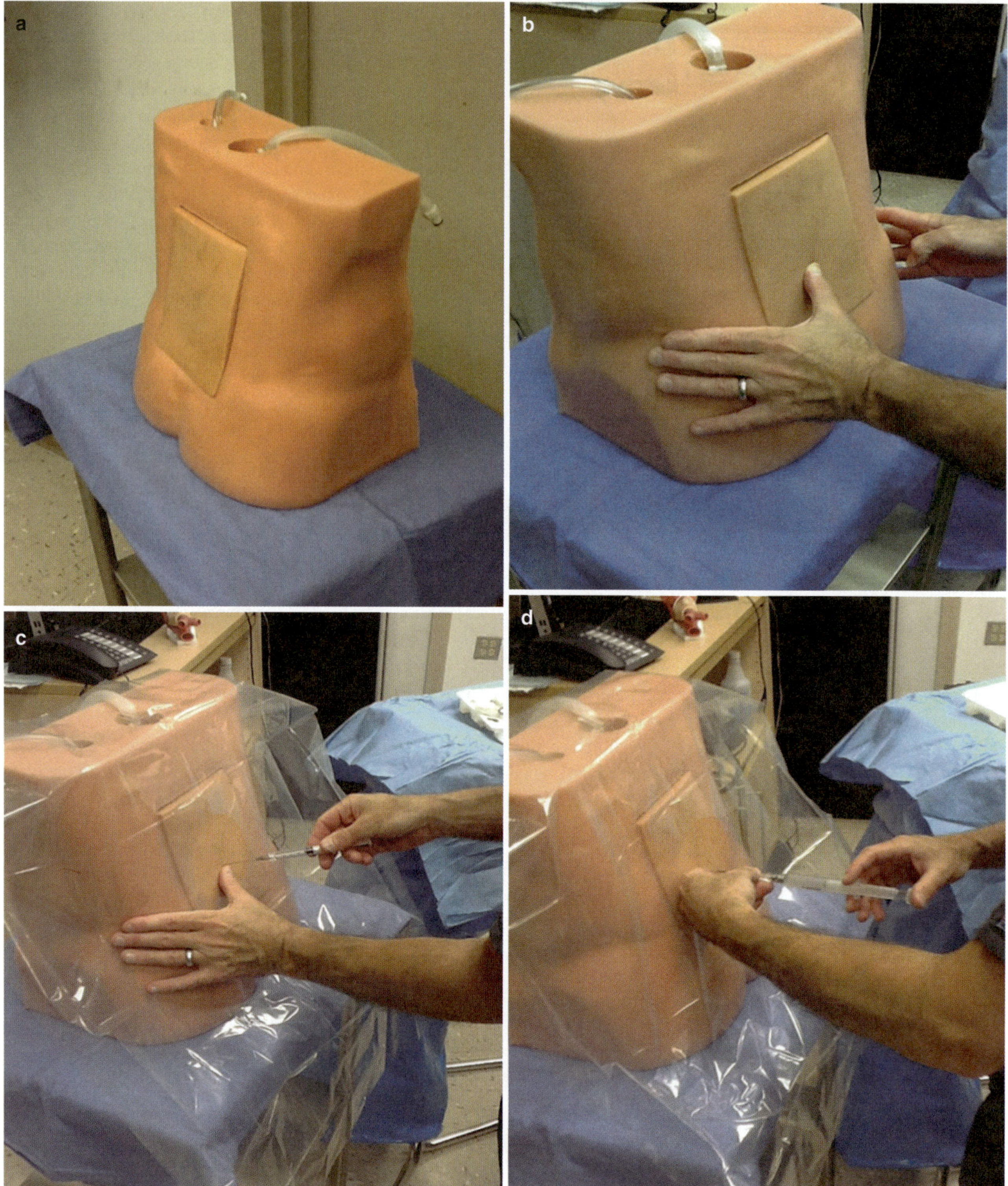

Fig. 17.7 (**a–e**) Neuraxial anesthesia simulator showing participant doing steps of epidural catheter placement

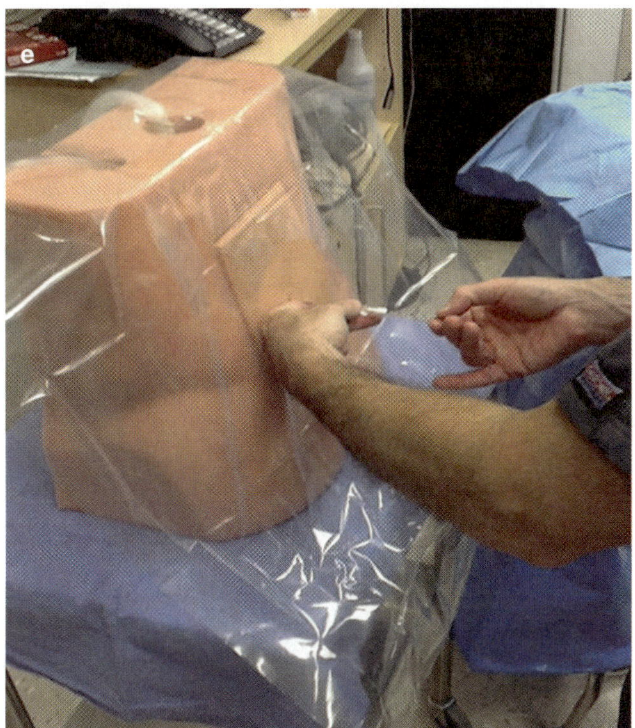

Fig. 17.7 (continued)

The Importance of Fidelity

Systematic analysis of simulation education calls for some meaningful method of classifying the levels of fidelity. Cumin and Merry [29] suggest a three-part scheme by which simulators are classified according to (1) how the learner interacts with them, (2) what determines their represented physiology, and (3) what can best be taught by their use.

Three major groups based on type of interaction are hardware-based (mannequin or hands-on task trainer), screen-based (computer-based system in which interaction takes place by keyboard or mouse on a nonspecialized computer), and virtual reality-based (interaction with the simulated environment via headsets and haptics). The physiologic behavior of a simulator may be script-controlled in which an operator prescribes the changes in physiology, or model-driven in which a mathematical model of a physiological system determines the physiology observed. Finally, different simulators are best suited to teaching knowledge, cognitive skills, and psychomotor skills. Not every feature from "real life" has to be present in a simulation; it may even be better for nonessential items and representations to be removed to limit complexity, decreasing cognitive load and enhancing focus on the learning task at hand.

Scenario design is ultimately the bottom line of purchasing any simulators. A well-constructed scenario should have fidelity and be reproducible, that is, able to provide essentially the same experience to a number of learners. Reproducibility is especially important if summative assessment is planned. Full environment or full-scale simulation can be used to provide the experience of medical catastrophes; the emotion engendered may enhance learning by decreasing extinction/forgetting and facilitating learning [30]. Role-play with standardized patients can also elicit an authentic emotional experience and offer practice in handling these emotions.

Simulation exercises can show the difference in skill levels between experienced and less experienced providers with experienced practitioners performing better than less experienced trainees [31, 32]. Simulation can also differentiate between experienced anesthesia providers who have and have not undergone ACLS training [33].

Fundamental Competencies in Anesthesiology

Anesthesia-Specific Equipment

Errors in anesthesia machine checks and fault identification, even by experienced anesthesia providers, continue to be a problem [34–36]. In a recent investigation, experiential training in machine checkout was found to be superior to didactic teaching; in fact, junior residents exhibited machine-check skills superior to those of graduating senior residents who had not received experiential training. In addition, the skills were retained for at least 2 years [37]. Fischler et al. [38] compared a screen-based schematic teaching model of the anesthesia machine with a photorealistic screen-based teaching model of the anesthesia machine as teaching tools on machine function. They found that learners who used the schematic model understood the function of the machine more thoroughly as assessed by written examination than those who used the photorealistic model. The photorealistic model was the higher-fidelity offering, showing that improving realism by itself does not always lead to better retention and understanding.

Crisis Resource Management (CRM), Human Factors, and Nontechnical Skills

While Chap. 8 provides a more comprehensive treatment of the subject of CRM, its importance in anesthesiology as it pertains to simulation deserves special mention. Emphasis on team skills or nontechnical skills was pioneered in the aviation industry as the contribution of dysfunctional teams to aviation accidents was recognized. Anesthesia training has traditionally focused on cognitive knowledge (knowing facts) and psychomotor skills (learning tasks, e.g., endotracheal intubation, placement of an axillary nerve block). Team skills, effective communications, and handoffs, although

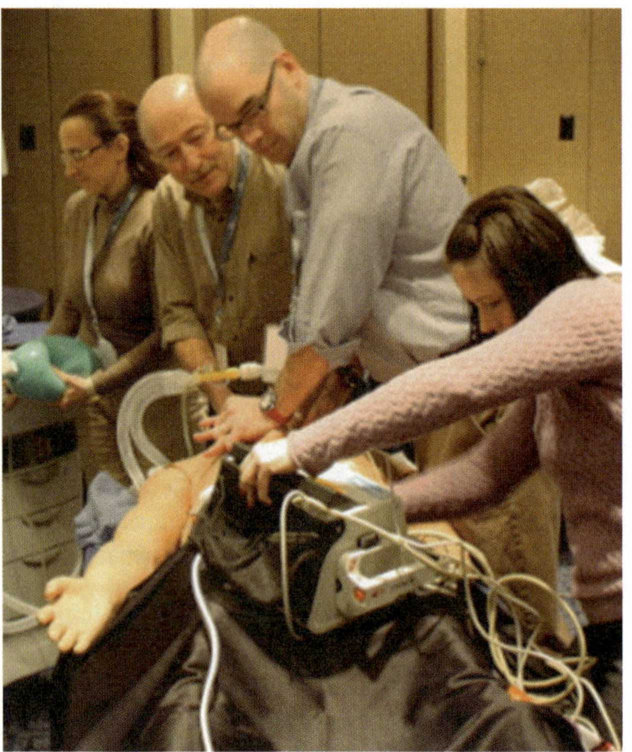

Fig. 17.8 Critical events management course in progress

always a part of medical practice, have not been specifically taught and rehearsed. Gaps in these skills are frequently cited as contributing to sentinel events. Simulation provides an opportunity to see good team and human factors skills as well as the consequences of weaknesses in this realm. It also provides an opportunity to rehearse the skills (Fig. 17.8).

Anesthesia Nontechnical Skills (ANTS) is a nontechnical skills framework specifically designed for anesthesia that provides the taxonomy and tools to rate anesthesia behaviors [39–41]. It evaluates task management, teamwork, situational awareness, and decision-making, with well-developed criteria for each. Other frameworks customized for particular perioperative fields include NOTSS for surgeons and SPLINTS for scrub nurses [40, 42]. These tools focus on the performance of the individual in executing nontechnical skills. Other tools have been developed to evaluate the function of the team rather than that of individual members. TeamSTEPPS® is a toolkit, funded by the Agency for Healthcare Research and Quality (AHRQ), that both measures teamwork function and provides a strategy for improving it [43]. The Mayo High Performance Teamwork Scale also evaluates team performance [44]. Both examples highlight strengths and weaknesses of the team that could be analyzed for the contributions of individual team members to that strength or weakness.

Johnson et al. [45] compared the effects of task training and variable priority training in a simulator, to the effects of standard training, on first year anesthesiology residents' subsequent management of simulated adverse airway and respiratory events. Variable priority training emphasizes dividing attention appropriately among multiple competing factors. Participants in both groups showed improvement in all metrics after a year of residency. The experimental group was able to complete more tasks and answered more comprehension questions correctly, although both managed the case appropriately and had a similar perceived workload, suggesting that both approaches to teaching novices airway management were effective.

Park et al. [64] studied the use of simulation in novice anesthesia residents who underwent training for initial intraoperative management of either hypoxia (group 1) or hypotension (group 2) in a crossover study. In a simulated scenario of intraoperative hypotension, group 2 outperformed group 1, while group 1 outperformed group 2 in a hypoxia scenario. The groups then completed the simulation training on the other topic. At 6 weeks there was no difference between the groups, thus supporting the effectiveness and efficiency of simulation training for novices, particularly in hypoxia and hypotension scenarios.

Airway Management

In developing an airway management curriculum, one must recognize that airway management is considered a fundamental skill within an anesthesiology training program that is reinforced nearly every day through clinical practice; however, for non-anesthesia personnel, airway management is seen as a low-frequency/high-risk event. For non-anesthesia personnel, airway simulation training tends to focus on bag/mask ventilation and more straightforward laryngoscopy and intubation; simulation training for anesthesia personnel is more concerned with management of the difficult airway.

A recent survey of anesthesia residency programs found that half of respondents had a formal airway rotation as part of the anesthesia residency. More than two-thirds of programs used a combination of lecture and practice on a mannequin [46]. An Australian study found that anesthesia trainee exposure to alternative methods of airway management in clinical practice was minimal—1.2 fiberoptic intubations, 0.5 mask-only cases, and 3.7 endobronchial double lumen tubes per year on average were reported [47].

Simulation training can improve the technical skills and confidence of non-anesthesia junior house staff in the basic airway management of effective mask seal, bag-mask ventilation, and use of oral airways in adults [48–50]. Non-operating room intubation skills were shown to improve in adult patients after simulation training [51–54]. In those studies, utilization of checklists and team management were also found to be improved in emergent airway management. Similarly in pediatric emergency airway management, simulation training improved both technical and nontechnical skills [55], although adding just-in-time training for pediatric intubation, before a pediatric ICU shift, in addition to usual airway training, did not improve clinical airway management skills [56].

After simulation training of difficult airway management , anesthesia personnel demonstrated a more organized approach to managing the difficult airway with improved confidence, which was sustained for 6 months after training [57, 58]. Interestingly, those anesthesia providers who did not follow the ASA algorithm before simulation training for a difficult airway scenario did not follow it even after training [59], suggesting that previous experience of the learners affected how they perceived and responded to the simulation session. Olympio et al. [60] noted that simulation training did not improve the detection of esophageal intubations in follow-up simulation scenarios. The authors did note that this may illustrate a problem with the design of their scenarios, a lack of deliberate practice, or long duration between scenarios.

Further studies have examined anesthesiologists' performance of surgical cricothyrotomy. After a single simulation session, improvements in performing cricothyrotomy on a simulator were retained for at least 1 year [61]. Siu et al. [62] showed that anesthesiologists improved their skills in surgical cricothyrotomy after completing a structured simulation session; however, older anesthesiologists (>45 years) were not only less adept at baseline than the younger group but remained less adept after undergoing the same structured training program.

Fiberoptic bronchoscopy skills for intubation can be enhanced with simulation task training. Even a virtual bronchoscopic training session in which learners used an interactive DVD before bronchoscopy training improved performance in the clinical setting [63]. Utilization of low-fidelity bronchoscopy trainers prior to clinical exposure significantly improved the clinical performance of the trainee [21]. There did not seem to be an incremental improvement in clinical performance when moving from a low- to a high-fidelity bronchoscopic task trainer [22].

Placement of supraglottic airways such as laryngeal mask airways and combined esophagotracheal tubes can be practiced on commercially available mannequins as can complex and lifesaving procedures such as needle cricothyroidotomy with jet ventilation to allow trainees comfort with these devices (Fig. 17.9a–c).

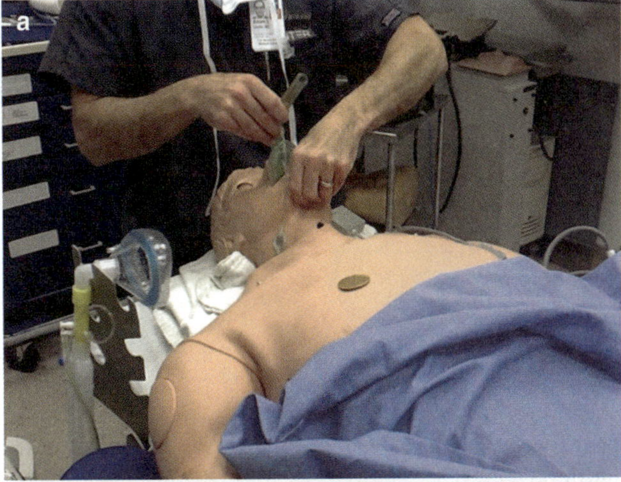

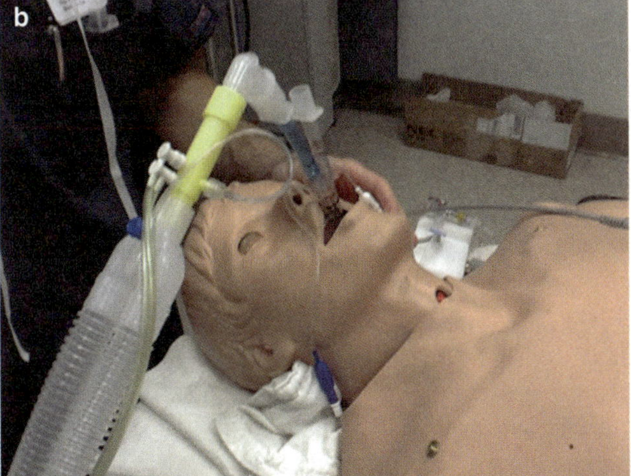

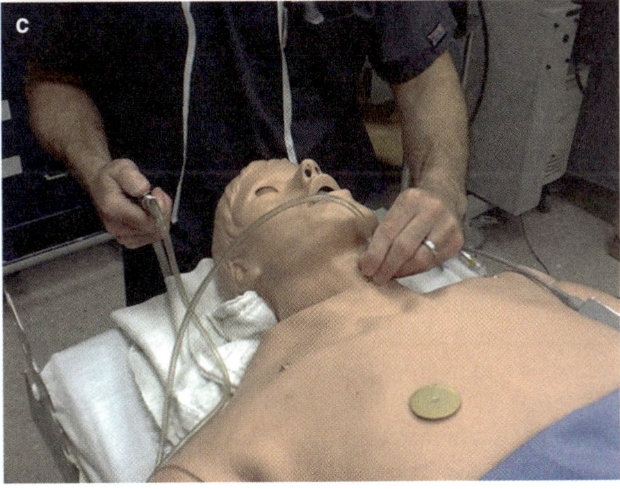

Fig. 17.9 Placement of (**a**) an LMA and (**b**) combitube on the METI HPS. (**c**) Placement of an angiocatheter with jet ventilation on the mannequin

Neuraxial and Peripheral Nerve Blocks

Simulation has been recommended as part of a comprehensive regional anesthesia curriculum [65, 66] using task training to learn technical skills as well as full-scale simulation management of associated crises such as high spinal and local anesthetic systemic toxicity (LAST). Most of the literature on regional anesthesia task trainers consists of descriptions of the trainers and the technology involved, but there is far less on the actual effectiveness of the trainers.

There are a number of task trainers available for teaching lumbar puncture (LP), epidural, and spinal anesthesia techniques as mentioned earlier in this chapter. There is little data showing definitive effect of these trainers in clinical care, although Kessler et al. [67] showed that pediatric residents who had trained on a pediatric LP trainer had a higher success rate with their first LP in clinical practice. Friedman et al. [68] showed that learners who received epidural placement training with a low-fidelity epidural simulation model [24] consisting of a banana wrapped in foam performed as well as those who utilized an expensive commercial high-fidelity epidural task trainer. Spinal and epidural trainers are becoming increasingly sophisticated, incorporating haptic feedback to simulate the tactile sensations of the needle passing through various tissue types [69, 70]. It remains to be seen if the increased fidelity has any influence on the educational outcome.

Ultrasound-guided regional anesthesia requires both familiarity with the sonoanatomy and skill with needle manipulation under ultrasound guidance. Niazi et al. [71] showed that residents training on a task trainer consisting of targets in a gel, in addition to didactic lessons, when compared to a cohort who received didactic training only, had a higher rate of successful blocks as well as had a higher degree of proficiency when assessed using a standardized checklist. In contrast Cheung did not see an improvement in skills when a high-fidelity ultrasound-guided regional anesthesia simulator was added to a training program [72]. Increasingly sophisticated regional anesthesia simulators, which are in essence interactive anatomy models, continue to be developed, some of which can build a virtual model of an individual patient with reconstructions from MRI [73], although the contribution of such a model to attainment of regional anesthetic skills remains to be seen.

Simulation for LAST is a popular subject. Smith et al. [74] describe rapid and successful management of LAST in an actual patient shortly after participants had undergone simulation training. Utilization of the American Society of Regional Anesthesia LAST checklist, as a cognitive aid, has been shown to improve performance in simulated resuscitations of LAST [75]. Simulation training for LAST has been suggested as a component of a regional anesthesia curriculum [65, 66]. Scenarios for LAST have been published and are now in the public domain [76].

Central Line and Invasive Monitor Placement

Reducing and/or eliminating central line-associated bloodstream infections (CLABSI) is an important national patient safety imperative, and the Agency for Healthcare Research and Quality (AHRQ) has funded a national effort to prevent CLABSI. Along with infection, central line placement can be complicated by arterial puncture, pneumothorax, brachial plexus injury, and inability to place the line. Although simulation training for central line placement was embraced, its introduction coincided with the use of other safety measures, including procedure standardization, timeouts, checklists, and team member empowerment to speak up if protocols are breached; therefore, it is impossible to separate the effects of simulation training specifically from these measures. However as simulation-based central line training has been introduced into practice, there has been a documented improvement in actual clinical performance measures including a decrease in time to complete the procedure [77], a decrease in arterial puncture, and an increase of line placement success [78] as well as decreased catheter-related blood stream infections [79]. Consequent cost savings [80] have been demonstrated. Some of the improvement in infection rate may be due to improved sterile technique noted in participants after simulation learning [81]. Simulation training was shown to be superior to didactics in teaching sterile technique [82]. These skills learned appear to be retained at least 1 year [83]; however, if the learners are in an environment in which central lines are frequently placed, by the end of a month, those who underwent simulation training showed similar skills to those who had not [84]. In a meta-analysis of studies of simulation training and central line placement, Ma et al. reviewed 25 studies and showed improved learner performance on simulated exercises (fewer needle passes and pneumothoraces) and improved knowledge and confidence [85].

Anesthesiology Subspecialties

Cardiovascular Anesthesia

Cardiopulmonary Bypass Management

Bruppacher showed that among cardiothoracic anesthesia learners training to wean patients from cardiopulmonary bypass, those randomized to simulation training showed improved performance in an actual clinical environment compared to trainees randomized to an interactive seminar on the material [86]. In an accompanying editorial, Steadman outlined the importance of connecting what is learned in the simulator to actual clinical practice; many studies demonstrate only improvement in performance in the simulated setting, and the questions arise as to whether such improvement is simply the result of "teaching to the test" [87].

Transesophageal Echocardiography (TEE)

Learning transesophageal echocardiography (TEE) can be challenging. In order to become proficient, one needs to master both technical and cognitive skills in order to manipulate the echo probe and the console controls while interpreting the images obtained. It is also challenging to assure that there is adequate exposure to both normal and abnormal anatomy. Simulation can be an educational adjunct that can be used to enrich the learning opportunities in the actual clinical environment. Bose et al. [88] showed simulation-based training in TEE to be a more effective education modality than the more traditional approach using textbooks and Web-based materials in terms of learners' anatomic correlations, identification of structures, and manual skill in acquiring suitable images. Further studies validating the commercially available simulators are under way.

Obstetric Anesthesia

Simulation's role in obstetric anesthesia includes acquisition of technical, communication, and teamwork skills; assessment of provider and team performance; and evaluation of the safety of the care systems and environment [89]. As the use of regional anesthesia on the labor floor has prevailed, there is concern that trainees will have limited opportunity to become familiar, let alone proficient, at conducting an emergent general anesthetic for delivery. It has been postulated that simulation would be an effective tool to fill this clinical void for anesthesiology residents. Scavone developed a checklist to assess resident performance in simulated induction of general anesthesia for cesarean section and showed improved performance after simulation training when assessed in a simulated setting [90, 91].

Daniels et al. [92] studied labor and delivery teams consisting of two to three nurses, one anesthesia resident, and one to two OB residents, who participated in a high-fidelity simulation of an obstetric patient who develops epidural-induced hypotension followed by an amniotic fluid embolism. Gaps identified included poor communication with pediatrics, poor leadership skills during the code, poor distribution of workload, and lack of proper use of low outlet forceps. The study identified key areas of need for focused learning in both patient management and team skills. An indication of the key role that anesthesiologists play on the labor unit is evidenced by several comments by the authors on the key role played by anesthesiologists in critical emergencies and the need for obstetricians to practice similar management skills [92]. Several organizations strongly encourage regular participation in practice sessions or drills for on-site emergencies, focused on events such as maternal hemorrhage, eclampsia, shoulder dystocia, failed intubation, and cardiac arrest. In addition to focus on provider function, these in situ scenarios may reveal latent errors in the environment and sessions that potentially could hamper care or harm a patient [93].

Recently, Lipman et al. [94] identified a number of deficiencies in simulated intrapartum cardiac arrest on the labor unit. In another study of resuscitation of simulated intrapartum cardiac arrest [95], teams were randomized to either stay in the labor room or to move the patient to the operating room; only 14% of teams moving to the OR were able to make incision for cesarean by 5 min. In addition, the teams that moved to the OR had more often performed poorer quality basic cardiopulmonary resuscitation, delayed intubation, and failed to call for pediatrics.

Pediatric Anesthesia

Pediatric anesthesia is an area of training in which duty-hour restrictions may have had particularly negative effects on case exposure. In the United Kingdom, for example, caseloads for pediatric anesthesia trainees have decreased below recommended levels [5]. In addition, anesthesiologists may only occasionally be called on to care for children and then in an emergent or urgent setting. Since the outcomes of pediatric cardiac arrest are related to number of cases and experience, it is important for both trainees and practicing physicians to have access to simulated experience. In the pediatric literature a 4-year exposure to mock codes on a pediatric service using simulation improved resuscitation outcomes from 32 to 50% survival [96]. This has not yet been demonstrated specifically for anesthesiology providers.

Edler et al. developed a portable system for in situ pediatric anesthesia simulation. Participants evaluated the course as useful, enjoyable, and felt their expectations were met, and the scenarios were realistic [97]. Fehr et al. developed ten simulation scenarios reflecting those encountered in clinical pediatric anesthesia for use in assessment of residents and fellows. More experienced subjects generally outperformed those less experienced. Score variance attributable to raters was low, yielding a high inter-rater reliability. There was a wide range of performance among the participants, even among those at equivalent levels of training [8]. Howard-Quijano et al. studied anesthesia residents' management of a simulated pediatric perioperative pulseless electrical activity arrest. Though chest compressions were initiated promptly, and epinephrine given, dosing was erroneous, and the differential diagnosis was often limited. The simulation evaluations were not compared to any other type of assessment [98].

Malignant hyperthermia (MH) management is a common topic for pediatric simulation. Gardi et al. [99] showed that while studying experienced anesthesiologists managing a simulated MH crisis, diagnosis was established quickly, dantrolene was effectively delivered, but hyperventilation was not carried out even though participants recognized it was needed, illustrating that simulation may uncover practical shortcomings in performance that are not necessarily knowledge related. MH scenarios have also illustrated shortcomings in team management as well as the value of cognitive aids in crisis management [100, 101]. These kinds of studies and scenarios can be used to inform training modules after they uncover important knowledge gaps in a particular area.

Simulation for Anesthesia Allied Health Professionals

Certified Registered Nurse Anesthetists (CRNA) and Student CRNAs (SRNA)

Like anesthesiologists, CRNAs have naturally embraced the use of simulation for education and training [39, 102–104], and much of the discussion concerning anesthesiologist and anesthesia trainee simulation-based education and assessment contained in this chapter has direct application to CRNAs [7, 105] and SRNAs. Unlike the ASA and ABA, the American Association of Nurse Anesthetists (AANA) has not established requirements for the use of simulation for primary or maintenance of certification. One CRNA training program has however adopted the use of high-fidelity simulation as one part of their admissions process for their CRNA school [106].

Simulation for Anesthesia Assistants (AA)

Very little can be found in the literature concerning the use of simulation for training and evaluating anesthesia assistants, but like anesthesiologists, anesthesiology residents, CRNAs, and SRNAs, the application and value of simulation-based education and evaluation for AAs can be inferred. There are currently only seven AA programs in the United States offering the degree of Master of Science in Anesthesia, and the majority of them list simulation-based courses in their curriculum (i.e., physiology model-based simulation, anesthesia nontechnical skills). Although the use of simulation for AA certification was discussed at the 2009 annual national conference conducted by the American Academy of Anesthesiologist Assistants (AAAA), they, like the AANA, have made no formal statements about the use of simulation for AA training, evaluation, or certification.

Given the AAs unique role and training, the AAAA adheres to and maintains the importance of the Anesthesia Care Team model. In fact, AAs practice exclusively under the supervision of anesthesiologists. Naturally, simulation would be an important training tool to foster care team effectiveness. Although AAs can perform technical aspects of the practice of anesthesia, like regional anesthesia and invasive line placements, when performed they must be carried out under the supervision, and with the express consent, of the attending anesthesiologist. It is logical to assume that the use of regional and invasive line part-task training would be valuable to the AA trainee and those in practices where experience may be limited.

Simulation for Non-anesthesia Providers

Sedation Nurses. Non-anesthesia personnel undergoing introduction to anesthesia training are common in most academic or training centers. Nurses are often expected to provide sedation, and the Joint Commission has tasked departments of anesthesia to be involved with personnel credentialing to provide sedation in a safe and appropriately monitored setting. The role of anesthesiologists is further demonstrated by the recent release of education materials to assist anesthesiologists in providing this type of training by the American Society of Anesthesiologists (ASA). Shavit et al. [107] showed that non-anesthesiologists who had undergone simulation training in pediatric sedation performed more safely in subsequent patient encounters, as measured by a checklist of safety standards, than did those who had not undergone the simulation training. Farnsworth et al. [108] showed that adding a simulation component to a sedation course for nurses improved scores on postexercise written exam; the effect on clinical practice was not assessed.

Medical Students. Hallikainen et al. [109] compared the outcomes of teaching anesthesia induction to medical students in full-scale simulation versus supervised teaching in the operating theater. The simulation group not only did significantly better than the OR group but five to six students could be trained together in the simulator, while only one was trained at a time in the OR. This shows that simulation may be more efficient as well as more effective than intraoperative teaching of novices.

Simulation for Assessment

Although competency assessment, that is, summative assessment, is covered in great detail in Chap. 11 and high-stakes assessment, for licensure and professional certification, is covered in detail in Chap. 12, for completeness it is worth briefly discussing simulation-based assessment within this chapter.

Assessment is commonly divided into formative (part of the learning process, allowing response and improvement, feedback, educational, or learner-centered in focus) and summative (sums up and applies terminology to the status of ability at a point in time, resulting in certification, licensure, or simply passing a course).

The effective use of simulation in assessment requires that appropriate metrics be developed. In scoring performance in anesthesia simulation, two types of process have been identified, explicit and implicit. Checklists exemplify explicit process or key action lists. A scoring rubric is developed from these lists. However, there are several criticisms of this type of assessment. Despite the seemingly objective nature, there is inherent subjectivity in the construction of a checklist. Experts will disagree about what belongs on a checklist, how important it is, in what order the tasks should be undertaken, and what items are "must do" (failed if absent) or "must not do" (failed if present). Checklists can encourage a rote or cookbook approach to management. Finally, timing/sequencing is difficult to incorporate into a checklist. Implicit process evaluation is demonstrated by the use of global or holistic ratings. In particular, complex competencies may be better evaluated using a rating scale than by partitioning into concrete behaviors on a checklist. Providing a rating rather than describing concrete steps calls for expert judgment. This type of assessment provides useful information on performance, including the nontechnical skills.

Adequate training and quality assessment of raters is critical to ensuring the data developed is meaningful, yet such training and calibration is often overlooked even when extensive time and effort have been devoted to developing the scale to be used. Many medical teachers find assigning a global score of 1–5 to a learner for "professionalism" or "communication" daunting. While psychometrics may be superior, and checking a number is certainly quicker than writing narrative content, such ratings fail to provide either the learner or program director with information sufficient to define steps for improvement.

A checklist, even if every expert would not follow every step, can be used to teach an acceptable approach to a skill such as placing an epidural catheter. Such a tool when completed and discussed with the learner presents detailed and specific feedback that could be used to improve skills.

Many teachers see the oral examination as a demonstration of what a learner would do in a given clinical situation. It is the demonstration that he or she knows what to do with the cognitive knowledge successfully demonstrated in a written exam (a prerequisite to advancing to the oral examination stage). However, this supposition has never been definitively demonstrated. Oral examination and simulation assessments measure different things—the oral exam lets the candidate demonstrate that he "knows how," but the simulation exercise lets him "show how" he would manage the case. Savoldelli et al. [110] used standardized evaluation tools to assess the performance of senior anesthesia residents who discussed an oral exam question then managed a different case with a similar degree of difficulty in a simulated setting. The authors found that the simulation trial assessed clinical judgment and skills with reliability equivalent to that of the oral exam. They noted that the simulation exercise allowed the examiners to observe suboptimal performance likely not detectable with the oral exam format, such as delay in performing chest compression after detecting loss of pulse and failure to perform a needle decompression of tension pneumothorax. The simulation exercise also allowed the examiners to observe the precise timing and sequencing of care. Of note, every participant who received a "fail" in the simulation exercise also received a "fail" in portions of the oral exam.

Israeli Anesthesia Board Examinations have incorporated simulation stations as an adjunct to their oral exams since 2003 [111]. Candidates go through five stations, each 15–20 min long. Trauma and resuscitation stations evaluate concepts of Advanced Trauma Life Support (ATLS) and Advanced Cardiac Life Support (ACLS), respectively. A CRM station demonstrates nontechnical CRM skills during a scenario in which the examinee is called in to assist a colleague with a difficult clinical situation. A ventilation station lets the candidate manage a ventilator attached to an artificial lung and make changes as needed in response to compliance and arterial blood gas changes. Finally a regional anesthesia station allows the candidate to demonstrate, with a standardized patient, surface anatomy landmarks, needle location, direction, dosing, and management of complications for various regional techniques [112]. Development of these simulations stations required the creation of detailed checklists of observable behaviors, standardization of the scenarios, and training of examiners. Examinees are oriented to the scenario types and the environment 3–4 weeks in advance of the actual exam. For successful completion of the examination, the candidates must pass both the simulation stations and the oral exam. Examinees' assessment of the difficulty of the simulation stations varied, but they reported that the simulation stations were preferable to the oral exam portion. While no such system is currently used in the UK, the ABA has announced the inclusion of Objective Structured Clinical Examinations (OSCEs) to the 2016 oral examination.

Continuing Professional Development and Maintenance of Certification in Anesthesiology (MOCA)

Since 2000, anesthesiologists in the United States have earned a time-limited (10-year) board certification from the American Board of Anesthesiology (ABA). In order to renew board certification, anesthesiologists must participate in the Maintenance of Certification in Anesthesiology (MOCA) program administered by the ABA [12]. MOCA consists of four components: I—professional standing, II—lifelong learning and self-assessment, III—cognitive examination, and IV—practice performance assessment and improvement. A simulation exercise is required at least once in every 10-year cycle as a component of part IV, practice performance assessment. The candidate participates in a simulated critical event and debriefing and through subsequent reflection, develops and executes a plan for improving knowledge, skills, or practice. These exercises must occur at simulation centers endorsed by the American Society of Anesthesiology (ASA) to ensure a quality offering [113]. Fellow participants in a MOCA simulation exercise are all board certified anesthesiologists. During the 6- to 8-h day of simulation, scenario/debrief exercises cover topics that must include hemodynamic and respiratory instability and crew resource management. Scenarios should not be subspecialty-based and should consist of cases that any board certified anesthesiologist should be able to manage. In addition, MOCA for anesthesia subspecialties (MOCA SUBS), in critical care and pain, are available at centers specifically endorsed for those MOCA SUBS. Some centers may offer a MOCA simulation day with a specific emphasis, for example, pediatric anesthesia, but are required to clearly notify registrants of the specific focus.

A MOCA simulation is not a summative assessment, that is, it is not a test, and a score is not generated. All feedback is formative, that is, constructive feedback to let the individual and teams function more effectively. At the end of the simulation exercise, participants develop a practice improvement plan that lists the changes or enhancement to their skill set, knowledge, or changes in practice processes he/she desires to make. Between 30 and 90 days after that initial report, the participant will provide a progress report on their initial plan in order to earn credit for the simulation portion of MOCA.

The ABA is the first of the American medical specialty boards to make simulation part of its maintenance of certification requirements. The ASA endorsement program for simulation centers is one of three (ASA, American College of Surgery, and Society for Simulation in Healthcare) that are currently available in the USA.

The "Art" of Simulation in Anesthesia

Scenario Design

It is important to recognize that simulation is a powerful educational technique that should not be expected to supplant or replace an entire curriculum of lectures, problem-based learning, self-study, and clinical contact. Simulation exercises are meant to enhance and supplement those other learning experiences by filling knowledge and ability gaps and by addressing skills and topics that are ineffectively taught with other approaches. Simulation can also be used to create a safe structured experiential learning for cases that occur infrequently in clinical practice but for which management expertise is still expected.

When considering creating a scenario, simulation-based course, or an entire simulation-based curriculum in a training program, it is important to first identify several key fundamental elements that must be considered. In the text below we outline our approach to simulation-based curriculum development.

Identify Your Audience

Audience identification is critical when developing your simulation-based curriculum. Although the same simulation can be used for a variety of audiences with various levels of training, the goals and objectives, performance expectations, and debriefing curriculum will vary greatly. For example, when developing a scenario of anaphylaxis-specific expectations for performance, skill set and management would depend on the learners. Goals for medical students might simply be the recognition of a critical incident and calling for help. A junior resident would be expected to recognize the critical event, call for help, but also manage the physiologic perturbations. Senior residents and practitioners would also be expected to recognize and manage the patient in an expeditious manner but would also be expected to work the patient up after the reaction, manage the patient should they come to the OR, and effectively educate and counsel the patient and other healthcare providers involved in the case. Even though the scenario might be ostensibly the same in all three situations, the objectives and the debriefing curriculum would, therefore, be very different for each audience.

For junior learners, simulation provides an opportunity to recognize a critical problem, initiate management, and be the principle operator or team leader. In clinical practice junior trainees are often relegated to a peripheral role in management of actual critical situations. Simulation is a unique opportunity for junior trainees to actually plan and carry out their care and experience the successes, pitfalls, limitations, and potential errors of their decision-making. What happens if one under-resuscitates a patient prior to induction? What if your dose of anesthetic agents is too high or too low? What if you forget to cross-check blood products before transfusion, or proceed with surgery without confirming that blood is available? Frequently at the junior level, the technical performance of the trainee is emphasized. At the more senior learner level, increasing emphasis is placed on human factors or nontechnical skills of management (e.g., communicating the problem to others in the room, managing the team, recognition of and management of emotional stressors) in addition to practicing management of critical events.

Medical Students. Developing appropriate educational objectives for medical students not headed into a career in anesthesiology can be challenging. The medical student is usually far more interested in "doing" procedures and less in the processes and science of anesthesiology. Providing their early exposure to anesthesia practice in a simulated setting offers students the opportunity to manage a case and practice its attendant skill set without the pressures of time or risk to patients. Simulation allows pausing at key moments to discuss how and why decisions are made in patient management. Task training with airway models, spinal models, and IV trainers can also give the very junior person opportunity to experience the basics of those skills.

Our introduction to anesthesia course is offered in the second year of medical school to students who have had a modest amount of patient contact but no exposure to acute care. In the simulation center, faculty guide small groups of students through an anesthetic induction, breaking it down into the component steps: preoperative evaluation of the patient, setup of the room and equipment, anesthesia machine check, induction of general anesthesia including choice of drugs, bag-and-mask ventilation, intubation and confirmation of endotracheal tube placement, and finally maintenance of anesthesia. The first simulated patient is healthy and responds to management as expected; the scenario is then repeated in a hypovolemic patient to highlight the consequences of volume depletion and show management of the subsequent hypotension. We pause the scenario at each step to discuss what has happened, anticipate what is likely to happen next, and to formulate a plan of action.

Another exercise appropriate for this level of learner treats the mannequin as a lab modeling the physiologic effects of hypovolemia, hypervolemia, hyperventilation, and hypoventilation. Another exercise is to play "name that drug" in which the mannequin is given a drug, the effects are observed, and the learners speculate on the class and identity of the drug administered.

Sedation Nurses. Designing a curriculum to educate nurses to safety provide sedation must effectively meet cognitive and psychomotor skills needs. Necessary cognitive knowledge includes drug effects and dosing, common problems that may be encountered (hypoventilation, agitation, nausea, vomiting), record keeping, and familiarity with the procedure being performed. Technical skills needed include placing intravenous access, airway management, recognition of hypoventilation, and operation of the monitoring equipment. Finally proficiency in nontechnical skills is important, including leadership and communications skills adequate to respond to challenges and problems during sedation, deal professionally and safely with pressure to over-sedate a patient, and maintain situation awareness. The cognitive knowledge items are probably as well learned through self-study or with Web-based products. The technical and nontechnical skills as well as the ability to apply the cognitive knowledge in a clinical setting can be practiced in simulation with reflection and improvement.

Anesthesiology Residents and Other Trainees. Simulation should be used strategically to enhance the current residency curriculum. If an area is already effectively covered by other means, it is redundant to put resources into creating simulation for that area. Since July 1, 2011, the Accreditation Council for Graduate Medical Education (ACGME) has required anesthesia residents to participate in at least one simulation education exersise each year of training. Training programs are not required to have or use formal simulation centers for these experiences. The ACGME encourages multidisciplinary simulation when possible, endorses the scenario/debrief model, and recommends that exercises incorporate the core competencies of medical knowledge, communication skills, professionalism, systems-based practice, and practice-based learning and improvement [11].

Table 17.2 Key problems that need to be managed by novice anesthesia residents

Problem
Hypotension
Hypertension
Cardiac rhythm changes
ST segment changes
Decreasing oxygen saturation
Increased airway pressures
Increased patient temperature
Undesired patient movement

Education and assessment must be clearly and consistently kept separate and distinct. As soon as learners perceive they are being "tested," the safe environment that a simulation center strives to maintain is changed.

New residents may benefit from high-fidelity simulation to ingrain key behaviors needed for effective responses to common potentially adverse events. Novices need to reliably (1) recognize events are going awry, (2) call for help, and (3) manage the problem appropriately for 2 or 3 min until more definitive help arrives. This helps the novice become a safe in-room provider and allows them to practice communication with the surgical team while carrying out universal initial steps of resuscitation. This training has been called "drownproofing" which colorfully conveys the concept of teaching someone how to stay afloat until rescued. With this outcome in mind, the number of topics to be covered is relatively small (see Table 17.2).

Within our residency program, novice residents are introduced to CRM as outlined above as well as task training for airway, monitor usage, infusion pumps, and central line placement within the first 2 months. Subsequently, simulation education in more advanced subspecialty-specific topics is offered during the applicable clinical rotation. Learners are able to practice and apply the skills learned in the clinical rotation in more challenging formats in the simulator center with enhanced opportunity for reflection and feedback. The instructors are the same clinicians supervising the clinical rotations. Examples of simulation scenarios offered with specific subspecialty rotations are shown in Tables 17.3, 17.4, 17.5, and 17.6. Airway management techniques for both operative and nonoperative settings are reinforced with task trainer-based airway workshops on an annual basis.

Identify the Role Simulation Will Have in the Curriculum

We recommend that programs decide whether or not their simulation activities will focus on education, assessment, or both, since this determination will have significant ramifications

Table 17.3 Obstetric anesthesia rotation: simulation scenarios

Cesarean section under general anesthesia
Unanticipated difficult airway after induction of general anesthesia for cesarean delivery
Intrapartum maternal cardiac arrest
Local anesthetic systemic toxicity
Eclampsia
Postpartum hemorrhage
The impaired obstetrics provider

Table 17.4 Cardiovascular anesthesia rotation: simulation scenarios

Weaning from cardiopulmonary bypass
Straightforward
Complicated
Open abdominal aortic aneurysm repair—unclamping the aorta
Management of intraoperative arrhythmias
The cardiopulmonary bypass machine

Table 17.5 Regional anesthesia rotation: simulation scenarios

Task trainers: ultrasound + gel models
High-fidelity simulation of:
High/total spinal
Local anesthetic systemic toxicity
Over-sedation of the regional anesthetic patient
Anaphylaxis
Panic attack
Myocardial ischemia
Retrobulbar block with local anesthetic uptake along optic nerve sheath

Table 17.6 Pediatric anesthesia rotation: simulation scenarios

Induction of general anesthesia challenges:
Bradycardia
Laryngospasm
Difficult venous access
Airway management
Intraoperative pediatric cardiac arrest
Pediatric multiple trauma—emergency surgery

on scenario design and assessment tool development. It needs to be clear to learners whether or not a simulation exercise will be used for education, in which formative feedback will be given, that is, constructive feedback, or used for assessment, in which a summative evaluation or a "score" is given. In an exercise in which formative feedback will be given, the participant is in a safe environment, and mistakes should be seen as opportunities for discussion and improvement.

When simulation is used as part of a summative assessment, mistakes may no longer serve as opportunities for participant improvement but may in fact be educational obstacles to the participant. Scoring tools for both technical skills and nontechnical skills must be developed and validated. Finally the scenarios themselves must be completely reproducible so that each participant truly does have the same case [13, 111]. Challenges in developing reproducible, validated scenarios and assessment tools have led many simulation centers to primarily focus on using simulation as an educational tool with formative assessment. This is not to say that summative assessments cannot be used; however, their use is complex and controversial to say the least.

Curriculum Development and Knowledge Gap Identification

Topics or cases for simulation should arise from a gap in the current curriculum. Examples are topics that have not traditionally been taught, for example, crew/crisis resource management, leadership and effective communication skills, and the management of rare and critical events, in which timely care can make the difference between life and death, including difficult airway management, malignant hyperthermia, operating room fires, blood transfusion reactions, anaphylaxis, tension pneumothorax, pulmonary embolus, cardiac and respiratory arrest, and local anesthetic toxicity. If a particular knowledge or skill is successfully taught in the current curriculum, there is little incentive to invest the time and resources needed to develop a redundant simulation exercise. For each topic one needs to identify the knowledge gap being filled as well as a set of specific goals and objectives taught. This will ensure that the scenario development will remain focused.

Conducting and observing participants' performance in simulated scenarios will itself highlight common errors and may reveal a gap in training not previously appreciated. For example, we developed a simulation exercise focusing on the management of an emergent cesarean section under general anesthesia. After a few run-throughs it became clear that the learners had a poorly organized approach to managing the difficult airway. We used this gap as the impetus to rewrite the scenario so that the main objective was mastering the management of the difficult airway with less emphasis on the other aspects of the case (see Fig. 17.10). Once the airway objectives were achieved, subsequent scenarios focused on the other important aspects of emergent cesarean section management.

Some gaps or educational goals may not require high-fidelity simulation exercises to be filled. For example, specific knowledge gaps such as the dosing of resuscitation medications may be learned effectively with self-study or use of cognitive aids. Task trainers or screen-based simulators may be an equally effective mode to fill the gap, for example, confusion about operation of a new defibrillator could be remedied

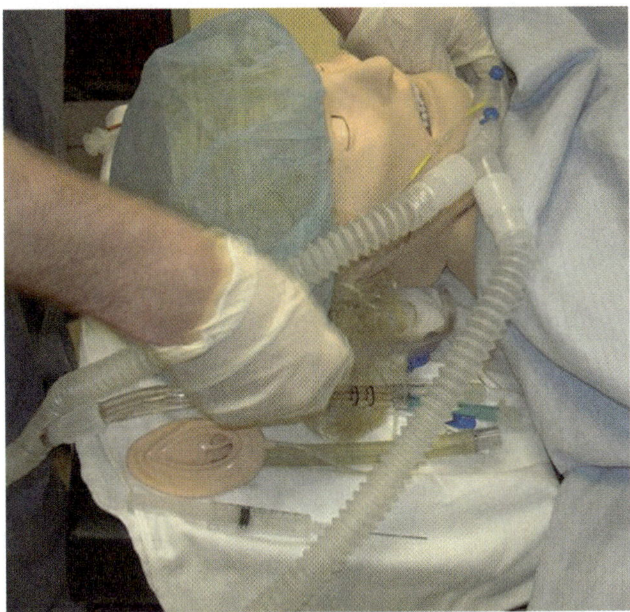

Fig. 17.10 Example of final securing of the airway in a patient with a difficult airway at the time of cesarean section under general anesthetic. The learner has attempted direct laryngoscopy, laryngeal mask, and combi-tube and finally did a surgical cricothyrotomy

by practicing the operation of the defibrillator in a small group without mobilizing all the other resources of a high-fidelity simulation. There is a maxim in the airline simulation industry that you only use as much sophistication in your simulation as is necessary to meet your objectives.

Utilization of Simulation Resources

Time in simulation is a finite resource, so scenario topics must be prioritized. Should one create a scenario around the extremely rare events of line swap of medical gases, a bioterrorism attack, or intraoperative electrical power loss if you have not already covered more fundamental events? Planning should take into account how much simulation time each learner has and use that time wisely. Still, some fundamental rules apply.

Keep It Simple. There is a temptation to build scenarios around interesting cases, rather than finding the curricular gaps that call for simulation techniques. Often as a scenario is created, it is made more complex than necessary, with the addition of dramatic shifts and multiple distracters, including a screaming family member, simply to stress the learner. Unnecessarily complex scenarios increase cognitive load for everyone. These scenarios are not only difficult to stage and reproduce, they are confusing to participants and possibly the instructors, increasing the risk that a scenario will go down an unexpected pathway and spin out of control and fail miserably. We have observed that as simulation authors become more skilled, the scenarios become increasingly simple and straightforward. Every ingredient in the scenario is there for a specific purpose tied to the learning objectives, not simply "to make the case more challenging" or "cooler." If the learners finish the exercise and cannot identify the learning objectives, it is unlikely that these goals were met at all. Simplicity allows the set goals and objectives to be clear to all by the debriefing.

Ok. Do Not Keep It Simple. There are times (e.g., with senior trainees or attending anesthesiologists) where the complexity of a scenario is deliberately increased to allow for the introduction of finite skills and knowledge that would only be expected of this group. If a specific task, like chest tube placement, is to be part of a high-fidelity simulation, we recommend that the learner should be familiar with the task before starting the scenario. If not, then a hands-on exercise focused on the skill should be completed before the scenario. Full-scale simulation should integrate that skill or task into the total picture of case management, working through its indications, contraindications, and potential consequences and complications. For example, one might start the day with a task trainer session on needle decompression of the chest for pneumothorax and perhaps even chest tube placement. Subsequently the learner manages a scenario in which a tension pneumothorax develops, and they are required to recognize the need for needle decompression and perform it. The final scenario might present findings suggestive of tension pneumothorax; however, needle decompression of the chest does not solve the problem, forcing the learner to widen the differential diagnosis and enact another plan.

Many of these principles can be seen when reviewing an example scenario (see Table 17.7). We observed that our residents were not considering an adequate differential diagnosis of increasing agitation in patients undergoing regional anesthesia. We identified specific objectives including recognition and management of agitation and dyspnea in a patient undergoing cystoscopy. The patient does not deteriorate to a malignant rhythm, seize, or develop any other of the more dramatic potential outcomes since the objective is management of agitation and respiratory distress.

Multidisciplinary Versus Single Discipline Simulation

The practice of anesthesiology is seldom done in isolation. The practice setting typically includes surgeons, other OR personnel, and recovery room and ICU staff, all with different backgrounds and roles. In an ideal world, simulation training would involve a variety of personnel from different disciplines. If the objectives of a simulation are very specialty specific, there is probably less to be gained from the multidisciplinary approach. One of the challenges with this approach is that the other roles in the scenario, for example, scrub nurse, surgeon, patient, and family member, will likely be played by anesthesia participants although some centers use medical

Table 17.7 An example of an anesthetic scenario with objectives identified and the actions of the scenario specifically tailored to achieve those objectives

Title: Cystoscopy with bladder perforation			
Audience: Anesthesia resident, SRNA			
Objectives-Medical Knowledge: Identify potential problems associated with cystoscopy			
Patient care: Management of unexpected agitation in a patient with spinal anesthesia and management of intraoperative dyspnea			
Communication: Utilize crew resource management skills to successfully manage an intraoperative emergency			
Case stem: Mr. Jones is a 70-year-old male with stable CAD, taking metoprolol and daily ASA and presenting for cystoscopy and fulguration for bladder cancer. Previous anesthetics have been uneventful. Spinal anesthesia has been successfully placed by your colleague with 1.5 ml of 0.5% bupivacaine with 25 mcg of fentanyl and solid T6 block. Patient is resting comfortably with propofol infusion of 25 mcg/kg/min running. The cystoscopy has been under way for 5 min			
Room setup: OR with patient in lithotomy position. Cystoscopy equipment with an irrigation bag. Patient covered with drapes.			
Patient will have O_2 by nasal cannula, single IV with normal saline running, and propofol infusion. He will have ECG, BP cuff, pulse oximeter, and temperature probe			
An anesthesia machine will be at the head of the bed with induction drugs and airway equipment available			
State	**Patient status**	**Learner actions**	
Baseline	Drowsy but responsive	After handoff, introduces himself to the patient and surgeon, checks IVs, infusions and monitor	If learner does not introduce himself within 1 min, the surgeon will initiate intros
	HR 60, NSR; RR 10, BP 115/84, Sat 100%, T 37	Inquire of the surgeon what the problem is	After 2 min the surgeon will complain that he is having trouble seeing and will ask that the irrigation be turned up higher
Agitation	Patient gets agitated and would not lay still. He will not answer questions	Generates a differential diagnosis of agitation and confusion	Surgeon complains that he cannot work with the patient moving all around but states he has increased bleeding in bladder
	VS as above except BP 150/90, RR 15, Sat 95%	Draws Na Asks surgeon if anything has changed on his end	Asks for irrigation to be increased
Dyspnea	Patient continues to be confused and agitated. HR 85, BP 175/90, RR 30, Sat 89%	Recognition of respiratory failure Assist breathing, consider conversion to GA and intubation: if intubates, go to stabilizes Tell surgeon and room that there are problems	If he does not intubate within 2 min, go to deterioration
Deterioration	Patient is unresponsive but gasping. HR 100, BP 84/60, RR 35, Sat 70%, NSR with PVC's	Assists ventilation and intubation Consider pressors, e.g., ephedrine or phenylephrine	Surgeon and OR nurse ask if there is a problem Will stay in this state if nothing is done until the patient is intubated or instructor decides to help the learner
Stabilizes	Patient is intubated, HR 90, BP 100/70, Sat 95%, decreased compliance	Articulates induction drugs Anticipates hemodynamic instability with induction Generates Ddx for decompensation and shares it with surgeon	Surgeon comments on tense abdomen If learner does not consider it, surgeon will offer that he may have perforated bladder Develop a plan for abdominal exploration
Discussion points: Ddx for agitation in sedated patient under functioning regional anesthesia (hypoxia, hypercapnia, high block, electrolyte abnormality, hypoglycemia, disinhibition with sedation, surgical stimulation moving beyond blocked area)			
Any special considerations for cystoscopy (bladder perforation, hyponatremia with systemic absorption of irrigation solution)?			
Why did the patient become dyspneic (abdominal pain, abdominal distension and displacement of diaphragm)?			
Did the hypoxia come first and then the dyspnea or the other way around?			
Were the surgeon and OR crew aware of your problems—what was the help that you needed (labs, lights on, someone to assist with induction/intubation, info that the surgeon could share)?			
What special concerns are there for converting this case to general anesthesia (decreased venous return and risk of post-induction hypotension, decreased FRC and risk of desaturation with apnea, airway management during suboptimal circumstances, e.g., airway assessment, draped patient)?			
What could be done to mitigate these challenges (tell surgeon and OR staff of need to convert, designate one of the OR staff to assist you with induction, move drapes back for patient, check of induction drugs and airway equipment, adequate preoxygenation assisting patient with his ventilation, having pressors immediately at hand?)			

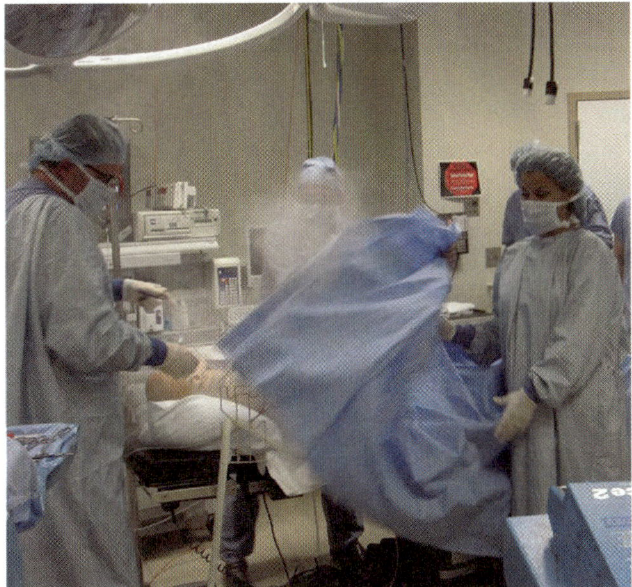

Fig. 17.11 Scenario of a drape fire moments after it ignites in patient who is undergoing a superficial surgery of his right neck under sedation. The anesthesiologist has just discontinued oxygen, and he and the scrub nurse are removing the drapes

students, educators, and actors to portray other roles (confederates) in the scenario. It is imperative that the confederates have a clear understanding of their purpose, their limitations, and how helpful they should be and that they must forget that they are anesthesiologists. On the other hand if the objectives include management of problems where input from different disciplines is critical, the effort to develop a multidisciplinary exercise may well be worth the effort.

An example of multidisciplinary simulation training that we found to be very successful centered on an OR fire. In this scenario, anesthesiology personnel are working side by side with OR personnel. A simulated fire breaks out and management requires stopping excess oxygen, removing burning drapes, ensuring that the fire is in fact out, activating a call for help, and subsequently caring for any injuries to the patient (see Fig. 17.11).

During the debrief, fire prevention and management were covered, but a rich discussion ensued around each person's responsibilities in the OR and how each can assist the other. It also provided an opportunity to explore how our fire management policies are drafted and to identify both misconceptions and unclear areas in the drafted policy.

Simply getting a team together outside of their usual clinical setting to meet and discuss problems can often be team building in addition to the richness associated with the simulation exercise. Breaking through the barriers of hierarchy and learning to know one another as individuals is often easier outside of the usual workspace.

Logistics: Dedicated Simulation Center Versus Simulation In Situ

Dedicated Simulation Center

High-fidelity simulation exercises may be carried out in a dedicated simulation center, in which simulated clinical space and equipment as well as the mannequin are all available. Advantages of this approach include complete control over the setting, equipment, staffing, and scheduling. Audio and video recording capabilities tend also to be more sophisticated. Finally, participants and instructors will be less likely to be interrupted and called away for clinical duties if they are in a separate nonclinical setting. Disadvantages include difficulty in getting people to the simulation center, particularly if it is far from the clinical areas. Finally, in spite of best efforts and significant resources, a simulation center simply cannot recreate the clinical work space in precise and exact detail.

Simulation In Situ

An alternative approach is "simulation in situ," in which simulation equipment is brought to a clinical area. Advantages include that the clinical and training spaces are exactly alike (enhancing suspension of disbelief), and it is quicker and easier to get participants to the simulation location, particularly important for short exercises and multidisciplinary participation. In addition to seeing how participants perform, simulation in situ also reveals how the system and physical space function and allows participants hands-on experience with new equipment if that is the goal of the simulation (e.g., new anesthesia workstation, IV pumps).

In situ simulation can also allow for "just-in-time" task training, for example, rehearsal of a task on a trainer, just prior to completing the task in a clinical setting. In situ simulation provides the opportunity to do short quick exercises between clinical responsibilities or even reenact clinical scenarios that have just played out. However, scenarios that are done on an impromptu basis will have limited sophistication due to the inability to plan in detail and assemble a simulation team quickly. Simulation in a more public setting will increase visibility of a simulation program for other departments, learners, clinicians, and leaders as well.

Simulation in situ does have some disadvantages compared to a dedicated simulation center: support personnel and equipment may not work as smoothly in non-dedicated space, "ownership" of equipment and responsibility for its use and maintenance is less clear, and scheduling simulation exercises as clinical activity and staffing varies can be challenging. Learners and instructors may be less able to focus and engage with the simulation if distracted by clinical responsibilities, patients/families/other staff may be disturbed, and finally, assuring psychological safety in a multidisciplinary exercise in one's daily work site can be problematic due to public exposure and imbedded hierarchies and cultural expectations.

Logistics: Running the Scenario and Putting It All Together

Consider the Simulator's Capabilities in Your Scenario Design

Once one has decided on a topic, objectives, audience, and location and drafted a clinical story that will form the basis of the scenario, the simulation equipment and personnel required will need to be considered. Ensure the scenario takes into account the strengths and weaknesses of the equipment and physical space. For example, if heart sounds are difficult to hear and interpret on a particular mannequin, do not create a scenario in which noticing changes in heart sounds is critical to successful management. To make successful management of a scenario contingent on recognition of clinical signs that are poorly replicated on the mannequin is frustrating both for learners and instructors. Develop plausible alternatives that get clinical findings across to the participants: create other clinical evidence that would accompany the clinical condition being portrayed or use a confederate to pass the information to them. For example, suppose you wanted to portray a seizure and your mannequin does not have "seizure capabilities." One could have the mannequin stop responding to the learners, close its eyes, change its respiratory pattern, and increase its heart rate, all features that may accompany a seizure, and ultimately have one of the confederates in the room comment on seizure activity, perhaps shaking the mannequin's leg or bumping the bed. Ultimately one needs to ask how much fidelity is needed to achieve the objectives of the exercise.

Programming the Simulator

Preprogrammed. Control of the mannequin as its physiology changes throughout the case may be completely preprogrammed, in which physiologic changes occur based on activities sensed by the mannequin, for example, pulse checks, ventilation, or at predetermined times. Preprogramming is advantageous if you want multiple physiological changes to occur simultaneously, for example, a rise in heart rate and respiratory rate, with a fall in blood pressure and oxygen saturation, or if the scenario should be consistent each time it is run, important if summative assessments will be made. Unfortunately, the sensing mechanisms on many of the mannequins can be inconsistent leading to erroneous movement from physiological state to state. This can mislead the participants and send the scenario down an unexpected pathway. In addition, it does not permit you to adjust the scenario on the fly in response to the participants' performance.

On the Fly. The opposite extreme is to have all physiological changes controlled manually by an operator. Advantages to operator control include the ability to respond to unanticipated actions by the learners, nudge them toward desired pathways, and emphasize findings not being noticed, as you directly observe their actions and respond accordingly. However, disadvantages include the challenge of making many changes quickly, possibly missing some actions of learners, and making changes that are inconsistent from group to group doing the same scenario.

We recommend a hybrid approach in which predefined physiological sets of physiological changes are defined, but the operator controls the transition from state to state based on the learners interventions and fine-tuning the mannequin's responses as needed.

Defining the Role of Confederates and Participants

In addition to describing how the mannequin reacts as the case progresses, one needs to prospectively identify the roles of the people who will be in the room and what they should do. We will usually have at least one "confederate" in the scenario room from the simulation center staff. They are in communication with the simulation control room, prompt the participants as needed, provide supplies, and act as the eyes and ears of the control room for interactions that would otherwise be missed. Other roles in the scenario are frequently assigned to participants in the simulation session; however, it is necessary that they have a clear description of their role, including dialogue, how helpful they should be, what their skill set is, and their emotional state. In a multidisciplinary simulation scenario, we will usually assign participants to roles that mimic their regular duties.

One must explicitly decide what information to provide to the participant leading the case, the "hot-seat" person or "star," before he/she enters the room. We will typically do this as a handoff from another caregiver (usually a confederate). The adequacy of the handoff depends on the objectives, for example, it may be complete and thorough or too brief or misleading.

Before Starting

The Dress Rehearsal. Ultimately, prior to running the scenario with actual learners, a dry run with simulation center staff can help to highlight potential problem areas. A common error on the part of novice instructors is to think that a good teacher can walk into a simulator and create a good learning experience on the fly. Not only is this unlikely to provide a good learning opportunity for the residents, it is extremely challenging for simulation center staff to facilitate a smooth running scenario with necessary supplies and equipment available.

Orientation Is Critical. Typically a simulation session will consist of a number of simulation scenarios/debrief exercises. Prior to beginning the exercise, learners are thoroughly introduced to the setting, made aware of the rules of the simulation center, especially confidentiality, and are assured that this is a safe place for learning—errors are common and expected. Learners should be introduced to the technology that they will be using, including the use and limitations of the clinical equipment available, as well as the salient features of the mannequin. When learners come to the simulation center for the first time, we give them an opportunity to see the mannequin prior to any scenario, encouraging them to feel the pulses, listen to heart and breath sounds, see him breathing, and interact with him. We have found that rather than saying "here is the mannequin, feel here for a pulse," we introduce the learners to the mannequin as if it were a patient, including introducing him by name, having the mannequin respond, asking permission to listen to his chest and so on. This helps to set the expectation of interacting with the mannequin as if it were a patient, with respect and consideration.

Strategies to Contend with Hyper-vigilance, Pattern Matching, and Other Behaviors Common in the Simulated Environment

When participants are in a simulation session, they expect the worst to happen and are frequently hyper-vigilant, overreacting to minor changes in physiology. There is also the risk of "pattern matching" after a scenario, in which the learners may come away from the scenario with a bias that every instance of a particular physiological change is the clinical problem that they saw in the scenario rather than considering a differential diagnosis after initial resuscitation. One strategy is to build a session around a theme with a number of scenarios, each starting out with the same clinical situation going down different pathways. An example is a simulation session in which a patient who is undergoing peri-lumbar or psoas nerve block becomes unstable [76], but from that point the simulation evolves into different scenarios including local anesthetic-induced seizure, local anesthetic-induced cardiac toxicity, tachycardia and myocardial ischemia (unrelated to local anesthetic), high spinal, and panic attack—all from the same initial case—reinforcing the necessity of developing differential diagnoses, avoiding pattern matching, and recognizing the similarities and differences of the therapy for each. It also provides an opportunity to discuss the consequences of proceeding down the wrong pathway and methods of recovery from that wrong step. Another strategy, which presents some logistical challenges, is simulation roulette [114] in which the course of the scenario from its stem is determined by chance from a number of different possibilities, some of which may be completely benign. This can avoid some of the over-vigilance and excessively aggressive therapy that is seen in simulation. The case shown in Table 17.7, in which a patient undergoing cystoscopy suffers a bladder perforation and requires conversion to general anesthesia, was part of a series of scenarios that were staged one after another around the theme of the agitated patient.

Troubleshooting a Scenario or Rescuing a Scenario Gone Awry

Despite everyone's best efforts in developing a well-thought-out and rehearsed scenario, there are a variety of reasons why a scenario might fail to go as planned, and educators and staff need to be prepared with strategies to rescue the derailed or failing scenario. The reasons a scenario can go off course include issues with the learners, the scenario, and technical problems. Below is a discussion of each and effective ways to contend with and learn from the "failed scenario."

Learner Issues. A scenario may go awry when the learners go down a management pathway that the scenario author did not anticipate [115]. This can occur when learners do not understand what the scenario portrays. Gaps in the participants' knowledge base, missing important signs, or faults in the scenario design may contribute. During the scenario, the exercise may be "rescued" if the confederate "nudges" the participants in the correct direction by commenting on findings that the participants have overlooked or misinterpreted ("I don't think the patient's chest is moving; what do you think?") or even suggesting therapies ("I've often seen the senior people in the department give epinephrine in this case"). Another confederate ("the nursing supervisor") may be sent into the room to "help out" and guide the scenario onto the right track. Both of these strategies can maintain some sense of realism while effectively bringing the scenario back to the objectives. A final approach is the "voice from above" in which the scenario director announces into the room what they want the participants to see, with the scenario functionally being paused for a moment and then restarted.

A participant in the scenario may do something completely unanticipated. Occasionally one of the participants who is in a supporting role may go "off script." For example, a participant assigned the role of an anesthesia assistant in one of our scenarios went "off script" and acted sullen and unhelpful to the learner on the hot seat, much to the instructor's dismay. The instructor worried that the learner on the hot seat, managing an unanticipated inability to intubate or ventilate after induction of general anesthesia for cesarean section, would not have a good learning experience due to this additional stressor. However, close observation showed that the learner was taking his colleague's improvisation completely in stride. During debriefing, this offered an unexpected learning opportunity as possible management and communication strategies in the face of unhelpful team members were discussed. These unexpected events may signal to the scenario author that the script for a given role needs clarification and firmer boundaries. Still, the ability to recognize and smoothly exploit these unanticipated opportunities during the debriefing is a skill to be developed in instructors.

Controlling the "mood" of the scenario, particularly with first-time simulation participants, may be challenging. Buy-in of the participants to the whole simulation experience is critical; this can be enhanced with a thoughtful introduction that lays out the ground rules of the simulation activity. It is frustrating to see learners joking or bantering with each other at the beginning of the scenario. A confederate may need to tweak the emotional atmosphere in the scenario by challenging them as he might if people were acting inappropriately in front of patients, for example, "the patient seems to be getting upset with your remarks" or "who are you?" The mannequin/patient may begin to cry or comment on the unprofessionalism of the caregivers, giving a wake-up call for the team that they need to think of the mannequin as a living patient, bringing them back into the scenario. We have found that reminding participants of the vulnerability of patients, with a sad or worried patient comment, is usually more effective than a confrontational patient who challenges them on their behavior. Instructors need to recognize though that levity at the beginning of a scenario may reflect anxiety on the part of the learner and this should not be negatively perceived.

Occasionally one may encounter a difficult learner who resists engaging and participating as expected. During the introductory remarks, it is important to emphasize the need for all members of the session to embrace the experience in order that the entire group is able to make the most of the learning opportunities; an uncooperative learner not only limits his or her own learning but may disrupt the scenario for all. When a learner is not performing as expected, one approach is to have the scenario progress as it would in real life: a cursory exam, rude or dismissive behavior, or failure to inject medications results in logical consequences such as misdiagnosis, an uncooperative team member or angry patient, or worsening vital signs or pain. Thus, the learner and the team are forced to deal with the outcomes, reinforcing the "fictional contract." During the debriefing, one needs to let the difficult learner vent and then acknowledge perceived shortcomings of the scenario while keeping the focus on learning from the scenario. The difficult learner and his or her concerns must be dealt with proactively to avoid contaminating the entire debrief. This "bump in the road" may also provide an opportunity during debriefing to discuss issues related to professionalism.

A learner may become upset during or immediately after his performance during a scenario. This may be due to a disappointing performance or because the scenario itself is traumatic or uncovers painful past experiences. The emotion should be gently acknowledged during the debrief: "I sense that you are upset." Usually the others in the learner group are very supportive of their colleague, and can be asked if they have experienced similar situations, moving the focus away from one individual's performance and toward developing solutions to improve management in the future.

Scenario Issues. Shortcomings in the design and staging of a scenario may also lead to the scenario unfolding in unintended ways. The scenario should be matched to the level of the participants—too simple or, more commonly, too complex a scenario may cause participants to be distracted by a single task or concept that is not one of the objectives. This can be a problem when a simulation center has a library of scenarios and an instructor uses one without appreciating the audience's unique needs. If a scenario is not perceived as "believable," for instance, if the case presented is unusual or implausible, buy-in can be a problem. Basing a scenario, or at least core theme of a scenario, on actual cases can be helpful when the "plausibility" of the scenario comes up in the debrief session. A good approach during the debrief is to ask, "Has anyone seen a case similar to this?"

Technical Issues. Major technical failure, for example, the mannequin fails, is inevitable and will usually mean the scenario needs to stop. We have found that halting the scenario until the issue is resolved and then trying to restart the scenario from that point usually does not work well, since the buy-in and momentum have been lost. We will often abandon that scenario, but debrief about what has happened up to that point and discuss how the scenario might progress, so the partial scenario and debrief evolves into a problem-based learning discussion. We have a post-simulation debriefing with the simulation center staff and instructors after every simulation session to address technical failures and develop solutions.

At the end of a scenario that did not go as anticipated, the short-term goal is deciding how to utilize what transpired in the debrief. The longer-term goal is to decide how to modify the scenario and its execution so that the scenario will run in a more predictable manner in the future.

Debriefing

Participating in a high-fidelity simulation without a debrief is simply playing in the sandbox. The debrief gives participants an opportunity to analyze their behaviors in a guided fashion to develop the skills of self-reflection as well as to specifically develop a plan or strategy to improve future performance. Debriefing is a critical component of simulation and thus is covered in great detail in Chaps. 6 and 7, but for completeness a brief discussion will be included here as well.

During the debriefing session that follows a scenario, the "hot-seat" participant, as well as the other learners involved, discusses what occurred. The debriefing allows the participants to reflect upon the case, identify points of strength, opportunities for improvement, and uncover the thought processes and events that led to key management decisions. The emotional aspects of the scenario performance must also be acknowledged. This is usually most effective if done before any other analysis of performance occurs.

Debriefing Techniques

Holistic

This approach is arguably best. The learner is asked how the scenario went and his or her emotional state is taken into account. Then a thorough discussion of the good and the bad during the scenario is done with an emphasis on areas for improvement as well as the "victories" that may have occurred during the scenario. Models for this sort of debriefing are discussed elsewhere in the text.

The Checklist Approach

The checklist approach to debriefing, in which a list of expected best behaviors is compared with the observed behavior, is probably best suited to technical skills, for example, airway management and less experienced practitioners. The challenge with developing a checklist for more complicated clinical situations is deciding what actually constitutes best behaviors given the multitude of ways to solve a clinical problem. Scavone [90] described the development of a checklist for management of cesarean section under general anesthesia, using a rigorous approach. Each clinical problem or complex task will require a separate checklist. Checklists for nontechnical or human factors skills have been developed, for example, the Anesthesia Nontechnical Skills (ANTS) [39, 41], evaluating task management, teamwork, situational awareness, and decision-making, with well-developed criteria for each.

The debriefing faculty may primarily facilitate learners' reflection upon the scenario to uncover performance issues both technical and nontechnical in nature. When multidisciplinary simulation exercises occur, the debriefer must take into account the different roles of people around the table and encourage input by all. In addition to covering the objectives of a scenario, it is an opportunity to demonstrate and reinforce the skills of reflection, analysis, and for the generation of a plan for improvement. This is the rationale for integrating simulation into part IV, the practice performance assessment and improvement portion of MOCA.

The Start-Stop Technique

Another model that presents an alternative to that of scenario followed by debrief is a start-stop technique. An instructor is in the simulation room; when the case comes to a point requiring a decision, the scenario pauses while the instructor and learners discuss options and determine the next action; the scenario then proceeds ahead to its conclusion. We use this technique with medical students who have minimally developed clinical skills. There is evidence that learners, even very junior ones, do not care for the start-stop approach, and think they benefit more from debriefing after a completed scenario [116].

Barriers and Challenges to Simulation Utilization in Anesthesia

Skepticism about the utility of simulation in anesthesia training and practice is being pushed to the wayside by regulatory requirements for simulation in anesthesia residencies [11] and MOCA [12]. Residency programs will be required to either develop their own simulation programs or contract the simulation training of their residents out to established simulation centers.

A bigger barrier to building a simulation program is recognition that it is a very personnel and resource-intensive undertaking. In budgeting for the operation of a simulation program, the capital expenditure for space and equipment is only part of the success of a program. Support for simulation personnel and instructors must be part of budgeting. Developing a simulation exercise requires time not only to author it but time needs to be budgeted for communication with the simulation center for programming, practicing, and staging, making for a far larger commitment of time for an instructor than authoring a presentation for lecture.

Scheduling time away from clinical duties for simulation can be challenging. Unlike other educational experiences where participants can arrive late or can break away to take calls, a simulation exercise requires participants' uninterrupted attention. A learner might "catch" part of a lecture and reap a partial benefit, but attending only a part of a scenario (minus briefing, context, and debriefing) is unlikely to have much value and may destroy the experience for the other participants. Organizing multidisciplinary simulations presents even greater challenges as schedules must be coordinated across multiple groups, for example, anesthesia OR timetables, surgical departments, and nursing departments. In fact, we have found scheduling challenges to be our biggest obstacle to multidisciplinary simulation. Only by convincing the leadership of each involved group of the value of simulation experiences will the necessary changes in scheduling occur.

Another barrier is participant's reluctance to attend, which may be due to perception that simulation is not a good learning experience, fear of embarrassment, or concern about a negative effect on evaluations and grades. Well-designed and executed exercises that respond to learner feedback, establish a safe learning environment, and emphasize learning outcomes are important. Thoughtful review of policies and practices within the simulation center is in order to ensure that all instructors keep the simulation center "safe" and that introductory comments emphasize the commitment to keeping the simulation center a "safe" place. Finally maintaining a barrier between assessment sessions and learning sessions will also help to foster the idea of "safety."

Novel Uses of Simulation in Anesthesia

Simulation allows new policies, protocols, and procedures to be "test-driven" in a simulated clinical setting with enhanced ability to analyze impact. New equipment can be explored in a simulated setting to identify design flaws or find problems in the user-device interactions that may require additional training. For example, we began a new service in which sedation nurses would provide sedation services at the bedside. The nurse would bring a sedation cart that had monitoring and resuscitation equipment, medications, and other supplies. A number of simulation exercises using these carts were conducted with the initial intention of practicing critical event management. However, during these sessions accessing emergency supplies was seen to be difficult due to the placement of equipment on the cart. The carts were reorganized and further simulation exercises showed improved performance. Without the simulation exercise, the suboptimal cart layout would likely not have been identified until a clinical emergency occurred.

Simulation in situ can be used to "test" a physical space as well. Simulation exercises revealed that being able to quickly reach a face mask in our ICU was challenging due to its location. In daily practice the respiratory therapists put the masks and equipment together and so were providing a work-around that hid the underlying problem.

Conclusions

Strong evidence supporting the superiority of simulation to other education modalities in changing clinical outcomes is growing slowly. Clearly there is a role for simulation in ensuring that learners are exposed to a core set of clinical situations and have an opportunity to manage them independently. It allows instructors to observe and provide feedback on that management and can assist in identifying gaps in performance or systems.

The challenge comes with providing firm evidence that simulation training is more effective than other forms of training in changing patient outcomes within anesthesia. Researchers have consistently shown that simulation training is more effective than didactic training or no training at all if the measure of success is performance on a simulated case. They have consistently shown that more experienced people manage simulated crises more effectively than less experienced personnel. In addition, people "enjoy" simulation and feel more confident after a simulation session. Translating these observations into showing that simulation is actually improving clinical outcomes, making our hospitals safer places, making teams function more effectively, helping learners to succeed more quickly, and helping professionals continue to grow more effectively is where the future focus of simulation research must concentrate. We need research showing simulation is effective higher up the levels of educational evaluation as outlined in Table 17.1.

Simulation is just one of many tools in the educator's armamentarium. One must thoughtfully plan for what parts of a curriculum are most effectively delivered by simulation. To simply try to move an entire curriculum to a simulation-based program may not utilize resources efficiently.

Multidisciplinary simulation is exciting and enables learning with the teams you practice with; however, the logistics of scheduling can be challenging. Simulation may occur in a dedicated simulation center or in situ, and each location has its advantages and disadvantages.

Design of a scenario must take into account the audience served, the gaps that you are trying to meet, your predefined objectives, and the practicalities of what your simulation center can offer, taking into account both equipment and personnel. Simulations can fail because a scenario is not appropriate for the audience, depends too heavily on subtle signs and symptoms not well portrayed by the equipment, or is misinterpreted by participants who then take a management path unanticipated by the scenario author. Alternatively equipment may fail altogether. Flexibility on the part of the instructor both during the scenario and debrief can minimize the consequences of the scenario not running smoothly.

High-fidelity simulation can be used to address both technical-/knowledge-based topics through management of clinical problems and nontechnical skills using crew resource management concepts. The goal of a task trainer is not to make an expert out of a learner but rather move him through the novice phase more quickly. Hence, ultrahigh fidelity is not necessarily a requirement for all task trainers. Task trainers do not replace patient contact but rather make patient contact safer, more comfortable, and maximizes the learning opportunities. In addition to considering simulation as an educational tool to help providers improve, one can also consider it as a tool to help systems improve, with identification of procedural, equipment, or structural shortcomings.

References

1. Gaba DM. What makes a "good" anesthesiologist? Anesthesiology. 2004;101(5):1061–3.
2. Larsson J, Holmström I, Rosenqvist U. Professional artist, good Samaritan, servant and co-ordinator: four ways of understanding the anaesthetist's work. Acta Anaesthesiol Scand. 2003;47(7):787–93.
3. Sandberg J. Understanding human competence at work: an interpretative approach. Acad Manag J. 2000;43(1):9–25.
4. Dornan T. Osler, Flexner, apprenticeship and 'the new medical education'. J R Soc Med. 2005;98(3):91–5.
5. Fernandez E, Williams DG. Training and the European working time directive: a 7 year review of paediatric anaesthetic trainee caseload data. Br J Anaesth. 2009;103(4):566–9.
6. Bowhay AR. An investigation into how the European Working Time Directive has affected anaesthetic training. BMC Med Educ. 2008;8:41.
7. Henrichs BM, Avidan MS, Murray DJ, et al. Performance of certified registered nurse anesthetists and anesthesiologists in a simulation-based skills assessment. Anesth Analg. 2009;108(1):255–62.
8. Fehr JJ, Boulet JR, Waldrop WB, Snider R, Brockel M, Murray DJ. Simulation-based assessment of pediatric anesthesia skills. Anesthesiology. 2011;115(6):1308–15.

9. Dijksterhuis MGK, Voorhuis M, Teunissen PW, et al. Assessment of competence and progressive independence in postgraduate clinical training. Med Educ. 2009;43(12):1156–65.
10. Frank JR, Snell LS, Cate OT, et al. Competency-based medical education: theory to practice. Med Teach. 2010;32(8):638–45.
11. ACGME. Simulation: New Revision to Program Requirements. RRC News for Anesthesiology. 2011:6. http://www.acgme.org/acWebsite/RRC_040_news/Anesthesiology_Newsletter_Mar11.pdf. Accessed 30 Apr 2012.
12. Maintenance of Certification in Anesthesiology (MOCA). 2012. Description of MOCA requirements by the ABA. http://theaba.org/Home/anesthesiology_maintenance. Accessed 19 Mar 2012.
13. Boulet JR, Murray DJ. Simulation-based assessment in anesthesiology: requirements for practical implementation. Anesthesiology. 2010;112(4):1041–52.
14. Davis DA, Mazmanian PE, Fordis M, Van Harrison R, Thorpe KE, Perrier L. Accuracy of physician self-assessment compared with observed measures of competence: a systematic review. JAMA. 2006;296(9):1094–102.
15. Hodges B, Regehr G, Martin D. Difficulties in recognizing one's own incompetence: novice physicians who are unskilled and unaware of it. Acad Med. 2001;76(10 Supplement):S87–9.
16. Weller JM, Robinson BJ, Jolly B, et al. Psychometric characteristics of simulation-based assessment in anaesthesia and accuracy of self-assessed scores. Anaesthesia. 2005;60(3):245–50.
17. Plant JL, Corden M, Mourad M, O'Brien BC, van Schaik SM. Understanding self-assessment as an informed process: residents' use of external information for self-assessment of performance in simulated resuscitations. Adv Health Sci Educ. 2012:17(1):1–12.
18. Wenk M, Waurick R, Schotes D, Gerdes C, Van Aken HK, Pöpping DM. Simulation-based medical education is no better than problem-based discussions and induces misjudgment in self-assessment. Adv Health Sci Educ. 2009;14(2):159–71.
19. Cook DA. One drop at a time: research to advance the science of simulation. Simul Healthc. 2010;5(1):1–4.
20. Diedrich DA, personal communication. 2012:Consultant, Mayo Clinic Department of Anesthesia and Critical Care.
21. Naik VN, Matsumoto ED, Houston PL, et al. Fiberoptic orotracheal intubation on anesthetized patients: do manipulation skills learned on a simple model transfer into the operating room? Anesthesiology. 2001;95(2):343–8.
22. Crabtree NA, Chandra DB, Weiss ID, Joo HS, Naik VN. Fibreoptic airway training: correlation of simulator performance and clinical skill. Can J Anesth. 2008;55(2):100–4.
23. Toronto Uo. Bronchoscopy Simulator. http://www.thoracic-anesthesia.com/?page_id=2. Accessed 29 May 2012.
24. Leighton BL. A greengrocer's model of the epidural space. Anesthesiology. 1989;70(2):368–9.
25. Issenberg SB, McGaghie WC, Petrusa ER, Gordon DL, Scalese RJ. Features and uses of high-fidelity medical simulations that lead to effective learning: a BEME systematic review*. Med Teach. 2005;27(1):10–28.
26. Boet S, Bould MD, Bruppacher HR, Desjardins F, Chandra DB, Naik VN. Looking in the mirror: self-debriefing versus instructor debriefing for simulated crises. Crit Care Med. 2011;39(6):1377–81.
27. Savoldelli GL, Naik VN, Park J, Joo HS, Chow R, Hamstra SJ. Value of debriefing during simulated crisis management: oral versus video-assisted oral feedback. Anesthesiology. 2006;105(2):279–85.
28. Byrne AJ, Sellen AJ, Jones JG, et al. Effect of videotape feedback on anaesthetists' performance while managing simulated anaesthetic crises: a multicentre study. Anaesthesia. 2002;57(2):176–9.
29. Cumin D, Merry AF. Simulators for use in anaesthesia. Anaesthesia. 2007;62(2):151–62.
30. Bryson EO, Levine AI. The simulation theater: a theoretical discussion of concepts and constructs that enhance learning. J Crit Care. 2008;23(2):185–7.
31. Byrne AJ, Jones JG. Responses to simulated anaesthetic emergencies by anaesthetists with different durations of clinical experience. Br J Anaesth. 1997;78(5):553–6.
32. DeAnda A, Gaba DM. Role of experience in the response to simulated critical incidents. Anesth Analg. 1991;72(3):308–15.
33. Kurrek MM, Devitt JH, Cohen M. Cardiac arrest in the OR: how are our ACLS skills? Can J Anaesth. 1998;45(2):130–2.
34. Larson ER, Nuttall GA, Ogren BD, et al. A prospective study on anesthesia machine fault identification. Anesth Analg. 2007;104(1):154–6.
35. Ben-Menachem E, Ezri T, Ziv A, Sidi A, Berkenstadt H. Identifying and managing technical faults in the anesthesia machine: lessons learned from the Israeli Board of Anesthesiologists. Anesth Analg. 2011;112(4):864–6.
36. Lorraway PG, Savoldelli GL, Joo HS, Chandra DB, Chow R, Naik VN. Management of simulated oxygen supply failure: is there a gap in the curriculum? Anesth Analg. 2006;102(3):865–7.
37. Chiu M, Arab AA, Elliott R, Naik VN. An experiential teaching session on the anesthesia machine check improves resident performance. Can J Anaesth. 2012;59:280–7.
38. Fischler IS, Kaschub CE, Lizdas DE, Lampotang S. Understanding of anesthesia machine function is enhanced with a transparent reality simulation. Simul Healthc. 2008;3(1):26–32.
39. Fletcher G, Flin R, McGeorge P, Glavin R, Maran N, Patey R. Anaesthetists' Non-Technical Skills (ANTS): evaluation of a behavioural marker system. Br J Anaesth. 2003;90(5):580–8.
40. Flin R, Patey R. Non-technical skills for anaesthetists: developing and applying ANTS. Best Pract Res Clin Anaesthesiol. 2011;25(2):215–27.
41. ANTS – A Behavioural Marker System for Rating Anaesthetists' Non-Technical Skills. Industrial Psychology Research Center, University of Aberdeen. 2011; http://www.abdn.ac.uk/iprc/ants/. Accessed 22 Mar 2012.
42. Flin R, Patey R, Glavin R, Maran N. Anaesthetists' non-technical skills. Br J Anaesth. 2010;105(1):38–44.
43. Quality AHRQ. TeamSTEPPS: National Implementation. 2012; http://teamstepps.ahrq.gov/. Accessed 22 Apr 2012.
44. Malec JF, Torsher LC, Dunn WF, et al. The Mayo high performance teamwork scale: reliability and validity for evaluating key crew resource management skills. Simul Healthc. 2007;2(1):4–10.
45. Johnson KB, Syroid ND, Drews FA, et al. Part task and variable priority training in first-year anesthesia resident education: a combined didactic and simulation-based approach to improve management of adverse airway and respiratory events. Anesthesiology. 2008;108(5):831–40.
46. Pott LM, Randel GI, Straker T, Becker KD, Cooper RM. A survey of airway training among U.S. and Canadian anesthesiology residency programs. J Clin Anesth. 2011;23(1):15–26.
47. Clarke RC, Gardner AI. Anaesthesia trainees' exposure to airway management in an Australian tertiary adult teaching hospital. Anaesth Intensive Care. 2008;36(4):513–5.
48. Kory PD, Eisen LA, Adachi M, Ribaudo VA, Rosenthal ME, Mayo PH. Initial airway management skills of senior residents: simulation training compared with traditional training. Chest. 2007;132(6):1927–31.
49. Rosenthal ME, Adachi M, Ribaudo V, Mueck JT, Schneider RF, Mayo PH. Achieving housestaff competence in emergency airway management using scenario based simulation training: comparison of attending vs housestaff trainers. Chest. 2006;129(6):1453–8.
50. Kovacs G, Bullock G, Ackroyd-Stolarz S, Cain E, Petrie D. A randomized controlled trial on the effect of educational interventions in promoting airway management skill maintenance. Ann Emerg Med. 2000;36(4):301–9.
51. Batchelder AJ, Steel A, Mackenzie R, Hormis AP, Daniels TS, Holding N. Simulation as a tool to improve the safety of pre-hospital anaesthesia – a pilot study. Anaesthesia. 2009;64(9):978–83.

52. Frengley RW, Weller JM, Torrie J, et al. The effect of a simulation-based training intervention on the performance of established critical care unit teams. Crit Care Med. 2011;39(12):2605–11.
53. Chen PT, Huang YC, Cheng HW, et al. New simulation-based airway management training program for junior physicians: Advanced Airway Life Support. Med Teach. 2009;31(8):e338–44.
54. Mayo PH, Hegde A, Eisen LA, Kory P, Doelken P. A program to improve the quality of emergency endotracheal intubation. J Intensive Care Med. 2011;26(1):50–6.
55. Sudikoff SN, Overly FL, Shapiro MJ. High-fidelity medical simulation as a technique to improve pediatric residents' emergency airway management and teamwork: a pilot study. Pediatr Emerg Care. 2009;25(10):651–6.
56. Nishisaki A, Donoghue AJ, Colborn S, et al. Effect of just-in-time simulation training on tracheal intubation procedure safety in the pediatric intensive care unit. Anesthesiology. 2010;113(1):214–23.
57. Kuduvalli PM, Jervis A, Tighe SQM, Robin NM. Unanticipated difficult airway management in anaesthetised patients: a prospective study of the effect of mannequin training on management strategies and skill retention. Anaesthesia. 2008;63(4):364–9.
58. Russo SG, Eich C, Barwing J, et al. Self-reported changes in attitude and behavior after attending a simulation-aided airway management course. J Clin Anesth. 2007;19(7):517–22.
59. Borges BCR, Boet S, Siu LW, et al. Incomplete adherence to the ASA difficult airway algorithm is unchanged after a high-fidelity simulation session. Can J Anaesth. 2010;57(7):644–9.
60. Olympio MA, Whelan R, Ford RPA, Saunders ICM. Failure of simulation training to change residents' management of oesophageal intubation. Br J Anaesth. 2003;91(3):312–8.
61. Boet S, Borges BCR, Naik VN, et al. Complex procedural skills are retained for a minimum of 1 yr after a single high-fidelity simulation training session. Br J Anaesth. 2011;107(4):533–9.
62. Siu LW, Boet S, Borges BCR, et al. High-fidelity simulation demonstrates the influence of anesthesiologists' age and years from residency on emergency cricothyroidotomy skills. Anesth Analg. 2010;111(4):955–60.
63. Boet S, Bould MD, Schaeffer R, et al. Learning fibreoptic intubation with a virtual computer program transfers to 'hands on' improvement. Eur J Anaesthesiol. 2010;27(1):31–5.
64. Park CS, Rochlen LR, Yaghmour E, et al. Acquisition of critical intraoperative event management skills in novice anesthesiology residents by using high-fidelity simulation-based training. Anesthesiology. 2010;112(1):202–11.
65. Smith HM, Kopp SL, Jacob AK, Torsher LC, Hebl JR. Designing and implementing a comprehensive learner-centered regional anesthesia curriculum. Reg Anesth Pain Med. 2009;34(2):88–94.
66. Tan JS, Chin KJ, Chan VWS. Developing a training program for peripheral nerve blockade: the "nuts and bolts". Int Anesthesiol Clin. 2010;48(4):1–11.
67. Kessler DO, Auerbach M, Pusic M, Tunik MG, Foltin JC. A randomized trial of simulation-based deliberate practice for infant lumbar puncture skills. Simul Healthc. 2011;6(4):197–203.
68. Friedman Z, Siddiqui N, Katznelson R, Devito I, Bould MD, Naik V. Clinical impact of epidural anesthesia simulation on short- and long-term learning curve: high- versus low-fidelity model training. Reg Anesth Pain Med. 2009;34(3):229–32.
69. Kulcsár ZM, Lövquist E, Fitzgerald AP, Aboulafia A, Shorten GD. Testing haptic sensations for spinal anesthesia. Reg Anesth Pain Med. 2011;36(1):12–6.
70. Magill JC, Byl MF, Hinds MF, Agassounon W, Pratt SD, Hess PE. A novel actuator for simulation of epidural anesthesia and other needle insertion procedures. Simul Healthc. 2010;5(3):179–84.
71. Niazi AU, Haldipur N, Prasad AG, Chan VW. Ultrasound-guided regional anesthesia performance in the early learning period: effect of simulation training. Reg Anesth Pain Med. 2012;37(1):51–4.
72. Cheung JJH, Chen EW, Al-Allaq Y, et al. Acquisition of technical skills in ultrasound-guided regional anesthesia using a high-fidelity simulator. Stud Health Techol Inform. 2011;163:119–24.
73. Grottke O, Ntouba A, Ullrich S, et al. Virtual reality-based simulator for training in regional anaesthesia. Br J Anaesth. 2009;103(4): 594–600.
74. Smith HM, Jacob AK, Segura LG, Dilger JA, Torsher LC. Simulation education in anesthesia training: a case report of successful resuscitation of bupivacaine-induced cardiac arrest linked to recent simulation training. Anesth Analg. 2008;106(5):1581–4.
75. Neal JM, Hsiung RL, Mulroy MF, Halpern BB, Dragnich AD, Slee AE. ASRA checklist improves trainee performance during a simulated episode of local anesthetic systemic toxicity. Reg Anesth Pain Med. 2012;37(1):8–15.
76. Torsher LC, Craigo P, Lynch JJ, Smith HM. Regional anesthesia emergencies. Simul Healthc. 2009;4(2):109–13.
77. Evans LV, Dodge KL, Shah TD, et al. Simulation training in central venous catheter insertion: improved performance in clinical practice. Acad Med. 2010;85(9):1462–9.
78. Sekiguchi H, Tokita JE, Minami T, Eisen LA, Mayo PH, Narasimhan M. A prerotational, simulation-based workshop improves the safety of central venous catheter insertion: results of a successful internal medicine house staff training program. Chest. 2011;140(3):652–8.
79. Barsuk JH, Cohen ER, Feinglass J, McGaghie WC, Wayne DB. Use of simulation-based education to reduce catheter-related bloodstream infections. Arch Intern Med. 2009;169(15):1420–3.
80. Cohen ER, Feinglass J, Barsuk JH, et al. Cost savings from reduced catheter-related bloodstream infection after simulation-based education for residents in a medical intensive care unit. Simul Healthc. 2010;5(2):98–102.
81. Khouli H, Jahnes K, Shapiro J, et al. Performance of medical residents in sterile techniques during central vein catheterization: randomized trial of efficacy of simulation-based training. Chest. 2011;139(1):80–7.
82. Latif RK, Bautista AF, Memon SB, et al. Teaching aseptic technique for central venous access under ultrasound guidance: a randomized trial comparing didactic training alone to didactic plus simulation-based training. Anesth Analg. 2012;114(3):626–33.
83. Barsuk JH, Cohen ER, McGaghie WC, Wayne DB. Long-term retention of central venous catheter insertion skills after simulation-based mastery learning. Acad Med. 2010;85(10 Suppl):S9–12.
84. Smith CC, Huang GC, Newman LR, et al. Simulation training and its effect on long-term resident performance in central venous catheterization. Simul Healthc. 2010;5(3):146–51.
85. Ma IWY, Brindle ME, Ronksley PE, Lorenzetti DL, Sauve RS, Ghali WA. Use of simulation-based education to improve outcomes of central venous catheterization: a systematic review and meta-analysis. Acad Med. 2011;86(9):1137–47.
86. Bruppacher HR, Alam SK, LeBlanc VR, et al. Simulation-based training improves physicians' performance in patient care in high-stakes clinical setting of cardiac surgery. Anesthesiology. 2010;112(4):985–92.
87. Steadman RH. Improving on reality: can simulation facilitate practice change? Anesthesiology. 2010;112(4):775–6.
88. Bose RR, Matyal R, Warraich HJ, et al. Utility of a transesophageal echocardiographic simulator as a teaching tool. J Cardiothorac Vasc Anesth. 2011;25(2):212–5.
89. Pratt SD. Simulation in obstetric anesthesia. Anesth Analg. 2012;114(1):186–90.
90. Scavone BM, Sproviero MT, McCarthy RJ, et al. Development of an objective scoring system for measurement of resident performance on the human patient simulator. Anesthesiology. 2006;105(2): 260–6.
91. Scavone BM, Toledo P, Higgins N, Wojciechowski K, McCarthy RJ. A randomized controlled trial of the impact of simulation-based training on resident performance during a simulated obstetric anesthesia emergency. Simul Healthc. 2010;5(6):320–4.

92. Daniels K, Lipman S, Harney K, Arafeh J, Maurice D. Use of simulation based team training for obstetric crises in resident education. Simul Healthc. 2008;3(3):154–60.
93. Thompson S, Neal S, Clark V. Clinical risk management in obstetrics: Eclampsia drills. Br Med J. 2004;328(7434):269–71.
94. Lipman SS, Daniels KI, Carvalho B, et al. Deficits in the provision of cardiopulmonary resuscitation during simulated obstetric crises. Am J Obstet Gynecol. 2010;203(2):179.e171–e175.
95. Lipman S, Daniels K, Cohen SE, Carvalho B. Labor room setting compared with the operating room for simulated perimortem cesarean delivery: a randomized controlled trial. Obstet Gynecol. 2011;118(5):1090–4.
96. Andreatta P, Saxton E, Thompson M, Annich G. Simulation-based mock codes significantly correlate with improved pediatric patient cardiopulmonary arrest survival rates. Pediatr Crit Care Med. 2011;12:33–8.
97. Edler AA, Chen M, Honkanen A, Hackel A, Golianu B. Affordable simulation for small-scale training and assessment. Simul Healthc. 2010;5(2):112–5.
98. Howard-Quijano KJ, Stiegler MA, Huang YM, Canales C, Steadman RH. Anesthesiology residents' performance of pediatric resuscitation during a simulated hyperkalemic cardiac arrest. Anesthesiology. 2010;112(4):993–7.
99. Gardi TI, Christensen UC, Jacobsen J, Jensen PF, Ording H. How do anaesthesiologists treat malignant hyperthermia in a full-scale anaesthesia simulator? Acta Anaesthesiol Scand. 2001;45(8):1032–5.
100. Harrison TK, Manser T, Howard SK, Gaba DM. Use of cognitive aids in a simulated anesthetic crisis. Anesth Analg. 2006;103(3):551–6.
101. Berkenstadt H, Yusim Y, Katznelson R, Ziv A, Livingstone D, Perel A. A novel point-of-care information system reduces anaesthesiologists' errors while managing case scenarios. Eur J Anaesthesiol. 2006;23(3):239–50.
102. Fletcher JL. AANA journal course: update for nurse anesthetists–anesthesia simulation: a tool for learning and research. AANA J. 1995;63(1):61–7.
103. Lucisano KE, Talbot LA. Simulation training for advanced airway management for anesthesia and other healthcare providers: a systematic review. AANA J. 2012;80(1):25–31.
104. Turcato N, Roberson C, Covert K. Simulation-based education: what's in it for nurse anesthesia educators? AANA J. 2008;76(4):257–62.
105. Murray DJ, Boulet JR, Kras JF, McAllister JD, Cox TE. A simulation-based acute skills performance assessment for anesthesia training. Anesth Analg. 2005;101(4):1127–34, table of contents.
106. Penprase B, Mileto L, Bittinger A, et al. The use of high-fidelity simulation in the admissions process: one nurse anesthesia program's experience. AANA J. 2012;80(1):43–8.
107. Shavit I, Keidan I, Hoffmann Y, et al. Enhancing patient safety during pediatric sedation: the impact of simulation-based training of nonanesthesiologists. Arch Pediatr Adolesc Med. 2007;161(8):740–3.
108. Farnsworth ST, Egan TD, Johnson SE, Westenskow D. Teaching sedation and analgesia with simulation. J Clin Monit Comput. 2000;16(4):273–85.
109. Hallikainen J, Väisänen O, Randell T, Tarkkila P, Rosenberg PH, Niemi-Murola L. Teaching anaesthesia induction to medical students: comparison between full-scale simulation and supervised teaching in the operating theatre. Eur J Anaesthesiol. 2009;26(2):101–4.
110. Savoldelli GL, Naik VN, Joo HS, et al. Evaluation of patient simulator performance as an adjunct to the oral examination for senior anesthesia residents. Anesthesiology. 2006;104(3):475–81.
111. Berkenstadt H, Ziv A, Gafni N, Sidi A. Incorporating simulation-based objective structured clinical examination into the Israeli National Board Examination in Anesthesiology. Anesth Analg. 2006;102(3):853–8.
112. Ben-Menachem E, Ezri T, Ziv A, Sidi A, Brill S, Berkenstadt H. Objective Structured Clinical Examination-based assessment of regional anesthesia skills: the Israeli National Board Examination in Anesthesiology experience. Anesth Analg. 2011;112(1):242–5.
113. ASA Simulation Education Network. 2012; http://www.asahq.org/for-healthcare-professionals/education-and-events/simulation-education-network.aspx. Accessed 19 Mar 2012.
114. Frederick HJ, Corvetto MA, Hobbs GW, Taekman J. The "Simulation Roulette" game. Simul Healthc. 2011;6(4):244–9.
115. Dieckmann P, Lippert A, Glavin R, Rall M. When things do not go as expected: scenario life savers. Simul Healthc. 2010;5(4):219–25.
116. Van Heukelom JN, Begaz T, Treat R. Comparison of postsimulation debriefing versus in-simulation debriefing in medical simulation. Simul Healthc. 2010;5(2):91–7.
117. Beckman TJ, Cook DA. Developing scholarly projects in education: a primer for medical teachers. Med Teach. 2007;29(2–3):210–8.
118. McGaghie WC. Medical education research as translational science. Sci Transl Med. 2010;2(19):19cm8.
119. Miller GE. The assessment of clinical skills/competence/performance. Acad Med. 1990;65(9 Suppl):S63–7.

Simulation in Non-Invasive Cardiology

18

James McKinney, Ross J. Scalese, and Rose Hatala

Introduction

The diagnostic abilities associated with the practice of non-invasive cardiology are, in many ways, a set of fundamental skills that most healthcare providers are expected to possess. Indeed, one of the first physical diagnostic skills medical students are exposed to and expected to acquire is minimal competence with cardiac auscultation. Recently many healthcare educators believe that the ability to visualize the heart and determine its functional status may supplant the ability to listen to heart sounds. Some have gone so far to call the echo probe the "new stethoscope." In light of this development, basic echocardiography will likely find its way into early medical school curriculums and physical diagnosis courses. In any case the noninvasive cardiac exam has evolved over time, but fundamental physical diagnostic skills remain a core competency for the cardiologist as well as any provider. Although these skills can and will be taught on actual patients with limited risk or harm, the ability to predictably expose all students to a given set of normal and pathologic sounds and images makes simulation a powerful tool in the educator's armamentarium. This chapter focuses on non-invasive cardiology-based simulation for medical education. We begin with a focus on the simulation of the cardiac physical examination and conclude the chapter with an overview of echocardiography simulation.

J. McKinney, MD, MSC (✉)
Department of Cardiology, University of British Columbia, 301-2100 3rd. Ave. W., Vancouver U6R 1 LI, BC, Canada
e-mail: mckinney.jimmy@gmail.com

R.J. Scalese, MD, FACP
Division of Research and Technology, Gordon Center for Research in Medical Education, University of Miami Miller School of Medicine, PO Box 016960 (D-41), Miami, FL 33101, USA
e-mail: rscalese@med.miami.edu

R. Hatala, MD, MSc
Department of Medicine, University of British Columbia, Vancouver, BC, Canada

Department of Medicine, St. Paul's Hospital, Suite 5907, Burrard Bldg., 1081 Burrard St., Vancouver, BC V6Z 1Y6, Canada
e-mail: rhatala@mac.com

The Importance of Cardiac Physical Examination Skills

Proficiency in cardiac auscultation remains an important skill in clinical medicine [1]. Cardiac examination can accurately detect most structural cardiac conditions when performed correctly [2]. It is a noninvasive tool that can directly diagnose and assess severity of disease and guide further evaluation and therapeutic management [1]. Despite its role as an invaluable diagnostic tool, proficiency in this skill remains poor [2]. This was highlighted by Mangione and Nieman [3] who found that only 20% of audio-recorded auscultatory findings were recognized correctly by family practice residents, internal medicine residents, and medical students. Furthermore, there is minimal improvement with increasing levels of clinical experience, implying that trainees are not developing these skills as they progress through residency [2, 4].

Poor cardiac examination skills among trainees have been attributed to a number of factors: less formal teaching dedicated to the cardiac physical examination, less opportunity for trainees to encounter patients with cardiac pathology, and less time spent in direct patient contact yielding fewer opportunities to practice physical examination skills and receive feedback on performance [5]. This phenomena has also lead to a shortage of clinically oriented instructors proficient in cardiac examination, as even practicing physicians lack self-confidence in the physical examination [2]. The increasing reliance on imaging technology at the expense of physical examination may also play a role.

There is thus a clear need for better methods by which to teach cardiac auscultation and diagnostic skills for all levels of learners. The ideal learning environment would include the opportunity for students to examine real cardiac patients

A.I. Levine et al. (eds.), *The Comprehensive Textbook of Healthcare Simulation*,
DOI 10.1007/978-1-4614-5993-4_18, © Springer Science+Business Media New York 2013

with an opportunity to review each patient with an expert on repeated occasions [6]. Due to the constraints outlined previously, this is not possible in most clinical or educational environments. Thus, students are expected to learn cardiac examination skills from random, unstructured patient encounters during their clinical clerkship, an approach which is, given the evidence, inadequate [7].

Simulation provides an opportunity to address these deficiencies by recreating cardiac abnormalities for the express purposes of exposure, teaching, and repetition (i.e., deliberate practice) [6]. A simulator can provide standardized physical findings for a wide variety of conditions with options for titrating the severity and progression of the disease [5, 8]. Simulation also provides a safe, supportive environment where education and assessment can take place [9]. Furthermore, it allows learners at all levels to practice and develop skills with the knowledge that mistakes carry no penalties or harm to patients or learners [10].

Current Use of Cardiology Simulation in Medical Education

Medical educators have recognized that simulation can play a key role in the development and maintenance of proficiency in the cardiac physical examination. In a 2011 survey by the Association of American Medical Colleges, medical students at over 80% of responding institutions were exposed to some form of simulation (from standardized patients to technology-enhanced simulators) during medical school. Residents also had a high use of simulation early in their residency programs. Examining the content of the simulation-based teaching, approximately 30% of programs taught topics relevant to cardiology which would include physical examination [11]. Interestingly, this is quite similar to the prevalence of dedicated formal cardiac physical examination instruction reported by Mangione et al. in the 1990s [4].

The ultimate goal for simulation-based cardiac physical examination teaching is to facilitate learning of cardiac physical examination skills and diagnostic accuracy and for this to translate into improved skills and accuracy in clinical practice. In the following sections in this chapter, we examine the simulators available for cardiac physical examination teaching and explore effective methods for employing this technology.

Types of Simulators

A wide range of simulators have been developed to aid in the development of cardiac auscultation skills and knowledge. Examples include standardized patients, audio recordings, multimedia CD-ROMs, computer-assisted instruction, virtual patient encounters, electronic heart sound simulators, and mannequins. Each of these modalities has proposed theoretical and documented benefits and limitations as will be reviewed below.

Table 18.1 Exclusively audio simulators

Benefits
Portable and easily accessible. Learners can work through diagnoses at their own pace
Opportunity for self-practice and repetitive practice
Not constrained by patient or instructor availability
Multiple examples of a single diagnosis can be presented quickly and economically
Limitations
Unable to correlate sounds with tactile or visual patient cues. Lack of interaction with physical "patient" (real or simulation)
In the absence of instructor, lack of interaction and feedback regarding auscultatory abnormalities

Audio Simulations (Table 18.1)

Audio simulations, which typically consist of CD-ROMs but can include other sound file formats, present recordings of real or simulated patient heart sounds. The benefit of this approach is that the recorded audio sounds are free of contaminating background noise commonly found at the bedside, so it may be easier for the learners to hear the sounds [3]. This is unlike the difficulties encountered when listening to a patient's heart in a noisy setting, such as the emergency department, where a conventional acoustic stethoscope is unable to filter the additional environmental noise making auscultation more challenging. For novice learners, the absence of extra visual and tactile stimuli may simplify the task at hand and improve their auscultatory accuracy. Supporting this argument, Vukanovic-Criley et al. noted that learners and clinicians at all levels of experience would close or avert their eyes when auscultating a virtual patient that processed a combination of sights and sounds. This was done instinctively, despite the fact that doing so would mean the clinician would actively choose to ignore visual reference that could have assisted them the timing of sounds and murmurs [2].

The efficacy of the audio simulations has been demonstrated in at least two studies [12, 13]. Horiszny demonstrated that repetitive auscultation of heart sounds and murmurs with interactive discussion about pathophysiology with an instructor improved the cardiac auscultatory proficiency of family medicine residents [13]. Auscultatory diagnostic accuracy improved from 36 to 62% after three 45-min sessions, as tested using the simulated sounds. A similar study confirmed the utility of the audio recordings for medical students after a 2½-h session with an instructor [12]. These studies demonstrate the effectiveness of repetitious listening to heart sounds when enhanced by the

Table 18.2 Multimedia simulators

Benefits
Able to present interactive cases with additional supportive history, laboratory tests, and explanations of pathophysiology
Incorporation of visual stimuli, such as ECG tracings, pulse waveforms, videos of carotid pulses, JVP, and precordium, to help correctly locate and identify heart sounds and murmurs
Opportunity for self-practice and repetitive practice
Not constrained by patient or instructor availability
Limitations
In the absence of instructor, limited feedback from computer (absence of feedback with non-CAI multimedia formats)
Lack of interaction with physical "patient" (real or simulation)
More expensive and less accessible than exclusively audio simulations

presence of an instructor providing feedback and guiding group discussion.

Another study powerfully demonstrated the importance of repetitive listening to heart sounds and murmurs [14]. Third-year medical students either listened to 500 repetitions of 6 simulated heart sounds and murmurs, recorded on a 1-h CD, or were not exposed to any recorded sounds. Those students who engaged in repetitive practice had significantly higher diagnostic accuracy on both simulated and real patient heart sounds.

These studies support the efficacy of pure auscultatory simulations in improving diagnostic accuracy, at least as tested on auscultatory simulations. These types of simulators are well suited to novice learners and require only a few hours of repetitive practice to demonstrate significant learning gains.

Multimedia Simulations (Table 18.2)

CD-ROM

It has been hypothesized that the lack of information regarding location, intensity, and radiation of the murmur may limit the utility of the exclusively audio simulations [14]. Critics of these simulators suggest that listening to heart sounds and murmurs in isolation without visual and tactile stimuli is not reflective of auscultation at the bedside [3]. Multimedia cardiac simulation typically involves audio recordings of heart sounds with visual stimuli in the form of graphics, ECG tracings, phonocardiograms, and video recordings of the jugular venous pulsation (JVP), carotid arteries, and precordium. Additionally, some of these simulations have supplementary history, imaging (e.g., CXR, echocardiogram), and teaching points. The primary characteristic of multimedia cardiac simulations is the ability to identify systole and diastole through the visual modality, allowing the user to properly time auscultatory findings within the cardiac cycle.

Multimedia CD-ROMs have been shown to improve cardiac auscultation knowledge and skill [3, 6, 15, 16]. The study designs include a single-group pre-post study [16], cohort studies comparing multimedia to classroom teaching [15, 16], and multimedia plus traditional clerkship to clerkship alone [6, 15]. For example, Stern et al. [6] found that students who were exposed to CD-ROM cases demonstrated improved diagnostic accuracy when tested on simulated sounds compared to students who only experienced the traditional clerkship instruction. Furthermore, the subset of students who had the full intervention (reviewing in-depth CD-ROM cases and 20 mini-cases) had a preservation of auscultatory skill when retested 9 months later.

In the study by Stern et al., and in another study by Finley et al. [6, 15], students used the multimedia simulations either on their own or in the presence of an instructor. Both studies demonstrated similar diagnostic accuracy on simulated heart sounds between both instructor present and instructor absent groups. These studies suggest that students can use these simulations independently and demonstrate significant gains in skills. However, from the students' perspective, they felt that a combination of both classroom and computer learning would be preferable to either modality alone [15].

Computer-Assisted Instruction

For our purposes, computer-assisted instruction (CAI) is defined as a multimedia simulation program that uses computer programs or Web-based learning as the central means of information delivery *but* is also interactive. Within cardiology, considerable interest in CAI has led to the development of CAI modalities for teaching cardiac physiology and cardiac physical examination skills. Conceptually complex, visually intense, and detail-oriented tasks such as understanding the pathophysiology behind a murmur are well suited to CAI [15]. An interactive computer screen can show animations of anatomy, ECG tracings, pressure-volume curves, and echo images, in addition to supplementary text or audio instruction to help the learner acquire the necessary background knowledge. This can then be coupled with heart sound recordings and videos of physical examination to serve as a comprehensive presentation of a particular cardiac condition. Similar to the multimedia CD-ROMs, CAI allows the student to engage in self-directed learning in a nonthreatening environment [17]. Both multimedia modalities generally do not require immediate direct supervision from the instructor, thus reducing the geographical and time constraints on both students and instructors [17].

Perhaps the best studied example of a cardiology-specific CAI is the UMedic system (University of Miami medical education development system for instruction using computers) [18, 19]. Developed to be used in conjunction with Harvey® The Cardiopulmonary Patient Simulator, UMedic is a multimedia program that presents an extensive cardiovascular curriculum, incorporating cardiac auscultation and

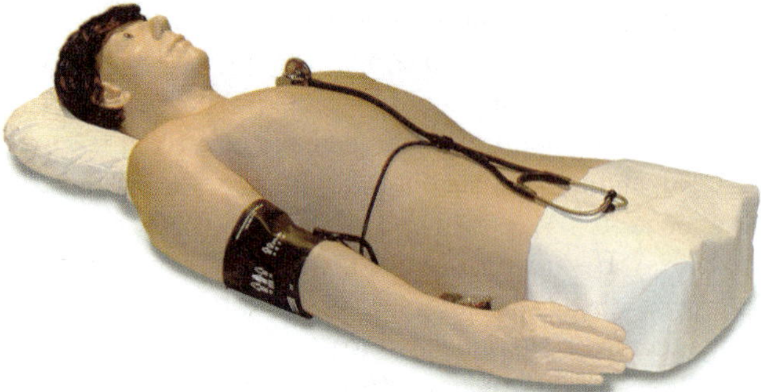

Fig. 18.1 Harvey® The Cardiopulmonary patient simulator (Photo courtesy of Laerdal)

cardiovascular imaging in its presentation [20] (Fig. 18.1). It has been shown to improve diagnostic accuracy on simulated cardiac findings, for clerkship students, compared to a traditional clerkship rotation [19].

Sverdrup et al. [21] addressed whether traditional bedside teaching versus training with CAI would lead to differences in diagnostic accuracy with real patients. Two groups of third-year medical students received a 2-h instructional session focused on cardiac examination and physiology. One group received an additional 2-h traditional bedside teaching session, while the other group went through a series of cases with the multimedia simulation. Both groups had equal diagnostic accuracy when tested with real patients.

Virtual Patient Encounters

Virtual patient encounters (VPE) are defined as "a specific type of computer program that simulates real-life clinical scenarios; allowing learners to obtain a history, conduct/view a physical exam, assess diagnostic tests and make diagnostic and therapeutic decisions" [21, 22].

These interactive multimedia teaching programs use real or standardized patients filmed at the bedside with supplemental animations, demonstrations of anatomy, ECG tracings, echocardiogram images, and text or audio instruction. In addition to the ancillary information, actual recorded heart sounds and actual video recordings of a live patient are presented. The VPEs permit the learner to move the virtual stethoscope over the virtual patient's precordium while observing pulses, respiration, and/or postural maneuvers [7].

Virtual patient encounters can improve the cardiac examination competency of medical students [7]. In one study, 24 medical students received eight 90-min sessions with a VPE in addition to their baseline core curriculum and were compared to 52 students receiving no additional instruction. The VPE group improved their diagnostic accuracy when tested on the VPE compared to the control group. Moreover, a subset of students in the intervention group was tested 14 months later and had a sustained increase in accuracy compared to the control group. VPEs have also been used to assess the knowledge and auscultation skills of medical students, residents, fellows, and clinicians [2].

Despite the appeal of multimedia simulations, whether CD-ROM, CAI, or VPE, there still exists a need for more well-designed studies examining how best to use these simulation modalities. The majority of studies employ nonrandomized designs, add multimedia simulators to instruction received by both groups as opposed to comparing two interventions that require equal time, and test learners using the multimedia simulator as opposed to real patients. Without stronger research designs, and particularly without demonstrating the translation of skills from simulation to real patients, the benefits of multimedia simulations remain under-explored.

Table 18.3 Standardized patients

Standardized patients
Benefits
Real person with which to interact
Ability to learn the techniques and cardiac findings of the normal cardiac physical examination
Patient and/or instructor present to provide feedback on performance
Potential for "hybrid" simulations, combining the normal physical examination of the patient with any of the simulation modalities presenting the cardiac abnormalities
Limitations
Typical standardized patient does not have cardiac abnormalities, thus unable to present abnormal physical findings
Inefficient, as only a few students can examine the patient at any one time
Not conducive to repetitive practice or available for independent practice
Cost and time intensive to recruit and train appropriate standardized patients

Standardized Patients (Table 18.3)

A standardized patient (SP) (see Chap. 13) is an actor or patient who has received training to present his or her history in a standardized, reliable manner and who sometimes mimics physical signs [10]. The use of SPs for teaching the basics of cardiac physical examination is widespread in North American undergraduate medical education, as is their use in assessment [11]. SPs may be helpful for teaching normal physical exam findings and instructing learners in physical exam technique. However, the SP's normal physical exam poses a problem when assessing learners' ability to recognize abnormal clinical signs and to apply and integrate knowledge [23]. There is a low correlation between clinicians' physical examination technique and their ability to diagnose cardiac abnormalities [24].

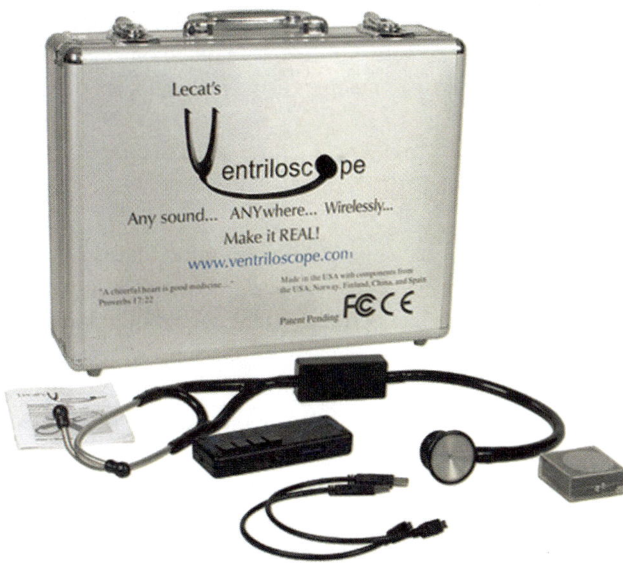

Fig. 18.2 Lecat's Ventriloscope (Picture courtesy of Limbs & Things ©2012 www.limbsandthings.com)

Lecat's Ventriloscope, manufactured by Limbs & Things, is a modified stethoscope that allows prerecorded sounds (activated wirelessly) to be integrated with a standardized patient [23]. It is designed to overcome some of the limitations of the SP with normal physical findings. The Ventriloscope allows for projection of abnormal auscultatory signs onto a healthy person, requiring students to recognize and interpret such signs within the wider context of a clinical encounter [25]. The learner also benefits by completing the cardiac examination on a live person. Additionally, the same SP can have a number of cardiac conditions that can be interchanged with ease (Fig. 18.2).

Limitations of early Ventriloscope models included lack of synchronization of cardiac auscultatory findings with the SP's pulse and lack of respiratory variation of the heart sounds. Technology is being developed to track the pulse (by having the SP wear a heart rate monitor) and trigger the recorded sounds simultaneously. A foreseeable limitation to the Ventriloscope is that it simulates auscultatory abnormalities, but cannot simulate associated physical examination findings, such as JVP or pulse abnormalities. The Ventriloscope is a relatively new technology, and comparative effectiveness studies are not presently available.

For teaching cardiovascular physical examination, perhaps the ideal use of the SP is to combine the teaching of the normal cardiac examination with recognition of auscultatory abnormalities using any one of the simulation modalities. Although such "hybrid" or integrated simulations are being used in other domains, especially invasive procedural skills training [20, 23, 26–29], and despite the prevalent use of SPs in the medical education system, there is little research examining how best to use them for cardiac physical examination teaching.

Table 18.4 Cardiopulmonary simulators

Benefits
Simulate physical patient, with palpable pulses, JVP waveforms, precordial movements, and simulated heart sounds. Facilitates comprehensive physical examination as would be performed on a real patient
Allows for repetitive practice and can provide opportunity for self-practice
Typically, instructor present to provide feedback on performance
Multiple learners can listen to and examine the simulator at the same time, without the issues of real patient fatigue
Limitations
More expensive and less accessible than other simulator modalities. A single institution may have only one cardiopulmonary simulator, thus limiting learner access to the simulator
Typically only have one or two examples of each diagnosis
Although self-study modes are available, typical presence of instructor is faculty intensive

Cardiopulmonary Simulators (CPS) (Table 18.4)

Cardiopulmonary simulators (CPS) are mannequin-based simulators that have palpable pulses, JVP waveforms, precordial movements, and simulated heart sounds. Conceptually, CPS have great potential as tools to enhance the education of learners' cardiac examination skills. By more closely mimicking a real patient, CPS allow a full cardiac examination, integrating all sensory information. Cardiopulmonary simulators can replicate abnormal pathology and can be reviewed at the instructor's and learner's convenience, thus alleviating the constraints of patient and pathology availability. Unlike real patients who may tire from being examined by multiple trainees, multiple learners can listen to and examine the simulator at the same time, thus increasing the efficiency of teaching.

Almost all of the research into the effectiveness of CPS as a teaching modality has been undertaken using Harvey®. Across multiple studies, it has been demonstrated that instruction with Harvey®, either in isolation or in conjunction with the UMedic multimedia system, can improve novice and resident learners' diagnostic accuracy on Harvey® and on real patients [20, 23, 26–29]. Typically, these are single-group studies, but one was a cohort design comparing a fourth-year medical student cardiology elective focused on Harvey® examination in addition to real patients to a traditional elective focused on real patients. There was a small but statistically significant superiority in diagnostic accuracy with real patients for the Harvey®-trained students [28].

There has only been one study that compared CPS to another simulation modality for teaching cardiac physical examination skills [30]. This study suggested that instruction with Harvey® was no more effective than instruction using CD-ROMs [30], but limitations of the study design including no pretest to establish equivalence of the two groups at baseline and difficulty establishing equivalence of the post-tests done with real patients limit interpretation of the results. In one study using only CPS, medical students demonstrated a transfer of skills from CPS to real patients for a cardiac murmur presented on the CPS but a lack of transfer from simulated murmurs that were different from the real patient's diagnosis [31]. Thus, the comparative benefit of CPS over other simulation modalities remains largely unexplored.

Overall, it appears as though most forms of cardiac physical examination simulation can provide effective instruction in cardiac physical examination skills. There is a perceived relationship between greater physical fidelity of a simulator and better learning outcomes [30]. Kneebone has suggested that developers and educators have primarily focused on creating lifelike simulators and have forgotten to ask whether low-cost, low-fidelity simulators are able to produce similar results in teaching and learning [32]. Likely of more importance than the specific simulator is how the simulator is incorporated into any teaching session. As shown by Barrett et al., repetitively listening to cardiac abnormalities can significantly improve diagnostic accuracy [14]. The exclusively auditory and multimedia simulations are able to present many examples of the same diagnosis conveniently and economically, whereas the CPS may only have one or two representations of a particular diagnosis [30].

As outlined in a review of effective instructional design features for simulation-based medical education, the instructional session should incorporate the principles of feedback to learners on their performance, integration of the teaching session into the curriculum and deliberate practice and mastery learning [32]. Mastery learning describes an instructional approach wherein learners must "pass" a learning unit before proceeding on to the next unit. In cardiac physical examination, this was implemented by Butter et al. who taught medical students using mastery learning principles with a multimedia tutorial and CPS [29]. Using this approach, trained third-year medical students had better diagnostic accuracy examining real patients compared to fourth-year students who did not experience the course.

There is little doubt that in this era of reduced in-hospital patient volumes, larger medical school class sizes, and reduced faculty availability for teaching, simulation-based education for cardiac physical examination is a necessity. Simulation affords an opportunity for learners to work independently and at their own pace, to teach large numbers of learners multiple cardiac abnormalities, and to reserve teaching with real patients to learners with a basic skill set. Not only is patient contact opportunistic, it may not be the most efficacious method for students to learn an essential competency.

The field of simulation-based education for cardiac physical examination would benefit from more rigorous educational studies. Our understanding of how to use these potentially expensive resources would be strengthened through randomized, controlled study designs, examining different instructional approaches, comparing different simulation modalities directly, and assessing outcomes using real patients.

Echocardiography

Echocardiography is one of the most important diagnostic tools in cardiology and has an ever-growing role in perioperative anesthesia and in critical care. Echocardiography provides detailed information about cardiac structure and function. Clinically important information can be provided in real time to assist clinical decision making [34]. The two forms of echocardiography commonly used are transthoracic echocardiography (TTE) and transesophageal echocardiography (TEE). Proper interpretation of either modality requires extensive knowledge of cardiac anatomy, cardiac physiology, and visualization of image planes. Although both TTE and TEE employ the same echocardiographic principles to assess cardiac structure and function, each modality has its strengths and limitations.

Transthoracic Echocardiography (TTE)

Transthoracic echocardiography involves placing the ultrasound probe on the surface of the chest in various locations to obtain different image planes of the heart. Transthoracic echocardiography is noninvasive and has the ability to dynamically monitor cardiac function and accurately estimate intracardiac chamber pressures [35].

A limitation of TTE is the significant technical skill that is required to obtain adequate images, which can be difficult even in the hands of experienced echocardiographers [35]. The acquisition of high-quality, clinically relevant images requires precise angulations of the TTE probe and knowledge of how to improve image acquisition. The transthoracic approach is noninvasive but often yields unsatisfactory images because of obstacles limiting the acoustic window [30, 36].

Transesophageal Echocardiography (TEE)

Transesophageal echocardiography involves the placement of the echo probe into the esophagus (or stomach) when the patient is sedated or unconscious, to view cardiac structures and assess function [37]. Transesophageal echocardiography generally provides clearer images of the endocardium, specifically the mitral valve, and is also superior at visualizing the left atrial appendage, aortic root, and interatrial septum.

Transesophageal echocardiography is a standard imaging tool used during cardiac surgery to facilitate the assessment of cardiovascular anatomy and function without surgical interruption [34, 37]. Furthermore, TEE is playing an increasing role during percutaneous valve interventions; positioning of closure devices for atrial septal defects, patent foramen ovale, and ventricular septal defects; and for electrophysiological procedures [38]. TEE is also used in the intensive care unit, to evaluate hypotensive patients, provide an accurate estimate of left ventricular function, and help assess preload [39]. A number of studies have also shown its safety among critically ill patients [36].

The Need for Simulation-Based Echocardiography Training

Extensive hands-on training is necessary to develop echocardiography skills [40]. For example, in the 2003 American College of Cardiology Foundation/American Heart Association (ACCF/AHA) Clinical Competence Statement on Echocardiography, the board suggested that minimum competence as an adult TTE echocardiographer requires 75 patient examinations and 150 echocardiogram interpretations [41]. Although the merit of establishing competence based on an absolute number of examinations as opposed to a competency-based approach is debatable, there is little doubt that higher levels of proficiency require increased training time and number of patient examinations.

With either echocardiography modality, there are common barriers to the development of proficiency. First, echocardiography requires significant cognitive and technical skills. The echocardiographer needs extensive knowledge of cardiac structure and function and must be able to visualize the heart in different acoustic planes. Parceled with this visual-spatial knowledge is the technical ability required to manipulate the ultrasound probe in order to produce quality images that are amenable to interpretation. Second, there is a paucity of formal training opportunities for learners to acquire these skills. Practice is limited because of patient and situational factors. For the awake patient in the echo laboratory undergoing TEE, there is limited time to practice given the potential physical discomfort. During surgical procedures in the operating room, practice is limited because of the need for prompt diagnosis, image interference from the use of electrocautery, and the initiation of cardiopulmonary bypass.

The traditional teaching model consists of the use of textbook reading and echocardiogram interpretation sessions combined with supervised practical experience in the echocardiography lab or in the operating room. In the case of TTE, trainees can learn from technicians and echocardiographers in a clinic or hospital setting and have the opportunity for independent practice. However, hands-on TEE experience is acquired during higher-risk clinical situations in the company of advanced echocardiographers. Regardless of modality (TTE or TEE), novices face a steep initial learning curve where basic image acquisition is dependent on simultaneously mastering probe manipulation.

Echocardiography simulators are ideally suited to overcome these learning obstacles. The simulator can accurately represent the various cardiac structures in an infinite number of image planes to help master the visualization of the heart during various manipulations of the probe. Some simulators have the ability to show real-time real-life and animated depictions of the heart relative to the ultrasound probe. There may be enhanced graphical features that allow the user to see the plane in which their echo beam is cutting through relative to the heart. Simulators can incorporate both normal and pathological findings. However, the ability to practice for extended periods of time in a nonthreatening zero-risk environment is arguably the most enticing feature of echo simulators. The use of simulation technology provides an opportunity to create a virtual training environment to offset the initial learning curve and shorten the eventual duration of training with patients [35].

Types of Echocardiography Simulators

At present there are three types of echo simulators designed to help improve the acquisition of knowledge and technical skill for TTE and TEE. These range from Web-based simulations to part-task heart models to part-task mannequins that incorporate virtual reality echocardiography.

Web-Based Echocardiography Simulators

The Web-based echocardiography simulators have been developed to aid in learning TEE. They use a 3-dimensional heart model, constructed from serial computer tomography slices of a real heart, with a virtual probe that the learner manipulates via their computer keyboard. These simulators allow the learner to visualize the cardiac structures in different planes, which is critical in the early stages of acquiring TEE knowledge [31, 40].

The effectiveness of one of these Web-based TEE simulators was evaluated with a pre- and posttest design [34]. After using the simulator for an average of 130 min, ten postgraduate fellows in anesthesia, cardiology, and cardiac surgery demonstrated a significant increase in their posttest scores on a video-based multiple choice test.

These simulators provide learners with the opportunity to develop structure identification and the visual-spatial correlation of echo plane and cardiac structure that is necessary for competency in TEE. Their benefits include the low cost (free) and the ability for the trainee to become familiar with the standard TEE views with the opportunity for unlimited practice. However, it remains to be seen if the knowledge gains translate to clinical practice.

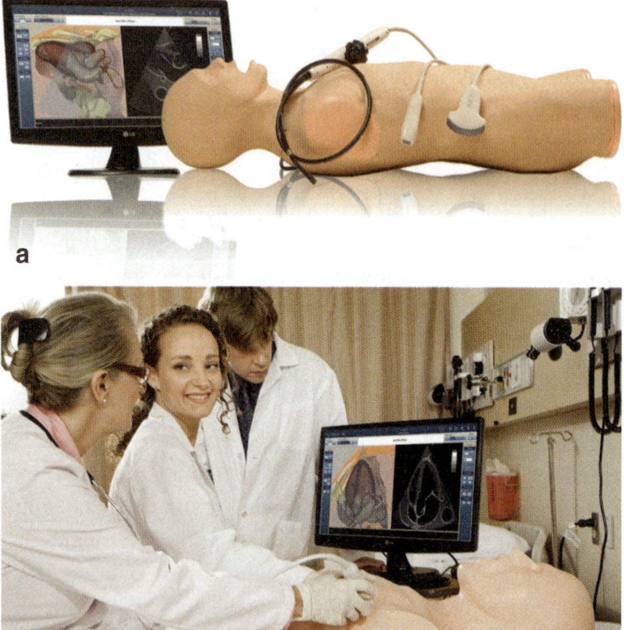

Fig. 18.3 (**a** and **b**) CAE Vimedix echocardiography simulator (Photo courtesy of CAE Healthcare ©2012 CAE Healthcare)

Part-Task Trainers

The simplest of the part-task trainers is an echocardiography simulator that consists of a full-body mannequin fitted with a physical, static, non-beating model of a human heart as well as lungs, ribs, and pericardial fluid (Blue Phantom™, USA). The heart model can be visualized and interrogated with either a TTE or TEE probe. This trainer allows the learner to become familiar with working a probe, working with the ultrasound machine, and obtaining images from all the relevant planes. However, because it is a static model, this trainer does not yield a realistic TTE experience for the operator.

The latest development in echocardiography part-task trainers is to combine a mannequin and dummy echo probe with virtual reality display of echocardiography images. In this setting, the learner moves the probe along the mannequin and views the echocardiographic images displayed on a computer screen. Manipulation of the probe changes the corresponding digital image, as in a real patient. These have been developed for both TTE and TEE, and their visual display combines both the echocardiographic image and a second screen displaying the three-dimensional virtual heart [35, 37, 42, 43]. Two commercially available simulators are CAE Vimedix (CAE Healthcare Inc, Montreal Canada) and HeartWorks (Inventive Medical Ltd, London, UK) (Figs. 18.3 and 18.4). The potential benefits of this type of trainer are the link between the transducer, the plane of the heart, and the echocardiographic image which may aid learners in acquiring knowledge and skills. The simulators have the capability to mimic both normal and abnormal cardiac exams (Fig. 18.5).

Aside from assessing user satisfaction, only one of these augmented simulators has been studied in a randomized, controlled trial to assess its educational effectiveness [44]. Fourteen first-year anesthesia residents were randomized either to a 90-min simulator-based teaching session with an instructor or to a control group consisting of self-study without the simulator. There was a statistically significant improvement in posttest scores for the simulator group compared to controls, on a video-based multiple choice questionnaire.

At the present time, the development of echocardiography simulators has outpaced the evaluation of their educational effectiveness. Theoretically, these simulators have many practical advantages to facilitate knowledge and skill acquisition. Acceptance of training in TEE and TTE with simulators has been shown to be very high among both novice and experienced echocardiographers [42, 43]. However, without studies comparing different approaches to echocardiography training, it is impossible to ascertain the relative benefits of the various simulation approaches. This is not to say that simulator-based training can or should replace the need for patient exposure, but it may supplement the traditional approaches to education and allow for development of basic knowledge and skills prior to practice on real patients. These technologies certainly hold the potential to address the barriers of time, patient exposure, and a steep learning curve that are associated with traditional echocardiography training methods.

Implementing a Noninvasive Simulation Curriculum

For any of the simulation modalities outlined in this chapter, a number of principles will facilitate the implementation of a simulation-based curriculum for noninvasive cardiology. First, a needs assessment of the learners is important, in order to develop appropriate learning objectives for the simulation sessions. This should take into account the current learning environments, with consideration of where the simulation modalities may best be used. For example, for novice learners of cardiac physical examination, adding time spent with simple heart sound or multimedia simulators prior to patient contact is a very efficient way of quickly improving learners' skills in heart sound recognition. The CPS can then be used to augment patient encounters that occur in the early clinical years, reinforcing the sounds heard at the bedside.

Second, the simulation-based modalities should be incorporated into the curriculum, as opposed to being stand-alone sessions. Third, whenever the simulation modality is in use, there may be a role for learners having time by themselves engaging in deliberate practice with the simulator. But of great importance is the presence of faculty, at some point in the learning session, to provide feedback and guidance to the learner. Finally, learning is consolidated if the session concludes with a skills test that requires the learner to achieve a certain level of competence before proceeding with the rest

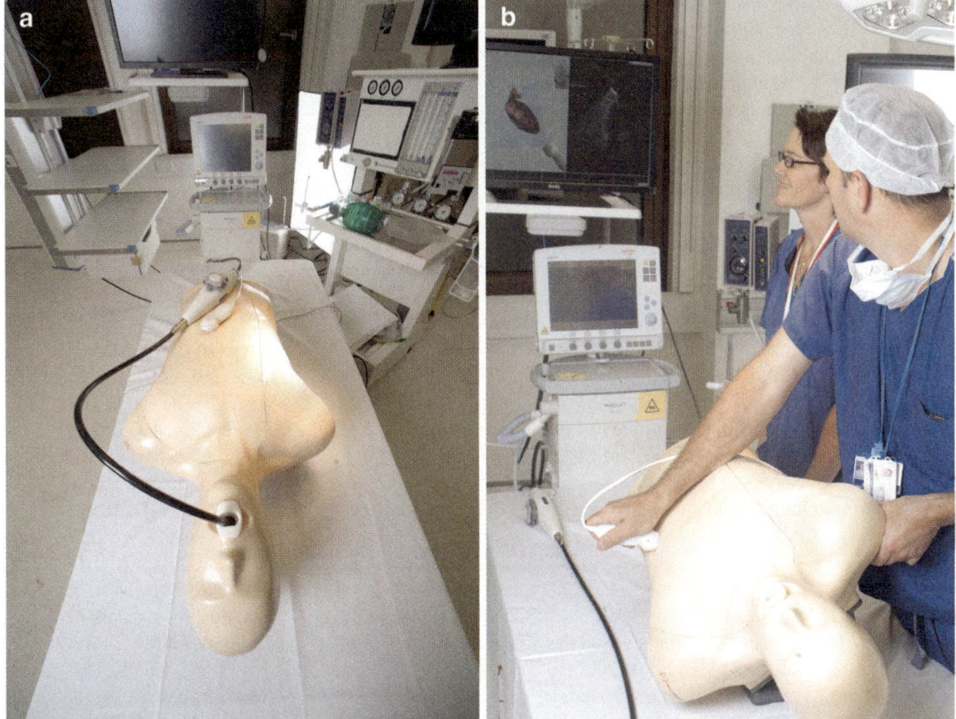

Fig. 18.4 (a and b) HeartWorks echocardiography simulator (Photo courtesy of HeartWorks)

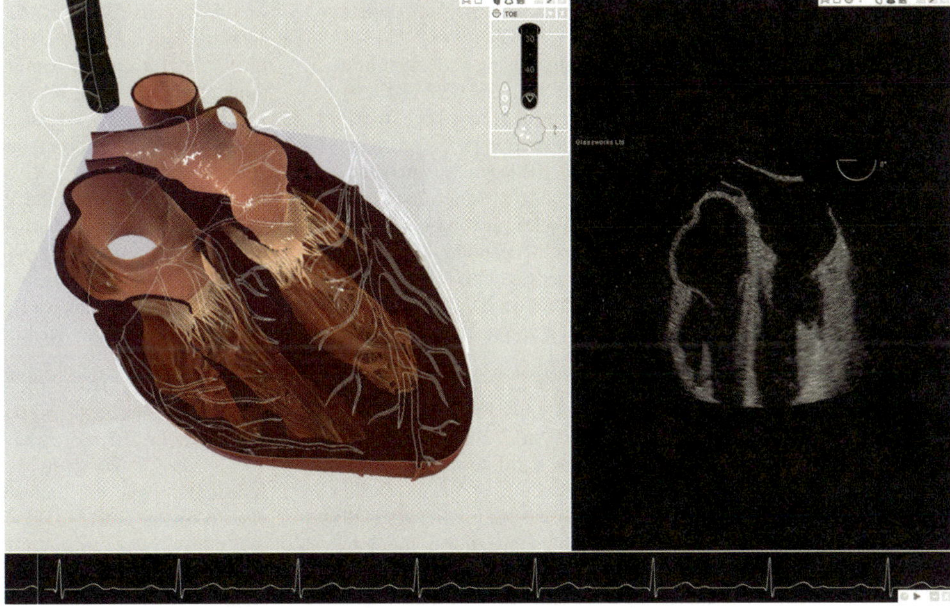

Fig. 18.5 Screenshot from HeartWorks TEE (Photo courtesy of HeartWorks)

of the curriculum. Layering different simulation modalities at different places in the curriculum can help learners scaffold their learning along a continuum of simple concepts to complex heart sounds.

Conculsion

Invasive cardiology skills are a vital to evaluate all patients specifically those with known cardiac disease. Auscultation has been shown to be under developed in our recent medical school graduates cardiac visualization skills seem to be supplanting Auscultation but this certainly require extensive training. Simulation may play a growing role in the aquisition and mastery of these auditory and visual skills.

References

1. Conn RD, O'Keefe JH. Cardiac physical diagnosis in the digital age: an important but increasingly neglected skill (from stethoscopes to microchips). Am J Cardiol. 2009;104(4):590–5.

2. Vukanovic-Criley JM, Criley S, Warde CM, et al. Competency in cardiac examination skills in medical students, trainees, physicians, and faculty: a multicenter study. Arch Intern Med. 2006;166(6):610–6.
3. Mangione S, Nieman LZ. Cardiac auscultatory skills of internal medicine and family practice trainees. A comparison of diagnostic proficiency. JAMA. 1997;278(9):717–22.
4. Mangione S, Nieman LZ, Gracely E, Kaye D. The teaching and practice of cardiac auscultation during internal medicine and cardiology training: a nationwide survey. Ann Intern Med. 1993;119(1):47.
5. Kern DH, Mainous III AG, Carey M, Beddingfield A. Simulation-based teaching to improve cardiovascular exam skills performance among third-year medical students. Teach Learn Med. 2011;23(1):15–20.
6. Stern DT, Mangrulkar RS, Gruppen LD, Lang AL, Grum CM, Judge RD. Using a multimedia tool to improve cardiac auscultation knowledge and skills. J Gen Intern Med. 2001;16(11):763–9.
7. Vukanovic-Criley JM, Boker JR, Criley SR, Rajagopalan S, Criley JM. Using virtual patients to improve cardiac examination competency in medical students. Clin Cardiol. 2008;31(7):334–9.
8. Gordon MS, Ewy GA, DeLeon AC, et al. "Harvey", the cardiology patient simulator: pilot studies on teaching effectiveness. Am J Cardiol. 1980;45(4):791–6.
9. Gordon MS, Ewy GA, Felner JM, et al. Teaching bedside cardiologic examination skills using "Harvey", the cardiology patient simulator. Med Clin North Am. 1980;64(2):305–13.
10. Bradley P. The history of simulation in medical education and possible future directions. Med Educ. 2006;40(3):254–62.
11. Passiment M, Sacks H, Huang G. Medical simulation in medical education: results of an AAMC survey. Washington: Association of American Medical Colleges; 2011. p. 1–48.
12. Ostfeld RJ, Goldberg YH, Janis G, Bobra S, Polotsky H, Silbiger S. Cardiac auscultatory training among third year medical students during their medicine clerkship. Int J Cardiol. 2010;144(1):147–9.
13. Horiszny JA. Teaching cardiac auscultation using simulated heart sounds and small-group discussion. Fam Med. 2001;33(1):39–44.
14. Barrett M, Kuzma M, Seto T, et al. The power of repetition in mastering cardiac auscultation. Am J Med. 2006;119(1):73–5.
15. Finley JP, Sharratt GP, Nanton MA, Chen RP, Roy DL, Paterson G. Auscultation of the heart: a trial of classroom teaching versus computer-based independent learning. Med Educ. 1998;32(4):357–61.
16. Roy D, Sargeant J, Gray J, Hoyt B, Allen M, Fleming M. Helping family physicians improve their cardiac auscultation skills with an interactive CD-ROM. J Contin Educ Health Prof. 2002;22(3):152–9.
17. Greenhalgh T. Computer assisted learning in undergraduate medical education. BMJ. 2001;322(7277):40–4.
18. Waugh RA, Mayer JW, Ewy GA, et al. Multimedia computer-assisted instruction in cardiology. Arch Intern Med. 1995;155(2):197–203.
19. Issenberg SB, Petrusa ER, McGaghie WC, et al. Effectiveness of a computer-based system to teach bedside cardiology. Acad Med. 1999;74(10 Suppl):S93–5.
20. Issenberg SB, Gordon MS, Greber AA. Bedside cardiology skills training for the osteopathic internist using simulation technology. J Am Osteopath Assoc. 2003;103(12):603–7.
21. Sverdrup Ø, Jensen T, Solheim S, Gjesdal K. Training auscultatory skills: computer simulated heart sounds or additional bedside training? A randomized trial on third-year medical students. BMC Med Educ. 2010;10(1):3.
22. AAMC. Effective use of educational technology in medical education. Washington: Association of American Medical Colleges; 2007. p. 1–19.
23. Verma A, Bhatt H, Booton P, Kneebone R. The Ventriloscope® as an innovative tool for assessing clinical examination skills: appraisal of a novel method of simulating auscultatory findings. Med Teach. 2011;33(7):e388–96.
24. Hatala R, Issenberg SB, Kassen BO, Cole G, Bacchus CM, Scalese RJ. Assessing the relationship between cardiac physical examination technique and accurate bedside diagnosis during an objective structured clinical examination (OSCE). Acad Med. 2007;82(10 Suppl):S26–9.
25. Criley JM, Criley D, Zalace C. Multimedia instruction of cardiac auscultation. Trans Am Clin Climatol Assoc. 1997;108:271–84; discussion 284–5.
26. Issenberg SB, McGaghie WC, Gordon DL, et al. Effectiveness of a cardiology review course for internal medicine residents using simulation technology and deliberate practice. Teach Learn Med. 2002;14(4):223–8.
27. Frost DW, Cavalcanti RB, Toubassi D. Instruction using a high-fidelity cardiopulmonary simulator improves examination skills and resource allocation in family medicine trainees. Simul Healthc. 2011;6(5):278–83.
28. Ewy GA, Felner JM, Juul D, Mayer JW, Sajid AW, Waugh RA. Test of a cardiology patient simulator with students in fourth-year electives. J Med Educ. 1987;62(9):738–43.
29. Butter J, McGaghie WC, Cohen ER, Kaye M, Wayne DB. Simulation-based mastery learning improves cardiac auscultation skills in medical students. J Gen Intern Med. 2010;25(8):780–5.
30. de Giovanni D, Roberts T, Norman G. Relative effectiveness of high- versus low-fidelity simulation in learning heart sounds. Med Educ. 2009;43(7):661–8.
31. Fraser K, Wright B, Girard L, et al. Simulation training improves diagnostic performance on a real patient with similar clinical findings. Chest. 2011;139(2):376–81.
32. Kneebone RL, Kidd J, Nestel D, et al. Blurring the boundaries: scenario-based simulation in a clinical setting. Med Educ. 2005;39(6):580–7.
33. McGaghie WC, Issenberg SB, Petrusa ER, Scalese RJ. A critical review of simulation-based medical education research: 2003–2009. Med Educ. 2010;44(1):50–63.
34. Jerath A, Vegas A, Meineri M, et al. An interactive online 3D model of the heart assists in learning standard transesophageal echocardiography views. Can J Anaesth. 2011;58(1):14–21.
35. Matyal R, Bose R, Warraich H, et al. Transthoracic echocardiographic simulator: normal and the abnormal. J Cardiothorac Vasc Anesth. 2011;25(1):177–81.
36. Heidenreich PA, Stainback RF, Redberg RF, Schiller NB, Cohen NH, Foster E. Transesophageal echocardiography predicts mortality in critically ill patients with unexplained hypotension. J Am Coll Cardiol. 1995;26(1):152–8.
37. Bose R, Matyal R, Panzica P, et al. Transesophageal echocardiography simulator: a new learning tool. J Cardiothorac Vasc Anesth. 2009;23(4):544–8.
38. Flachskampf FA, Badano L, Daniel WG, et al. Recommendations for transoesophageal echocardiography: update 2010. Eur J Echocardiogr. 2010;11(7):557–76.
39. Tousignant CP, Walsh F, Mazer CD. The use of transesophageal echocardiography for preload assessment in critically ill patients. Anesth Analg. 2000;90:351–5.
40. Kempny A, Piórkowski A. CT2TEE – a novel, internet-based simulator of transoesophageal echocardiography in congenital heart disease. Kardiol Pol. 2010;68(3):374–9.
41. Quiñones MA, Douglas PS, Foster E, et al. ACC/AHA clinical competence statement on echocardiography. J Am Coll Cardiol. 2003;41(4):687–708.
42. Weidenbach M, Wild F, Scheer K, et al. Computer-based training in two-dimensional echocardiography using an echocardiography simulator. J Am Soc Echocardiogr. 2005;18(4):362–6.
43. Weidenbach M, Drachsler H, Wild F, et al. EchoComTEE – a simulator for transoesophageal echocardiography. Anaesthesia. 2007;62(4):347–53.
44. Bose RR, Matyal R, Warraich HJ, et al. Utility of a transesophageal echocardiographic simulator as a teaching tool. J Cardiothorac Vasc Anesth. 2011;25(2):212–5.

Simulation in Cardiothoracic Surgery

19

James I. Fann, Richard H. Feins, and George L. Hicks

Introduction

Changes to surgical training, patient safety concerns, and the emergence of complex procedures in high-risk patients have generated greater interest in simulation-based learning in cardiothoracic surgical education [1–16]. Surgical simulation, defined as any skills training or practice outside of the operating room, can provide practice in a less stressful environment and enable graduated training of technical skills and crisis management. Further, this modality may be one means by which proficiency can be assessed [2–6, 9, 13, 17–22]. In general, cardiothoracic surgery simulation has been directed at the technical aspects of procedures, with emphasis on unique requirements of this specialty, such as performing small vessel anastomosis in a moving environment with time constraints (i.e., off-pump coronary artery bypass grafting), or implanting a cardiac valve with limited exposure. For the simulation exercises, the trainee needs to understand and articulate the correct way to use instruments, how to handle tissue and suture, and the relevant surgical anatomy. Additionally, scenarios for crisis management in cardiothoracic surgery are being developed and employed in simulation training.

As evidenced by laboratories investigating surgical techniques and the use of explanted porcine hearts in "wet-lab" environments, simulation, while not originally termed as such, has been widely employed in the history of cardiothoracic surgery. For instance, the technique of cardiac transplantation was extensively evaluated in the animal laboratory prior to clinical application. In the 1990s, synthetic cardiac surgery simulators for training attracted attention in the educational arena [23–26]. Stanbridge et al. and Reuthebuch et al. described beating heart simulators intended for training residents and surgeons [23, 24]. Bashar Izzat et al. and Donias et al. developed plastic and tissue-based beating heart models and noted that trainees became more proficient in their ability to perform beating heart anastomoses [25, 26]. In general, the focus and educational goals of these models were limited, and these efforts did not result in widespread adoption. Reported in 2005, Ramphal and colleagues employed a high-technology, high-fidelity porcine heart model to address the shortage of cardiac surgery cases for training in Jamaica [7]. To enhance cardiac surgical education in Europe, an important simulation effort was initiated over 10 years ago using a tissue-based approach by the Wetlab Ltd facility in the United Kingdom [8, 27].

Along with local efforts, the leadership in cardiothoracic surgery has provided focused programs to advance and formalize simulation-based learning, including the Thoracic Surgery Foundation for Research and Education Visioning Conference and the "Boot Camp" and "Senior Tour" supported by the Thoracic Surgery Directors Association, American Board of Thoracic Surgery, and the Joint Council on Thoracic Surgery Education [1, 3–5, 14, 15]. These efforts have increased our understanding of the type of simulators required, led to the development of performance assessment, and provided a venue to address barriers to

J.I. Fann, MD (✉)
Department of Cardiothoracic Surgery, Stanford University, 300 Pasteur Drive, Stanford, CA 94305, USA
e-mail: jfann@stanford.edu

R.H. Feins, MD
Division of Thoracic Surgery, University of North Carolina, 3031 Burnett Womack Building, CB 7065, Chapel Hill, NC 27599, USA
e-mail: richard_feins@med.unc.edu

G.L. Hicks MD
Division of Cardiothoracic Surgery, University of Rochester Medical Center, 601 Elmwood Avenue, Rochester, NY 14642, USA
e-mail: george_hicks@urmc.rochester.edu

A.I. Levine et al. (eds.), *The Comprehensive Textbook of Healthcare Simulation*,
DOI 10.1007/978-1-4614-5993-4_19, © Springer Science+Business Media New York 2013

adoption [3–5]. The emphasis at the Boot Camp has been on five basic aspects of training, including cardiopulmonary bypass and aortic cannulation, coronary anastomosis, aortic valve surgery, pulmonary resection, and bronchoscopy and mediastinoscopy. At the meeting of the Senior Tour, comprised of senior (retired or semiretired) cardiothoracic surgical educators, 12 cardiothoracic surgical simulators are employed along with proposed assessment tools [4]. Concurrent with these initiatives has been the development of cardiothoracic surgical simulators at many centers [2–4, 6, 7, 9–12, 28].

Simulator Development

Because procedures in surgery can be partitioned into components leading to the development of partial-task trainers, one emphasis in cardiothoracic surgery simulation has been to provide the trainee with models that can be used for deliberate and distributed practice [2, 4, 9]. Synthetic simulators, considered "low-tech and low to moderate fidelity," can be useful in developing basic surgical skills, whereas tissue-based simulators such as the "wet-lab" experience can be considered "low-tech, high fidelity", since they are readily available and provide good anatomic representation and appropriate tissue or haptic response.

Cardiac Surgery Simulators

Coronary Artery Bypass Surgery

The technical tasks and procedures include coronary artery anastomosis, proximal anastomosis, and beating heart coronary anastomosis [2–4, 9]. Generally, coronary artery anastomoses can be performed using synthetic or tissue-based vessels attached to an apparatus. Synthetic models and simulators in coronary artery and vascular anastomosis are commercially available, and simpler models can be constructed (e.g., anastomosis "block") (Fig. 19.1a). The HeartCase model (Chamberlain Group, Great Barrington, MA) has a vessel anastomosis attachment which permits sewing an end-to-side anastomosis at different angles using 3–4 mm synthetic target vessels (Fig. 19.1b) [4]. For the tissue-based or "wet-lab" component, porcine hearts are prepared and positioned so as to expose the left anterior descending artery in a container (Wetlab Ltd, Kenilworth, Warwickshire, England) (Fig. 19.1c) [8, 27]. Synthetic tissue grafts from the Chamberlain Group and LifeLike BioTissue (Toronto, Ontario) can be used as grafts for the anastomosis. These grafts and target vessel thus offers some degree of realism, but its importance is in teaching the mechanics of anastomosis [4].

Beating Heart Surgery

The technical challenge of off-pump coronary artery bypass grafting is to expeditiously perform accurate coronary anastomoses on constantly moving target vessels, typically 1–2 mm in diameter. Understanding the stabilization devices is critical as is the various methods of optimizing exposure of the target vessel [2]. Commercially available synthetic beating heart model includes a simulator from the Chamberlain Group, which includes a compressor and controller (Fig. 19.2a), and one developed by EBM, which is motor driven (EBM, Tokyo). Tissue-based models using explanted porcine hearts include the Ramphal simulator, which is a high-fidelity, computer-controlled simulator that can be employed in many aspects of training (Fig. 19.2b). This educational approach permits the surgeon to become familiar and achieve some degree of proficiency before attempting this technique in the clinical setting.

Aortic Cannulation

One part-task simulator for aortic cannulation is the HeartCase model with the synthetic thoracic aortic attachment. Using a syringe or a pressure bag, normal saline can be instilled into the synthetic aorta for pressurization. A tissue-based model used at the Boot Camp is a porcine heart in which the coronary sinus, coronary arteries, and aortic arch vessels are oversewn (Fig. 19.3a) [5, 28]. The ascending aorta with the arch and a portion of the descending aorta is pressurized with a bag of saline. Another model utilizes the porcine descending thoracic aorta, which is prepared by oversewing the intercostal vessels, securing it in a plastic container, and pressurizing it using saline (Fig. 19.3b) [4]. The tissue-based models are realistic, permitting multiple cannulations. Also, they can serve as thoracic aortic surgery anastomosis simulators [4].

Atrial Cannulation

Right atrial or bicaval cannulation for cardiopulmonary bypass is simulated using the porcine heart model placed in a container. Understanding the anatomy, suture placement, and cannulation are the primary objectives. Ideally, atrial cannulation is performed as part of other procedures, such as aortic cannulation. In order to simulate atrial cannulation in a more realistic, beating heart setting, the Ramphal simulator can be used.

Cardiopulmonary Bypass

Used in the training of perfusionists and surgeons, cardiopulmonary bypass simulators are intended to be highly interactive [4, 5]. The simulators provide multiple physiologic conditions and permit the trainee to manage the steps preceding and during cardiopulmonary bypass, including intraoperative crisis management. The Ramphal simulator is thus well suited for cardiopulmonary bypass simulation. Other "high-tech, high-fidelity" cardiopulmonary bypass simulators, such as the Orpheus perfusion simulator (ULCO

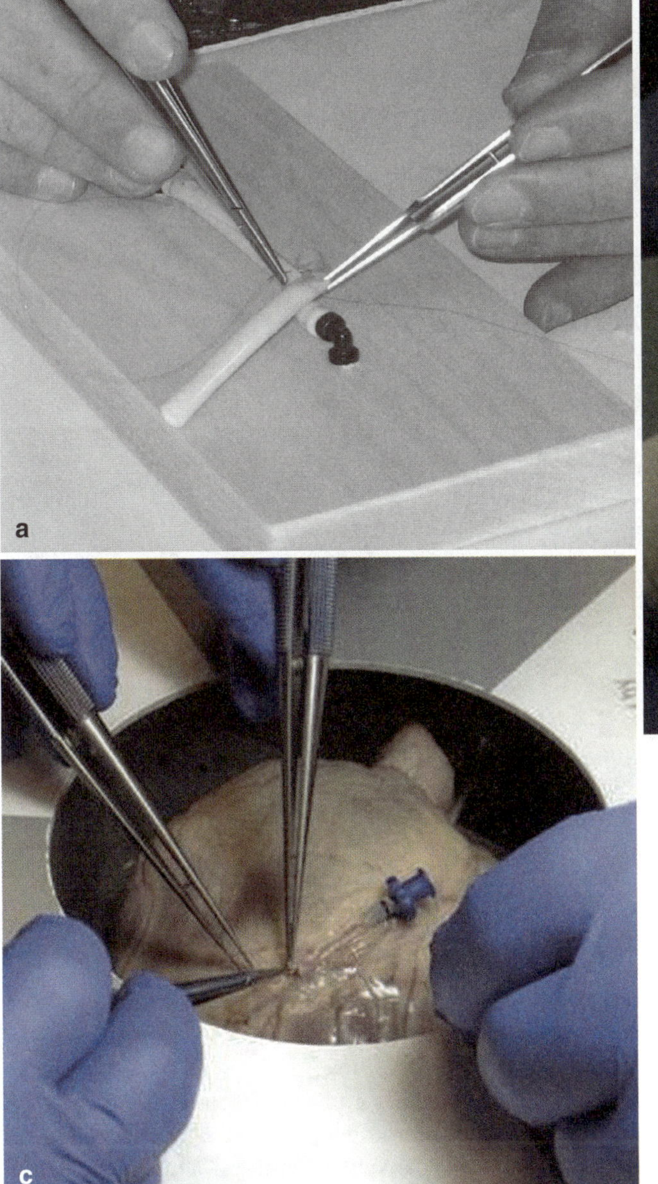

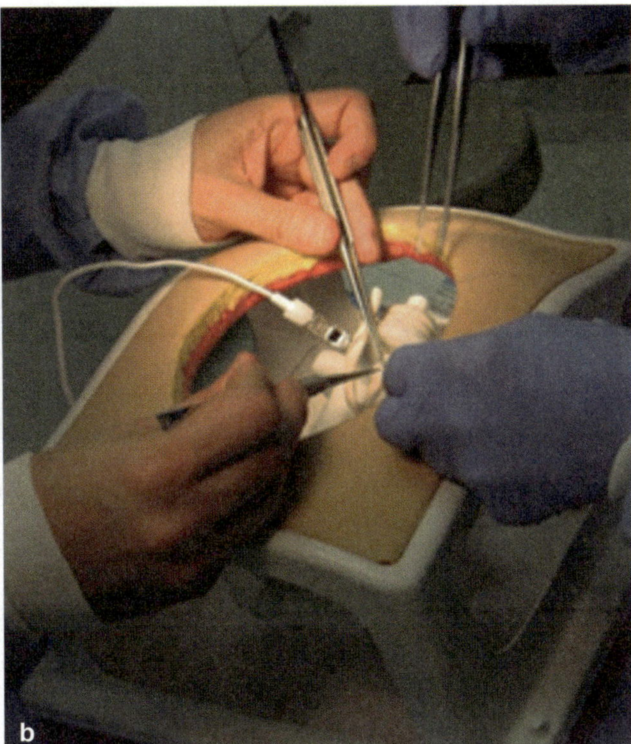

Fig. 19.1 Small vessel anastomosis: (**a**) An anastomotic block can be constructed using a wood block on which are mounted ¼ in. angled irrigation connectors. A synthetic graft can be positioned in place using the connectors (Reprinted from Fann et al. [3], with permission from Elsevier). (**b**) Mounted in the portable chest model is a synthetic target vessel; to simulate vein graft for anastomosis, another synthetic vessel is used. (**c**) For the tissue-based or "wet-lab" component, porcine hearts are prepared and positioned so as to expose the left anterior descending artery in a container

Medical), are commercially available with assessment modules, recognizing that such simulators are expensive (Fig. 19.4). A commonly employed method to learn about cardiopulmonary bypass circuit is to have access to a perfusion pump and arrange a tutorial with the perfusionist.

Aortic Valve Replacement

Synthetic models are adequate in teaching important components such as surgical anatomy and approach to placing annular sutures [4]. The aortic root model is available from the Chamberlain Group and can be attached to the HeartCase simulator (Fig. 19.5a). The objectives are to train proper needle angle for suture placement, effective knot tying in a deep confined space, placing sutures in the valve sewing cuff, and seating the valve prosthesis. For tissue-based simulation, porcine hearts are placed in a container and situated so as to present the ascending aorta and aortic root (Fig. 19.5b) [4]. The aortotomy is made followed by excision of the leaflets and the muscle bar under the right coronary cusp. Interrupted sutures are placed followed by the

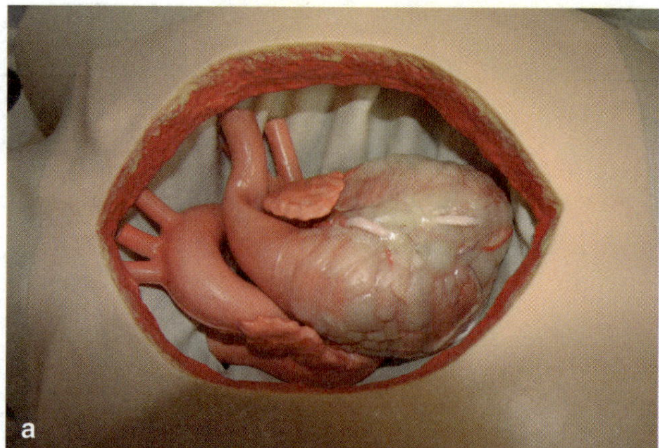

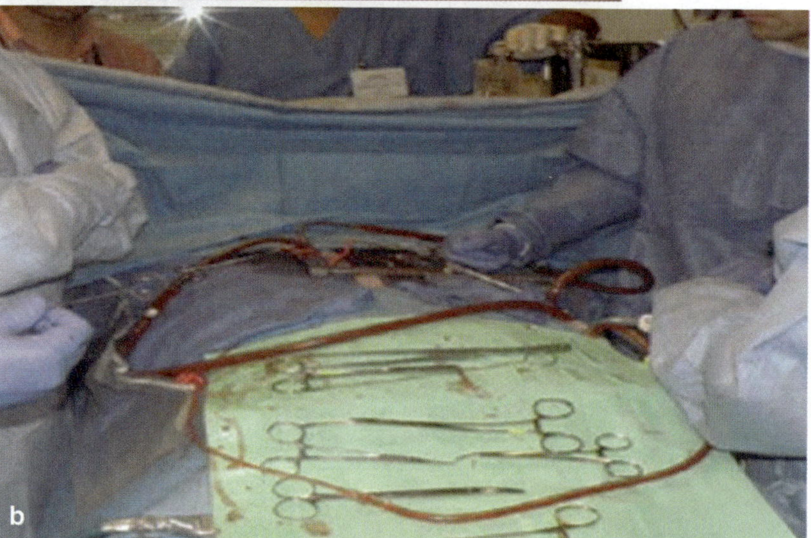

Fig. 19.2 Beating heart simulator: (**a**) The beating heart model is constructed of silicone and connected to a controller and external compressor. Partially embedded in the myocardium are 2-mm target coronary arteries. The heart is placed in a plastic torso simulating the pericardial well. (**b**) The Ramphal cardiac surgery simulator is a high-fidelity computer-controlled tissue-based simulator that allows the trainee to perform tasks such as beating heart and arrested heart surgery. Additionally, it provides cardiopulmonary bypass simulation and crisis management

placement and seating of the prosthesis. This model lends itself to standardized training, as it is currently used in many centers [4].

Mitral Valve Repair

The synthetic mitral valve attachment is a silicone-based cylinder placed in the portable HeartCase model (Fig. 19.6a) [4, 6]. The synthetic model provides a method to learn basic components of mitral valve surgery, such as exposure techniques and needle angles, but it is limited in its fidelity [4]. To more accurately simulate the mitral leaflets and annulus requires the use of a porcine heart model, which is placed in the container and situated so as to present the left atrium and mitral annular plane. The left atrium is opened and the mitral valve and annulus exposed in an "anatomically correct" configuration (Fig. 19.6b) [4, 6]. Interrupted annular sutures are placed and annuloplasty ring situated and secured. The porcine model is realistic but can pose some challenges with anterior-posterior orientation in the setup [4].

Aortic Root Replacement

For the tissue-based aortic root replacement simulator, explanted porcine hearts are placed in the container and situated so as to present ascending aorta and aortic root [4]. The porcine aorta and root are resected after creation of the coronary ostial buttons. A composite valve graft (or just a Dacron graft) or an expired aortic homograft (CryoLife, Inc. Kennesaw, GA), if available, is prepared and anastomosed as a root replacement using polypropylene sutures for coronary button reimplantation [4]. This realistic, tissue-based model has been helpful in familiarizing the trainee with the complexity of this procedure [4].

Thoracic Surgery Simulators

Hilar Dissection and Pulmonary Resection

A porcine heart-lung block placed within the chest cavity of a mannequin simulates the necessary maneuvers of hilar dissection and pulmonary resection through a thoracotomy incision

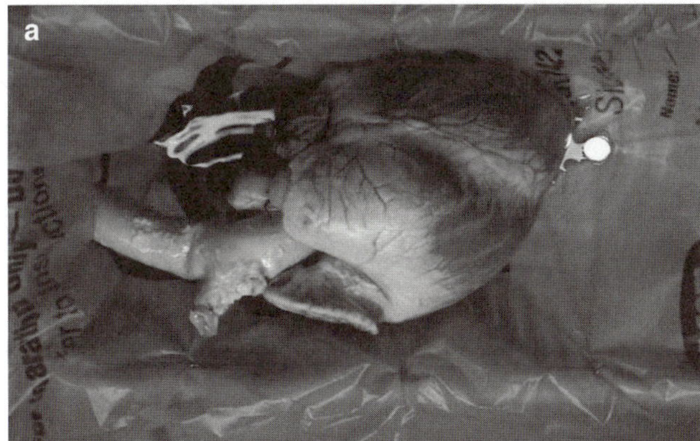

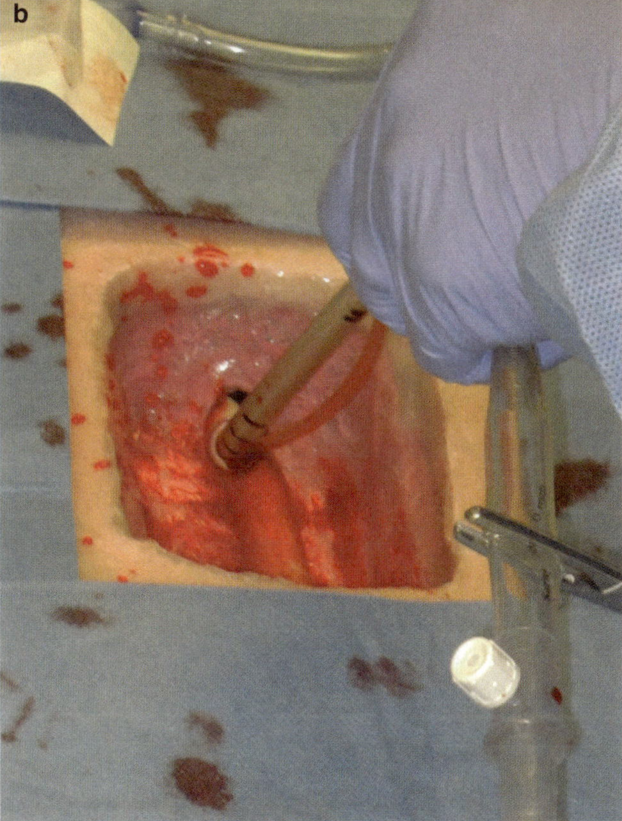

Fig. 19.3 Aortic cannulation: (**a**) For the perfused non-beating porcine heart placed in a container, the arch vessels are oversewn, and a portion of the descending aorta in continuity with the ascending aorta provides a long segment to practice multiple aortic and cardioplegia cannulations. (**b**) A porcine descending thoracic aorta is secured in a plastic thoracic model. The pressurized aorta allows placement of purse-string sutures and multiple aortic cannulations (Reprinted from Fann et al. [4], with permission from Elsevier)

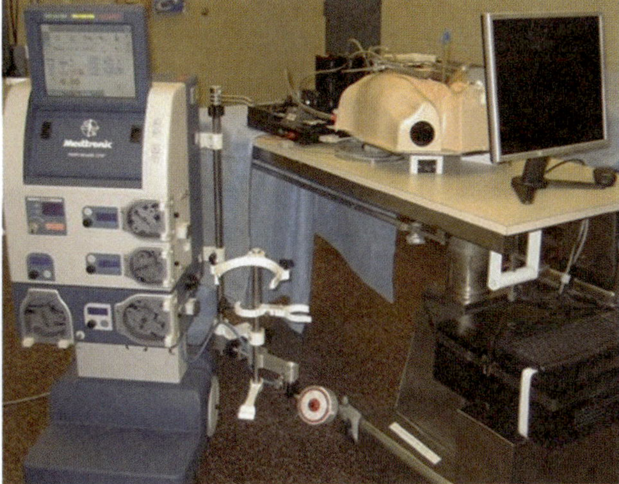

Fig. 19.4 Cardiopulmonary bypass: The Silastic heart model is placed in a plastic thorax and attached to the Orpheus cardiopulmonary bypass simulator. This simulation exercise allows the trainee to understand the cardiopulmonary bypass circuit and to participate in emergency and crisis management (Reprinted from Hicks et al. [5], with permission from Elsevier)

(Fig. 19.7) [4, 11]. Either the right or left lung can be used. This tissue-based simulator replicates the confined space in which pulmonary resections are performed and provides a method to practice hilar dissection and resection skills. The objectives are to identify anatomic landmarks, dissect and encircle the hilar vessels and bronchus, and ligate and divide vascular structures using sutures and staplers. This model is moderately realistic recognizing variability of porcine anatomy relative to human anatomy and the fragility of the vascular structures [4].

Esophageal Anastomosis

Placed within a thoracic mannequin, a porcine heart-lung-esophagus block simulates the thoracotomy providing access to the posterior mediastinum [4]. The esophagus, positioned and secured in the posterior cavity, is isolated and transected. The two free ends are re-approximated in either one or two layers. This model permits alignment and approximation of the esophageal ends, proper placement of sutures within the esophageal wall, and securing the sutures following placement [4]. By including the stomach in the tissue block, esophago-gastric anastomosis can be simulated. Additionally, providing and resolving tension on the anastomosis can be introduced, and creating longitudinal incision (with longer mucosal than muscular incision) would simulate esophageal rupture requiring the trainee to perform appropriate repair [4].

Rigid Bronchoscopy

Using conventional bronchoscopic equipment, the TruCorp AirSim simulator (Belfast, N. Ireland) is a model of the oral pharynx, larynx, and the tracheobronchial tree out to the segmental anatomy (Fig. 19.8) [4]. The model also allows simulation of awake bronchoscopy, bronchial stent placement, and removal of foreign body [4]. Since the image of the bronchoscope can be projected and the position of the light on the bronchoscope can be visualized through the wall of the model, assessment of resident performance in navigation is possible.

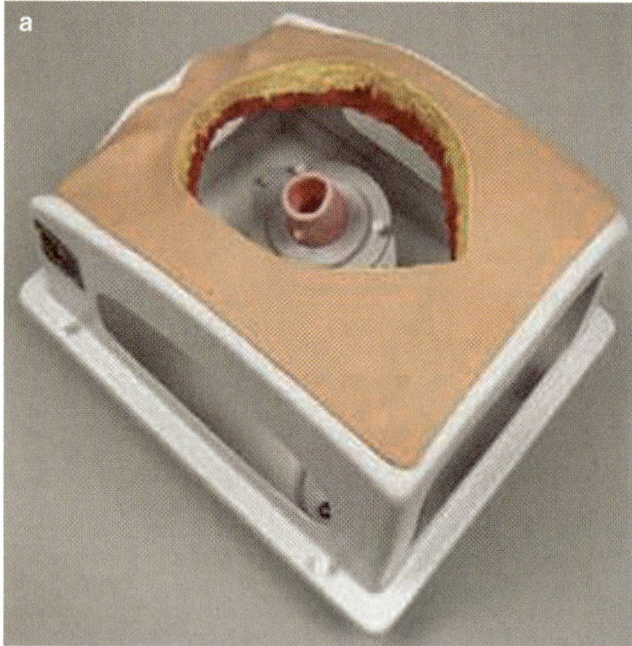

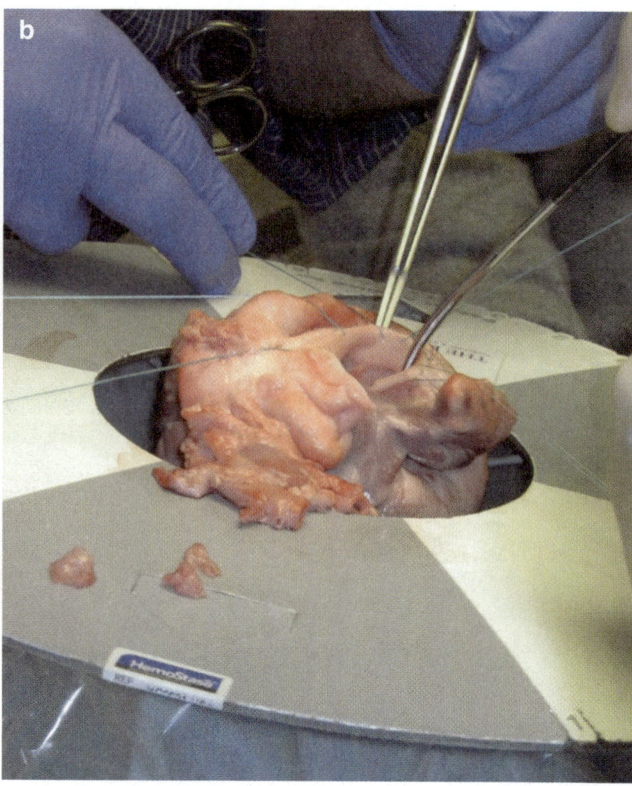

Fig. 19.5 Aortic valve replacement: (**a**) Mounted in a portable HeartCase chest model is a silicone-based aortic valve model which requires the trainee to understand proper needle angles, working in a deep, confined space, and seating the prosthesis. (**b**) For the tissue-based aortic valve replacement model, a porcine heart is placed in a container and situated so as to present the ascending aorta and aortic root. The aortotomy is made followed by excision of the leaflets and implantation of the aortic valve (Reprinted from Fann et al. [4], with permission from Elsevier)

Another bronchoscopic simulator is the CAE Accutouch EndoscopyVR Surgical Simulator (CAE, Montreal, Quebec), which is a highly sophisticated virtual reality simulator.

Video-Assisted Thoracoscopic Surgery (VATS) Lobectomy

A left porcine heart-lung block placed within the chest cavity of a mannequin is accessed via working ports to allow for video-assisted resection (Fig. 19.9) [4]. This exercise replicates the confined thoracic space in which pulmonary resections are performed and also provide a model to practice hilar dissection and resection skills. This simulator allows for identifying anatomic landmarks, maneuvering the thoracoscope and pulmonary structures, dissecting and encircling hilar vessels and bronchus, and dividing the structures using the endoscopic staplers. Recognizing interspecies differences, this model may be more complex than a case in the clinical setting, but it does provide simulation of many advanced maneuvers [4].

Tracheal Resection

A porcine tracheal-esophageal segment placed within the open neck of a mannequin simulates tracheal resection and anastomosis (Fig. 19.10) [4]. This realistic exercise reproduces the confined space in which tracheal resections are performed and provides a model to practice such resection and anastomosis. Given the shorter period of time required for this exercise, additional procedures, such as tracheostomy and tracheal release maneuvers, can be added [4].

Sleeve Resection

As an extension of the pulmonary resection simulator, a porcine heart-lung block placed within the chest cavity of a mannequin simulates the necessary maneuvers of sleeve resection via a thoracotomy (Fig. 19.11) [4]. This exercise replicates the confined thoracic space in which sleeve resections are performed. This realistic model permits airway mobilization and understanding the principles of bronchial anastomosis [4].

Pleural and Mediastinal Disorders

To date, simulation with pleural and mediastinal disorders has been limited to mediastinoscopy, anterior mediastinotomy, and video-assisted thoracoscopic procedures. Simulators used at the Boot Camp include a mediastinoscopy model made of the head, neck, and thorax of a mannequin with a synthetic airway and mediastinal structures strategically placed in the anterior aspect of the upper thorax (Fig. 19.12). Mediastinoscopy is performed with conventional instrumentation and video monitor.

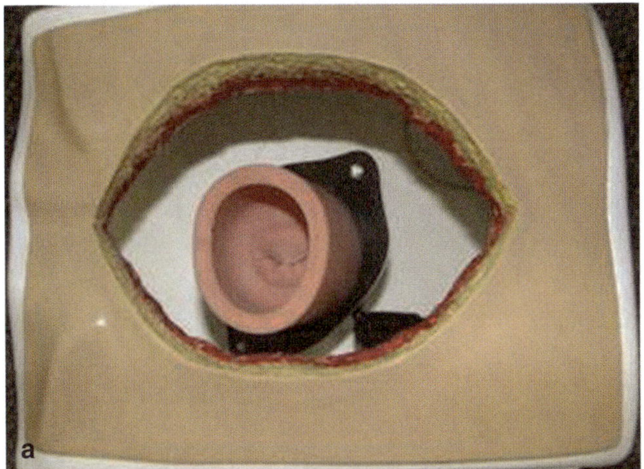

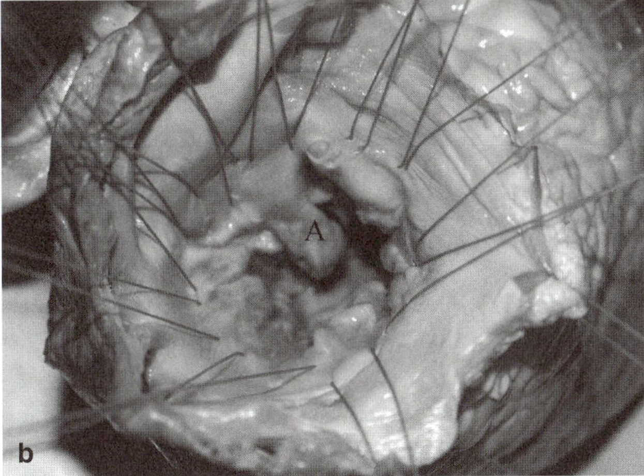

Fig. 19.6 Mitral valve repair: (**a**) The synthetic mitral valve model is placed in portable chest model. (**b**) For the tissue-based simulator, porcine hearts are placed in the container and situated so as to present the mitral valve. The left atrium is retracted so as to expose the mitral valve and annuloplasty performed. *A* anterior leaflet (Reprinted from Joyce et al. [6], with permission from Elsevier)

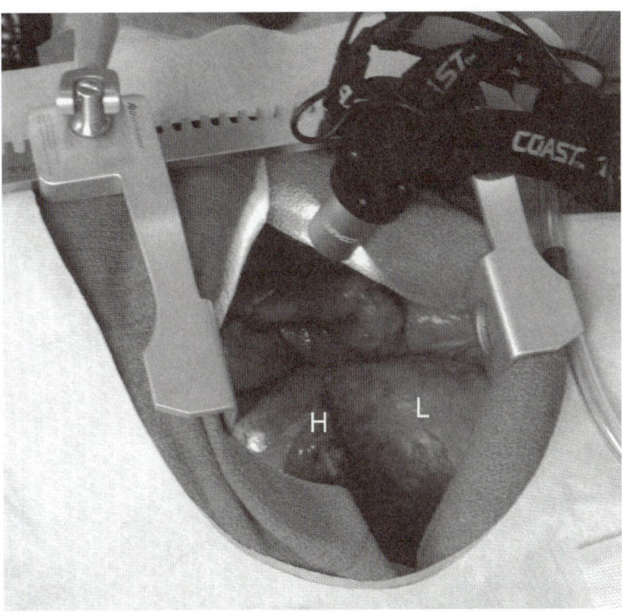

Fig. 19.7 Hilar dissection: a porcine heart-lung block placed within the chest cavity of a mannequin simulates the necessary maneuvers of hilar dissection through a thoracotomy incision. *H* hilum, *L* lung (Reprinted from Fann et al. [4], with permission from Elsevier)

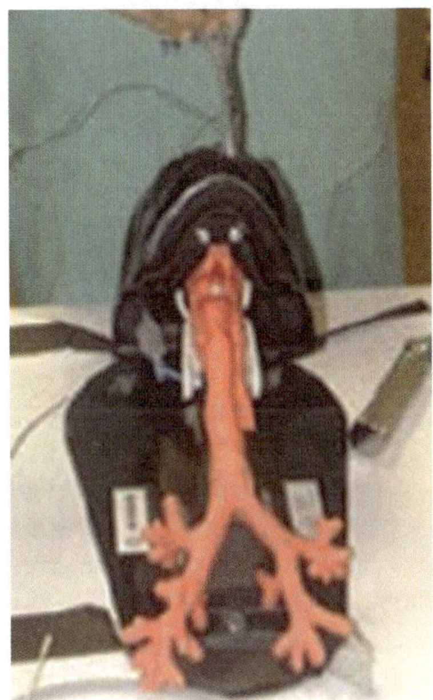

Fig. 19.8 Bronchoscopy: using conventional bronchoscopic equipment, the TruCorp AirSim model simulates the tracheobronchial tree

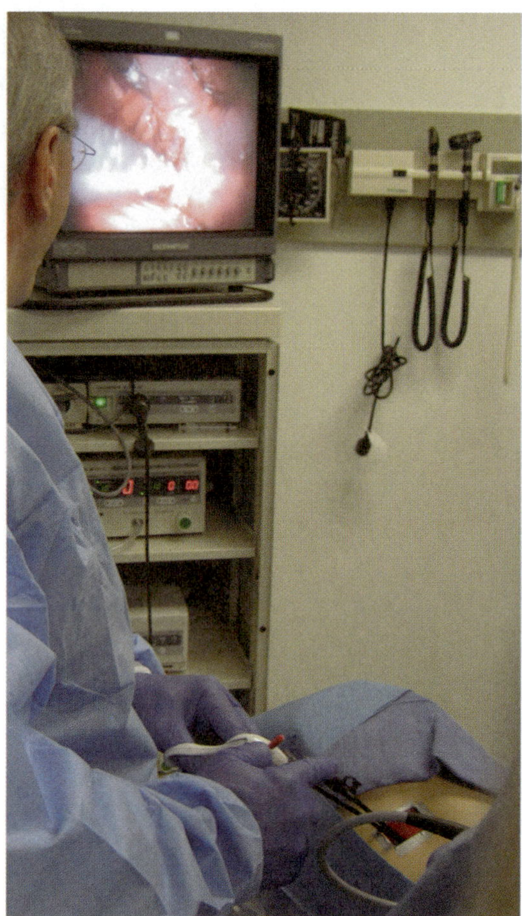

Fig. 19.9 Video-assisted thoracoscopic surgery (VATS) lobectomy: a left porcine heart-lung block placed within the chest cavity of a mannequin is accessed via working ports to allow for video-assisted resection (Reprinted from Fann et al. [4], with permission from Elsevier)

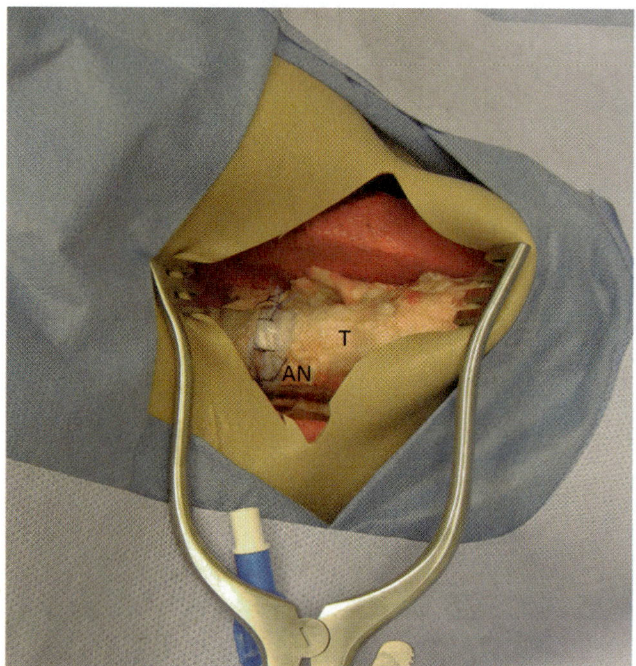

Fig. 19.10 Tracheal resection: a porcine tracheal-esophageal segment placed within the open neck of a mannequin simulates tracheal resection and anastomosis (*T* trachea, *An* anastomosis) (Reprinted from Fann et al. [4], with permission from Elsevier).

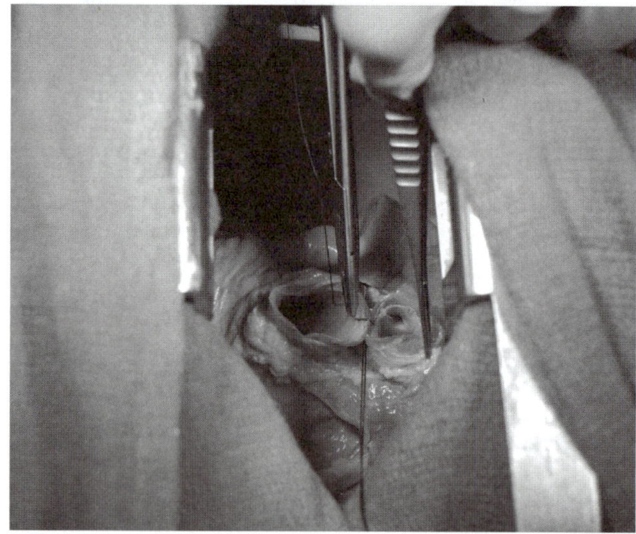

Fig. 19.11 Sleeve resection: a porcine heart-lung block placed within the chest cavity of a mannequin (similar to the hilar dissection model) simulates the necessary maneuvers of sleeve resection (Reprinted from Fann et al. [4], with permission from Elsevier)

Performance Assessment

Because surgical residents at the same training level may be at different technical proficiency levels, simulation-based learning is one means to assess performance and provide practice and remediation [2–6, 9, 16–19, 29–32]. Ultimately, surgery training may be competence based and not solely determined by the number of years in training or the number of procedures performed. Reliable and valid methods of assessment and passing standards for skills performance must be defined if such criterion-based system is to be implemented. Current and evolving assessment tools are based on direct observation and video recordings of a particular simulated procedure and include the use of task-specific checklists and global rating scales, such as the Objective Structured Assessment of Technical Skills (OSATS) developed at the University of Toronto and the Southern Illinois University Verification of Proficiency [2–6, 9, 16–19, 29–32]. To date, performance assessment in cardiothoracic surgery simulation has been reported for coronary anastomosis, cardiopulmonary bypass, mitral valve surgery, and pulmonary surgery [2–6, 9, 10]. Proposed rating scales for performance assessment created for the simulators used at the Senior Tour will require further modifications, including comprehensive anchoring points [4].

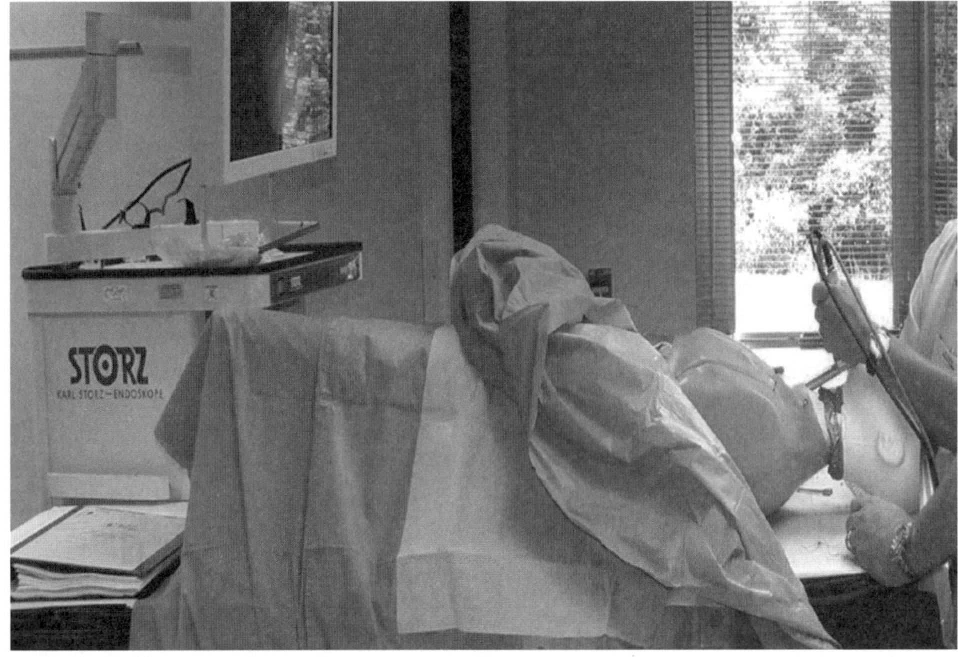

Fig. 19.12 Mediastinoscopy: developed at the Boot Camp, a mediastinoscopy simulator is constructed of the head, neck, and thorax of a mannequin with a synthetic airway and mediastinal structures strategically placed in the anterior aspect of the upper thorax. Mediastinoscopy is performed with conventional instrumentation and video monitor

For coronary anastomosis, Fann et al. evaluated distributed practice using a portable task station and a beating heart model in training coronary anastomosis [2]. With eight cardiothoracic surgery residents, times to completion for anastomosis on the task station decreased 20% after 1 week of practice (351 ±111 to 281±53 s), and times to completion for beating heart anastomosis decreased 15% at 1 week (426± 115 to 362±94 s). Distributed practice using the task station resulted in improvement in ability to perform the anastomosis as assessed by times to completion and 5-point rating scale (Table 19.1). Not all residents improved, however, consistent with a "ceiling effect" with the simulator and a "plateau effect" with the trainee [2]. To assess the value of focused training or massed practice, 33 first-year cardiothoracic surgery residents at the first Boot Camp participated in a 4-h coronary anastomosis session [3]. During the session, components of anastomosis were assessed using a 3-point rating scale. Performance was video recorded and reviewed by three surgeons in a blinded fashion. There was significant improvement from the initial assessment compared to the end of session, which were confirmed with video recordings [3]. Thus, the 4-h focused training using porcine model and task station resulted in improved ability to perform an anastomosis. In evaluating vascular anastomosis, Price et al. assessed 39 surgery trainees randomized to expert-guided tutorial alone versus expert-guided tutorial with self-directed practice [9]. Those who had the opportunity for self-directed simulator practice performed anastomoses more adeptly, more quickly, and at a higher quality [9]. Consistent with previous findings, simulator training should be incorporated into the curriculum, and trainees should have access to this modality for independent practice.

Joyce et al. evaluated simulation-based learning in skill acquisition in mitral valve surgery [6]. Eleven cardiothoracic surgery residents performed mitral annuloplasty in the porcine model. The video-recorded performance was reviewed by an attending surgeon providing audio formative feedback superimposed on video recordings; these recordings were returned to residents for review. After a 3-week practice period using the plastic model, residents repeated mitral annuloplasty in the porcine model. The time to completion improved from a mean of 31±9 to 25±6 min after the 3-week period. At 3 weeks, improvement in the technical components was achieved in all residents (Table 19.2) [6]. Thus, simulation-based learning employing formative feedback results in overall improved performance in a mitral annuloplasty model.

At the Boot Camp in 2009, Hicks et al. evaluated a modular approach to skills mastery related to cardiopulmonary bypass and crisis scenarios [5]. Thirty-two first-year cardiothoracic surgery residents were trained for four consecutive hours in cardiopulmonary bypass skills using a perfused non-beating heart model, computer-controlled simulator, and perfused beating heart simulator. Based on their performance using the cardiopulmonary bypass simulator, each resident was assessed using a checklist rating score on perfusion management and one crisis scenario (Table 19.3) [5]. For initiation and termination of cardiopulmonary bypass, most residents performed the tasks and sequence correctly. Some elements were not performed correctly. For instance, three

Table 19.1 Coronary artery anastomosis assessment

Resident name ______________________ **Year of training** ______________ **Date** ____________

Evaluator________________________ **Time to completion**________________

	Poor		Average		Excel
1. Arteriotomy (porcine model: able to identify target, proper use of blade, single groove, centered)	1	2	3	4	5
2. Graft orientation (proper orientation for toe-heel, appropriate start and end points)	1	2	3	4	5
3. Bite appropriate (entry and exit points, number of punctures, even and consistent distance from edge)	1	2	3	4	5
4. Spacing appropriate (even spacing, consistent distance from previous bite, too close vs. too far)	1	2	3	4	5
5. Use of Castroviejo/Jacobson needle holder (finger placement, instrument rotation, facility, needle placement, pronation and supination, proper finger and hand motion, lack of wrist motion)	1	2	3	4	5
6. Use of forceps (facility, hand motion, assist needle placement, appropriate traction ontissue)	1	2	3	4	5
7. Needle angles (proper angle relative to tissue and needle holder, consider depth of field, anticipating subsequent angles)	1	2	3	4	5
8. Needle transfer (needle placement and preparation from stitch to stitch, use of instrument and hand to mount needle)	1	2	3	4	5
9. Suture management/tension (too loose vs. tight, use tension to assist exposure, avoid entanglement)	1	2	3	4	5

Definitions:

5. Excellent, able to accomplish goal without hesitation, showing excellent progress and flow
4. Good, able to accomplish goal deliberately, with minimal hesitation, showing good progress and flow
3. Average, able to accomplish goal with hesitation, discontinuous progress and flow
2. Below average, able to partially accomplishgoal with hesitation
1. Poor, unable to accomplish goal; marked hesitation

Modified from Fann et al. [2]

Table 19.2 Mitral valve repair

Resident name________________ **Year of training**________ **Date** ________

Evaluator________________

	Poor		Average		Excel
1. Identify posterior mitral annulus (demonstrate annulus, i.e., decussation or junction of leaflet and atrial wall, for suture placement)	1	2	3	4	5
2. Identify anterior mitral annulus (demonstrate annulus, i.e., junction of leaflet and fibroskeleton, for suture placement)	1	2	3	4	5
3. Needle angles (proper angle to permit needle point to puncture orthogonal to tissue plane; consider depth of field, and space constraints)	1	2	3	4	5
4. Needle removal from annulus (follow curve of the needle to minimize tissue trauma)	1	2	3	4	5
5. Tissue handling (gentle manipulationwithout excessive tension and tissue trauma)	1	2	3	4	5
6. Depth of bite (proper depth of entry and exit points; proper and consistent depth of needle and suture)	1	2	3	4	5
7. Suture advance along annulus (proper distance of suture travel in annulus, not too small or large)	1	2	3	4	5
8. Spacing between sutures (even spacing; consistent distance from previous bite, not too close or too far)	1	2	3	4	5
9. Situating mitral ring (proper orientation relative to the annulus; proper suture placement from edge; proper suture spacing)	1	2	3	4	5
10. Knot-tying (adequate tension, facility; follow for finger and hand to secure knots, not too loose or tight)	1	2	3	4	5
11. Suture management/tension (avoid entanglement; use tension and traction to assist exposure)	1	2	3	4	5

Definitions:

5. Excellent, able to accomplish goal without hesitation, showing excellent progress and flow
4. Good, able to accomplish goal deliberately, with minimal hesitation, showing good progress and flow
3. Average, able to accomplish goal with hesitation, discontinuous progress and flow
2. Below average, able to partially accomplish goal with hesitation
1. Poor, unable to accomplish goal; marked hesitation

Reprinted from Joyce et al. [6], with permission from Elsevier

Table 19.3 Cardiopulmonary bypass

Assessment

Resident name ________________ **Year of training** __________ **Date** ________

Evaluator ________________

Steps	**Satisfactory**		**Comments**
Initiation:			
Assure adequate activated clotting time	Y	N	
Communicate with perfusionist	Y	N	
Check line pressure	Y	N	
Assess venous drainage	Y	N	
Vent placement	Y	N	
Cardioplegia	Y	N	
Cross-clamp	Y	N	
Termination:			
Removal of cross-clamp	Y	N	
De-airing procedures	Y	N	
Vent removal	Y	N	
Weaning CPB:			
Ventilator is on	Y	N	
Temperature satisfactory	Y	N	
TEE to assess intracardiac air	Y	N	
TEE to assess cardiac function	Y	N	
No bleeding in inaccessible areas	Y	N	
Acceptable rhythm / pacing wires	Y	N	
Need for inotropic support	Y	N	
Termination of bypass	Y	N	
Decannulation	Y	N	

Economy of time and motion	1	2	3	4	5
	1= many unnecessary/ disorganized movements		3=organized time/motion, some unnecessary movement		5=maximum economy of movement and efficiency

Final rating (circle one) Demonstrates competence Needs further practice

Additional comments:

Reprinted from Hicks et al. [5], with permission from Elsevier

CPB Cardiopulmonary bypass, *TEE* Transesophageal echocardiography

residents did not verify the activated clotting time prior to cardiopulmonary bypass initiation. Four residents demonstrated inadequate communication with the perfusionist, including lack of assertiveness and unclear commands. In crisis scenarios, management of massive air embolism was challenging with the most errors; poor venous drainage and high arterial line pressure scenarios were managed with fewer errors. For the protamine reaction scenario, all residents identified the problem, but in three cases, heparin was not re-dosed prior to resuming cardiopulmonary bypass for right ventricular failure. Based on a modular approach, technical skills and knowledge of cardiopulmonary bypass can be acquired and assessed using simulation, but further work employing more comprehensive educational modules will lead to mastery of these critical skills [5].

Initiatives in Cardiothoracic Surgery

Despite progress to date, educational and logistical concerns of cardiothoracic surgery simulation training remain [3–5]. Identified barriers to adoption include but are not limited to faculty time and commitment, facility and personnel cost, cost of equipment and supplies, trainee's time away from clinical activity, identifying appropriate simulators, defining comprehensive curriculum, and, perhaps the most challenging, organizational or specialty "buy-in" [4]. By defining the educational objectives, simulation can be incorporated formally in the residency program with scheduled courses and a means to provide adequate materials. Development of a technical skills curriculum at the national level has been through the Joint Council on Thoracic Surgery Education and locally by a number of institutions supported by institutional and national grants [1–6, 10–12, 33]. Incorporated into the skills training is emphasis on practice in the laboratory with formative feedback and at home using portable simulators. Weekly modular components, including coronary anastomosis, valve surgery, cardiopulmonary bypass, and crisis management, are directed at application of graduated skills with assessment. This project will require the continued, dedicated efforts of cardiothoracic surgical educators.

The Thoracic Surgery Directors Association and the American Board of Thoracic Surgery organized the first Boot Camp at the University of North Carolina in August 2008 to provide focused simulation-based training for approximately one-third of all first-year cardiothoracic surgery residents in the United States [3, 5, 14, 15]. In the ensuing 3 years, the Boot Camp, with support from the Joint Council on Thoracic Surgery Education, has emphasized training of essential components of cardiothoracic surgery, directed resources to development of assessment tools, and established a venue to educate faculty in the utility of simulation-based learning. Along with basic surgical skills training for cardiothoracic surgery residents, the directive of the Boot Camp has been to evaluate and develop surgical simulators and to explore novel approaches to the surgical training using simulation.

To increase the group of expert educators in training residents and to disseminate novel training methods to residency programs were the basis for the development of the Senior Tour, which originally comprised 13 senior cardiothoracic surgical educators [4]. The intent of the initial Senior Tour session was to introduce the members to simulation-based learning and to provide them with an opportunity to train residents using these modalities. At the meeting in January 2011, Senior Tour members evaluated the current simulators and identified methods to improve the training exercises, addressed constraints to simulation-based learning, and defined the process of starting simulation programs. Although many simulators stressed important concepts of a certain task, they do not fully simulate the clinical operative experience (Table 19.4). Along with simulator development, rating scales for performance assessment were proposed for nine simulators [4]. By providing the necessary tools, such as task trainers and assessment tools, Senior Tour members can assist in initiating surgical simulation efforts locally and provide regular programmatic evaluation to ensure that proposed simulators are of value. The Senior Tour continues to expand and currently comprises over 20 retired cardiothoracic surgeons who are committed to surgical education.

One important issue in the implementation of skills session in all specialties is whether time should be taken from clinical activity and directed into the simulation laboratory. Although some educators contend that such an approach would provide a favorable teaching experience in a controlled, laboratory environment, it is not clear that clinical hours should be redirected into a simulated environment. Some institutions have already mandated scheduled time in the simulation laboratory. Other efforts have been made to customize the training so that a resident can focus on certain skills at a time not disruptive to clinical care. Many institutions have employed physician extenders and technicians to provide access to and training in the simulation laboratory when the resident has clinical "downtime." As the benefits of simulation-based skills training become better defined, we anticipate that there will be scheduled time in the laboratory that minimizes clinical conflicts.

The cost of developing a surgical simulation laboratory remains challenging. Along with the requirement for space and equipment, such as operating room table, overhead lighting, and surgical instruments, unique to cardiothoracic surgery is the reliance on tissue-based simulators and the need for refrigeration. Although many of the simulators have been developed by local surgical educators, important is allocation of resources for the purchase of disposables and the maintenance costs required with many simulators.

Table 19.4 Summary evaluation of simulators used at the Senior Tour

	Time required to set up	Time required to complete	Complexity of simulator	Degree of perceived realism	Stressed important technical skills	Compared to operative experience
Small vessel anastomosis						
Synthetic	+	+	+	+	+++	+
Tissue-based	++	+	+	+++	+++	++
Aortic cannulation	++	+	+	++	++	++
Cardiopulmonary bypass	++	+++	+++	+++	+++	+++
Hilar dissection	++	++	++	+++	+++	++
Esophageal anastomosis	++	++	++	+++	+++	++
Rigid bronchoscopy	+	+	++	++	+++	++
Aortic valve replacement	++	++	+	+++	+++	++
Mitral valve repair						
Synthetic	+	++	+	+	++	+
Tissue-based	++	++	+	++	+++	++
Aortic root replacement	++	+++	++	+++	+++	+++
VATS lobectomy	++	++	++	++	+++	++
Tracheal resection	++	++	++	++	++	++
Sleeve resection	++	++	++	++	++	++

Reprinted from Fann et al. [4], with permission from Elsevier

+ less time, low level, or less agreement, ++ moderate time, mid level, moderate agreement, +++ longer time, high level, or more agreement

VATS video-assisted thoracoscopic surgery

Conclusion

Surgical simulation can provide a less stressful environment for graduated training of technical skills and training in crisis management; additionally, such an approach may be one means by which proficiency can be assessed. The leadership in cardiothoracic surgery has provided focused programs to advance and formalize simulation-based learning, including the Thoracic Surgery Foundation for Research and Education Visioning Conference and the Boot Camp and Senior Tour supported by the Thoracic Surgery Directors Association, the American Board of Thoracic Surgery, and the Joint Council on Thoracic Surgery Education. These efforts have increased our understanding of the utility of simulators in education, resulted in the development of performance assessment, and provided a venue to address barriers to adoption. Because procedures in surgery can be partitioned into components, one emphasis in cardiothoracic surgery simulation has been to provide the trainee with models that can be used for deliberate and distributed practice. Ultimately, it is recognized that cardiothoracic surgery training must be proficiency based. One challenge of a competence-based system of education is how to establish passing standards for technical skills ability; also, reliable and valid methods of assessment need to be developed if such a system is to be implemented. Thus, simulation-based learning may not only provide an opportunity to identify the methods for training and remediation but also help to define the competence levels for each stage of training.

References

1. Carpenter AJ, Yang SC, Uhlig PN, Colson YL. Envisioning simulation in the future of thoracic surgical education. J Thorac Cardiovasc Surg. 2008;135:477–84.
2. Fann JI, Caffarelli AD, Georgette G, Howard SK, Gaba DM, Youngblood P, et al. Improvement in coronary anastomosis with cardiac surgery simulation. J Thorac Cardiovasc Surg. 2008;136:1486–91.
3. Fann JI, Calhoon JH, Carpenter AJ, Merrill WH, Brown JW, Poston RS, et al. Simulation in coronary artery anastomosis early in residency training: the Boot Camp experience. J Thorac Cardiovasc Surg. 2010;139:1275–81.
4. Fann JI, Feins RH, Hicks Jr GL, Nesbitt J, Hammon J, Crawford F, et al. Evaluation of simulation training in cardiothoracic surgery: the Senior Tour perspective. J Thorac Cardiovasc Surg. 2012;143:264–72.
5. Hicks Jr GL, Gangemi J, Angona Jr RD, Ramphal PS, Feins RH, Fann JI. Cardiopulmonary bypass simulation and assessment at the Boot Camp. J Thorac Cardiovasc Surg. 2011;141:284–92.
6. Joyce DL, Dhillon TS, Caffarelli AD, Joyce DD, Tsirigotis DN, Burdon TA, et al. Simulation and skills training in mitral valve surgery. J Thorac Cardiovasc Surg. 2011;141:107–12.
7. Ramphal PS, Coore DN, Craven MP, et al. A high fidelity tissue-based cardiac surgical simulator. Eur J Cardiothorac Surg. 2005;27:910–6.
8. Munsch C. Establishing and using a cardiac surgical skills laboratory (monograph). Leeds: Wetlab Ltd., The Royal College of Surgeons of England; 2005.
9. Price J, Naik V, Boodhwani M, Brandys T, Hendry P, Lam BK. A randomized evaluation of simulation training on performance of vascular anastomosis on a high-fidelity in vivo model: the role of deliberate practice. J Thorac Cardiovasc Surg. 2011;142:496–503.
10. Carter YM, Marshall MB. Open lobectomy simulator is an effective tool for teaching thoracic surgical skills. Ann Thorac Surg. 2009;87:1546–50.
11. Tesche LJ, Feins RH, Dedmon MM, Newton KN, Egan TM, Haithcock BE, et al. Simulation experience enhances medical students' interest in cardiothoracic surgery. Ann Thorac Surg. 2010;90:1967–74.

12. Solomon B, Bizekis C, Dellis SL, Donington JS, Oliker A, Balsam LB, et al. Simulating video-assisted thoracoscopic lobectomy: a virtual reality cognitive task simulation. J Thorac Cardiovasc Surg. 2011;141:249–55.
13. Lodge D, Grantcharov T. Training and assessment of technical skills and competency in cardiac surgery. Eur J Cardiothorac Surg. 2011;39:287–93.
14. Feins RH. Expert commentary: cardiothoracic surgical simulation. J Thorac Cardiovasc Surg. 2008;135:485–6.
15. Hicks Jr GL, Brown JW, Calhoon JH, Merrill WH. You never know unless you try. J Thorac Cardiovasc Surg. 2008;136:814–5.
16. Hance J, Aggarwal R, Stanbridge R, Blauth C, Munz Y, Darzi A, et al. Objective assessment of technical skills in cardiac surgery. Eur J Cardiothorac Surg. 2005;28:157–62.
17. Reznick RK, MacRae H. Teaching surgical skills—changes in the wind. N Eng J Med. 2006;355:2664–9.
18. Reznick R, Regehr G, MacRae H, Martin J, McCulloch W. Testing technical skill via an innovative "bench station" examination. Am J Surg. 1996;172:226–30.
19. Reznick RK. Teaching and testing technical skills. Am J Surg. 1993;165:358–61.
20. Palter VN, Grantcharov T, Harvey A, Macrae HM. Ex vivo technical skills training transfers to the operating room and enhances cognitive learning: a randomized controlled trial. Ann Surg. 2011;253:886–9.
21. Beard JD, Jolly BC, Newbie DI, Thomas WEG, Donnelly TJ, Southgate LJ. Assessing the technical skills of surgical trainees. Br J Surg. 2005;92:778–82.
22. Martin JA, Regehr G, Reznick R, MacRae H, Murnaghan J, Hutchison C, et al. Objective structured assessment of technical skill (OSATS) for surgical residents. Br J Surg. 1997;84:273–8.
23. Stanbridge RD, O'Regan D, Cherian A, Ramanan R. Use of pulsatile beating heart model for training surgeons in beating heart surgery. Heart Surg Forum. 1999;2:300–4.
24. Reuthebuch O, Lang A, Groscurth P, Lachat M, Turina M, Zund G. Advanced training model for beating heart coronary artery surgery: the Zurich heart-trainer. Eur J Cardiothorac Surg. 2002;22: 244–8.
25. Bashar Izzat M, El-Zufari H, Yim APC. Training model for "beating-heart" coronary artery anastomoses. Ann Thorac Surg. 1998; 66:580–1.
26. Donias HW, Schwartz T, Tang DG, et al. A porcine beating heart model for robotic coronary artery surgery. Heart Surg Forum. 2003; 6:249–53.
27. WetLab, Ltd, website in the United Kingdom. http://www.wetlab.co.uk. Accessed 20 Mar 2013.
28. Schiralli MP, Hicks GL, Angona RE, Gangemi JJ. An inexpensive cardiac bypass cannulation simulator: facing challenges of modern training. Ann Thorac Surg. 2010;89:2056–7.
29. Moulton CA, Dubrowski A, MacRae H, Graham B, Grober E, Reznick R. Teaching surgical skills: what kind of practice makes perfect? Ann Surg. 2006;244:400–9.
30. Seymour NE, Gallagher AG, Roman SA, O'Brien MK, Bansal VK, Andersen DK, et al. Virtual reality training improves operating room performance. Ann Surg. 2002;236:458–64.
31. Sidhu RS, Park J, Brydges R, MacRae HM, Dubrowski A. Laboratory-based vascular anastomosis training: a randomized controlled trial evaluating the effects of bench model fidelity and level of training on skill acquisition. J Vasc Surg. 2007; 45:343–9.
32. Southern Illinois University Verification of Proficiency website. http://www.siumed.edu/surgery/surgical_skills/verification_of_proficency.html. Accessed 20 Mar 2013.
33. Verrier ED. Joint council on thoracic surgical education: an investment in our future. J Thorac Cardiovasc Surg. 2011;141:318–21.

Simulation in Emergency Medicine

20

Steve McLaughlin, Sam Clarke, Shekhar Menon, Thomas P. Noeller, Yasuharu Okuda, Michael D. Smith, and Christopher Strother

Introduction

Emergency medicine is a specialty with a high decision load, and the decisions are typically high stakes. In addition, emergency physicians work in an environment where effective communications and teamwork are essential to patient safety. These two factors combined with the wide range of uncommon yet critical illnesses and breadth of procedures make simulation training in emergency medicine a necessity. Driven by these demands, the emergency medicine simulation community has been at the forefront of simulation-based assessment and education over the last 10 years. This chapter will provide a description of the state of the art in emergency medicine simulation which is applicable to both emergency medicine educators and educators from other specialties. Much of what has been done well in emergency medicine can be easily applied to a variety of clinical disciples.

Simulation allows both practitioners and students to safely practice medical decision-making and procedural skills without incurring risk to patients [1]. This allows critical learning to occur for the emergency medicine practitioner outside of the uncontrolled and chaotic environment of the emergency department. Initially described and used in the military and in aviation, simulation techniques have been used in the healthcare industry for over 40 years. In 1966 Dr. Stephen Abrahamson and Dr. Judson Denson developed "Sim One" at the University of Southern California [2, 3]. Gaba and DeAnda took the next steps in development of this technology and educational techniques in the 1980s [4]. These initial efforts at lifelike human simulation lead to the now widespread adoption of the technique. In 1999, the first published use of simulation training for the specialty of emergency medicine appeared, detailing an advanced airway course which taught rapid sequence intubation (RSI) [5]. Based on the crew resource model, another landmark study was published in 1999 that described a simulation course to "improve EM clinician performance, increase patient safety, and decrease liability" [6]. Some of the initial descriptions of the use of simulation in emergency medicine education included a description of team training principles [6, 7], a discussion of human responses to the simulated environment [8], and a description of a simulation-based medical education service [9]. Since 2000, the specialty of emergency medicine has been a leader in the development of simulation

S. McLaughlin, MD (✉)
Department of Emergency Medicine, University of New Mexico, MSC 10 5560, Albuquerque, NM 87131, USA
e-mail: smclaughlin@salud.unm.edu

S. Clarke, MD
Department of Emergency Medicine, Harbor-UCLA Medical Center, 1000 West Carson St, Box, 21, 90509 Torrance, CA, USA
e-mail: sclarke@emedharbor.edu

S. Menon, MD
Division of Emergency Medicine, Northshore University Healthsystem, 3650 Ridge Ave., Room G909, Evanston, IL, USA
e-mail: shekharmenon@gmail.com

T.P. Noeller, MD, FAAEM, FACEP
Department of Emergency Medicine, Case Western Reserve University School of Medicine, 2500 MetroHealth Dr, 44109 Cleveland, OH, USA

Department of Emergency Medicine, MetroHealth Simulation Center, MetroHealth Health Medical Center, 2500 MetroHealth Dr, 44109 Cleveland, OH, USA

Y. Okuda, MD
Department of Emergency Medicine, SimLEARN, Simulation Learning Education & Research Network, Veterans Health Administration, University of Central Florida College of Medicine, Orlando, FL, USA
e-mail: haru.okuda@gmail.com

M.D. Smith, MD, FACEP
Department of Emergency Medicine, Case Western Reserve University, MetroHealth Medical Center, 2500 MetroHealth Drive, 44109 Cleveland, OH, USA
e-mail: msmith2@metrohealth.org

C. Strother, MD
Departments of Emergency Medicine and Pediatrics, Mount Sinai Hospital, 1601 3rd Ave., Apt. 31A, 10128 New York, NY, USA
e-mail: christopher.strother@mountsinai.org

A.I. Levine et al. (eds.), *The Comprehensive Textbook of Healthcare Simulation*,
DOI 10.1007/978-1-4614-5993-4_20, © Springer Science+Business Media New York 2013

techniques, faculty training, systems integration, research, and policy. There is currently a strong national simulation community in emergency medicine that continues to work on future applications of simulation to high-stakes assessment, maintenance of certification, patient safety, and quality. Indeed, as anesthesiology introduced the use of simulation, emergency medicine quickly helped advance the field in tandem.

Emergency Medicine Simulation History and Organization

Simulation in emergency medicine was first organized through the *Society for Academic Emergency Medicine* (SAEM). In 2002, in response to a growing number of members interested in simulation, the SAEM Simulation Interest Group was formed. The emphasis of this group was to increase collaboration and advance the emerging field of medical simulation. Its inaugural chair, Bill Bond, MD, also served as the EM representative to the national exploratory committee for the establishment of the Society for Medical Simulation, later renamed the Society for Simulation in Healthcare (SSH). As simulation matured within the field of emergency medicine, the SAEM Board of Directors established the Simulation Task Force to represent and support the organizational direction within the field of medical simulation. This group, originally chaired by Jim Gordon, MD, was established in 2005 and elevated to a standing committee in 2007, the SAEM Technology in Medical Education Committee. In 2008, the two groups worked together to sponsor an Agency for Healthcare Research and Quality (AHRQ) funded Consensus Conference entitled "The Science of Simulation in Healthcare: Defining and Developing Clinical Expertise" [10], which was held at the SAEM Annual Meeting in Washington DC. In 2009, the Simulation Interest Group and Technology in Medical Education Committee were combined to form the SAEM Simulation Academy, encompassing the goals, membership, leadership, and direction of both groups. This effort was spearheaded by Steve McLaughlin, MD. Rosemarie Fernandez, MD, was named the inaugural chair. The current focus of the Simulation Academy is to enhance education, research, and patient safety through the use of simulation. Recent Simulation Academy programs include consultative services for academic EM departments establishing simulation programs, establishing collaborative research projects, and administering the SimWars competition, created and developed in 2007 by Yasuharu Okuda, MD, Steven. A. Godwin, MD, and Scott Weingart, MD, at national and international meetings. The *Council of Emergency Medicine Residency Directors*, another EM national organization, set up a task force to create an oral board/simulation case bank. The simulation case development began in 2009, in collaboration with the Simulation Academy and the Clerkship Directors in Emergency Medicine, and currently has over 75 assigned cases. The *American College of Emergency Physicians* (ACEP) has a Simulation Subcommittee under the broader Education Committee. The focus of the ACEP Simulation Subcommittee is to investigate and create opportunities in the use of simulation for continuing medical education. Lastly, SSH has a Special Interest Group (SIG) in emergency medicine, which is dedicated to improving the quality of emergency care using simulation. This interdisciplinary group works together to support programs at the International Meeting on Simulation in Healthcare (IMSH) as well as liaises with other leading EM organizations to the SSH.

The Science of Simulation in Emergency Medicine

Medical Students

With the growth of simulation in emergency medicine (EM) resident education as described in other sections of this chapter, it follows naturally that these programs would bring simulation to their medical student clerkships as well. However, a complete description of the current state of EM-focused simulation in medical schools is difficult as we have incomplete data from which to draw. Descriptions of medical student use of all varieties of simulation exist, such as standardized patients, computer-based training, procedural trainers, and mannequin-based simulation. Chakravarthy et al. published the most comprehensive review of simulation in medical student EM education to date [11], which examined the prevalence and research behind simulation in EM education focused on students.

Wide variation in the methods and use of simulation exists in medical schools, and EM education is no exception. A recent survey gathered data about the current state and challenges in simulation for EM clerkships [12]. In 60 institutions surveyed, 83% reported simulation was available to students during preclinical years. The majority of clerkships included some simulation, including 79% using high-fidelity simulation, 55% using task trainers, and 30% using low-fidelity simulations. The majority of programs spend less than 25% of their core curriculum hours in simulation exercises, but actual time reported varied widely. When asked about barriers to increased simulation in their clerkships, 88% reported faculty time as a barrier, with available time and financial considerations being the next largest barriers reported by 47 and 42% of respondents, respectively. Another survey of 32 clerkship directors with EM rotations that include third-year medical students reported that 60% included some simulation exposure, including one that used simulation as an evaluation tool for the students [13].

While we have increasing data demonstrating the use and effectiveness of simulation in graduate emergency medicine programs, data on EM simulation in medical schools remains sparse. Most outcome data in medical student simulation has been completed in other specialties such as anesthesiology and obstetrics, but some of the skills studied, such as resuscitation and airway management, apply directly to EM. Simulation has been well described for use in teaching resuscitation skills to medical students [14, 15].

Over the past few years, there has been a growth in articles relevant to EM clerkship use, and these are well reviewed in the Chakravarthy article [11]. Some focus on demonstrating positive student perceptions of simulation exercises [16–18], others on simulation as a superior teaching tool versus traditional methodologies [19–22]. Not all studies have demonstrated positive outcome studies favoring simulation. One study by Schwartz et al. showed no difference in examination scores between a Human Patient Simulator group and a Case-Based Learning group [23]. Another showed no difference in posttest scores between groups randomized to simulation exercises versus lecture on two subjects [24]. These mixed but promising studies show a need for more high-quality research into the effectiveness of simulation versus other modalities in EM student education and a need to examine which subjects and competencies are best taught by simulation. In addition, studies describing which students may benefit most from this sort of learning are also needed, as it is entirely possible that simulation is not a "one size fits all" teaching modality.

Simulation as a patient safety and patient satisfaction tool has also been explored in at the medical student level. It has been demonstrated that emergency department patients' perceptions of students and their willingness to allow students to perform a procedure on them are improved if the patients are told the students have shown competence in that procedure on a simulator [25]. Procedural training eventually requires practice on real patients and improving the patients' comfort, and willingness to allow students to learn procedures on them is important. Patients also deserve students who are prepared in the most thorough way before being subjected to procedures to reduce the likelihood for error and harm. As the majority of research and published descriptions of successful simulation in EM has been completed with residents, a real opportunity exists for future research looking at using simulation for EM education in medical students. This position is reflected in statements from the SAEM Simulation Task Force research agenda from 2007 [26].

In summary, there are variations in the use of simulation in undergraduate EM education but growing evidence that it can be successful. The majority of undergraduate EM programs are using some simulation although the amount and types of simulation are not standardized and vary from completely replacing all didactics to nonexistent. Simulation would likely be used more if not for some well-described barriers such as faculty time and financial considerations. There is evidence that simulation can be a superior teaching tool to some more traditional methods for teaching students EM concepts and competencies, but further study is still needed in this area.

Graduate Medical Education

Simulation has been increasingly used in Graduate Medical Education (GME) programs for emergency medicine resident training. During the time period from 2003 to 2008, emergency medicine training programs reported that the use of some form of simulation increased from 29 to 91% [27]. Simulation has been shown to be an effective means of EM resident education and evaluation along the entire spectrum, from clinical knowledge and skill acquisition to teamwork training and development of interpersonal skills and professionalism. A comprehensive review of simulation in graduate medical education for emergency medicine was published in 2008 [28].

Most EM programs offering simulation-based teaching have added selected simulation modalities to their existing curriculum. Binstadt et al. described a revamped EM curriculum utilizing a comprehensive approach to simulation-based teaching [29]. McLaughlin et al. also describe a comprehensive 3-year curriculum that includes graduated complexity to match advancing PGY levels [30]. The Emergency Medicine Residency at the Mayo Clinic has also transitioned 20% of the core curriculum to simulation-based teaching without segregating junior and senior residents for the cases or debriefing sessions [31].

The standard educational conference is also being improved through the incorporation of simulation as an educational tool. Emergency medicine residents generally rate simulation-based training sessions higher than traditional lectures [32]. There are existing models which demonstrate how to include simulation scenarios, standardized patients, task trainers, and small-group sessions within the format of a 5-h resident conference [33]. Simulation has also been shown as an effective alternative for morbidity and mortality (M&M) resident conferences [34]. In a simulation-based M&M conference, the clinical scenario in question is actually re-created using simulation. The audience then actively evaluates the case in real time which increases learner involvement.

Simulation also appears to be an effective assessment tool for residency training programs [35]. The studies validating assessment tools for use in simulation in emergency medicine are increasing [35–38]. A study of pediatric residents found that high-fidelity medical simulation can assess a resident's ability to manage a pediatric airway [39]. A study by McLaughlin et al. used simulation-based assessment as part of a comprehensive assessment program to demonstrate competence of emergency medicine residents in the care of victims of sexual assault [40]. This type of study is an example of how simulation can be used effectively along with other assessment tools to capture a more full picture of a learner's performance. Simulation-based assessment has the potential to revolutionize competence assessment and may serve as a critical tool to accomplish the objectives of the ACGME Outcomes Project. Bond et al. identified that simulation was most useful for addressing the patient care, system-based practice (SBP), and interpersonal skills portions of the core competencies [41]. The system-based practice competency addresses the enormous variety of medical and social conditions as well as medical and nonmedical interactions that an emergency physician will encounter on a daily basis. This specific competency was addressed via a simulation-based curriculum by Wang and Vozenilek [42]. Using direct observation by attending physicians and coresidents, checklist evaluation of competency criteria, and videotape-based debriefing, this curriculum emphasized SBP objectives such as appropriate consultation, patient disposition, and resource utilization. Simulation has also been shown to be an effective way to assess multiple scenarios and procedures, encompassing the medical knowledge competency [43]. Professionalism in EM residents can also be assessed using a simulated environment as demonstrated by Gisondi et al. [36]. They evaluated residents by observing a scenario that focused on patient confidentiality, informed consent, withdrawal of care, practicing procedures on the recently deceased, and the use of do-not-attempt resuscitation orders. With direct observation, potential weaknesses and areas for improvement were identified in different classes of residents, as well as demonstrating improved professionalism as they progressed during the training.

Caring for multiple patients simultaneously is also an important skill for emergency medicine physicians and represents a high-risk aspect of their practice. Simulation scenarios with two or more simultaneous patients are being used to develop multitasking, crew resource management, and decision-making skills without risk to actual patients [44]. Simulation-based assessments should also reliably discriminate between novice and experienced clinicians. Evaluation tools previously developed for emergency medicine oral examinations appear to be effective when used in a simulator-based testing environment [35]. Crisis resource management in critically ill patients was assessed in residents using a novel rating scale and found significant differences between first-year and third-year residents [45]. Another study of residents in a pediatric training program found that simulation can reliably measure and discriminate competence [46]. A study of 44 emergency medicine residents found significant differences between novice and experienced resident physicians who were tested on a patient care competency using time-based goals for decision-making [37]. These studies suggest that well-designed simulation-based assessment is an effective way to monitor the progress of residents through the training program. Developing guidelines for training that are geared towards outcomes rather than processes will be essential under the new accreditation model for GME.

There are opportunities for simulation-based education to satisfy specific training requirements for emergency medicine. Currently, the chief complaint competency, resuscitation competency, and procedural competency requirements can all be effectively assessed using a simulation model. Although simulation is potentially well suited to such high-stakes assessment until it is validated as described above, it should only be used in combination with other metrics with proven performance [46–49]. Currently, in emergency medicine, simulation-based assessment is used more often and very effectively for formative assessment. Simulation helps provide a medium by which faculty can objectively identify areas in which a learner needs improvement. When used for formative feedback, the goal is to improve performance through deliberate practice.

Simulation has become an integral part of emergency medicine graduate medical education in the last 10 years showing growth in both numbers of programs using simulation and the sophistication of the curriculum and assessments. The future of simulation in GME will likely include an increased role in high-stakes assessment as well as more robust research programs.

Continuing Medical Education

Nationally, the role of simulation in continuing medical education (CME) has developed at a slower pace than that of GME and undergraduate medical education (UME). Currently, there is very little data on the role of simulation in CME for emergency medicine. However, there are a number of courses for practicing emergency physicians, which use simulation-based training to teach particular skills such as airway management, procedural sedation, or ultrasound. Most of these courses are independent and not organized into a comprehensive quality-focused CME program. In addition, there are some courses that have used simulation to develop teamwork in practicing emergency physicians. Some medical education companies offer *AMA PRA Cat 2 CME™* for completion of screen-based simulation training online. This limited application of simulation to CME in emergency medicine is beginning to change as it is increasingly seen as a tool to address the identification and closure of many performance gaps for the practicing emergency physician. This change is partially driven by the maintenance of certification (MOC)/licensure (MOL) processes and hospital credentialing requirements. Emergency medicine would be a likely candidate to develop simulation-based MOC requirements similar to anesthesiology.

Recently, a review of the literature, evidence, and best practices in CME was completed by the AHRQ [50]. This was followed up with a review article discussing the future of simulation in CME and lessons from GME/UME [51]. The conclusions of the AHRQ study were that the evidence is limited but does point to the effectiveness of simulation-based teaching of psychomotor and communications skills. It also noted that current assessment tools are limited and that simulation is hindered by its somewhat high cost. Emergency medicine educators should take away from these studies the message that quality simulation-based education in CME requires prepared teachers, integrated curriculum, quality assessment tools, and strong alignment with other patient safety and quality efforts. CME providers should also build curricula that foster mastery learning, deliberate practice, and recognition and attention to cultural barriers within the medical profession.

Interprofessional Education and Emergency Medical Services

The Institute of Medicine recommends that "all health professionals should be educated to deliver patient-centered care as members of an interdisciplinary team, emphasizing evidence-based practice, quality improvement approaches, and informatics" [52]. The emergency department is rich with opportunities to implement simulation-based interprofessional education (IPE) for teams of physicians, nurses, pre-hospital personnel, respiratory therapists, social workers, pharmacists, radiology technicians, other allied health professionals, and administrative support personnel.

Simulation provides an effective modality to enable interprofessional teams to improve knowledge and attitudes regarding teamwork and to identify effective team skills [53]. Integrating IPE principles with simulation methods allows innovative educators to pull from the strengths of each to design realistic programs that have significant potential to affect the clinical environment [54].

Simulation scenarios can and should be designed with each of the many involved disciplines in mind. Using both familiar and unusual case scenarios, ideas are generated directly from the real experiences of all disciplines, although it is important to develop a sustainable curriculum to address the long-term goals of the educational program [29]. Several scenarios can be linked to simulate a "regular workday" both to identify systems issues and to develop procedures addressing patient surges and disaster response.

At the inception of a program, representatives should collaborate to develop the desired learning objectives. Scenarios, as well as evaluation tools and metrics, should include elements specific to each discipline while simultaneously incorporating shared goals that bridge professional boundaries. Immediate debriefing incorporating facilitators from each professional group will serve to involve all individuals as active learners. A longitudinal collaborative evaluation process, addressing evolving objectives and program improvements, will help assure the sustainability of IPE programs. There are numerous examples of simulation-based team training in emergency medicine which are discussed in detail in one of the following sections.

There is also a growing body of literature to support simulation-based training and assessment in the emergency medicine services (EMS) community. Simulation has been used effectively for new skills acquisition [55], for identification of gaps in knowledge or skills [56], and for assessment [57]. Simulation has also been demonstrated to be an effective tool for teaching advanced disaster management skills and response to weapons of mass destruction [58]. Paramedic students are similar to other learners in that they find current simulation technology to be adequately realistic and effective [59, 60]. Simulation can effectively address many of the barriers to EMS education including exposure to serious but uncommon events, skills maintenance, and recertification. It should be considered a critical tool in modern EMS education.

The Art of Simulation in Emergency Medicine

Case Development and Scenario Design

There have been a variety of different approaches to case development in emergency medicine. The overall theme has been one of collaboration across the national emergency medicine organizations. Two specific pathways to case development include (1) creating tools and techniques for local/institutional level case development and (2) organized larger initiatives to create peer-reviewed case banks for use by multiple programs. For local case development there are a large number of different approaches, models, and templates. One approach used at several centers is the "Eight-Step Model" of scenario design [28] (Table 20.1). This model was developed at the University of New Mexico and is one example of a structured approach to case development. Often case development is supported by the use of a structured template for recording the case material, objectives, and assessment tools. Emergency medicine educators have also successfully used a second approach detailed below.

Starting in 2010 there was an initiative by the Council of Residency Directors in emergency medicine and the Simulation Academy of the Society of Academic Emergency Medicine to update and revise an existing bank of cases used for oral examination practice. This initiative focused on building

Table 20.1 The eight steps of scenario design

1. Objectives: Create learning/assessment objectives
2. Learners: Incorporate background/needs of learners
3. Patient: Create a patient vignette to meet objectives which also must elicit the performance you want to observe
4. Flow: Develop flow of simulation scenario including initial parameters, planned events/transitions, and response to anticipated interventions
5. Environment: Design room, props, and script and determine simulator requirements
6. Assessment: Develop assessment tools and methods
7. Debriefing: Determine debriefing issues and mislearning opportunities
8. Debugging: Test the scenario, equipment, learner responses, timing, assessment tools, and methods through extensive pilot testing

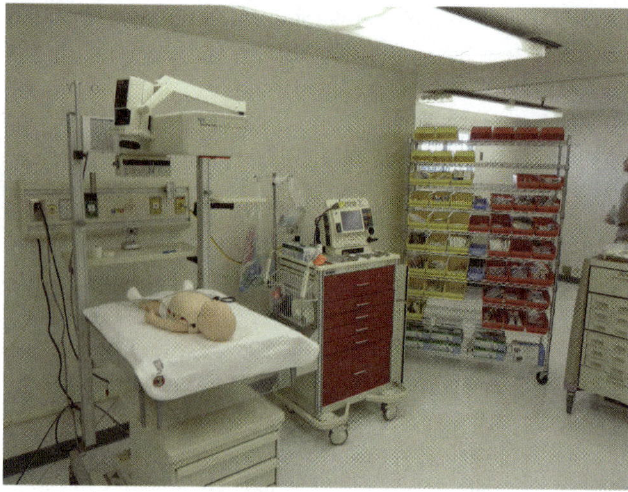

Fig. 20.1 Pediatric simulation lab

a shared bank of cases following a standard template which could be used by residency programs for simulation-based education, mock oral cases, or as an assessment resource. Each case was submitted by experienced simulation faculty and went through a rigorous peer-review process. The cases are accessible to all residency program members from emergency medicine. There are secure cases designed to be used for resident assessment as well as open-access cases which can be used to teaching or practice. This open-access portion of the website is available at www.cordem.org.

Equipment and Space

There has been strong growth in the use of simulation technology in emergency medicine since 2000, with the majority of accredited residency programs in the United States currently using some form of mannequin-based simulation [27]. Along with this trend has come a proliferation of simulation centers with technological resources and space dedicated to high-end clinical and procedural simulation, videoconferencing, and standardized patient encounters. Of the three professional organizations that have created accreditation standards for simulation programs (the American Society of Anesthesiologists, the American College of Surgeons, and the Society for Simulation in Healthcare), only the American College of Surgeons lists specific space and technological requirements for simulation centers. The SAEM Simulation Academy does not emphasize hardware or space requirements for simulation programs, recognizing that these are highly dependent on the educational goals and the resources available to individual programs [61]. Additionally, as high-fidelity simulators become increasingly portable and require less supporting equipment, it becomes less clear that a "fixed" simulation center is advantageous in every setting [28]. Successful in situ simulation can be conducted even within the confines of an ambulance, and its use in the clinical environment may indeed represent the natural evolution of the technology [62]. The following example provides a description of a dedicated space used for emergency medicine simulation but is not intended to be prescriptive.

For high-fidelity patient care scenarios, the space used for simulation should match the clinical environment in terms of equipment, patient monitoring, and available personnel as closely as possible (Fig. 20.1). For emergency medicine-specific simulation, this includes a basic cardiac monitor capable of displaying simulated vital signs and which can be manipulated remotely, IV supplies (IV catheters and start-kits, tubing, fluids, and an IV pole), equipment for managing airway emergencies (wall-mounted suction, bag–valve–mask, intubation tray), and a defibrillator and code cart. The added value of having functional equipment (e.g., suction, supplemental oxygen, defibrillator capable of delivering shocks) is debatable and should not be viewed as requisite for successful simulation. Additional equipment such as ventilators lends heightened realism to scenarios but at considerable cost and need for additional storage space. In situ simulation can mitigate many of these challenges, as scenarios can be conducted in the clinical environment with actual equipment.

In addition to the simulation space, consideration should be given to a control area from which to conduct the scenario. Ideally, this should include a "line of sight" (such as a one-way mirror) to the simulation area in order to facilitate quick adjustments during scenarios in progress, as well as adequate sound proofing to prevent interference from those conducting the scenario (Fig. 20.2). This may require some creativity in the case of in situ simulation, where the ability to create adequate distance for those conducting the simulation can be difficult. In these instances, a well-placed curtain or an adjacent doorway may be the best option. An area for observation and debriefing, ideally in a location adjacent or close to the simulation area,

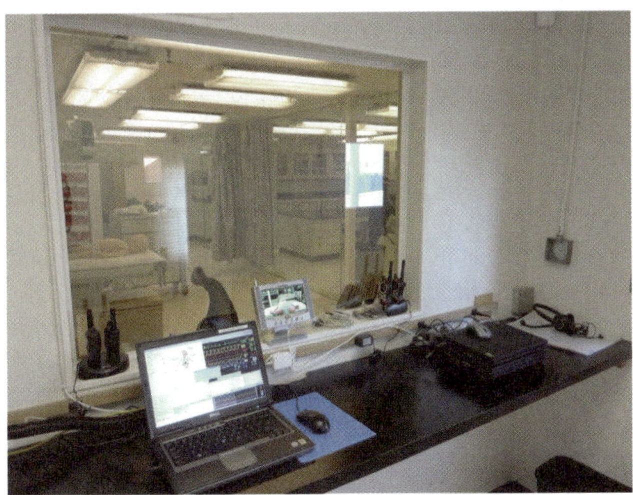

Fig. 20.2 Control room showing view of simulation area

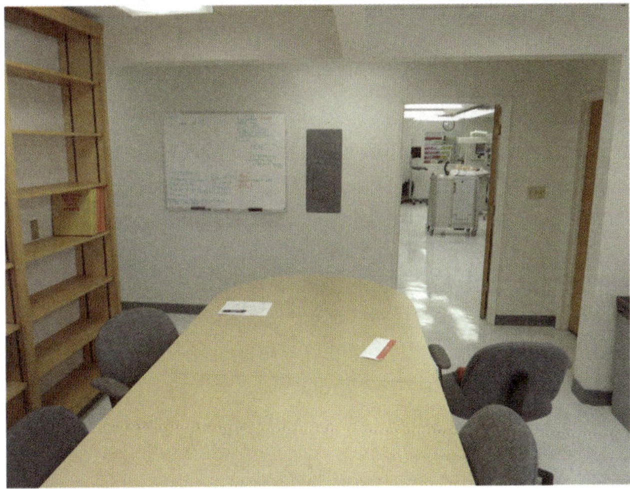

Fig. 20.3 Debriefing room

should also be available (Fig. 20.3). Depending on the audiovisual capabilities of the facility, this space can be used for video monitoring of ongoing simulation as well as post hoc review for debriefing. Finally, it should be emphasized that dedicated space for equipment storage, as well as for fabrication and repair of materials used in simulation, is essential to any simulation program and may be underestimated or overlooked in initial design.

Debriefing

Debriefing is a critical component of simulation education and is discussed extensively in Chaps. 6 and 7. For debriefing to be successful, it needs to be timely, focused, task based, and linked to established goals and objectives. The first part of developing a simulation program is identifying the learning objectives, which will be closely linked to the debriefing content. It is important that the faculty debrief to the task/learning objective rather than focusing on the learner being debriefed. In emergency medicine, video-assisted debriefing immediately after the scenario is used frequently. Most often team performances are debriefed with the entire team, and this is especially important in simulations that include a variety of healthcare professionals.

The specific debriefing model varies widely across different programs and with different learners. One common technique is the "Plus/Delta" model (what went well, the Plus vs. what can be improved, the Delta), which is useful for relatively straightforward discussions [63]. The WISER Simulation program uses a model referred to as "GAS" which stands for Gather–Analyze–Summarize. This three-step technique focuses on active listening followed by facilitating learner reflection and analysis of their actions and finally a summary of lessons learned [64]. A third technique is the "Debriefing with Good Judgment" model, which uses an advocacy–inquiry model to assist in the discovery of the participants' "frame" or understanding of the situation that underlies the visible action [65]. This technique is useful to understand more complex individual and team behaviors. Emergency medicine educators have strongly embraced debriefing because of its important role in deliberate practice and the development of mastery skills.

Funding

Simulation programs require substantial initial investments of capital and robust sources of operational funding for both personnel and equipment [66]. To successfully cultivate an array of funding sources, the leadership team should make use of all available resources within an institution. A combination of internal and external funding sources is necessary in many cases. Fortunately, simulation training appeals to a broad audience and tends to easily address the needs and goals of administrators, department chairs, program directors, hospital and university governing boards, governmental granting agencies, private foundations, and individual philanthropists. The concepts of patient safety, healthcare quality, and efficient training and evaluation of providers resonate widely. When it is recognized that funding a simulation center is a "win–win" situation for the institution, the providers', and most importantly the patients', funding tends to follow.

Those in a position to initiate a simulation program will need to advocate for the utility of simulation training and the ability of well-designed programs to serve the needs of the individuals, programs, and the institution. As the center matures, the need to maintain funding will require proof of effectiveness. Robust data collection and tracking will demonstrate that a simulation center can help the institution efficiently meet its requirements from the Joint Commission, American Nurses Credentialing Center (ANCC), and the Accreditation Council for Graduate Medical Education (ACGME) [43, 45, 67–69].

Beyond even these requirements, consistent training and evaluation of providers to maintain skills and improve quality helps to justify financial outlay from administration. Reducing medical errors and improving quality through simulation may lead to a reduction in healthcare delivery costs and even a reduction in medical liability premiums [70]. Additional drivers such as maintenance of board certification make simulation a necessary element in ongoing training and provider evaluation [71]. Simulation funding should be viewed as an investment in quality, efficiency, and safety.

Budget Allocations

An investment in a simulation program pays dividends regardless of the clinical environment. Whether serving a small contract group, a large multihospital group, or an academic program with a residency, budgetary allocations will provide the most consistent source of funding. Centers have been started and even operated for several years with funding from a single large grant, but sustainability relies on consistent funding both for personnel and equipment. It becomes the job of the simulation leadership team to reveal the benefits of simulation and leverage the many drivers to generate budget allocations. As a simulation center develops a consistent source of funding, directors and staff can focus more of their energies on simulation program development and dissemination. Because simulation is increasingly being shown to improve real patient outcomes and even decrease healthcare costs, it has demonstrable value to all those who control operational and capital budgets. Those who control operational budgets often are the same individuals who will benefit from the data generated in a simulation center, helping them to fulfill training, reporting, and accreditation requirements.

Philanthropy

Foundations and individual donors are a critical source of funding for both capital and operational budgets. Capital purchases tend to be more appealing to donors, but the goals of various foundations differ. It takes a firm understanding of the development process to work with potential donors to achieve mutually beneficial goals. This almost always requires that the simulation team work with a skilled and experienced development staff. These individuals can help identify potential donors, prepare presentations, generate publications, and facilitate the donation process. This involves balancing the needs of a simulation center with those of an entire institution, but often the appeal of simulation attracts considerable interest. Smaller groups or those without development personnel may identify donors on their own. A grateful patient or family, a local foundation with a shared mission, or even personal connections can provide fruitful opportunities. It is important to recognize these very important contributions with naming rights, donor recognition displays, publications, and sponsorship materials.

Corporate donors can potentially provide funding through a variety of mechanisms. A company may be interested in providing discounted clinical equipment since it is to their advantage to have their product used by a large audience. They may be willing to rent space to train their sales representatives and healthcare providers, or provide sponsorship for CME programs. Lastly, they may be willing to provide donations outright for naming rights to a simulation space.

Those with a direct stake in simulation training, including current faculty, physicians, and nurses, are often willing to make contributions through a giving campaign. Many programs have alumni funds that are used for education. Alumni easily recognize the importance of quality training opportunities for current trainees. A simulation center provides such tangible benefits. When a donor sees a simulator, a task trainer, or a named simulation room, they know that their money is having a direct impact on training and patient care.

Granting Agencies

Federal agencies largely under Health and Human Services including NIH, HRSA, and AHRQ make specific calls for funding proposals. Writing a federal grant application requires a significant level of experience and sophistication, a task made much easier if a support staff is available. Novice grant writers should seek to develop a track record of peer-reviewed publication and smaller grants before pursuing federal funding. State funding from EMS agencies can be a fruitful place to start, as can specialty-specific granting bodies including the Society for Academic Emergency Medicine and the Emergency Medicine Foundation. Grants targeted not only at simulation but any program that involves patient safety, reduction of medical errors, and healthcare quality improvement may be suitable for simulation-based applications.

Fee Generation

Attempts are being made at some centers to operate on a fee-for-service business model. The success of such a model depends on potential client mix and the ability of these client groups to establish and operate their own programs rather than turning to a third party. Medium to large groups, hospitals, universities, and academic departments have the resources to seek funding in a number of areas, making an investment in creating a simulation program worthwhile. Individual practitioners and small groups may not be able create and operate their own simulation programs, thus are likely to be potential clients of a fee-for-service center. Future market conditions and an increasing desire for courses that incorporate simulation may lead some fee-for-service simulation centers to a greater likelihood of sustainability.

Few centers are currently able to cover all operating expenses with fees alone. For most centers, fee generation from CME and maintenance of certification courses will be most effective if viewed as a way to defray the cost of capital improvements and operations rather than a method to cover all operating costs or generate profits.

Faculty Development in Simulation

Emergency medicine faculty are similar to all simulation educators in that they should be familiar with the advantages and disadvantages of simulation as an educational tool. Simulation will not be effective unless it is used as a well-planned and thoughtful part of the entire curriculum [72]. Faculty time constraints and lack of training were the top two barriers to simulation use in a recent study of emergency medicine simulation users [27, 73]. Faculty members who are interested in providing educational sessions for physicians in residency training must therefore be supported with adequate release time and training. General educational competencies such as objective writing, feedback, and assessment are required skills in simulation [74–76]. All faculty should also be experts in the clinical content area. Finally, the faculty member must develop expertise in simulation-specific skills such as scenario design, debriefing, and some technical knowledge about simulator operation, capabilities, limitations, and programming. These skills can be gained through institutional level training programs or by attending specialty-specific meetings where simulation is a focus. Some examples of these include the AEM Consensus Conference, the Council of Emergency Medicine Program Directors Annual Meeting, or the ACEP Teaching Fellowships and Simulation Courses. Many emergency physicians have also received training at simulation-specific national courses such as the Institute for Medical Simulation at the Center for Medical Simulation or at the International Meeting for Simulation in Healthcare. Simulation skills should be seen as a core competency for emergency medicine faculty along with the more traditional teaching techniques.

Fellowships

With the almost universal use of simulation in emergency medicine training programs [27], there is growing need for educators trained in how to use the teaching method effectively. This has led to rapid growth in non-ACGME approved fellowships in simulation at a variety of simulation centers, many with active ED participation or leadership. As there is no recognizing body or regulation of such fellowships, so their content and focus varies widely. Many include master's degree coursework in adult education or certificates. These fellowships are often conducted at interdisciplinary centers and with interdisciplinary leadership that reflect the composition of their simulation centers which often merge educators from different specialties. Funding can be provided by part-time clinical work, department funds, grants, or institutional budgets [28].

The Society for Academic Emergency Medicine lists six simulation fellowships (http://www.saem.org/fellowship-directory): Alpert Medical School of Brown University, Massachusetts General, St. Luke's-Roosevelt Hospital Center, Stanford University School of Medicine, Summa Akron City Hospital, and University of California, Davis. Each of these fellowships has their own unique strengths and design that are described below. Additional fellowships are being added every year, so this list is meant to provide a sample and is not a comprehensive catalog.

The MGH Fellowship in Medical Simulation in Boston is a tailored program over 1–2 years and includes an established curriculum in the Harvard Macy Institute and the Institute for Medical Simulation. Fellows here run the "On-Demand Medical Education Service" which has been previously published [1, 9]. Certificates in teaching and learning and other advanced certificates are available. Fellows work approximately half time clinically as an EM attending at MGH or an affiliate. The St. Luke's-Roosevelt program is one of the newest fellowships listed at SAEM and is located in New York City. Taking two people per year as about 20 h clinical, it is a 1-year fellowship and is a joint effort with other departments including critical care.

The Stanford University fellowship in California is one of the oldest and most established fellowships. It is a 1-year fellowship with work at four separate simulation centers. Fellows attend in the hospital emergency department. The Summa Akron City fellowship is a 1–2-year program in Akron, Ohio, and accepts up to two fellows per year. Fellows work in several simulation laboratories and attend in the emergency department at one of three local EDs. The University of California, Davis, simulation fellowship is a 1- or 2-year program, and fellows participate both at the center and in local disaster preparedness training. Fellows work part-time as attending physicians in the emergency department at the UC Davis Medical Center. The STRATUS Center for Medical Simulation Brigham and Women's Hospital has a 2-year fellowship that includes matriculation into Harvard Graduate School of Education for a master's degree in education.

Simulation-Based Education

Team Training

High-quality healthcare in essentially all clinical specialties requires a high level of team performance. Nowhere is this more apparent than in emergency medicine where rapid, accurate decision-making and communication must all operate efficiently and effectively to provide optimal care. Errors in communication and inefficiencies in team dynamics can lead to delays, incorrect treatment, and adverse outcomes [77]. By creating a structure to deliberately practice critical team skills in a systematic fashion, dissecting and debriefing all elements of a complex team dynamic, simulation training provides an opportunity that cannot be accomplished easily in a real-world setting.

The principles of team dynamics have evolved largely from other fields, most notably the flight industry. Crew resource management (CRM) principles are widely used in simulator-based exercises for pilots and flight crews [78]. CRM formed the basis for the development of the TeamSTEPPS® program by the Agency for Healthcare Research and Quality, a program that has come into wide usage for healthcare team training [79]. The elements of effective team training include team structure, leadership, situation monitoring, mutual support, and communication. Each of these elements is further subdivided to include key components that can be easily incorporated into simulation scenarios.

It is important to recognize that team training should itself form the simulation case objectives, leading to a delineation of the critical actions and development of evaluation tools. Often, learners will naturally focus on the medical management elements of a case, but when team training is the goal, it becomes the role of the scenario author and director to clearly define the goals, design the scenario to incorporate the critical elements, and focus on these elements in the debriefing.

Robust observation and evaluation tools such as the TeamSTEPPS® performance observation tool, the Behaviorally Anchored Rating Scale (BARS), and Behavioral Assessment Tool (BAT) can be useful adjuncts to scenario design, learner evaluation, and debriefing [79, 80]. Using such tools importantly focuses the objectives on the critical elements of team function.

Assembling the team to perform simulation training can present some challenges. Creating "buy in" and convincing administrators to allocate funds for training requires identifying discipline-specific drivers. Administrators easily recognize the value of simulation training once they become familiar with the ways in which it can help them train and evaluate staff, collect data for reporting requirements (e.g., Joint Commission, ACGME, ANCC), address patient safety goals, and contribute to the reduction of medical errors. Evidence is building in the literature to support these assertions [81]. Additionally, offering CME and CE credit often helps to serve the needs of both the simulation program and individual providers. Building team dynamics and esprit de corps in the real clinical setting has intrinsic value. "If we practice how we play, we play how we practice" resonates with both providers and departmental leaders.

Emergency medicine is uniquely positioned to take advantage of multidisciplinary and multispecialty team training opportunities, interacting with virtually every clinical specialty and often intersecting at the point where well-developed team skills can affect patient outcome. A trauma resuscitation bay, for example, is a nexus of interdisciplinary care requiring physicians, nurses, paramedics, and ancillary staff to function together efficiently and expertly. In the real clinical environment, team members change regularly. A single team with consistent individual members familiar with each other may be elusive. Incorporating standardized team training on a regular basis with all members of a department leads to more clearly defined expectations and greater consistency in care.

In an OR setting, team training has been shown to decrease patient mortality [82]. In the emergency department, team training can be applied to an array of multidisciplinary clinical scenarios. The high-intensity, low-frequency events such as mass casualty situations, pediatric arrest, emergent obstetrical delivery, and neonatal resuscitation all provide an opportunity to bring providers from several specialties and healthcare disciplines together for team training. Beyond the low-frequency events, using simulation to drill the more routine intradepartmental scenarios can improve team dynamics. ST-elevation myocardial infarction, stroke, respiratory distress, status asthmaticus, status epilepticus, and toxicologic emergencies are just some of the contexts within which such team training can take place.

Simulation can be used to develop and troubleshoot new protocols and systems that require a highly efficient team function. "Code STEMI," "Code Stroke," and sepsis response protocols, for instance, incorporate an array of moving parts, personnel, and equipment that must function seamlessly. A change in one or two variables may impact the delivery of essential interventions – door-to-balloon time, door-to-drug, or time-to-antibiotics. Rather than altering variables in the real clinical setting, changing them in a simulated setting can allow examination of their impact and help troubleshoot systems and provide an efficient, safe avenue to explore quality improvement. Team training is an essential part of quality healthcare delivery and patient safety, and simulation programs can clearly impact the many facets of healthcare team dynamics to optimize patient outcomes.

Procedural Training

The use of simulation to train practitioners to perform both routine and rare or high-risk procedures has gained traction among virtually every procedure-based specialty. This approach to training is founded not only on pragmatic considerations of patient safety but also on the concept of skill acquisition through deliberate practice [83–85]. Advanced surgical simulators have been developed for training in endoscopy and laparoscopy and have demonstrated a high degree of transfer of training to the clinical setting [86]. Likewise, obstetric simulators have been linked to improved technical proficiency, self-reported confidence and teamwork, and decreased incidence of complications such as shoulder dystocia [87].

Task trainers have become commercially available for a wide array of emergency department procedures. Products that offer a high degree of physical fidelity appear to be of greatest utility for procedures (e.g., intubation) that require complex motor movements and precise navigation of anatomic structures. Medical students trained on simulators can achieve proficiency with uncomplicated intubation in as little as 75–90 min [88], and clinicians trained on simulators perform equally well on fresh cadavers and live patients [89]. Procedures such as cricothyrotomy and chest tube placement are frequently taught with either commercially available products such as TraumaMan (Simulab Corp., Seattle, WA) or improvised synthetic or tissue-based task trainers. While these techniques are employed widely, the evidence for their efficacy in knowledge transfer to the clinical setting is limited. Additionally, there is sparse and conflicting data as to the comparative effectiveness of commercial task trainers versus tissue-based simulation for invasive procedure training [89, 90].

Psychological fidelity, or the degree to which a simulation incorporates the constituent elements of a targeted task, is of greater importance for skill acquisition than physical fidelity [91]. This is especially true for novice learners and for less complex tasks. Procedure training should emphasize the cognitive and motor elements involved in a given procedural skill and should seek a high degree of physical fidelity only for complex tasks or those performed by experienced users. While commercial task trainers have been designed for many diagnostic and resuscitative procedures encountered in the emergency department, some can be realistically simulated via the creative application of conventional materials. Task trainers for cricothyrotomy, venous cutdown, and chest tube placement, among others, can be performed using a combination of conventional medical equipment and either simulated or actual (animal or cadaver) tissue (Figs. 20.4 and 20.5). Given the high cost of many commercial task trainers, these creative solutions provide an appealing option for training in basic procedures. A number of procedure-based simulation curricula have been designed for healthcare providers at all levels of training. Those seeking curricula targeted towards a specific procedure (e.g., lumbar puncture) or learner group (e.g., medical students) often face the question of whether curricula already exist and have been used successfully by other institutions. While there is currently no comprehensive resource for simulation curricula, a number of useful resources do exist. MedEdPORTAL (www.mededportal.org), an online, peer-reviewed educational resource created by the AAMC, is widely used for the dissemination of simulation curricula. For emergency medicine-specific content, the Council of Emergency Medicine Residency Directors (CORD-EM), along with the Simulation Academy of the Society for Academic Emergency Medicine (SAEM), has created an online bank of peer-reviewed simulation cases which is discussed above. Both resources are available to simulation educators free of charge.

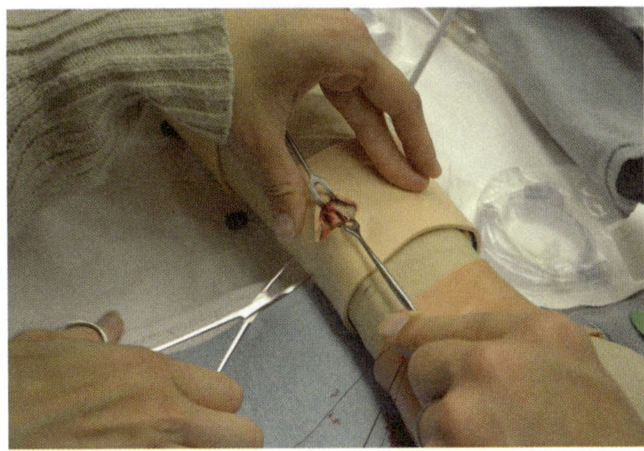

Fig. 20.4 Venous cutdown simulation

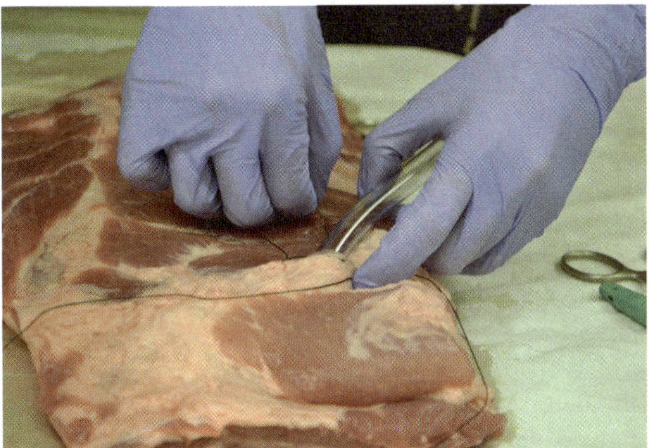

Fig. 20.5 Chest tube simulation

Integrated Simulation Curriculum

When selecting or designing a simulation curriculum, attention should be paid to the specific goals and objectives of the simulation experience, the training and experience level of the target audience, and the number of contact hours required to complete the curriculum. Table 20.2 demonstrates one sample of a curriculum which is designed as a 1-year introduction to core procedures for PGY I emergency medicine residents. The curriculum takes place over ten sessions of 2 h each, and each session includes reading material, a pretest, and hands-on practice in the simulation lab. The sessions are taught in small groups with only the PGY-1 residents present. The other residents participate in their own level-specific training during the same time.

Procedure training is a cornerstone of emergency medicine simulation, and those seeking to incorporate it into their training programs should not feel constrained by lack of funding or access to commercially available task trainers. Successful curricula for the vast majority of clinical procedures can be created by emphasizing the psychological fidelity of the experience to the procedure being taught,

Table 20.2 Sample procedure curriculum

Session number	Core procedures	Location
#1 – August	1. Regional blocks 2. Arterial line 3. Lumbar puncture	Simulation lab
#2 – September	1. CT interpretation 2. Central venous line placement 3. Ultrasound	Simulation lab
#3 – October	1. Slit lamp exam 2. Rust ring removal 3. Tono-pen use 4. Nasal packing 5. I+D of auricular hematoma 6. Foreign body removal	Simulation lab and in situ simulation in emergency department
#4 – November	1. Thoracentesis 2. Pericardiocentesis 3. Transvenous pacing	Simulation lab
#5 – December	1. Orthopedic reductions 2. Splinting 3. Extremity radiology	In situ simulation in emergency department
#6 – January	1. Fiber-optic laryngoscopy 2. Awake intubation 3. Difficult airways	Simulation lab and in situ simulation in emergency department
#7 – February	1. Communication skills lab 2. Ultrasound	Simulation lab
# 8 – March	1. Normal delivery 2. Complicated delivery 3. C-section 4. Third trimester bleeding	Simulation lab
#9 – April 18	1. Communication skills lab 2. Palliative care	Simulation lab
#10 – June	1. Leadership in critical care 2. Medical and trauma resuscitation	Simulation lab and in situ simulation in emergency department

having clearly defined goals and objectives for learners, and understanding the baseline experience level of trainees.

Conclusion

The use of simulation-based education and assessment is robust in emergency medicine for medical students and housestaff. It is a matter of time when faculty level education and assessment will catch up as simulation is engrained in the fabric of emergency medicine education, assessment and maintenace of certification, during the last decade emergency medicine has been at the forefront of simulation and is poised to be leaders of the field in the future.

References

1. Gordon JA, Oriol NE, Cooper JB. Bringing good teaching cases "to life": a simulator-based medical education service. Acad Med. 2004;79(1):23–7.
2. Abrahamson S, Denson JS, Wolf RM. Effectiveness of a simulator in training anesthesiology residents. J Med Educ. 1969;44(6):515–9.
3. Cooper JB, Taqueti VR. A brief history of the development of mannequin simulators for clinical education and training. Qual Saf Health Care. 2004;13 Suppl 1:i11.
4. Gaba DM, DeAnda A. A comprehensive anesthesia simulation environment: re-creating the operating room for research and training. Anesthesiology. 1988;69(3):387–94.
5. Ellis C, Hughes G. Use of human patient simulator to teach emergency medicine trainees advanced airway skills. J Acad Emerg Med. 1999;16(6):395–9.
6. Small SD, Wuerz RC, Simon R, Shapiro N, Conn A, Setnik G. Demonstration of high-fidelity team training for emergency medicine. Acad Emerg Med. 1999;6(4):312–23.
7. Reznek M, Smith-Coggins R, Howard S, et al. Emergency Medicine Crisis Resource Management (EMCRM): pilot study of a simulation-based crisis management course for emergency medicine. Acad Emerg Med. 2003;10(4):386–9.
8. Gordon JA, Wilkerson WM, Shaffer DW, Armstrong EG. "Practicing" medicine without risk: students' and educators' responses to high-fidelity patient simulation. Acad Med. 2001; 76(5):469–72.
9. Gordon JA, Pawlowski J. Education on-demand: the development of a simulator-based medical education service. Acad Med. 2002; 77(7):751–2.

10. Gordon J, Vozenilek J. 2008 Academic Emergency Medicine Consensus Conference – the science of simulation in healthcare: defining and developing clinical expertise. Acad Emerg Med. 2008;15: 971–7.
11. Chakravarthy B, Harr ET, Bhat SS, McCoy CE, Denmark TK, Lotfipour S. Simulation in medical school education: review for emergency medicine. West J Emerg Med. 2011;12(4):461–6.
12. Heitz C, Ten Eyck R, Smith M, Fitch M. Simulation in medical student education: survey of clerkship directors in emergency medicine. West J Emerg Med. 2011;12(4):455–60.
13. Mulcare MR, Suh EH, Tews M, Swan-Sein A, Pandit K. Third year medical student rotations in emergency medicine: a survey of current practices. Acad Emerg Med. 2011;18:S41–7.
14. Robak O, Kulnig J, Sterz F, et al. CPR in medical schools: learning by teaching BLS to sudden cardiac death survivors: a promising strategy for medical students? BMC Med Educ. 2006;6:27.
15. Weller J, Robinson B, Larsen P, et al. Simulation based training to improved acute care skills in medical undergraduates. N Z Med J. 2004;117:U1119.
16. Takayesu JK, Farrell SE, Evans AJ, et al. How do clinical clerkship students experience simulator-based teaching? A qualitative analysis. Simul Healthc. 2006;1:215–9.
17. Nguyen HB, Daniel-Underwood L, Van Ginkel C, et al. An educational course including medical simulation for early goal directed therapy and the severe sepsis resuscitation bundle: an evaluation for medical student training. Resuscitation. 2009;90:674–9.
18. Smolle J, Prause G, Smolle-Juttner FM. Emergency treatment of chest trauma: an e-learning simulation model for undergraduate medical students. Eur J Cardiothorac Surg. 2007;32:644–7.
19. Steadman RH, Coates WC, Huang YM, et al. Simulation based training is superior to problem based learning for the acquisition of critical assessment and management skills. Crit Care Med. 2006;34:151–7.
20. Ten Eyck RP, Tews M, Ballester JM. Improved medical student satisfaction and test performance with a simulation–based emergency medicine curriculum: a randomized controlled trial. Ann Emerg Med. 2009;54:684–91.
21. Frank-Law JM, Ingrassia PL, Ragazzoni L, et al. The effectiveness of training with an emergency department simulator on medical student performance in a simulated disaster. CJEM. 2010;12:27–32.
22. McCoy CE, Menchine M, Anderson C, et al. Prospective randomized crossover study of simulation versus didactics for teaching medical students the assessment and management of critically ill patients. J Emerg Med. 2000;40:448–55.
23. Schwartz LR, Fernandez R, Kouyoumjian SR, et al. A randomized comparison trial of case-based learning versus human patient simulation in medical student education. Acad Emerg Med. 2007;14: 130–7.
24. Gordan JA, Shaffer DW, Raemer DB, et al. A randomized controlled trial of simulation based teaching versus traditional instruction in medicine: a pilot study among clinical medical students. Adv Health Sci Educ Theory Pract. 2006;11:33–9.
25. Graber MA, Wyatt C, Kasparek L, et al. Does simulator training for medical students change patient opinions and attitudes toward medical student procedures in the emergency department? Acad Emerg Med. 2005;12:635–9.
26. Bond WF, Lammers RL, Spillane LL, et al. The use of simulation in emergency medicine: a research agenda. Acad Emerg Med. 2007;14:353–63.
27. Okuda Y, Bond W, Bonfante G, et al. National growth in simulation training within emergency medicine training programs, 2003–2008. Acad Emerg Med. 2008;15(11):1113–6.
28. McLaughlin S, Fitch MT, Goyal DG, Hayden E, Kauh CY, Laack TA, et al. Simulation in graduate medical education 2008: a review for emergency medicine. Acad Emerg Med. 2008;15(11):1117–29.
29. Binstadt ES, Walls RM, White BA, Nadel ES, Takayesu JK, Barker TD, et al. A comprehensive medical simulation education curriculum for emergency medicine residents. Ann Emerg Med. 2007; 49(4):495–504.
30. McLaughlin SA, Doezema D, Sklar DP. Human simulation in emergency medicine training: a model curriculum. Acad Emerg Med. 2002;9:1310–8.
31. Goyal DG, Cabrera DT, Laack TA, Luke A, Sadosty AT. Back to the bedside: a redesign of emergency medicine core curriculum content delivery. Poster presentation at ACGME Educational meeting in Orlando; 2007.
32. Wang EE, Beaumont J, Kharasch M, Vozenilek JA. Resident response to integration of simulation-based education into emergency medicine conference. Acad Emerg Med. 2008;15(11):1207–10.
33. Noeller TP, Smith MD, Holmes L, Cappaert M, Gross AJ, Cole-Kelly K, et al. A theme-based hybrid simulation model to train and evaluate emergency medicine residents. Acad Emerg Med. 2008;15(11):1199–206.
34. Vozenilek J, Wang E, Kharasch M, Anderson B, Kalaria A. Simulation-based morbidity and mortality conference: new technologies augmenting traditional case-based presentations. Acad Emerg Med. 2006;13:48–53.
35. Gordon JA, Tancredi D, Binder W, Wilkerson W, Shaffer DW, Cooper J. Assessing global performance in emergency medicine using a high-fidelity patient simulator: a pilot study. Acad Emerg Med. 2003;10(5):472.
36. Gisondi MA, Smith-Coggins R, Harter PM, Soltysik RC, Yarnold PR. Assessment of resident professionalism using high-fidelity simulation of ethical dilemmas. Acad Emerg Med. 2004;11(9): 931–7.
37. Girzadas Jr DV, Clay L, Caris J, Rzechula K, Harwood R. High fidelity simulation can discriminate between novice and experienced residents when assessing competency in patient care. Med Teach. 2007;29(5):472–6.
38. Gaba DM, Howard SK, Flanagan B, Smith BE, Fish KJ, Botney R. Assessment of clinical performance during simulated crises using both technical and behavioral ratings. Anesthesiology. 1998;89(1): 8–18.
39. Overly FL, Sudikoff SN, Shapiro MJ. High-fidelity medical simulation as an assessment tool for pediatric residents' airway management skills. Pediatr Emerg Care. 2007;23(1):11–5.
40. McLaughlin SA, Monahan C, Doezema D, Crandall C. Implementation and evaluation of a training program for the management of sexual assault in the emergency department. Ann Emerg Med. 2007;49(4):489–94.
41. Bond WF, Spillane L. The use of simulation for emergency medicine resident assessment. Acad Emerg Med. 2002;9(11):1295–9.
42. Wang EE, Vozenilek JA. Addressing the systems-based practice core competency: a simulation- based curriculum. Acad Emerg Med. 2005;12(12):1191–4.
43. Wagner MJ, Thomas Jr HA. Application of the medical knowledge general competency to emergency medicine. Acad Emerg Med. 2002;9(11):1236–41.
44. Kobayashi L, Shapiro MJ, Gutman DC, et al. Multiple encounter simulation for high-acuity multipatient environment training. Acad Emerg Med. 2007;14(12):1141–8.
45. Kim J, Neilipovitz D, Cardinal P, Chiu M, Clinch J. A pilot study using high-fidelity simulation to formally evaluate performance in the resuscitation of critically ill patients: the University of Ottawa CriticalCare Medicine, High-Fidelity Simulation, and Crisis Resource Management I Study. Crit Care Med. 2006;34(8):2167–74.
46. Adler MD, Trainor JL, Siddall VJ, McGaghie WC. Development and evaluation of high-fidelity simulation case scenarios for pediatric resident education. Ambul Pediatr. 2007;7(2):182–6.
47. Morgan PJ, Cleave-Hogg D, Guest CB. A comparison of global ratings and checklist scores from an undergraduate assessment using an anesthesia simulator. Acad Med. 2001;76(10):1053–5.
48. Schwid HA, Rooke GA, Carline J, Steadman RH, Murray WB, Olympio M, et al. Evaluation of anesthesia residents using

mannequin-based simulation: a multiinstitutional study. Anesthesiology. 2002;97(6):1434–44.
49. Boulet JR, De Champlain AF, McKinley DW. Setting defensible performance standards on OSCEs and standardized patient examinations. Med Teach. 2003;25(3):245–9.
50. Evidence Report/Technology Assessment Number 149. Effectiveness of continuing medical education prepared for: agency for healthcare research and quality U.S. Department of Health and Human Services.
51. Myers J, McGaghie WC, Siddall VJ, Mazmanian PE. Guidelines physicians evidence-based educational education: American College of Chest effectiveness of continuing medical and Graduate Medical Education: from simulation research in undergraduate lessons for continuing medical education. Chest. 2009;135: 62S–8.
52. Greiner AC, Knebel E, Institute of Medicine, editors. Health professions education: a bridge to quality. Washington: National Academies Press; 2003. p. 45.
53. Robertson B, Kaplan B, Atallah H, Higgins M, Lewitt MJ, Ander DS. The use of simulation and a modified TeamSTEPPS curriculum for medical and nursing student team training. Simul Healthc. 2010;5:332–7.
54. Robertson J, Bandali K. Bridging the gap: enhancing interprofessional education using simulation. J Interprof Care. 2008;22(5):499–508.
55. Hall R, Plant J, Bands C, Wall A, Kang J, Hall C. Human patient simulation is effective for teaching paramedic students endotracheal intubation. Acad Emerg Med. 2005;12:850–5.
56. Lammers R, Byrwa M, Fales W, Hale R. Simulation-based assessment of paramedic pediatric resuscitation skills. Prehosp Emerg Care. 2009;13(3):345–56.
57. Regener H. A proposal for student assessment in paramedic education. Med Teach. 2005;27(3):34–241.
58. Subbarao I, Bond W, Johnson C, Hsu E, Wasser T. Using innovative simulation modalities for civilian bases, chemical, biological, radiological, nuclear and explosive training in the acute management of terrorist victims: a pilot study. Prehosp Disaster Med. 2006; 21(4):272–5.
59. Bond W, Kostenbader M, McCarthy J. Prehospital and hospital based healthcare providers experience with a human patient simulator. Prehosp Emerg Care. 2001;5(3):284–7.
60. Wyatt A, Archer F, Fallows B. Use of simulators in teaching and learning: paramedics' evaluation of a patient simulator? J Emerg Prim Health Care. 2007;5(2):72–88.
61. Fernandez R, Wang E, Vozenilek JA, Hayden E, et al. Simulation center accreditation and programmatic benchmarks: a review for emergency medicine. Acad Emerg Med. 2010;17(10):1093–103.
62. Kobayashi L, Patterson M, Overly F, Shapiro M, et al. Educational and research implications of portable human patient simulation in acute care medicine. Acad Emerg Med. 2008;15:1166–74.
63. http://academiclifeinem.blogspot.com/2010/08/incorporating-debriefing-into-clinical.html. Accessed 9 Feb 2012.
64. http://www.wiser.pitt.edu/sites/wiser/ns08/day1_PP_JOD_DebriefingInSimEdu.pdf. Accessed 10 Feb 2012.
65. Rudolph JW, Simon R, Dufresne RL, Raemer D. There's no such thing as "nonjudgmental" debriefing: a theory and method for debriefing with good judgment. Simul Healthc. 2006;1(1):49–55.
66. Kurrek MM, Devitt JH. The cost for construction and operation of a simulation centre. Can J Anaesth. 1997;44:1191–5.
67. The Joint Commission National Patient Safety Goals. http://www.jointcommission.org/standards_information/npsgs.aspx. Accessed 9 Feb 2012.
68. American Nurses Credentialing Center: Magnet recognition program. http://www.nursecredentialing.org/Magnet.aspx. Accessed 9 Feb 2012.
69. ACGME Outcomes Project. Accreditation Council for Graduate Medical Education. http://www.acgme.org/acWebsite/navPages/nav_110.asp. Accessed 9 Feb 2012.
70. Hanscom R. Medical simulation from an Insurer's perspective. Acad Emerg Med. 2008;15:984–7.
71. Maintenace of Certification Events. http://www.asahq.org/For-Members/Education-and-Events/Simulation-Education.aspx. Accessed 9 Feb 2012.
72. Issenberg SB, McGaghie WC, Petrusa ER, Lee Gordon D, Scalese RJ. Features and uses of high-fidelity medical simulations that lead to effective learning: a BEME systematic review. Med Teach. 2005;27(1):10–28.
73. McLaughlin SA, Bond W, Promes S, Spillane L. The status of human simulation training in emergency medicine residency programs. Simul Healthc. 2006;1:18–21.
74. Bransford JD, Brown AL, Cocking RR, editors. How people learn: brain, mind, experience, and school: expanded edition. Washington: DC; National Academy Press; 2000. http://en.wikipedia.org/wiki/National_Academy_Press.
75. Mager RF. Preparing instructional objectives. 2nd ed. Belmont: David S. Lake; 1984.
76. Fink LD. Creating significant learning experiences: an integrated approach to designing college courses. San Francisco: Wiley; 2003.
77. The Joint Commission. Sentinel event data – root causes by event type. http://www.jointcommission.org/sentinel_event.aspx. Accessed 9 Feb 2012.
78. Seamster TL, Boehm-Davis DA, Holt RW, Schultz K. Developing advance crew resource management (ACRM) Training: a training manual. Federal Aviation Administration, Office of the Chief Scientific and Technical Advisor for Human Factors. 1998. Available at www.hf.faa.gov/docs/dacrmt.pdf.
79. Team STEPPS Training Program. http://teamstepps.ahrq.gov/. Accessed 9 Feb 2012.
80. Anderson JM, LeFlore J, Cheng A, et al. Validation of a behavioral scoring tool for simulated pediatric resuscitation: a report from the EXPRESS pediatric research collaborative. Simul Healthc. 2009;4(4):A131.
81. Cook DA, Hatala R, Brydges R, et al. Technology-enhanced simulation for health professions education – a systematic review and meta-analysis. JAMA. 2011;306(9):978–88.
82. Neily J, Mills PD, Young-Xu Y, Carney BT, West P, Berger DH, et al. Association between implementation of a medical team training program and surgical mortality. JAMA. 2010;304(15):1693–700.
83. Maran NJ, Glavin RJ. Low- to high-fidelity simulation- a continuum of medical education? Med Educ. 2003;37(S1):22–8.
84. Ericsson KA. Deliberate practice and acquisition of expert performance: a general overview. Acad Emerg Med. 2008;15:988–94.
85. Hochmitz I, Yuviler-Gavish N. Physical fidelity versus cognitive fidelity training in procedural skills acquisition. Hum Factors. 2011;53:489–501.
86. Van Sickle K, Ritter E, McClusky III D, Baghai L, et al. Attempted establishment of proficiency levels for laparoscopic performance on a national scale using simulation: the results from the 2004 SAGES minimally invasive surgical trainer – virtual reality (MIST-VR) learning center study. Surg Endosc. 2007;21:5–10.
87. Okuda Y, Bryson E, DeMaria S, Jacobson L, et al. The utility of simulation in medical education: what is the evidence? Mt Sinai J Med. 2009;76:330–43.
88. Owen H, Plummer JL. Improving learning of a clinical skill: the first year's experience of teaching endotracheal intubation in a clinical simulation facility. Med Educ. 2002;36:635–42.
89. Wang E, Quinones J, Fitch M, Dooley-Hash S, et al. Developing technical expertise in emergency medicine – the role of simulation in procedural skill acquisition. Acad Emerg Med. 2008;15(11): 1046–57.
90. Hall AB. Randomized comparison of live tissue training versus simulators for emergency procedures. Am Surg. 2011;77(5):561–5.
91. Fernandez R, Vozenilek J, Hegarty C, Motola I, et al. Developing expert medical teams: toward an evidence-based approach. Acad Emerg Med. 2008;15(11):1025–36.

Simulation in Dentistry and Oral Health

21

Riki Gottlieb, J. Marjoke Vervoorn, and Judith Buchanan

Introduction

Simulation has been a great asset to many fields, perhaps most notably aviation. Defining simulation as any artificial item or method that mimics in some way a body part or a Real Life situation, the field of dentistry has employed simulation almost since the inception of the first dental college, which was chartered in 1840 [1]. Since these early times, simulation in dental education has progressed from the use of oversized models of teeth, to simulated patients, high-fidelity virtual reality [2], haptics [3–7], and most recently robotics [8].

Importance of Simulation to Dental Education

Although a variety of medical specialties, such as surgery, involve substantial expertise in technical or psychomotor skills, virtually all fields of dentistry are very reliant on the ability of the dentist to have well-developed surgical and psychomotor skills. Much of what a dentist does involves the use of instruments, like high-speed dental drills (handpiece), that have the capacity to cut through and potentially harm any tissue in contact with the device. In addition, these instruments are used in environments that present access challenges, offer less than optimal light, are mobile, and are often obscured by blood and saliva. Skill and confidence using these instruments are paramount for the protection of the patient.

Due to the nature of the practice, the reliance on simulation for dental education is quite mature and may actually exceed other healthcare specialties, to the surprise of many. Dental students must achieve an acceptable level of competence prior to actual patient care since most procedures on teeth are irreversible, and learning these skills solely on patients is not an acceptable practice. Other dental procedures such as endodontics (root canal therapy) [9], oral surgery [10, 11], and periodontal surgery are likewise irreversible, and patient harm can occur if procedures are not performed by students with acceptable levels of skills. Although some dental techniques such as suturing [12], impressions, or calculus removal can be learned on patients, for optimal patient care, a certain level of skill should be obtained in almost all clinical procedures prior to the start of patient care. Hence, most psychomotor skills are first learned in a simulated manner before students progress to direct patient care. Simulation is essential since it allows procedures to be repeated many times thus assuring the student demonstrates a consistent, acceptable level of skill and procedural competence.

Patient Simulation

Mannequins

Mannequins are a relatively new addition to the armamentarium for teaching dental skills, but are now commonly found in most dental schools. In order to simulate a patient, mannequins of the head which include the simulated

R. Gottlieb, DMD, FAGD (✉)
Virtual Reality Simulation Laboratory,
International Dentist Program,
Virginia Commonwealth University School of Dentistry,
520 N 12th St, Richmond, VA, USA

Department of General Practice, Admissions,
Virginia Commonwealth University School of Dentistry,
520 N 12th St, Richmond, VA, USA
e-mail: rgottlieb@vcu.edu

J.M. Vervoorn, PhD, DDS
Educational Institute, Academic Centre
for Dentistry Amsterdam (ACTA),
Gustav Mahlerlaan 3004, 1081 LA, Amsterdam,
The Netherlands
e-mail: j.vervoorn@acta.nl

J. Buchanan, MS, PhD, DMD
School of Dentistry, University of Minnesota,
15-209 Moos Tower, 515 Delaware St. SE,
Minneapolis, MN, 55455, USA
e-mail: buchanan@umn.edu

A.I. Levine et al. (eds.), *The Comprehensive Textbook of Healthcare Simulation*,
DOI 10.1007/978-1-4614-5993-4_21, © Springer Science+Business Media New York 2013

masticatory system, sometimes including the upper torso (Figs. 21.1 and 21.2), can be used in conjunction with simulated arches containing plastic teeth (dentoforms) [13, 14]. Students can perform dental procedures in the simulated mouth and the presence of the head and torso adds to the reality of the simulation and is very helpful in developing good ergonomic skills. Simulation labs of this type are becoming quite popular in preclinical education in the USA and are often coupled with other technology such as computers. It is unclear, however, if the use of this type of simulation laboratory improves student learning or prepares students better for direct patient care [15, 16].

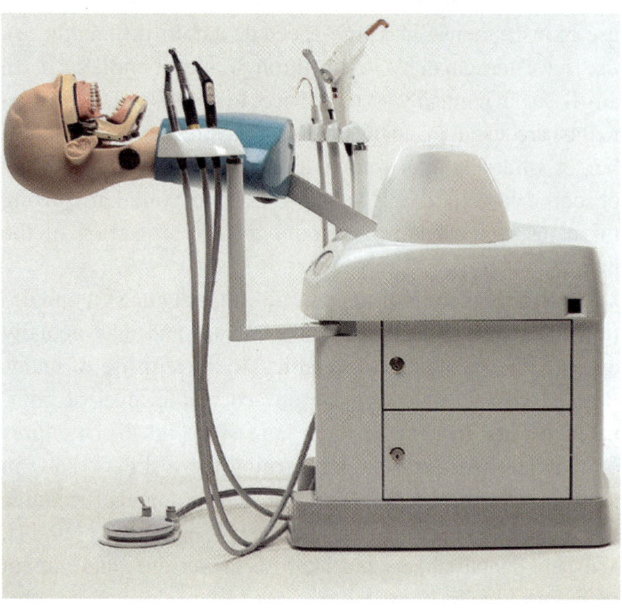

Fig. 21.1 Simulated head with torso (Used with permission from the KaVo Group)

Standardized Patients

Standardized patients [17] (see Chap. 13) have been used in medical education since the early 1960's and were first reported in dental education in 1990 [18]. Standardized patients are very helpful in developing appropriate communication and interpersonal skills for dental students, eliciting a thorough medical and dental history, completing a head and neck exam, and completing accurate and appropriate record keeping. Unfortunately, standardized patients are not available at many health science centers and if available, may be cost prohibitive for many dental schools.

Web-Based and Computer-Based Simulation

Case-Based Simulations

Computers can be extremely helpful in simulating patients or presenting case scenarios [19–22]. In case-based computer programs, students are presented a narrative that represents a patient encounter. The students can interact with the program that provides responses to a variety of interventions including answers to a series of questions relating to medical history, diagnostic test results, orders, possible diagnoses, and the development of appropriate treatment plans. These programs are becoming more and more interactive, allowing for more pertinent feedback to the student.

Simulation-Based Assessment

Since the early 1990s, computer simulations have been considered for dental licensure examinations or other evaluations and testing applications; however, when used for these

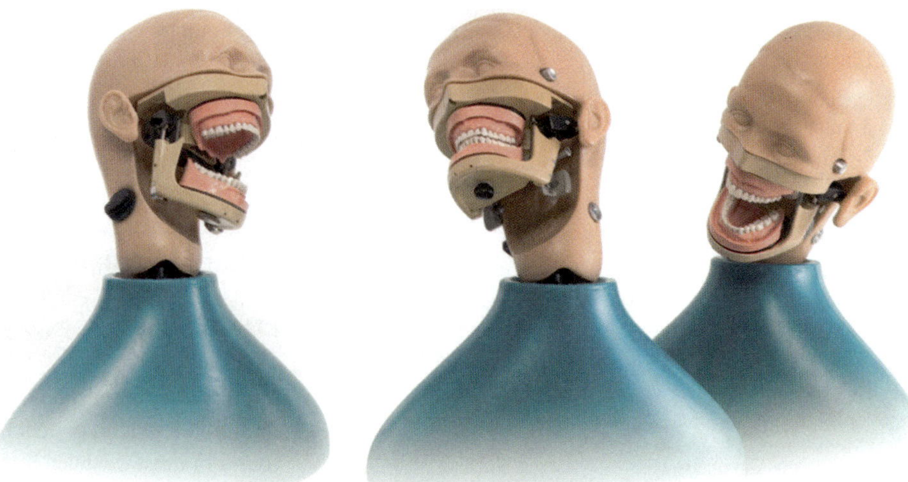

Fig. 21.2 Simulated head and torso with masticatory system (Used with permission from the KaVo Group)

purposes, reliability and validity are of utmost concern [23]. The goal when using simulation for education is to achieve performance improvement, whereas simulation for dental licensure examinations is used to ensure that the provider has reached competency. This requires that simulation for these high-stakes assessments must meet a higher standard in reliability and criterion validity. The advantages, however, of using simulation for dental examinations, assuming the level of reliability and validity is sufficient, are compelling. Simulation may have a greater potential validity, is safer in comparison to using live patients, and may be less expensive and easier. Some schools use simulation to assess students during their education, but advanced simulation is not currently used in any clinical examination for state licensure. As simulations in dentistry become more and more advanced, their use in dental licensure examinations will receive more consideration.

Computer Imaging

Recent advances in computer imaging have allowed for the production of very accurate 3D dental models of the oral apparatus by destructive scanning, laser scanning, or direct imaging of teeth [24–27]. Also imaging systems have been used to capture 3D images of mandibular motion [25]. The technology of computer imaging is important in the educational component of dentistry since it can dictate the relation to reality. Computer imaging is instrumental in simulations using virtual reality and/or haptics. Accurate and detailed imaging is critical because dental procedures require measurements in the tenths of millimeters; hence, virtual images must have very high resolution to order to evaluate such precise detail.

Virtual Reality-Based Technology (VRBT)

DentSim System

Mannequin-based simulation has become the standard of preclinical teaching in dental schools as described at the beginning of this chapter. Over a decade ago, a computerized dental simulator was developed by DenX Ltd. (presently owned by Image Navigation Ltd., Fig. 21.3). This new virtual reality simulator allows students to receive immediate, three-dimensional, audio, and written feedback of their work on artificial teeth (such as cavity, crown, and endodontic access preparations) and to review their work on video. This computerized simulator can be installed on an existing traditional mannequin, with the addition of a computer, camera, a special handpiece (dental drill), and a reference body that functions as the tracking device [2].

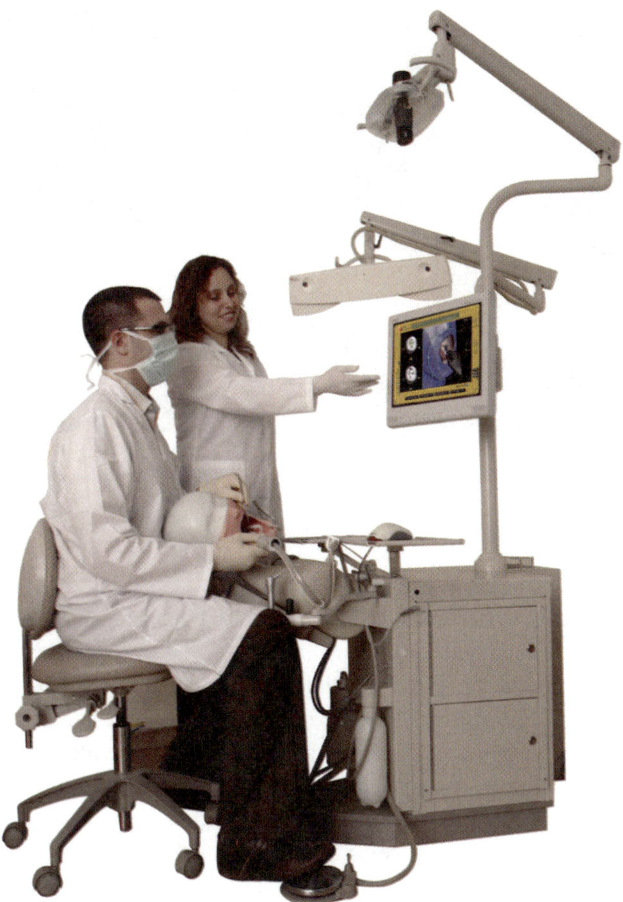

Fig. 21.3 Virtual reality-based simulator (DentSim™, Image Navigation Ltd. Used with permission)

The DentSim tracking system technology is based on the principles of GPS (global positioning system) technology. The optical system uses a camera to track a set of light-emitting diodes (LED), located on the dental handpiece and on the simulator's jaw. The LEDs send infrared signals that are picked up by the camera which is located above the workstation. The handpiece LEDs provide data indicating the motions of the user, while the LEDs attached to the jaw provide data regarding the location of the teeth. Once the camera has picked up the signals, the exact location of the tip of the bur (dental drill bit) in relation to the tooth may be calculated. This information is transferred to the computer and displayed through virtual simulation and as a color-coded, three-dimensional, tooth image.

Using the virtual reality simulator, the student's work is recorded and compared to an ideal preparation that is predesigned or selected by the course director from the software database. The students can view an accurate image of the ideal preparation, the student's preparation, and the exact measurements of each preparation in every dimension.

Several studies have been conducted to test the validity of the DentSim system. This is the only technology of its kind that has

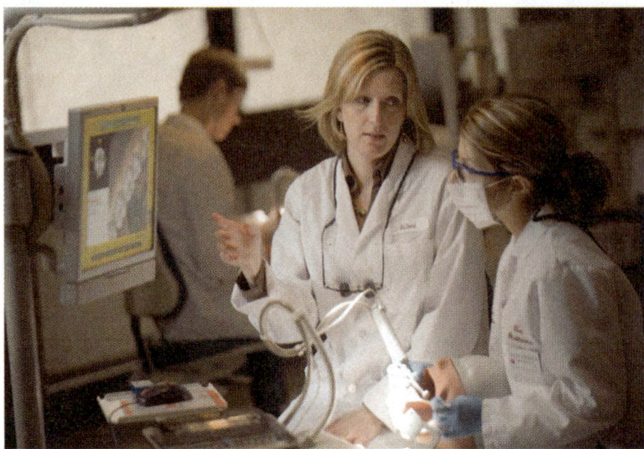

Fig. 21.4 Advanced Simulation Clinic, University of Minnesota, School of Dentistry

been evaluated in the scientific literature. One study demonstrated that when trained with the virtual reality simulator, starting at a minimum of 6 h dental, students learn faster than their peers in the traditional preclinical course, arrive at the same level of performance as expected of students trained in a traditional manner, accomplish more practice procedures per hour, and request more evaluations per procedure or per hour than in the traditional preclinical laboratories [28]. Another study suggested that virtual reality technology has the potential to provide an efficient and more self-directed approach for learning clinical psychomotor skills. That study showed that students using only traditional instruction received five times more instructional time from faculty than did students who used the virtual reality simulation system. There were no statistical differences in the quality of the preparations [29]. Several studies have shown an improvement in course performance through higher examination and course scores [30–32] as well as a decrease in overall course failure rate and elimination of student remediation by more than 50% [31, 32]. In addition, studies have shown the advantage of dental students using virtual reality simulators to learn psychomotor skills, as well as examined faculty members' evaluation and expectations of employing this relatively new technology [33]. Results for other studies support the use of VRS in a preclinical dental curriculum. This virtual reality-based technology is currently being used in several dental schools around the world (Fig. 21.4). This system has many capabilities which allow specific adaptation and curricular integration based on the individual school's requirements.

EPED System

EPED stands for efficiency, professionalism, education, and dependability. EPED's main product is the Computerized Dental Simulator (CDS-100), which combines a simulation system, an evaluation system, and 3D virtual reality technology [34]. CDS-100 system is based on exactly the same approach as the DentSim and comprised of a dental handpiece for drilling a cavity in a plastic tooth; a three-dimensional sensor with six degrees of freedom attached to the dental handpiece, which provides the system with the position and orientation of the handpiece; and a data processing and display unit for displaying the procedure [34, 35] (Fig. 21.5). There is no scientific evidence of its use at this time; however, it is expected to have similar educational benefits as the DentSim system.

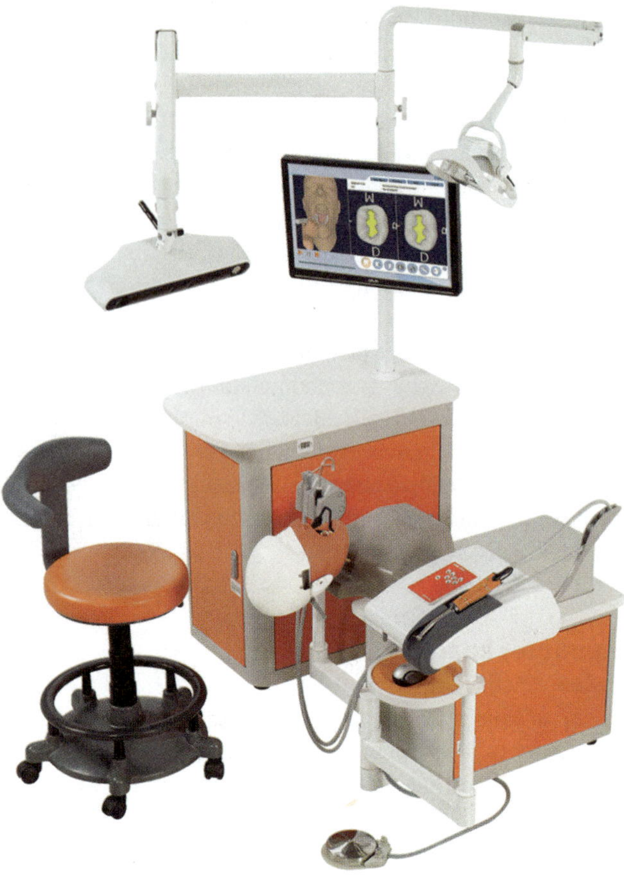

Fig. 21.5 CDS 100 virtual reality simulator by EPED (Imaged used with permission)

Second Life

Dental education has been assessing the value of distance education and the steps required to deliver technology-based learning while providing high-quality patient care teaching methods for dental and dental hygiene students. *Second Life* (SL) is a three-dimensional technology that provides simulation-based virtual settings. Activities in SL provide a way to combine new simulation technologies with role-plays to enhance instruction in diagnosis and treatment planning. Case studies and role-plays have been used as effective evaluation mechanisms to foster decision-making and problem-solving

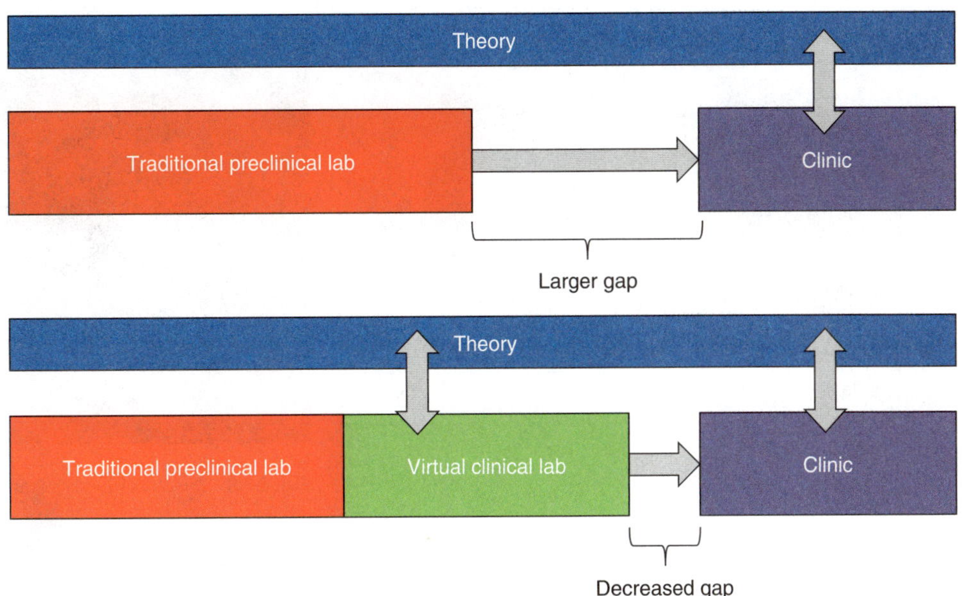

Fig. 21.6 The virtual clinical lab integrates theory and decreased the gap to the clinic

strategies in the delivery of patient care. It is a newly emerging technology and its benefits are yet to be reported in the scientific literature [36].

Technology with Haptic Focus

The growth of computer hardware and software has led to the development of virtual worlds that support the field of advanced simulation. Virtual reality (VR) creates virtual worlds using mathematical models and computer programs, allowing users to move in the created virtual world in a way similar to real life. Adding haptic technology to the VR world provides users with the ability to interact with virtual objects within the virtual environment via feel and touch. A dental training system using a haptic interface requires haptic rendering to generate force feedback and drilling simulation for the material cutting behavior from the virtual tooth model.

Haptic dental trainers enable students to learn and practice in a safe and almost real environment. Whereas traditional simulation laboratories restrict skill development to practicing on unrealistic plastic teeth, a virtual simulation lab offers the opportunity to let students learn in a realistic, pathology-oriented basis. A large variety of realistic clinical problems can be simulated in the virtual environment to assure the acquisition of the essential competencies to manage a multitude of pathologies. Problem solving, treatment planning, as well as performing treatment can also be learned in this environment before the students encounter actual patients in the dental clinics. Introduction of a virtual clinical lab decreases the gap between the traditional preclinical curriculum and the clinics (Fig. 21.6) by adding more realistic scenarios in the preclinical training environment. The realistic scenarios embed integration of the theory in the preclinical phase and stimulate further theoretical inquiry as a result of virtual clinical experiences.

In the virtual clinical lab, students can encounter and provide treatment to a variety of simulated patients with dental pathology. Although the use of actual extracted teeth in the preclinical simulation lab may add some reality and pathology, it is impossible to offer students similar cases and scenarios without virtual capabilities. Besides, it becomes clear that current restrictions on the use of extracted teeth as well as their limited availability in some regions make their use more difficult. Because of this shortage of suitable extracted teeth, it is hard for students to train and assess all skills taught in the preclinics.

Another advantage of the virtual clinical lab is the ability to combine the standardization of exercises, as the students would experience in the present preclinical environment, with the realistic scenarios as encountered in the clinic. This ability provides an excellent environment for competency development. Other VR-related advantages include the ability to assess complete processes instead of the end result, while allowing students the opportunity to practice exercises without limits and without the need to use exhaustible materials like drills and plastic teeth (Fig. 21.7).

The virtual lab also has some limitations. Not all procedures are equally suitable for training in a virtual clinical lab. For instance, applying filling material, matrix band, and wedge procedures might be hard to train virtually. Also feeling and handling of teeth in virtual reality is not as rich and versatile as it is in the real world. The virtual clinical lab

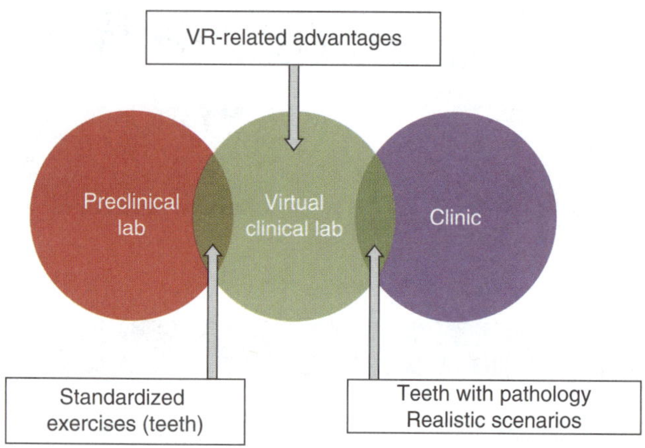

Fig. 21.7 The virtual clinical lab features advantages of both the preclinical lab and the clinic

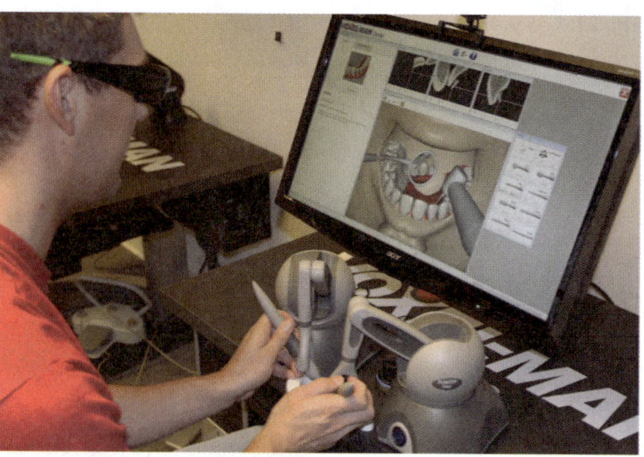

Fig. 21.8 The VOXEL-MAN tabletop system

should be considered an adjunct to the learning potential of the existing preclinical lab, not a replacement. Combining them provides the opportunity to use the best of both worlds in preparing for the clinics.

Recently, VR simulators using haptic feedback have been introduced into the dental curriculum as training devices for manual dexterity acquisition in tooth probing and preparation tasks. Various systems have been developed of which a few are on the market or entering the market [37–40].

PerioSim is an example of a haptic technology system that uses a periodontal probe [37]. It was developed at the University of Illinois at Chicago through joint efforts of the College of Dentistry and the College of Engineering. The system consists of a high-end computer workstation, a haptic device, and a stereoscopic computer monitor with stereo glasses. It was developed for training and evaluation of performance by students in periodontal probing and detecting the feel of a caries-active white spot lesion.

A realistic 3D human mouth is shown in real time, and the user can adjust the model position, viewpoint, and transparency level. The haptic device allows the student to feel the sensations in the virtual mouth. The instrument pressure (in grams of force being applied to the gingival area) can be viewed and recorded. A control panel is available for fine control of a variety of parameters such as instrument and model selection, degree of model transparency, navigation, haptic fidelity of tissues, and tremor modulation.

The system allows instructors to create short scenarios of periodontal procedures, which can be saved and replayed at any time. The 3D component permits students to replay the procedure from any angle. This allows the user a unique advantage to observe different views of the placement of the instrument and gingival relationships during a given procedure. It appears that the PerioSim is considered as highly realistic with proper feedback for teeth and instrument [41].

VOXEL-MAN Dental [38] was developed by the VOXEL-MAN group within the University Medical Center Hamburg-Eppendorf. The VOXEL-MAN Dental (Figs. 21.8 and 21.9) is a compact unit that comes in a variety of configurations including a tabletop system, a stand-alone system, or attached to a conventional dental training unit. With this device teeth and instruments are computer generated via high-resolution modeling displayed on a 3D screen. The high-resolution tooth models were derived from real teeth by microtomography. The dental handpiece can be moved in three dimensions and is represented by a force feedback device. This interface provides a very lifelike and convincing sense of touch. Impressively the differences in feel between enamel, dentin, pulp, and carious tissue have been faithfully reproduced.

Instruments available with this system include a selection of foot pedal-controlled high- and low-speed burs of different shapes. The dental mirror function permits the inspection of the virtual teeth from all sides using multiple magnifications. A unique cross-sectional view is also available.

The hapTEL [39] is a 4-year collaborative project involving Kings College London, University of London, and the University of Reading. The overall aim of the hapTEL™ project was to design, develop, and evaluate a virtual learning system that includes haptic and synthetic devices.

The hapTEL virtual system was intended to be used initially in dentistry with the design focused on enhancing learners' 3D perceptions, manipulations, and skills and to relate these to concepts needed in preparing 3D virtual tooth cavities. In 2011 the "curriculum beta version" of the haptic mouth was launched. The system allows dental students to practice drilling teeth in a 3D touch-sensitive simulation. Students perform virtual operations on a three-dimensional reconstruction of the anatomy of teeth and jaw. The cutting of different tooth tissues can be felt as a result of the tactile feedback provided through a real dental drill attached to a modified gaming device.

The MOOG Simodont Dental Trainer [40] (Fig. 21.10) was developed in cooperation between MOOG Nieuw-Vennep, the Netherlands and the Academic Centre for Dentistry Amsterdam (ACTA), the Netherlands. The haptics of the Simodont Dental

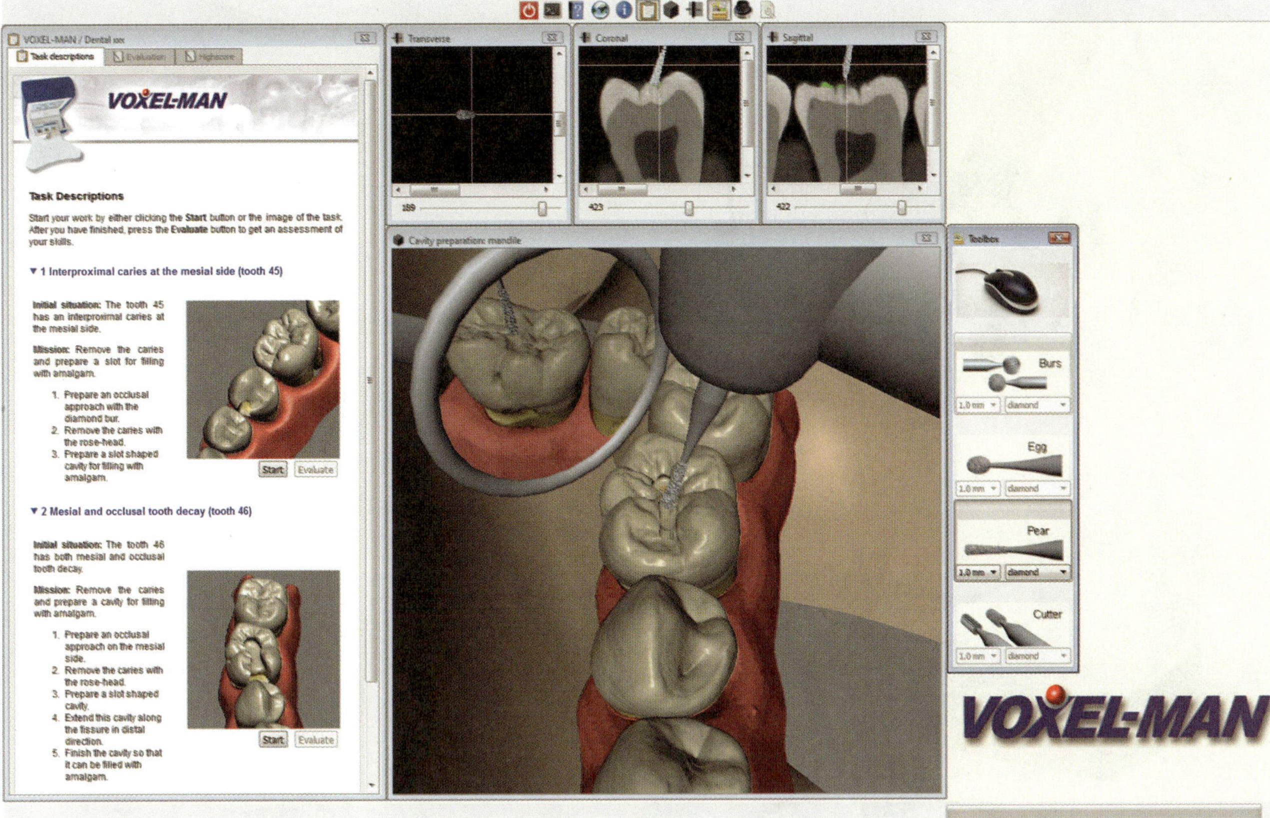

Fig. 21.9 Screen shot of the VOXEL-MAN system. (Used with permission from Springer)

Trainer are based on the MOOG-patented admittance control paradigm of the HapticMaster [40]. The dental tool has six degrees of freedom positional sensing, generating three degrees of freedom force feedback. Collision detection and tooth cutting simulation are running along with the haptic loop in such a way that it allows computing realistic force feedback and simulating tooth cutting within 1 ms. A high-resolution stereo, true-size colocated visual display approaches the acuity limits of the human eye. Three-dimensional projection and mirror technology allow the full-resolution, full stereo image to be seen "in" the physical workspace of the handpiece. A realistic model of the behavior of the drill speed, under the control of a foot pedal and the force exerted by the operator on the handpiece, drives a built-in sound module which faithfully renders the sound of a dental drill. 3D glasses provides stereo imaging.

The Simodont Dental Trainer allows dental students to be trained in operative dental procedures in a dedicated immersive virtual reality environment while receiving haptic, visual, and audio sensory information. By incorporating pathological dental conditions within the system, it offers the opportunity to train from a problem-based perspective. The operation of the Simodont is accompanied by courseware, providing the educational context of the training [42]. Prior to the introduction of the Simodont in dental education, a pilot study has been carried out to investigate whether skills developed on the Simodont are transferred to the present simulation phantom head lab. It appeared that students that had practiced either on the Simodont or on plastic material performed equally well during a standard test on plastic teeth [43]. This indicated that skills learned on the Simodont were transferred to real practice. The first lab of six Simodont units was installed at ACTA in 2009. Now in 2012, approximately 100 Simodont units worldwide are being installed in various dental schools.

Some studies and reports suggest the possible application and promising opportunities of haptic systems in dental education [44–46].

Robotics

Parallel to the development of more realistic teeth and tools in virtual reality, a development exists focused on more realistic mannequins. These mannequins are able to simulate jaw movements and verbal expression of emotions like pain while participants work in the device's mouth. Instructors can direct the expressions and movements of the mannequin by remote control to teach the students to anticipate patient's behavior while working [8].

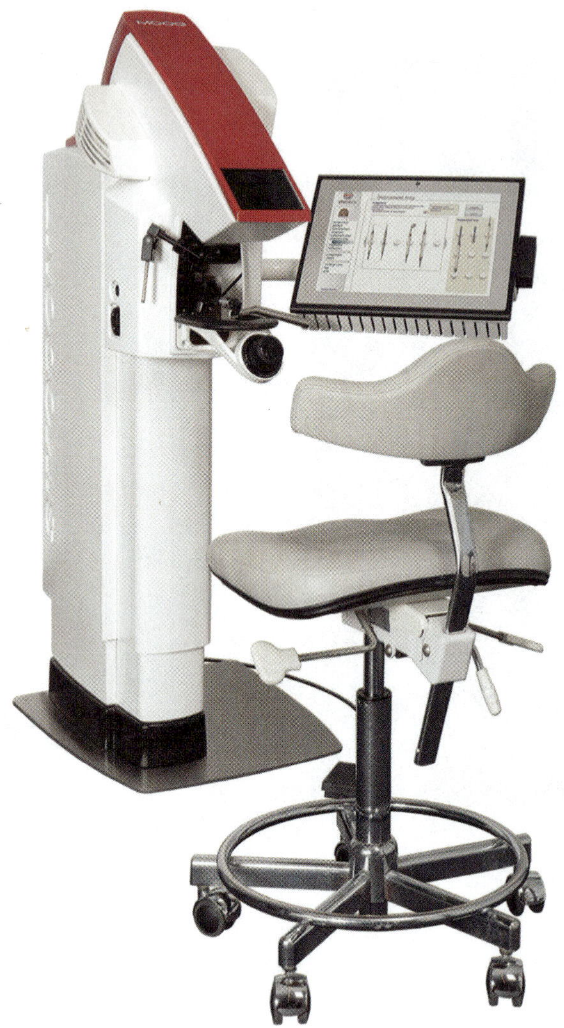

Fig. 21.10 MOOG Simodont Dental Trainer (Image Navigation Ltd. Used with permission)

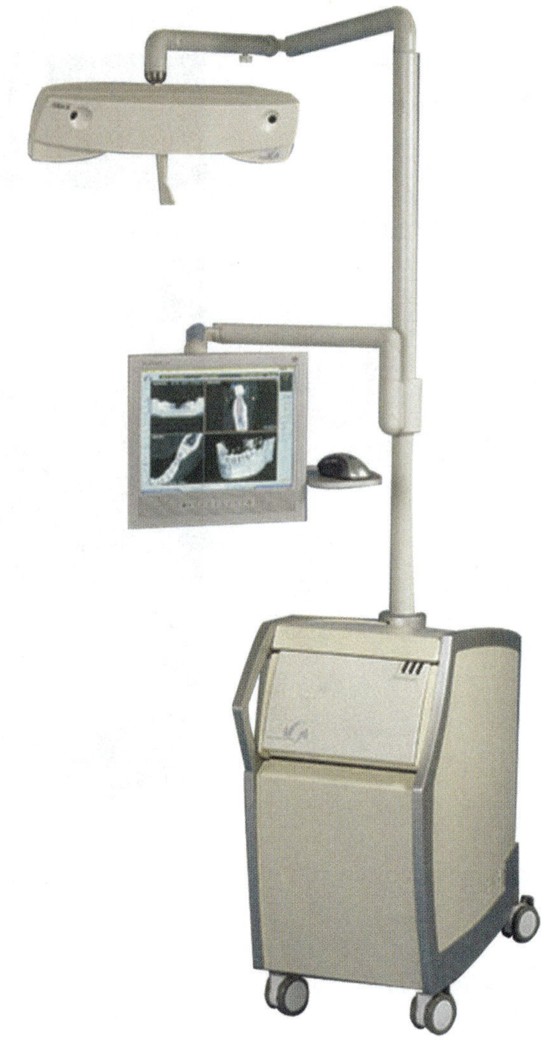

Fig. 21.11 Image-guided implantology unit (IGI, Image Navigation Ltd. Used with permission)

Game-Based Simulation

Game-based simulation is being used in medical education with increased frequency [47, 48]. In 2009, a leading developer of game-based technology (Breakaway) partnered with a university to develop a game-based dental implant training simulation. It is anticipated that games of this nature will be engaging and help students learn in a highly immersive, virtual, and three-dimensional environment [48]. The objective of this partnership is to improve dental student learning outcomes in the area of diagnostics, decision-making, and treatment protocols for enhanced patient therapy outcomes and risk management.

Advanced Navigational Simulation (Global Positioning-Type Systems)

Computerized navigation surgery is a surgical modality in which the surgical instruments are accurately tracked and targeted to a preplanned location within the surgical field. This technology is based on the synchronization of the intraoperative position of the instruments with the imaging of the patient's anatomy previously obtained by computed tomography (CT) or magnetic resonance imaging (MRI). Originally implemented in neurosurgery, this technology has subsequently been introduced into other surgical disciplines where it enables intraoperative localization and augments the surgeon's orientation within the surgical field [49].

In dentistry, there is only one computerized navigation system based on the description above, named image-guided implantology (IGI) system (Fig. 21.11) [50]. The IGI is an optical-based computerized navigation system that uses an infrared camera to detect and track the intraoperative position of a contra-angled dental surgical handpiece. The handpiece (dental drill) is equipped with a distinctive array of light-emitting diodes (LEDs) that signal its real-time position to the camera. The fiducial markers are 3-mm ceramic spheres that are embedded within a plastic U-shaped

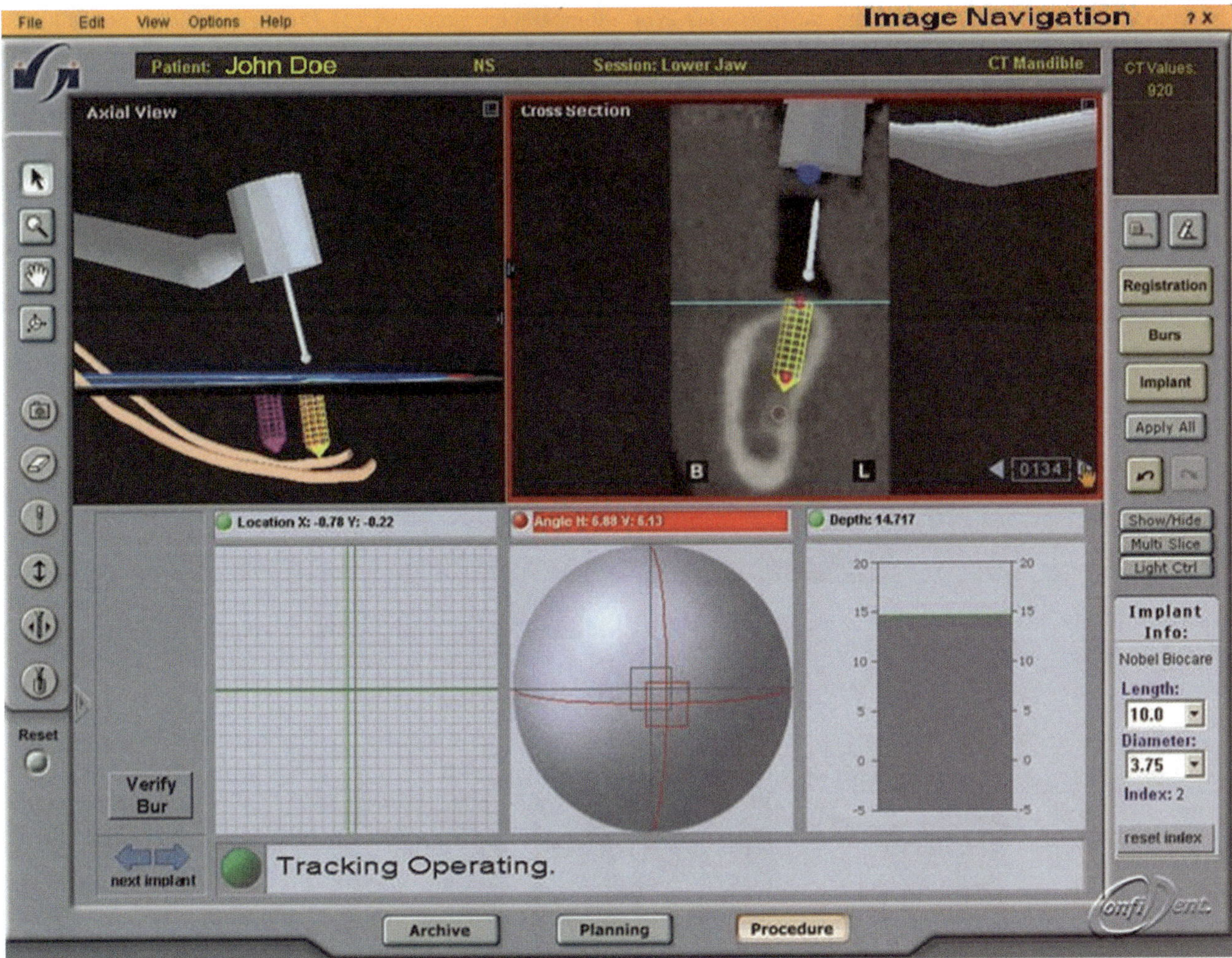

Fig. 21.12 Residents in the VCU Department of Periodontics placing implants with the help of IGI technology

registration mold. This mold is attached to a tooth-supported removable acrylic occlusal template that allows the mounting of the registration mold intraorally on the operated jaw. At the beginning of surgery, the dental handpiece is used as a probe for registration of the fiducial markers, the position of which is subsequently used for the synchronization of the jaw's position with the three-dimensional reconstructed CT model. Intraoperative movements of the operated jaw that occur after the coregistration are accurately compensated for by a special reference sensor frame that mounts on the jaw via the above-mentioned removable occlusal template. Therefore, the jaw can be allowed to move during the surgery, while its synchronization with the CT model is maintained [50–52].

IGI is a computerized navigation system designed to guide the placement of dental implants in real time (Figs. 21.12 and 21.13). IGI offers freehand implant navigation, highly accurate motion tracking technology that tracks the positions of the dental drill and the patient throughout the surgery [50–52].

IGI has been used in private dental offices, as well as by highly experienced dental professionals for complex restorative cases. One study evaluated the benefits of the system in a predoctoral educational system, for teaching basic concepts of implant placement. There was no clear advantage over traditional teaching methods [51]. According to recent publications, the IGI system has an advantage in clinical cases involving immediate restoration of multiple implants, flapless surgery, and treatment of completely edentulous patients and patients with complex anatomical features or tumors requiring removal of hard and soft tissues [52–56].

This computerized navigation system is different from other existing image-guided implantology systems, referred to as computer-driven implantology systems. The computer-driven implantology systems provide a means with which to control the placement of implants with a high degree of accuracy, without real-time computer tracking of implant placement. In computer-driven implant dentistry, a scan template is a radiologic template that permits visualization of the prosthetic plan prior to treatment and determines the course of implant treatment from the perspective of esthetics [57]. For example, the SimPlant software program (Materialise) [58] allows implants to be planned in two and three dimensions using data received from a computerized tomographic scan (Fig. 21.14). The resulting implant plan can be transferred to the mouth and implemented by means of a stereolithographic surgical guide. Another data transfer system is then used for guided implant placement. It is associated with dedicated drilling devices and can be used in combination with surgical guides (plastic and metal devices fabricated by a CAD/CAM system or with traditional acrylic resin guides manufactured by the dental lab on a synthetic plaster cast [58]).

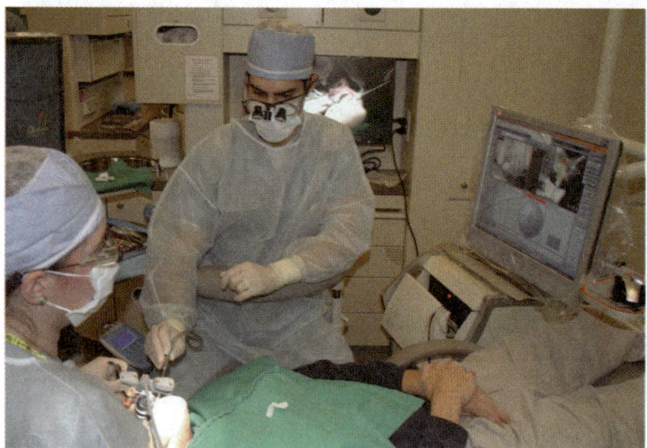

Fig. 21.13 IGI clinical screen view showing real-time drilling using patient's CT scan

Resources Needed for Simulation

Further development of advanced simulation in dentistry is somewhat hampered by the specialized use of this type of simulation. Although the need is great in the area of dental education, the technology currently available cannot be easily used in medicine, nursing, pharmacy, etc. The cost of the technology for this type of simulation is high and the number of dental schools worldwide is limited. Hence, simulation

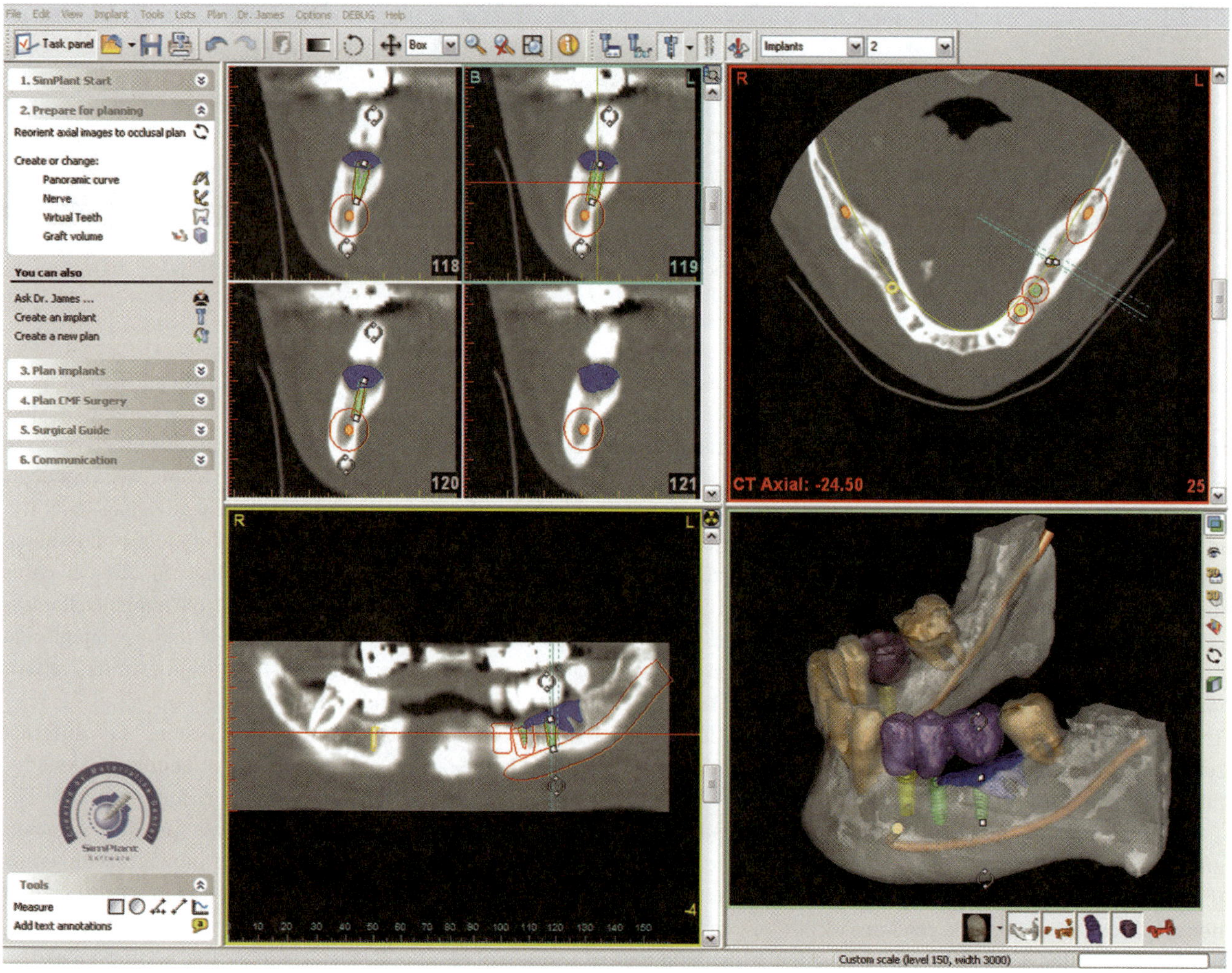

Fig. 21.14 Simplant planning software (Used with permission from Springer)

that is based on software development rather than specialized hardware may be more economically attractive to future investors in the area of simulation.

Conclusion

Simulation use in dentistry began soon after the establishment of dental education and, because of the nature of the profession and its high dependency on surgical psychomotor skills, one can assume that it will not disappear in the foreseeable future. From all possible indicators, the field of simulation in the health professional schools will move forward and adapt to the demands of the professions. Advanced simulation has made an impact in dentistry. It would seem wise for all of the health professions to listen and learn from each other and when possible collaborate. Given the importance of learning critical skills in a safe environment, simulation should be one of education's highest priorities.

References

1. Ring ME. Dentistry: an illustrated history. New York: Abradale Press/Harry N. Abrams, INC, Publishers/Mosby-Year Book; 1985. p. 274, 277.
2. Buchanan J. Use of simulation technology in dental education. J Dent Educ. 2001;65:1225–31.
3. Konukseven EL, Onder ME, Mumcuoglu E, Kisnisce TS. Development of a visio-haptic integrated dental training simulation system. J Dent Educ. 2010;74(8):880–91.
4. Suebnukarn S, Haddawy P, Rhienmora P, Jittimanee P, Viratket P. Augmented kinematic feedback from haptic virtual reality for dental skill acquisition. J Dent Educ. 2010;74(12):1357–66.
5. Yoshida Y, Yamaguchi S, Kawamoto Y, Noborio H, Murakami S, Sohmura T. Development of a multi-layered tooth model for the haptic dental training system. Dent Mater J. 2011;30(1):1–6. Epub 2011 Jan26.
6. Bal GB, Wiess EL, Gafne N, Ziv A. Preliminary assessment of faculty and student perception of a haptic virtual reality simulator for training dental manual dexterity. J Dent Educ. 2011;75(4): 496–504.
7. Urbankova A, Engebretson SP. Computer-assisted dental simulation as a predictor of preclinical operative dentistry performance. J Dent Educ. 2011;75(9):1249–55.
8. Tanzawa T, Futaki K, Tani C, et al. Introduction of a robot patient into dental education. Eur J Dent Educ. 2011;15:1–5.
9. Al-Jewair TS, Qutub AF, Malkhassian G, Dempster LJ. A systematic review of computer-assisted learning in endodontics education. J Dent Educ. 2010;74(6):601–11.
10. Gateno J, Xia JJ, Teichgraeber JF, et al. Clinical feasibility of computer-aided surgical simulation (CASS) in the treatment of complex cranio-maxillofacial deformities. J Oral Maxillofac Surg. 2007;65(4):728–34.
11. Lund B, Fors U, Sejersen R, Sallnas EL, Rosen A. Student perception of two different simulation techniques in oral and maxillofacial surgery undergraduate training. BMC Med Educ. 2011;11:82. doi:10.1186/1472-6920-11-82.
12. Shi HF, Payandeh S. Suturing simulation in surgical training environment. Intell Robot Syst. 2009;10:422–3. doi:10.1109/IROS.2009.5354595.
13. Frasaco. http://www.frasaco.com/index.php?seite=arbeitsmodelle_en&navigation=12891&root=11485&kanal=html. Accessed 3 Mar 2012.
14. Kavo. http://www.kavousa.com/US/Other-Products/Dental-Training/Teeth-and-study-models.aspx. Accessed 3 Mar 2012.
15. Clancy JMS, Lindquist TJ, Palik JF, Johnson LA. A comparison of student performance in a simulation clinic and a traditional laboratory environment: three-year results. J Dent Educ. 2002;66:1331–7.
16. Chan DC, Pruzler KB, Caughman WF. Simulation with preclinical operative dentistry courses – 3 year retrospective results. J Dent Educ. 2000;64:224.
17. Wagner J, Arteaga S, D'Ambrosio J, et al. A patient-instructor program to promote dental students' communication skills with diverse patients. J Dent Educ. 2007;71(12):1554–60.
18. Johnson JA, Kipp KC, Williams RG. Standardized patients for the assessment of dental students' clinical skills. J Dent Educ. 1990;54: 331–3.
19. Messer LB, Kan K, Cameron A, Robinson R. Teaching paediatric dentistry by multimedia: a three-year report. Eur J Dent Educ. 2002;6:128–38.
20. Abbey LM. Interactive multimedia patient simulation in dental and continuing dental education. Dent Clin N Am. 2002;46:575–87.
21. Zary N, Johnson G, Fors U. Web-based virtual patients in dentistry: factors influencing the use of cases in the Web-SP system. Eur J Dent Educ. 2009;13:2–9.
22. Kamyab S, Kamya S, Uijtdehaage S, Gordon C, Roos K. Cardiovascular simulation cases for dental students. MedEdPortal 2009. Available from: www.mededportal.org/publication/1722.
23. Alessi SM, Johnson LA. Simulations for dental licensure examinations: reliability and validity. Simul/Games Learn. 1992;22:286–307.
24. Encisco R, Memon A, Mah J. Three dimensional visualization of the craniofacial patient: volume segmentation, data integration and animation. Orthod Craniofac Res Suppl. 2003;6:66–71.
25. Langenbach GEJ, Ahang F, Herring SW, Hannam AG. Modelling the masticatory biomechanics of a pig. J Anat. 2002;201:383–93.
26. Hannam AG. Dynamic modeling and jaw biomechanics. Orthod Craniofac Res Suppl. 2003;6:59–65.
27. eHuman. http://www.ehuman.org. Accessed 3 Mar 2012.
28. Buchanan JA. Experience with virtual reality-based technology in teaching restorative dental procedures. J Dent Educ. 2004;68(12): 1258–65.
29. Jasinevicius R, Landers M, Nelson S, Urbankova A. An evaluation of two dental simulation systems: virtual reality versus contemporary non-computer-assisted. J Dent Educ. 2004;68(11):1151–62.
30. Leblanc VR, Urbankova A, Hadavi F, Lichtenthal RM. A preliminary study in using virtual reality to train dental students. J Dent Educ. 2004;68(3):378–83.
31. Maggio MP, Buchanan JA, Berthold P, Gottlieb R. Virtual reality-based technology (VRBT) training positively enhanced performance on preclinical examinations. J Dent Educ. 2005;69(1):Abstract 161.
32. Maggio MP, Buchanan JA, Berthold P, Gottlieb R. Curriculum changes in preclinical laboratory education with virtual reality-based technology training. J Dent Educ. 2005;69(1):Abstract 160.
33. Gottlieb R, Lanning S, Gunsolley J, Buchanan J. Faculty impressions of dental students' performance with and without virtual reality simulation. J Dent Educ. 2011;75:1443–51.
34. EPED. http://www.eped.com.tw/html/front/bin/ptlist.phtml?ategory=309143. Accessed 3 Mar 2012.
35. Walsh LJ, Chai L, Farah C, Ngo H, Eves G. SLE in dentistry and oral health: final report 2010. https://www.hwa.gov.au/sites/uploads/sles-in-dentistry-oral-health-curricula-201108.pdf. Accessed 3 Mar 2012.
36. Phillips J, Berge ZL. Second life for dental education. J Dent Educ. 2009;73(11):1260–4.
37. Kolesnikov M, Steinberg A, Zefran M, Drummond J. PerioSim: haptics-based virtual reality dental simulator. Digital Dental News 2008;6–12.
38. The VOXEL-MAN Dental. www.voxel-man.de/simulator/dental/. Accessed 3 Mar 2012.

39. HapTEL (Haptic Technology Enhanced Learning). www.haptel.kcl.ac.uk/. Accessed 3 Mar 2012.
40. Moog Simodont dental haptic trainer. http://www.simodont.org/. Accessed 3 Mar 2012.
41. Steinberg AD, Bashook PG, Drummond J, Ashrafi S, Zehran M. Assessment of faculty perception of content validity of PerioSim, a haptic 3-D virtual reality dental training simulator. J Dent Educ. 2007;71:1574–82.
42. Koopman P, Buijs J, Wesselink P, Vervoorn M. Simodont, a haptic dental training simulator combined with course ware. Bio-Algorithms Med-Systems. 2012;6:117–22.
43. Bakker D, Lagerweij M, Wesselink P, Vervoorn M. Transfer of manual dexterity skills acquired on the Simodont, a haptic dental trainer with a virtual environment to reality; a pilot study. Bio-Algorithms Med-Systems. 2010;6:21–4.
44. Kim L, Park SH. Haptic interaction and volume modeling techniques for realistic dental simulation. Vis Comput. 2006;22: 90–8.
45. Marras I, Nikolaidis N, Mikrogeorgis G, Lyroudia K, Pitas I. A virtual system for cavity preparation in endodontics. J Dent Educ. 2008;72(4):494–502.
46. Suebnukarn S, Hataidechadusadee R, Suwannasri N, Suprasert N, Rhienmora P, Haddawy P. Access cavity preparation training using haptic virtual reality and microcomputed tomography tooth models. Int Endod J. 2011;44:983–9.
47. Amer RS, Denehy GE, Cobb DS, Dawson DV, Cunningham-Ford MA, Bergeron C. Development and evaluation of an interactive dental video game to teach dentin bonding. J Dent Educ. 2011; 75(6):823–31.
48. eurekalert. http://www.eurekalert.org/multimedia/pub/14584.php?from=138734. Accessed 3 Mar 2012; http://www.physorg.com/news163937088.html. Accessed 3 Mar 2012; http://www.breakawaygames.com/serious-games/solutions/healthcare/. Accessed 3 Mar 2012.
49. Casap N, Wexler A, Eliashar R. Computerized navigation for surgery of the lower jaw: comparison of 2 navigation systems. J Oral Maxillofac Surg. 2008;66(7):1467–75.
50. Image Navigation Ltd. http://image-navigation.com/IGI/overview.html. Accessed 3 Mar 2012.
51. Casap N, Nadel S, Tarazi E, Weisss EL. Evaluation of a navigational system for dental implantation as a tool to train novice dental practitioners. J Oral Maxillofac Surg. 2011;69(10):2548–56. Epub 2011 Aug 6.
52. Casap N, Wexler A, Persky N, Schneider A, Lustmann J. Navigation surgery for dental implants: assessment of accuracy of the image guided implantology system. J Oral Maxillofac Surg. 2004;62 Suppl 2:116–9.
53. Casap N, Laviv A, Wexler A. Computerized navigation for immediate loading of dental implants with a prefabricated metal frame: a feasibility study. J Oral Maxillofac Surg. 2011;69(2):512–9.
54. Casap N, Tarazi E, Wexler A, Sonnenfeld U, Lustmann J. Intraoperative computerized navigation for flapless implant surgery and immediate loading in the edentulous mandible. Int J Oral Maxillofac Implants. 2005;20(1):92–8.
55. Casap N, Wexler A, Tarazi E. Application of a surgical navigation system for implant surgery in a deficient alveolar ridge postexcision of an odentogenic myxoma. J Oral Maxillofac Surg. 2005;63(7): 982–8.
56. Elian N, Jalbout ZN, Classi AJ, Wexler A, Sarment D, Tarnow DP. Precision of flapless implant placement using real-time surgical navigation: a case series. Int J Oral Maxillofac Implants. 2009;23: 1123–7.
57. Tardieu PB, Vrielinck L, Escolano E, Hanne M, Tardieu AL. Computer-assisted implant placement: scan template, simplant, surgiguide and SAFE system. Int J Periodontics Restorative Dent. 2007;27(2):141–9.
58. Materialise. http://www.materialise.com/Dental. Accessed 3 Mar 2012.

Simulation in Family Medicine

22

James M. Cooke and Leslie Wimsatt

Introduction

In this chapter, we review the use of simulation-based training in family medicine. Much of the research in this field has focused on training for specific procedural skills and the use of simulation as an evaluative tool. Some of the evidence comes to us from the fields of anesthesiology, cardiology, obstetrics, and surgery, with direct implications for the extension to physician training in family medicine. This body of inquiry has sought to estimate the impact of clinical simulation on a variety of broad-based outcomes, including learner satisfaction, perceived value, and clinical competency. Within the primary care literature, clinical simulation is frequently devoted to procedural skill development and competency measurement. However, simulation can also be used to develop skills related to clinical decision-making and the delivery of team-based care to patients. For this reason, simulation is appealing and gaining traction for specialties such as family medicine.

We begin with a brief discussion of how the practice of family medicine is uniquely suited to take advantage of clinical simulation training. We then undertake a synthesis of the literature to explore the types of content material and instructional strategies currently integrated within the clinical simulation learning environment, the potential benefits and challenges to successful implementation, and the outcome measures used to assess the impact of simulator use on clinical performance. Finally, we discuss the "art" of simulation for family medicine, that is, how does one apply the evidence and principles available to effectively implement simulation into training programs.

J.M. Cooke, MD (✉)
Department of Family Medicine, University of Michigan, L2003 Women's Hospital, 1500 E. Med Ctr Dr. SPC 5239, Ann Arbor 48109-5239, MI, USA
e-mail: cookej@med.umich.edu

L. Wimsatt, PhD
Department of Family Medicine, University of Michigan, 1018 Fuller St, Ann Arbor, MI 48104-1213, USA
e-mail: lwimsatt@umich.edu

A Unique Opportunity for Family Medicine

The emergence of clinical simulation in medical education is particularly exciting for those engaged in training family physicians and allied healthcare professionals functioning in the family practice environment. Such equipment can simulate a variety of conditions and present learners with a broad array of scenarios commonly and uncommonly encountered in clinical practice. This is especially important in family medicine where trainees must master an ever-increasing array of clinical skills in order to prepare for practice, while working under the constraints of curtailed duty hours. The delivery of services is complex, often requiring knowledge of a wide variety of interventions and methods of caring for diverse patient populations [1]. In addition, providers must be able to implement emergent healthcare delivery models as proposed by leadership within the field, including the American Academy of Family Physicians (AAFP). The patient-centered medical home (PCMH) model has emerged, for example, as an innovative framework on which to base family medicine practice improvement [2], and clinical simulation shows promise in addressing many of the competencies that are required to train physicians to successfully practice medicine within the PCMH environment.

The PCMH model is designed as a way of improving access to care, disease prevention, chronic disease and population management, care coordination, teamwork, and patient-centeredness [3–8]. It emphasizes the use of clinical technology systems and ongoing provider training to improve patient communication and a variety of clinical outcomes [9]. Demonstration projects show promising results, with early data suggesting a linkage between care coordination and cost reductions plus better quality of care for patients with chronic illnesses [3–5]. Continuity of care may significantly predict use of preventive services [10], but

A.I. Levine et al. (eds.), *The Comprehensive Textbook of Healthcare Simulation*,
DOI 10.1007/978-1-4614-5993-4_22,

research findings on primary care teams and knowledge of the skills needed for successful team-based care are just beginning to surface in the literature [11, 12].

The demand for patient safety, competency-based evaluation, and an ever-changing "basket of services" as advocated by the AAFP [13] also motivates many primary care educators to consider how simulation can be used to effectively teach and document mastery of a variety of required skills and competencies. Simulation can be a powerful tool for rapid skill acquisition and competency assessment. As an instructional approach, it offers a way to clearly define and standardize learning goals. It also can present a wide range of medical conditions. These considerations are particularly salient in family medicine where educators face increasing pressure to develop more effective and efficient educational approaches. Patient demographics and the medical conditions encountered by trainees vary within and across family medicine programs; therefore, it is often difficult for educators to maintain consistency in the provision of clinical training experiences. At most medical schools, third-year family medicine clerkships are relatively brief in duration, and recent changes in accreditation requirements have shortened the work week for residents while expanding the curriculum in many Accreditation Council for Graduate Medical Education (ACGME) competency areas (i.e., systems-based practice, interpersonal/communication skills, professionalism, practice-based learning, and improvement). Hence, a large volume of knowledge and skills must be acquired despite reductions in contact hours. Simulation is one of several new educational modalities with the potential to facilitate more effective and efficient procedural, inpatient, and outpatient skill development.

To date, the use of simulation in medical education is isolated within a small number of educational institutions. Only one-third of US hospital-based clerkships and 54% of medical school-based clerkships incorporate use of simulators within the curriculum. While only a small percentage of teaching hospitals (12%) expose family medicine residents to clinical simulation, the rate is much higher for programs located within academic health centers where over half of the family medicine residency programs (58%) deliver at least some simulator-based instruction [14].

Among published studies, educational applications relevant to family medicine include high-fidelity simulation for the acquisition of endoscopic competency [15], perineal birth trauma repair [16], and pediatric advanced life support (PALS) skills [17] as well as enhancement of resident confidence in managing obstetric emergencies [18], evaluation of endotracheal intubation skills [19], and general medical decision-making [20, 21]. While the results appear promising, our understanding of the implications remains limited to a narrow range of study contexts, learner populations, and programmatically driven educational experiences.

The Science: Status of Existing Applications

Medical School

In the medical school setting, family medicine educators have primarily used standardized patients (SPs) to prepare clerkship students with the skills necessary to assume the role of a family doctor with expertise in diagnostics, the provision of acute care services, and chronic disease management (e.g., history taking, physical diagnosis, medical decision-making, health maintenance). These skills, while by no means exclusive to family medicine, are typically taught by family medicine educators and represent traditional areas of excellence within most medical school curricula.

Cardiac examination simulators, such as the Harvey® Cardiopulmonary Patient Simulator (Laerdal Medical Corporation, Wappingers Falls, NY), have been available for many years and accurately simulate a wide variety of heart sounds, lung sounds, jugular venous waves, and point of maximal impulse locations. Studies evaluating educational efficacy of this simulator have expanded from reports of learner acceptance and perceived benefits to translational studies that link simulation-based curricula to actual improvements in diagnostic accuracy [22]. Instruction that integrates use of clinical vignettes with cardiopulmonary examination scenarios translates particularly well to family medicine. Such approaches challenge learners to not only accurately recognize and cogently describe physical findings but also to synthesize important points of the history and physical exam to develop a differential diagnosis. Blended methods of instruction can offer medical students a robust learning experience while providing faculty with a valuable tool for evaluating the development of diagnostic and medical decision-making skills. Utilizing simulators to support training in physical examination skills, such as bimanual pelvic exam, also allows students greater opportunity for practice than would be possible during patient encounters in clinic, or within a standardized patient setting. Studies indicate that instructors are able to offer more discrete evaluations of student performance and that simulation is often less costly and more convenient than using standardized patients for the delivery of physical examination skills training [23].

In lieu of animal labs, patient simulators can be used for teaching cardiac and pulmonary physiology [24]. Patient simulators such as METI's Human Patient Simulator (HPS)® (Medical Education Technologies Inc. CAE Healthcare, Sarasota, FL) are capable of processing complex algorithms and calculating outputs such as arterial and pulmonary pressures. Inputs can be modified by instructors to demonstrate simple and complex physiologic responses. Some educators have found it useful to engage learners in developing and implementing their own scenarios, a method found effective in increasing learner satisfaction and extending student understanding of core content knowledge [25].

Three-dimensional anatomy programs, initially used by students as supplementary study tools, have significantly advanced in recent years and may soon replace the traditional cadaveric anatomy lab experience. Obstetrical and procedural simulators are also being used prior to clinical experiences at some institutions for additional hands-on learning experiences and to focus novice skill acquisition so that learners and teachers can concentrate on higher-level skills during patient encounters. Some examples include the use of obstetric simulators for teaching proper delivery technique, perineal protection, shoulder dystocia maneuvers [26], and placenta delivery. Students can also learn higher-risk procedures typically managed by residents or faculty, including manual rupture of membranes, intrauterine pressure catheter placement, fetal scalp electrode placement, perineal laceration repair, and vacuum-assisted vaginal delivery. Similar applications have been well received by medical students and faculty, with documented improvements in medical knowledge, risk assessment ability, medical decision-making, and communication skills with laboring patients based on post-simulation testing [27, 28].

On-demand learning programs using simulation, although relatively costly due to instructor time, have been piloted with similar levels of student acceptance [29]. Small groups of students can incorporate problem-based learning cases into a simulated environment, such as those involving congestive heart failure, chronic obstructive pulmonary disease, or diabetic ketoacidosis. This allows learners to engage in a variety of predetermined, sequential exercises that progress from history taking and physical exam/diagnosis to discussions with the patient, treatment planning, and the monitoring of initial treatment outcomes. Using this approach, medical students are able to blend their case discussions with active engagement in patient management learning activities.

Many organizations are beginning to design and implement web-based simulations to address clinical issues commonly encountered by primary care providers. Cases derived from the Society of Teachers of Family Medicine (STFM) Clerkship Curriculum [30] feature acute complaints (e.g., insomnia, low back pain, vaginal bleeding, dyspnea) and management of chronic diseases such as diabetes, hypertension, obesity, and dementia. Compared with traditional formats for discussing patient case scenarios, the STFM applications create a more realistic clinical decision-making dynamic. Students obtain a history through a series of linked questions, elicit physical exam findings, retrieve relevant empirical studies, and make a diagnosis based on the information provided. The cases include a series of embedded pre- and posttest questions as well as patient education materials that can be downloaded (Fig. 22.1).

Residency Programs

At the residency level, the use of simulator-based training has expanded in recent years, moving beyond procedural instruction to address a more complex array of patient management topics and skills that relate to the delivery of team-based care to patients (e.g., professional communication, team leadership). Clinical simulation has been embraced by some programs for advanced cardiac life support, neonatal advanced life support, and advanced life support for obstetrics as well as for procedural and critical care training (Figs. 22.2, 22.3, 22.4, and 22.5). Advancements in team training, team management, ethics, and other complex patient care issues are emerging [31, 32]. Table 22.1 contains a comprehensive list of modalities applicable to family medicine. Table 22.2 provides an overview of published curricula that can be tailored to the needs of individual programs and learner needs.

Educators can shape simulation exercises to address program-specific, organizational, or community-based needs. If a residency curriculum lacks certain procedural training opportunities, simulation can be used as an adjunct to expand residency skill development. Hospitals may choose to use simulation during staff orientation as a method of promoting uniformity in first-responder skills and transfer protocols. Travel or in situ simulation programs can enhance multidisciplinary training of residents, nurses, pharmacists, respiratory therapists, and other healthcare team members because they can be physically located in or near patient care areas where team communication, supervision, and performance takes place. Given the large number of clinical care environments encountered by family medicine residents and the large number of colleagues and staff with whom the residents must interact, it is essential that they learn and apply standard concepts in team resource management to optimize patient safety and clinical outcomes. Simulation provides an ideal tool for such training.

The simulation center is, in many ways, becoming the bench lab for educators, with significant potential for impact on family medicine. Many residency programs have been studying simulation-based training to determine best practices for training as well as formative and summative evaluation. A hybrid approach to procedural skills training, using both standardized patients and simulators, has been used for obstetrics and endoscopy training to incorporate interpersonal communication skills. Large group simulation for pandemic planning and mass casualty scenarios have been advocated by emergency medicine and military physician groups and will likely prove well suited to the training of primary care providers in the coming years.

Within family medicine, the number of research studies and national conference presentations has increased in recent years, with a focus on topics such as resident perceptions and acceptance of simulation for critical care training [33],

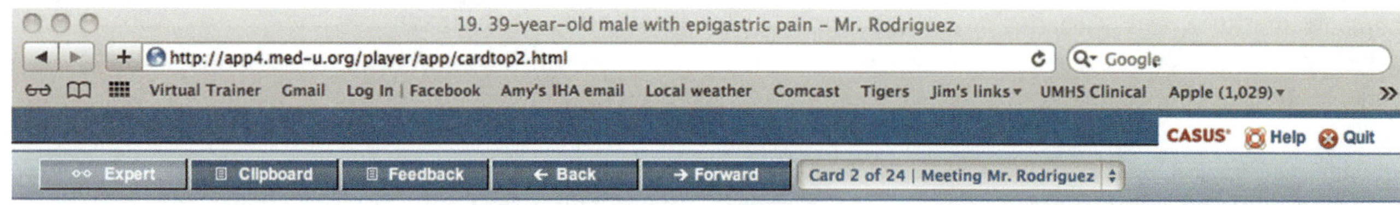

As you walk down the hall, Lola, the Spanish-speaking interpreter asks if you have worked with interpreters before.

You reply, "Well, an older patient I saw in the emergency room last month had a family member help out and translate. But I haven't really thought about it. What do you recommend?"

After checking in with Lola about the reason for Mr. Rodriguez's visit, you enter the room and greet him. You introduce yourself as a medical student working with Dr. Medel and Lola today and ask the patient's permission to talk with him.

You sit directly across from Mr. Rodriguez, with Lola sitting just off to your left and facing him. You sense that Mr. Rodriguez seems anxious about coming to the physician today.

You ask him, "How are you doing today?"

"Is there anything that makes the pain better or worse?"

You ask, "What worries you the most about your symptoms?"

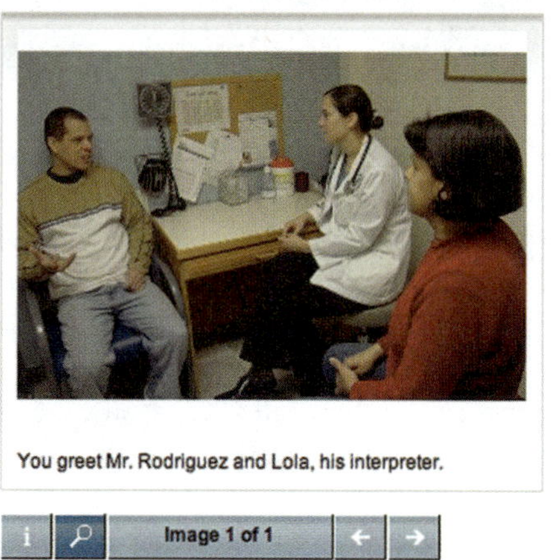

You greet Mr. Rodriguez and Lola, his interpreter.

Image 1 of 1

Thinking about some of the common causes of abdominal pain, you conduct a focused review of systems.

References:
American Association of Medical Colleges. Guidelines for use of medical interpreter services, https://www.aamc.org/44826/search.html?q=guidelines+for+use+of+medical+interpreter+services&x=0&y=0, Accessed March 8, 2011.

Fig. 22.1 Web-based, interactive scenario designed for use by medical students during their third-year clinical clerkship in family medicine. The dyspepsia case (shown) addresses several learning objectives embedded within the Society for Teachers of Family Medicine (STFM) Family Medicine Clerkship Curriculum. Image used with permission of the author, Dr. Joel Heidelbaugh, and available at http://www.med-u.org/virtual_patient_cases/fmcases

improvement in endoscopy skills [15], pediatric life support [17], adult intubation [19], and medical decision-making. We anticipate more discussion of best practices and validation studies of assessment tools linked to clinical competencies as simulators are more widely utilized. We also anticipate that incoming residents will begin to factor the availability of simulation experiences into their selection of residency programs during the match process especially as more students have exposure to simulator training during medical school.

Certification Examinations and Renewals

The American Board of Family Medicine has recognized the importance of translating knowledge into practice by adopting case-based, computer simulations as part of its certification and recertification examinations and annual maintenance of certification (MOC) modules. Beginning in 2004, the MOC modules were modified to include a wide variety of inpatient and outpatient medical scenarios, from well child care and maternity care to care of the vulnerable elderly (see Table 22.3). Diplomates are expected to complete one module per year. Each module contains a knowledge test, evidence-based competency measures, and a computer-simulated patient scenario that extends from an initial visit through ongoing management of a chronic medical condition. Physicians receive an image of a patient and a presenting complaint. After entering free-text diagnostic questions into the module program, they elicit and review physical exam findings. The simulator sequence allows physicians to order office-based studies and laboratory tests, utilize a working problem and diagnosis list, and recommend treatment. Follow-up visits are sometimes embedded in the module sequence and require that physicians engage in additional history taking, physical examinations, diagnostics, and/or therapeutic recommendations. At the end of each simulation, the physician receives a performance evaluation and evidenced-based feedback based on published data and guidelines.

To date, research on the use of simulators for physician certification has focused primarily on perceptions of the certification process and estimation of its impact on future practice behavior [34]. Additional outcomes data will become available as the volume of family medicine physicians who have completed the annual self-assessment module (SAM) increases.

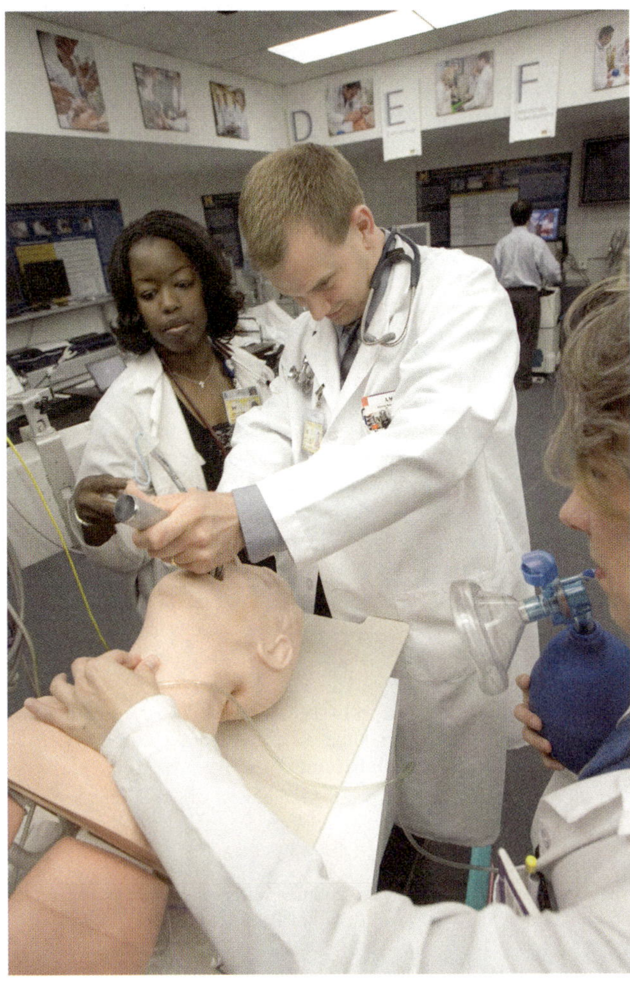

Fig. 22.2 Family medicine residents work as a group on manual endotracheal intubation skills prior to rapid sequence intubation team training

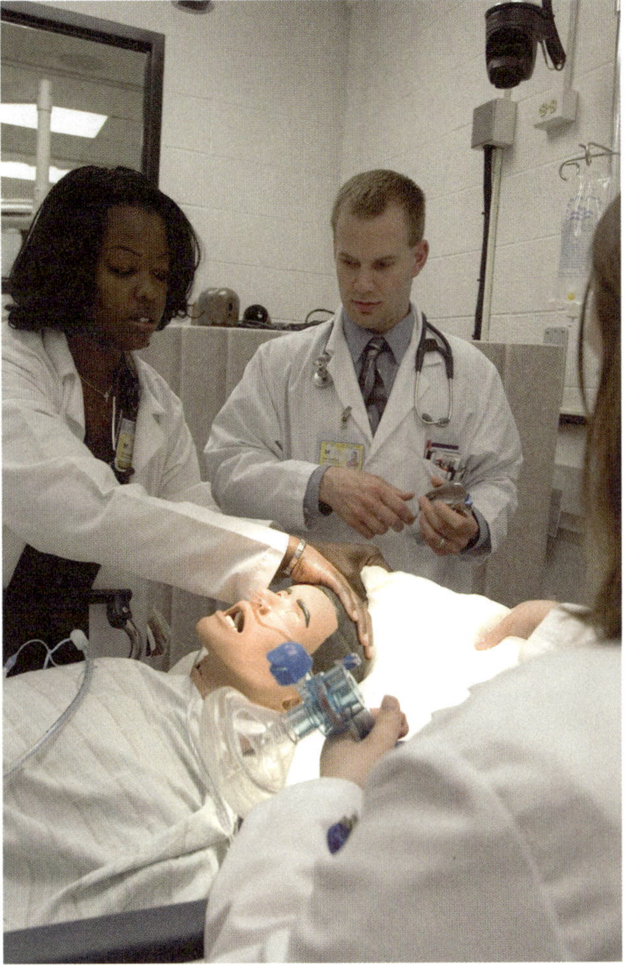

Fig. 22.3 Residents participate in a simulated respiratory distress scenario to demonstrate team communication skills, delegation of tasks, supervision, and efficient diagnosis and treatment

Continuing Medical Education

The use of simulation for continuing medical education (CME) is limited. Some research supports the integration of clinical simulation with traditional learning techniques at CME courses to allow physicians to practice newly introduced techniques and concepts [35]. Such training could involve longitudinal experiences using scenarios that replicate a clinical practice setting to promote deeper learning and better application to patient care.

While simulation is used in the delivery of bioterrorism and disaster training for healthcare providers, it could also be quite useful for retraining physicians who have had an extended leave of absence from medical practice. The benefits of retraining are probably most applicable to higher-risk care, such as hospital care, critical care, obstetrics and procedural training. Other educational and safety initiatives using patient simulation include: realistic reenactments of critical events [36], multidisciplinary in-hospital mock codes, and education on the use of new medical equipment or new skills [37]. Despite lack of supporting evidence, several hospitals, medical groups, and malpractice insurers are beginning to mandate such training based solely on its perceived benefits. Some malpractice insurers now provide financial incentives

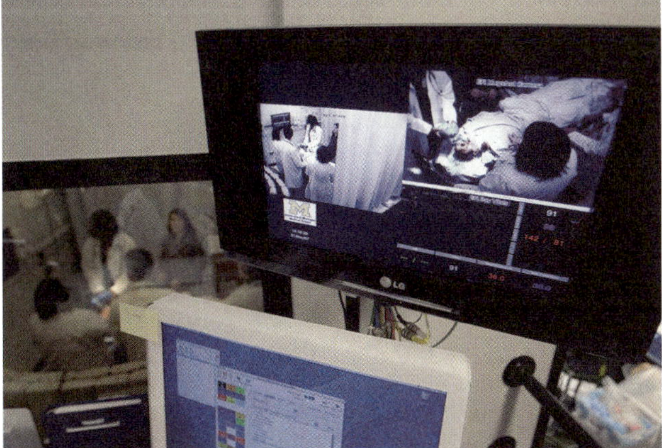

Fig. 22.4 The instructors view from the control room of a simulation center

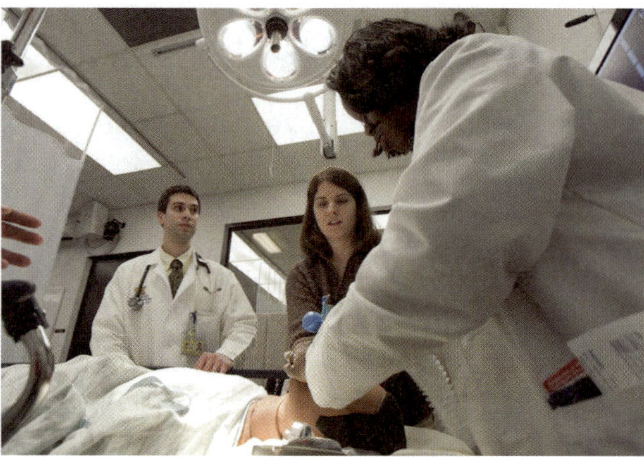

Fig. 22.5 The realism, or fidelity, of the simulation suite, materials, and scenario can promote a high level of learner activation and engagement

Table 22.1 Topics and simulation modalities applicable to family medicine

Clinical skills
History (standardized patient)
Physical examination (heart, lung, breast, prostate, cervical dilation)
Diagnostic ultrasound (obstetric, vascular, abdominal)
Medical knowledge
Case-based medical and surgical scenarios (ABFM self-assessment modules, EKG evaluation, radiology)
Team-based training
Mobile training in native clinical environments
Respiratory failure
Code or rapid-response team leadership and communication
Cardiac arrhythmia and arrest
Shock (anaphylactic, cardiogenic, septic, hemorrhagic, neurogenic)
Disaster preparedness (multiple trauma, terrorism, biological and chemical warfare)
Conscious sedation
Neonatal resuscitation
Obstetric emergencies
Assisted vaginal delivery
Procedures
Basic life support
Airway management (endotracheal, nasotracheal, or non-visualized intubation, cricothyroidotomy, tracheostomy)
Vascular access (IV, arterial puncture, arterial cutdown, umbilical, intraosseous, or central line)
Endoscopy (colonoscopy, sigmoidoscopy, EGD, endoscopic biopsy)
Nasolaryngoscopy
Laparoscopy
Arthrocentesis
Thoracentesis/paracentesis with or without ultrasound guidance
Lumbar puncture
Chest tube placement
Circumcision
Other
Ethics (post-intubation DNR discovery, withdrawal of care)
Toxicology
Managing differences of medical opinion in critical situations
Wilderness medicine or rural trauma

Table 22.2 On-line resources for family medicine simulation scenarios and curricula

American Board of Family Medicine Self-Assessment Modules (SAMs) for on-line outpatient-based knowledge assessment simulations available to family medicine residents and certified attending physicians at www.theabfm.org
Family Medicine Digital Resource Library at www.fmdrl.org (maintained by the Society for Teachers of Family Medicine)
Critical Care Simulation Curriculum, by James Cooke, M.D. www.fmdrl.org/794
Simulation Scenarios (OB), by Douglas Maurer, D.O. et al. http://www.fmdrl.org/2145
Cardiac Exam Simulation Curriculum, by James Cooke, M.D. http://www.fmdrl.org/3179
A Foundation for Procedure Acquisition and Competence using On-line Resources, Individualized Education, and Simulation, by Beth Fox, M.D. http://www.fmdrl.org/3368
Role of simulation laboratory in medical student's education during family medicine clerkship, by Wessam Labib, M.D., M.P.H. http://www.fmdrl.org/3388
fmCASES – Family Medicine Computer-Assisted Simulations for Educating Students, on-line case-based simulations for clerkship students www.med-u.org/virtual_patient_cases/fmcases
MedEdPortal www.mededportal.org (maintained by the Association of American Medical Colleges) – 191 listed simulation curricula, scenarios, and web-based modules as of 2011 including medical and dental cases at every level of training
Society for Academic Emergency Medicine (SAEM) Simulation Case Library http://www.emedu.org/sim

Table 22.3 Self-assessment modules offered for maintenance of certification by the American Board of Family Medicine

Care of the vulnerable elderly
Cerebrovascular disease
Childhood illness
Coronary artery disease
Depression
Diabetes
Health behavior
Heart failure
Hypertension
Maternity care
Pain management
Preventive care
Well child care

to physicians who complete simulations that emphasize error avoidance and team communication. This is encouraged due to the perceived safety benefits for patients as well as the potential financial benefit to the insurers [32].

Assessment and Evaluation

To review the use of simulation as a vehicle for assessment and evaluation, we must consider the smaller studies in family medicine in combination with those from other medical specialties. In a recent meta-analysis that included 609 eligible studies enrolling 35,226 healthcare professional trainees, Cook and colleagues found that the use of technology-enhanced simulation training had large effects on measured knowledge, skills, and behaviors and moderate effects for patient-related outcomes when compared to no intervention [38]. This argues for the increased use of simulation, but family medicine educators still need to determine which knowledge, skills, or attitudes are best suited to simulation and the extent to which this varies by learner education level.

Evidence from the surgical specialties has validated several measures of resident procedural competence, such as cecal intubation time for colonoscopy and efficiency of movement and procedure time for laparoscopic cholecystectomy using high-fidelity endoscopic and laparoscopic simulators. These procedural skills are relatively easy to isolate and evaluate in a controlled simulation environment. In contrast, evaluating primary care resident competency in the management of respiratory distress is a much more complex undertaking. To determine competence, one must simultaneously assess multiple communication, physical exam, diagnostic reasoning, therapeutic decision-making, and procedural skills. Validated checklists have been developed to assess the evaluation and management of apnea, asthma, supraventricular tachycardia, and sepsis by pediatric residents [39], but the challenge remains to define a core group of skills and develop valid assessments for the wide variety of patients and medical conditions encountered in family medicine.

The value of providing standardized scenarios linked to validated evaluation tools holds significant promise in primary care in general and family medicine residency in particular because traditional observational methods employed in the clinical setting are fraught with potential bias and inaccuracy. This is due, in part, to time constraints placed on faculty and residents attributable to competing needs and demands in the clinical environment. It is also due to a lack of standardized faculty training in direct observation.

Studies are underway to help define clinical simulation competencies using several objective measures, including diagnostic accuracy and length of time from diagnosis to the delivery of effective treatment [40, 41]. Future research on validity will be needed as we begin to adopt standardized competency measures instead of simply using prior experience as an indicator of skill acquisition. While documentation of the number of cases managed (e.g., congestive heart failure or acute MI) or number of surgical procedures performed (e.g., sigmoidoscopy) traditionally served as indicators of skill competency, we may soon be able to use measures such as time to diagnosis a medical condition or percent of mucosa visualized during endoscopic procedures as more accurate determinants of clinical competence or procedural expertise.

Indeed, one can imagine future physicians reporting their simulation-based procedures to augment their actual case numbers or simulator-measured metrics to document competency for procedures or hospital credentialing. Validated assessment tools are needed to measure the impact of simulation-based learning on clinical practice behavior across a range of clinical competencies, care settings (e.g., inpatient, outpatient, home, skilled nursing facility), and patient populations (e.g., geriatric, adult, pediatric, obstetric). Family medicine educators should be prepared for the eventual incorporation of clinical simulation competency milestones into residency program accreditation requirements.

The Art: Addressing Challenges and Maximizing Benefits

Challenges for Implementation

To date, relatively few articles on simulator-based education have been published in the primary care literature [42] despite demonstrated interest and the previously proven benefit of standardized patients in medical education [43, 44]. Similarly, no requirements for the incorporation of simulation into medical school and residency education have been articulated by the Liaison Committee on Medical Education (LCME) or the ACGME. This apparent deficit in the literature is likely due to a combination of factors. Many faculty members lack personal experience with (or exposure to) clinical simulation training, and access to simulation center facilities is not yet widely available [14]. Because the use of simulation-based training in family medicine is a relatively recent development, fully elaborated curricula are just beginning to emerge and data on instructional outcomes remain scarce. Also, many family medicine programs lack access to a clinical simulation center, the establishment of which comes at a high cost that likely falls outside of many program budgets. Although reported annual operating expenses for teaching hospital-based or medical school-based simulation centers vary widely (ranging from less than $250,000 to over one million dollars), these estimates do not include the initial start-up costs [14].

Over the past several years, family medicine educators have published and presented several lessons learned when implementing simulation-based or simulation-supplemented curricula. A common theme among these articles and presentations is the value of specialized training prior to implementation. Due to the nature of the medical school admissions process and the traditions within graduate education, most physicians come to medical school with a science rather than an education background. Teaching skills among academic faculty are typically gained through mentoring and a series of progressive teaching responsibilities from individual, to small group, to large group venues. Some physicians supplement this with targeted faculty development programs or fellowships, but the majority of these individuals develop teaching skills through experience.

Simulation, despite offering a compelling instructional delivery system for learners, presents a unique set of challenges to faculty. Faculty must possess an understanding of the clinical simulation environment, simulation design, simulator use, and debriefing, not withstanding a possible lack of previous exposure during medical training. Fortunately, there are a growing number of simulator instructor training courses offered through national organizations and individual simulation centers as well as national conferences, journals, and on-line resources. Any program considering the incorporation of simulation into its curriculum should provide specialized training for a core group of faculty members who can, in turn, share their knowledge and experience with others engaged in simulation-based education.

Experienced instructors recognize that there is always a chance that things might not go according to plan during a simulation-based scenario, so instructor adaptability is key to a positive and productive session. When such errors occur, it can be frustrating for both the instructor and learners. Trained instructors know how to reframe unexpected "glitches" in the planned scenario in a manner that may actually enhance the learning experience, sometimes by taking the learning experience in an entirely new direction.

Despite the potential for improvements in safety and educational efficacy, use of simulator training has potential risks. If the clinical environment is not accurately replicated, or if the learner is not adequately prepared or supervised, there is potential for lack of "buy-in" by the learner, inaccurate presentation of material, and/or reinforcement of errors. There also exists a possibility for emotional or psychological harm if the simulation is especially difficult, traumatic, or reminiscent of a previous experience. These risks should be anticipated and effectively addressed by instructors prior to launching the simulation or during the critical post-simulation debriefing. In general, it is advisable to establish ground rules prior to starting any simulation exercise (especially if the learners are new to the environment). Participants need to understand that things may go poorly, but that this often happens by design.

Needless to say, simulation is not immune from common instructional pitfalls such as oversaturating learners with information, inappropriately applying educational technology, and failing to examine the efficacy of skills transfer, instructional delivery methods, assessment approaches, and overall implementation costs. However, proper needs assessment, thoughtful design, pilot testing, and ongoing program evaluation can overcome many of these potential pitfalls.

Potential Benefits

Simulation offers an experiential learning opportunity in which participants can make errors in a controlled and safe instructional environment [42]. For family medicine educators, one of the most compelling arguments for the use of simulator training is enhanced safety. As educators, we know that medical students and residents can potentially harm patients during the process of learning new skills regardless of the safeguards and protocols put into place to avoid such occurrences. In addition to patient risk, injuries to the learners and to other healthcare staff are possible. It has been suggested that simulation is an ethical imperative given the possible safety benefits to patients, learners, and professional colleagues without the inherent risks of actual patient care. As a training methodology, it is certainly safer than many traditional approaches for learning the complex skills required in modern medical practice [45]. For family medicine trainees, simulation holds promise for reversing the decreased hands-on experience and procedural competence documented among medical students in recent years and attributed to increases in supervisory requirements imposed by accrediting bodies. For example, clinical procedures that pose higher risks such as lumbar puncture, endotracheal intubation, central line placement, normal or assisted vaginal delivery, and neonatal circumcision may be well suited to be taught and evaluated using simulation.

In addition to the safety benefits, there are many other notable benefits to learning through simulation. Several studies have found it to be a more enjoyable [46], a more valuable [47, 48], and a more effective way to learn than traditional approaches [49, 50]. Specific surgical skills such as suturing can be broken down into small components to allow for the measurement of time to completion and accuracy. Some studies of training in procedural skills document the effectiveness of clinical simulation as an instructional strategy as measured in terms of performance outcomes [15, 50]. One recent study provides a useful illustration in describing the process used by a learner to tie three 2-handed throws of a square knot in less than 10 seconds with no errors, thereby qualifying for a rating of "expert" for that component of the suturing curriculum [51].

Simulation can be used by more experienced or advanced learners to develop competency in systems-based practice, professionalism, and interpersonal communication. Such scenarios might involve the management of incompetent clinical team members or support staff, malfunctioning equipment, or environmental cofounders such as a fire, environmental disaster, or chemical weapons attack. Ethical dilemmas (e.g., the discovery of a patient's wish not to be resuscitated after successful intubation and mechanical ventilation) can also be embedded. For assessment, time to correct diagnosis or the time to implementation of appropriate treatment can be used as efficient proxies for the synthesis of effective communication, physical examination, data collection and decision-making.

Simulator training can be customized to present learners with a range of difficulty levels, and it provides learners with the opportunity to perform tasks repeatedly. Moreover, the

Table 22.4 Example of a respiratory distress scenario utilizing multiple end points for use by learners at various levels of training

Ethics case #1: "post-intubation DNR discovery"
Narrative: A 55 kg elderly female, former smoker with a history of COPD, comes to the ER with progressive shortness of breath and cough. She has been using albuterol without improvement. She has not had fevers or chest pain. She has the following vital signs: HR = 85 bpm, BP = 154/83 mmHg, RR = 10, SpO_2 = 88%, and body temperature = 36 °C. After initial evaluation, her blood gas is pH = 7.32, PaO_2 = 51 mmHg, and $PaCO_2$ = 55 mmHg.
Notes for Instructor: After intubation, notify the team in person or by intercom that the patient's husband arrived and notified the staff that the patient is DNR/DNI and that he would like to talk with them. Note the response to the news and the medical management from that point. The best response by the team is to call the husband (instructor in the booth) and explain the situation. They should also discuss continuing care or withdrawing care with the husband.
Scenario: Baseline Bag with oxygen (event—hypopnea) Sedate with Versed Paralysis with succinylcholine Intubate Vagal reaction (bradycardia recognition and management) Give atropine Awake but paralyzed (tachycardia recognition and management) Give Versed PVC's 25% V tach with pulse (arrhythmia recognition and management) Give lidocaine
Debriefing session about ethical issues, topics include: Proper identification of DNR orders Proper discussion of DNR wishes with patients and families Halting or continuing life-sustaining treatment Managing team input into care Managing the feelings of healthcare workers through code debriefing

breadth of possible scenarios and ability to teach and evaluate multiple competencies at the same time in an environment that very closely resembles the work environment is a very compelling argument in support of incorporating simulation into family medicine curricula. While standardized patients are often not thought of as simulators, they still represent the most commonly used modality for primary care physician instruction. They are covered elsewhere in this text (see Chap. 12) but in brief, procedural (e.g., rectal and pelvic exams) and "softer" skills such as history and physical exam skills are honed using simulated encounters of this nature. Standardized patient care scenarios provide teachers and learners with the opportunity to set multiple end points in series for both formative and summative evaluation of complex tasks. For example, in a respiratory distress scenario, evaluators can halt a scenario after three learning points in the case of a formative scenario, or three errors in the case of a summative evaluation (see Table 22.4)—from the data gathering stage through any or all of the following: diagnostic test selection, determination of critical patient status, gathering of endotracheal intubation materials, peri-intubation support and monitoring, intubation, confirmation of tube placement, stabilization maneuvers, management of complications, and safe transfer. This ability to interrupt the simulation allows for a much more manageable debriefing session and an evaluation with a much higher level of discrimination (i.e., learners correctly completing a large number of correct medical decisions and interventions in series).

Conclusion

There are many challenges facing the specialty of family medicine as a whole, and family medicine educators, in particular. Trainees must master an ever-increasing array of clinical skills in order to prepare for practice while working under the constraints of curtailed work hours. The diversity of patients and medical conditions encountered in clinical practice makes it challenging for educators to maintain consistency in the provision of clinical training experiences. Simulation has the potential to help mitigate many of these challenges. Simulators provide opportunities for extended practice, performance benchmarking, and experience in developing a broad array of less frequently encountered and higher-risk procedural skills. Associated costs include equipment, faculty training and the time required to develop and integrate appropriate curricula and assessment protocols. Simulation can be a powerful tool for rapid skill acquisition and competency assessment. Our goals over the coming decade should be to better understand the concepts underlying the effective delivery of simulation-based teaching, to more widely incorporate best practices in simulation-based education within the family medicine curricula, and to study and disseminate our findings.

References

1. Katerndahl D, Wood R, Jaen CR. Family medicine outpatient encounters are more complex than those of cardiology and psychiatry. J Am Board Fam Med. 2011;24(1):6–15.
2. American Academy of Family Physicians, American Academy of Pediatrics, American College of Physicians, American Osteopathic Association. Joint principles of the patient-centered medical home. 2007. Available from: http://www.pcpcc.net/content/joint-principles-patient-centered-medical-home. Accessed 21 Jan 2012.
3. Iglehart J. No place like home—testing a new model of care delivery. N Engl J Med. 2008;359(12):1200–2.
4. Boult C, Reider L, Frey K, et al. Early effects of "Guided Care" on the quality of health care for multimorbid older persons: a cluster-randomized controlled trial. J Gerontol A Biol Sci Med Sci. 2008; 63(3):321–7.
5. Steiner BD, Denham AC, Ashkin E, Newton WP, Wroth T, Dobson Jr LA. Community Care of North Carolina: improving care through community health networks. Ann Fam Med. 2008;6(4):361–7.
6. Miller WL, Crabtree BF, Nutting PA, Stange KC, Jaén CR. Primary care practice development: a relationship-centered approach. Ann Fam Med. 2010;8 Suppl 1:S68–79.
7. Martin JC, Avant RF, Bowman MA, et al. The future of family medicine: a collaborative project of the family medicine community. Ann Fam Med. 2004;2 Suppl 1:S3–32.
8. Green LA, Graham R, Bagley B, et al. Task force 1: report of the task force on patient expectations, core values, reintegration, and the new model of family medicine. Ann Fam Med. 2004;2 Suppl 1:S33–50.
9. Nutting PA, Miller WL, Crabtree BF, Jaen CR, Stewart EE, Stange KC. Initial lessons from the first national demonstration project on practice transformation to a patient-centered medical home. Ann Fam Med. 2009;7(3):254–60.
10. Ferrante JM, Balasubramanian BA, Hudson SV, Crabtree BF. Principles of the patient-centered medical home and preventive services delivery. Ann Fam Med. 2010;8(2):108–16.
11. Crabtree BF, Nutting PA, Miller WL, Stange KC, Stewart EE, Jaen CR. Summary of the national demonstration project and recommendations for the patient-centered medical home. Ann Fam Med. 2010;8 Suppl 1:S80–90.
12. Jaén CR, Crabtree BF, Palmer RF, et al. Methods for evaluating practice change toward a patient-centered medical home. Ann Fam Med. 2010;8 Suppl 1:S9–20.
13. Martin JC, Avant RF, Bowman MA, Bucholtz JR, Dickinson JR, Evans KL, et al. The future of family medicine: a collaborative project of the family medicine community. Ann Fam Med. 2004;2 Suppl 1:S3–32.
14. Passiment M, Sacks H, Huang G. Medical simulation in medical education: results of an AAMC survey. Washington D.C.: American Association of Medical Colleges; 2011.
15. Tuggy ML. Virtual reality flexible sigmoidoscopy simulator training: impact on resident performance. J Am Board Fam Pract. 1998; 11(6):426–33.
16. Cain JJ, Shirar E. A new method for teaching the repair of perineal trauma of birth. Fam Med. 1996;28(2):107–10.
17. Gerard JM, Thomas SM, Germino KW, Street MH, Burch W, Scalzo AJ. The effect of simulation training on PALS skills among family medicine residents. Fam Med. 2011;43(6):392–9.
18. Pliego JF, Wehbe-Janek H, Rajab MH, Browning JL, Fothergill RE. OB/GYN boot cAMP using high-fidelity human simulators: enhancing residents' perceived competency, confidence in taking a leadership role, and stress hardiness. Simul Healthc. 2008;3(2): 82–9.
19. Stausmire JM. Interdisciplinary development of an adult intubation procedural checklist. Fam Med. 2011;43(4):272–4.
20. Curran VR, Butler R, Duke P, et al. Evaluation of the usefulness of simulated clinical examination in family-medicine residency program. Med Teach. 2007;29(4):406–7.
21. Terry R, Hiester E, James GD. The use of standardized patients to evaluate family medicine resident decision making. Fam Med. 2007;39(4):261–5.
22. Fraser K, Wright B, Girard L, Tworek J, Paget M, et al. Simulation training improves diagnostic performance on a real patient with similar clinical findings. Chest. 2011;139(2):376–81.
23. Pugh CM, Heinrichs WL, Dev P, Srivastava S, Krummel TM. Use of a mechanical simulator to assess pelvic examination skills. JAMA. 2001;286:1021.
24. Euliano TY. Teaching respiratory physiology: clinical correlation with a human patient simulator. J Clin Monit Comput. 2000;16(5–6): 465–70.
25. Zvara DA, Olympio MA, MacGregor DA. Teaching cardiovascular physiology using patient simulation. Acad Med. 2001;76(5):534.
26. Draycott TJ, Crofts JF, Ash JP, et al. Improving neonatal outcome through practical shoulder dystocia training. Obstet Gynecol. 2008;112:14–20.
27. Posner G, Nakajima A. Development of an undergraduate curriculum in obstetrical simulation. Med Educ. 2010;44(5):520–1.
28. Siassakos D, Draycott T, O'Brien K, Kenyon C, Bartlett C, Fox R. Exploratory randomized controlled trial of hybrid obstetric simulation training for undergraduate students. Simul Healthc. 2010; 5(4):193–8.
29. Gordon JA, Oriol NE, Cooper JB. Brining good teaching cases "to life": a simulator-based medical education service. Acad Med. 2004;79(1):23–7.
30. Chumley H, Chessman A, Clements D, et al. The society of teachers of family medicine family medicine clerkship curriculum. Available from: http://www.stfm.org/initiatives/fmcurriculum.cfm. Accessed 16 Jan 2012.
31. Blum RH, Raemer DB, Carroll JS, Dufresne RL, Cooper JB. A method for measuring the effectiveness of simulation-based team training for improving communication skills. Anesth Analg. 2005;100(5):1375–80.
32. Blum RH, Raemer DB, Carroll JS, Sunder N, Felstein DM, Cooper JB. Crisis resource management training for an anesthesia faculty: a new approach to continuing education. Med Educ. 2004;38(1):45–55.
33. Cooke JM, Larsen J, Hamstra SJ, Andreatta PB. Simulation enhances resident confidence in critical care and procedural skills. Fam Med. 2008;40(3):165–7.
34. Hagen MD, Ivins DJ, Puffer JC, et al. Maintenance of certification for family physicians (MC-FP) self-assessment modules (SAMs): the first year. J Am Board Fam Med. 2006;19(4):398–403.
35. Green L, Seifert C. Translation of research into practice: why we can't "just do it". J Am Board Fam Med. 2005;18:541–5.
36. Cooper JB, Barron D, Blum R, et al. Video teleconferencing with realistic simulation for medical education. J Clin Anesth. 2000; 12(3):256–61.

37. Lampotang S, Good ML, Westhorpe R, Hardcastle J, Carovano RG. Logistics of conducting a large number of individual sessions with a full-scale patient simulator at a scientific meeting. J Clin Monit. 1997;13(6):399–407.
38. Cook DA, Hatala R, Brydges R, et al. Technology-enhanced simulation for health professions education, a systematic review and meta-analysis. JAMA. 2011;306(9):978–88.
39. Adler MD, Trainor JL, Siddall VJ, McGaghie WC. Development of an evaluation of high-fidelity simulation case scenarios for pediatric resident education. Ambul Pediatr. 2007;7(2):182–6.
40. Murray DJ, Boulet JR, Kras JF, McAllister JD, Cox TE. A simulation-based acute skills performance assessment for anesthesia training. Anesth Analg. 2005;101(4):1127–34.
41. Devitt JH, Kurrek MM, Cohen MM, Cleave-Hogg D. The validity of performance assessments using simulation. Anesthesiology. 2001;95(1):36–42.
42. Issenberg BS, McGaghie WC, Petrusa ER, Lee GD, Scalese RJ. Features and uses of high-fidelity medical simulations that lead to effective learning: a BEME systematic review. Med Teach. 2005;27(1):10–28.
43. Epstein RM, Hundert EM. Defining and assessing professional competence. JAMA. 2002;287(2):226–35.
44. Carney PA, Dietrich AJ, Freeman Jr DH, Mott LA. A standardized-patient assessment of a continuing medical education program to improve physicians' cancer-control clinical skills. Acad Med. 1995;70(1):52–8.
45. Ziv A, Wolpe PR, Small SD, Glick S. Simulation-based medical education: an ethical imperative. Acad Med. 2003;78(8):783–8.
46. Morgan PJ, Cleave-Hogg D, McIlroy J, Devitt JH. Simulation technology: a comparison of experiential and visual learning for undergraduate medical students. Anesthesiology. 2002;96(1):10–6.
47. Gordon JA, Wilkerson WM, Shaffer DW, Armstrong EG. "Practicing" medicine without risk: students' and educators' responses to high-fidelity patient simulation. Acad Med. 2001;76(5): 469–72.
48. Bond WF, Kostenbader M, McCarthy JF. Prehospital and hospital-based health care providers' experience with a human patient simulator. Prehosp Emerg Care. 2001;5(3):284–7.
49. Nackman GB, Bermann M, Hammond J. Effective use of human simulators in surgical education. J Surg Res. 2003;115(2): 214–8.
50. Gerson LB, Van Dam J. Technology review: the use of simulators for training in GI endoscopy. Gastrointest Endosc. 2004;60(6): 992–1001.
51. Scott DJ, Goova MT, Tesfay ST. A cost-effective proficiency-based knot-tying and suturing curriculum for residency programs. J Surg Res. 2007;144(1):7–15.

Simulation in General Surgery

23

Dimitrios Stefanidis and Paul D. Colavita

Introduction

Surgical training, traditionally governed by the Halstedian apprenticeship model [1], has recently undergone a paradigm shift. Patient safety and ethical concerns of learning new procedures on patients, changing technology, and the need for a more objective assessment of resident skill [2] have shifted the focus of surgical training outside the operating room. This has been made possible by the development of simulators that allow deliberate practice of technical procedures and training on clinical scenarios in a safe, low-stakes environment with the opportunity for constructive performance feedback.

In general surgery, the biggest impetus for implementation of simulator training has been the advent of laparoscopic surgery. This technique creates several challenges otherwise not present in traditional "open" surgeries: the reliance on a two-dimensional display to interpret the three-dimensional operative field, the fixed trocar sites that create a fulcrum effect, the reduced tactile feedback, and the limited range of instrument motion. These techniques require surgeons to overcome a significant learning curve when adopting laparoscopy [3]. The initial experience in the early 1990s with laparoscopic cholecystectomy produced a greater incidence of bile duct injuries compared to open procedures [4]. This initial increase in morbidity was attributed to inadequate training of surgeons adopting the technique and led to the development of laparoscopic simulators for training outside the operating room [1]. Since that time, many improvements have been made in the field of surgical simulation. This chapter presents the current status and future directions of simulation use in general surgery.

Simulators for General Surgery

Given the enormous variety of technical and nontechnical skills required of a general surgeon, a variety of methods and simulator models are used for general surgery training inside and outside the operating room. The two main and distinct methods used include task/procedural and scenario-based training with a clear tendency in recent years to combine the two in hybrid forms to more closely approximate the actual OR environment. For scenario-based training, high-fidelity mannequins and occasionally standardized patients are used as described in other chapters of this book. For task and procedural training, a number of models are available, which in the literature appear with variable names leading to confusion for those unfamiliar with the field. To simplify, surgical simulators can be divided into realistic, virtual reality, and hybrid models. In addition, such models may offer training in specific surgical tasks and/or whole procedures and may have variable levels of fidelity. Nevertheless, a man-made model is not always required, as traditionally animals or human cadavers or parts thereof have also been used as models for training. The latter have comprised the backbone of training models for practicing surgeons being introduced to new techniques and procedures, as they offer high levels of fidelity (Fig. 23.1). Despite their value, their high cost, resource intensive nature, and ethical considerations make these models less than ideal for training [5]. The ongoing

D. Stefanidis, MD, PhD, FACS, FASMBS (✉)
Department of General Surgery,
University of North Carolina–Charlotte,
Charlotte, NC, USA

Department of General Surgery,
Carolinas Simulation Center,
Carolinas HealthCare System, 1025 Morehead Medical Drive,
Suite 300, Charlotte, NC 28203, USA
e-mail: dimitrios.stefanidis@carolinas.org

P.D. Colavita, MD
Department of Gastrointestinal and Minimally Invasive Surgery,
Carolinas Medical Center,
Charlotte, NC, USA

Department of General Surgery,
Carolinas Medical Center,
1025 Morehead Medical Drive,
Charlotte, NC 28204, USA
e-mail: paul.d.colavita@carolinas.org

A.I. Levine et al. (eds.), *The Comprehensive Textbook of Healthcare Simulation*,
DOI 10.1007/978-1-4614-5993-4_23,

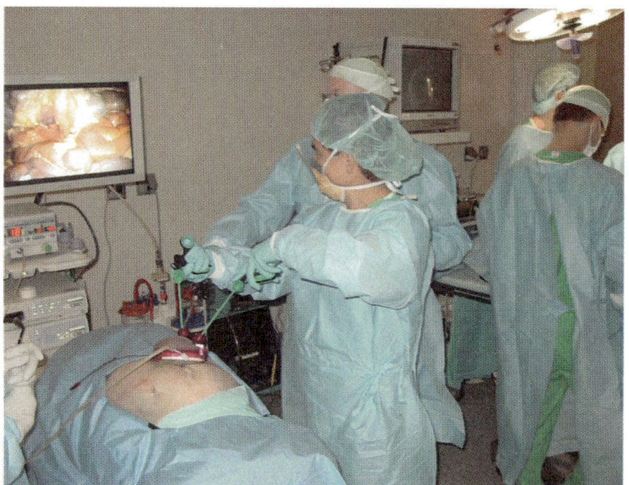

Fig. 23.1 Surgery residents and attendings practicing laparoscopic colectomy on a cadaver model

development and refinement of simulators is expected to minimize, if not eliminate, the need for such models. Still, animal parts such as pig's feet or chicken breasts that can be used to practice suturing are fairly inexpensive and easy to acquire. These are likely to continue providing a popular "low-tech" platform for training in these tasks.

Physical Part-Task Trainers

Popular part-task trainers used in general surgery include a variety of models that allow training in chest tube placement, cricothyroidotomy, central line placement (subclavian, jugular, and femoral), arterial line placement, thoracentesis and paracentesis, ultrasound techniques, and several biopsy techniques. Examples of these products include: the Focused Abdominal Sonography in Trauma (FAST) Exam Real Time Ultrasound Training Model (Blue Phantom, Redmond, WA, USA), Arterial Puncture Wrist (Limbs & Things, Bristol, UK), IOUSFAN (Kyoto Kagaku, Kyoto, Japan), SimMan (Leardal, Wappingers Falls, NY, USA), TraumaMan (see Fig. 23.2), CentraLineMan, and FemoraLineMan (Simulab Corporation, Seattle, WA, USA). Home-made models are not uncommon to address skills for which a commercial product is not available. Examples include, but are not limited to, a laparotomy model using foam, bubble wrap, plastic wrap, and various fabrics to inexpensively replicate the peritoneal contents and abdominal wall [6], which has been adapted in the ACS/APDS surgical skills curriculum [7]; an abscess model using mock purulent material injected into a chicken breast [8]; and a laparoscopic common bile duct exploration model using vesical catheters [9].

For training in laparoscopy, the most commonly used and widely available simulators are realistic part-task trainers, also known as benchtop, video, box, or pelvic trainers. These trainers have been developed to provide inexpensive and reproducible training in laparoscopy and generally include a confined space (box) that resembles the abdominal cavity, an imaging system (video camera, light source, and monitor), access ports, and laparoscopic equipment (see Fig. 23.3). Historically, the Yale Top Gun laparoscopic skills and suturing course developed the first task trainer and included three tasks: the rope pass, cup drop, and triangle transfer drill [3]. Several other models and tasks have been developed subsequently with variable penetration in the market. The Southwestern stations were an expansion of the Top Gun tasks and included a suturing task with foam and a task for placing numbered and lettered blocks on a checkerboard [10]. Laparoscopic models for simulation include the Fundamentals of Laparoscopic Surgery (FLS) Laparoscopic Trainer Box (Venture Technologies, North Billerica, MA, USA), Portable Laparoscopic Task Trainers (Ethicon, Somerville, NJ, USA), Helago Laparoscopic Trainer (Limbs & Things, Bristol, UK), and the Minimally Invasive Training System (3-Dmed, Franklin, OH, USA).

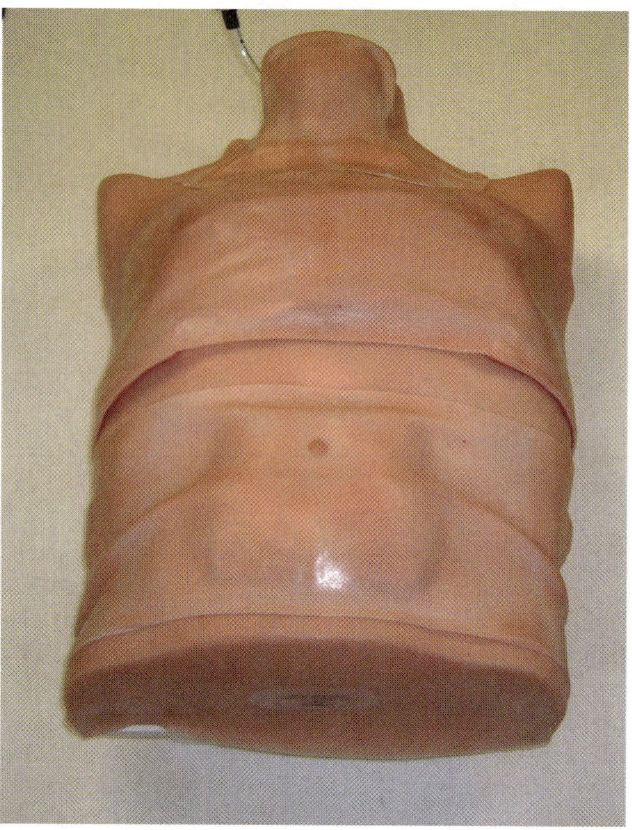

Fig. 23.2 TraumaMan (Simulab Corporation, Seattle, WA, USA) allows trainees to practice cricothyroidotomy, chest tube insertion, pericardiocentesis, needle decompression, percutaneous tracheostomy, diagnostic peritoneal lavage, and IV cutdown (Photo from authors' collection)

The Fundamentals of Laparoscopic Surgery (FLS) program deserves special mention. This program was developed under the auspices of the Society of American Gastrointestinal and

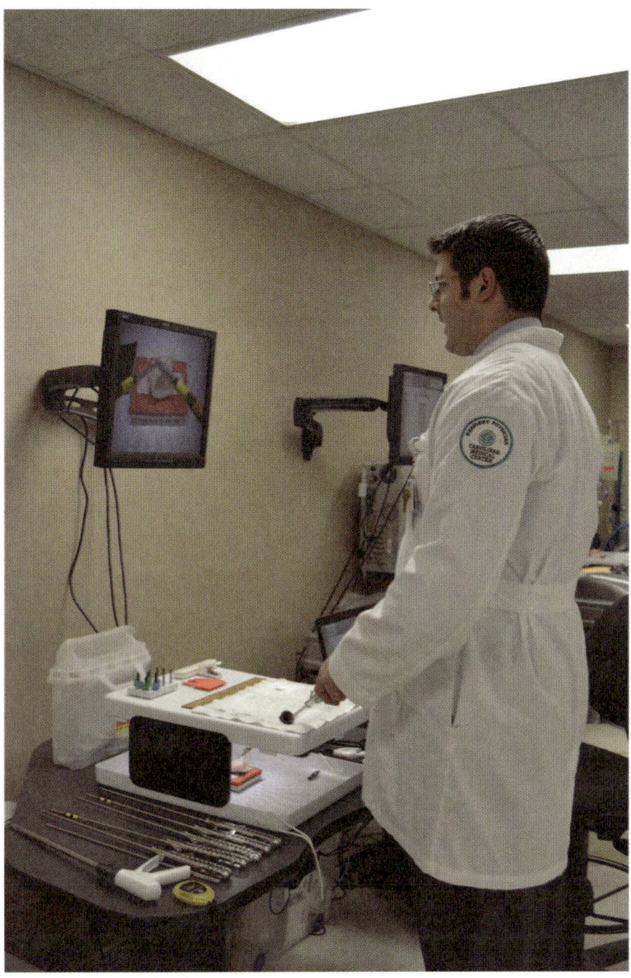

Fig. 23.3 Surgery resident practices laparoscopic suturing on a box trainer

Endoscopic Surgeons (SAGES) and the American College of Surgeons (ACS) and was based on the prior work of McGill University researchers [11–14]. FLS is an Internet-based program designed to provide and verify the fundamental skills and knowledge necessary for effective and safe laparoscopic surgery and includes knowledge and skills components. It includes modules on preoperative, intraoperative, and postoperative considerations during basic laparoscopic procedures and potential complications, as well as manual skill practice on five tasks: peg transfer, precision cutting, placement of a ligating loop, and suturing using extracorporeal and intracorporeal knot tying [15] (see Fig. 23.4). This program has undergone rigorous validation [16] and is currently available to all general surgery residency programs in the USA through an industry-supported grant [17]. Importantly, general surgery residents are now required to obtain FLS certification to be eligible to take the qualifying examination for the American Board of Surgery [16]. This is the first inclusion of simulation as a component of board certification in general surgery.

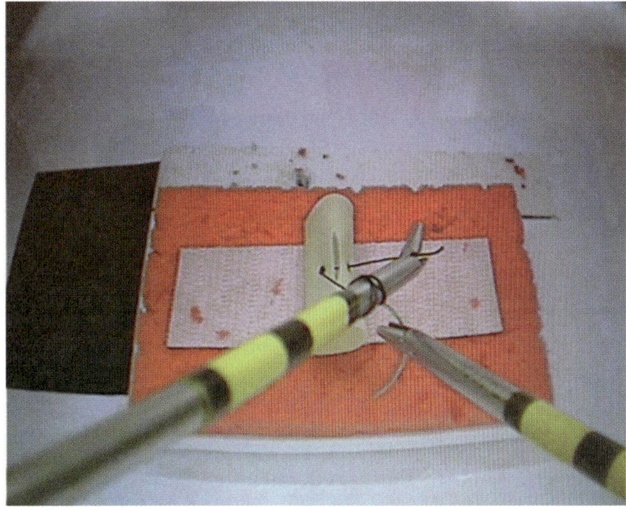

Fig. 23.4 Screenshot of intracorporeal knot tying on a box trainer

Virtual Reality Part-Task Trainers

Compared with realistic simulators, virtual reality (VR) simulators offer different advantages to the learner. These systems are configurable (different levels of difficulty), allow for multiple anatomic variations to simulate pathology and aberrant anatomy [3], and enable repetitive practice of procedures at minimal cost (i.e., the same task/procedure can be performed an infinite number of times without the need for supplies or disposables). Additionally, VR simulators do not require the presence of an instructor as they often provide built-in tutorials and multiple metrics that can be used for learner performance assessment and feedback. Their disadvantages include high acquisition and maintenance costs, the need for periodic software and hardware updates, suboptimal realism, and the potential for learning bad habits in the absence of an instructor to give feedback.

The first and best validated VR simulator, the Minimally Invasive Surgical Trainer-Virtual Reality (MIST-VR; Mentice, Gothenburg, Sweden), is currently available as part of LapSim. Popular VR systems include the LapMentor (Simbionix, Cleveland, OH, USA), CAE LaparoscopyVR (CAE Healthcare, Montreal, Canada), and LapSim (Surgical Science, Göteborg, Sweden) and offer a variety of laparoscopic procedures that extend beyond general surgery. Virtual reality simulators also exist for training in flexible endoscopy including upper endoscopy, colonoscopy, and bronchoscopy and are addressed in other chapters. Examples include the CAE EndoscopyVR Simulator (CAE Healthcare, Montreal, Canada), the GI Mentor (Simbionix, Cleveland, OH, USA), the Surgical Science colonoscopy simulator (Surgical Science, Göteborg, Sweden), and the Endo TS-1 (Olympus Keymed, Southend, UK). Basic endoscopic skills as well as biopsy, polypectomy, and bleeding control techniques can be practiced on these devices. At the time of writing this chapter, SAGES is developing the Fundamentals of Endoscopic Surgery (FES), which is a VR-based program similar to FLS that aims to teach and assess the endoscopic skills of surgery residents. The authors anticipate that FES, like FLS, will eventually become an integral part of the general surgery resident curriculum.

Other VR systems available for training in general surgery involve endovascular techniques and procedures. Systems such as the Procedicus VIST (Mentice, Göteborg, Sweden), ANGIO Mentor (Simbionix, Cleveland, OH, USA), and SimSuite (Medical Simulation Corporation, Denver, CO, USA) provide the opportunity to practice endovascular procedures and a means of skill assessment. Moreover, some of these systems allow for the import of actual patient imaging data that can then be used for practice of a planned intervention before its actual performance on the patient. Evidence suggests that patient-specific practice may be superior to generic practice when using these simulators [18].

Other VR simulators that deserve mention include the CAE VIMEDIX ultrasound simulator (CAE Healthcare, Montreal, Canada), which besides providing an excellent platform for training in echocardiography also offers FAST modules that are very useful for training surgery residents to recognize intra-abdominal injuries in trauma patients. In addition, laparoscopic ultrasound compatible models (e.g., IOUSFAN, Kyoto Kagaku, Kyoto, Japan) are being developed, which can be combined with liver biopsy and radiofrequency ablation (RFA) techniques.

With the recent popularity of robotic surgery, especially in disciplines such as urology and gynecology, new VR simulators have emerged such as the Mimic dV-Trainer (Mimic Technologies Inc, Seattle, WA) available to the users of the da Vinci robotic system. Other home-made training systems in robotic surgery exist as well, using FLS-type tasks [19]. Multidisciplinary efforts in surgery are currently ongoing to create the Fundamentals of Robotic Surgery (FRS). Hybrid simulators, such as the ProMIS (CAE Healthcare, Montreal, Canada), which combine realistic instruments and imaging with a virtual reality interface and metrics (motion tracking), are also popular.

Finally, while the majority of available simulators focus on laparoscopy, the increasing dominance of laparoscopic procedures over their open counterparts has created a need for training in open procedures. To address this need, open-surgery VR platforms have been developed such as the SurgSim Trainers (SimQuest LLC, Silver Springs, MD, USA), the Phantom Desktop (SensAble Technologies, Wilmington, MA, USA), and the CyberGlove II (Meta Motion, San Francisco, CA, USA). Initial experience indicates that the creation of VR systems for open surgery is considerably more difficult than for laparoscopic procedures [5].

Evidence in Support of Simulation in General Surgery

In a landmark 2000 study, Scott and colleagues [10] demonstrated that simulator-acquired skill successfully transferred to the operating room. In this randomized controlled study, junior general surgery residents trained on basic laparoscopic tasks using the five UT-Southwestern video trainers, and their performance during a laparoscopic cholecystectomy was compared with a control group. Simulator-trained residents performed better in the OR than controls demonstrating the value of simulator training for the acquisition of laparoscopic skill [10]. In 2002, another landmark, randomized, double-blinded study demonstrated transferability of laparoscopic skill acquired on the MIST-VR simulator to the operating room. Virtual reality-trained residents were 29% faster and six times less likely to commit an error compared with non-VR-trained residents during gallbladder dissection. Additionally, the non-VR-trained residents were nine times more likely to transiently fail to make progress [20]. Since that time, several additional good quality studies have demonstrated the value of training on surgical simulators [21, 22].

A systematic review of ten randomized controlled trials [23] confirmed that simulator-acquired surgical skill transfers to the operating room but also recommended additional better quality studies. More recently, another randomized controlled trial demonstrated that junior surgery residents performed better in the operating room compared with controls after they trained to proficiency on the FLS tasks [24]. Importantly, after only 2.5 h of supervised practice and 5 h of individual practice, the FLS-trained first- and second-year residents performed in the OR at the level of third- and fourth-year residents as measured in a prior study [25]. Several other studies have demonstrated the value of available endoscopy and angiography simulators [26–29]. While the evidence documenting the impact of simulator training on clinical performance is adequate, the majority of published studies report T2 translational outcomes (impact of training on learner performance), and T3 outcomes (impact of training on patient outcomes) are sparse. A group from Northwestern University demonstrated that residents who received internal jugular and subclavian training on simulators inserted central lines in the medical intensive care unit with significantly fewer needle passes, catheter adjustments, arterial punctures, and with higher success rates than traditionally trained residents (historical controls) [30]. They then conducted a before/after observational study in the medical intensive care unit on the incidence of catheter-related and bloodstream infections over 32 months and found a 85% reduction in catheter-related bloodstream infections after the simulation-based trained residents entered the intensive care unit (0.50 infections per 1,000 catheter days) compared with both the same unit before the intervention (3.20 infections per 1,000 catheter days,

$P=0.001$) and a comparison intensive care unit in the same hospital throughout the study period (5.03 infections per 1,000 catheter days, $P=0.001$) [31].

While the previous studies were not done with surgery residents, the procedural task assessed clearly has relevance to surgery. A recently published, more surgery-specific study demonstrated improved operative performance and time, as well as improved patient outcomes regarding intraoperative and postoperative complications after laparoscopic inguinal hernia repair for residents who trained to expert levels on an inguinal hernia simulator compared with a control group in a randomized controlled trial [32]. It should be noted, however, that the transfer of skill acquired on surgical simulators to the clinical environment is not complete. Several studies have demonstrated that, when using a proficiency-based simulator training paradigm, while novices can achieve expert-derived performance criteria on the simulator, their performance lags that of experts in the OR [33–35]. This phenomenon is likely multifactorial and requires further investigation [35]. A comprehensive review of all the studies in support of simulation-based training is beyond the scope of this chapter, and readers are referred to excellent review articles [23, 36, 37]. Suffice it to say that the evidence for simulation in general surgery is mounting and as such, its use has expanded.

Performance Assessment Using Simulators

Besides providing an effective training tool, simulators make it possible to objectively assess learner performance. A variety of assessment tools and simulator performance metrics currently are used in general surgery, and efforts are ongoing to refine them. The most often used metrics in surgical simulation include task duration and performance error measurements. These metrics provide robust and relevant information and have been incorporated into the FLS program. In the latter, learners practice repetitively until they reach a level of efficient and error-free performance as defined by task-specific metrics of time and errors. Nevertheless, while these traditional metrics have stood the test of time and are easy to obtain, concerns exist that they may not be the ideal or the only metrics for performance assessment on simulators. The rationale is that these metrics do not provide insight regarding the effort the individual had to invest to achieve a specific level of performance or whether learning has been completed [38, 39].

Several research groups have therefore suggested that additional performance metrics be used. Limb kinematics (i.e., trajectory, velocity, and acceleration) have probably gathered the most attention and have been shown to distinguish performers of variable skill in several studies [40, 41]. Such metrics can be obtained on physical simulators using specialized recording systems, such as the Imperial College Surgical Assessment Device (ICSAD) that uses an electromagnetic tracking system for motion tracking [40] or the ProMIS simulator (CAE Healthcare, Montreal, Canada) that tracks motion from the instrument tips [41] and are readily available on virtual reality simulators. Unfortunately, there is limited evidence about the importance of such metrics for learning. In a prior prospective study, 60% of novices who trained to proficiency in a basic laparoscopic task were able to achieve motion metrics goals easier than time goals indicating that the incorporation of motion metrics into training goals had limited effectiveness for skill acquisition [42]. In a very recent study, the authors demonstrated in a randomized controlled trial that the use of motion metrics as performance goals did not lead to improved transfer of skill to the OR compared with time goals alone or in combination (Stefanidis et al., Does the Incorporation of Motion Metrics Into the Existing FLS Metrics Lead to Improved Skill Acquisition on Simulators? publication pending).

Besides the aforementioned metrics, additional metrics have been proposed for simulator performance assessment with promising results. These either reflect the effort that the learner had to invest to achieve a level of performance (such as the NASA-TLX workload assessment tool) [43], rely on the measurement of distinct expert characteristics (such as eye tracking) [44], or use secondary task measures that reflect multitasking ability [38, 45]. In a study by Stefanidis et al., training of novices to automaticity using secondary task performance as a training goal in addition to time and errors led to better transfer of simulator-acquired skill to the OR compared with traditional proficiency-based training alone [46]. Such metrics may prove important to augment skill acquisition on surgical simulators and minimize the incomplete transfer of skill to the OR environment.

Besides using these metrics, surgical performance can also be reliably assessed by an experienced observer. In fact, this type of assessment may be preferable for some skills, as it provides qualitative information on learner performance that can then be provided as summative and formative feedback to the learner [47, 48]. Furthermore, these instruments are versatile as they can often be used for similar tasks. This type of assessment is frequently criticized as it relies on subjective ratings, unclear operational definitions of performance, and ambiguity in responding [5]; it is therefore imperative that the reliability and validity of such instruments be proved before their use for evaluation [47]. Observer ratings are typically provided on global rating scales, visual analog scales, checklists, or a combination of these. When completed by experts, current evidence suggests that global rating scales are superior to checklists for the evaluation of technical skills [49, 50].

Some authors suggest that checklists and visual analog scales should not be included in technical skills assessment, as they fail to enhance the effectiveness of performance assessment compared with global rating scales alone [47, 49]. On the other hand, checklists may provide important, more specific information for formative feedback on learner performance that could augment learning. Validated rating scales for technical skill assessment have been developed for open, laparoscopic, and endoscopic skills. The objective structured assessment of technical skill (OSATS) [48], the global operative assessment of laparoscopic skills (GOALS) [47], and global assessment of gastrointestinal endoscopic skill (GAGES) [51] have been demonstrated to be valid and reliable measures of performance and have been used widely in the literature for this purpose. However, the exact relationship of observer ratings with other more objective performance metrics is not well understood and requires further study.

Skills Curriculum Development

Despite the evidence supporting simulation training in general surgery, the sole availability of a simulator does not guarantee its educational effectiveness. The most important ingredient is the curriculum. More importantly, most experts in the field advise that simulators are acquired or developed based on the objectives of the curriculum [52, 53]. Early experience with simulators in general surgery supports this notion, as in the absence of a structured curriculum, most simulators, no matter how expensive or sophisticated ended up collecting dust. Curriculum development starts with a needs assessment and gap analysis, a selection of objectives and instructional methods and ongoing evaluation of its effectiveness and optimization based on accumulated experiences [54]. It is also imperative to assess, at the beginning of the curriculum, the required resources for its successful implementation. Besides associated costs, equipment (including simulators), and supplies, the need for supervising faculty and/or other personnel should not be overlooked. Importantly, in the case of residents, this translates into identifying protected time and implementing external motivators for participation (both for residents and teaching faculty). In the authors' experience, the latter two factors have been the most challenging [55].

Several ingredients guarantee a successful skills curriculum; foremost is deliberate practice for the purpose of effectively improving specific aspects of an individual's performance [56]. According to Duvivier et al. [57], the characteristics of deliberate practice in medical education include: (a) repetitive performance of intended cognitive or psychomotor skills, (b) rigorous skills assessment, (c) provision of specific performance feedback, and (d) the ongoing effort to improve one's performance. The same authors suggest that the personal skills needed to successfully develop clinical skills include planning (organize work in a structured way), concentration/dedication (long attention span), repetition/revision (strong tendency to practice), and study style/self-reflection (tendency to self-regulate learning). The applicability and value of deliberate practice for surgical skill training has been demonstrated for surgical tasks on a virtual reality simulator [58]. Important ingredients for deliberate practice include internal and external motivation of learners. Internal motivation is the most important driving force for learning but is unique to each trainee and difficult to modify externally. Nevertheless, several external motivators can help improve learning on simulators. These may include practice time protected from other training responsibilities, healthy competition among trainees with performance goals and recognition of the best performers, rewarding excellent performance, and requiring the achievement of specific performance scores before the trainee is permitted to work in the clinical environment [59]. Mandatory participation of surgery residents in simulation training is critical to a curriculum, as resident participation has been shown to range from 7 to 14% in voluntary curricula [55, 60].

Feedback

Performance feedback helps learners improve, but the timing of its administration is also important. Several studies [61–65] have shown that external feedback versus no feedback leads to improved skill acquisition and retention, independent of the practiced task. Furthermore, the provision of summative feedback (at the end of performance) has been demonstrated to be superior to concurrent feedback (during practice trials) [61, 66]; the latter may in fact inhibit performance if excessive [61]. The benefit of video tutorials for surgical skill acquisition has also been well documented. CD-ROM tutorials have been shown to effectively transfer cognitive information for motor skill learning [67]. Video tutorial viewings have been shown to augment laparoscopic performance on simulators [68] and hasten the attainment of proficiency [61] especially when provided before and during training as needed [69]. Importantly, computer-based video instruction has been shown to be as effective as expert feedback for the retention of simulator-acquired laparoscopic suturing and knot-tying skills [62].

Training Intervals

Practice distribution can also be optimized to enhance learning. It has been established that practice can initiate neural processes that continue to evolve many hours after practice has ended [70]. Related to surgical skills, this has been supported in a randomized, controlled trial that revealed microvascular anastomosis skills to be better retained and transferred when taught in a distributed manner, as opposed to a massed (all training provided in one session) manner [71]. In a large meta-analysis, it was noted that simple tasks are better acquired with shorter inter-training intervals, while more complex tasks required longer intervals for optimal learning [72]. For the creation of an end-to-side vascular anastomosis, no difference in performance was demonstrated 4 months after training when the skill was acquired in weekly versus monthly training sessions [73].

Proficiency-Based Curricula

Proficiency-based curricula deserve special mention. Such curricula set training goals for learners that are derived from expert performance. Unlike traditional training paradigms that define training duration based on time or number of repetitions, proficiency-based curricula tailor training to individual needs and lead to homogenous skill acquisition. The superiority of proficiency-based training compared with these traditional training methods is well supported in the literature [5, 33, 53, 74, 75]. With known goals, the trainee can compare his or her performance to these targets for immediate feedback. This promotes deliberate practice, enhances motivation, and improves skill acquisition [69, 76]. In a randomized trial by Madan and colleagues, residents who trained with performance goals outperformed residents who practiced the same amount of time but without goals in eight simulated laparoscopic tasks [77]. In another study, Gauger and colleagues [78] demonstrated that the use of specific performance targets and feedback improved the ability of novice surgeons to attain high levels of proficiency in both simulated tasks and actual operative performance. They also demonstrated that if learners are left to determine their own proficiency targets and practice needs, less practice occurs and the level of accomplishment is lower [78]. Furthermore, the establishment of performance goals on simulators has been shown to increase resident attendance and participation in training programs [76] and proficiency-based training to lead to improved retention of simulator-acquired skill [34].

Examples of simulator-based curricula widely used in general surgery include the American College of Surgeons and the Association of Program Directors in Surgery (ACS/APDS) national surgical skills curriculum (Table 23.1) that addresses the needs of general surgery residents. This proficiency-based skills curriculum is web-based and readily accessible to all. It includes a variety of simulations to achieve the desired learning objectives and was introduced in three phases. Phase I includes 20 modules that address basic surgical skills, and phase II includes 15 advanced procedures modules. Each of these modules includes objectives, assumptions, suggested readings, descriptions of steps for specific skills and common errors, an expert performance video, recommendations for guided practice, and information on station setup and use. Many modules also include tools for the verification of proficiency to assess the readiness of individual residents for the operating room. A faculty guidebook provides descriptions of information on

Table 23.1 (ACS/APDS) National surgical skills curriculum

Phase 1: Basic/core skills and tasks
Advanced laparoscopy skills
Advanced tissue handling: flaps, skin grafts
Airway management
Asepsis and instrument identification
Basic laparoscopy skills
Bone fixation and casting
Central line insertion and arterial lines
Chest tube and thoracentesis
Colonoscopy
Hand-sewn gastrointestinal anastomosis
Inguinal anatomy
Knot tying
Laparotomy opening and closure
Stapled gastrointestinal anastomosis
Surgical biopsy
Suturing
Tissue handling, dissection, and wound closure
Upper endoscopy
Urethral and suprapubic catheterization
Vascular anastomosis
Phase 2: Advanced procedures
Gastric resection and peptic ulcer disease
Laparoscopic appendectomy
Laparoscopic inguinal hernia repair
Laparoscopic right colon resection
Laparoscopic sigmoid resection
Laparoscopic Nissen fundoplication
Laparoscopic ventral hernia repair
Laparoscopic ventral/incisional hernia repair
Laparoscopic/open bile duct exploration
Laparoscopic/open cholecystectomy
Laparoscopic/open splenectomy
Open inguinal/femoral hernia repair
Open right colon resection
Parathyroidectomy/thyroidectomy
Sentinel node biopsy and axillary lymph node dissection
Phase 3: Team-based skills
Laparoscopic crisis
Laparoscopic troubleshooting
Latex allergy anaphylaxis
Patient handoff
Postoperative hypotension
Postoperative MI (cardiogenic shock)
Postoperative pulmonary embolus
Preoperative briefing
Retained sponge on postoperative chest X-ray
Trauma team training

supplies, station design, vendors, products, and laboratory setup, as well as information on recommended teaching times. Phase III includes ten modules that address team-based skills, including scenarios in the OR, surgical ICU, and other settings. A faculty guidebook for team training is provided, and each module includes case information, patient data, faculty and resident information, and debriefing and assessment tools. Important concepts in team training are addressed, such as the development of expert team members versus expert teams, communication (critical language, closed loop), leadership, coping with stress, decision-making, and situational awareness [79, 80].

Another example is the Advanced Trauma Operative Management (ATOM) course. The ATOM course is grounded in social cognitive theory and is designed to increase students' knowledge, self-efficacy, and surgical skill to manage penetrating trauma for 12 injuries in a porcine model [81–83]. Developed in 1998, the ATOM program came under the auspices of the American College of Surgeons Committee on Trauma in 2008. The course consists of pre-course reading materials, a pre-and post-course examination, and a 1-day on-site curriculum of lectures and simulations. The pre-course materials include a textbook and a CD-ROM that demonstrate the surgical repair of penetrating injuries to the abdomen and chest. Students are expected to completely manage the injuries, which includes identifying the injuries, developing management plans, and using surgical repair techniques. During the 1-day session, six 30-min lectures about the repair of penetrating injuries to individual organs are presented in the morning. In the afternoon, the students participate in a simulation session of penetrating trauma scenarios in a porcine model. Students are evaluated on their knowledge, self-efficacy, and psychomotor ability [81, 82]. Table 23.2 contains an abbreviated skills curriculum outline, employed at the authors' institution for weekly 90-min training sessions. Performance criteria for PGY-I and PGY-II residents, as well as the curriculum structure for PGY-II residents, are included in Table 23.2.

Nontechnical Skills and Team Training

While most of the research and development in surgical simulation has focused on technical skills, simulation for the teaching of nontechnical skills and team training of surgeons has recently gained significant attention. Nontechnical skills consist of cognitive (decision-making, planning, and situation awareness) and interpersonal skills (communication, teamwork, and leadership). Nontechnical skills complement technical skills to create a safe operating room [84].

Poor nontechnical skills have been associated with increased technical skills errors [85], wrong-site surgery [86], and incorrect instrument and sponge counts [87]. Importantly, breakdowns in nontechnical skills have been shown to result in increased patient morbidity and mortality [88]. Poor timing of communication and exclusion of key team members from communication have been reported to contribute to the failure of nearly one-third of all operating room communications [89]. The current operating room culture has also been shown to discourage members from alerting other members to potential threats [90] with a negative impact on patient safety [91]. Many experts believe that the operating staff is not an expert team, but rather a team of experts who prefer multi-professional practice over interprofessional collaboration [92, 93]. Indeed, surgeons and anesthesiologists have been reported to view an operating room team as a group of specialists working within their own boundaries [94]. Furthermore, the perception of teamwork ability is flawed. A previous study showed that, in the same interaction, surgeons believed almost twice as often as nurses that quality teamwork occurred [95].

Similar to technical skills, nontechnical skills can also be acquired through training [96]. Simulation has been shown to be superior to lectures for the transfer of necessary teamwork behaviors to the clinical setting [97]. High-fidelity simulation has been shown to improve team-based attitudes in trainees, as well as teamwork within the operating room [98, 99]. High-fidelity simulation not only allows for practice and refinement of cooperative patient care but also provides the opportunity to manage rare events and learn the consequences of correct and incorrect management [100]. Surgical team training, in general, has been shown to improve cognitive, affective, process, and performance outcomes through many modalities [97, 101, 102].

High-fidelity patient simulators described in previous chapters of this book are also used for team training in general surgery (see Fig. 23.5). The ability to use these simulators, to replicate an immersive operating room, critical care, or trauma bay environment together with the opportunity to debrief the learner at the end of the simulation session provide a very effective teaching tool for surgeon educators. An example of team training scenarios used widely in general surgery is the phase III modules of the ACS/APDS national skills curriculum described previously in this chapter [103]. In addition, home-made scenarios allow teaching programs to expand their curriculum and focus on areas of resident weakness and need for improvement.

Several tools have also been developed and validated for the assessment of nontechnical skills in the operating room. Examples include the Oxford NOTECHS system [104–106] which was developed by an aviation instrument used to evaluate nontechnical skills (Fig. 23.6).

Table 23.2 CMC general surgery skills curriculum outline

The skills curriculum at Carolinas Medical Center consists of a combination of proficiency-based training in open, laparoscopic, and endoscopic skills on surgical simulators, scenario-based training on high-fidelity patient simulators, and hands-on interactive lectures.
PGY-I–III residents participate in both training and testing sessions. PGY-IV and PGY-V residents participate in testing sessions only unless their performance does not meet the set performance criteria; then they resume training. Residents who achieve the level assigned goals but fail to demonstrate proficiency during testing sessions are required to resume training until they demonstrate proficiency on simulators again.
Training is mandatory and tailored to year of training. Performance data are collected and analyzed on a quarterly basis. Residents are provided feedback on their progress and on how their performance relates to the average performance in their level.
Performance Criteria by Level
PGY-I
1. *Basic laparoscopic skills* (FLS tasks 1–3 and LapMentor VR basic Skills 1–8)
(a) Expert level + 2 standard deviations
2. *Open skills* (suturing and knot-tying tasks, APDS/ ACS skills curriculum modules and UTSW tasks)
(a) Expert level + 2 standard deviations
3. *Endoscopic skills* (basic skills and first 3 cases of EGD modules on VR endoscopy trainer)
(a) Completion of 10 repetitions on each module
4. *Performance during scenarios on patient simulator* (APDS/ACS skills curriculum modules and home-made modules, assessment using scenario specific checklists)
5. *Faculty evaluation forms for the following procedures* (direct observation, 20 total)
(a) Central/arterial line, chest tube placement, open inguinal hernia, lap/open appendectomy, skin and soft tissue procedures (excisions, biopsies)
6. *Traditional rotation evaluations by faculty*
PGY-II
1. *Advanced laparoscopic skills* (FLS tasks 4 and 5 suturing, Endostitch, VR suturing module, VR lap chole and VR lap ventral)
(a) Expert + 1 standard deviation
(b) Completion of 5 repetitions of VR lap chole and ventral (all 6 modules)
2. *Open skills* (difficult level)
(a) Expert level + 1 standard deviation
3. *Endoscopic skills* (colonoscopy, bronchoscopy)
(a) Completion of 10 repetitions on each module
(i) Expert levels (case 6 of colonoscopy)
4. *Performance during scenarios on patient simulator* (checklists)
5. *Faculty evaluation forms for the following procedures* (20 total)
(a) Lap chole/ IOC, bowel resection/anastomosis, open/lap ventral hernia, lap/open appy, EGD/colonoscopy (GAGES assessment form), breast procedures
6. *Traditional rotation evaluations by faculty*
Example of Skills Curriculum Structure: PGY-II
Cognitive Skills
Fundamentals of surgery curriculum (continued from PGY-I if not already completed)
Fundamentals of laparoscopic surgery (continued from PGY-I if not already completed)
SAGES procedural videos
Procedural Skills
Simulation Center: Procedural side
Proficiency-based training on the following skills:
FLS tasks 4 and 5 (suturing) and Endostitch (both in FLS box)
APDS-I Module 18: Advanced laparoscopy skills (complementary)
VR lap suturing modules (several) on LapMentor
Advanced open suturing and knot-tying curriculum (UTSW 6 tasks)
VR lap cholecystectomy 5 repetitions of each of the 6 modules on LapMentor
VR lap ventral hernia 5 repetitions of each of the 6 modules on LapMentor
Colonoscopy modules on VR endoscopic simulator
APDS I Module 16: Colonoscopy (complementary)
Bronchoscopy modules on VR endoscopic simulator
Also:
APDS-I Module 19: Hand-sewn gastrointestinal anastomosis

(continued)

Table 23.2 (continued)

APDS-I Module 20: Stapled gastrointestinal anastomosis
FAST exam (US simulator)
US-guided percutaneous biopsy of soft tissue lesions
Vivarium: Live workshop (animal/cadaver)
APDS-II Module 1: Lap ventral hernia repair
APDS-II Module 6: Intestinal stomas
APDS-II Module 9: Sentinel node biopsy and axillary lymph node dissection
APDS-I Module 10: Open inguinal/femoral hernia repair (repeat)
APDS-II Module 13: Laparoscopic/open cholecystectomy/liver biopsy
Lap/open lysis of adhesions
Simulation Center: Patient Simulation Side
APDS-III Module 1: Teamwork in the trauma bay
APDS-III Module 3: Laparoscopic crisis
APDS-III Module 5: Laparoscopic troubleshooting
APDS-III Module 10: Retained sponge on post-op X-ray
Hypoxemic ICU patient/ventilator management
Oliguric ICU patient
Skills Maintenance
If residents do not demonstrate proficiency in PGY-I tasks during OSCE testing, they will have to retrain to proficiency.

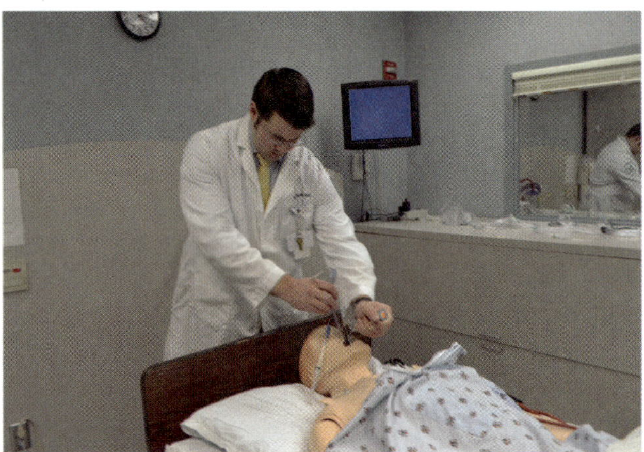

Fig. 23.5 Surgery resident practices intubation on a high-fidelity patient simulator

Work in Progress and Future Directions of Surgical Simulation

Medical Student Curriculum

As described in this chapter, simulation in general surgery has significantly advanced over the past decade. While most of these accomplishments have centered on the training of general surgery residents, there are several ongoing activities to address training needs across the educational spectrum. Such efforts include the development of the ACS/APDS/ASE (Association for Surgical Education) Entering Surgery Resident Prep Curriculum for graduating medical students who have matched with surgery residency programs. This curriculum aims to improve the knowledge and skill of fourth-year medical students transitioning to surgical residency programs [80]. In addition, the ACS/ASE Medical Student Simulation-Based Surgical Skills Curriculum for all medical students in years 1–3 is nearing completion. This curriculum addresses cognitive, clinical, and technical skills relative to surgery that all medical students should acquire, regardless of intended specialty, and should be available soon to medical schools [80].

Practicing Surgeon Curriculum and Assessment

Besides medical students and residents, efforts are also addressing the needs of practicing surgeons for the acquisition and maintenance of surgical knowledge and skills. These activities involve design and implementation of surgical skills courses, verification of knowledge and skills using valid and reliable assessment methods, and support for surgeons following participation in courses. While many of these activities traditionally have been industry-sponsored and conducted at institutions with adequate resources and available surgical expertise, simulation-based surgical skills courses focusing on new procedures are now offered to surgeons at the ACS annual clinical congresses.

For the assessment of knowledge and skills of the course participants, a 5-level verification model of the ACS Division of Education has been implemented: level I – verification of attendance; level II – verification of satisfactory completion of course objectives; level III – verification of knowledge and

Operating-theatre team Non-technical Skills (NOTECHS) assessment tool

Leadership and management	
Leadership	Involves/reflects on suggestions/visible/accessible/inspires/motivates/coaches
Maintenance of standards	Subscribes to standards/monitors compliance to standards/intervenes if deviates with team approval/ demonstrates desire to achieve high standards
Planning and preparation	Team participation in planning/plan is shared/understanding confirmed/projects/changes in consultation
Workload management	Distributes tasks/monitors/reviews/tasks are prioritised/allots adequate time/responds to stress
Authority and assertiveness	Advocates position/values team input/takes control/persistent/appropriate assertiveness
Teamwork and cooperation	
Team building/maintaining	Relaxed/supportive/open/inclusive/polite/friendly/use of humour/does not compete
Support of others	Helps others/offers assistance/gives feedback
Understanding team needs	Listens to others/recognises ability of team/condition of others considered/gives personal feedback
Conflict solving	Keeps calm in conflicts/suggests conflict solutions/concentrates on what is right
Problem-solving and decision-making	
Definition and diagnosis	Uses all resources/analytical decision-making/reviews factors with team
Option generation	Suggests alternative option/asks for options/reviews outcomes/comfirms options
Risk assessment	Estimates risks/considers risk in terms of team capabilities/estimates patient outcome
Outcome review	Reviews outcomes/reviews new options/objective, constructive and timely reviews/makes time for review/seeks feedback from others/conducts post-treatment review
Situation awareness	
Notice	Considers all team elements/asks for or shares information/aware of available of resources/encourages vigilance/ checks and reports changes in team/requests reports/updates
Understand	Knows capabilities/cross-checks above/shares mental models/speaks up when unsure/updates other team members/discusses team constraints
Think ahead	Identifies future problems/discusses contingencies/anticipates requirements

Below standard = 1	**Basic standard = 2**	**Standard = 3**	**Excellent = 4**
Behaviour directly compromises patient safety and effective teamwork	Behaviour in other conditions could directly compromise patient safety and effective teamwork	Behaviour maintains an effective level of patient safety and teamwork	Behaviour enhances patient safety and teamwork; a model for all other teams

Fig. 23.6 NOTECHS Assessment Tool (Reproduced from Mishra et al. [104]. With permission from BMJ Publishing Group Ltd)

skills, level IV – verification of preceptorial experience; and level V – demonstration of satisfactory patient outcomes [80, 107]. Efforts to further refine this verification model, design effective practical models for preceptoring, and focus on the impact of the courses on the short- and long-term performance of surgeons and on patient outcomes are underway.

Importantly, the Accredited Education Institutes of the ACS [108–110] have created a state-of-the-art simulation center network that offers training opportunities to practicing surgeons and trainees that also allows the implementation of a more objective assessment process for the initial certification, maintenance of certification, or reentry into the surgical field. In addition, the consortium of these institutes and its committees are actively exploring collaborative research opportunities among centers that will advance the field. They are also working on the development of standard-setting activities; the creation, broad dissemination, and adoption of standard curricula; the design of models to evaluate outcomes; and the provision of uniform certificates of verification [80].

Research in the field has exponentially grown over the past few years but has been limited in quality and focus by consisting of single-institution studies with small sample sizes. In an effort to provide guidance to researchers and funding agencies, the simulation committee of the Association for Surgical Education recently published a research agenda for surgical simulation generated using the Delphi process [111]. The same committee is working on determining performance benchmarks in laparoscopic and open skills for surgical residents across the USA. Such levels will inform residents and faculty about their standing at a national level and may influence curriculum design and resident advancement. Similar collaborative and multi-institutional research projects are likely to multiply and provide better quality evidence in the field.

Simulation for Surgical Credentialing

Simulation will also likely play a bigger role for the credentialing of surgeons. One example is the requirement by the ABS for FLS certification before graduation of general surgery residents. Given that simulators are great tools for objective assessment of performance, their increased use in credentialing is a matter of time.

Technologic advances are likely to improve existing simulators and lead to the creation of new ones. Simulators for open surgery in particular are expected to have the most growth. The teaching and assessment of nontechnical skills will continue to gain acceptance by the surgical community, and wider implementation of interdisciplinary and team training is on the horizon. Along with this, more emphasis will be placed on the development and training of the trainers and specific criteria established for instructors. Further research is also likely to determine the best metrics for performance assessment on technical and nontechnical skills. Better and more sensitive metrics of performance are likely to enhance skill acquisition on simulators and transfer to the operating room [46]. Better integration of simulation with clinical performance and patient outcomes will be pursued, and deficiencies in the clinical performance of surgeons will identify training needs in the simulation lab. Simulators may also be used to supplement the acquisition and maintenance of skills that are rarely encountered in clinical practice by trainees and practicing surgeons. It will not be surprising if programs low on some procedures use simulator-based training to supplement their resident experience and numbers. The creation of performance databanks that can inform learners, instructors, and programs and allow outcomes research is anticipated. The development of specific guidelines and standards for simulation training and assessment is also in sight. More collaborative work among disciplines and the exchange of ideas will bring simulation to the next level. One such example is the recent formation of the Alliance of Surgical Simulation in Education and Training (ASSET) group that aims to create common standardized curricula for all surgical specialties and a structure that will provide the forum for exchange of ideas and collaboration among surgical disciplines.

Conclusion

Simulation in general surgery has had many advances in recent years. From the development of a variety of simulators to the creation of national skills curricula, the establishment of the accredited education institute network, and the refinement of assessment tools and metrics, the progress achieved signals a very bright future for the field. Surgical simulation will continue bringing the education and assessment of surgical trainees and practicing surgeons to new levels and is destined to improve patient care and outcomes.

References

1. Martin RF. Simulation and surgical competency. Foreword. Surg Clin North Am. 2010;90(3):xiii–xv.
2. Reznick RK, MacRae H. Teaching surgical skills – changes in the wind. N Engl J Med. 2006;355(25):2664–9.
3. Choy I, Okrainec A. Simulation in surgery: perfecting the practice. Surg Clin North Am. 2010;90(3):457–73.
4. Strasberg SM, Hertl M, Soper NJ. An analysis of the problem of biliary injury during laparoscopic cholecystectomy. J Am Coll Surg. 1995;180(1):101–25.
5. Gallagher AG, Ritter EM, Champion H, et al. Virtual reality simulation for the operating room: proficiency-based training as a paradigm shift in surgical skills training. Ann Surg. 2005;241(2):364–72.
6. Ketchum J, Bartless J. Laparotomy model. ACS/APDS surgical skills curriculum for residents: phase I, module 12. American College of Surgeons; 2009.
7. Scott DJ, Dunnington GL. The new ACS/APDS skills curriculum: moving the learning curve out of the operating room. J Gastrointest Surg. 2008;12(2):213–21.
8. Heiner JD. A new simulation model for skin abscess identification and management. Simul Healthc. 2010;5(4):238–41.
9. Sanchez A, Rodriguez O, Benitez G, Sanchez R, De la Fuente L. Development of a training model for laparoscopic common bile duct exploration. JSLS. 2010;14(1):41–7.
10. Scott DJ, Bergen PC, Rege RV, et al. Laparoscopic training on bench models: better and more cost effective than operating room experience? J Am Coll Surg. 2000;191(3):272–83.
11. Fried GM, Feldman LS, Vassiliou MC, et al. Proving the value of simulation in laparoscopic surgery. Ann Surg. 2004;240(3):518–25; discussion 525–8.
12. Derossis AM, Fried GM, Abrahamowicz M, Sigman HH, Barkun JS, Meakins JL. Development of a model for training and evaluation of laparoscopic skills. Am J Surg. 1998;175(6):482–7.
13. Derossis AM, Bothwell J, Sigman HH, Fried GM. The effect of practice on performance in a laparoscopic simulator. Surg Endosc. 1998;12(9):1117–20.
14. Fraser SA, Klassen DR, Feldman LS, Ghitulescu GA, Stanbridge D, Fried GM. Evaluating laparoscopic skills: setting the pass/fail score for the MISTELS system. Surg Endosc. 2003;17(6):964–7.
15. Derossis AM, Antoniuk M, Fried GM. Evaluation of laparoscopic skills: a 2-year follow-up during residency training. Can J Surg. 1999;42(4):293–6.
16. Vassiliou MC, Dunkin BJ, Marks JM, Fried GM. FLS and FES: comprehensive models of training and assessment. Surg Clin North Am. 2010;90(3):535–58.
17. Fundamentals of Laparoscopic Surgery. http://www.flsprogram.org. Accessed 31 Dec 2011.
18. Willaert WI, Aggarwal R, Van Herzeele I, et al. Patient-specific endovascular simulation influences interventionalists performing carotid artery stenting procedures. Eur J Vasc Endovasc Surg. 2011;41(4):492–500.
19. Stefanidis D, Hope WW, Scott DJ. Robotic suturing on the FLS model possesses construct validity, is less physically demanding, and is favored by more surgeons compared with laparoscopy. Surg Endosc. 2011;25(7):2141–6.
20. Seymour NE, Gallagher AG, Roman SA, et al. Virtual reality training improves operating room performance: results of a randomized, double-blinded study. Ann Surg. 2002;236(4):458–63; discussion 463–4.
21. Ahlberg G, Enochsson L, Gallagher AG, et al. Proficiency-based virtual reality training significantly reduces the error rate for residents during their first 10 laparoscopic cholecystectomies. Am J Surg. 2007;193(6):797–804.
22. Grantcharov TP, Kristiansen VB, Bendix J, Bardram L, Rosenberg J, Funch-Jensen P. Randomized clinical trial of virtual reality simulation for laparoscopic skills training. Br J Surg. 2004;91(2):146–50.
23. Sturm LP, Windsor JA, Cosman PH, Cregan P, Hewett PJ, Maddern GJ. A systematic review of skills transfer after surgical simulation training. Ann Surg. 2008;248(2):166–79.
24. Sroka G, Feldman LS, Vassiliou MC, Kaneva PA, Fayez R, Fried GM. Fundamentals of laparoscopic surgery simulator training to proficiency improves laparoscopic performance in the operating room-a randomized controlled trial. Am J Surg. 2010;199(1):115–20.
25. McCluney AL, Vassiliou MC, Kaneva PA, et al. FLS simulator performance predicts intraoperative laparoscopic skill. Surg Endosc. 2007;21(11):1991–5.

26. Haycock A, Koch AD, Familiari P, et al. Training and transfer of colonoscopy skills: a multinational, randomized, blinded, controlled trial of simulator versus bedside training. Gastrointest Endosc. 2010;71(2):298–307.
27. Haycock AV, Youd P, Bassett P, Saunders BP, Tekkis P, Thomas-Gibson S. Simulator training improves practical skills in therapeutic GI endoscopy: results from a randomized, blinded, controlled study. Gastrointest Endosc. 2009;70(5):835–45.
28. Chaer RA, Derubertis BG, Lin SC, et al. Simulation improves resident performance in catheter-based intervention: results of a randomized, controlled study. Ann Surg. 2006;244(3):343–52.
29. Cohen J, Cohen SA, Vora KC, et al. Multicenter, randomized, controlled trial of virtual-reality simulator training in acquisition of competency in colonoscopy. Gastrointest Endosc. 2006;64(3):361–8.
30. Barsuk JH, McGaghie WC, Cohen ER, O'Leary KJ, Wayne DB. Simulation-based mastery learning reduces complications during central venous catheter insertion in a medical intensive care unit. Crit Care Med. 2009;37(10):2697–701.
31. Barsuk JH, Cohen ER, Feinglass J, McGaghie WC, Wayne DB. Use of simulation-based education to reduce catheter-related bloodstream infections. Arch Intern Med. 2009;169(15):1420–3.
32. Zendejas B, Cook DA, Bingener J, et al. Simulation-based mastery learning improves patient outcomes in laparoscopic inguinal hernia repair: a randomized controlled trial. Ann Surg. 2011;254(3):502–9; discussion 509–11.
33. Korndorffer Jr JR, Dunne JB, Sierra R, Stefanidis D, Touchard CL, Scott DJ. Simulator training for laparoscopic suturing using performance goals translates to the operating room. J Am Coll Surg. 2005;201(1):23–9.
34. Stefanidis D, Acker C, Heniford BT. Proficiency-based laparoscopic simulator training leads to improved operating room skill that is resistant to decay. Surg Innov. 2008;15(1):69–73.
35. Stefanidis D, Korndorffer Jr JR, Markley S, Sierra R, Heniford BT, Scott DJ. Closing the gap in operative performance between novices and experts: does harder mean better for laparoscopic simulator training? J Am Coll Surg. 2007;205(2):307–13.
36. McGaghie WC, Issenberg SB, Petrusa ER, Scalese RJ. A critical review of simulation-based medical education research: 2003–2009. Med Educ. 2010;44(1):50–63.
37. McGaghie WC, Issenberg SB, Cohen ER, Barsuk JH, Wayne DB. Does simulation-based medical education with deliberate practice yield better results than traditional clinical education? A meta-analytic comparative review of the evidence. Acad Med. 2011;86(6):706–11.
38. Stefanidis D, Scerbo MW, Korndorffer Jr JR, Scott DJ. Redefining simulator proficiency using automaticity theory. Am J Surg. 2007;193(4):502–6.
39. O'Donnell RD, Eggemeier FT. Workload assessment methodology. In: Boff KR, Kaufman L, Thomas JP, editors. Handbook of perception and performance, cognitive processes and performance, vol. 2. New York: Wiley; 1986. p. 1–49.
40. Datta V, Mackay S, Mandalia M, Darzi A. The use of electromagnetic motion tracking analysis to objectively measure open surgical skill in the laboratory-based model. J Am Coll Surg. 2001;193(5):479–85.
41. Pellen MG, Horgan LF, Barton JR, Attwood SE. Construct validity of the ProMIS laparoscopic simulator. Surg Endosc. 2009;23(1):130–9.
42. Stefanidis D, Scott DJ, Korndorffer Jr JR. Do metrics matter? Time versus motion tracking for performance assessment of proficiency-based laparoscopic skills training. Simul Healthc. 2009;4(2):104–8.
43. Yurko YY, Scerbo MW, Prabhu AS, Acker CE, Stefanidis D. Higher mental workload is associated with poorer laparoscopic performance as measured by the NASA-TLX tool. Simul Healthc. 2010; 5(5):267–71.
44. Wilson M, McGrath J, Vine S, Brewer J, Defriend D, Masters R. Psychomotor control in a virtual laparoscopic surgery training environment: gaze control parameters differentiate novices from experts. Surg Endosc. 2010;24(10):2458–64.
45. Stefanidis D, Scerbo MW, Sechrist C, Mostafavi A, Heniford BT. Do novices display automaticity during simulator training? Am J Surg. 2008;195(2):210–3.
46. Stefanidis D, Scerbo MW, Montero PN, Acker CE, Smith WD. Simulator training to automaticity leads to improved skill transfer compared with traditional proficiency-based training: a randomized controlled trial. Ann Surg. 2012;255(1):30–7.
47. Vassiliou MC, Feldman LS, Andrew CG, et al. A global assessment tool for evaluation of intraoperative laparoscopic skills. Am J Surg. 2005;190(1):107–13.
48. Martin JA, Regehr G, Reznick R, et al. Objective structured assessment of technical skill (OSATS) for surgical residents. Br J Surg. 1997;84(2):273–8.
49. Hodges B, Regehr G, McNaughton N, Tiberius R, Hanson M. OSCE checklists do not capture increasing levels of expertise. Acad Med. 1999;74(10):1129–34.
50. Regehr G, MacRae H, Reznick RK, Szalay D. Comparing the psychometric properties of checklists and global rating scales for assessing performance on an OSCE-format examination. Acad Med. 1998;73(9):993–7.
51. Vassiliou MC, Kaneva PA, Poulose BK, et al. Global Assessment of Gastrointestinal Endoscopic Skills (GAGES): a valid measurement tool for technical skills in flexible endoscopy. Surg Endosc. 2010;24(8):1834–41.
52. Satava RM. Disruptive visions: surgical education. Surg Endosc. 2004;18(5):779–81.
53. Fried GM. Lessons from the surgical experience with simulators: incorporation into training and utilization in determining competency. Gastrointest Endosc Clin N Am. 2006;16(3):425–34.
54. Kern DE, Thomas PA, Hughes MT. Curriculum development for medical education: a six-step approach, vol. 2. Baltimore: Johns Hopkins University Press; 2009.
55. Stefanidis D, Acker CE, Swiderski D, Heniford BT, Greene FL. Challenges during the implementation of a laparoscopic skills curriculum in a busy general surgery residency program. J Surg Educ. 2008;65(1):4–7.
56. Ericsson KA, Krampe RT, Tesch-Römer C. The role of deliberate practice in the acquisition of expert performance. Psychol Rev. 1993;100(3):363–406.
57. Duvivier RJ, van Dalen J, Muijtjens AM, Moulaert VR, Van der Vleuten CP, Scherpbier AJ. The role of deliberate practice in the acquisition of clinical skills. BMC Med Educ. 2011;11(1):101.
58. Crochet P, Aggarwal R, Dubb SS, et al. Deliberate practice on a virtual reality laparoscopic simulator enhances the quality of surgical technical skills. Ann Surg. 2011;253(6):1216–22.
59. Stefanidis D. Optimal acquisition and assessment of proficiency on simulators in surgery. Surg Clin North Am. 2010;90(3):475–89.
60. Chang L, Petros J, Hess DT, Rotondi C, Babineau TJ. Integrating simulation into a surgical residency program: is voluntary participation effective? Surg Endosc. 2007;21(3):418–21.
61. Stefanidis D, Korndorffer Jr JR, Heniford BT, Scott DJ. Limited feedback and video tutorials optimize learning and resource utilization during laparoscopic simulator training. Surgery. 2007;142(2): 202–6.
62. Xeroulis GJ, Park J, Moulton CA, Reznick RK, Leblanc V, Dubrowski A. Teaching suturing and knot-tying skills to medical students: a randomized controlled study comparing computer-based video instruction and (concurrent and summary) expert feedback. Surgery. 2007;141(4):442–9.
63. Porte MC, Xeroulis G, Reznick RK, Dubrowski A. Verbal feedback from an expert is more effective than self-accessed feedback about motion efficiency in learning new surgical skills. Am J Surg. 2007; 193(1):105–10.
64. Mahmood T, Darzi A. The learning curve for a colonoscopy simulator in the absence of any feedback: no feedback, no learning. Surg Endosc. 2004;18(8):1224–30.

65. Chang JY, Chang GL, Chien CJ, Chung KC, Hsu AT. Effectiveness of two forms of feedback on training of a joint mobilization skill by using a joint translation simulator. Phys Ther. 2007;87(4):418–30.
66. Schmidt RA, Wulf G. Continuous concurrent feedback degrades skill learning: implications for training and simulation. Hum Factors. 1997;39(4):509–25.
67. Rosser JC, Herman B, Risucci DA, Murayama M, Rosser LE, Merrell RC. Effectiveness of a CD-ROM multimedia tutorial in transferring cognitive knowledge essential for laparoscopic skill training. Am J Surg. 2000;179(4):320–4.
68. Pearson AM, Gallagher AG, Rosser JC, Satava RM. Evaluation of structured and quantitative training methods for teaching intracorporeal knot tying. Surg Endosc. 2002;16(1):130–7.
69. Magill RA. Motor learning and control. Concepts and applications. 7th ed. New York: McGraw-Hill; 2004.
70. Karni A, Meyer G, Rey-Hipolito C, et al. The acquisition of skilled motor performance: fast and slow experience-driven changes in primary motor cortex. Proc Natl Acad Sci USA. 1998;95(3):861–8.
71. Moulton CA, Dubrowski A, Macrae H, Graham B, Grober E, Reznick R. Teaching surgical skills: what kind of practice makes perfect? A randomized, controlled trial. Ann Surg. 2006;244(3):400–9.
72. Donovan J, Radosevich DJ. A meta-analytic review of the distribution of practice effect: now you see it, now you don't. J Appl Psychol. 1999;84(5):795–805.
73. Mitchell EL, Lee DY, Sevdalis N, et al. Evaluation of distributed practice schedules on retention of a newly acquired surgical skill: a randomized trial. Am J Surg. 2011;201(1):31–9.
74. Aggarwal R, Grantcharov T, Moorthy K, Hance J, Darzi A. A competency-based virtual reality training curriculum for the acquisition of laparoscopic psychomotor skill. Am J Surg. 2006;191(1):128–33.
75. Stefanidis D, Heniford BT. The formula for a successful laparoscopic skills curriculum. Arch Surg. 2009;144(1):77–82; discussion 82.
76. Walters C, Acker C, Heniford BT, Greene FL, Stefanidis D. Performance goals on simulators boost resident motivation and skills lab attendance. J Am Coll Surg. 2008;207(3):S88.
77. Madan AK, Harper JL, Taddeucci RJ, Tichansky DS. Goal-directed laparoscopic training leads to better laparoscopic skill acquisition. Surgery. 2008;144(2):345–50.
78. Gauger PG, Hauge LS, Andreatta PB, et al. Laparoscopic simulation training with proficiency targets improves practice and performance of novice surgeons. Am J Surg. 2010;199(1):72–80.
79. ACS/APDS Surgical Skills Curriculum for Residents. 2009. http://elearning.facs.org. Accessed 10 Jan 2012.
80. Sachdeva AK, Buyske J, Dunnington GL, et al. A new paradigm for surgical procedural training. Curr Probl Surg. 2011;48(12):854–968.
81. Jacobs LM, Luk S. Advanced trauma operative management: surgical strategies for penetrating trauma. 2nd ed. Woodbury: Ciné-Med Publishing, Inc; 2010.
82. Jacobs LM, Burns KJ, Kaban JM, et al. Development and evaluation of the advanced trauma operative management course. J Trauma. 2003;55(3):471–9; discussion 479.
83. Bandura A. Social foundations of thought and action: a social cognitive theory. Englewood Cliffs: Prentice Hall; 1986.
84. Fletcher GC, McGeorge P, Flin RH, Glavin RJ, Maran NJ. The role of non-technical skills in anaesthesia: a review of current literature. Br J Anaesth. 2002;88(3):418–29.
85. Mishra A, Catchpole K, Dale T, McCulloch P. The influence of non-technical performance on technical outcome in laparoscopic cholecystectomy. Surg Endosc. 2008;22(1):68–73.
86. Kwaan MR, Studdert DM, Zinner MJ, Gawande AA. Incidence, patterns, and prevention of wrong-site surgery. Arch Surg. 2006;141(4):353–7; discussion 357–8.
87. Greenberg CC, Regenbogen SE, Studdert DM, et al. Patterns of communication breakdowns resulting in injury to surgical patients. J Am Coll Surg. 2007;204(4):533–40.
88. Mazzocco K, Petitti DB, Fong KT, et al. Surgical team behaviors and patient outcomes. Am J Surg. 2009;197(5):678–85.
89. Lingard L, Espin S, Whyte S, et al. Communication failures in the operating room: an observational classification of recurrent types and effects. Qual Saf Health Care. 2004;13(5):330–4.
90. Helmrich RL, Davies JM. Team performance in the operating room. In: Bogner MS, editor. Human error in medicine. Hillside: Erlbaum; 1994. p. 225–53.
91. Belyansky I, Martin TR, Prabhu AS, et al. Poor resident-attending intraoperative communication may compromise patient safety. J Surg Res. 2011;171(2):386–94.
92. Burke CS, Salas E, Wilson-Donnelly K, Priest H. How to turn a team of experts into an expert medical team: guidance from the aviation and military communities. Qual Saf Health Care. 2004;13 Suppl 1:i96–104.
93. Bleakley A, Boyden J, Hobbs A, Walsh L, Allard J. Improving teamwork climate in operating theatres: the shift from multiprofessionalism to interprofessionalism. J Interprof Care. 2006;20(5):461–70.
94. Undre S, Sevdalis N, Healey AN, Darzi SA, Vincent CA. Teamwork in the operating theatre: cohesion or confusion? J Eval Clin Pract. 2006;12(2):182–9.
95. Makary MA, Sexton JB, Freischlag JA, et al. Operating room teamwork among physicians and nurses: teamwork in the eye of the beholder. J Am Coll Surg. 2006;202(5):746–52.
96. Baker DP, Day R, Salas E. Teamwork as an essential component of high-reliability organizations. Health Serv Res. 2006;41(4 Pt 2): 1576–98.
97. Fernandez R, Vozenilek JA, Hegarty CB, et al. Developing expert medical teams: toward an evidence-based approach. Acad Emerg Med. 2008;15(11):1025–36.
98. Paige JT, Kozmenko V, Yang T, et al. High-fidelity, simulation-based, interdisciplinary operating room team training at the point of care. Surgery. 2009;145(2):138–46.
99. Paige JT, Kozmenko V, Yang T, et al. High fidelity, simulation-based training at the point-of-care improves teamwork in the operating room. J Am Coll Surg. 2008;207(3):S87–8.
100. Beaubien JM, Baker DP. The use of simulation for training teamwork skills in health care: how low can you go? Qual Saf Health Care. 2004;13 Suppl 1:i51–6.
101. Wilson KA, Burke CS, Priest HA, Salas E. Promoting health care safety through training high reliability teams. Qual Saf Health Care. 2005;14(4):303–9.
102. Salas E, DiazGranados D, Weaver SJ, King H. Does team training work? Principles for health care. Acad Emerg Med. 2008;15(11):1002–9.
103. ACS/APDS surgical skills curriculum for residents: phase III, team-based skills. http://elearning.facs.org/course/view.php?id=10. Accessed 10 Jan 2012.
104. Mishra A, Catchpole K, McCulloch P. The Oxford NOTECHS System: reliability and validity of a tool for measuring teamwork behaviour in the operating theatre. Qual Saf Health Care. 2009; 18(2):104–8.
105. Sevdalis N, Davis R, Koutantji M, Undre S, Darzi A, Vincent CA. Reliability of a revised NOTECHS scale for use in surgical teams. Am J Surg. 2008;196(2):184–90.
106. Hull L, Arora S, Kassab E, Kneebone R, Sevdalis N. Observational teamwork assessment for surgery: content validation and tool refinement. J Am Coll Surg. 2011;212(2):234–243.e231–235.
107. Sachdeva AK. Acquiring skills in new procedures and technology: the challenge and the opportunity. Arch Surg. 2005;140(4):387–9.
108. Sachdeva AK, Pellegrini CA, Johnson KA. Support for simulation-based surgical education through American College of Surgeons – accredited education institutes. World J Surg. 2008;32(2):196–207.
109. Sachdeva AK. Credentialing of surgical skills centers. Surgeon. 2011;9 Suppl 1:S19–20.
110. Sachdeva AK. Establishment of American College of Surgeons-accredited Education Institutes: the dawn of a new era in surgical education and training. J Surg Educ. 2010;67(4):249–50.
111. Stefanidis D, Arora S, Parrack DM, et al. Research priorities in surgical simulation for the 21st century. Am J Surg. 2012;203(1): 49–53.

24 Simulation in Gastroenterology

Jenifer R. Lightdale

Introduction

Simulation is emerging as a critical tool for teaching and assessing skills in the field of gastroenterology. The use of simulation has had particular application to endoscopic procedures, as a fundamental component of gastrointestinal (GI) patient care, in an era when academic physicians are facing increasing clinical practice demands, and training regulations may limit time available to learn [1, 2]. Simulation has been well demonstrated to provide GI trainees a means to gain technical exposure and experience in basic procedural skills, without compromising patient comfort and safety [3–11]. For more experienced endoscopists, simulation lends itself to learning new techniques and to working with new technologies [12–14]. Ultimately, simulation is likely to become important as a means for measuring GI procedural competency, as well as for ensuring skill maintenance and retention over the lifetime of a gastroenterologist's career [15, 16].

As an integral part of gastroenterological care, GI endoscopy is a nonsurgical invasive procedure that is routinely performed using procedural sedation and analgesia to maintain patient comfort and safety [17]. The need to train gastroenterologists to master all skills involved in performing basic as well as advanced endoscopy is great. In accordance with CDC guidelines, all US adults over the age of 50 should undergo endoscopic screening for colorectal cancer [18]. An additional 200,000 US children annually undergo endoscopic exams for diagnostic and therapeutic purposes [19, 20]. To meet population demands, adult and pediatric gastroenterologists must reliably perform endoscopy safely, efficiently, and with maximum patient comfort.

To date, most emphasis on simulation in gastroenterology has focused on part-task simulators designed to promote technical skills [1, 3, 4, 9, 21, 22]. These procedural trainers provide few means for simulating nontechnical (behavioral) skills necessary for optimal patient care, including leadership and teamwork skills, as well as those involved in administering procedural sedation [23, 24]. Sedation is itself an inherently risky part of the procedure. Inadequately sedated patients may move excessively, increasing potential for adverse events, including perforation and hemorrhage [17]. Oversedation presents a host of patient risks, including hypoxia and cardiopulmonary arrest. With the high potential for both situations, gastroenterologists can benefit from training in crisis resource management [25]. Over time, it is likely that high-fidelity simulation of sedated gastrointestinal endoscopy will be emphasized in an effort to maximize technical and nontechnical skills required to successfully perform multiple tasks vital to safe GI procedures.

Training in GI Procedures

Formal training of physicians in gastroenterology includes both the supervised performance of procedures and the provision of patient sedation [26]. Although competency in the performance of GI procedures has remained a somewhat subjective issue, there is consensus that it requires certain core motor and cognitive skill elements [27]. Acquisition of teamwork skills required for competency is also acknowledged, but less defined [28]. Likewise, while a multi-society consensus curriculum has recently emerged for teaching sedation to gastroenterologists [29], it remains expected that endoscopists will learn both skills simultaneously [30, 31].

At a technical level, competency for performing procedures depends upon visual pattern recognition, hand-eye coordination, and manual dexterity. Societal guidelines state that the degree or extent of supervision may be adjusted as

J.R. Lightdale, MD, MPH
Department of Pediatrics,
Harvard Medical School, Boston, MA, USA

Department of Gastroenterology and Nutrition,
Children's Hospital Boston,
Boston, MA, USA
e-mail: jenifer.lightdale@childrens.harvard.edu

A.I. Levine et al. (eds.), *The Comprehensive Textbook of Healthcare Simulation*,
DOI 10.1007/978-1-4614-5993-4_24, © Springer Science+Business Media New York 2013

these skills mature [28]. Historically, the American Society for Gastrointestinal Endoscopy (ASGE) described three stages of endoscopic training [32]:

- Stage I—the stage of complete supervision during which indications, contraindications, and sedation practices are carefully reviewed and handling of the endoscope by the trainee is gradually increased
- Stage II—the stage at which partial supervision is necessary, with the teacher intervening only when difficulties are encountered
- Stage III—the stage at which a trainee has been declared competent to perform a particular procedure and no longer requires direct supervision, yet may at times request assistance or advice for unusual findings or difficult procedures

Most GI training guidelines have recommended threshold numbers (e.g., 130 upper endoscopies, 200 colonoscopies) of procedures that should be performed in patients before competency can be assessed [28]. These threshold numbers have been both criticized as being either too high or too low [26, 33]. To date, the debate about how best to achieve competency to preserve patient safety has assumed that the performance of GI endoscopy in actual patients is the only route to procedural mastery, although several studies have suggested that simulation may provide a credible adjunct [27, 34, 35].

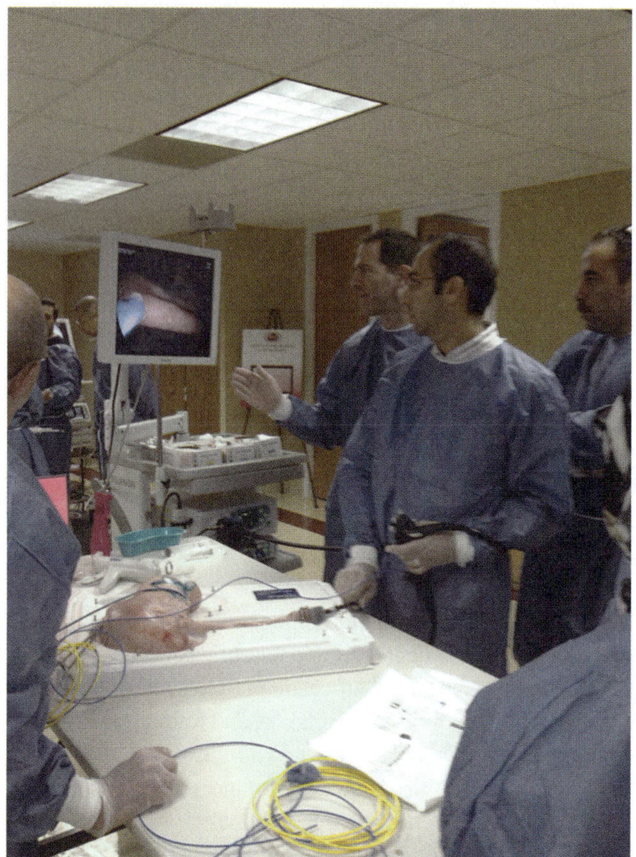

Fig. 24.1 Simulation teaching of thermal hemostasis using combined technology with harvested (ex vivo) porcine organs

Simulation and Gastrointestinal Procedures

Gastrointestinal endoscopy simulators can be broadly categorized as being animal, mechanical, or computerized. The use of simulation as a strategy to train gastrointestinal endoscopists in technical skills can be traced to the early 1970s when the use of anesthetized dogs, baboons, and pigs were introduced as expensive, yet effective models for teaching and acquiring skills [36, 37]. Mechanical simulators were developed subsequently and remain generally limited in applicability to the most beginning stages of training. The earliest of computer simulators in gastroenterology combined technology with harvested (ex vivo) porcine organs [38] (Fig. 24.1). More recently, entirely computerized simulators have been developed and have been demonstrated to be effective tools for teaching procedural skills to non-surgeons involved in performing upper and lower endoscopy [1, 3, 22, 39].

Gastroenterological Animal Models

To a certain extent, animal models remain the most realistic endoscopy simulators. Live animals, in specific, can provide a tactile and haptic experience that is remarkably similar to working with humans. Many live animal models favor juvenile pigs (approximately 35 kg in weight) and involve general anesthesia (Fig. 24.2). The use of such models on a wide basis is limited, appropriately, by the expense, facility requirements, and ethical considerations involved in their use.

Explanted animal models can also be used to simulate a number of important endoscopic interventions in a controlled setting, including polypectomy, endoscopic mucosal resection (EMR), endoscopic retrograde cholangiopancreatography (ERCP), and double-balloon enteroscopy. Generally speaking, the explanted organs must be situated in a mechanical device in a composite fashion (Fig. 24.3). The most commonly used composite simulator is the Erlangen Active Simulator for Interventional Endoscopy (EASIE) (ECE-Training, GmbH, Erlangen, Germany), which was developed specifically to provide training in therapeutic techniques, such as hemostasis. Modified, lighter-weight tabletop versions including the Erlangen compactEASIE, and the Endo X Trainer (Medical Innovations International, Rochester, MN) are designed to incorporate porcine organs (Fig. 24.4). Disadvantages of these models include complex preparatory routines, acquiring and disposing of explanted tissue and often unrealistic look, feel, and behavior of cadaveric tissues, which can detract from the experience.

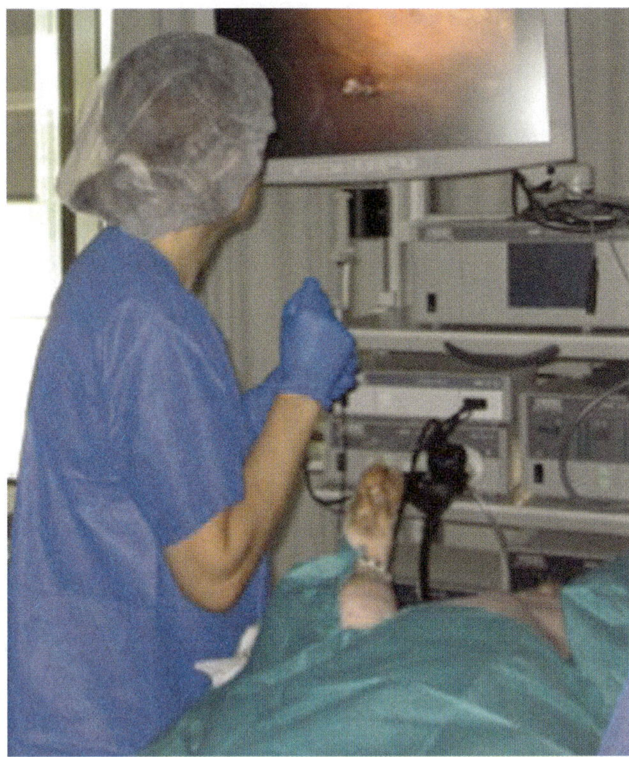

Fig. 24.2 Simulation training on an anesthetized pig serves as an effective model for teaching and acquiring skills

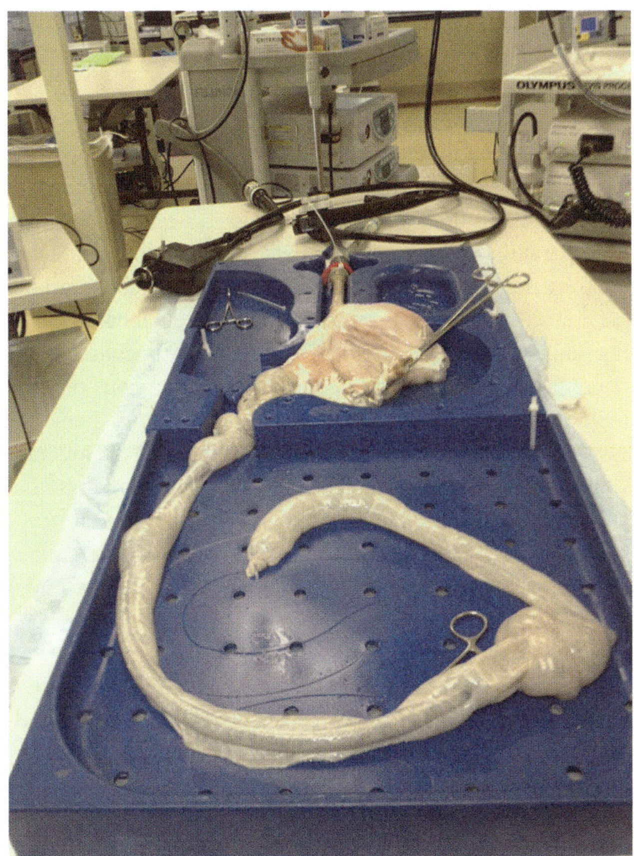

Fig. 24.3 Explanted porcine organs arranged for use in endoscopic simulation of small bowel double-balloon enteroscopy

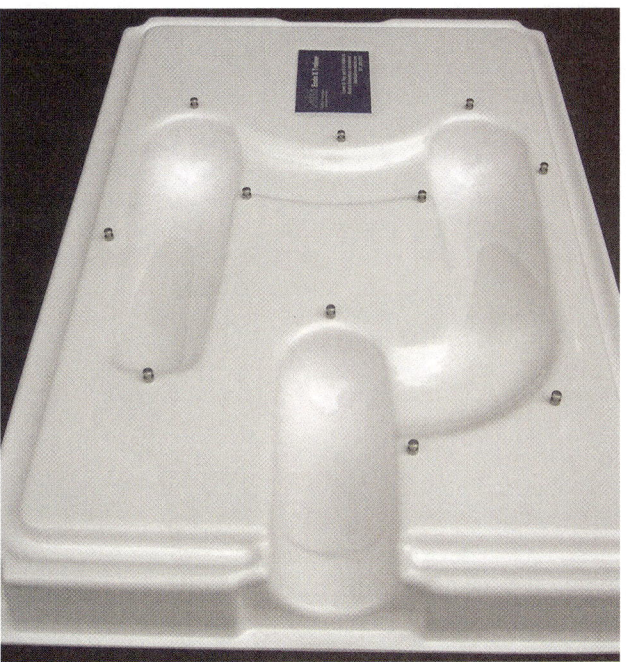

Fig. 24.4 Top and side view of the Endo X Trainer, a porcine endoscopy mold. The explanted porcine organs go in the mold for use in simulation (Image from http://www.medicalinnovations.com/text/endoscopic%20training%20device%20endo%20x%20trainer.html. Used with permission from Medical Innovations)

Computer-Based Endoscopic Simulators

Computer-based simulators for gastrointestinal procedures involve the insertion of a mock scope into an anatomically illustrative orifice to initiate a re-creation of visual and tactile sensations involved in using a flexible endoscope to examine and treat either the upper and lower gastrointestinal tract. Of two categories of computer-based simulators, virtual reality simulators and physical models, the virtual reality simulators are generally standalone systems that are specially equipped with dedicated monitors and endoscopes, while the physical model simulators (i.e., the Koken Colonoscopy Training Model Type 1-B (Koken C. Ltd., Tokyo, Japan)) are used in conjunction with real endoscopic equipment. One study by Hill et al. compared virtual reality endoscopic simulators with physical models and found little difference across simulators in terms of their overall realism, while only the virtual reality simulators provided more realistic auditory feedback regarding simulated patient discomfort [40].

There are currently two different virtual reality models of computer-based part-task endoscopic simulators that are commercially available: the GI Mentor (Simbionix USA, Cleveland, OH) and CAE Endoscopy VR simulator (CAE Healthcare, Montreal, Quebec, Canada). Both models provide diagnostic and therapeutic endoluminal experiences, record performance metrics of operators, and have been

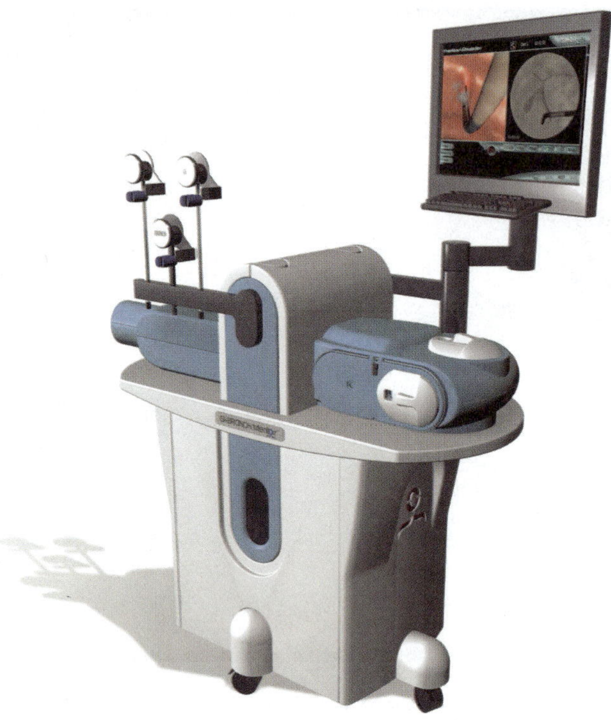

Fig. 24.5 Simbionix's GI Mentor is a virtual reality model for computer-based part-task endoscopic simulation. A modified endoscope can be inserted through one of the mannequin's two orifices while projecting the examination onto a monitor (Image used with permission from Simbionix)

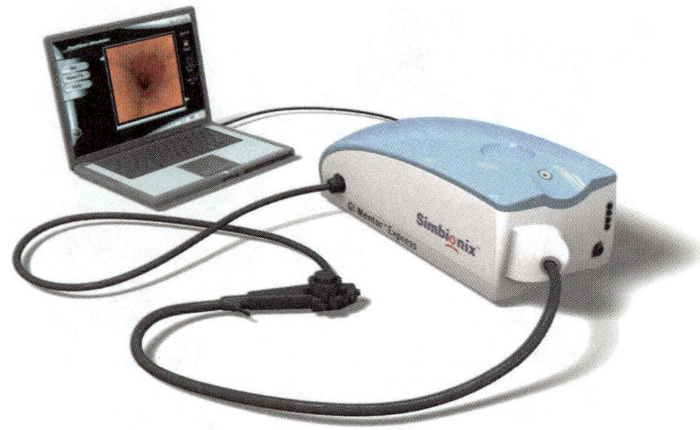

Fig. 24.6 The GI Mentor Express is a portable adapted version of the GI Mentor. A modified scope is inserted into orifices representative of mouth or anus to simulate live endoscopy (Image used with permission of Simbionix)

independently shown to have construct, content, and face validity [39, 41], as well as reliability [39, 42].

The GI Mentor simulator consists of a mannequin though which a modified endoscope (Pentax ECS-3840 F) can be inserted through one of two orifices that are representative of either a mouth or an anus [43]. The modified scope has an extremely high degree of realism and includes an air/water button, a suction button, and a working port that enables the simulation of diagnostic and therapeutic maneuvers, including biopsy examination, polypectomy, balloon dilation, and electrocautery. As with actual procedures, the examination is projected on a monitor located behind the patient (Fig. 24.5).

Rather than a mannequin and standard scope, the CAE Endoscopy VR system is a simulator platform that consists of a cart, CPU, monitor, and a specially made proxy scope [44]. As a scope insertion point, the CAE Endoscopy VR uses an "interface device" with an appropriate anatomical reference plate. The GI Mentor has recently been adapted in the GI Mentor™ Express, which includes all of the software, but is designed to be more elegant and portable (Fig. 24.6). As with the GI Mentor™ Express and the original GI Mentor™, insertion of the scope into the anatomical opening of the CAE Endoscopy VR initiates a computer program that allows a tactile, audio, and visual experience similar to live endoscopy.

In both models, insertion of the endoscope triggers a software program, which brings up sequential computer-generated images on the monitor of either the upper gastrointestinal tract or the rectum and colon, as appropriate to the insertion point. Sensors along the scope and within the torso of the mannequin track the motions of the endoscope resulting in computer-generated feedback in the form of tissue resistance, as well as insufflation of the intestine secondary to manipulation by the operator. Haptic feedback also reproduces the sensation of scope looping and resistance, and audio feedback occurs in the form of a computer-generated voice that simulates patient discomfort.

In addition to procedural simulation, the GI Mentor includes "game modules" for manual dexterity training that allow more novice endoscopists to develop skills controlling the endoscope dials and using torque. The simulator also incorporates a series of cases of varying pathology and technical difficulty. Instructors may delineate specific training programs, and trainees can receive immediate feedback during and after completing each simulated procedure. The computer generates auditory and visual expressions of pain, including moaning and distressed facial expressions, for overinsufflation, looping, and excessive force on the mucosal wall (Fig. 24.7). Performance is recorded, including number and types of errors made. The instructor can provide feedback to each trainee based upon a "videotape" of the simulated procedure and written procedure reports generated by the trainee that help to determine whether abnormalities were correctly detected.

Both systems record performance metrics while a simulated procedure is being performed. For the GI Mentor II, these consist of the following: adverse events (e.g., scope-to-bowel trauma, bleeding, and perforation), time required for the procedure, percentage of mucosa visualized, whether retroflexion was performed or not when appropriate (e.g., to visualize the cardia of the stomach or the distal rectum), the

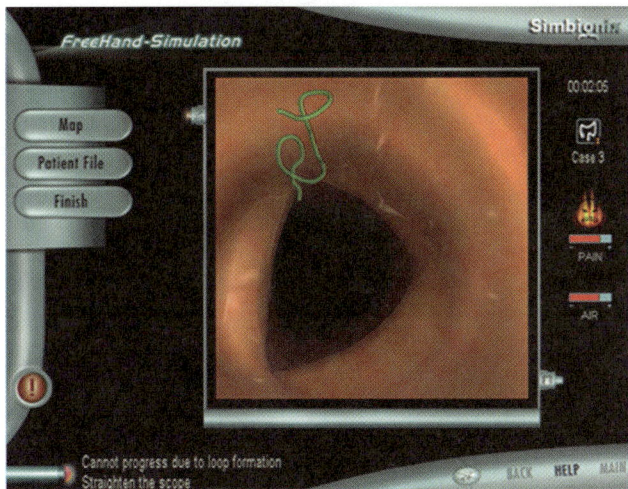

Fig. 24.7 The GI Mentor is capable of delivering immediate feedback to trainees and instructors during the simulated procedure. This figure shows the scenario in which the scope is unable to proceed due to loop formation (Image used with permission of Simbionix)

number of inappropriate (dangerous) retroflexions, the time spent with obscured visualization of the mucosa (i.e., because of touching the tip of the scope against the intestinal wall, not using water to clear the lens), and patient pain.

Validity of Part-Task Computer-Based Endoscopic Simulators

Several studies have determined the general validity of both models of gastrointestinal procedural simulators, defined as the extent to which measures are true to what they are designed to measure. There are several forms of validity that are relevant to gastrointestinal simulators. Several studies have examined *face validity*, defined as the degree to which the experience they evoke for the user is comparable to real procedures on actual patients [15, 45, 46]. Secondly, simulator *content validity* has been established in the sense that simulator activities adequately reflect subject matter encountered during live endoscopic procedures [1, 10, 15].

A number of other studies have examined the *construct validity* of gastrointestinal simulators, defined as the extent to which assessment by the simulator can discriminate between different ability or experience levels of endoscopists [10, 11, 39, 41, 47]. For example, Moorthy et al. divided physician participants into three groups according to prior experience (novices with none, intermediates with 10–50 prior, and experts endoscopists with >200 prior) and found that the more experienced endoscopists took less time to perform a complete upper gastrointestinal procedure on the GI Mentor, visualized more mucosa, and performed less inappropriate and dangerous maneuvers [39]. Similarly, Felsher et al. demonstrated the ability of the GI Mentor to discriminate between colonoscopists of varying experience and found that staff gastroenterologists took less procedural time, visualized more of the colonic mucosa, achieved a greater polypectomy rate, and spent a greater proportion of time with a clear view of the intestinal lumen than trainees [10].

Finally, several studies have sought to determine whether gastrointestinal simulators may offer *predictive validity*, defined as the extent to which performance on the system can be used to predict outcomes with other established assessment methods or during real procedures. Using a cohort of surgical trainees, Adamsen et al. investigated the correlation between laparoscopic surgical skills and flexible endoscopic skills and found that experienced laparoscopic surgeons performed significantly better than surgical trainees on both laparoscopic and endoscopic tasks in terms of time, errors, and economy of movement [11]. Using a different angle, Enochsson et al. found that medical residents who tested well on a well-validated visuospatial test (PicOr) scored more favorably on the GI Mentor's measures.

Simulation for Assessing Competency in Gastroenterology

It remains unknown whether endoscopic simulators can be used to assess procedural competence in trainees or to grant hospital privileges to qualified gastroenterologists [48]. To a certain extent, the uncertainty around the use of simulators for assessing endoscopic skills lies in the fact that no "gold standard" scale of procedural competency exists in gastroenterology. Strictly speaking, competence is the minimal level of skill and knowledge, derived through training and experience, required to safely and proficiently perform a task or procedure [49]. Competence in performing gastrointestinal endoscopy likely requires demonstrated proficiency in three domains: technical, cognitive (knowledge), and higher-order integrative competencies required for safe, intelligent performance in varied contexts (e.g., communication, judgment, clinical reasoning, and ethical integrity) [50]. Another possible marker of competence may be adverse events, although these may be too rare to track as a meaningful short-term indicators and may be influenced by patient characteristics [51].

Over the last two decades, there has been a growing appreciation in the field of gastroenterology that the addition of structure to components of the assessment process may provide objectivity, validity, and reliability to the global concept of endoscopic competence [26]. In turn, several measures of clinical ability in performing GI procedures have been developed [27, 33, 52, 53]. A few have been validated in a systematic and objective manner that would allow for widespread adoption in clinical practice. For example, the GAGES (Global Assessment of Gastrointestinal Endoscopic Skills) has been demonstrated to provide an objective measure of endoscopic skills during clinical procedures [33, 53].

Several studies have shown that simulators can improve novice skillsets [54]. In contrast, the long-term lasting benefit of using simulators to train in GI endoscopy remains uncertain. Transfer of endoscopic skills gained during simulation training to the clinical setting has also not been fully demonstrated. These facts appropriately leave the role of simulators to assess competence in credentialing processes for endoscopy still to be determined. Currently, credentialing in gastroenterology is still largely based on numbers of patient procedures performed and independent reviews of clinical performance fundamental to endoscopist assessments.

Simulation to Reduce Risks of Gastrointestinal Endoscopy

Simulation may represent a tool for improving patient safety during GI procedures. While endoscopy is generally considered safe, patients undergoing GI procedures are by definition placed in potentially harmful situations from inherent risks associated with instrumentation, as well as from sedatives. In many ways, the latter may represent the more salient risk. The risk of colonic perforation during scope insertion is estimated to lie between 0.3 and 1%, while the risk of esophageal perforation is estimated at 0.5% [55]. The risk of cardiopulmonary complications associated with sedation has been recently estimated to be as high as 1.1% during colonoscopy [56]. It has been estimated that >40% of all endoscopic complications are caused by sedatives [57]. Nevertheless, most patients undergoing gastrointestinal procedures *expect* to receive sedation, which is generally administered by endoscopists working in concert with specialized endoscopy nurses, but can involve anesthesiologists [17].

Sedation for GI endoscopy is defined as a drug-induced depression in patient consciousness that can range in levels from minimal anxiolysis to general anesthesia. The primary goals of sedation for gastrointestinal endoscopy are to ensure patient safety, comfort, and cooperation throughout procedures. Secondary goals of providing sedation for gastrointestinal endoscopy may include patient amnesia, immobility, and willingness to undergo repeat procedures.

Irrespective of who administers it, the ideal procedural sedation regimen for endoscopy should act predictably and rapidly and induce a level and duration of sedation appropriate to the procedure being performed [58]. A main barrier to risk reduction during endoscopy is that no ideal regimen exists. Instead, best practices for sedation during gastroenterology remain controversial [24]. General consensus dictates that it is cost prohibitive and inappropriate to perform diagnostic endoscopy in healthy patients with anesthesiologist assistance [59, 60]. In addition, levels of sedation achieved by anesthesiologists may be deeper than what is required for many procedures [61–63].

In upper endoscopy, a major goal of sedation may be to avoid gagging and increase patient cooperation; in colonoscopy, the goal of sedation is to avoid visceral pain associated with looping. Patient anxiety levels may also be different for different procedures. Generally speaking, endoscopy seems to be better tolerated by older than by younger individuals, by men than women, and by patients who have had a prior endoscopy [23]. The ability to tolerate procedures without sedation may be enhanced by older age and decreased pharyngeal sensitivity [64], while a history of poor tolerance of prior examinations may be predictive of patients who require deep sedation [65].

Recent Centers for Medicare & Medicaid Services (CMS) Guidelines published in 2010 have restricted the administration of deep sedation, in particular using propofol, without the presence of clinician trained in anesthesiology [66]. A major factor in this recent policy decision was the fact that non-anesthesiologists, such as gastroenterologists, have not been specifically trained in comprehensive skills required to care for patients with the potential to experience the entire continuum of sedation. Simulation may present an excellent tool for training gastroenterologists in all of the skills required for procedural sedation, as well as a means for assessing competencies in specific tasks such as airway management or cardiopulmonary resuscitation.

Simulation for Training in Technical and Nontechnical Endoscopy Skills

To a large extent, the successful development of simulation-based training to impact patient safety rests on the understanding that both technical and teamwork skills are critical components of endoscopy (see Table 24.1) [25]. Technical

Table 24.1 Technical and teamwork skills for GI endoscopy

Technical skills	Teamwork skills
Efficiently reaches anatomic landmarks	Knows the environment
Performs unassisted insertion	Anticipates and plans
Identifies landmarks	Assumes leadership role
Intubates esophagus/rectum	Communicates effectively
Adequately visualizes mucosa	Distributes workload optimally
Administers appropriate sedation	Allocates attention wisely
Appropriately interprets electronic monitors for patient monitoring	Utilizes all available information
Assess patient ventilation	Utilizes all available resources
	Calls for help early enough
	Maintains professional behavior

skills are defined as those tasks necessary to perform a procedure (e.g., for the MD use the endoscope, perform polypectomy, bag-mask ventilate an apneic patient, insert an endotracheal tube). Teamwork skills encompass all behaviors essential to effective individual and team performance, including the establishment of role clarity (e.g., leadership), communication skills (e.g., read back feedback of instructions), and decision-making skills (e.g., avoiding fixation errors). Research suggests that the great majority of all adverse events are related to teamwork skills [56].

The use of simulation as a strategy to educate gastroenterologists on tasks that are central to patients undergoing risk-inherent procedures is intuitively preferable to ensuring patient safety than traditional methods of teaching at the time of doing, especially if events where such skills are required are extremely infrequent. Through simulation, clinical teams are given the chance to learn and practice skills that may be vital, but are infrequently required. Training in crisis resource management (CRM), with its emphasis on principles of teamwork and critical event management, may also be useful in endoscopy [25]. This use of simulation-based training may be especially important for gastrointestinal procedures, which have low-frequency, high-stakes events.

There have been a few studies that have focused on the use of high-fidelity simulation for improving patient outcomes during GI procedures. One published in Germany combined a full-mannequin simulator with an animal-based simulator for the performance of endoscopy and evaluated endoscopic performance during critical events [21]. In an English abstract, the investigators describe the development of two different scenarios for trained endoscopists to use in developing CRM skills: gastrointestinal bleeding with significant blood loss and a medical error involving sedation overdose. "Patient vital signs," endoscopic skills, as well as personal interactions were recorded and graded for 100 participants with more than 12 months of endoscopic experience. After debriefing on an initial scenario, participants showed improvement in scores on the second one.

Another study by Sedlack et al. determined that randomizing trainees to simulator-based training (SBT) in *non-sedated* flexible sigmoidoscopy improved patient comfort [4]. Trainees self-rated their own performances in actual patients and were graded by supervising staff. In addition, patients who were not sedated during the procedure and could recall everything completed questionnaires grading the discomfort they experienced. Trainees rated themselves considerably more highly than supervising staff, who did not discern a difference in skill level between trainees who received SBT and those who received traditional patient-based training. On the other hand, patients did rate trainees with SBT significantly better in terms of comfort, suggesting that non-sedated patient comfort may be increased by practice on simulators.

Perceptions of Simulation by Endoscopy Clinicians at All Levels

Generally speaking, physicians and GI clinicians find simulation to be enjoyable, valuable, and realistic to their practice. In one study, nursing and technical staff involved in full-scale simulations (as described above) were prospectively invited to complete three short surveys regarding their perceptions of simulation-based training prior to engaging in simulation, immediately following participation in a session, and 1 month later [25]. Of survey responders, 42% had 5 or more years' experience in GI endoscopy; 83% had no previous experience with simulation-based training. Prior to participation in simulation, nurses with more than 5 years' experience in GI endoscopy rated their perceived enjoyment of simulation significantly lower than less experienced peers. However, when surveyed immediately after participation, nurses of both experience levels reported simulation to be highly useful, enjoyable, applicable, and realistic, with no significant differences between groups.

Comments elicited from clinicians after scenarios concluded included reports that simulation was "very interesting and useful," "very informative," and helped to "bring up [one's] awareness and skills." Specifically, CRM principles of teamwork and avoiding fixation were highlighted, with one technician noting that "from observing the simulation, [they] came to realize that instead of focusing on the biopsy [they] should focus on everything going on around [them] and [their] team." Debriefing was also noted to be a critical portion of simulation, with one participant noting that "debriefing was more beneficial than the actual simulation exercise."

Of course, simulation is also recognized to evoke stress in participants, no matter how nonthreatening the environment created or the scenarios encountered. In their study of clinicians practicing regularly in a GI endoscopy unit, Bong et al. found that physicians who underwent simulation-based training involving several scripted case scenarios experienced a significantly higher stress response—as evidenced by increases in both physiologic and biochemical markers—when compared to those who engaged in tutorial-based discussion and management of the same cases [67]. This response was similar in all team members who participated in simulation-based training, although when analyzed by clinical role, endoscopy technicians were found to experience a relatively smaller increase in salivary cortisol (1.1-fold vs. 2-fold) as compared to physicians and RNs. Additional findings included that measures of physiologic stress among caregivers were elevated from baseline even prior to engaging in (in anticipation of) simulation and also remained above baseline during debriefing.

Fortunately, all studies to date have suggested that gastroenterology physician trainees are enthusiastic about a simulation-based approach to their education and appreciate the value of simulation in their training. In one study of GI fellows in a large training center, computer-based endoscopic simulators (CBES) were reported by trainees to be valuable tools for increasing their skills and confidence [68]. This study found a direct relationship between time spent on the simulator and improved sense of skill and confidence. On the other hand, there were also "real-world" difficulties encountered. Indeed, despite best intentions of both training directors and fellows themselves, participants had difficulty incorporating simulator time into their daily activities. This issue may have important implications for programmatic development and integration of simulation into current gastroenterology training programs. In contrast with studies which have found that non-GI students and physicians were willing to spend time outside of their regular work hours to train on a simulator [69], GI fellows may require scheduled times for simulation training, if such educational tools are to be optimally employed.

In terms of the time that is to be spent on the simulator, fellows may particularly benefit from a mixture of attending guidance with solo practice time [68]. Attending presence during simulation instruction may not only enhance the value of a simulation curriculum but also allow new approaches to assessing procedural skills. Ultimately, it is likely that an understanding of how fellow skills on the simulator relate to procedural skills in actual patients will inform an active discussion of how simulation plays into endoscopy training.

Art of Simulating Gastrointestinal Endoscopy

Given the overall complexity of GI endoscopy as a procedure often performed with endoscopist-administered procedural sedation, high-fidelity simulation should be fully contextualized to include clinician interactions with the patient at the level of emotional, physiologic, and technical. To achieve this, our group and others have developed multimodal hybrid simulations that integrate both a part-task computer-based endoscopy simulator (i.e., GI Mentor, Simbionix USA) or a porcine endoscopy model with various realistic whole-body patient simulators (i.e., SimMan, Laerdal) [21, 67] (Fig. 24.8). In addition, professional actors are included to emphasize the "patient-doctor-parent triad" and thus round out the full-scale simulated environment. Finally, simulation courses are delivered to the point of care via mobile carts (aka in situ) directly to the endoscopy units, facilitating full "native" multidisciplinary team involvement as well as opportunities to study and promote rapid cycle improvements of the work environment itself (e.g., identify latent safety threats) [70].

In our experience, clinical scenarios are best designed around actual patient events, both common and rare (high risk). This allows a multidisciplinary team to learn from important cases that risk morbidity and mortality via a means

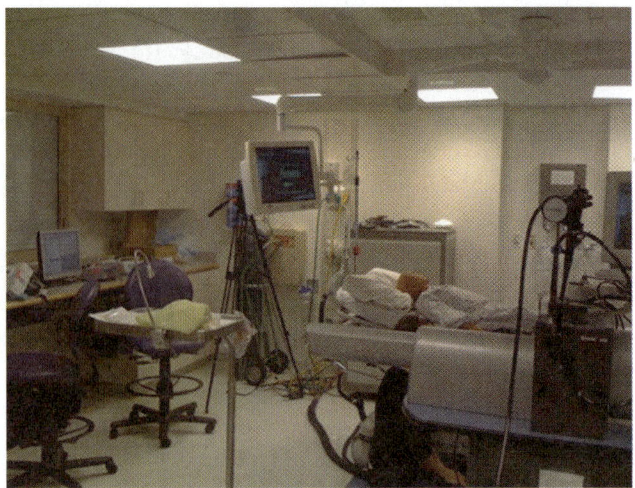

Fig. 24.8 Integrating part-task computer-based endoscopy simulators with whole-body patient simulators can provide a more realistic procedural training experience

that mitigates issues around time and chance. Clinical teaching objectives in our curriculum around procedural complications include unanticipated significant bleeding and perforation, while those around sedation include oversedation, apnea, agitation, and laryngospasm. We believe that simulation-based team training should balance clinical (airway management, bag-mask ventilation) and behavioral (CRM, role clarity, communication, and decision-making) objectives.

Sample Course Overview

All clinicians participating in simulation should be oriented to the procedural part-task and/or the full-mannequin simulator to assure their comfort during the scenarios. All simulated endoscopies should subsequently be staffed in a way that is typical in the unit undergoing training. Physicians and nurses not directly participating in the case can be assigned to be on hand to be called into the case by scenario participants if scenarios progress into emergency. Prior to each session, an expert simulation facilitator should review the principles of crisis resource management with all participants, guiding all participants to suspend disbelief and preserve a nonjudgmental, collegial atmosphere during training. Participants should be given time to review simulated patient medical records, complete routine sedation template orders, and fill out relevant paperwork prior to starting the case.

Structured debriefings should immediately follow each clinical scenario and ideally are guided by a trained facilitator using video-assisted playback. Debriefing sessions should include the entire team of participants and emphasize the principles of crisis resource management: role clarity, communication, teamwork, global assessment, and appropriate use of resources.

In our experience, we have found it quite effective for scenarios around GI endoscopy to begin with an awake patient using a live actor [25, 67]. Each simulation session ideally centers on a single scenario that is designed from clear learning goal objectives (based on formal prior needs assessment of participant pool) and metrics. It is often helpful if the start of the simulation requires the endoscopist to obtain informed consent and answer patient questions. This helps the team to "relax" into the scenario. Subsequent to obtaining consent, a timeout can be conducted and the endoscopist can lead the clinical team in initiating sedation. Some examples of scripted sedation scenarios for simulating endoscopy are listed below.

Example 1

In an *unanticipated GI bleeding scenario*, a 65-year-old man will undergo screening colonoscopy and a polyp will be encountered. During the polypectomy, blood will start to ooze at a brisk pace. The endoscopist will need to call for hemostatic equipment and to focus on hemostasis. The team will need to work together to assign roles, including event manager, appropriately.

Example 2

In an *excessive sedation and apnea scenario*, a 45-year-old woman will be quite anxious about undergoing colonoscopy until a combination of benzodiazepines and fentanyl are administered. The endoscopist will start the case and get past the hepatic flexure, and then the patient will become apneic. The team will need to recognize the apnea (e.g., by RN assessment and/or other monitoring options), stop the procedure, and act appropriately to treat the apnea.

Conclusion

Simulation of endoscopic procedures has become a routine means of enhancing training in the field of gastroenterology. A number of technological advances have improved the validity of animal, mechanical, and computerized models; in turn, simulation is gaining acceptance as a preferable means to teach gastroenterologists the skills required to perform diagnostic and therapeutic procedures. Although most emphasis to date has been on part-task simulators which are used to promote technical skills, high-fidelity full-scale simulation of gastrointestinal endoscopy may provide an important tool for teaching teamwork and other nontechnical skills critical to ensuring patient safety and comfort.

References

1. Gerson LB, Van Dam J. Technology review: the use of simulators for training in GI endoscopy. Gastrointest Endosc. 2004;60(6):992–1001.
2. McCashland T, Brand R, Lyden E, de Garmo P. The time and financial impact of training fellows in endoscopy. CORI Research Project. Clinical Outcomes Research Initiative. Am J Gastroenterol. 2000;95(11):3129–32.
3. Ferlitsch A, Glauninger P, Gupper A, et al. Evaluation of a virtual endoscopy simulator for training in gastrointestinal endoscopy. Endoscopy. 2002;34(9):698–702.
4. Sedlack RE, Kolars JC, Alexander JA. Computer simulation training enhances patient comfort during endoscopy. Clin Gastroenterol Hepatol. 2004;2(4):348–52.
5. Neumann M, Hahn C, Horbach T, et al. Score card endoscopy: a multicenter study to evaluate learning curves in 1-week courses using the Erlangen Endo-Trainer. Endoscopy. 2003;35(6):515–20.
6. Neumann M, Siebert T, Rausch J, et al. Scorecard endoscopy: a pilot study to assess basic skills in trainees for upper gastrointestinal endoscopy. Langenbecks Arch Surg. 2003;387(9–10):386–91.
7. Sedlack RE, Kolars JC. Colonoscopy curriculum development and performance-based assessment criteria on a computer-based endoscopy simulator. Acad Med. 2002;77(7):750–1.
8. Ladas SD, Malfertheiner P, Axon A. An introductory course for training in endoscopy. Dig Dis. 2002;20(3–4):242–5.
9. Sedlack RE, Kolars JC. Computer simulator training enhances the competency of gastroenterology fellows at colonoscopy: results of a pilot study. Am J Gastroenterol. 2004;99(1):33–7.
10. Felsher JJ, Olesevich M, Farres H, et al. Validation of a flexible endoscopy simulator. Am J Surg. 2005;189(4):497–500.
11. Adamsen S, Funch-Jensen PM, Drewes AM, Rosenberg J, Grantcharov TP. A comparative study of skills in virtual laparoscopy and endoscopy. Surg Endosc. 2005;19(2):229–34.
12. Sedlack RE, Petersen BT, Kolars JC. The impact of a hands-on ERCP workshop on clinical practice. Gastrointest Endosc. 2005; 61(1):67–71.
13. Matthes K, Cohen J. The Neo-Papilla: a new modification of porcine ex vivo simulators for ERCP training (with videos). Gastrointest Endosc. 2006;64(4):570–6.
14. Harewood GC, Yusuf TE, Clain JE, Levy MJ, Topazian MD, Rajan E. Assessment of the impact of an educational course on knowledge of appropriate EUS indications. Gastrointest Endosc. 2005;61(4):554–9.
15. Sedlack RE. Endoscopic simulation: where we have been and where we are going. Gastrointest Endosc. 2005;61(2):216–8.
16. Aslanian HR. Ain't nothing like the real thing? Simulators in endoscopy training. Gastrointest Endosc. 2012;75(2):261–2.
17. Lightdale JR. Patient preparation and sedation for endoscopy. In: Classen M, Tytgat GNJ, Lightdale CJ, editors. Gastroenterological endoscopy. 2nd ed. New York: Thieme; 2010. p. 57–67.
18. Seeff LC. Increased use of colorectal cancer tests – United States, 2002 and 2004. CDC. 2006;11:308–11.
19. Colletti RB, Di Lorenzo C. Overview of pediatric gastroesophageal reflux disease and proton pump inhibitor therapy. J Pediatr Gastroenterol Nutr. 2003;37 Suppl 1:S7–11.
20. Kugathasan S, Judd RH, Hoffmann RG, et al. Epidemiologic and clinical characteristics of children with newly diagnosed inflammatory bowel disease in Wisconsin: a statewide population-based study. J Pediatr. 2003;143(4):525–31.
21. Kiesslich R, Moenk S, Reinhardt K, et al. Combined simulation training: a new concept and workshop is useful for crisis management in gastrointestinal endoscopy. Z Gastroenterol. 2005;43(9):1031–9.
22. Kneebone RL, Nestel D, Moorthy K, et al. Learning the skills of flexible sigmoidoscopy – the wider perspective. Med Educ. 2003;37 Suppl 1:50–8.
23. Bell GD. Preparation, premedication, and surveillance. Endoscopy. 2004;36(1):23–31.

24. Lightdale JR. Sedation and analgesia in the pediatric patient. Gastrointest Endosc Clin N Am. 2004;14(2):385–99.
25. Heard LA, Fredette ME, Atmadja ML, Weinstock P, Lightdale JR. Perceptions of simulation-based training in crisis resource management in the endoscopy unit. Gastroenterol Nurs. 2011; 34(1):42–8.
26. Spier BJ, Benson M, Pfau PR, Nelligan G, Lucey MR, Gaumnitz EA. Colonoscopy training in gastroenterology fellowships: determining competence. Gastrointest Endosc. 2010;71(2): 319–24.
27. Sedlack RE. Training to competency in colonoscopy: assessing and defining competency standards. Gastrointest Endosc. 2011;74(2): 355–366.e351–2.
28. Adler DG, Bakis G, Coyle WJ, et al. Principles of training in GI endoscopy. Gastrointest Endosc. 2012;75(2):231–5.
29. Vargo JJ, Delegge MH, Feld AD, et al. Multisociety sedation curriculum for gastrointestinal endoscopy. Gastroenterology. 2012; 143(1):e18–41.
30. American Society of Anesthesiologists Task Force on Sedation and Analgesia by Non-Anesthesiologists. Practice guidelines for sedation and analgesia by non-anesthesiologists. Anesthesiology. 2002; 96(4):1004–17.
31. Rex DK, Overley CA, Walker J. Registered nurse-administered propofol sedation for upper endoscopy and colonoscopy: why? when? how? Rev Gastroenterol Disord. 2003;3(2):70–80.
32. Vennes JA, Ament M, Boyce Jr HW, et al. Principles of training in gastrointestinal endoscopy. American Society for Gastrointestinal Endoscopy. Standards of Training Committees. 1989–1990. Gastrointest Endosc. 1992;38(6):743–6.
33. Vassiliou MC, Kaneva PA, Poulose BK, et al. How should we establish the clinical case numbers required to achieve proficiency in flexible endoscopy? Am J Surg. 2010;199(1):121–5.
34. Leung JW, Lee JG, Rojany M, Wilson R, Leung FW. Development of a novel ERCP mechanical simulator. Gastrointest Endosc. 2007; 65(7):1056–62.
35. Haycock AV, Youd P, Bassett P, Saunders BP, Tekkis P, Thomas-Gibson S. Simulator training improves practical skills in therapeutic GI endoscopy: results from a randomized, blinded, controlled study. Gastrointest Endosc. 2009;70(5):835–45.
36. Heinkel K, Kimmig JM. Stomach models for training in gastrocamera examination and gastroscopy. Z Gastroenterol. 1971;9(5):331–40.
37. Falkenstein DB, Abrams RM, Kessler RE, Jones B, Johnson G, Zimmon DS. Endoscopic retrograde cholangiopancreatography in the dog: a model for training and research. Gastrointest Endosc. 1974;21(1):25–6.
38. Hochberger J, Neumann M, Hohenberger W, Hahn EG. EASIE-Erlangen Education Simulation Model for Interventional Endoscopy – a new bio-training model for surgical endoscopy. Biomed Tech (Berl). 1997;42 Suppl:334.
39. Moorthy K, Munz Y, Jiwanji M, Bann S, Chang A, Darzi A. Validity and reliability of a virtual reality upper gastrointestinal simulator and cross validation using structured assessment of individual performance with video playback. Surg Endosc. 2004;18(2):328–33.
40. Hill A, Horswill MS, Plooy AM, et al. Assessing the realism of colonoscopy simulation: the development of an instrument and systematic comparison of 4 simulators. Gastrointest Endosc. 2012;75(3):631–40.
41. Mahmood T, Darzi A. A study to validate the colonoscopy simulator. Surg Endosc. 2003;17(10):1583–9.
42. Carter FJ, Schijven MP, Aggarwal R, et al. Consensus guidelines for validation of virtual reality surgical simulators. Surg Endosc. 2005;19(12):1523–32.
43. http://www.simbionix.com/index.html. 2006; Accessed 21 Mar 2013.
44. https://caehealthcare.com/home/eng/product_services/product_details/endovr#. 2006; Accessed 21 Mar 2013.
45. Lightdale JR, Fishman LN, Newburg AR, Villegas L, Fox VF. Fellow perceptions of computer-based endoscopy simulators vs. actual procedures for training purposes. J Pediatr Gastroenterol Nutr. 2003;36:366.
46. Moorthy K, Munz Y, Orchard TR, Gould S, Rockall T, Darzi A. An innovative method for the assessment of skills in lower gastrointestinal endoscopy. Surg Endosc. 2004;18(11):1613–9.
47. Ritter EM, McClusky 3rd DA, Lederman AB, Gallagher AG, Smith CD. Objective psychomotor skills assessment of experienced and novice flexible endoscopists with a virtual reality simulator. J Gastrointest Surg. 2003;7(7):871–7; discussion 877–878.
48. Desilets DJ, Banerjee S, Barth BA, et al. Endoscopic simulators. Gastrointest Endosc. 2011;73(5):861–7.
49. Faigel DO, Baron TH, Lewis B, et al. 2006. Ensuring competence in endoscopy. Oak Brook/Bethesda: American Society for Gastrointestinal Endoscopy. American College of Gastroenterology. http://www.asge.org/WorkArea/showcontent.aspx?id=3384. Accessed Mar 2011
50. Armstrong D, Enns R, Ponich T, Romagnuolo J, Springer J, Barkun AN. Canadian credentialing guidelines for endoscopic privileges: an overview. Can J Gastroenterol. 2007;21(12):797–801.
51. Bjorkman DJ, Popp Jr JW. Measuring the quality of endoscopy. Am J Gastroenterol. 2006;101(4):864–5.
52. Verma D, Gostout CJ, Petersen BT, Levy MJ, Baron TH, Adler DG. Establishing a true assessment of endoscopic competence in ERCP during training and beyond: a single-operator learning curve for deep biliary cannulation in patients with native papillary anatomy. Gastrointest Endosc. 2007;65(3):394–400.
53. Vassiliou MC, Kaneva PA, Poulose BK, et al. Global Assessment of Gastrointestinal Endoscopic Skills (GAGES): a valid measurement tool for technical skills in flexible endoscopy. Surg Endosc. 2010;24(8):1834–41.
54. Van Sickle KR, Buck L, Willis R, et al. A multicenter, simulation-based skills training collaborative using shared GI Mentor II systems: results from the Texas Association of Surgical Skills Laboratories (TASSL) flexible endoscopy curriculum. Surg Endosc. 2011;25(9):2980–6.
55. Bini EJ, Firoozi B, Choung RJ, Ali EM, Osman M, Weinshel EH. Systematic evaluation of complications related to endoscopy in a training setting: a prospective 30-day outcomes study. Gastrointest Endosc. 2003;57(1):8–16.
56. Sharma VK, Nguyen CC, Crowell MD, Lieberman DA, de Garmo P, Fleischer DE. A national study of cardiopulmonary unplanned events after GI endoscopy. Gastrointest Endosc. 2007;66(1):27–34.
57. Radaelli F, Terruzzi V, Minoli G. Extended/advanced monitoring techniques in gastrointestinal endoscopy. Gastrointest Endosc Clin N Am. 2004;14(2):335–52.
58. Cohen LB, Delegge MH, Aisenberg J, et al. AGA Institute review of endoscopic sedation. Gastroenterology. 2007;133(2):675–701.
59. Baxter NN, Rabeneck L. Is the effectiveness of colonoscopy "good enough" for population-based screening? J Natl Cancer Inst. 2010; 102(2):70–1.
60. Thomson A, Andrew G, Jones D. Optimal sedation for gastrointestinal endoscopy: review and recommendations. J Gastroenterol Hepatol. 2010;25:469–78.
61. Lightdale JR, Valim C, Newburg AR, Mahoney LB, Zgleszewski S, Fox VL. Efficiency of propofol versus midazolam and fentanyl sedation at a pediatric teaching hospital: a prospective study. Gastrointest Endosc. 2008;67(7):1067–75.
62. Rex DK. Review article: moderate sedation for endoscopy: sedation regimens for non-anaesthesiologists. Aliment Pharmacol Ther. 2006;24(2):163–71.
63. Rex DK. The science and politics of propofol. Am J Gastroenterol. 2004;99(11):2080–3.
64. Abraham N, Barkun A, Larocque M, et al. Predicting which patients can undergo upper endoscopy comfortably without conscious sedation. Gastrointest Endosc. 2002;56(2):180–9.
65. Campo R, Brullet E, Montserrat A, et al. Identification of factors that influence tolerance of upper gastrointestinal endoscopy. Eur J Gastroenterol Hepatol. 1999;11(2):201–4.

66. DHHS, CMS. Clarification of the interpretive guidelines for the anesthesia services condition of participation. 2010. http://www.cms.gov/Regulations-and-Guidance/Guidance/Transmittals/downloads//R59SOMA.pdf. Accessed 21 Mar 2013.
67. Bong CL, Lightdale JR, Fredette ME, Weinstock P. Effects of simulation versus traditional tutorial-based training on physiologic stress levels among clinicians: a pilot study. Simul Healthc. 2010;5(5):272–8.
68. Lightdale JR, Newburg AR, Mahoney LB, Fredette ME, Fishman LN. Fellow perceptions of training using computer-based endoscopy simulators. Gastrointest Endosc. 2010;72(1):13–8.
69. Greene AK, Zurakowski D, Puder M, Thompson K. Determining the need for simulated training of invasive procedures. Adv Health Sci Educ Theory Pract. 2006;11(1):41–9.
70. Weinstock PH, Kappus LJ, Garden A, Burns JP. Simulation at the point of care: reduced-cost, in situ training via a mobile cart. Pediatr Crit Care Med. 2009;10(2):176–81.

Simulation in Genitourinary Surgery

25

Marjolein C. Persoon, Barbara M.A. Schout, Matthew T. Gettman, and David D. Thiel

Introduction

Surgical education has been traditionally based on the Halstedian methodology of see one, do one, teach one [1]. This model relies on volume as well as access to real-life patients in order to work. The field of urology involves a very broad array of surgical procedures, and teaching/learning this breadth of surgical disciplines is a challenge, especially with the Halstedian model. Contemporary urologists are expected to learn an array of surgical techniques and procedures including open abdominal surgery, complex endoscopic surgery, percutaneous surgery, and laparoscopic surgery and the principles of implant surgery. The shift of a significant number of urology procedures to "minimally invasive" techniques poses a challenge to surgeon and educator alike. The loss of tactile feedback and the often counterintuitive movements encountered in these procedures place a strain on training [2]. Residency work hour restrictions and the public focus on improved patient safety [3] result in the learning needs of trainees taking a backseat to the legal and ethical imperatives of patient safety [3]. These training limitations provide a framework for the necessity of simulation training in urology.

The depth and breadth of urology practice combined with the introduction of new technologies have given rise to concerns regarding certification and recertification. Task training for technical skills may help improve manual dexterity, but training for situational awareness, decision making, communication, and teamwork is also vital [4]. The nontechnical skills of urology are seldom assessed or clarified [4]. The current certification/recertification process relying on written and oral exams needs revising in light of the advances and complexities of modern urology practice. The development of valid urology simulators will eventually play a role in the certification/recertification of urologists. The development of these same simulators will also no doubt provide a breakthrough for continuing medical education (CME).

Simulation will never be able to replace clinical experience and hands-on training; however, currently available urology simulation may help decrease the initial stages of the learning curve in a forgiving environment without compromising patient safety [5]. This level of simulation is adequate for beginning and even intermediate trainees but is not supported for the more advanced surgeon/urologist. The effectiveness of this training together with the transfer of skills gained on a simulator to the real environment also remains unproven [3]. Still, the role of simulation in surgical disciplines is growing, and rightfully so. Urology is no different and is perhaps better suited than most fields to have simulation take an important educational role by nature of the competencies required.

Simulation of Basic Urologic Procedures and Exams

Medical students have come to expect that they are no longer required to perform common bedside procedures such as urethral catheter placement because many of the procedures are performed by ancillary hospital personnel [6]. In fact, only 9–13% of fourth year acting interns will place a urethral cath-

M.C. Persoon, MD (✉)
Department of Urology, Catharina Hospital Eindhoven, Eindhoven, The Netherlands

Department of Surgery, Jeroen Bosch Ziekenhuis, 's-Hertogenbosch, Noord-Brabant, The Netherlands
e-mail: mleinpersoon@hotmail.com

B.M.A. Schout, MD, PhD
Urology Department, VU University Medical Center, Amsterdam, Noord Holland, The Netherlands
e-mail: bschout.uro@gmail.com

M.T. Gettman, MD
Department of Urology, Mayo Clinic, 200 1st St. SW, Rochester, MN 55905, USA
e-mail: gettman.matthew@mayo.edu

D.D. Thiel, MD
Department of Urology, Mayo Clinic Florida, 4500 San Pablo Road, Jacksonville, FL 32224, USA
e-mail: thiel.david@mayo.edu

A.I. Levine et al. (eds.), *The Comprehensive Textbook of Healthcare Simulation*,
DOI 10.1007/978-1-4614-5993-4_25,

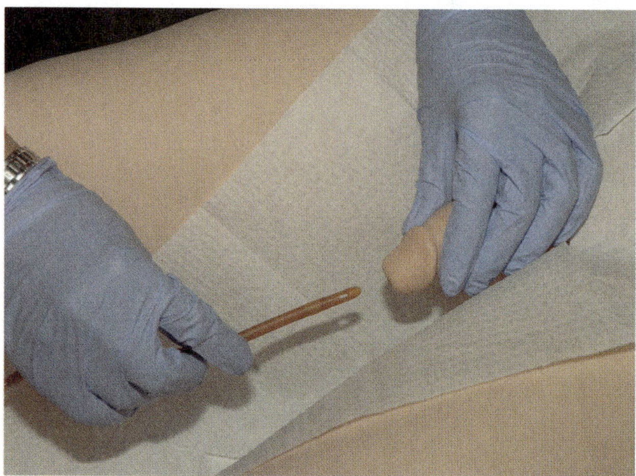

Fig. 25.1 Foley catheter task trainer. This penile task trainer aids in simulating proper urethral catheter insertion

eter during their rotations, but 82% feel competent performing the procedure without supervision [6]. The Medical School Objectives Project (MSOP) was designed to develop a standard curriculum of core procedures to be completed by graduating medical students [7]. Foley catheterization was one of the routine medical procedures to have competency established by graduating medical students. First year residents who completed a dedicated procedure course in medical school were more likely to report competency and adequacy in performing such procedures such as urethral catheterization [7]. It has been shown that didactic procedural skill sessions for urethral catheter placement utilizing task trainers (Fig. 25.1) increase medical student participation in the hospital and lead to demonstrable competence when performing the task [8].

Medical students perceive genital and rectal examinations as threatening [9]. Standardized patients have been used to teach rectal examinations for decades, although the use of mannequins has been proposed [10, 11]. Randomized controlled trials have demonstrated that medical students who trained using mannequin-based simulation had better bedside confidence and rapport for female pelvic exams as well as some benefit in male digital rectal exams [10, 11]. Siebeck et al. [11] evaluated the effect of low-fidelity simulation (mannequins) versus high-fidelity simulation (standardized patients) on student inhibition and acquisition of knowledge for male digital rectal examination. Both types of simulation were found to facilitate the acquisition of knowledge, but the standardized patients reduced inhibition more than low-fidelity simulation. The study focused on the social skills required to perform rectal examination. The authors did note that the low-fidelity simulator may aid in acquiring skills to detect pathology on rectal examination.

One problem with learning the digital rectal examination (DRE) is that the procedure being performed is hidden from instructor view. Low-Beer et al. [12] attempted to overcome this problem by cutting away the proximal portion of rectum from a standard benchtop male DRE simulator. They then recorded the learners' technique. This allowed the authors to deconstruct the procedure into 49 procedural steps and aided in teaching the steps that may be omitted during standard teaching of digital rectal examination. In general, there is a small but useful place for these sorts of simulations in medical education.

Transurethral Resection of Prostate (TURP) and Bladder Tumor (TURBT) Simulation

Transurethral resection techniques are commonly used in urology. With these techniques, one is able to resect prostate (TURP) or bladder tumor (TURBT) tissue, using a transurethral approach and an electrocoagulatory knife.

TURP

The goal of performing a TURP is to resect benign prostatic hyperplastic tissue, aiming to reduce the bulk of the prostatic tissue causing the bladder outlet obstruction and lower urinary tract symptoms. Several new, minimally invasive prostate resection techniques have been developed in the past years, including holmium laser enucleation of the prostate, photoselective vaporization, transurethral needle ablation, and transurethral microwave therapy. Although these new techniques have demonstrated safety and short-term efficacy, data on long-term efficacy are currently lacking, and the conventional transurethral resection of the prostate remains the gold standard [13]. Common complications are: bleeding, undermining the bladder neck, inadvertent peritoneal puncture during suprapubic catheter insertion, and capsular perforation with entry into the periprostatic venous plexus causing TURP syndrome [14].

A number of TURP simulators have been described in the literature [15–17]. Some of these were early prototypes of current simulators or were simulators which, to our knowledge, were not further developed and are not available on today's market [18–20]. In Table 25.1, a list of simulators is shown. The AMS/CREST simulator does not actually replicate TURP, but contains a photoselective vaporization of the prostate (PVP) module, where endoscopic instrument tracking, haptic rendering, and a web/database curriculum management modules are integrated into the system [21]. The development is based on the same prototype as the University of Washington TURP trainer. The Uro Trainer includes a TURBT module as well.

Validation studies have been performed to investigate the educational value of the available simulators. Most validation studies used the definitions of face, content, construct, and criterion validity similar to those described by McDougall [22]. Table 25.1 summarizes TURP simulators and validity described in literature.

Table 25.1 Simulators for transurethral resection of prostate (TURP) and investigated validity

Simulator	Alias	Face validity	Content validity	Construct validity	Criterion validity
METI/CAE SurgicalSIM	University of Washington TURP trainer	Y	Y	Y	Y
VirtaMed	TURPSim Simbionix trainer	N	N	N	N
CREST	AMS/PVP	Y	N	N	N
Uro Trainer	Storz trainer	Y	Y	N	N
PelvicVision	Melerit Medical trainer	Y	Y	Y	Y
Tupper™	Homemade TUR trainer	N	N	N	N
Dr. Forke's resection trainer	Samed GmbH	N	N	Y	N

Of the available TURP simulators, the METI/CAE Healthcare SurgicalSIM (alias: the University of Washington TURP trainer) has been most frequently described and most comprehensively investigated [23–29]. The simulator has been developed and improved over several years, and several prototypes of the simulator have been validated in the stages of development. Validation studies have been performed by the developers [23–27, 29] as well as by an external research group [28]. Studies included between 19 and 136 participants. However, this simulator is not available on the commercial market anymore.

The Uro Trainer (Storz, Germany) has been investigated for face and content validity by two study groups, which included 19 and 97 participants, respectively [30, 31]. Both groups concluded that face and content validity of this simulator could not yet be established, and further modification of the Uro Trainer was recommended before initiating further experimental validity studies. The virtual reality VirtaMed simulator has recently been developed and face, content, and construct validation studies are currently underway.

The PelvicVision trainer has been developed and evaluated by one Swedish study group; their face, content, construct, and criterion studies included 9–24 participants [32–35]. Based on these results, the authors conclude that criterion-based training of the TURP procedure on the PelvicVision trainer significantly improves operative performance and raises the level of skill dexterity of inexperienced urology residents compared to no training at all [32].

The Tupper™ simulator consists of 7 cm of a 30 ft garden hose, a suprapubic tube, a Tupperware™ box, three catheter plugs, and silicone gel [36]. Costs are below $40 US. Different transurethral procedures, such as mono- and bipolar resection, as well as laser vaporization, can be carried out on the model [36].

Dr K. Forke's resection trainer (LS 10-2/S) is a mobile device, consisting of a penis simulator, featuring a urethra, a specifically constructed device for the insertion of a different training prostate, a bladder chamber, and simulated suprapubic access, as well as optional intermittent or continuous-flow irrigation [37]. Two different training prostates are offered: one with and one without anatomical structures. In their construct validity study, the resection results of the one non-experienced resident showed a distinct learning curve during supervised training on the model. Also, the trained residents showed a more constant progress rate in the post-training phase compared to the results of three non-trained experienced residents. In the past, the company Limbs & Things produced a TURP and TURBT model for resection skill training. This device however was most commonly used by industry to demonstrate endoscopic equipment, and not for residency training. No validation studies were ever published on the model, which is currently off the market.

TURBT

Bladder tumors are very common tumors of the genitourinary system; therefore, transurethral resection of such tumors is often performed [14]. The goal is to remove the tumors, as well as to determine depth of invasion. Common complications are bleeding and perforation. Although several endourologic training models, such as animal models, virtual reality models, and synthetic models, have been developed for transurethral resection of the prostate and for urethrocystoscopy, only a few models or modules exist for the TURBT procedure. The Uro Trainer described in the TURP section also contains a TURBT module. In the past, the company Limbs & Things has also developed a TURBT module using synthetic materials, which is, however, no longer on the market. Furthermore, three low-cost, low-fidelity models have been described in the literature, but they were not validated (Table 25.2).

Validity studies have only been performed for the Uro Trainer (Storz, Germany). Study participants varied from 12 to 150 medical students, residents, or urologists. Conclusions of face and content validity investigations of this simulator differed between the two research groups. Reich et al. found an overall positive opinion of urologists towards the simulator with scores of 5.0–8.0 on a scale of 0–10 (0, insufficient/very unrealistic; 10, very good/extremely realistic) [38], whereas Schout et al. concluded that, measured against face and content criteria of other studies, only 3, 5, and 8% of the parameters could be interpreted as positive, moderately acceptable, and good, respectively [31]. Construct validity investigations showed improvement of medical students' results, but no improvement of residents' performances on the simulator [38].

Table 25.2 Simulators for transurethral resection of bladder tumor (TURBT) and investigated validity

Simulator	Alias	Face validity	Content validity	Construct validity	Criterion validity
Uro Trainer	Storz trainer	Y	Y	Y	N
Glass globe		N	N	N	N
Pig bladder model		N	N	N	N
Tupper™	Homemade TUR trainer	N	N	N	N

The financial costs of the virtual reality simulators are not clearly stated in the literature. In general, virtual reality simulators account for some tens of thousands of US dollars, whereas the box pig bladder model costs $160 US [39], the Tupper™ costs below $40 US, and the glass globe costs around $10 US [40].

Ureteroscopy Simulation

Adequate performance of basic endourological skills is of crucial importance in urological practice. Ureterorendoscopy (URS) is a widely used procedure that has diagnostic and therapeutic purposes in ureteric stone management and other abnormalities of the urinary tract [41]. For URS training outside the operating room, several models have been developed in past years ranging from low- to high-fidelity models. Simulators of animate and inanimate materials are available for various prices. Practicing on live animals or animate models has limitations, since it requires strict hygiene and can only be done in specialized laboratories. In general, animate models can be reused less frequently than inanimate ones, leading to increased financial costs. Moreover, ethical considerations increasingly restrict the use of animal models.

In 2008, Schout et al. published a review of the literature concerning existing training models in endourology [39]. More recent updates on training in ureteroscopy are described by Skolarikos and Olweny et al. [42, 43]. The most frequently described models are listed in Table 25.3.

Virtual Reality Simulators

In the last decade, computerized models, including virtual reality (VR) simulators, have been further developed and used for training surgical skills. A URS model which has often been described is the URO Mentor (Simbionix, Israel), a computer-based virtual reality (VR) model offering semi-rigid and flexible URS modules as well as rigid and flexible urethrocystoscopy (UCS) modules. In addition, a percutaneous access simulator can be added to the URO Mentor platform.

A personal computer is linked to a male mannequin with lifelike endoscopes. Computer-based graphics provide realistic images of the male genitourinary system. Various learning modules are included, which contain virtual patients with background, laboratory, and radiographic information. Trainees can choose appropriate instruments and record their performance for later evaluation. Several performance parameters like time, minutes of X-ray exposure, occurrence of perforations, and percentage of laser misfires are measured to evaluate a trainees performance.

The URO Mentor has proven effective as a tool for learning endoscopic skills. Parameters of performance on this VR simulator can distinguish inexperienced urologists from experienced ones. Furthermore, training on the URO Mentor has shown to improve real-time performance of URS and UCS procedures on patients and cadavers, although the number of studies and participants are limited [44–55].

Bench Models

Low-Fidelity Bench Models

Matsumoto et al. described a low-fidelity ureteroscopy model which consisted of a Penrose drain, an inverted cup, molded latex in a portable plastic case and two straws approximately of 8 mm. in diameter as substitutes for urethra, bladder dome, bladder base and bilateral ureters, respectively. Openings were cut midway up straws to facilitate placement of mid ureteral stones. It costs CAD$20 to manufacture [50].

High-Fidelity Bench Models

The Uro-Scopic Trainer (Limbs & Things, United Kingdom) is a high-fidelity bench model that offers training with real-time instruments [51, 53, 56, 57]. There was no difference in the performance of a basic ureteroscopic stone management procedure between trainees who trained on the URS training model from Limbs & Things and the URO Mentor VR simulator [53]. On the other hand, in the study described by Matsumoto et al., there was no difference in performance between trainees who trained on the low-fidelity bench model and the trainees who trained on the high-fidelity Uro-Scopic Trainer, measured in a laboratory environment using a checklist, global ratings score, pass rating, and time needed to perform the procedure [57].

Another bench model for URS is the Scope Trainer, which is developed by Mediskills Limited (United Kingdom). This model has an expandable bladder with vessels and contains a few bladder tumors. It has life-size ureters, and two anatomically accurate kidneys with renal pelvises and calyces. Through a tap from the bladder, irrigation fluid can be

Table 25.3 Most frequently described Ureterorendoscopy (URS) training models

Simulator	Manufacturer	Material	Fidelity	Content validity	Construct validity	Criterion validity	Virtual instructor
URO Mentor	Simbionix	Computerized	High	Y	Y	Y	Y
Adult Ureteroscopy Trainer	Ideal Anatomic Modeling	Inanimate	High	Y	Y	N	N
Uro-Scopic Trainer	Limbs & Things	Inanimate	High	Y	Y	N	N
Scope Trainer	Mediskills	Inanimate	High	Y	Y	N	N
Bench model	Liske et al.	Animal	High	Y	N	N	N
Bench model	Matsumoto et al.	Inanimate	Low	Y	Y	N	N

infused, and the bladder can be emptied [44, 58]. In a study by Brehmer et al., the performance of 26 urology residents was assessed on the bench model before and after training on this model. The participants were assessed by an experienced endourologist who used a task-specific checklist and global score. The study was performed in an operating room using the same instruments as in real life, and the model was covered with drapes to make the experience more realistic. The participants performed significantly better on the model after training, and the authors concluded that training on this bench model in a realistic setting enhanced the manual dexterity as well as familiarity with the method among urology residents [59].

More recently, in 2010, White et al. reported on the Adult Ureteroscopy Trainer (Ideal Anatomic Modeling, USA) [60]. This high-fidelity model has not been fully validated; however, results suggest face, content, and construct validity after the evaluation of 46 participants. The model claims to have anatomical accuracy, durability, and portability. In addition to inanimate bench simulators, porcine models have also been used for training ureteroscopic skills [61, 62]. In 2009, Liske et al. describe a bench model using a porcine urinary tract on which 150 urologists have trained; however, reports on validation studies are not available [63].

Costs of high-fidelity models range from $3,000 to $60,000 US [60]. Costs of the adult ureteroscopy trainer are $485 US. However, the costs and maintenance of the ureteroscope, basket retrieval devices, and phantom stones remain unclear. Most models require the presence of an instructor, since there is no virtual instructor, as in the URO Mentor. This could add to the overall cost of the simulation training.

Since all types of simulators have been shown to improve trainees' performance, it can be assumed that animate, inanimate, and virtual reality simulators, separately or in combination, can all be suitable for training purposes. Since high-fidelity models are not necessarily superior to low-fidelity models in all situations, the usefulness of a model may be better defined using the concept of functional fidelity, indicating the extent to which the skills required for the real task are performed during the simulated tasks [64].

Studies concerning the effect of simulator training on patient outcome are limited for the URS procedure. Furthermore, not all simulators have been validated. The choice for a particular model will partly depend on the instructors and resources, which are available in a hospital or training institution. Whether a low- or high-cost simulator is purchased, it is of paramount importance to provide optimal learning conditions for the trainee. A first step for structured implementation of simulator training for URS is to define which learning goals should be achieved and to create opportunities for trainees to practice skills on a regular basis. More research is needed to determine the optimal interval training scheme for simulator training for URS to achieve sustained learning. Conditions to optimize learning include feedback to the learner, repetitive practice, integration in the curriculum, different levels of difficulty, the use of multiple learning strategies, variety of clinical conditions, a controlled environment, individualized learning, the presence of clearly stated goals, and the use of validated simulators [2].

Transrectal Ultrasound Simulation

Ultrasound is an important diagnostic imaging modality in many areas of clinical medicine. In transrectal ultrasound (TRUS), the prostate can be visualized by introducing the ultrasound probe into the rectum. This technique is widely used for diagnosing benign prostate hyperplasia, performing volumetry, and enabling transrectal prostate biopsies to diagnose prostate cancer [65–68]. A standardized procedure for taking prostate biopsies is needed since the presence of prostate cancer may not always be visible in ultrasound images. There is no standard for the number of prostate biopsies required to diagnose prostate cancer accurately. However, most authors recommend an extended biopsy scheme of >10 biopsies [65, 68, 69]. The procedure for TRUS-guided prostatic biopsies is not without complications. The most frequently reported complications are hematuria, hematochezia, hematospermia, fever, sepsis, urinary retention, and prostatitis [70, 71].

The performance of TRUS requires several skills. Two-dimensional images have to be mentally related to a 3D environment, and there has to be adequate hand-eye coordination of the clinician performing the procedure. Visual input and haptic feedback must be combined with knowledge of anatomy and prostate pathology, to reach satisfying diagnostic

Table 25.4 Simulators for transrectal ultrasound (TRUS)

Author	Year	Material	Biopsies Y/N	Theoretical module	Content validity	Construct validity	Criterion validity
Cos	1990	Inanimate	N	N	N	N	N
Sclaverano	2009	Computerized	Y	N	Y	N	N
Persoon	2010	Computerized	N	N	Y	N	N
Chalasani	2011	Computerized	Y	N	Y	Y	N
Janssoone	2011	Computerized	Y	Y	Y	N	N

and biopsy results. Education and training are, therefore, key elements for successful application of ultrasound technology in patient care. Furthermore, TRUS and, especially, taking biopsies are uncomfortable for patients, and prolonging procedure time for educational purposes is not desirable. A training method with the use of simulators could help overcome these drawbacks of clinical training and improve efficiency and safety of the operator.

Little research has been done on TRUS simulators, and the simulators that have been described in literature are of limited validity, using the definitions of face, content, construct, and criterion validity described by McDougall [22]. Table 25.4 summarizes TRUS simulators described in the literature [72–76].

A 1990 paper describes a TRUS simulator in which the prostate was simulated by a Foley catheter balloon. This simple and inexpensive model can be used to learn the principles of ultrasound and to learn how to make a 3D mental composition from a 2D ultrasound image of the prostate, since it does not include real prostate images [74]. More recent simulators focus on the aspects of the prostate tissue itself. By using real patient data, it is possible for trainees to learn about normal and pathological aspects of the prostate, as well as practicing to adequately visualize all parts of the prostate [73, 75, 76]. In 2009, Sclaverano et al. described the first version of a simulator for ultrasound-guided prostate biopsy. The same simulator was described in 2011 and has been further developed. In addition to several technical improvements, the theoretical application in which exercises, knowledge, and feedback are included is of importance [72, 76]. Studies on construct and criterion validity of this simulator have not yet been described. In fact, none of the simulators described are criterion validated. Chalasani et al. describe a TRUS simulator in which construct validity is studied; however, a theoretical module was not described [75]. Other currently available ultrasound simulators used for medical training offer no option for TRUS, though developments are ongoing [77–82].

The financial costs of the TRUS simulators are not clearly stated in the literature and depend on several aspects. The simulator described by Persoon et al. is estimated to be $64,000 US, and optional devices are not included (Fig. 25.2). On the other hand, the relatively simple model, as described by Cos in 1990, seems less expensive but actually requires a real-time working ultrasound machine [73, 74]. To date, there is no accurate calculation on the financial benefits of simulator-based training for TRUS.

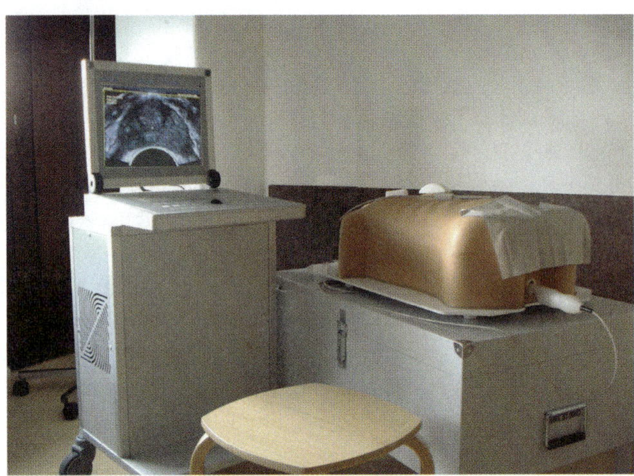

Fig. 25.2 TRUS simulator (MedCom, Germany). This virtual simulator allows the learner to place an ultrasound probe in a simulated rectum and practice coronal and axial viewing of the prostate

Simulator-based training for TRUS could be a helpful addition in the traditional apprenticeship-type training, especially for beginners, since all the simulators described offer basic training options for TRUS. Developments of the simulators for TRUS are ongoing and more extensive validation studies must follow before TRUS simulator training will likely be a standard part of resident training.

Laparoscopic Simulation in Urology

Despite the proven benefits of laparoscopic surgery as a surgical method for the kidney and prostate, widespread adoption by urologists has been lacking. Three-dimensional intervention with two-dimensional viewing, lack of haptic feedback, the fulcrum effect of the pubic bone and ribs for prostate and kidney surgery respectively, and the difficulty of intracorporeal suturing required for prostate and kidney surgery are reasons for the lack of widespread incorporation of laparoscopy into urology practice. A review of 2,407 laparoscopic urology surgeries demonstrated that the complication rate decreases from 13.3 to 3.6% after 100 cases. This demonstrates the inadequacy of laparoscopic training prior to entering the operating room [83, 84].

Autorino et al. [83] divided laparoscopic simulators into three types: mechanical, hybrids, and virtual reality. Mechanical simulators are boxes in which organs/objects are placed and manipulated. This type of simulator is relatively inexpensive and teaches the basic laparoscopic principles including instrument manipulation and hand-eye coordination. Hybrid simulators are similar to mechanical simulators with performance being monitored by a computer that is able to give guidance on how to perform the tasks and objective feedback to the trainee. Virtual reality (VR) simulation is based on computer-generated images of organs/objects linked to a human-computer interface. VR simulation also provides objective feedback to the trainee and may provide the option of training in advanced laparoscopic skills. VR simulation has been shown in several randomized trials to improve operating room performance of surgical trainees [83]. However, there is a lack of randomized studies assessing the predictive validity in laparoscopic urology as reported in general surgery for cholecystectomy, likely because the most frequently performed laparoscopic procedures in urology involve complex surgical steps [83].

Hybrid Simulators

Various substances have been injected into animal kidneys in an attempt to replicate partial nephrectomies. Improved renal pelvic anastomosis scores (laparoscopic pyeloplasty) have been noted with a training regiment consisting of a crop and esophagus of a chicken inside a training box [85]. Chicken skin has been used in a laparoscopic box to simulate the urethrovesical anastomosis required for laparoscopic prostatectomy. This training has led to improved manual dexterity and faster anastomosis times among trainees learning laparoscopic prostatectomy [86]. A 2009 study compared the use of VR simulation to a pelvic laparoscopic box trainer in 20 medical students learning laparoscopic suturing and knot-tying [87]. The students were randomized to the VR trainer or the box trainer. A 1-h didactic session and video was followed by 2 h of training on the assigned simulator. The students then all performed laparoscopic cystotomy closure on a porcine model. All students were able to complete the cystorrhaphy. There was no difference in time to complete the task or objective assessment of skills between the two groups. The authors concluded that there was no difference between the box trainer and VR simulation for simple laparoscopic tasks and that the box trainer may be more user-friendly for novice learners.

VR Simulators

Virtual reality nephrectomy simulation has been developed but is still in its infancy. Mentice (Gothenburg, Sweden) developed a VR simulator for laparoscopic nephrectomy that simulates a number of steps of the real-time procedure [88]. A 2010 study evaluated 22 novices, 32 intermediates, and 10 experienced urologists on the simulator performing similar tasks of laparoscopic nephrectomy [88]. The simulator did not differentiate between intermediate and experienced participants and learning curves were flat in all groups. The authors concluded that the simulator lacked construct validity. In addition, it was the authors' opinion that trainees' improvements on measured dexterity on the simulator were learned skills specific to the simulator rather than an improvement in operative skills. Simbionix (Cleveland, OH, USA) has developed a laparoscopic nephrectomy software package for use on the Lap Mentor II device. No validation studies are available to date for this software. Haptic feedback has been lacking from many VR simulators. However, the addition of haptic feedback software to VR simulators has not contributed to the improvement of accuracy, economy, or speed of hand movement to simulations performed with novice learners to date [89]. Better haptic feedback may be required for VR simulation to more accurately reflect real-life urologic surgery, and whether or not that would translate to "better" simulators is unclear.

Robotic Simulation in Urology

There is a steady increase in the number of urologists incorporating robotic-assisted laparoscopic prostatectomy (RALP) into practice. Related to this, the robotic training background of these urologists is becoming more varied and diverse as RALP utilization continues to increase. There remains no standardized credentialing system to evaluate surgeon competency and safety with regards to robotic surgery [90]. Most medical malpractice claims surrounding robotic surgeries are secondary to systems malfunctions, and 75% of those malfunctions arise intraoperatively [91]. The most common cause of these intraoperative systems malfunctions is due to inexperience or lack of technical competence with the instrumentation/surgical device [90, 91].

Multiple avenues exist to attain postgraduate robotic training including urologic oncology fellowships, laparoscopic/endourology fellowships, and robotic fellowships [92]. These fellowships vary in their length (1–3 years of duration) and accreditation. It is not known if one form of training is superior to another. What appears to be consistently successful in robotic training is a three-phase approach to learning surgical robotics and the guidance of an experienced mentor. The first phase involves learning the robotic technology including port placement, arm clutching, and overall familiarization with the robot. The second phase is assisting laparoscopically at the bedside; the third phase is completing individual steps of the RALP while sitting at the console [93, 94]. The role that formal robotic simulation plays in these steps remains to be determined.

Training on the robotic console can be difficult due to the expense of simulators and the difficulty of allowing untrained learners on the console in a clinical setting. The residency training program at Indiana University demonstrated the success of incorporating robotic tasks during training on inanimate models with the da Vinci robot [95]. New residents completed four Saturday sessions consisting of drills on inanimate objects (i.e., pegboard, letter board, string running, pattern cutting, and suturing). Trainees demonstrated significant improvements in terms of accuracy and time to completion regardless of level of experience or number of robotics cases completed. The residents preferred the weekend training over weekday training as well and noted an overall increase in their self-reported mean preparedness for live surgery.

There are currently three virtual reality robotic simulators commercially available. The Robotic Surgical Simulator (RoSS) is a novel virtual reality simulator of the da Vinci Surgical System (Simulated Surgical Systems; Williamsville, NY, USA) [96]. The console of the trainer consists of two, six degrees of freedom input devices; a stereo head-mounted display; pedals for clutch and camera controls; and pinch components to simulate the EndoWrist of the standard da Vinci surgical system console. The urology group from Roswell Park Cancer Institute divided simulation users into three groups: novice (no robot experience), intermediate (fewer than 149 cases), and expert (at least 150 robot cases). All study subjects rated the clutch control as "good" or "excellent," but 22% rated the device "poor" for object placement realism (ball placement drill). Thirteen percent rated the needle control simulation as poor, and only 27% rated needle control drills as excellent. While the simulator appeared to have its flaws, 75% recommended the simulator for training and 79% thought it could play a role in future privileging or certification for robotic surgery.

The Mimic dV-Trainer (MdVT) was developed by Mimic Technologies, Inc. (Seattle, WA). It includes foot pedals, side pods, EndoWrist, and high-definition stereoscopic display that functions similarly to the console components of the da Vinci surgical system (Fig. 25.3) [97]. Lerner et al. [97] evaluated use of the MdVT in a novice group of learners (medical students and residents) compared to a more experienced group of urology residents that trained utilizing the robot and inanimate objects. The MdVT group improved in pattern cutting and pegboard times, but only the group trained using inanimate objects improved in the knot-tying time and pegboard accuracy. The authors commented that the Mimic device lacked an adequate suturing exercise. Two recent publications have confirmed the face and content validity of the MdVT utilizing novice and experienced robotic subjects [98, 99]. Each study noted the realism of the tasks available and the validity of teaching what the drills were intended to teach. The experts were noted to outperform the novices with regard to time and accuracy in all assigned tasks.

Mimic Technologies also offers a backpack that attaches to the back of the da Vinci Si console. The software is the same as the MdVT and the drills are similar. Hung et al. [100] confirmed the face, content, and construct validity of the backpack among 16 novices, 32 intermediates, and 15 experts. The experts outperformed the intermediates and novices in almost every metric. All of the expert surgeons noted the device to be an excellent training tool for residents and fellows.

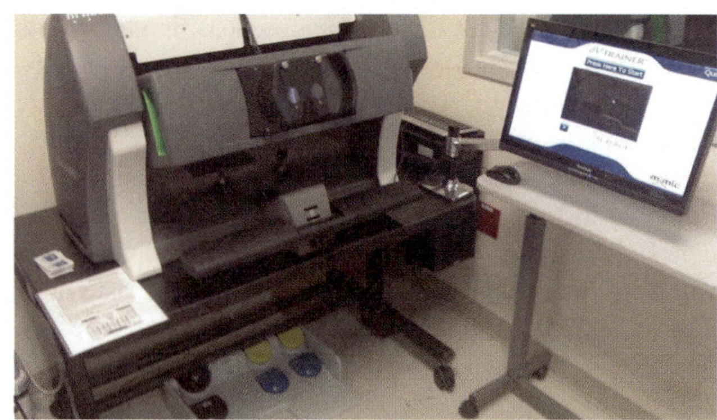

Fig. 25.3 Mimic virtual reality robotic simulator (Mimic Technologies, Inc., Seattle, WA). The Mimic virtual reality simulator offers a console and foot pedals that mimic the actual da Vinci surgical robot. The simulator relies on software-based drills to accommodate the learner to the three-dimensional robotic environment

All of the systems attempt to give immediate performance feedback after the completion of the exercise via software that interfaces with the virtual environment. The RoSS and MdVT are stand-alone devices that can be placed in an actual simulation center and be under the supervision of the simulation staff. The Si console backpack must be used on the actual da Vinci Si surgical console and, therefore, can only be used when the console is available in the operating room. Another limitation of the backpack is that it is used mostly in the operating room and, therefore, in most cases, not under the watchful eye of the simulation staff. The benefit to the backpack is that the learner participates on the actual da Vinci Si surgical console and not on a simulate interface.

Current robotic simulation is limited to simulating basic robotic tasks. Actual steps of robotic surgery (e.g., dissection) cannot currently be simulated or adequately replicated. However, having trainees learn basic robotic skills in a simulated environment (camera movement, clutching, hand movements, foot pedal coordination, and suturing) can decrease surgical risk and prepare the learner for more advanced tasks (prostate apical dissection, nerve sparing, etc.). What is still unknown is how much simulated learning is needed to improve safety and outcome and which simulated program provides the best pathway to the desired results [95].

High-Fidelity Simulation in Urology

Structured intraoperative communication and teamwork simulation has been limited for urology trainees. Gettman et al. [101] provided the first urology evaluation of teamwork, communication, and laparoscopic skills in a simulated environment. Nineteen residents participated in simulated scenarios involving insufflator failure and CO_2 embolus. The simulated mannequin was set up for laparoscopic renal surgery, and learners were videotaped gaining laparoscopic access. The scenario involving insufflator failure relied on the operating room team to troubleshoot the problem while activating a patient deterioration scenario if too much attention was diverted away from the patient. A majority of the participants noted that the scenarios were realistic and that they prompted realistic responses. The participants noted the lower realism of the simulated abdominal wall compared to a standard patient's abdomen. They also noted that the debriefing session was extremely helpful. The authors concluded that while some aspects of immersive OR simulation are lacking, the scenario and equipment did not need to be perfect to achieve the stated goals.

The same group utilized the Mayo Clinic Multidisciplinary Simulation Center to deliver an unexpected death scenario to 19 urology residents [102]. The resident was called to an unstable patient's bedside following cystectomy for evaluation. The authors assessed verification of code status before calling a code. Once a code was activated, the patient's wife was sent to a quiet room. Once the patient died, the resident was assessed for their ability to deliver the bad news. The group was unsatisfactory with verification of codes status before calling a code and resident performance was unsatisfactory when it came to choice of words used to deliver the news of death. Only 3 of 19 residents used the words "died" or "death" in their delivery. All residents found the simulation useful and provided adequate realism and most thought the simulation should be incorporated into their standard curriculum. Undre et al. [103] demonstrated that crisis management simulation in an operating room environment during a scenario of uncontrolled bleeding from a TURP or TUR syndrome was feasible for training with good learner feedback. The authors noted that this type of simulation builds situational awareness and improves team communication. The benefit of high-fidelity crisis simulation lies in the fact that it involves not only the surgeon but the entire operating room team, and therefore, the boundaries between technical and nontechnical performance can become blurred [4].

Implementing Simulation Training into Urology Training

Implementation of all of the above training into a program is an overwhelming task. The limitations of physician-instructor availability due to heavy patient loads, the ACGME work hour limitations, and overall clinical duties preclude implementation of all of the above simulation exercises into resident training. The cost of much of the above technology is also prohibitive to widespread incorporation into training programs. Many programs are relegated to offering simulation in 1- or 2-h blocks during set education time during the week. It is not practical to offer formal week-long laparoscopic training courses to each new resident as they enter a program. A 2007 study of American residency program directors demonstrated that simulators were good educational tools that allowed practice in a controlled environment, but there was disagreement about the cost-effectiveness, validity, and ability of the simulators to replace hands-on operative training [104]. Much of the current literature on simulation in urology focuses on residents in training. An overlooked aspect of simulation training is in the allied health involved in bedside assisting during major laparoscopic/abdominal operations as well as postoperative patient care.

With these limitations, programs must pick and choose areas of focus. Many programs will also feel obligated to utilize equipment that has already been purchased. For instance, a program that has a robotic simulator will preferentially focus on robotic simulation training due to their ownership of the technology. A common theme of all of the above-mentioned simulation equipment is its value for beginning surgeons yet limited value for more experienced surgeons. For instance, an experienced robotic surgeon may find little value in commercially available robotic simulators, due to the lack of advanced software mimicking difficult scenarios (e.g., bleeding during robotic prostatectomy).

Standards for certification and recertification of urologists vary by region of the world [5]. General surgeons have incorporated the Fundamentals of Laparoscopic Surgery (FLS) into the surgical licensure process for residents in training [105]. This program has been modified for urologists and termed BLUS (Basic Laparoscopic Urologic Surgery) [106]. BLUS has modified the didactic portion to be more urocentric and has eliminated the endoloop and extracorporeal knot-tying psychomotor exercises. BLUS has good acceptability and evidence of construct validity for assessment of basic laparoscopic skills for urologists but has not yet been utilized in the licensing process. The American Board of Medical Specialties (ABMS) identifies six components of competency. Simulation-based training or recertification may play a role in all six ABMS competencies but is especially relevant in the patient care, communication, and practice-based learning modules. Currently, there is no formal requirement for simulation or hands-on demonstration of skills in the licensure or recertification process for urologists.

Conclusion

The need for simulation in urology is inherent. Numerous simulation techniques and equipment have been developed for the different aspects of urology from laparoscopic/robotic surgery to endoscopic surgery. Training for the nontechnical aspects of urology (i.e., team training/communication) lag behind simulation for the technical aspects of urology. The cost-effectiveness of this simulation-based training as it transfers to the operating theater and relates to patient safety outcomes needs further assessment, but it is likely that as more evidence points towards improved patient safety via simulation-based training, the widespread adoption will be inevitable.

References

1. Barnes RW, Lang NP, Whiteside MF. Halstedian technique revisited. Innovations in teaching surgical skills. Ann Surg. 2010;1989:118–21.
2. Issenberg SB, McGaghie WC, Petrusa ER, Lee Gordon D, Scalese RJ. Features and uses of high-fidelity medical simulations that lead to effective learning: a BEME systematic review. Med Teach. 2005;27(1):10–28.
3. Ahmed K, Jawad M, Abboudi M, et al. Effectiveness of procedural simulation in urology: a systematic review. J Urol. 2011;186(1):26–34.
4. Arora S, Lamb B, Undre S, Kneebone R, Darzi A, Sevdalis N. Framework for incorporating simulation into urology training. BJU Int. 2011;107(5):806–10.
5. Ahmed K, Jawad M, Dasgupta P, Darzi A, Athanasiou T, Khan MS. Assessment and maintenance of competence in urology. Nat Rev Urol. 2010;7(7):403–13.
6. Coberly L, Goldenhar LM. Ready or not, here they come: acting interns' experience and perceived competency performing basic medical procedures. J Gen Intern Med. 2007;22(4):491–4.
7. Promes SB, Chudgar SM, Grochowski CO, et al. Gaps in procedural experience and competency in medical school graduates. Acad Emerg Med. 2009;16 Suppl 2:S58–62.
8. Meyers MO, Meyer AA, Stewart RD, et al. Teaching technical skills to medical students during a surgery clerkship: results of a small group curriculum. J Surg Res. 2011;166(2):171–5.
9. Rochelson BL, Baker DA, Mann WJ, Monheit AG, Stone ML. Use of male and female professional patient teams in teaching physical examination of the genitalia. J Reprod Med. 1985;30(11):864–6.
10. Norman G, Barrows H, Gliva G, Woodward C. Simulated patients. In: Neufeld V, Norman G, editors. Assessing clinical competence. New York: Springer; 1985. p. 219–29.
11. Siebeck M, Schwald B, Frey C, Roding S, Stegmann K, Fischer F. Teaching the rectal examination with simulations: effects on knowledge acquisition and inhibition. Med Educ. 2011;45(10):1025–31.
12. Low-Beer N, Kinnison T, Baillie S, Bello F, Kneebone R, Higham J. Hidden practice revealed: using task analysis and novel simulator design to evaluate the teaching of digital rectal examination. Am J Surg. 2011;201(1):46–53.
13. Kacker R, Williams SB. Endourologic procedures for benign prostatic hyperplasia: review of indications and outcomes. Urol J. 2011;8(3):171–6.
14. Hohenfellner R, Stolzenburg JU. Manual endourology. Training for residents. Heidelberg: Springer Medizin Verlag; 2008.
15. Sweet RM. Review of trainers for transurethral resection of the prostate skills. J Endourol. 2007;21(3):280–4.
16. Schout BM, Hendrikx AJ, Scherpbier AJ, Bemelmans BL. Update on training models in endourology: a qualitative systematic review of the literature between January 1980 and April 2008. Eur Urol. 2008;54(6):1247–61.
17. Wignall GR, Denstedt JD, Preminger GM, et al. Surgical simulation: a urological perspective. J Urol. 2008;179(5):1690–9.
18. Gomes MP, Barrett AR, Timoney AG, Davies BL. A computer-assisted training/monitoring system for TURP structure and design. IEEE Trans Inf Technol Biomed. 1999;3(4):242–51.
19. Ballaro A, Briggs T, Garcia-Montes F, MacDonald D, Emberton M, Mundy AR. A computer generated interactive transurethral prostatic resection simulator. J Urol. 1999;162(5):1633–5.
20. Kumar PV, Gomes MP, Davies BL, Timoney AG. A computer assisted surgical trainer for transurethral resection of the prostate. J Urol. 2002;168(5):2111–4.
21. Shen Y, Konchada V, Zhang N, et al. Laser surgery simulation platform: toward full-procedure training and rehearsal for benign prostatic hyperplasia (BPH) therapy. Stud Health Technol Inform. 2011;163:574–80.
22. McDougall EM. Validation of surgical simulators. J Endourol. 2007;21(3):244–7.
23. Sweet RM, McDougall EM. Simulation and computer-animated devices: the new minimally invasive skills training paradigm. Urol Clin North Am. 2008;35(3):519–31, x.
24. Sweet R, Kowalewski T, Oppenheimer P, Weghorst S, Satava R. Face, content and construct validity of the University of Washington virtual reality transurethral prostate resection trainer. J Urol. 2004;172(5 Pt 1):1953–7.
25. Sweet R, Porter J, Oppenheimer P, Hendrickson D, Gupta A, Weghorst S. Simulation of bleeding in endoscopic procedures using virtual reality. J Endourol. 2002;16(7):451–5.
26. Rashid HH, Kowalewski T, Oppenheimer P, Ooms A, Krieger JN, Sweet RM. The virtual reality transurethral prostatic resection trainer: evaluation of discriminate validity. J Urol. 2007;177(6): 2283–6.
27. Kishore TA, Beddingfield R, Holden T, Shen Y, Reihsen T, Sweet RM. Task deconstruction facilitates acquisition of transurethral resection of prostate skills on a virtual reality trainer. J Endourol. 2009;23(4):665–8.
28. Hudak SJ, Landt CL, Hernandez J, Soderdahl DW. External validation of a virtual reality transurethral resection of the prostate simulator. J Urol. 2010;184(5):2018–22.
29. Oppenheimer P, Gupta A, Weghorst S, Sweet R, Porter J. The representation of blood flow in endourologic surgical simulations. Stud Health Technol Inform. 2001;81:365–71.
30. Mishra S, Kurien A, Ganpule A, Veeramani M, Sabnis RB, Desai M. Face and content validity of transurethral resection of prostate on Uro Trainer: is the simulation training useful? J Endourol. 2010;24(11):1839–43.
31. Schout BM, Bemelmans BL, Martens EJ, Scherpbier AJ, Hendrikx AJ. How useful and realistic is the uro trainer for training transurethral prostate and bladder tumor resection procedures? J Urol. 2009;181(3):1297–303; discussion 1303.
32. Kallstrom R, Hjertberg H, Svanvik J. Impact of virtual reality-simulated training on urology residents' performance of transurethral resection of the prostate. J Endourol. 2010;24(9):1521–8.
33. Kallstrom R, Hjertberg H, Kjolhede H, Svanvik J. Use of a virtual reality, real-time, simulation model for the training of urologists in transurethral resection of the prostate. Scand J Urol Nephrol. 2005;39(4):313–20.
34. Kallstrom R. Construction, validation and application of a virtual reality simulator for the training of transurethral resection of the prostate. Linkoping University medical dissertations No.11672010.
35. Kallstrom R, Hjertberg H, Svanvik J. Construct validity of a full procedure, virtual reality, real-time, simulation model for training in transurethral resection of the prostate. J Endourol. 2010;24(1):109–15.
36. Bach T, Geavlete B, Herrmann TR, Gross AJ. "Homemade" TUR-simulator for less than $40 U.S.? The "Tupper" experience. J Endourol. 2009;23(3):509–13.
37. Ebbing J, Schostak M, Steiner U, et al. Novel low-cost prostate resection trainer-description and preliminary evaluation. Int J Med Robot. 2011. [Epub ahead of print].
38. Reich O, Noll M, Gratzke C, et al. High-level virtual reality simulator for endourologic procedures of lower urinary tract. Urology. 2006;67(6):1144–8.

39. Schout B, Dolmans V, Bemelmans B, Schoot D, Scherpbier A, Hendrikx A. Teaching diagnostic and therapeutic procedures of bladder pathology using a newly developed pig bladder model. J Endourol. 2008;22(11):2547–53.
40. Persoon MC, Schout BM, Muijtjens AM, Hendrikx AJ, Witjes JA, Scherpbier AJ. The effect of a low-fidelity model on cystoscopic skill training: a single-blinded randomized controlled trial. Simul Healthc. 2010;5(4):213–8.
41. Preminger GM, Tiselius HG, Assimos DG, et al. 2007 Guideline for the management of ureteral calculi. Eur Urol. 2007;52(6): 1610–31.
42. Skolarikos A, Gravas S, Laguna MP, Traxer O, Preminger GM, de la Rosette J. Training in ureteroscopy: a critical appraisal of the literature. BJU Int. 2011;108(6):798–805; discussion 805.
43. Olweny EO, Pearle MS. Update on resident training models for ureteroscopy. Curr Urol Rep. 2011;12(2):115–20.
44. Watterson JD, Denstedt JD. Ureteroscopy and cystoscopy simulation in urology. J Endourol. 2007;21(3):263–9.
45. Schout BM, Muijtjens AM, Hendrikx AJ, et al. Acquisition of flexible cystoscopy skills on a virtual reality simulator by experts and novices. BJU Int. 2010;105(2):234–9.
46. Schout BM, Ananias HJ, Bemelmans BL, et al. Transfer of cysto-urethroscopy skills from a virtual-reality simulator to the operating room: a randomized controlled trial. BJU Int. 2010;106(2):226–31; discussion 231.
47. Ogan K, Jacomides L, Shulman MJ, Roehrborn CG, Cadeddu JA, Pearle MS. Virtual ureteroscopy predicts ureteroscopic proficiency of medical students on a cadaver. J Urol. 2004;172(2):667–71.
48. Nedas T, Challacombe B, Dasgupta P. Virtual reality in urology. BJU Int. 2004;94(3):255–7.
49. Michel MS, Knoll T, Kohrmann KU, Alken P. The URO Mentor: development and evaluation of a new computer-based interactive training system for virtual life-like simulation of diagnostic and therapeutic endourological procedures. BJU Int. 2002;89(3): 174–7.
50. Matsumoto ED, Pace KT, D'A Honey RJ. Virtual reality ureteroscopy simulator as a valid tool for assessing endourological skills. Int J Urol. 2006;13(7):896–901.
51. Laguna MP, Hatzinger M, Rassweiler J. Simulators and endourological training. Curr Opin Urol. 2002;12(3):209–15.
52. Gettman MT, Le CQ, Rangel LJ, Slezak JM, Bergstralh EJ, Krambeck AE. Analysis of a computer based simulator as an educational tool for cystoscopy: subjective and objective results. J Urol. 2008;179(1):267–71.
53. Chou DS, Abdelshehid C, Clayman RV, McDougall EM. Comparison of results of virtual-reality simulator and training model for basic ureteroscopy training. J Endourol. 2006;20(4):266–71.
54. Hoznek A, Salomon L, de la Taille A, et al. Simulation training in video-assisted urologic surgery. Curr Urol Rep. 2006;7(2):107–13.
55. Knoll T, Trojan L, Haecker A, Alken P, Michel MS. Validation of computer-based training in ureterorenoscopy. BJU Int. 2005;95(9):1276–9.
56. Matsumoto ED, Hamstra SJ, Radomski SB, Cusimano MD. A novel approach to endourological training: training at the Surgical Skills Center. J Urol. 2001;166(4):1261–6.
57. Matsumoto ED, Hamstra SJ, Radomski SB, Cusimano MD. The effect of bench model fidelity on endourological skills: a randomized controlled study. J Urol. 2002;167(3):1243–7.
58. Brehmer M, Tolley D. Validation of a bench model for endoscopic surgery in the upper urinary tract. Eur Urol. 2002;42(2):175–9; discussion 180.
59. Brehmer M, Swartz R. Training on bench models improves dexterity in ureteroscopy. Eur Urol. 2005;48(3):458–63; discussion 463.
60. White MA, Dehaan AP, Stephens DD, Maes AA, Maatman TJ. Validation of a high fidelity adult ureteroscopy and renoscopy simulator. J Urol. 2010;183(2):673–7.
61. Hammond L, Ketchum J, Schwartz BF. Accreditation council on graduate medical education technical skills competency compliance: urologic surgical skills. J Am Coll Surg. 2005;201(3): 454–7.
62. Strohmaier WL, Giese A. Porcine urinary tract as a training model for ureteroscopy. Urol Int. 2001;66(1):30–2.
63. Liske P, Ober P, Aguilar Y, Zimmermanns V, Lahme S. Training of upper urinary tract endoscopy – experience with a new model using porcine urinary tract. J Endourol. 2009;23 suppl 1:A224.
64. Matsumoto ED. Low-fidelity ureteroscopy models. J Endourol. 2007;21(3):248–51.
65. Eichler K, Hempel S, Wilby J, Myers L, Bachmann LM, Kleijnen J. Diagnostic value of systematic biopsy methods in the investigation of prostate cancer: a systematic review. J Urol. 2006;175(5):1605–12.
66. Shapiro A, Lebensart PD, Pode D, Bloom RA. The clinical utility of transrectal ultrasound and digital rectal examination in the diagnosis of prostate cancer. Br J Radiol. 1994;67(799): 668–71.
67. Fuchsjager M, Shukla-Dave A, Akin O, Barentsz J, Hricak H. Prostate cancer imaging. Acta Radiol. 2008;49(1):107–20.
68. Chun FK, Epstein JI, Ficarra V, et al. Optimizing performance and interpretation of prostate biopsy: a critical analysis of the literature. Eur Urol. 2010;58(6):851–64.
69. Karakiewicz PI, Perrotte P, McCormack M, et al. Early detection of prostate cancer with ultrasound-guided systematic needle biopsy. Can J Urol. 2005;12 Suppl 2:5–8.
70. Kakehi Y, Naito S. Complication rates of ultrasound-guided prostate biopsy: a nation-wide survey in Japan. Int J Urol. 2008;15(4): 319–21.
71. Gallina A, Suardi N, Montorsi F, et al. Mortality at 120 days after prostatic biopsy: a population-based study of 22,175 men. Int J Cancer. 2008;123(3):647–52.
72. Sclaverano S, Chevreau G, Vadcard L, Mozer P, Troccaz J. BiopSym: a simulator for enhanced learning of ultrasound-guided prostate biopsy. Stud Health Technol Inform. 2009;142: 301–6.
73. Persoon MC, Schout B, Martens EJ, et al. A simulator for teaching transrectal ultrasound procedures: how useful and realistic is it? Simul Healthc. 2010;5(5):311–4.
74. Cos LR. Simulator for transrectal ultrasound of prostate. Urology. 1990;35(5):450–1.
75. Chalasani V, Cool DW, Sherebrin S, Fenster A, Chin J, Izawa JI. Development and validation of a virtual reality transrectal ultrasound guided prostatic biopsy simulator. Can Urol Assoc J. 2011;5(1):19–26.
76. Janssoone T, Chevreau G, Vadcard L, Mozer P, Troccaz J. Biopsym: a learning environment for trans-rectal ultrasound guided prostate biopsies. Stud Health Technol Inform. 2011;163:242–6.
77. Weidenbach M, Drachsler H, Wild F, et al. EchoComTEE – a simulator for transoesophageal echocardiography. Anaesthesia. 2007; 62(4):347–53.
78. Terkamp C, Kirchner G, Wedemeyer J, et al. Simulation of abdomen sonography. Evaluation of a new ultrasound simulator. Ultraschall Med. 2003;24(4):239–44.
79. Maul H, Scharf A, Baier P, et al. Ultrasound simulators: experience with the SonoTrainer and comparative review of other training systems. Ultrasound Obstet Gynecol. 2004;24(5):581–5.
80. Ehricke HH. SONOSim3D: a multimedia system for sonography simulation and education with an extensible case database. Eur J Ultrasound. 1998;7(3):225–300.
81. d'Aulignac D, Laugier C, Troccaz J, Vieira S. Towards a realistic echographic simulator. Med Image Anal. 2006;10(1):71–81.
82. Knudson MM, Sisley AC. Training residents using simulation technology: experience with ultrasound for trauma. J Trauma. 2000;48(4):659–65.

83. Autorino R, Haber GP, Stein RJ, et al. Laparoscopic training in urology: critical analysis of current evidence. J Endourol. 2010; 24(9):1377–90.
84. Fahlenkamp D, Rassweiler J, Fornara P, Frede T, Loening SA. Complications of laparoscopic procedures in urology: experience with 2,407 procedures at 4 German centers. J Urol. 1999;162 (3 Pt 1):765–70; discussion 770–1.
85. Ramachandran A, Kurien A, Patil P, et al. A novel training model for laparoscopic pyeloplasty using chicken crop. J Endourol. 2008;22(4):725–8.
86. Katz R, Nadu A, Olsson LE, et al. A simplified 5-step model for training laparoscopic urethrovesical anastomosis. J Urol. 2003; 169(6):2041–4.
87. McDougall EM, Kolla SB, Santos RT, et al. Preliminary study of virtual reality and model simulation for learning laparoscopic suturing skills. J Urol. 2009;182(3):1018–25.
88. Wijn RP, Persoon MC, Schout BM, Martens EJ, Scherpbier AJ, Hendrikx AJ. Virtual reality laparoscopic nephrectomy simulator is lacking in construct validity. J Endourol. 2010;24(1): 117–22.
89. Salkini MW, Doarn CR, Kiehl N, Broderick TJ, Donovan JF, Gaitonde K. The role of haptic feedback in laparoscopic training using the LapMentor II. J Endourol. 2010;24(1):99–102.
90. Zorn KC, Gautam G, Shalhav AL, et al. Training, credentialing, proctoring and medicolegal risks of robotic urological surgery: recommendations of the society of urologic robotic surgeons. J Urol. 2009;182(3):1126–32.
91. Rogers Jr SO, Gawande AA, Kwaan M, et al. Analysis of surgical errors in closed malpractice claims at 4 liability insurers. Surgery. 2006;140(1):25–33.
92. Guzzo TJ, Gonzalgo ML. Robotic surgical training of the urologic oncologist. Urol Oncol. 2009;27(2):214–7.
93. Thiel DD, Francis P, Heckman MG, Winfield HN. Prospective evaluation of factors affecting operating time in a residency/fellowship training program incorporating robot-assisted laparoscopic prostatectomy. J Endourol. 2008;22(6):1331–8.
94. Rashid HH, Leung YY, Rashid MJ, Oleyourryk G, Valvo JR, Eichel L. Robotic surgical education: a systematic approach to training urology residents to perform robotic-assisted laparoscopic radical prostatectomy. Urology. 2006;68(1):75–9.
95. Lucas SM, Gilley DA, Joshi SS, Gardner TA, Sundaram CP. Robotics training program: evaluation of the satisfaction and the factors that influence success of skills training in a resident robotics curriculum. J Endourol. 2011;25(10):1669–74.
96. Seixas-Mikelus SA, Stegemann AP, Kesavadas T, et al. Content validation of a novel robotic surgical simulator. BJU Int. 2011;107(7):1130–5.
97. Lerner MA, Ayalew M, Peine WJ, Sundaram CP. Does training on a virtual reality robotic simulator improve performance on the da Vinci surgical system? J Endourol. 2010;24(3):467–72.
98. Sethi AS, Peine WJ, Mohammadi Y, Sundaram CP. Validation of a novel virtual reality robotic simulator. J Endourol. 2009; 23(3):503–8.
99. Kenny PA, Wszolek MF, Gould JJ, Libertino JA, Monizadeh A. Face, content, and construct validity of dV-Trainer, a novel virtual reality simulator for robotic surgery. Urology. 2009;73:1288–92.
100. Hung AJ, Zehnder P, Patil MB, et al. Face, content and construct validity of a novel robotic surgery simulator. J Urol. 2011;186(3): 1019–24.
101. Gettman MT, Pereira CW, Lipsky K, et al. Use of high fidelity operating room simulation to assess and teach communication, teamwork and laparoscopic skills: initial experience. J Urol. 2009;181(3):1289–96.
102. Gettman MT, Karnes RJ, Arnold JJ, et al. Urology resident training with an unexpected patient death scenario: experiential learning with high fidelity simulation. J Urol. 2008;180(1):283–8; discussion 288.
103. Undre S, Koutantji M, Sevdalis N, et al. Multidisciplinary crisis simulations: the way forward for training surgical teams. World J Surg. 2007;31(9):1843–53.
104. Le CQ, Lightner DJ, VanderLei L, Segura JW, Gettman MT. The current role of medical simulation in American urological residency training programs: an assessment by program directors. J Urol. 2007;177(1):288–91.
105. Fried GM, Feldman LS, Vassiliou MC, et al. Proving the value of simulation in laparoscopic surgery. Ann Surg. 2004;240(3):518–25; discussion 525–8.
106. Sweet RM, Beach R, Sainfort F, et al. Introduction and validation of the American Urological Association Basic Laparoscopic Urologic Surgery skills curriculum. J Endourol. 2012;26(2):190–6.

Simulation in Internal Medicine

26

Paul E. Ogden, Courtney West, Lori Graham, Curtis Mirkes, and Colleen Y. Colbert

Introduction

Simulation-based medical education (SBME) offers several benefits that make it an excellent instructional tool and a good fit for Internal Medicine education. SBME, which includes both low-fidelity and high-fidelity simulation modalities, has the potential to shorten the learning curve for trainees, improve patient safety, standardize the curriculum, assess all six of the Accreditation Council for Graduate Medical Education (ACGME) [1] competencies, and offer observations of real-time clinical decision making [2, 3]. SBME offers significant advantages in teaching medical students and Internal Medicine residents, as SBME methodology ensures comparable learning experiences [2]. SBME is also important for Internal Medicine physicians, as it offers opportunities to learn and practice new technical skills and remediate skills required for clinical practice in controlled, safe environments [4].

SBME has increased exponentially over the last few years and has gained acceptance in many medical fields [5, 6]. Internal Medicine, was not an early adopter of simulation [2]. In the past, Internal Medicine did not use simulation with residents as extensively as departments of Anesthesiology and Emergency Medicine [13, 14], due to questions about its value and sustainability [6, 12]. However, Internal medicine is now one of the disciplines most commonly utilizing simulation [7]. The increasing use of SBME methodologies may be a result of patient safety and quality initiatives [6–8]; the shift to ambulatory medicine, which tends to limit types of clinical encounters; the focus on outcomes-based education [3]; and duty-hour restrictions. For example, Internal Medicine residency training has become shorter due to duty-hour restrictions, despite the fact that residents have more to learn. Since trainees are spending fewer hours in the hospital setting [9], simulation provides an efficient and effective way for residents to interact with a variety of patients and various clinical scenarios. SBME shortens learning time [2], increases confidence [10, 11], and can improve the assessment of general competencies.

Widespread support by students [12] and faculty members is making SBME a common instructional method in Internal Medicine clerkship curricula [7, 15], as well as in Graduate Medical Education (GME), Continuing Medical Education (CME), and recertification. In this chapter, SBME initiatives in the field of Internal Medicine will be described and future implications discussed. Simulation is vital in facilitating lifelong learning, problem solving, self-assessment [16], and critical thinking [12]. We believe it is a critical component throughout the educational continuum [2].

P.E. Ogden, MD (✉)
Department of Internal Medicine, Academic Affairs,
Texas A&M University System – HSC College of Medicine,
8447 State Hwy. 47, Bryan, TX 77807-3260, USA
e-mail: ogden@medicine.tamhsc.edu

C. West, PhD • L. Graham, PhD
Office of Medical Education, Internal Medicine,
Texas A&M HSC College of Medicine,
8447 State Hwy. 47, Bryan, TX 77807-3260, USA
e-mail: west@medicine.tamhsc.edu; graham@medicine.tamhsc.edu

C. Mirkes, DO
Department of Internal Medicine,
Scott & White Healthcare/Texas A&M HSC College of Medicine,
2401 S. 31st St., Temple, TX 76508, USA
e-mail: csmirkes@swmail.sw.org

C.Y. Colbert, PhD, MA
Office of Medical Education, Evaluation & Research Development,
Department of Internal Medicine,
Texas A&M HSC College of Medicine/Scott & White Healthcare,
2401 S. 31st St., Temple, TX 76508, USA
e-mail: cycolbert@swmail.sw.org

A.I. Levine et al. (eds.), *The Comprehensive Textbook of Healthcare Simulation*,
DOI 10.1007/978-1-4614-5993-4_26, © Springer Science+Business Media New York 2013

Undergraduate Simulation

Preclinical Courses

Basic Science Correlations

Internal Medicine faculty members frequently participate in basic science courses and provide clinical correlations. Simulation used at the preclinical level tends to focus on medical knowledge [7]. For example, high-fidelity mannequin simulators can be used to teach physiology and pharmacology, especially cardiovascular physiology and response to medications [6]. The use of mannequins, rather than the recruitment and training of real patients, can provide a feasible way to demonstrate clinical correlations. Via et al. [17] used simulators to demonstrate cardiac output, heart rate, and systemic vascular resistance to second-year medical students. Gordon et al. [18] showed that a high-fidelity mannequin can be used to demonstrate physiological changes during myocardial infarction to second-year medical students. It is also possible to teach basic neuroscience concepts to large groups using a simulator [19].

The utilization of virtual patients and avatars for basic clinical encounters is in its infancy, but these types of virtual simulation options show promise. While the benefits of simulation are apparent (see Fig. 26.1 and Table 26.1), challenges with faculty development, faculty numbers, space, time, cost, and equipment are limiting factors.

Physical Diagnosis

The Harvey cardiology patient simulator (CPS), developed by Dr. Michael Gordon in 1968, has been shown to be an efficient and effective tool for teaching cardiac physical exam skills to medical students and Internal Medicine residents [21, 22]. Students using CPS mannequins can develop the ability to recognize normal and abnormal findings with breath sounds, heart sounds, pulses, jugular venous pulsations, and precordial movements. Harvey mannequins have enabled Internal Medicine clerkships to teach and assess medical students' cardiac physical diagnosis skills [23]. Simulators which demonstrate other physical examination findings are not readily available, but computer-generated simulations can reproduce visual findings well. Virtual reality simulations such as Second Life and other similar products may be helpful in physical examination training and assessment in the future.

Clinical Clerkships

Overall Use

According to the AAMC [24], approximately 76% of medical schools indicated that simulation is used within Internal Medicine clerkships, and approximately 57% of teaching hospitals indicated it is a part of the Internal Medicine

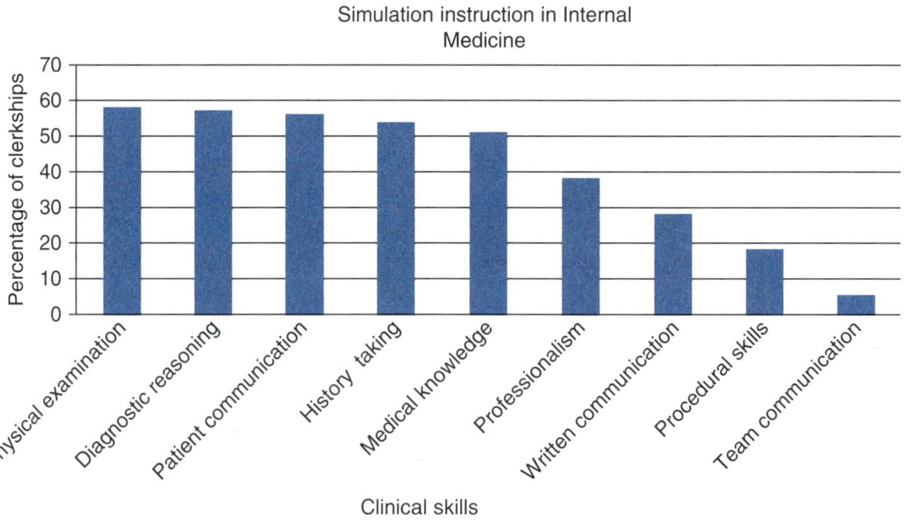

Fig. 26.1 Simulation in Internal Medicine clerkships (Based upon data provided within Torre et al. [15] study)

Table 26.1 Simulation advantages

Scenarios	Instruction and assessment	Learner	Patient safety and care
Consistent and reproducible	Supervised instruction	Tailored to learner's level	No risk to patient
Realistic problems	Deliberate feedback	Reflective practice	Error-forgiving clinical experience
Uncommon events	Outcome-based assessment	Practice to point of automaticity	Increases patient confidence

Based upon "Learning Through Simulation," Mayo Clinic Multidisciplinary Simulation Center [20]

clerkship. This places Internal Medicine within the top three disciplines in its use of simulation within medical school and teaching hospital settings [7].

Torre et al. [15] in a survey of US and Canadian clerkship directors found that SBME was used by 84% of survey respondents ($n=76/110$), with 39% reportedly using it for teaching, 49% for formative assessment, and 38% for summative assessment. For example, partial task trainers (rectal exam, lumbar puncture, venipuncture, arterial blood gas draw) are often used to teach technical skills to third-year medical students during Internal Medicine clerkships [25]. As a result, Graber et al. [25] reported that patients were more willing to allow medical students to perform procedures such as venipuncture, lumbar puncture, or central lines on them after the students had undergone simulation training.

Standardized patients (SPs) were used by approximately 54% of clerkship respondents. About one-third of clerkships responding reported using SPs for summative evaluations, presumably OSCE exams. Comprehensive simulation programs with evaluation of teamwork (5.6%) and procedural skills (18%) are less common [15]. Survey respondents represented 61% of all eligible schools surveyed.

Cases

Several companies have developed virtual cases, which are in common use during third-year clerkships. Virtual cases are often used as supplements or substitutes for actual cases to fulfill clerkship requirements [15]. Software, such as Laerdal MicroSim, is similar to gaming software and allows students to play the role of a physician in emergency or intensive care situations. For example, the software can time student responses during an emergency scenario and give students grades based upon timeliness of responses and ability to follow standard patient protocols. Students may find this software useful when they lack opportunities to practice decision making with seriously ill patients [25].

Cases involving mannequins are effective for teaching and assessing core curriculum topics during the Internal Medicine clerkship [2]. McMahon et al. have shown that simulators can help students compare and contrast different presentations of similar cases, thus enhancing reflective and metacognitive learning [26].

Assessment of Technical Skills

Technical skills are typically formatively assessed during clerkships, but students often finish the third and fourth year of medical school without establishing proficiency in many of the skills outlined by the AAMC in its Medical Schools Objectives Project initiative [27, 28]. Technical skills such as airway management, central lines, and ACLS skills are usually formatively assessed, as well, but often not until residency [6]. Objectives related to these skills can easily be added to a medical simulation curriculum.

Assessment: Objective Structured Clinical Exams (OSCEs)

OSCEs, first introduced in the UK by Ronald Harden, MD and FA Gleeson in the 1970s, are used in medical schools around the world to formatively and summatively assess clinical skills of medical students. While the use of OSCEs is widespread in US medical schools, Iqbal et al. [29] and Troncon [30] noted that OSCE use is limited in resource-constrained countries, which may not have standardized patient programs or skills labs. Troncon [30] also pointed out that without competency requirements mandated by accreditation agencies, the case for resource-intense, objective, simulation-based exams may not be there.

While reliability and validity evidence for OSCE-derived scores tends to be strong [31, 32], the psychometric properties related to scores use (reliability and validity) are highly dependent upon the standardization of SP training. As no tool or measure contains reliability or validity [33, 34], OSCEs are not inherently valid or reliable. Like any other tools dependent upon rater training, when SPs or faculty vary in the way they rate learners, reliability and validity of score use suffers [35]. In terms of formative assessment, standardized patient scenarios are also used by medical schools to assess medical students' communication and history and physical examination skills in preparation for OSCEs and licensure exams. There is evidence that data derived from standardized patient (announced and unannounced) evaluations may be more reliable and valid than faculty observer or patient evaluation data [35].

Graduate Medical Education

Overview

The number of residency programs offering simulation curricula has increased dramatically since the ACGME began mandating simulation learning experiences for all Internal Medicine residents. Across the specialties, approximately 90% of medical schools and teaching hospitals use simulation during the first 3 years of postgraduate training [7]. Once again, Internal Medicine is one of the most common disciplines utilizing simulation instruction in residency training [7].

The addition of core competencies by the ACGME has provided opportunities to utilize simulation for competency evaluation in a structured environment. Some of the competencies can be difficult to evaluate and remediate, including interpersonal and communication skills, professionalism, and systems-based practice [36–38]. With SBME, residents have opportunities to practice in risk-free environments and engage in patient encounters which would have high procedural risks or are infrequent events (i.e., ACLS code, weapons of mass destruction, mass causality scenarios) in real clinical settings.

Procedural Skills

Procedural skills have traditionally been taught within a "see one, do one, teach one" paradigm, which places patients at significant risk for complications and may increase frustration with operators and/or procedures. Standardized patients have allowed certain bedside procedures (starting an IV, phlebotomy, and electrocardiogram) to be performed on them for medical education, but most of these are examples of low-risk, frequently utilized procedures for hospitalized patients. The more complex procedures (lumbar puncture, central venous catheterization, paracentesis, and thoracentesis) all have a higher risk associated with them and are infrequently performed by general Internal Medicine physicians.

SBME allows trainees to improve their performance with procedures prior to clinical practice. Central venous catheterization (CVC) has been one of the most studied procedures within simulation, and studies that have shown improvement with ultrasound-guided SBME training was superior to traditional training [39, 40]. Evans et al. [41] showed postgraduate year 1 and 2 (PGY-1 and PGY-2) physicians, when given a structured, competency-based simulation training protocol, improved CVC insertion performance with regard to success at first cannulation [16]. Simulation-based curricula for CVC has also been associated with improvement in catheter-related bloodstream infection [42]. Barsuk et al. [43] found that SBME-trained residents had fewer catheter-related bloodstream infections within the intensive care unit after participating in a central venous catheter insertion skills simulation curriculum [9]. Simulation with partial task trainer models allows trainees the opportunity to learn the overall procedure with sterile techniques in an environment which will not interfere with patient safety or quality of care. Procedural skills activities can be used to evaluate resident competencies such as medical knowledge, patient care, systems based practice and communication skills with the addition of trained SPs to evaluate informed consent or delivery of bad news.

Hospital Teams and Infrequent Events

SBME also allows graduate trainees to practice infrequent events (i.e., ACLS code, weapons of mass destruction, mass causality scenarios) in a controlled environment, allowing for adaptation according to the skill level of the learner. As the learner advances within her/his medical training, simulation allows for diversity of experiences and complexity of the simulation scenario. Starting residency training can be a challenging period for individuals and specifically being on the code team increases trainee anxiety. The American Board of Internal Medicine requires residents to be competent in advance cardiac life support (ACLS) for certification. Simulation allows trainees to become more competent with ACLS while decreasing the stress associated with infrequent events which have life-altering consequences [44]. In addition, the utilization of multidisciplinary teams during code training can improve a trainee's competency in teamwork skills [45], an aspect of systems-based practice, and improve learner's professionalism and communication skills [45]. Multidisciplinary teams often consist of members who are responsible for the code teams within the institution (i.e., nurses, pharmacists, respiratory therapists, and physicians). Evaluation of team dynamics can be performed with tools such as the Mayo High Performance Teamwork Scale [10, 46]. This team training helps to improve technical skills of the practitioner but also works to emphasize teamwork within the institution.

Competency Evaluation

In GME, other uses of SBME include the teaching and assessment of patient communication. Simulation scenarios can be developed to highlight the physician-patient relationship. Learning objectives and learning activities can target ethical dilemmas, including those encountered when dealing with advanced directives [47] and breaking bad news. Unannounced standardized patient visits to the resident clinic have been used within a number of GME programs, including the University of Texas Medical School at Houston. The scenarios can be viewed in real time or videotaped so that the resident has the opportunity to later watch their interactions with standardized patients. This gives residents some insight into their own medical interviewing and physical examination skills. Simulated scenarios are somewhat unique because they can be designed to include and evaluate all six competencies (patient care, medical knowledge, practice-based learning, interpersonal and communication skills, professionalism, and systems-based practice).

Internal Medicine residency programs have struggled with teaching and assessing systems-based practice [36], practice-based learning and improvement, and communication skills and professionalism [47]. McGaghie et al. [48] have used medical simulation to teach systems-based practice skills to Internal Medicine residents and have discovered that the simulation experience is irreplaceable. Simulation education offers an excellent opportunity to perform observed competency-based education and assessment.

GME Final Thoughts

The utilization of SBME within graduate medical education is increasing [7], with numerous opportunities for improvement in patient care. Studies have shown not only the improvement of resident procedural skills performance but also improved communication and professionalism within multidisciplinary teams [49–51]. The number of programs offering simulation curricula has increased dramatically since the ACGME began mandating simulation learning experiences for all Internal Medicine residents.

Practicing Physicians and CME

The field of continuing medical education (CME) has also embraced SBME to enhance education during CME conferences. A review of CME activities by Marinopoulos et al. [52] showed that effective CME includes live conferences, conferences with multiple media offerings, multiple opportunities to build new knowledge through repeated exposure to new information, and opportunities to interactively engage in new practices [8]. SBME utilizes all four effective CME approaches during most scenarios. The American College of Physicians (ACP) utilizes simulation activities during their annual meeting by offering the Waxman Clinical Skills stations. These sessions are well attended and have been a popular addition to the annual meeting since 2001. Simulation stations engage participants in a variety of procedural skills; physical exam improvement stations including cardiac, breast, or pelvic exam; and a variety of standardized patient scenarios. Simulation has become a strong and integral part of medical education and will continue to be a critical element in physician education, not only during medical school or residency training but also for lifelong learning.

Internal Medicine: Certification

While Internal Medicine has been relatively slow to adopt simulation for high-stakes testing when compared with the field of anesthesiology [5, 53], its use is increasing. Simulation is used in high-stakes testing for Internal Medicine specialty certification in Canada. Physicians are required to rotate through and pass a standardized patient physical exam station and an ethics and communication skills station [4]. In the USA, simulation-based virtual reality (VR) training for cardiac stenting was approved by the Society for Cardiovascular Angiography and Interventions, the Society for Vascular Medicine, and the Society for Vascular Surgery [54]. The American Board of Internal Medicine (ABIM) [55] also utilizes VR simulation; VR simulation is used for self-evaluation of medical knowledge within its maintenance of certification program for interventional cardiology diplomats (ABIM web site). A number of studies have been completed in recent years regarding the use of virtual reality training for carotid stenting [54, 56, 57]. In these studies, there was a significant part of the learning curve that could be accomplished using virtual reality training. The shift in procedural skills training to include the virtual reality format offers significant opportunities for acquiring these technical skills and providing enhanced patient care.

Practical Considerations

Faculty Development

As SBME is such a powerful tool for educating learners and observing performance, it would be logical to assume that SBME is used frequently within Internal Medicine faculty development. Yet, it is not incorporated to the degree we might expect. Significant barriers to adoption include cost of equipment and space, especially for resource-poor medical schools, and the time it takes to prepare for training. Although many faculty members support simulation training, another barrier is resistance that some faculty may have toward new ways of teaching. Seasoned Internal Medicine physicians may be less familiar with technology and as a result be apprehensive about incorporating high-fidelity mannequins, virtual reality, virtual patients, and other technology-driven simulation. These faculty members, who were taught within traditional apprenticeship models, often lack experience working with simulation equipment and/or computers and would rather not rely on new equipment when training young physicians.

The development of realistic clinical scenarios is also time-consuming for faculty and can be very expensive for institutions [58]. There may be technical limitations in terms of what can be simulated with current simulation mannequins, without the addition of standardized patients. Many of the current mannequins work best for anesthesia and ACLS-type scenarios. Faculty may be more inclined to embrace SBME as a teaching modality and the required faculty development if they can understand the utility of SBME for teaching patient safety and the newer more difficult general competencies [58]. Faculty who embrace SBME must be supported by their academic institutions and offered faculty development to be effective in developing advanced skills [59].

McGaghie et al. [48] emphasized that one of the areas of greatest need is faculty expertise. In order to be successful, there are several key components, including faculty training in the use of equipment, institutional support, and faculty motivation to succeed [48]. Research groups have emerged in many specialties studying best practices for the use of simulation [60]. With all the rapid changes in medical education, one thing remains constant and is evident in the research related to SBME: the need for faculty development to move faculty learners from novice to expert levels [60]. While physicians might agree with that concept in practice, not all are willing to acknowledge the value of experiential learning through the use of simulation. In our opinion, the lack of experts, age of Internal Medicine faculty, need for faculty development, and distrust of technology are major barriers that must be overcome. For Internal Medicine to improve its education of medical students, residents, and practicing physicians, Internal Medicine faculty must embrace SBME and learn the skills necessary to teach SBME effectively.

Finding a Champion

Successful programs have a faculty person who is passionate about SBME. SBME requires planning, imagination, and a willingness to experiment with new ideas and new technology. Many times, faculty champions are junior faculty members who are innovative and adaptable enough to appreciate the potential of SBME and be comfortable with the technology. However, this person must have enough authority to make curricular changes and time dedicated to program enhancement. This does not exclude the more seasoned faculty member, but the skill set does need to match the job. The person in charge needs to be a champion and must be given the time and resources to ensure program success.

Curriculum Development

The course administrator for the overall educational unit (e.g., clerkship director, residency program director) must be involved in planning the simulation curriculum or be willing to delegate planning to the simulation director. The overall goals and objectives of the program must fit with the objectives of the clerkship and/or residency program and align with institutional objectives.

The best place to start is with the current curriculum. Our institution utilized the CDIM clerkship curriculum to evaluate the Internal Medicine clerkship curriculum. Our review of that curriculum revealed medical problems and procedures which were not consistently taught. Those problems formed the basis of the first undergraduate simulation curriculum. For example, students were not consistently performing supervised IM recommended procedures, so those procedures were targeted for teaching at the simulation lab. In the lab, we could observe techniques and ensure students understood the indications, contraindications, and complications of the procedures. These procedures are now commonly tested on our OSCE. We also believed our students were not being observed performing history and physical examination skills and that bedside cardiac skills needed to be improved. One day devoted to standardized patient scenarios was added to the SBME curriculum. The sessions allow us to review history and physical skills and give faculty and standardized patient feedback to students. A progressive course utilizing the Harvey mannequin was incorporated into the clerkship's simulation curriculum as well.

The SBME curriculum should be structured developmentally, with advanced skills that are targeted as trainees progress. During the Internal Medicine clerkship, students do basic procedures, learn advanced cardiac physical diagnosis using Harvey, and run team-based scenarios. Students are expected to know ACLS, and scenarios are used to place students in the role of team leader, do real-time airway management, and reinforce curricular objectives. Internal Medicine interns practice code team training and basic procedures (Table 26.2). As residents advance, we introduce more complex cases, which allow us to formatively assess professionalism, communication, and skills involved in practice-based learning and improvement. For example, standardized patients playing the role of family members allow us to add complexity to cases and force residents to demonstrate skills in all six competencies in a controlled environment. Cases can come from personal experience and/or departments of risk management. Adverse events can be extremely useful for scenario building. Hybrid simulation cases, using high-fidelity mannequins and standardized patients, can be utilized to allow residents to explore ethical dilemmas in medicine. Representatives from risk management are often willing to assist during debriefing sessions. At our institution, hybrid cases have been developed and include a patient who has been hospitalized and has an out-of-hospital DNR on file; a case where family members have revoked a do-not-resuscitate order; and a scenario involving a patient with a reversible condition, where family members wish to withdraw care [47].

Debriefing

According to instructors at the Center for Medical Simulation of Harvard Medical School, simulation is just an excuse for debriefing. Debriefing should take about twice as long as the length of any scenario. Faculty must participate in faculty development training prior to leading debriefing sessions. Advocacy inquiry, a technique taught at the Center for Medical Simulation, is designed to allow participants to teach themselves by asking key questions. The faculty person makes an observation, such as "I noticed during the scenario that this happened." This is followed by a concern or a question about what was observed. The concept is to avoid being judgmental, but make the observation and frame the question in such a way as to get the trainee to think out loud

Table 26.2 Simulation-based medical education (SBME) activities

Examples of SBME activities by training level				
Activity	Training level	Format	Scenarios	Contact hours/ resident per activity (h)
Procedural skills Paracentesis Thoracentesis Central line placement Peripherally inserted central catheter (PICC) Lumbar puncture Intubation techniques	PGY-1 Available for additional training for PGY-2/PGY-3 residents	Journal article and video review Partial task trainers	Solo training simulation activities are focused on acquisition of medical knowledge of the procedure, related complications, consent, documentation, and laboratory interpretation of any results from the procedure. The resident obtains consent on the procedure with the patients and/or family members in a simulated environment. All activity is observed by faculty	4 (2 Sessions)
Harvey cardiac physical exam	PGY-1	High-fidelity simulation	Team discussions regarding venous wave forms, arterial pulsations, precordial movements, and cardiac auscultation to occur with reviewing the physical exam skills on the simulator	3
ACLS code scenarios	PGY-1	High-fidelity simulation	Team scenarios include patients who develop PEA, asystole, ventricular fibrillation, atrial fibrillation with rapid ventricular response, sinus tachycardia, sinus bradycardia, and second- and third-degree atrioventricular block Clinical scenarios monitored: residents must not only adhere to guidelines but also reinforce communication between team members	4 (2 Sessions)
Multidisciplinary code team training	PGY-1 and PGY-2	High-fidelity simulation	Team scenarios include patients who develop PEA, asystole, ventricular fibrillation, atrial fibrillation with rapid ventricular response, sinus tachycardia, sinus bradycardia, and second- and third-degree atrioventricular block Teams consist of Internal Medicine residents, pharmacy, and ICU nursing. All team members are part of the Dr. Blue team within hospital Clinical scenarios monitored: residents must not only adhere to guidelines but also reinforce communication between team members	3
Breaking bad news simulation	PGY-1	High-fidelity simulation and standardized patients	Team and solo training where the PGY-1 obtains medical consent from the patient and/or family member prior to a procedure taking place. A complication occurs during the procedure and the patient develops ventricular fibrillation. The code team resuscitates the patient with the original PGY-1 running the simulated code. The patient survives and the original PGY-1 informs the patient's family about the complication and the patient's condition following the complication	3
Night float simulation	PGY-1 and PGY-2	High-fidelity simulation and standardized patients	Solo training scenarios for the PGY-1 group developed by PGY-2 residents. The scenarios include patients who develop PEA, ventricular fibrillation, sinus bradycardia, and second- and third-degree atrioventricular block. Interactions between patients, family members, and physicians allow the PGY-1 to experience a night float environment prior to rotating on the ICU night float experience	3
Procedure skills Advanced airway	PGY-2	Journal article and video review High-fidelity simulation	Team training covering all techniques with advance airway, topics from LMA, Combitube insertion, surgical cricothyroidotomy, fiber optics, lighted stylet, glide scope	4 (2 Sessions)

(continued)

Table 26.2 (continued)

Examples of SBME activities by training level				
Activity	Training level	Format	Scenarios	Contact hours/resident per activity (h)
Advanced airway scenarios	PGY-2	High-fidelity simulation	Team scenarios include patients who develop PEA, asystole, ventricular fibrillation, and respiratory distress. These patients will have some difficulties with the airway – bronchospasm, rheumatoid arthritis, Down's syndrome, micrognathia, and late-term pregnancy	4 (2 Sessions)
Advance directive scenarios	PGY-2	High-fidelity simulation and standardized patients	Team scenarios include patients who develop PEA, asystole, ventricular fibrillation, and respiratory distress. The simulated patients have advance directive issues with power of attorney (POA) and do-not-resuscitate (DNR) orders and/or family controversy with medical care of the family member. Both standardized patients and high-fidelity simulation are utilized to optimize the experience for the participants	4 (2 Sessions)
Ethical scenarios	PGY-3	High-fidelity simulation and standardized patients	Team training covering a variety of ethical issues, e.g., blood transfusion advance directive in a Jehovah's Witness patient and discussions concerning physician-assisted suicide, elderly neglect, and the impaired colleague	4 (2 Sessions)
Advanced procedure skills Cardiac catheterization Esophagogastroduodenoscopy (EGD) Colonoscopy Bronchoscopy	PGY-3	High-fidelity simulation	Solo training for residents with pending fellowships. Residents have the opportunity to work on high-fidelity simulators. Curriculum has been developed to allow residents knowledge and understanding of the procedures and any potential complications	10 (3.5 Sessions)

and discuss what was happening internally during the scenario. After trainees begin talking, the goal is to keep the discussion focused and ensure that key teaching points are covered.

Session Planning

Trainees' views about simulation vary. The more junior the trainee, the more likely the trainee is to be engaged and enjoy simulation. Medical students usually like simulation, whereas the upper-level residents and faculty are often more skeptical. This is probably natural based upon what each person is expected to know. This factor can be overcome by telling the group up front that the scenario, or task, is difficult and we expect mistakes. The simulation center is a safe place to make mistakes, so that acknowledgement should be voiced up front.

As SBME requires active participation, groups should be relatively small, with less than ten participants under most circumstances. Large groups can interfere with active learning. Sessions also have to be focused with excellent use of time. Since student and resident time is valuable to many, you will have to negotiate for every minute of time. Residents often need to return to the hospital so resident sessions generally should be no longer than 3 hours.

A critical issue in curriculum development is establishing the purpose of the session. Simulation can be used for instruction, practice, or assessment. Medical students and residents need to know the purpose at the beginning, and it must be clear. Otherwise, buy-in from trainees may be compromised if the session is used for evaluation, and this was not established initially. Incorporating SBME does require a significant amount of planning, but when incorporated effectively, reciprocal benefits for learners and patients are immeasurable.

Conclusion

In summary, the power of SBME is rooted in its experiential and multimodal nature. Well-crafted simulated scenarios, offering multimodal learning experiences [61], can engage and challenge learners in ways that traditional instruction cannot. Compared with lecture-based instruction, simulation offers learners the opportunity to engage parallel or convergent learning pathways [61] to master skills and concepts. Hybrid simulations, can provide unique opportunities for learners to hear, see, touch, smell, and even emotionally experience a crisis. We believe SBME will continue to play a significant and expanding role in all levels of Internal Medicine education, from medical student to practicing physician education.

References

1. Accreditation Council for Graduate Medical Education (ACGME) 2001–2011. GME Information. http://www.acgme.org/acWebsite/resEvalSystem/reval_list.asp. Accessed 13 July 2011.
2. Ogden PE, Cobbs LS, Howell MR, Sibbitt SJ, DiPette DJ. Clinical simulation: importance to the internal medicine educational mission. APM perspectives. Am J Med. 2007;120:820–4.
3. Scalese RJ, Obeso VT, Issenberg SB. Simulation technology for skills training and competence assessment in medical education. J Gen Intern Med. 2007;23(supp 1):46–9.
4. Hatala R, Kassen BO, Nishikawa J, Cole G, Issenberg SB. Incorporating simulation technology in a Canadian Internal Medicine specialty examination: a descriptive report. Acad Med. 2005;80:554–6.
5. Berkenstadt H, Ziv A, Gafni N, Sidi A. The validation process of incorporating simulation-based accreditation into the anesthesiology Israeli national board exams. Isr Med Assoc. 2006;8:728–33.
6. Okuda Y, Bryson EO, DeMaria S, et al. The utility of simulation in medical education: what is the evidence? Mt Sinai J Med. 2009;76:330–43.
7. Passiment M, Sacks H, Huang G. Medical Simulation in Medical Education: results of an AAMC Survey. 2011; Association of American Medical Colleges (AAMC).
8. O'Flynn S, Shorten G. Simulation in undergraduate medical education. Eur J Anaesthesiol. 2009;26:93–5.
9. Di Francesco L, Pistoria MJ, Auerbach AD, Nardino RJ, Holmboe ES. Internal Medicine training in the inpatient setting. A review of published educational interventions. J Gen Intern Med. 2005;20:1173–80.
10. Morgan PJ, Cleave-Hogg D. Comparison between medical students' experience, confidence and competence. Med Educ. 2002;36:534–9.
11. Barnsley L, Lyon PM, Ralston SJ, et al. Clinical skills in junior medical officers: a comparison of self-reported confidence and observed competence. Med Educ. 2004;38:358–67.
12. Brim NM, Venkatan SK, Gordon JA, Alexander EK. Long-term educational impact of a simulator curriculum on medical student education in an Internal Medicine clerkship. Simul Healthc. 2010;5:75–81.
13. Boulet JR, Murray DJ. Simulation-based assessment in anesthesiology: requirements for practical implementation. Anesthesiology. 2010;112:1041–52.
14. McLaughlin D, Fitch MT, Goyal DG, et al. Simulation in graduate medical education 2008: a review for emergency medicine. Acad Emerg Med. 2008;15:1117–29.
15. Torre DM, Aagaard E, Elnicki DM, Durning SJ, Papp KK. Simulation in the internal medicine clerkship: a national survey of internal medicine clerkship directors. Teach Learn Med. 2011;23:215–22.
16. Issenberg SB, McGaghie WC, Petrusa ER, Gordon D, Scalese RJ. Features and uses of high-fidelity medical simulations that lead to effective learning: a BEME systematic review. Med Teach. 2005;27:10–28.
17. Via DK, Kyle RR, Trask JD, Shields CH, Mongan PD. Using high-fidelity patient simulation and an advanced distance education network to teach pharmacology to second-year medical students. J Clin Anesth. 2004;16:144–51.
18. Gordon JA, Hayden EM, Ahmed RA, Pawlowski JB, Khoury KN, Oriol NE. Early bedside care during preclinical medical education: can technology-enhanced patient simulation advance the Flexnerian ideal? Acad Med. 2010;85:370–7.
19. Fitch MT. Using high-fidelity emergency simulation with large groups of preclinical medical student in a basic science course. Med Teach. 2007;29:261–3.
20. Mayo Clinic Multidisciplinary Simulation Center. Learning through simulation. Available at http://www.mayo.edu/simulationcenter/. Accessed 2013.
21. Mangione S, Nieman LZ, Gracely E, Kaye D. The teaching and practice of cardiac auscultation during internal medicine and cardiology training. A nationwide survey. Ann Intern Med. 1993;119:47–54.

22. Mangione S, Nieman LZ. Cardiac auscultatory skills of Internal Medicine and family practice trainees A comparison of diagnostic proficiency. JAMA. 1997;278:717–22 (Published erratum appears in JAMA 1998;279:1444).
23. Ewy GA, Felner JM, Juul D, Mayer JW, Sajid AW, Waugh RA. Test of a cardiology patient simulator with students in fourth-year electives. J Med Educ. 1987;62:738–43.
24. Association of American Medical Colleges (AAMC). Medical School Objectives Project. Available at https://www.aamc.org/initiatives/msop. Accessed 1998.
25. Graber MA, Wyatt C, Kasparek L, Xu Y. Does simulator training for medical students change patient opinions and attitudes toward medical student procedures in the emergency department? Acad Emer Med. 2005;12:635–9.
26. McMahon GT, Monaghan C, Falchuk K, Gordon JA, Alexander EK. A simulator-based curriculum to promote comparative and reflective analysis in an internal medicine clerkship. Acad Med. 2005;80:84–9.
27. Coberly L, Goldenhar LM. Ready or not, here they come: acting interns' experience and perceived competency performing basic medical procedures. J Gen Intern Med. 2007;22:491–4.
28. Vukanovic-Criley JM, Criley S, Warde CM, et al. Competency in cardiac examination skills in medical students, trainees, physicians, and faculty: a multicenter study. Arch Intern Med. 2006;166:610–6.
29. Iqbal M, Khizar B, Zaidi Z. Revising an objective structured clinical examination in a resource-limited Pakistani Medical School. Educ Health (Abingdon). 2009;22:209.
30. Troncon LE. Clinical skills assessment: limitations to the introduction of an "OSCE" (Objective Structured Clinical Examination) in a traditional Brazilian medical school. Sao Paulo Med J. 2004;122:12–7.
31. Auewarakul C, Downing SM, Jaturatamrong U, Praditsuwan R. Sources of validity evidence for an internal medicine student evaluation system: an evaluative study of assessment methods. Med Educ. 2005;39:276–83.
32. Carraccio C, Englander R. The objective structured clinical examination: a step in the direction of competency-based evaluation. Arch Pediatr Adolesc Med. 2000;154:736–41.
33. American Educational Research Association, American Psychological Association, National Council on Measurement in Education. Standards for Educational and Psychological Testing. Washington, D.C.: American Educational Research Assoc.; 1999.
34. Beckman TJ, Cook DA. Developing scholarly projects in education: a primer for medical teachers. Med Teach. 2007;29:210–8.
35. Holmboe ES, Ward DS, Reznick RK, et al. Faculty development in assessment: the missing link in competency-based medical education. Acad Med. 2011;86:460–7.
36. Colbert CY, Ogden PE, Ownby AR, Bowe C. Systems-based practice in graduate medical education: systems thinking as the missing foundational construct. Teach Learn Med. 2011;23:179–85.
37. Englander R, Agostinucci W, Zalneraiti E, Carraccio CL. Teaching residents systems-based practice through a hospital cost-reduction program: a "win-win" situation. Teach Learn Med. 2006;18:150–2.
38. Varkey P, Karlapudi S, Rose S, Nelson R, Warner M. A systems approach for implementing practice-based learning and improvement and systems-based practice in graduate medical education. Acad Med. 2009;84:335–9.
39. Miller AH, Roth BA, Mills TJ, Woody JR, Longmoor CE, Foster B. Ultrasound guidance versus the landmark technique for the placement of central venous catheters in the emergency department. Acad Emerg Med. 2002;9:800–5.
40. Sekiguchi H, Tokita JE, Minami T, Eisen LA, Mayo PH, Narasimhan M. A prerotational, simulation-based workshop improves the safety of central venous catheter insertion: results of a successful internal medicine house staff training program. Chest. 2011;140:652–8.
41. Evans LV, Dodge KL, Shah TD, et al. Simulation training in central venous catheter insertion: improved performance in clinical practice. Acad Med. 2010;85:1462–9.
42. Centers for Medicare & Medicaid Services (CMS). US Department of Health and Human Services. https://www.cms.gov/home/medicare.asp. Accessed 13 July 2011.
43. Barsuk JH, Cohen ER, Feinglass J, McGaghie WC, Wayne DB. Use of simulation-based education to reduce catheter-related bloodstream infections. Arch Intern Med. 2009;169:1420–3.
44. Rodgers DL, Securro S, Pauley RD. The effect of high-fidelity simulation on educational outcomes in an advanced cardiovascular life support course. Simul Healthc. 2009;4:200–6.
45. Wehbe-Janek H, Lenzmeier C, Ogden PE, et al. Nurses' Perceptions of a simulation-based interprofessional training program for rapid response and code blue events. J Nurs Care Qual. 2012;27(1):43–50.
46. Malec JF, Torsher LC, Dunn WF, et al. The Mayo high performance teamwork scale: reliability and validity for evaluating key crew resource management skills. Simul Healthc. 2007;2:4–10.
47. Colbert CY, Mirkes C, Ogden PE, et al. Enhancing competency in professionalism: targeting resident advance directive education. J Grad Med Educ. 2010;2:278–82.
48. McGaghie W, Issenberg S, Petrusa E, Scalese RJ. A critical review of simulation-based medical education research: 2003–2009. Med Educ. 2010;44:50–63.
49. MacDowall J. The assessment and treatment of the acutely ill patient – the role of the patient simulator as a teaching tool in the undergraduate programme. Med Teach. 2006;28:326–9.
50. Wayne DB, Didwania A, Feinglass J, Fudala MF, Barsuk JH, McGaghie WC. Simulation-based education improves quality of care during cardiac arrest team responses at an academic teaching hospital: a case–control study. Chest. 2008;133:56–61.
51. Wayne DB, Siddall VJ, Butter J, et al. A longitudinal study of internal medicine residents' retention of advanced cardiac life support skills. Acad Med. 2006;81(10 suppl):S9–12.
52. Marinopoulos SS, Dorman T, Ratanawongsa N, et al. Effectiveness of continuing medical education. Evid Rep Technol Assess (Full Rep). 2007;(149):1–69.
53. Ziv A, Rubin O, Sidi A, Berkenstadt H. Credentialing and certifying with simulation. Anesthesiol Clin. 2007;25:261–9.
54. Gallagher AG, Cates CU. Approval of virtual reality training for carotid stenting: what this means for procedural-based medicine. JAMA. 2004;292:3024–6.
55. American Board of Internal Medicine. ABIM to use Medical Simulation Technology to Evaluate Physician Competence. http://www.abim.org/news/medical-simulation-technology-evaluate-physician-competence.aspx. Accessed 13 July 2011.
56. Aggarwal R, Black S, Hance JR, Darzi A, Cheshire NJ. Virtual reality simulation training can improve inexperienced surgeons' endovascular skills. Eur J Vasc Endovasc Surg. 2006;31:588–93.
57. Cates CU, Patel AD, Nicholson WJ. Use of virtual reality simulation for mission rehearsal for carotid stenting. JAMA. 2007;297:265–6.
58. Murphy JG, Cremonini F, Kane GC, Dunn W. Is simulation based medicine training the future of clinical medicine? Eur Rev Med Pharmacol Sci. 2007;11:1–8.
59. Murray DJ, Boulet JR, Kras JF, Woodhouse JA, Cox T, McAllister JD. Acute care skills in anesthesia practice: a simulation-based resident performance assessment. Anesthesiology. 2004;101:1084–95.
60. Benor DE. Faculty development, teacher training and teacher accreditation in medical education: twenty years from now. Med Teach. 2000;22:503–12.
61. Friedlander MJ, Andrews L, Armstrong EG, et al. What can medical education learn from the neurobiology of learning? Acad Med. 2011;86:415–20.

Simulation in Military and Battlefield Medicine

27

COL Robert M. Rush Jr.

Introduction

Between wars and combat deployments, the US military simulates combat scenarios better than any other military in the world. This is critical since combat cannot be learned on the job and therefore must be simulated ahead of time. There is no real-time "practice" during actual combat like there is in the "practice" of medicine [practice here meaning the actual care of patients]. In fact, entire military bases exist to support combat simulation and training. In contrast, simulation for military healthcare provider preparedness, up until a short while ago, was not thought necessary since their daily civilian or military base job, caring for patients, would be similar to that which would be encountered during deployment. However, it is now well known and appreciated that there are clear and significant differences between peacetime and wartime military practice and that training for one does not imply proficiency in practicing the other.

The differences of peacetime or US-based military practice and that of battlefield and combat medicine include providing care in mobile units and hospitals, trauma medicine, and preventive medicine and the treatment of exotic diseases, is apparent. Unfortunately, except for Advanced Trauma Life Support (ATLS) and a few other courses that allowed deployed surgical teams to train at civilian trauma centers, it was considered unnecessary to simulate anything beyond what was practiced in mobile medical units [1]. This included technical skills such as assembly, breakdown, and transport of tent-based medical facilities. These "field" exercises provided some experiential team and mass casualty training by incorporating moulaged (Fig. 27.1a–d) patients in immersive simulated environments (Fig. 27.2a, b). However, there was a paucity of experiences outside of the occasional medical school and special operations simulation-based training. These included live tissue labs, advanced individual training for medics, life-support courses (such as Basic Life Support [BLS], Advanced Cardiac Life Support [ACLS], Pediatric Advanced Life Support [PALS], ATLS and Pre-Hospital Trauma Life Support [PHTLS]), and unit-based ad hoc training.

While the military is just scratching the surface in medical simulation, some heroic efforts are currently underway. The military is helping to lead this change both in recognizing gaps in education that can be fulfilled by simulation and in improving the technology and the breadth of application of simulation platforms. For example, depicted in Fig. 27.3a, b are the newest versions of the vehicle rollover trainers used by all personnel deployed to combat zones. These simulators are excellent for improving ability and confidence in egressing from the vehicles especially after rollover accidents. Implementation of these simulators reduced fatalities and actual rollover incidents by over 60% from 2005 to 2007 [2]. Curriculum employed involved 1 h of vehicle safety training and then two to three rollover events on each vehicle simulator. This relatively simple, but expensive (each simulator costs between \$10 and \$20 million), deployment of simulation has made a tremendous impact on clinical outcomes. In this chapter, we describe the application of simulation for military and battlefield medicine in terms of deployment, wartime practice, and reentry into a civilian medical career.

C.R.M. Rush Jr., MD, FACS
Department of Surgery and the Andersen Simulation Center, Madigan Army Medical Center, Tacoma, WA 98431, USA

Central Simulation Committee, US Army Medical Department, Andersen Simulation Center, Madigan Army Medical Center, Tacoma, WA 98431, USA

Department of Surgery, University of Washington, Seattle, WA, USA

Department of Surgery, USUHS, Bethesda, MD, USA
e-mail: robert.rush1@us.army.mil, robert.m.rush4.mil@mail.mil

The opinions and statements made herein are solely those of the author and do not represent official policy or statements of the Department of Defense or the US Government.

A.I. Levine et al. (eds.), *The Comprehensive Textbook of Healthcare Simulation*, DOI 10.1007/978-1-4614-5993-4_27, © Springer Science+Business Media New York 2013

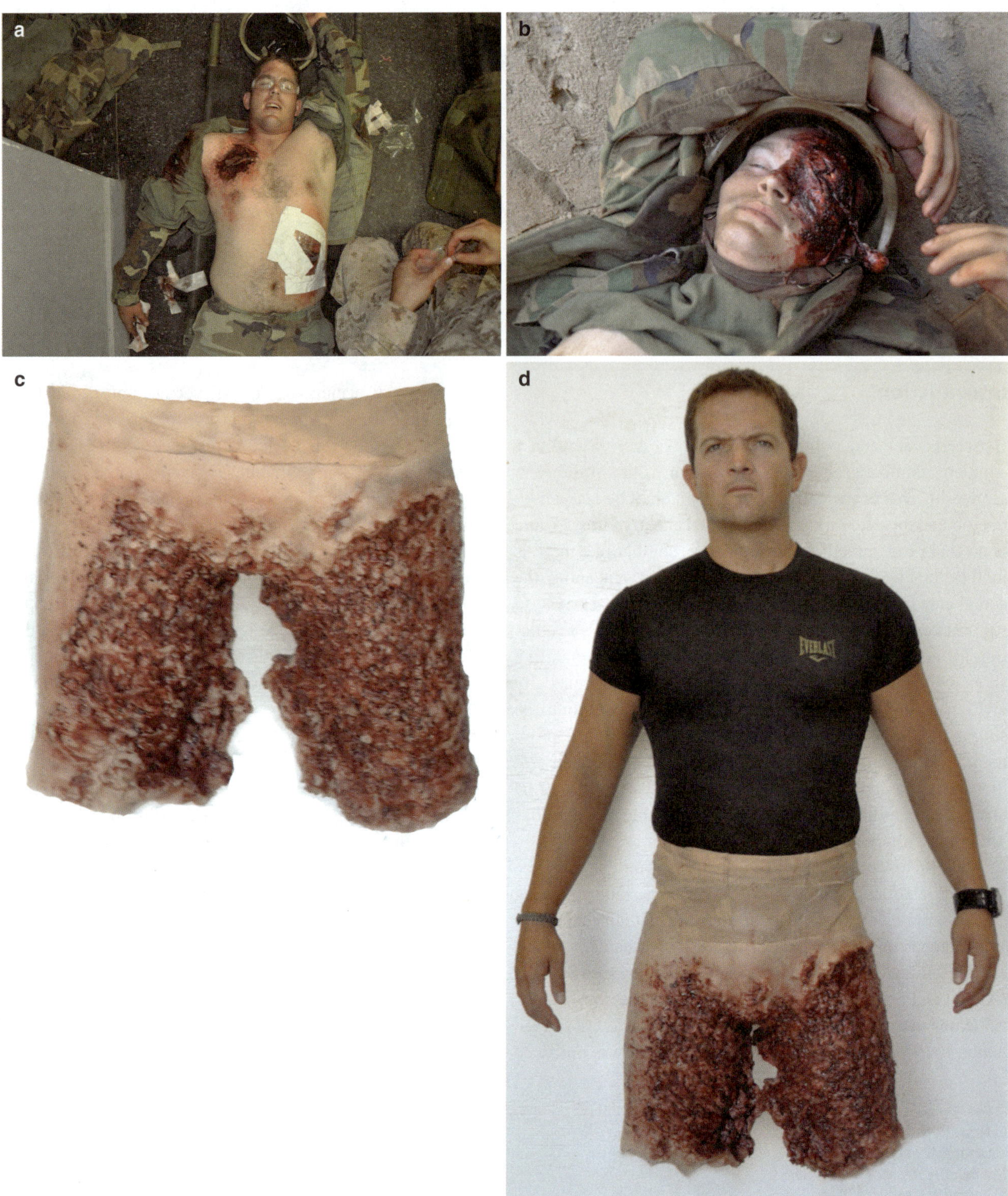

Fig. 27.1 Hyperrealistic moulage: (**a**) chest and abdominal wounds, (**b**) severe facial trauma, (**c**) reusable shorts to simulate leg wounds, (**d**) leg wound shorts (Photos courtesy of Strategic Operations, Inc.)

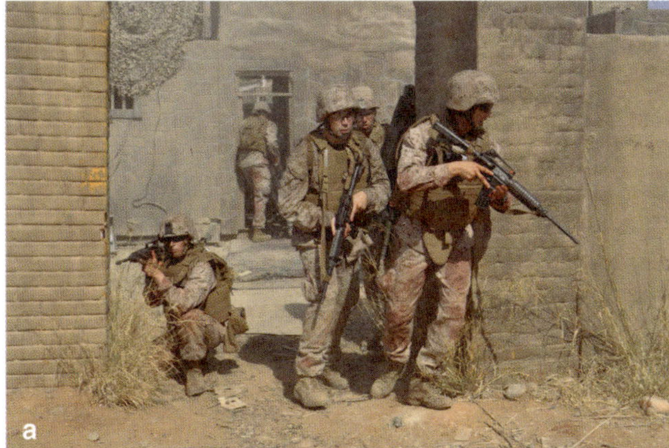

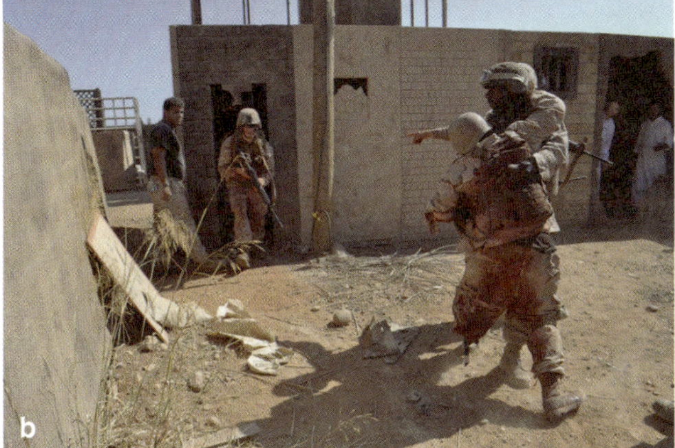

Fig. 27.2 Hyperrealistic (**a**) urban battle environment (**b**) with casualties (Photos courtesy of Strategic Operations, Inc.)

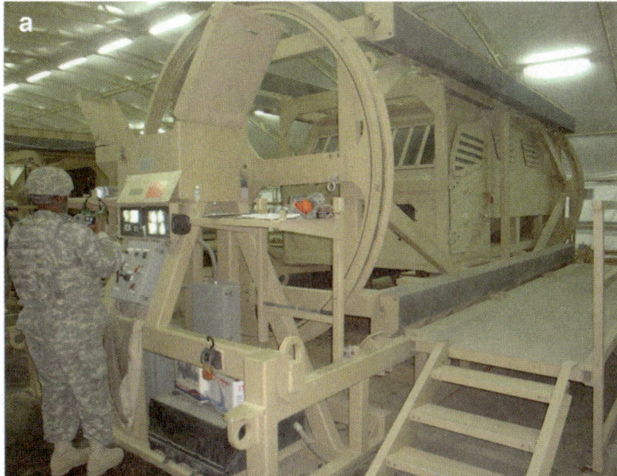

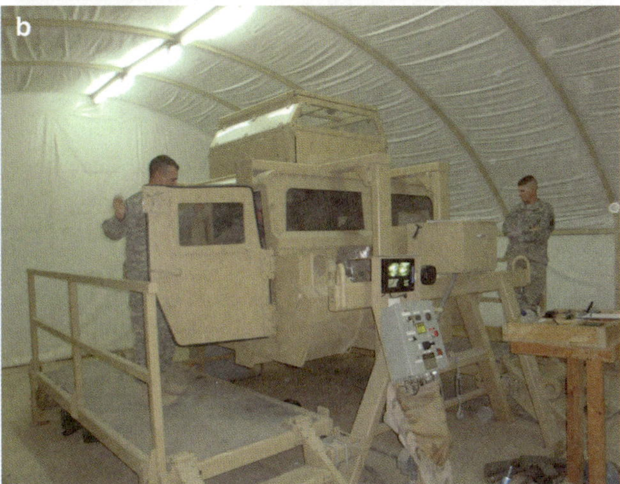

Fig. 27.3 The ultimate part-task and team trainers: (**a**) MRAP (Mine-Resistant, Ambush Protected) and (**b**) HMMWV (High-Mobility Multipurpose Wheeled Vehicle) rollover simulators. Instituting these simulators led to a marked decline in drowning and other rollover-related injuries during combat maneuvers in Iraq

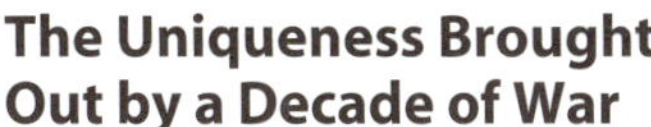

The Uniqueness Brought Out by a Decade of War

The War on Terror has meant that military medical personnel are more likely to be forward deployed and that the modern civilian medicine push towards subspecialization is opposite the needs of military healthcare. Military healthcare personnel are expected to be able to switch into "generalist mode" when deployed. The unique nature of military medicine is centered around the arduous deployment cycle. Massive numbers of active duty and reserve medical personnel are "mobilized" from their routine practice and placed in locations of varying austerity to perform in a different way than they are normally accustomed. When finished with deployment after 3–15 months in this environment, they are then expected to return to their routine practice without missing a beat—a tall order.

Many military healthcare providers expected their practice to cycle in this manner—that is, to practice at home in times of peace and to perform battlefield trauma care in support of our troops in times of war. What could be more heroic and fulfilling? Self-sacrifice during wartime has been the hallmark of our military medical services during all of our country's conflicts. However, how does one prepare a general surgeon to make the transition from elective hernia repairs at their local hospital to successfully performing lifesaving, complex damage control procedures for horribly injured soldiers on the battlefield? How then does one transition back to routine practice after this experience? This challenge relies on general medical officers that are capable of treating anyone for any reason, as well as general surgeons who are able to do any operation. These omni-capable medical professionals are diminishing [3]. The utilization of curricula augmented by simulation-based educational techniques is key to conquering this problem.

The systems the Department of Defense uses to allow for medical personnel to practice at home base and simultaneously be available for combat support missions are twofold. The system for assigning active duty military personnel to combat units is called the PROFIS (Professional Officer

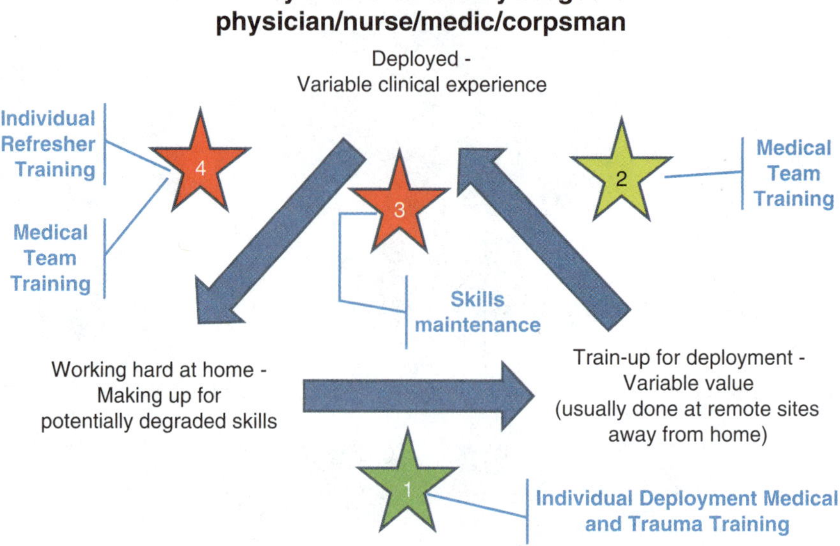

Fig. 27.4 The deployment cycle of military medical professionals. The *stars* represent potential interdiction points where curricula augmented with simulation in a hybrid model can make the transitions efficient

Filler System) system, mainly an Army Medical Department Program. The other system is that of the US Army, Navy, and Air Force Reserves. Regardless of the system, the cycle is similar and is depicted in Fig. 27.4. Deployment intervals vary depending on specialty. For instance, general surgeons, nurse anesthetists, and physician assistants deploy about every 2 years. Deployment length can also vary from 3 to 15 months for most PROFIS personnel, 6–12 months being the most common [4].

The Cycle

There are few instances outside of the military where vast numbers of healthcare professionals repeatedly rotate in and out of their everyday "practice" of medicine for significant lengths of time. There are civilian programs now available at universities and nonprofit volunteer organizations where healthcare providers visit underserved areas of the world in which their practice of medicine can vary from that in which they practice at home [5–7]. In the case of military surgeons and healthcare providers, the caseload and actual medical/surgical work can be highly variable and differ significantly between home and deployment. Although there are many reports from deployed units describing varied operative experiences and demonstrating robust cases, there are many days when few if any patients are seen or cases performed [8, 9]. To make up for this gap and to fill in this downtime, many units have incorporated host-nation humanitarian care into their routine when not caring for large numbers of combatant casualties [10]. Most credentialing bodies have established a minimum number of cases needed to be performed over a defined time period, a number based on consensus, as there have been no studies other than survey data showing skills degradation in seasoned surgeons or providers [4]. There is a push by some states and accrediting bodies to include simulation testing into overall certification. Interjecting this type of recertification prior to and just after deployments for all military personnel is an onerous task. However, there are some interdiction points where simulation and specific, efficient curricula can and are being used to improve transition, maintain skill levels, and monitor progress (Fig. 27.4).

Pre-deployment Training

Figure 27.4 depicts the cycle of most military healthcare professionals. Starting at home station after residency or schooling, most military providers work very hard to build their "practice" in a variety of settings from small isolated medical clinics at remote bases/posts to highly technical academic teaching centers with a host of subspecialties. In order to deploy, most providers participate in trauma and deployment refresher training. These programs provide training for medical including combat trauma (Fig. 27.5) and troop preventative medicine and nonmedical skills (Fig. 27.6). Currently, the military does well in this area (green-colored star #1 in Fig. 27.4). The available courses are listed in Table 27.1 along with the simulation formats used to support each effort.

Of the many training opportunities available in the pre-deployment phase, most focus on combat trauma care. Simulators for pre-deployment combat training range from part-task trainers that allow for the practice of specific, limited range of procedures (Fig. 27.7a–c) to full mannequins that are incorporated into more complex multisystem trauma scenarios for both individual and team training

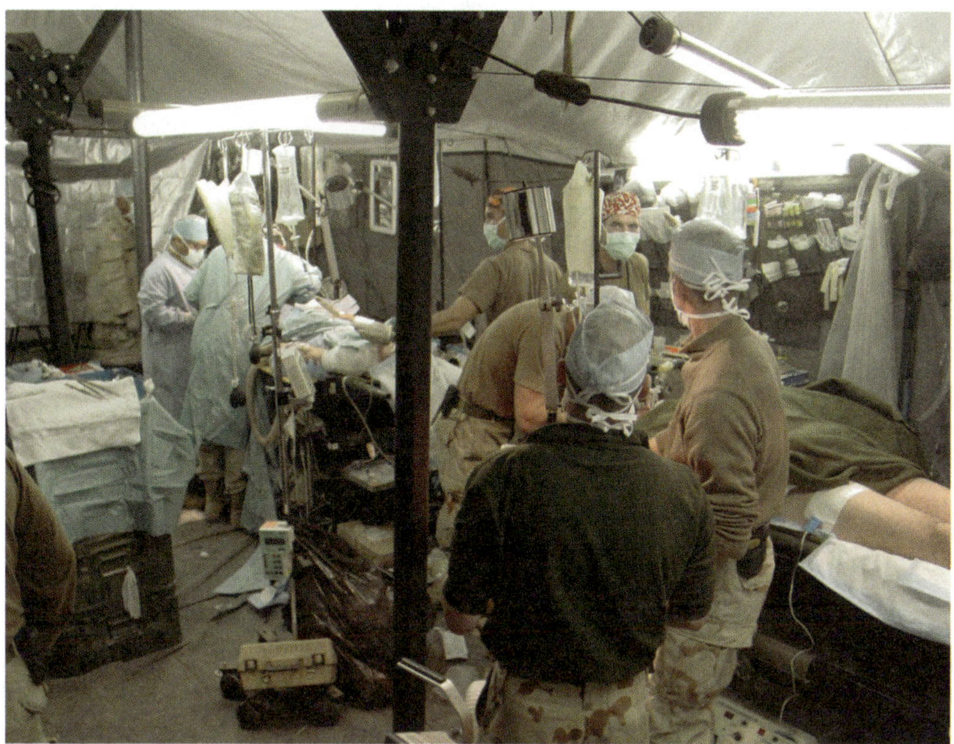

Fig. 27.5 Combat surgery at a forward surgical team in Afghanistan

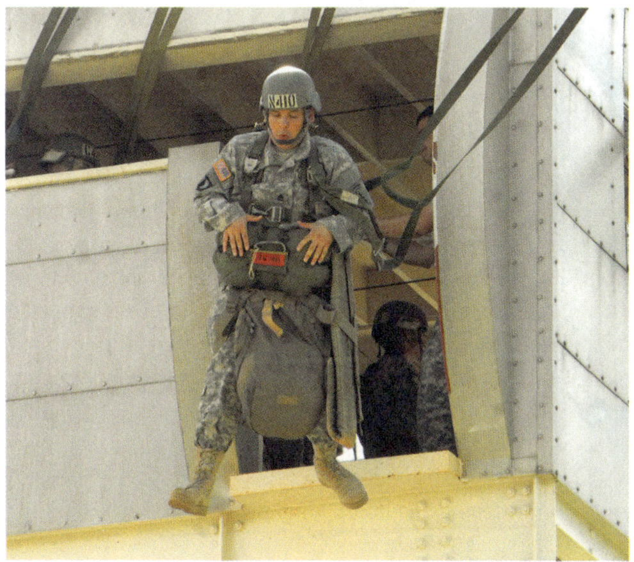

Fig. 27.6 Parachute training: Staff Sgt. Antonio Dipasquate, a trainee with 1st Battalion (Airborne), 507th Parachute Infantry Regiment, jumps with his combat gear. The students first conduct single jumps from the 34-ft towers and then moved on to mass exits with combat gear and the addition of "malfunctions" (Photo Credit: Cheryl Rodewig. Used courtesy of the United States Army)

(Fig. 27.8a–c). The Human Worn Partial Task Surgical Simulator (a.k.a. Cut Suit) from Strategic Operations [11] in Fig. 27.9a–g is a wearable simulated torso that an actor or moulaged team member dons to combine total patient injury management with actual procedural skill practice. (Table 27.2 lists the procedures available with the Cut Suit.)

These devices and actors can be placed in elaborate Hollywood-type sets (with pyrotechnics, sounds, and battlefield smells) for a "hyperrealistic" experience (Fig. 27.10a, b). While simulators are incorporated into specific courses with standardized curricula in order to support the learning of key concepts, they are also used on their own to support just-in-time and ad hoc training, practice, and assessment [12–14]. This is especially true for individual and small-unit team training just prior to deployment when there may not be enough time to fit in full courses that may involve unit travel or complex coordination.

Pre-deployment Team Training

Pre-deployment team training has markedly improved over the last decade but still lacks the standardized curricula and assessment tools that are necessary for reliable medical unit deployment (star #2 in Fig. 27.4). The Army Trauma Training Center at the Ryder Trauma Center in Miami does however prepare personnel of forward surgical teams and combat support hospitals both in terms of individual trauma and team skills, which are necessary to bring together for deployment [15, 16]. Brigade Tactical Combat Casualty Care (BTC3) provided by the Army Medical Department for all branches of service (Army, Navy, Air Force, Marines) furnishes this training for line unit medics.

Table 27.1 Sample courses, simulators used, and locations of training that are available for pre-deployment trauma refresher training

Course	Locations	Learners	Simulators
Combat Lifesaver	Most US Army posts	All service members	Part-task trainers and various mannequin-based simulators
BTC3 (Brigade Tactical Combat Casualty Care)	Fort Sam Houston, TX	All DoD healthcare providers	Part-task trainers for procedures, SimMan 3 G, Trauma Man, live tissue
Army Trauma Training Center (ATTC) Forward Surgical Team Training	Ryder Trauma Center, Miami, FL	Army forward surgical team members	Part-task trainers, live tissue, cadaver, Sawbones, TraumaMan, live patients (under trauma center oversight)
STAT Training	Any location	All team members	Moulaged unit members with scripts, SimMan 3 G
Combat Casualty Care Course (C4)	Camp Bullis, San Antonio, TX	Physicians, nurses, physician assistants new to the Army Medical Department	Part-task trainers
Combat Extremity Surgery Course	AMEDD Center and School and the Defense Medical Readiness Training Institute, Fort Sam Houston, TX	Surgeons	Sawbones, cadaver, part-task trainers
Emergency War Surgery Course	AMEDD Center and School and the Defense Medical Readiness Training Institute, Fort Sam Houston, TX	Surgeons	Live tissue, cadaver, part-task trainers
ATOM (Advanced Trauma Operative Management)	Various level I and II trauma centers	Surgeons	Live tissue model
ASSET (Advanced Surgical Skills for Exposure in Trauma)	Various level I trauma centers throughout USA	Surgeons	Cadaver
CSTARS	University of Cincinnati and other locations (colocated with university hospitals' ICUs and trauma centers)	Critical Care Air Transport Teams (CCATT), other Air Force personnel	SimMan 3 G, C-130 and C-17 aeromedical evacuation platforms

Currently, there are limited standardized training packages that take into account and incorporate the PROFIS to efficiently prepare medical professionals to work in deployed environments. The training ranges from being almost nonexistent to that which is often stretched into a month or more and is of variable utility (author's experience). Venues for joint operations training (those involving Army, Navy, and Air Force personnel) can be found however at Fort Indiantown Gap in Pennsylvania. This training center focuses on pre-deployment medical unit team training similar to the Joint Readiness Training Center (JRTC) in Louisiana and the National Training Center (NTC) in California for combat arms units. Cost of unit travel to these locations is a potential drawback. To circumvent this, virtual reality combat trainers similar to aviation flight simulators are used as a primer prior to large unit exercises. Casualty scenarios can be interjected into the virtual convoy episode to include point of injury care and evacuation practice. Using this venue, medical units can practice all aspects of a local medical clinic or hospital site mission prior to deployment including planning security elements, interpreter support, supply ordering, task execution, and combat casualty care.

The Air Force medical system provides pre-deployment trauma training to medical personnel similar to that of the Army Trauma Training Center. CSTARS (Centers for Sustainment for Trauma and Readiness Skills) is located at select civilian university hospitals. This training incorporates simulators to enhance the primary mission of aeromedical evacuation of casualties from the theater of war, through staging facilities, and ultimately to a final destination in the USA. Transporting critically wounded forces over long distances with no operative support is a monumental task. Coordination and care of patients must be practiced. Some of the specific elements practiced include the ability to conduct care in the hostile environment of an aircraft with turbulence, oppressive noise, limited visibility, and extremes of motions. On-loading and offloading patients must also be practiced as in Fig. 27.11a, b.

Deployment

On the Battlefield

Trauma refresher training while deployed is needed in some locations that are not experiencing high or even moderate casualty volumes. Trauma resuscitations and mass casualties can become rare events in deployed settings involving stability and low-intensity combat operations where coalition forces are more engaged in security details rather than force-on-force battles and where civilian trauma and medical care

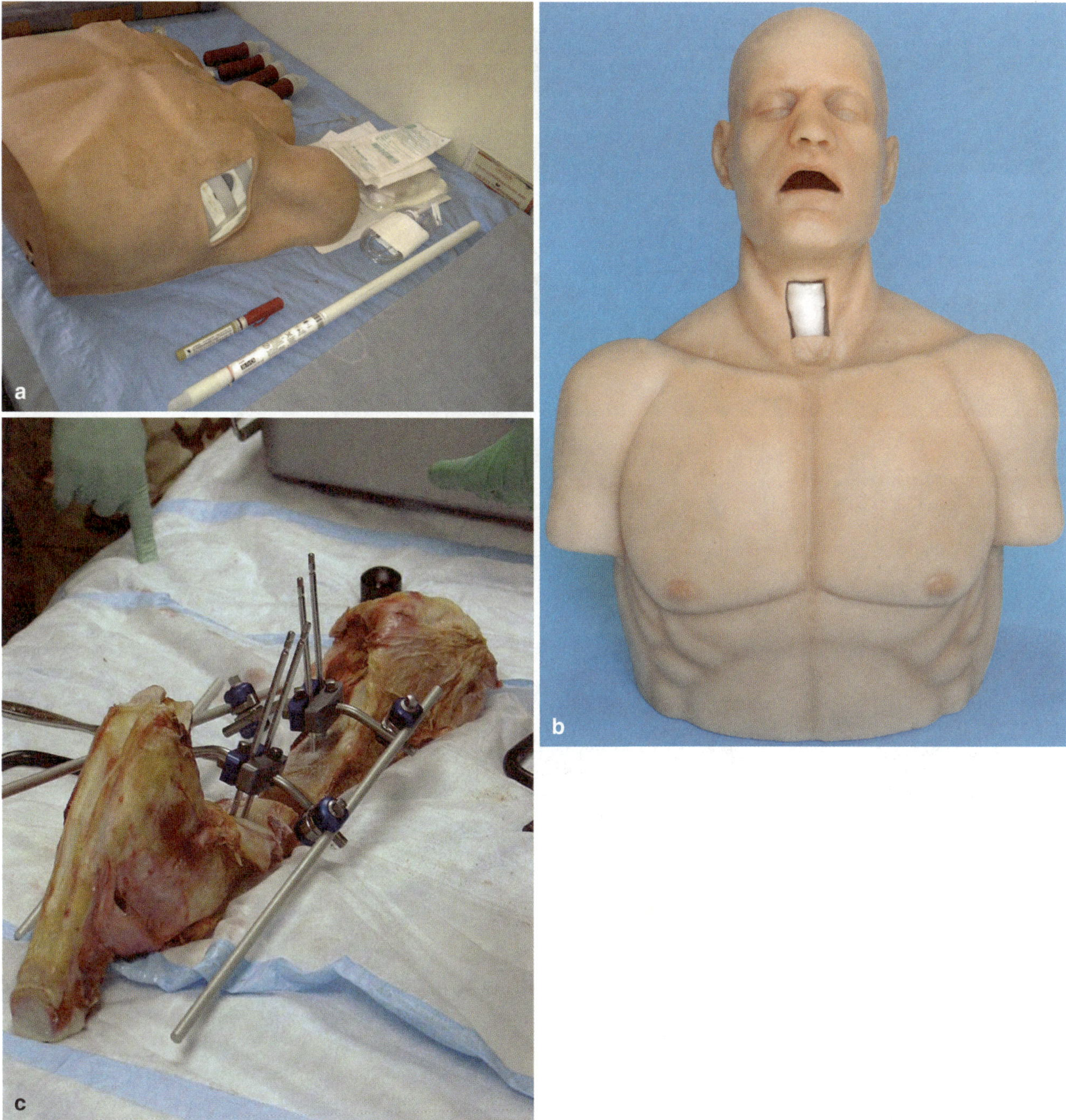

Fig. 27.7 Part-task trainers for (**a**) chest tube insertion; (**b**) 6 in 1 torso for tracheostomy placement, needle decompression, and chest tube placement; and (**c**) external fixator placement (Photo b courtesy of Strategic Operations, Inc.)

has been transitioned back to the host nation. These events must be practiced so that the vital individual and team trauma skills are maintained. This can be a difficult task in a deployed setting since other tasks take priority (especially if it is assumed that deployed units are adequately prepared for the trauma care mission regardless of patient volumes). The newly developed Surgical Team Assessment Tool/Training (STAT) and TeamSTEPPS™ courses provide a framework for training, team integration, and assessment of both patient care team and supporting team roles (Fig. 27.12). These programs are easily transportable throughout the battlefield and rely on moulaged unit members as standardized patients and low-fidelity mannequin simulators. Preliminary studies have shown that it is imperative that these events not only be practiced by the unit but also involve up-to-date training, standardized evaluation, and feedback by an experienced cadre to insure uniformity of readiness and capability throughout a battlespace (personal communication from COL Peter

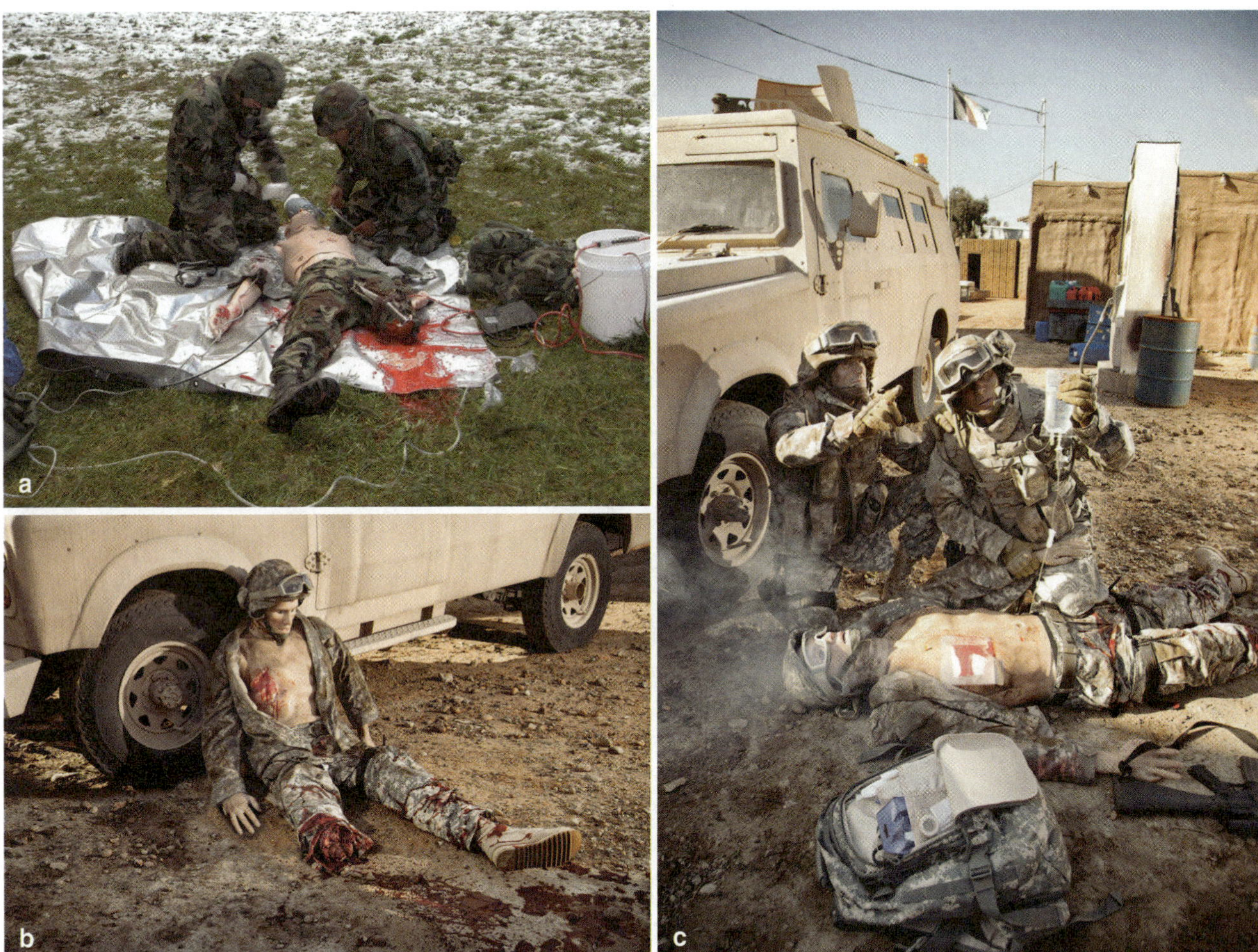

Fig. 27.8 (**a**) Team management of multiply injured simulated patient (Laerdal SimMan) at point of injury and (**b**, **c**) Caesar, a wireless, tetherless mannequin simulator by CAE (Photo courtesy of CAE Healthcare ©2012 CAE Healthcare)

Nielsen, Deputy Commander for Clinical Services, 86th Combat Support Hospital, August 2011).

Post-deployment (Returning Home)

Although this phase of the military cycle does not get as much notoriety, upon returning from deployment, many new and different stressors become evident for the military healthcare provider. Besides the obvious stressors all post-deployed military personnel encounter (reintegrating with family, friends, posttraumatic stressors), the healthcare provider must also reestablish a peace practice. While there is a perceived deficit in clinical and technical skills upon redeployment, it has not been measured or proven yet for seasoned board-certified and board-eligible clinicians [4]. Although there is no current standardized training for the post-deployed healthcare provider, many simulators are available for honing ones technical surgical skills both virtually as outlined in other sections of this book and with complete real-time haptic feedback (such as the Fundamentals of Laparoscopic Surgery, Fig. 27.13a, b). Also, hybrid cognitive/technical evaluations using simulators such as the Surgical Chloe™ from Gaumard (Fig. 27.14a–c) or the Cut Suit are in the evaluation phase and may be incorporated in surgical and physician refresher training after deployment. These, in combination with a knowledge assessment tool or test, are also being considered by state medical boards when evaluating physicians returning to practice after administrative jobs or other prolonged absences from clinical care. For these purposes, the instruction and evaluation phase must include both technical and cognitive portions, as well as hybrid scenarios where both critical thinking and precise execution of skills are performed.

What We Do Well: The Army Medical Department Center and School, the Central Simulation Committee, and Medical Simulation Training Centers

The military, in general, has been at the forefront of performance-based standardized courses for decades. Military training relies heavily on the achievement of specific step-by-step performance objectives. General military assessment is fairly straightforward. It is a pass/fail model. Passing implies that the trainee accomplished all tasks necessary in the correct order.

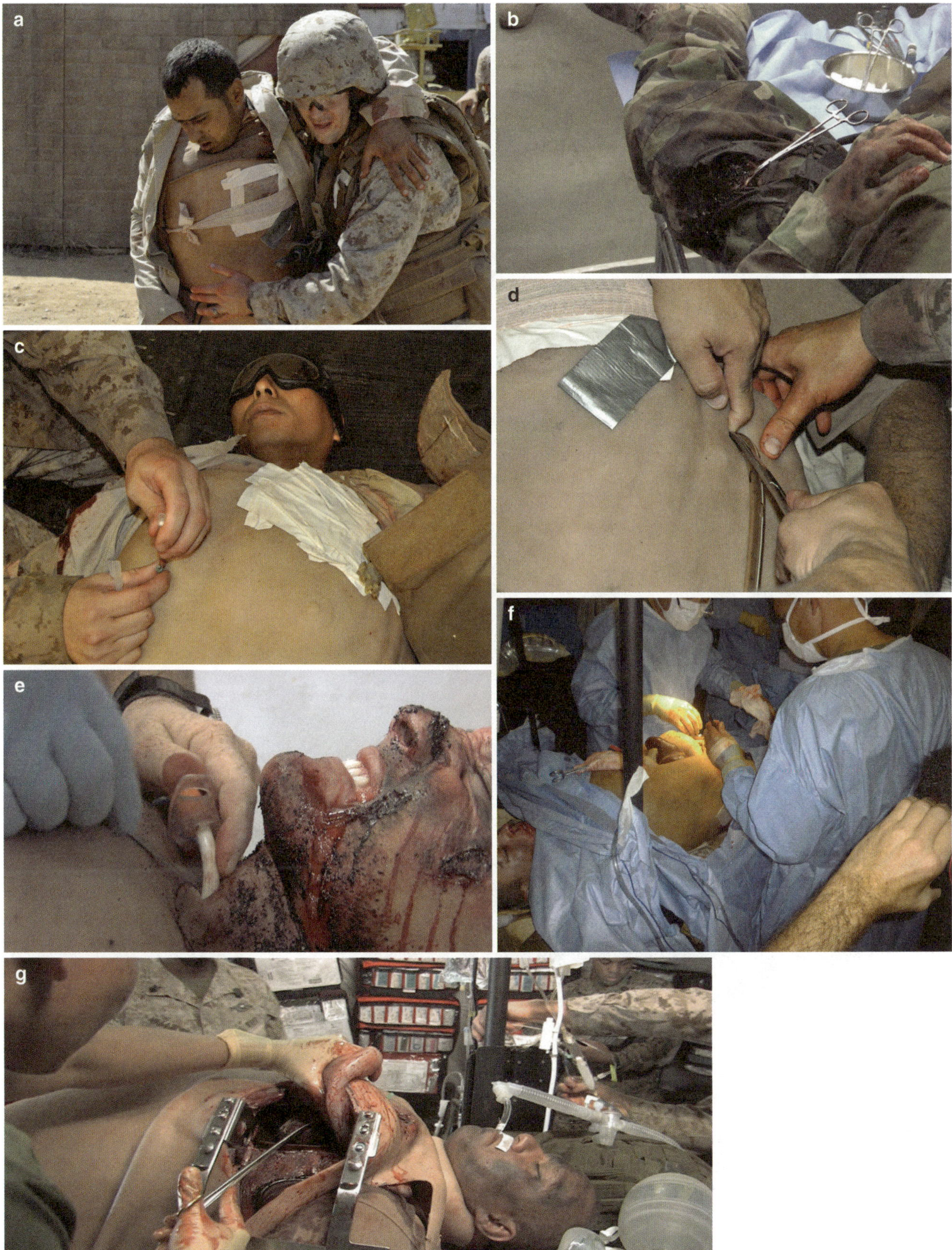

Fig. 27.9 (a) Cut Suit with simulated chest wounds in hyperrealistic environment, (b) Cut Suit with simulated leg wounds, (c) Cut Suit with pneumothorax needle decompression capability (d) and chest tube placement, (e) Cut Suit with tracheostomy placement, (f) Cut Suit with simulated hyperrealistic resuscitative, intraoperative abdominal surgery, and (g) thoracotomy using the Cut Suit at a Marine Forward Resuscitative Surgical Suite (FRSS) team exercise (Photos courtesy of Strategic Operations, Inc.)

Table 27.2 Medical procedures currently available on the Cut Suit

Extremity tourniquet application and hemorrhage control
Extremity arterial hemorrhage clamping
Needle and surgical cricothyroidotomy
Bilateral chest needle thoracentesis
Surgical chest tube thoracotomy
Surgical incisions to the thoracic and abdominal cavity with venous bleeding
Thoracotomy and intrathoracic exploration and hemorrhage control of gross organ structures
Laparotomy and intra-abdominal exploration and hemorrhage control of gross organ structures
Suturing or stapling of gross organs and skin in all locations
Urinary catheterization and bladder tap
Peripheral IV access

Source: http://www.strategic-operations.com/products/cut-suit

Omitting steps or deviating from the accepted correct order results in failure and may require a trainee to either repeat the entire course, or worse, be dismissed without attaining certification. This traditional model places the onus of sustained competence on the individual or on the unit, without a centralized mechanism for maintenance of certification. This has all changed significantly in the last 2 decades.

The Army Medical Department Center and School (AMEDD C&S)

Known as the "School House" throughout the Army Medical Department and colocated with Brooke Army Medical Center in San Antonio, TX, this is the place where standardized

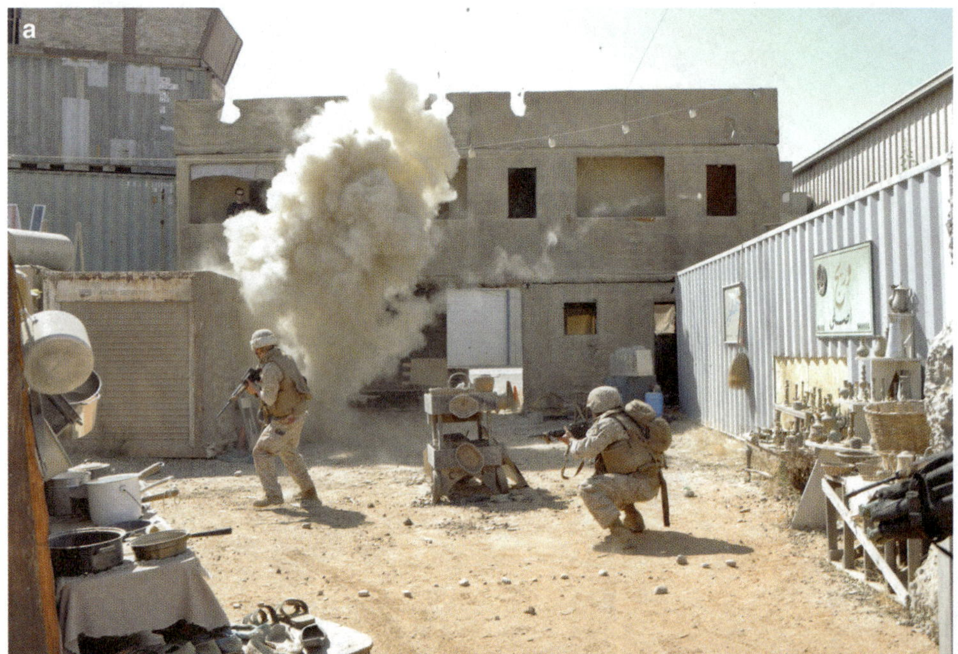

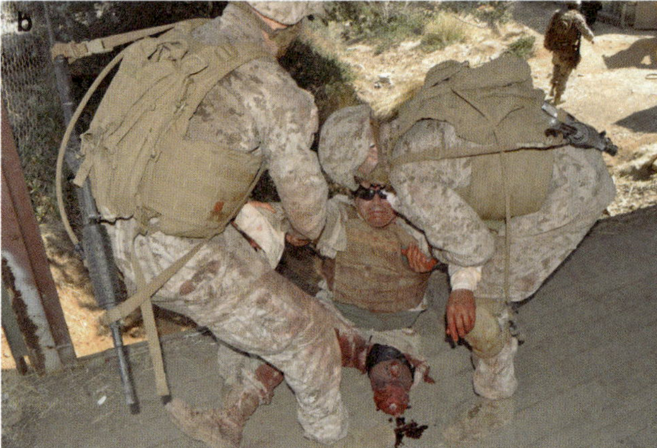

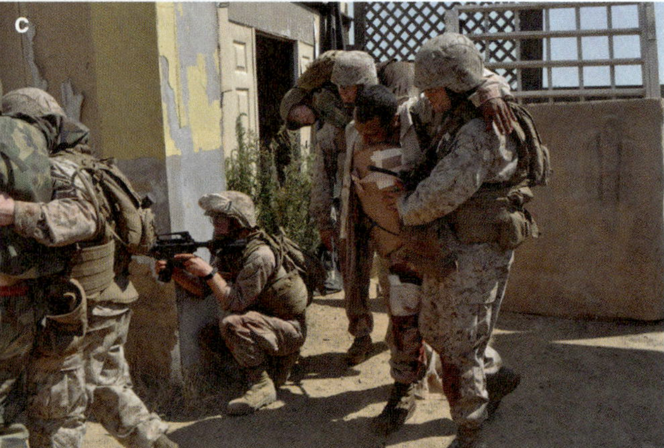

Fig. 27.10 (**a**) Hyperrealistic battle scene with pyrotechnics and (**b**, **c**) causalities (Photos courtesy of Strategic Operations, Inc.)

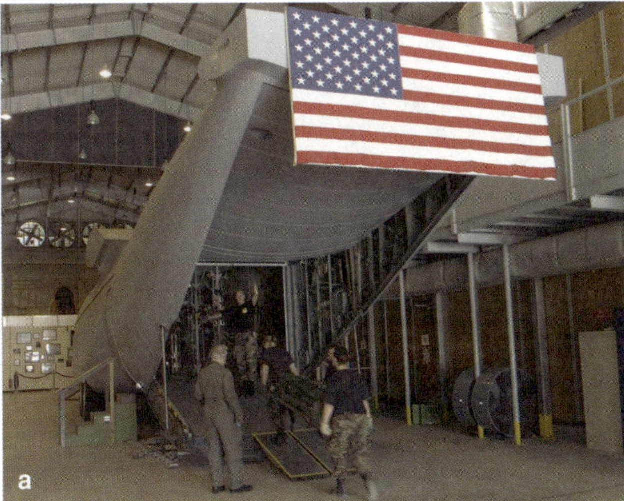

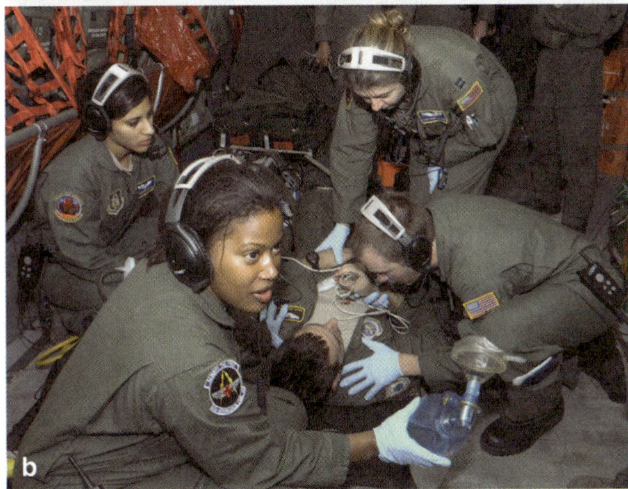

Fig. 27.11 (**a**) Evacuation platform simulators are used for practicing loading and unloading of patients and (**b**) in-flight care, where aircraft vibration and noise conditions are replicated

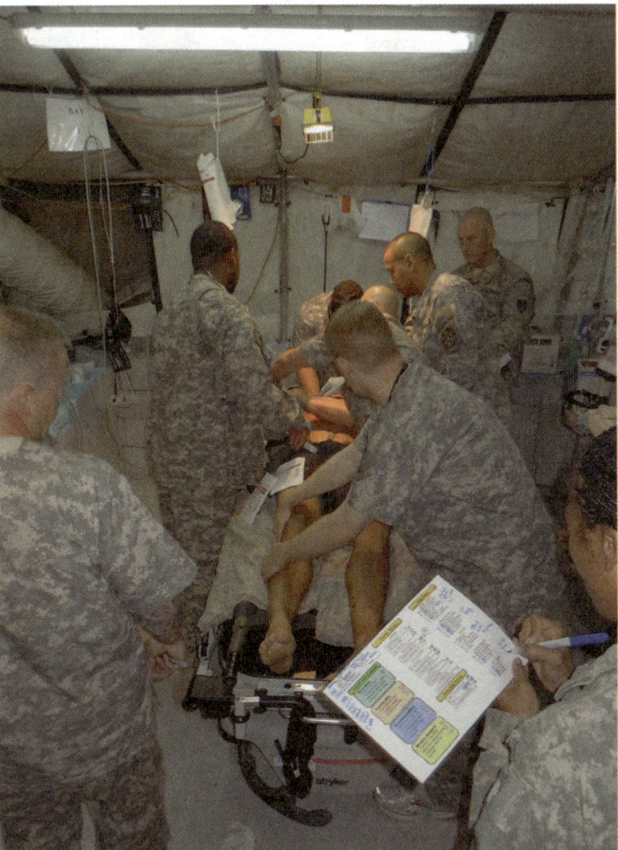

Fig. 27.12 STAT (Surgical Team Assessment Training) is used with moulaged simulated casualties during lulls in action in Iraq. Note the formal assessment document in the forefront that is used to insure that unit and personnel readiness goals are met

curricula are finalized and put into a format enabling rollout to the rest of the Army and the Department of Defense. It is the largest medical education and training center in the world, graduating over 35,000 students per year from various courses, schools, and certifying programs. Simulation here is the norm—and has been for decades. As in combat arms, the AMMED C&S injects simulation at every level—from the individual skills of combat medic training using part-task trainers and sophisticated wireless mannequins to force-on-force tabletop computerized war gaming scenarios that involve leadership teams guiding implementation of combat support hospitals and other health service support units into battles and humanitarian disaster relief efforts.

The Central Simulation Committee

Graduate medical education is strictly governed by the ACGME and each specialty's residency review committee, and this governance is stovepiped into each institution's individual residency teaching programs. While each residency, nursing specialty course, and technologist course have caseload and knowledge requirements for performance, all share similar working environments and "practice" subjects—the patients. Hospital simulation centers provide assets and curricula that cross between these program boundaries, the most obvious of which are the mannequin simulators, fundamentals of laparoscopic surgery MISTELs trainers, and other virtual reality laparoscopic/endoscopic simulators that can be used by urology, general surgery, OB/GYN, family practice, internal medicine, cardiology, and gastroenterology to name a few. This multidisciplinary approach also allows the Department of Defense to address issues corporately such as catheter-related central line blood stream infections, of which the standard central line curriculum is an excellent example.

Funding equipment centrally through a system-wide approach also allows for the oversight on where to place simulation assets, as some of the simulators can cost in the hundreds of thousands of dollars. Each facility in the Army to include USUHS has at least three to four members on the committee as either the director of the center, the graduate

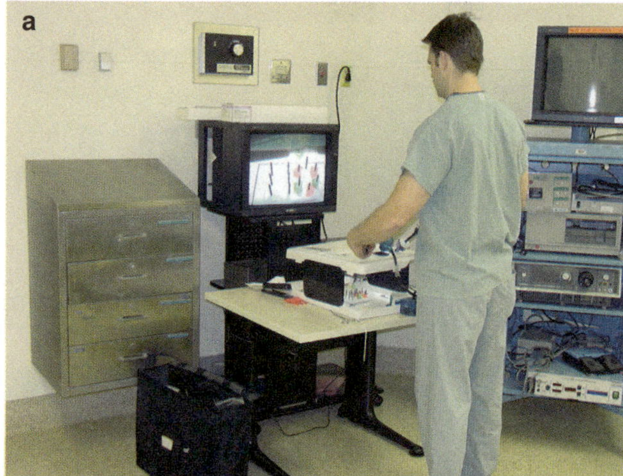

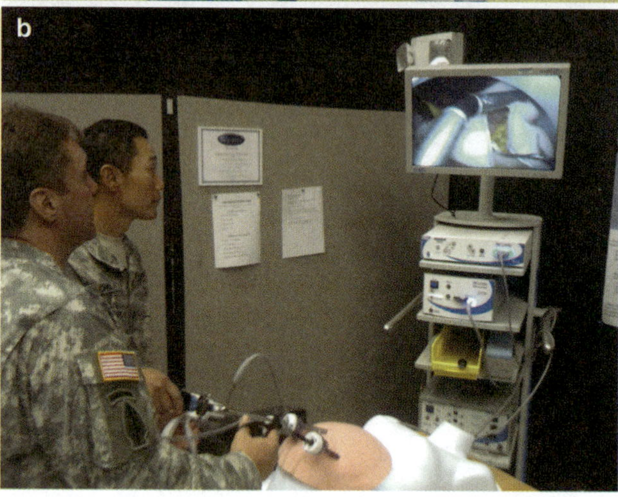

Fig. 27.13 (**a**) Fundamentals of laparoscopic surgery skills practice and (**b**) surgeons practicing bariatric surgery (sleeve gastrectomy) after returning from deployment using actual OR instruments and a stomach and intestinal model manufactured by Simulab

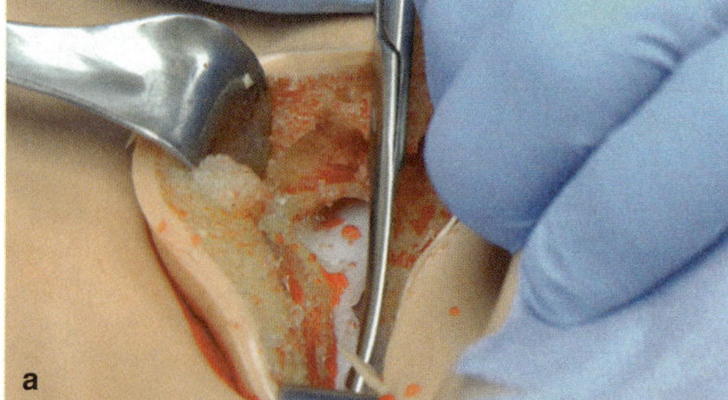

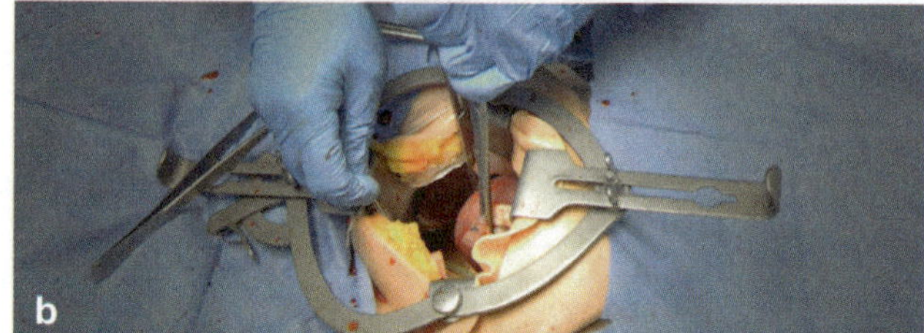

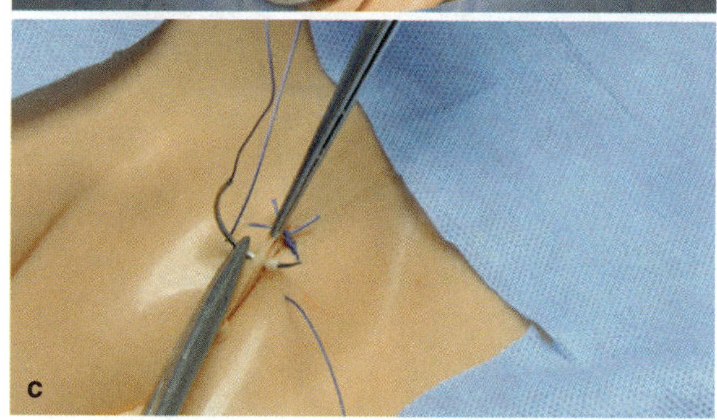

Fig. 27.14 Surgical simulator Chloe™ from Gaumard: (**a**) abdominal incision, (**b**) surgery, and (**c**) skin closure (Photo courtesy of Gaumard Scientific 2012. All rights reserved)

medical education director, the administrator of each center or the technical expert (and in many cases, all four of those represent the education centers). Each hospital's director is part of the graduate education committee at each center as well so that they have oversight of the needs of the specific residency or fellowship programs. This allows for top-down oversight and accountability of equipment needs and use as well as bottom-up requests from the users and students. Providing a common core management and administrative framework with a defined budget is essential for a large organization.

Medical Simulation Training Centers

There was a gap in the wartime experience of line medics (those frontline medical care providers who are equivalent to emergency medical technicians (EMTs) and paramedics) at the beginning of the War on Terrorism. While combat arm (infantry, armor, field artillery) specific units have always had huge simulation assets, there was a paucity of facilities and resources dedicated to training medical personnel on an ongoing basis. That has changed now as every large base has a medical training simulation center, known as the MSTC (pronounced "mistic"). MSTCs conduct EMT, paramedic, and lifesaving combat skills training and maintenance of certification, in addition to standardized pre-deployment training of line unit medics, nurses, and physician assistants. MSTCs are the key element in keeping US Army medics up to date on vital combat and noncombat lifesaving skills.

Navy, Air Force, and Marine Medical Simulation Training

US Navy Medicine also has a central simulation committee very similar to the Army's version. In combination with the marines and Strategic Operations, Inc., they have conducted some of the most exciting and realistic combat trauma training to date, combining line units on patrol through "Hollywood"-staged sets, full of special effects, and casualty scenarios including evacuation protocols back to surgical elements. The US Air Force equivalent to the Army's CSC is the Air Force Medical Modeling and Simulation Training (AFMAST) program. This program has ten Centers of Excellence at major bases throughout the world, each being responsible for subordinate units for simulation-based medical training. Another task of the AFMAST is to develop and enhance virtual training environments and medical gaming models to enhance retention and acquisition of vital medical skills.

Civilian Comparisons and Applications

There are rare similarities to the military deployment cycle that can be found in the civilian setting. Volunteer work in underserved areas depending on the location and time away from practice, physicians and nurses who have entered non-clinical administrative or leadership roles wishing to return to direct patient care and those professionals needing to exhibit improved skills due to disciplinary actions prior to re-engaging in patient care may also fit into this cycle at some point. Many states already have physician and nurse reentry programs to regain licensure, many of which are incorporating simulation for evaluation purposes.

Conclusion

Simulation in both military and civilian medical practice relies on curricula-based simulation platforms that involve a variety of techniques and technologies including part-task training, hybrid teaching models, and immersive environments that include corporately managed education centers to insure efficient and timely acquisition and maintenance of vital and perishable patient care skills. While we have not measured the skill decay in seasoned providers, cycling from deployed environments to US-based practices allows for unique training opportunities and the need for multidisciplinary and inter-professional simulation-based curricula to refresh and enhance skills for maximal performance. When injected efficiently into this cycle, the roll of simulation will continue to expand into frontiers unseen.

References

1. Place RJ, Porter CA, Azarow K, Beitler AL. Trauma experience comparison of army forward surgical team surgeons at Ben Taub Hospital and Madigan Army Medical Center(2)(2). Curr Surg. 2001;58(1):90–3.
2. Jennings J. Humvee rollover trainer: an officers quest to save lives on the battlefield. Professional Safety. 24–30 July 2010. Available from: http://www.asse.org/professionalsafety/docs/F1Jenni_0710.pdf. Cited 4 Mar 2012.
3. Cassel CK, Reuben DB. Specialization, subspecialization, and subsubspecialization in internal medicine. N Engl J Med. 2011;364(12):1169–73.
4. Deering SH, Rush Jr RM, Lesperance RN, Roth BJ. Perceived effects of deployments on surgeon and physician skills in the US Army Medical Department. Am J Surg. 2011;201(5):666–72.
5. Mitchell KB, Tarpley MJ, Tarpley JL, Casey KM. Elective global surgery rotations for residents: a call for cooperation and consortium. World J Surg. 2011;35(12):2617–24.
6. Ozgediz D, Chu K, Ford N, Dubowitz G, Bedada AG, Azzie G, et al. Surgery in global health delivery. Mt Sinai J Med. 2011;78(3):327–41.
7. Riviello R, Ozgediz D, Hsia RY, Azzie G, Newton M, Tarpley J. Role of collaborative academic partnerships in surgical training, education, and provision. World J Surg. 2010;34(3):459–65.
8. Rush Jr RM, Stockmaster NR, Stinger HK, Arrington ED, Devine JG, Atteberry L, et al. Supporting the Global War on Terror: a tale of two campaigns featuring the 250th Forward Surgical Team (Airborne). Am J Surg. 2005;189(5):564–70.
9. Place RJ, Rush Jr RM, Arrington ED. Forward surgical team (FST) workload in a special operations environment: the 250th FST in Operation ENDURING FREEDOM. Curr Surg. 2003;60(4):418–22.
10. Causey M, Rush Jr RM, Kjorstad RJ, Sebesta JA. Factors influencing humanitarian care and the treatment of local patients within the deployed military medical system: casualty referral limitations. Am J Surg. 2012;203(5):574–7.
11. Strategic Operations website. http://www.strategic-operations.com/. Assessed 23 Aug 2012.
12. Sohn VY, Runser LA, Puntel RA, Sebesta JA, Beekley AC, Theis JL, et al. Training physicians for combat casualty care on the modern battlefield. J Surg Educ. 2007;64(4):199–203.
13. Sohn VY, Miller JP, Koeller CA, Gibson SO, Azarow KS, Myers JB, et al. From the combat medic to the forward surgical team: the Madigan model for improving trauma readiness of brigade combat teams fighting the Global War on Terror. J Surg Res. 2007;138(1):25–31.
14. Sohn VY, Eckert MJ, Martin MJ, Arthurs ZM, Perry JR, Beekley A, et al. Efficacy of three topical hemostatic agents applied by medics in a lethal groin injury model. J Surg Res. 2009;154(2):258–61.
15. Pereira BM, Ryan ML, Ogilvie MP, Gomez-Rodriguez JC, McAndrew P, Garcia GD, et al. Predeployment mass casualty and clinical trauma training for US Army forward surgical teams. J Craniofac Surg. 2010;21(4):982–6.
16. Schulman CI, Graygo J, Wilson K, Robinson DB, Garcia G, Augenstein J. Training forward surgical teams: do military-civilian collaborations work? US Army Med Dep J. 2010;17–21.

Simulation in Neurosurgery and Neurosurgical Procedures

28

Ali Alaraj, Matthew K. Tobin, Daniel M. Birk, and Fady T. Charbel

Introduction

For over 100 years, observational learning has been the pillar of surgical education. The exponential growth of information technologies in recent decades has fueled a revolution in training in diverse fields, and medical education has been a major benefactor of this revolution. Recently, due to work hour restrictions, cost of operating room (OR) time, and concern for patient safety, neurosurgery resident training programs have come under increasing pressure to impart the necessary skills needed to perform competently as practicing surgeons. Given access to rapidly advancing simulation and virtual reality technology, there is increasing interest in developing neurosurgical simulation technologies to enhance surgical skill acquisition and proficiency.

Practicing neurological surgery requires consistent preparation in order to refine the necessary coordinated motor skills. Historically, the most widely accepted method for training and proficiency was to participate in as many surgeries as possible. This approach, however, poses a number of challenges to the healthcare team and can increase the risk of complications for the patient. For residents, learning new techniques requires one-on-one instruction, a practice that is limited by the number of instructors, the number of cases, and, more often, the amount of time available for learning. For the patient, intraoperative teaching during surgery results in a longer procedure and increases the period of time the patient remains under anesthesia, which can increase the overall risk to the patient. Mistakes made by surgical trainees can have catastrophic consequences. A controlled environment, such as a virtual reality (VR) simulator, allows surgeons the ability to practice their skills and learn through trial and error without fear of harm to a patient. New technologies offer a reliable means to safely and confidently refine surgical skills and learn advanced techniques while also decreasing the number of poor outcomes for the patient. Whether via stereolithographic modeling [1, 2] or virtual reality (VR) [3–9], hospitals throughout the world are turning to these rapidly advancing technologies to both help teach basic skills to young surgeons and new techniques to established neurosurgeons. Following the training model for commercial airline pilots, VR simulators have been developed and made available to train for endoscope-based procedures as well as endovascular treatments and other specialized interventions. Recently, VR simulators have been developed to model complex neurosurgical procedures including tumor debulking and cauterization [5], ventriculostomy [3, 10–14], aneurysm clipping [2], brain retraction modeling [4–6], skull base surgery [15], and endoscopic transsphenoidal pituitary surgery [16].

A. Alaraj, MD (✉) • D.M. Birk, MD • F.T. Charbel, MD
Department of Neurosurgery, University of Illinois at Chicago and University of Illinois Hospital and Health Science Systems, 912 S. Wood St., MC-799, Chicago, IL 60612, USA
e-mail: alaraj@uic.edu; dmbirk@uic.edu; fcharbel@uic.edu

M.K. Tobin, BS
College of Medicine, University of Illinois at Chicago, 912 S. Wood St., MC-799, Chicago, IL 60612, USA
e-mail: mktobin2@uic.edu

Simulation for Preoperative Planning

Preoperative planning is a crucial component of every operation. This is especially true for neurosurgical procedures. Neurosurgeons address complex and small-scale anatomy, with overlapping structures in three dimensions, both in the brain and spinal cord. Complex cranial and spine surgeries cannot be approached from a simple two-dimensional perspective that is characterized by standard imaging techniques such as CT and MRI display modalities. Therefore, computer-based visualization systems and VR systems that integrate standard patient imaging to create easily manipulated, three-dimensional (3D) representations of patient data are invaluable tools in order to optimize patient care. Neurosurgeons can plan the most effective surgical approach by creating 3D images that can be manipulated in a VR environment prior to operating, allowing them to fully

A.I. Levine et al. (eds.), *The Comprehensive Textbook of Healthcare Simulation*,
DOI 10.1007/978-1-4614-5993-4_28, © Springer Science+Business Media New York 2013

understand the consequences of the proposed surgical intervention on the surgical targets and surrounding viable tissues.

Interactive 3D Visualization

In the last 20 years, various computer-based systems have been developed to make preoperative planning easier, thus helping create beneficial patient outcomes. At the basic level is the University of Virginia's "Props" interface [17] and Netra [18]. These two systems incorporate a 3D user interface with a two-handed physical manipulation system. Essentially, the user controls one object with each hand, typically a miniature head in one hand and a variety of tools, such as a cross-sectioning plane or a stylus, in the other. Depending on the orientation of the two objects in the user's hands, the on-screen images are digitally manipulated to correspond with the physical objects in the user's hands. For example, if the user holds the mannequin head in one hand and the cross-sectioning plane tool in the other, the patient's diagnostic image displayed on screen will show a slice corresponding to the directionality of the cutting plane that the user selected (Fig. 28.1).

New technologies have emerged from the "Props" interface and Netra that not only offer the ability to physically manipulate objects in space but also incorporate immersive VR systems. These new systems allow for computer-based head-tracking as well as the physical manipulation of objects and tools. Stoakley et al. [19] introduced a system called "Words in Miniature (WIM)" that offers a second dynamic viewport that allows for manipulation via head-tracking. Now, not only can the user operate on-screen images through physical manipulation of objects in space but he or she can also control images through simple head motions (Fig. 28.2).

Stereotactic surgery is one area of neurosurgery in which preoperative planning is critical for a successful outcome. The ability to precisely calculate and localize surgical coordinates is paramount to successful stereotactic, frame-based functional neurosurgery. The first product introduced for this purpose was StereoPlan by Radionics (now Integra LifeSciences). Integra has numerous commercially available products [20] to aid functional neurosurgeons in their preoperative planning. These systems not only provide precise coordinate information but also have the ability to incorporate multiple image sets together, provide multiple measurement lines, and afford the surgeon the ability to track the entire trajectory through the anatomy that will be encountered during surgery. Therefore, a more complete analysis of patient data is possible, and multiple surgical approaches can be rehearsed and considered.

Adams and Wilson [21] developed a 3D simulation model of the cerebral ventricular system using commercially available computer software. This model was developed for the purposes of neuroanatomical education; however, it can also be applied for preoperative planning purposes. The team's main concern was that most anatomical education is based on either 2D images or on artist renderings of what the "ideal" brain should look like. Consequently, they developed a virtual anatomical model based on postmortem MRI analysis to develop an anatomically accurate ventricular and cerebral model. This model can be projected stereoscopically to allow the user a more realistic setting in which they view and manipulate the structures. In addition to the anatomical structures, Adams et al. modeled the flow of CSF through the ventricular system. These two abilities not only allow for

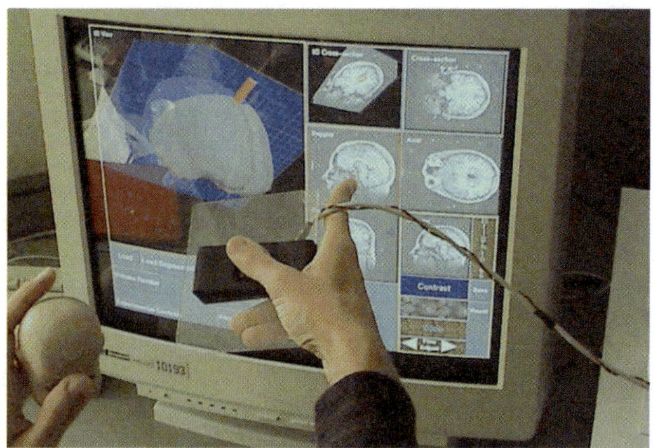

Fig. 28.1 The simulator interface allows neurosurgeons to explore a 3D MRI scan of a patient's brain during presurgical planning. From the surgeon's perspective, the interface is analogous to holding a miniature head in one hand which can be "sliced open" or "pointed to" using a cross-sectioning plane or a stylus tool, respectively, held in the other hand (Reprinted from Publication Hinckley et al. [17]. With permission from IOS Press)

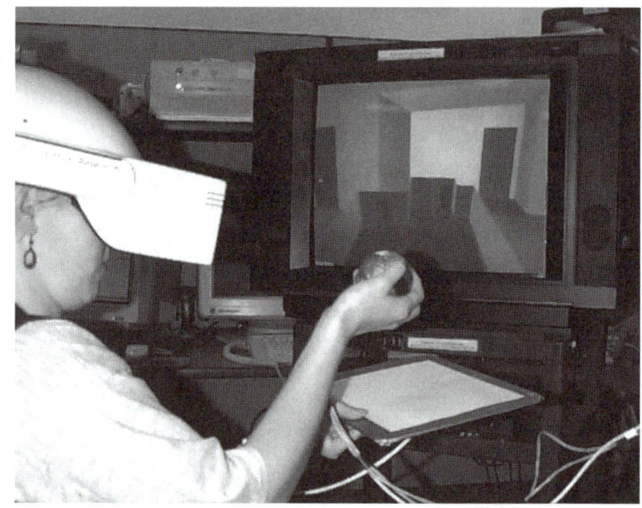

Fig. 28.2 Immersive VR system. The WIM graphics attached to the clipboard are a miniature copy of all the surrounding graphics in the immersive environment. Each of the objects in the WIM copy is tied to their counterparts in the immersive environment through pointers and vice versa at the point of WIM creation. The user can manipulate the objects in the WIM, and the objects in the world will follow (Reprinted from Stoakley et al. [19]. With permission ACM Press/Addison-Wesley Publishing Co.)

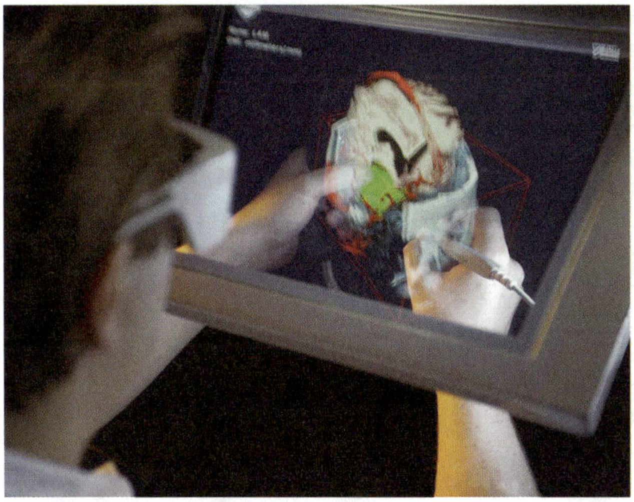

Fig. 28.3 Working with the Dextroscope, the user's hands are collocated with the virtual stereoscopic objects displayed as a reflection behind a mirror (Reprinted from Kockro et al. [24]. With kind permission from Wolters Kluwer Health)

proper education on relevant anatomy but can be used for successful preoperative planning. Using accurate models gives the surgeon the ability to create 3D models of abnormal anatomy such as shifted or slit ventricles and abnormal CSF flow as seen in noncommunicating hydrocephalus. This system provides a very good preoperative planning model for diseases involving the ventricular system.

Additionally, two other high-fidelity VR simulators are available that greatly improve the ability of the surgeon to plan preoperatively. The Virtual Workbench [22] and the Dextroscope [23] create a very fluid, 3D representation of patient data that is easily manipulated, allowing the surgeon to visualize patient anatomy in any orientation before operating. Although these systems are modeled on the binocular microscope, they remain "hands-on" in a way that microscopes cannot. Because of the binocular glass platform, users control the system with their hands and 3D images co-localized in the same position in real time. Consequently, the VR simulation mirrors that of a true OR situation. These systems are designed to incorporate and fuse together multiple patient image sets (magnetic resonance imaging, magnetic resonance angiography and venography, and computed tomography) so that a 3D representation of patient data is created. As a result, the user has the ability to manipulate this 3D model in real time and visualize the exact anatomy that will be encountered during the surgical procedure (Fig. 28.3). Without these VR systems, users are forced to plan procedures using standard techniques of looking at patient images in a two-dimensional, slice-by-slice fashion. Both the Virtual Workbench and the Dextroscope eliminate this problem by integrating all relevant data, ultimately presenting the surgeon with as complete a picture as possible. Users of this technology believe that this is helpful in the surgical planning, which is an abstract process that relies mainly on displaying and viewing certain key structures, combined with an ability to interact with those structures quickly and intuitively. Yet there is no data that rehearsing of the actual surgery was beneficial in decreasing the complication rates or shortening the surgical procedure. At this point this surgical planning software is still experimental and is mostly used in group conferences and teaching courses [24–26].

The potential advantages of these products are that they afford surgeons the ability to see all potential complications of surgery before actually operating. Users have the ability to plan the best surgical approach for each patient without facing concerns about the problems that may arise during surgery. As a result, intraoperative mistakes can be minimized, operating time can be reduced, and the overall safety of the patient can be ensured. Because this field is in its infancy, there is no data to support this potential benefit.

Stereolithographic Modeling

In addition to all of the VR simulation systems developed for preoperative planning, a more simplistic approach can also be utilized: stereolithographic modeling (Fig. 28.4) [1, 2]. This procedure has been used to model cerebral vasculature for the study of aneurysms and its application in microsurgical clipping. Physical modeling, though not as comprehensive as VR simulation, provides a few unique benefits for preoperative planning that VR simulation does not. First, it provides a physical model of patient data that surgeons can use for multiple purposes, one of which is to explain the complexities and intricacies of the procedure to the patient and their families. Because neurosurgical procedures tend to be very complex, it is difficult for the surgeon to explain the intricacies of the operation to patients and families. However, by having a physical model that a surgeon can manipulate, patient and family education becomes much easier, and any confusion the patient may have is inevitably reduced. Additionally, this type of modeling allows the surgeon to practice aneurysm clipping and aides in the process of choosing what surgical clip or clips will be appropriate for successful treatment.

Despite the benefits of stereolithography, many disadvantages remain in using this technique: primarily the inflexibility of the material used to create the model. Researchers have yet to find a model that realistically resembles in vivo vasculature – most of the material currently in use is frequently too rigid to approximate real human tissue. Consequently, preoperative planning is difficult because the surgeon does not have a completely realistic model on which to practice technique. Additionally, the process of making these models is both costly and time consuming. As the manufacturing process takes 3–7 days [2], it would take too long to create patient-specific models even if the equipment was on site. Additionally, since cerebral aneurysms are very

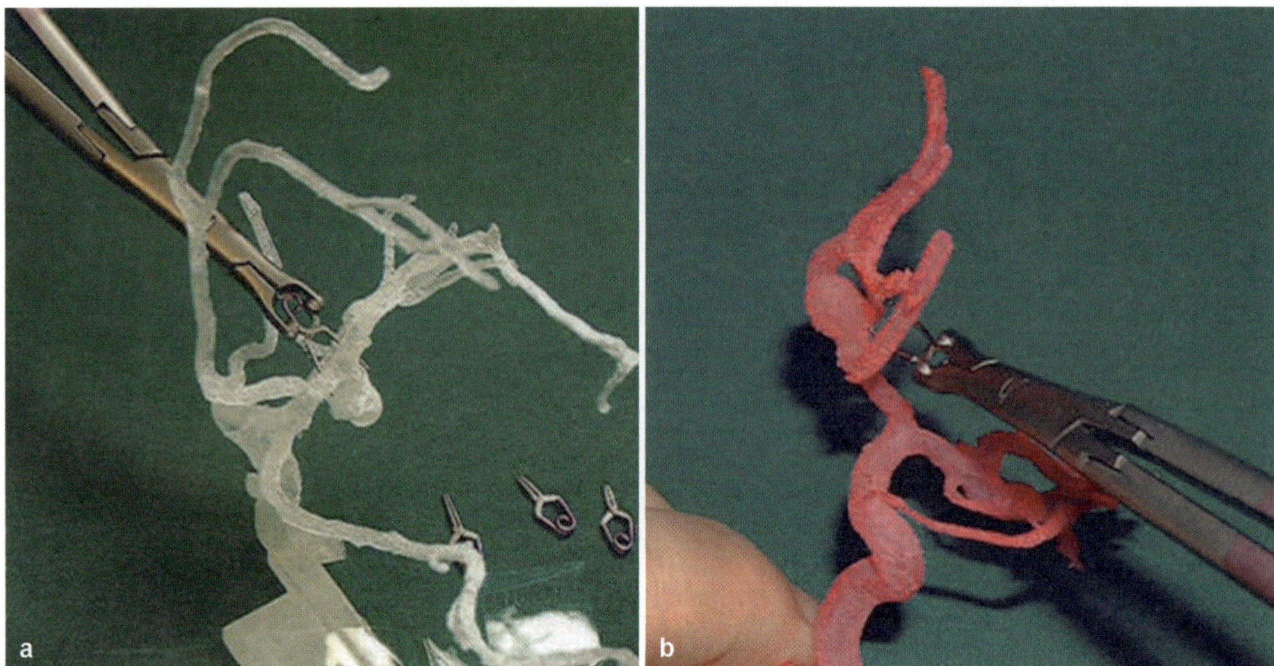

Fig. 28.4 Photographs of an MCA aneurysm clipping model. (**a**, **b**) different MCA aneurysm models detailed view of the aneurysm with the parent and branching vessels (Reprinted from Wurm et al. [1]. With kind permission from JNS publishing group)

unpredictable and ruptured aneurysms require emergency surgery, there is not enough time to create a planning model prior to surgery. While these models are beneficial for select purposes, mainly patient education, their overall usefulness is questionable until new models can be developed that both approximate human tissue more appropriately and take significantly less time to manufacture. Because there are no virtual reality aneurysm clipping modules available at this point, there are no comparative results to evaluate these two techniques.

Reality Training Applications

As stated above, preoperative planning is, without question, a fundamental part of any operation. However, when the time arrives for surgical execution, no amount of planning can compensate for an untrained, inexperienced surgeon. Various restrictions on work hours and clinical obligations can limit residents' training time and make new techniques necessary to help teach residents and allow established surgeons to practice and hone their skills. Simulation provides surgeons with a new immersive VR world that not only simulates patient data in 3D but provides tactile feedback to the system user. This affords the surgeons the ability to manipulate patient data as well as "perform" the operation using the immersive VR simulator. Therefore, the user feels as if he or she is actually performing the operation because the VR simulator provides both visual and haptic sensory feedback. The main requirements of a good VR simulator are that the user not only has a realistic sense of the visual world in which they will be working but also has appropriate tactile feedback that simulates a real operation. To date, many systems (Table 28.1) are available that provide a good approximation of real neurosurgery via VR simulation.

Table 28.1 A list of the virtual environments discussed in this chapter

Author	Year	VR	Surgical modules
Burtscher	1999	3D virtual images	Virtual endoscopy
Luciano	2005	Tactile haptics	Ventriculostomy
Chui	2006	Tactile haptics	Vertebroplasty
Tsang	2008	Tactile haptics	Endovascular surgery
Schulze	2008	2D visual	Endoscopy
Banerjee	2011	Tactile haptics	Thoracic pedicle screw placement
Delorme	2012	Tactile haptics	Craniotomy and tumor debulking/cauterization

Ventriculostomy

In 2006, Luciano et al. [3] developed what is perhaps the most widely used VR simulator for ventriculostomy: ImmersiveTouch. It is an augmented VR system and is the first of its kind to integrate a haptic device with a high-resolution stereoscopic display. The haptic device includes both head- and hand-tracking capabilities. Therefore, the

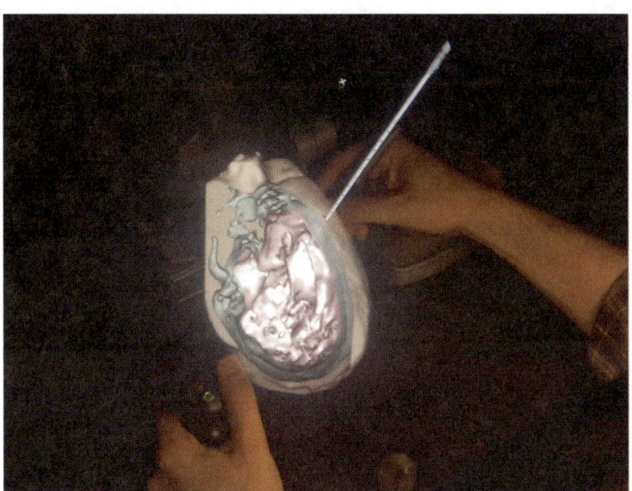

Fig. 28.5 A ventriculostomy simulation. The trainee is inserting the ventricular catheter according to skull landmarks. A virtual cranial window is shown to check the location of the tip of the ventricular catheter (Image courtesy of ImmersiveTouch)

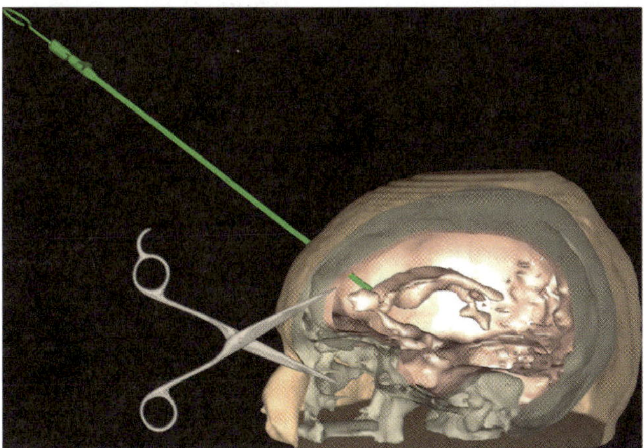

Fig. 28.6 Checking the location of the ventricular catheter at the end of the procedure. The catheter color changes *green* if the tip is within the ventricular system (Image courtesy of ImmersiveTouch)

user can control the on-screen images by either manipulating the hand controllers or by moving their head in space. This approximates real OR situations where the surgeon has the ability to do both of these maneuvers: manipulate surgical instruments and position his or her body and head in space to best visualize the surgical field. The haptic system was developed to provide multiple sensory modalities including visual, aural, tactile, and kinesthetic. Additionally, the system was developed so that different tissue types (e.g., CSF, parenchyma, ependymal lining) provide different haptic feedback responses. As a result, the user receives feedback similar to that in real surgery (Figs. 28.5 and 28.6).

In theory, ImmersiveTouch could be used for many different types of surgical interventions, but the device was validated for a simple ventriculostomy procedure that is often learned during the first year of residency. Luciano et al. [3] used patient data to develop a VR module based upon normal anatomy and had neurosurgery faculty, residents, and medical students test the system. All of the users found the platform to have realistic visual, tactile, and handling characteristics. Additionally, it was found to be a viable alternative to standard training. Lemole et al. [13] sought to prove that the system could be used with abnormal anatomy as well. After several attempts, ImmersiveTouch users were able to properly cannulate the abnormal virtual ventricle demonstrating proof of concept in a different spectrum of pathological scenarios.

Additionally, ImmersiveTouch was tested and validated by neurosurgery residents on numerous occasions [13, 14, 27], all of which validated the use of VR simulators. At the 2006 annual meeting of the American Association of Neurological Surgeons (AANS), 78 neurosurgical fellows and residents were tested on ImmersiveTouch during the 3-day-long Top Gun competition. ImmersiveTouch was used to demonstrate VR simulation of ventriculostomy. Banerjee et al. [14] showed that the ImmersiveTouch system allowed for accurate catheter placement that is comparable to retrospective evaluation of freehand ventriculostomy catheter placement as measured by mean distance of catheter tip from the foramen of Monro.

Furthermore, VR simulators have been used for training of catheter placement in abnormal ventricle anatomy [27]. Yudkowsky et al. [27] demonstrated, via the use of multiple image libraries, that ImmersiveTouch was a beneficial system for ventriculostomy training. They tested neurosurgery residents' ability to successfully place a ventricular catheter into normal, shifted, and slit ventricles using image libraries derived from patient data. Residents were allowed to practice on the ImmersiveTouch system with each type of ventricle before being tested with novel image libraries. Yudkowsky et al. [27] demonstrate that not only did practice on the ImmersiveTouch improve the residents' ability to successfully place catheters on the simulation post-intervention but also that residents' live-procedure outcomes showed improvement in the rate of successful cannulation on first pass. Residents felt that ImmersiveTouch provided appropriate tactile feedback and that it was a realistic alternative to actual ventriculostomy procedures.

Spinal Applications

One area of neurosurgery in which VR simulation would greatly benefit is spinal procedures. These include, but are not limited to, vertebroplasty [28], pedicle screw placement during fusion surgery [29], and spinal cord stimulation [30]. Properly executed vertebroplasty requires the surgeon to rely on both sight and touch. The critical step in this procedure is the injection of polymethylmethacrylate (PMMA) into the vertebra. Incorrect injection or reflux of PMMA can have very harmful clinical consequences for the patient. Therefore, if a surgeon trains for this procedure using a VR simulator, surgical errors can be minimized. Chui et al. [28] developed the Immersion CyberGrasp – a VR system designed to simulate PMMA injections during surgery. Utilizing patient CT images and a specially designed glove, surgeons can simulate the injection technique with appropriate haptic feedback. The glove is designed to provide realistic variable resistance felt during needle injection. All these elements together provide a realistic VR simulation.

Discussed above for its applications in ventriculostomy, Luciano et al. [29] recently described the use of their ImmersiveTouch system for thoracic pedicle screw placement. The system allows the user to continuously monitor drill projection via anterior/posterior, transverse, and lateral fluoroscopic views (Figs. 28.7 and 28.8). For more advanced training, the user can also turn the different views off. Additionally, ImmersiveTouch provides haptic feedback and vibration feedback to represent the natural vibration of the drill with corresponding changes in vibration feedback depending on the speed of the drill. Furthermore, like the Top Gun competition held at the 2006 AANS annual meeting, another competition was held at the 2009 AANS annual meeting in which thoracic pedicle screw placement was one of the tasks that residents and fellows had to perform. Luciano et al. [29] described the results from the ImmersiveTouch system and showed that accuracy of thoracic pedicle screw placement using the ImmersiveTouch system correlated with actual placement via a retrospective evaluation of OR screw placements.

In addition to vertebroplasty and pedicle screw placement, there is a commercially available VR simulation system from SimSuite, called Neurostimulation Simulator [30], that is used for the simulation of spinal cord stimulator placement. This system offers many features that allow for the most realistic simulation setting as possible. Among other features, it includes the following: virtual fluoroscopy for 3D needle tracking, the ability to manipulate needle and lead wire, programmable complications including addition of scar tissue and gutter complication, and allows for suturing practice. Additionally, it provides haptic feedback for all procedure simulations and gives the user the ability to map the spinal cord to optimize pain management.

Endoscopy

Endoscope-based procedures are becoming more and more common as they provide significant advantages over more traditional procedures. A disadvantage to this approach, however, is that the surgeon has a limited surgical field and relies upon projected images to guide the surgery. Because of the restricted tactile feedback and limited motion of endoscopic instruments, VR simulation of these procedures is a fairly easy task and has proved to be a very popular application of simulated training. To date, most VR simulators, for both neurosurgical and non-neurosurgical applications, relate to some form of endoscopic surgery [31–35]. The most common application of such a system used for neurosurgery is simulation of endonasal transsphenoidal pituitary surgery [16, 31].

Despite the limited use of VR simulators for neurosurgical procedures, endoscope-based VR simulators have been used for numerous other applications mainly those involving a laparoscopic approach in urologic surgery [9], abdominal surgery [35], and laparoscopic suturing [36]. For example, McCaslin et al. [36] show that after training on a VR simulator, medical students not only become proficient at suturing but develop automaticity in the task defined by the ability to multitask (pressing a foot pedal after presentation of an image on a screen) while suturing. Additionally, these abilities transferred well to a live porcine model of laparoscopic suturing. Furthermore, Laguna et al. [9] demonstrated that VR training improved surgeons' ability to perform vesicourethral suturing, and Devarajan et al. [35] showed an improved ability to perform laparoscopic cholecystectomy. While none of these are neurosurgical procedures, the findings suggest that endoscope-based VR simulators do work to train novice surgeons indicating that these systems could be applied to neurosurgery residents and fellows.

Endovascular Simulation

Despite the success of open surgical procedures such as microsurgical aneurysm clipping and carotid endarterectomy,

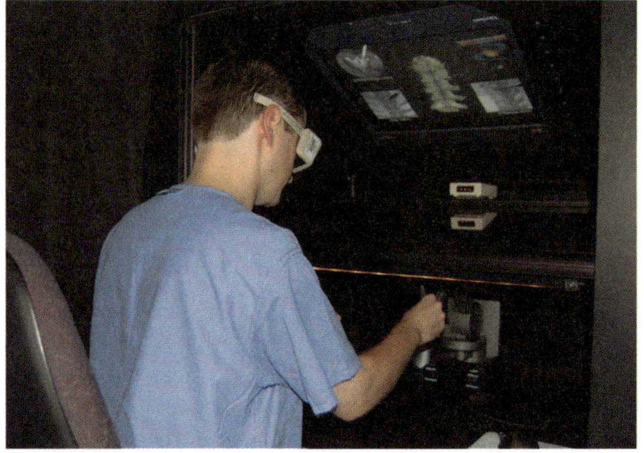

Fig. 28.7 A neurosurgical resident performing a virtual task of a pedicular screw instrumentation in a model of thoracic spine. A real-time virtual X-ray image of the spine is displayed on the screen while performing the procedure (Image courtesy of ImmersiveTouch)

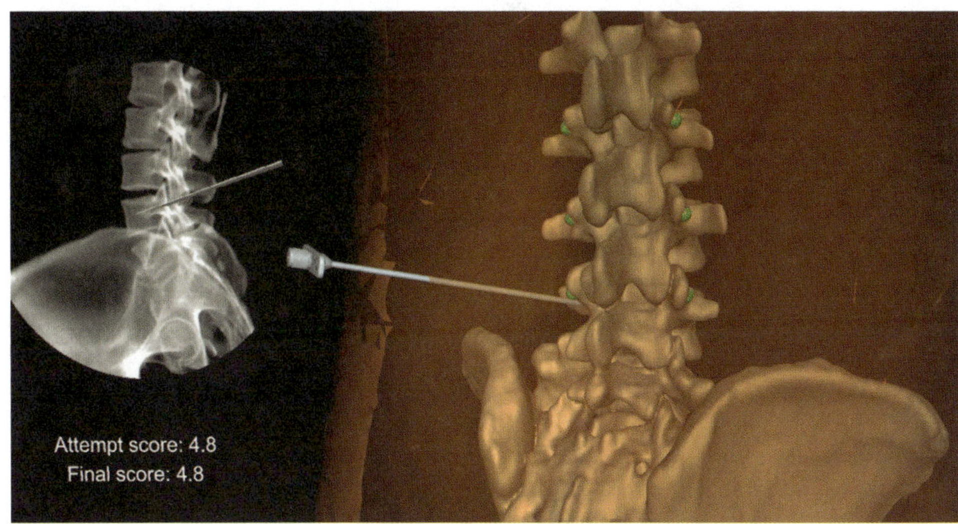

Fig. 28.8 A percutaneous model for lumbar vertebroplasty. The needle is advanced under fluoroscopic guidance through the pedicle into the vertebral body. A final score is given to the trainee at the end of the procedure (Image courtesy of ImmersiveTouch)

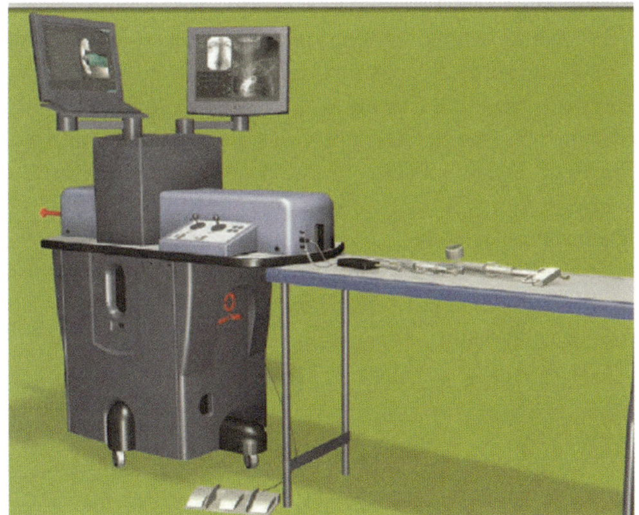

Fig. 28.9 The Simbionix endovascular simulator used for training for various neuro-endovascular techniques (Reprinted from Jason et al. [46]. With kind permission from Elsevier)

minimally invasive, endovascular procedures are becoming a preferred method of treatment because of the reduced risk for complications and the short amount of time they take to complete. However, the success of the operation is dependent upon the experience of the operator. Extensive training and practice is needed to ensure adequate expertise of the surgeon. As such, VR simulation is becoming a more utilized technique for training future interventionalists.

Currently, there are several commercially available endovascular simulators, all of which provide haptic, aural, and visual feedback. These include the ANGIO Mentor from Simbionix [37], the VIST training simulator from Mentice AB [38, 39], and the Simantha system from SimSuite [40]. Training on these devices includes cerebral angiography and stenting [37, 38], carotid artery angiography and stenting [39, 41–45], and endovascular aneurysm coiling [38, 40] (Fig. 28.9).

Several VR simulators are currently available that focus on training surgeons in carotid angiography and stenting. Mentice AB offers multiple VR simulator systems, most notably the VIST system. This system has the ability to run both a carotid intervention program [39] and a neuro-intervention program, discussed below [38]. The carotid intervention program allows for carotid angiography with subsequent carotid stenting. Certain cases even allow for the application of procedural complications. Based on the largest collection of data to date, Patel et al. [43] demonstrated that the VIST system from Mentice AB was able to improve surgeons' ability to perform these procedures and was also the first to establish the internal consistency of the VIST system and its test-retest reliability across several measured metrics. In addition to the Mentice AB systems, Simbionix developed the ANGIO Mentor system [37], which allows for VR training of both carotid applications and neurosurgical applications similar to those of the VIST system from Mentice AB. The ANGIO Mentor allows for training in carotid angiography and stenting as well intracranial aneurysm coiling and intracranial stenosis stenting.

Paramount to neurosurgeons is the endovascular simulation options for neurosurgical interventions. Generally, these should include cerebral angiography and stenting as well as cerebral aneurysm coiling. As mentioned above, Mentice AB developed a neuro-intervention program that can be run on the VIST system [38]. The program allows for simulation of cerebral angiography and stenting as well as intracranial aneurysm coiling. Additionally, SimSuite developed their Simantha system [40] to provide simulation training for endovascular procedures throughout the body. This system can be used for carotid procedures as well as neurosurgical procedures including angiography, stenting, and aneurysm coiling.

Craniotomy, Tumor Debulking, and Tumor Cauterization

The newest, and perhaps most comprehensive VR simulator to date, is the NeuroTouch system developed by Delorme et al. [5] in 2012. This system is designed to simulate craniotomy-based procedures and is currently limited to simulating two tasks: tumor debulking and tumor cauterization (Fig. 28.10). This system not only incorporates the most advanced 3D representations of anatomical imaging but also allows the use of multiple handheld instruments (surgical aspirator, CUSA, bipolar, and microscissors) and realistically simulates human tissues. Realistic tissues are displayed on all visible surfaces and are also displayed on new surfaces following tissue removal. Furthermore, vasculature is represented as distinct textures on the surface of the image and throughout the tissue volume, brain and tumor surface pulsate to represent basal heartbeat, and blood oozes a rate proportional to the size of the blood vessel supplying the surrounding tissue. In addition to deformable tissue, surgical drapes, skin, cranium, dura, and surgical hooks are all represented as rigid and fixed. Additionally, NeuroTouch approximates a true OR setting better than any other system now in use. All these components make the NeuroTouch simulation system the most realistic system available at this time.

There is currently no integrated program of virtual reality simulation into neurosurgical residency training. We are in the process of developing a virtual reality curriculum of different cranial and spinal modules. Those modules will include different procedures like ventriculostomy insertion, bone drilling, percutaneous vertebral vertebroplasty, and spinal instrumentation. Junior residents will be exposed to such modules before they start their hands-on surgical experience. Senior residents will use such modules to refine and improve on their surgical skills. Feedback from residents will be used to improve on those modules.

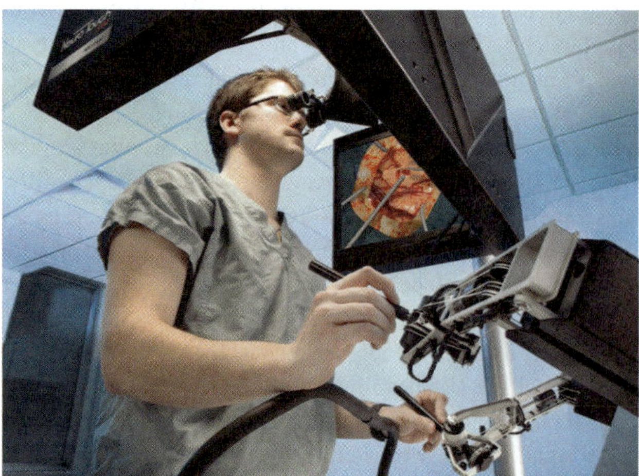

Fig. 28.10 The NeuroTouch Simulator; the trainee is using both hands to dissect a cortical brain tumor. The cranial opening, tumor removal, coagulation, and suction steps are all simulated (Reprinted from Delorme et al. [5]. With kind permission from Wolters Kluwer Health)

Conclusions

In the last 10 years, surgical training has been challenged by both legal and ethical concerns regarding patient safety, work hour restrictions, and the cost of operating room time. Organizations are requiring surgeons to maintain their skills and techniques in addition to learning new and more advanced ones to maintain technical competency. Furthermore, in a field such as neurosurgery where the majority of learning is done observing more senior surgeons, work hour restrictions make it increasingly difficult to learn and master all the necessary surgical techniques.

While all of the simulators discussed here provide a new approach to training residents, there still remains one important question: How does VR training translate to real life, surgical situations? The answer, not surprisingly, is that VR training has time and again proven to be an effective alternative to observational learning and, in some cases, has proven to be a more efficient educational system [14, 47–53]. Therefore, it would seem that VR simulation is the logical next step for properly educating neurosurgery residents and is an excellent platform from which established faculty can practice and maintain their skills.

References

1. Wurm G, Tomancok B, Pogady P, Holl K, Trenkler J. Cerebrovascular stereolithographic biomodeling for aneurysm surgery. Technical note. J Neurosurg. 2004;100(1):139–45.
2. Kimura T, Morita A, Nishimura K, et al. Simulation of and training for cerebral aneurysm clipping with 3-dimensional models. Neurosurgery. 2009;65(4):719–25; discussion 725–26.
3. Luciano C, Banerjee P, Lemole Jr GM, Charbel F. Second generation haptic ventriculostomy simulator using the ImmersiveTouch system. Stud Health Technol Inform. 2006;119:343–8.
4. Larsen O, Haase J, Hansen KV, Brix L, Pedersen CF. Training brain retraction in a virtual reality environment. Stud Health Technol Inform. 2003;94:174–80.
5. Delorme S, Laroche D, Diraddo R, Del Maestro R. NeuroTouch: a physics-based virtual simulator for cranial microneurosurgery training. Neurosurgery. 2012;71(1 Suppl Operative):32–42.
6. Wang P, Becker AA, Jones IA, et al. A virtual reality surgery simulation of cutting and retraction in neurosurgery with force-feedback. Comput Methods Programs Biomed. 2006;84(1):11–8.
7. Ferroli P, Tringali G, Acerbi F, Aquino D, Franzini A, Broggi G. Brain surgery in a stereoscopic virtual reality environment: a single institution's experience with 100 cases. Neurosurgery. 2010;67(3 Suppl Operative):ons79–84; discussion ons84.
8. Aggarwal R, Hance J, Darzi A. The development of a surgical education program. Cir Esp. 2005;77(1):1–2.
9. Laguna MP, de Reijke TM, Wijkstra H, de la Rosette J. Training in laparoscopic urology. Curr Opin Urol. 2006;16(2):65–70.
10. Lemole Jr GM, Banerjee PP, Luciano C, Neckrysh S, Charbel FT. Virtual reality in neurosurgical education: part-task ventriculostomy

simulation with dynamic visual and haptic feedback. Neurosurgery. 2007;61(1):142–8; discussion 148–9.
11. Brown N, Natsupakpong S, Johannsen S, et al. Virtual environment-based training simulator for endoscopic third ventriculostomy. Stud Health Technol Inform. 2006;119:73–5.
12. Çakmak H, Maaß H, Trantakis G, Strauß G, Nowatius E, Kühnapfel U. Haptic ventriculostomy simulation in a grid environment. Comp Anim Virtual Worlds. 2009;20:25–38.
13. Lemole M, Banerjee PP, Luciano C, et al. Virtual ventriculostomy with 'shifted ventricle': neurosurgery resident surgical skill assessment using a high-fidelity haptic/graphic virtual reality simulator Haptic ventriculostomy simulation in a grid environment. Neurol Res. 2009;31(4):430–1.
14. Banerjee PP, Luciano CJ, Lemole Jr GM, Charbel FT, Oh MY. Accuracy of ventriculostomy catheter placement using a head- and hand-tracked high-resolution virtual reality simulator with haptic feedback. J Neurosurg. 2007;107(3):515–21.
15. Kockro RA, Hwang PY. Virtual temporal bone: an interactive 3-dimensional learning aid for cranial base surgery. Neurosurgery. 2009;64(5 Suppl 2):216–29; discussion 229–30.
16. Wolfsberger S, Neubauer A, Buhler K, et al. Advanced virtual endoscopy for endoscopic transsphenoidal pituitary surgery. Neurosurgery. 2006;59(5):1001–9; discussion 1009–10.
17. Hinckley K, Pausch R, Downs JH, et al. The props-based interface for neurosurgical visualization two-handed spatial interface tools for neurosurgical planning. Stud Health Technol Inform. 1997;39(7):552–62.
18. Goble J, Hinckley K, Snell J, Pausch R, Kassell N. Two-handed spatial interface tools for neurosurgical planning. IEEE Comput. 1995;28:20–6.
19. Stoakley R, Conway M, Pausch R, Hinckley K, Kassell N. Virtual reality on a WIM: interactive worlds in miniature. Paper presented at: CHI'95, Denver; 1995.
20. Integra. For the neurosurgeon. http://www.integralife.com/Neurosurgeon/Neurosurgeon-Product-List.aspx?ProductLine=8&ProductLineName=Stereotaxy. Accessed 17 Mar 2012.
21. Adams CM, Wilson TD. Virtual cerebral ventricular system: an MR-based three-dimensional computer model. Anat Sci Educ. 2011;4(6):340–7.
22. Poston T. The Virtual Workbench: Dextrous VR. Paper presented at: ACM VRST'94 – Reality Software and Technology, Singapore; 1994.
23. Bracco. Dextroscope – 3D interactivity. http://dextroscope.com/interactivity.html. Accessed 17 Mar 2012.
24. Kockro RA, Stadie A, Schwandt E, et al. A collaborative virtual reality environment for neurosurgical planning and training. Neurosurgery. 2007;61(5 Suppl 2):379–91; discussion 391.
25. Kockro RA, Serra L, Tseng-Tsai Y, et al. Planning and simulation of neurosurgery in a virtual reality environment. Neurosurgery. 2000;46(1):118–35; discussion 135–7.
26. Stadie AT, Kockro RA, Reisch R, et al. Virtual reality system for planning minimally invasive neurosurgery. Technical note. J Neurosurg. 2008;108(2):382–94.
27. Yudkowsky R, Luciano CJ, Banerjee PP, et al. Ventriculostomy practice on a library of virtual brains using a VR/haptic simulator improves simulator and surgical outcomes. Paper presented at: 12th annual international meeting on simulation in healthcare (IMSH), San Diego; 2012.
28. Chui CK, Teo J, Wang Z, et al. Integrative haptic and visual interaction for simulation of PMMA injection during vertebroplasty. Stud Health Technol Inform. 2006;119:96–8.
29. Luciano CJ, Banerjee PP, Bellotte B, et al. Learning retention of thoracic pedicle screw placement using a high-resolution augmented reality simulator with haptic feedback. Neurosurgery. 2011;69(1 Suppl Operative):ons14–9; discussion ons19.
30. SimSuite. NEUROSTIMULATION. http://www.medsimulation.com/NeurostimulationSimulator.asp. Accessed 31 Mar 2012.
31. Schulze F, Buhler K, Neubauer A, Kanitsar A, Holton L, Wolfsberger S. Intra-operative virtual endoscopy for image guided endonasal transsphenoidal pituitary surgery. Int J Comput Assist Radiol Surg. 2010;5(2):143–54.
32. Burtscher J, Dessl A, Maurer H, Seiwald M, Felber S. Virtual neuroendoscopy, a comparative magnetic resonance and anatomical study. Minim Invasive Neurosurg. 1999;42(3):113–7.
33. Buxton N, Cartmill M. Neuroendoscopy combined with frameless neuronavigation. Br J Neurosurg. 2000;14(6):600–1.
34. Dumay AC, Jense GJ, Poston T, et al. Endoscopic surgery simulation in a virtual environment the Virtual Workbench: Dextrous VR virtual reality on a WIM: interactive worlds in miniature. Comput Biol Med. 1995;25(2):139–48.
35. Devarajan V, Scott D, Jones D, et al. Bimanual haptic workstation for laparoscopic surgery simulation. Stud Health Technol Inform. 2001;81:126–8.
36. McCaslin AF, Aoun SG, Batjer HH, Bendok BR. Enhancing the utility of surgical simulation: from proficiency to automaticity. World Neurosurg. 2011;76(6):482–4.
37. Simbionix. ANGIO mentor. http://simbionix.com/simulators/angio-mentor/library-of-modules/cerebral-intervention-module/. Accessed 31 Mar 2012.
38. Mentice. Neuro intervention. http://www.mentice.com/default.asp?viewset=1&on='Procedures'&id=&initid=98&heading=Procedures&mainpage=templates/05.asp?sida=84. Accessed 31 Mar 2012.
39. Mentice. Carotid intervention. http://www.mentice.com/default.asp?viewset=1&on='Procedures'&id=&initid=98&heading=Procedures&mainpage=templates/05.asp?sida=84. Accessed 31 Mar 2012.
40. SimSuite. SIMANTHA. http://www.medsimulation.com/Simantha.asp. Accessed 31 Mar 2012.
41. Tsang JS, Naughton PA, Leong S, Hill AD, Kelly CJ, Leahy AL. Virtual reality simulation in endovascular surgical training. Surgeon. 2008;6(4):214–20.
42. Van Herzeele I, Aggarwal R, Choong A, Brightwell R, Vermassen FE, Cheshire NJ. Virtual reality simulation objectively differentiates level of carotid stent experience in experienced interventionalists. J Vasc Surg. 2007;46(5):855–63.
43. Patel AD, Gallagher AG, Nicholson WJ, Cates CU. Learning curves and reliability measures for virtual reality simulation in the performance assessment of carotid angiography. J Am Coll Cardiol. 2006;47(9):1796–802.
44. Dayal R, Faries PL, Lin SC, et al. Computer simulation as a component of catheter-based training. J Vasc Surg. 2004;40(6):1112–7.
45. Dawson DL. Training in carotid artery stenting: do carotid simulation systems really help? Vascular. 2006;14(5):256–63.
46. Jason T et al. The utility of endovascular simulation to improve technical performance and stimulate continued interest of preclinical medical students in vascular surgery. J Surg Educ. 2009;66(6):367–73.
47. Aggarwal R, Black SA, Hance JR, Darzi A, Cheshire NJ. Virtual reality simulation training can improve inexperienced surgeons' endovascular skills. Eur J Vasc Endovasc Surg. 2006;31(6):588–93.
48. Chaer RA, Derubertis BG, Lin SC, et al. Simulation improves resident performance in catheter-based intervention: results of a randomized, controlled study. Ann Surg. 2006;244(3):343–52.
49. Aggarwal R, Ward J, Balasundaram I, Sains P, Athanasiou T, Darzi A. Proving the effectiveness of virtual reality simulation for training in laparoscopic surgery. Ann Surg. 2007;246(5):771–9.
50. Gurusamy K, Aggarwal R, Palanivelu L, Davidson BR. Systematic review of randomized controlled trials on the effectiveness of virtual reality training for laparoscopic surgery. Br J Surg. 2008;95(9):1088–97.
51. Jakimowicz JJ, Cuschieri A. Time for evidence-based minimal access surgery training – simulate or sink. Surg Endosc. 2005;19(12):1521–2.
52. Thijssen AS, Schijven MP. Contemporary virtual reality laparoscopy simulators: quicksand or solid grounds for assessing surgical trainees? Am J Surg. 2010;199(4):529–41.
53. Dawson DL, Meyer J, Lee ES, Pevec WC. Training with simulation improves residents' endovascular procedure skills. J Vasc Surg. 2007;45(1):149–54.

Simulation in Nursing

29

Kim Leighton

Introduction

High-fidelity patient simulation is utilized in a variety of ways in the nursing profession. Students at all levels and in all types of educational programs are being exposed to simulated clinical experiences (SCE) as they learn patient care and management. While simulation was slow to enter nursing education, beginning late in the 1990s, simulation use took even longer to reach the nurses already practicing in healthcare environments. Growth has steadily increased, though many nurses and nursing students still lack exposure to this valuable teaching strategy.

As with most technological advances, the cost of patient simulators has decreased over the past decade. The first simulators were expensive, with some being over $200,000, making their purchase unattainable for most nursing schools. Initial use of patient simulators, in the late 1990s and early 2000s, for nursing education occurred as the result of grant programs and visionary leaders. Few other colleges had the vision or the money at that time.

Many nursing educators were hesitant to move forward with adopting simulation technology not only because of the cost but also because of the perception of technological expertise required to manage the equipment. Early simulators were created with physiological modeling that required changes to the software in order to achieve accurate physiological responses. Later models featured programmable vital signs but lacked physiological accuracy. Today's models have features of both, potentially diminishing the need for extensive facilitator expertise in managing computer programming (Figs. 29.1a, b and 29.2).

Hospitals are now using patient simulation more frequently with practicing nurses, likely as a result of publications such as the Institute of Medicine's report [1], *To Err is Human*, followed in 2003 by *Keeping Patients Safe* [2]. In addition, focus on safe patient care through programs such as TeamSTEPPS [3] and Quality and Safety Education for Nurses (QSEN) [4] furthers the demand for training programs using high-fidelity patient simulation.

This chapter will focus on the benefits and challenges of using high-fidelity patient simulation to educate students and staff, assess competency, develop teamwork, enhance communication, and affect patient care outcomes. Examples of how simulation is used to facilitate learning at a variety of levels will be offered. Immediate research needs and opportunities will be discussed as nurses continue to work toward integration of best practices into their work using patient simulation.

Overview of Nursing Education

While some countries have a standardized curriculum in their nursing colleges (e.g., Canada), the USA has a variety of methods for nurses to obtain their education. Prelicensure nursing programs last 2, 3, or 4 years; however, all graduates take the same licensing exam (NCLEX-RN). Curricula are approved by each individual State Board of Nursing (SBON) and no two schools are required to have the same topic order, the same amount of time dedicated to each topic, the same number of clinical and observational hours, nor the same number of hours in the laboratory environment. In addition, each SBON determines how many hours of clinical time can be completed utilizing patient simulation. The percentage currently ranges from 0 to 50%. This has resulted in confusion among the nursing programs as to how simulation can best be used to facilitate learning. It also sets the scene for nursing students to receive inequitable education.

Countries with standardized curricula do not have the problems identified in the USA; however, there are numerous other concerns that are shared by programs worldwide, including access to clinical sites and patients, ability to

K. Leighton, PhD, RN, CNE
DeVry University,
Simulation Center of Excellence,
3005 Highland Parkway, Downers Grove, IL 60515-5683, USA
e-mail: kleighton@devry.com

A.I. Levine et al. (eds.), *The Comprehensive Textbook of Healthcare Simulation*,
DOI 10.1007/978-1-4614-5993-4_29, © Springer Science+Business Media New York 2013

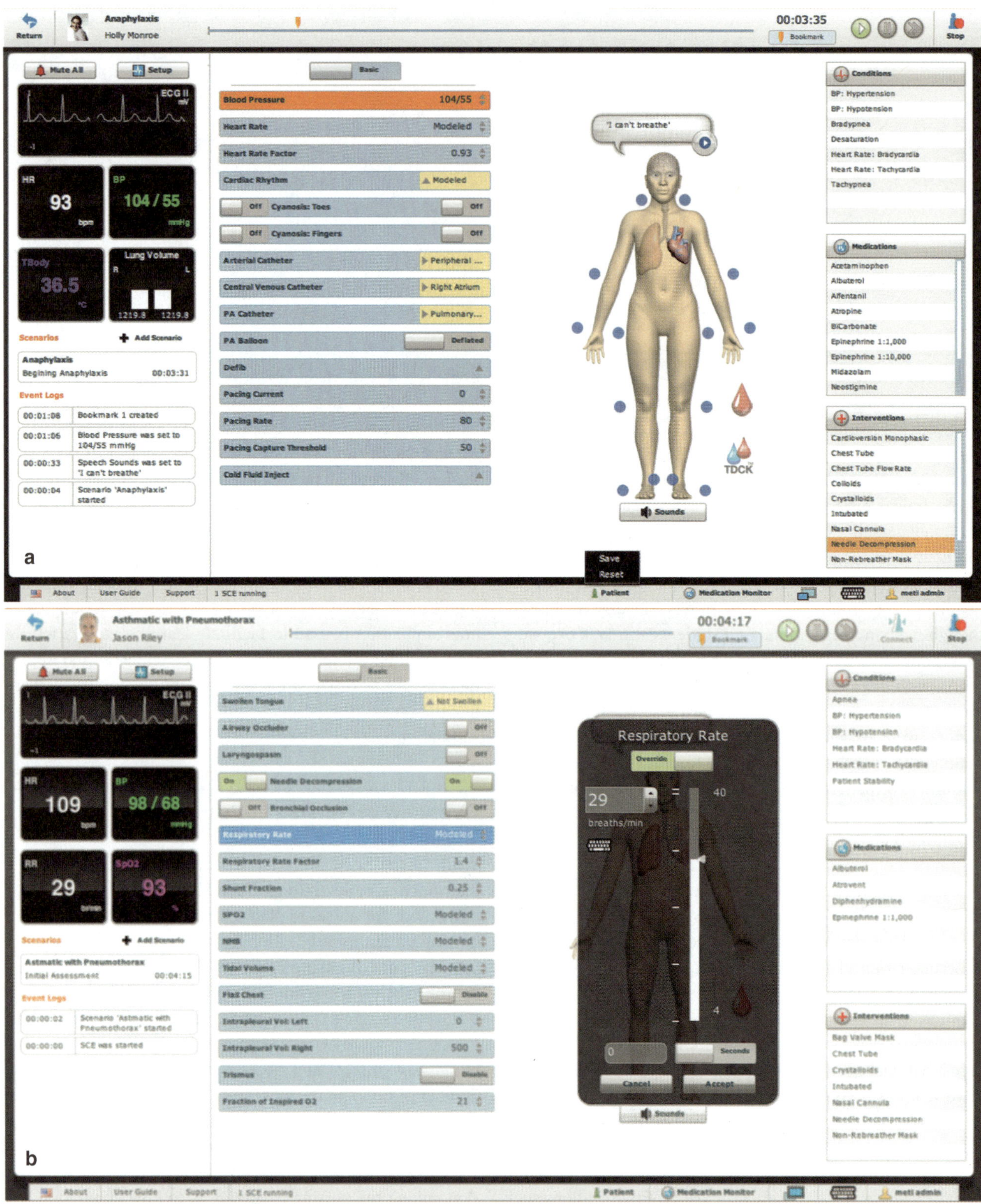

Fig. 29.1 (**a**) CAE Muse software screenshot of main screen interface and (**b**) CAE Muse software screenshot showing respiratory rate adjustment (Photos courtesy of CAE Healthcare ©2012 CAE Healthcare)

perform certain procedures or provide specific cares, nurse, and faculty shortages, and the complexity of today's patients, to name but a few.

Acute care clinical sites are available at a finite number in most communities, with relatively few new hospitals built each year. Nursing programs have been pushed to increase

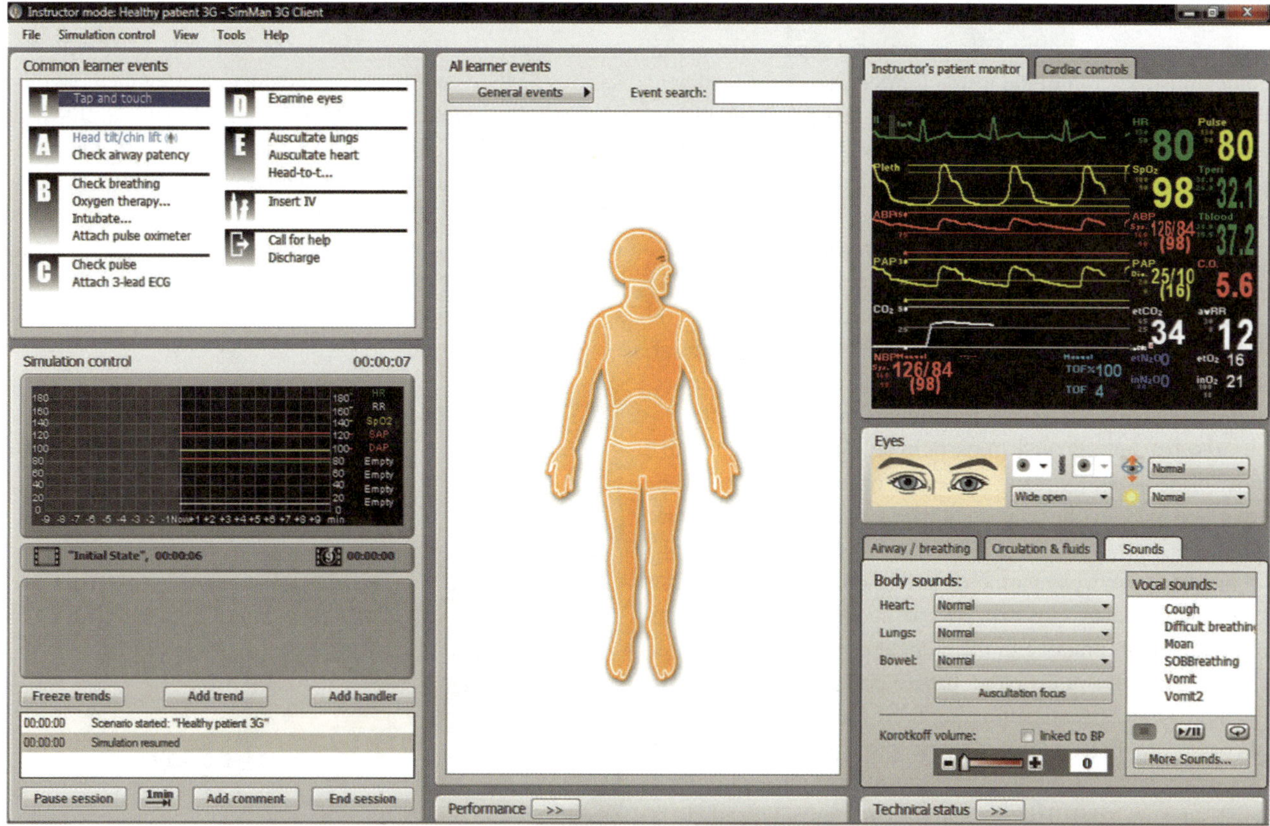

Fig. 29.2 Laerdal 3G screenshot of main screen interface (Photo courtesy of Laerdal Medical. All rights reserved)

enrollments to assuage the nursing shortage; however, clinical sites typically limit the number of students that can be on each unit at any given time. Novice students tend to be assigned clinical hours in the mornings when the majority of care and physician interactions occur. As they progress along the novice to expert continuum [5] and incorporate past experiences into their decision-making, they become more flexible in their thinking and ability to perform skills, allowing the students to be assigned to evening hours and creating additional clinical opportunities. Many programs use preceptors who are hospital staff to guide more advanced students so that faculty do not need to be present. The use of preceptors and of observational experiences is important due to the current nursing faculty shortage, which is concurrent to the overall nursing shortage.

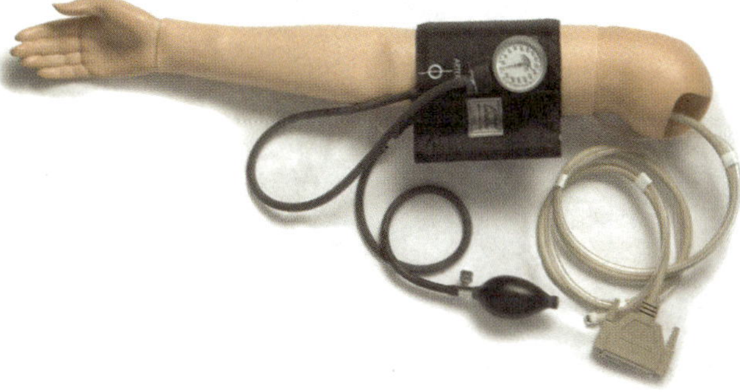

Fig. 29.3 Laerdal noninvasive blood pressure part-task trainer (Photo courtesy of Laerdal Medical. All rights reserved)

Nursing Students

Students in many programs visit their patient the day before providing their care so that they can review the chart; talk with the physician, nurses, family, and patient; and learn what medications and treatments they will need to understand in order to provide safe care. Unfortunately, it is not uncommon for that same patient to be discharged before the student returns to provide their care. For the advanced student, it may not be difficult to reassign them a new patient with a similar condition, for example, a patient who had abdominal surgery but for a different reason. It is not that easy for the novice student who is very focused on the specifics of providing care and is unable to generalize that care to patients with similar problems.

Nursing students learn psychomotor skills either at the beginning of their program of study or at intervals throughout their program (Figs. 29.3 and 29.4). Once competency is assessed in the skills laboratory, the student is typically allowed to perform those skills under direct supervision of the clinical instructor until the instructor deems them safe to perform on their own. Sadly, it is not uncommon for students to reach the point of graduation without ever having performed some skills, such as urinary catheter insertion or nasogastric tube insertion, on a live patient.

Students are also required to have cardiopulmonary resuscitation (CPR) certification before clinically caring for patients (Fig. 29.5); however, when a crisis does arise, students are often asked to leave the patient room to allow for the response team to enter or, due to fear or anxiety, remove themselves from the situation. Students may be permitted to observe but not allowed to participate. Therefore, even the most basic of skills may not be performed in school. This creates a gap in the expectations of those who hire new graduates.

In addition to psychomotor skills, there are procedures that new graduates are expected to know, but that they are often unable to practice in the clinical environment while in school. Many hospitals either have electronic health records (EHR) or are currently initiating their use. Due to the complexity of the EHR and staff's perception of the difficulty of use, many hospitals no longer allow student nurses to document care on the EHR. When students are allowed, it is difficult to orient them to the EHRs, as they are often different at every institution. The same concerns exist with the various methods of obtaining and documenting medications, particularly narcotics and other scheduled medications. Due to the perceived complexity of the variety of systems utilized, students are often not allowed to give medications, or if they do, their instructor is expected to sign for them (Fig. 29.6), which breaks the medication rules in place to prevent error and ensure documentation by the correct person. In addition to procedural restrictions, students have also

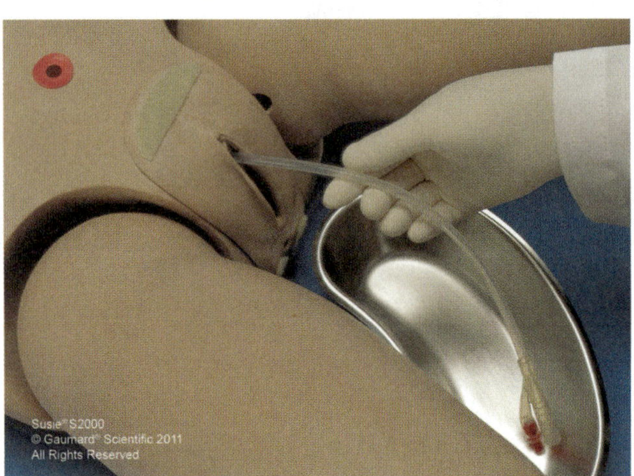

Fig. 29.4 Use of Gaumard Suse S2000 urinary catheterization part-task trainer (Photo courtesy of Gaumard® Scientific 2012. All rights reserved)

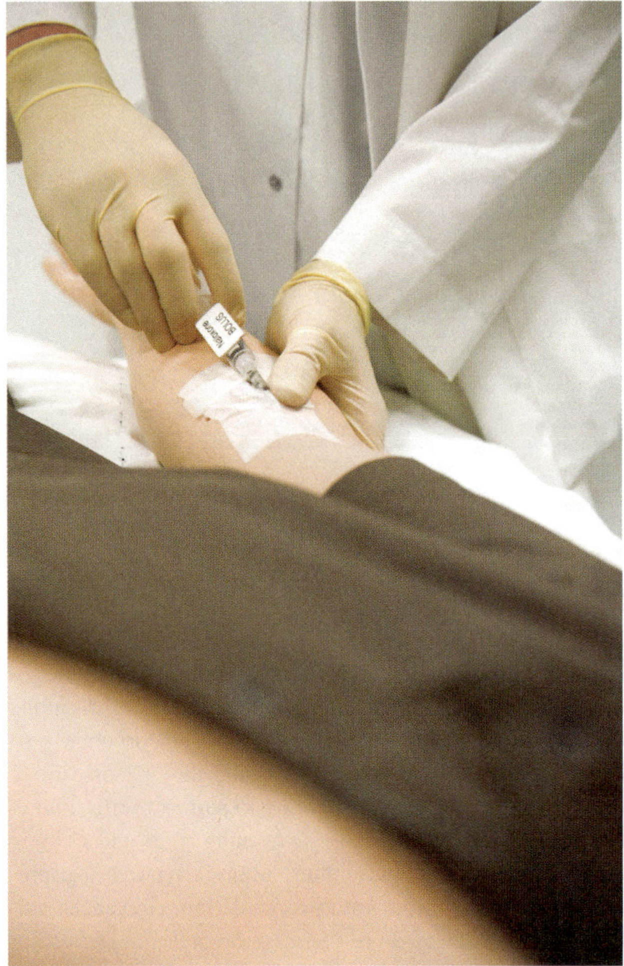

Fig. 29.6 IV drug administration through a drug recognition system (Laerdal SimMan) (Photo courtesy of Laerdal Medical. All rights reserved)

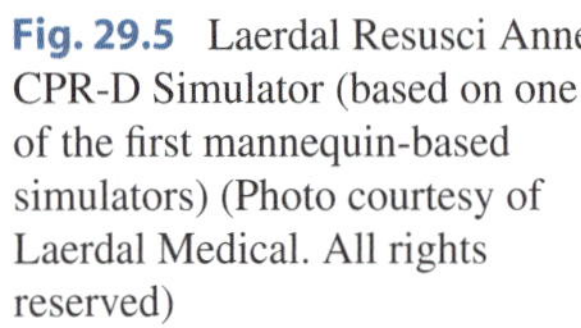

Fig. 29.5 Laerdal Resusci Anne CPR-D Simulator (based on one of the first mannequin-based simulators) (Photo courtesy of Laerdal Medical. All rights reserved)

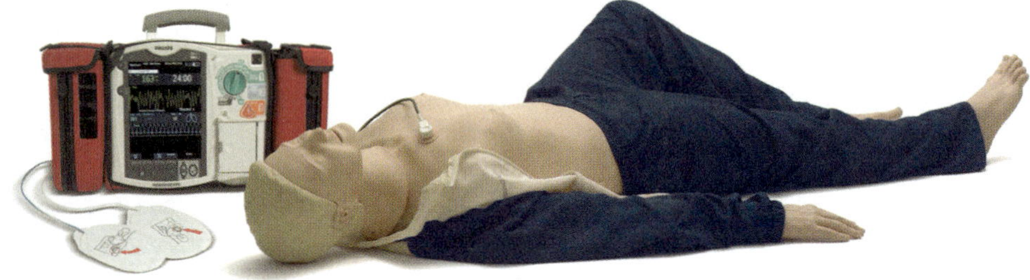

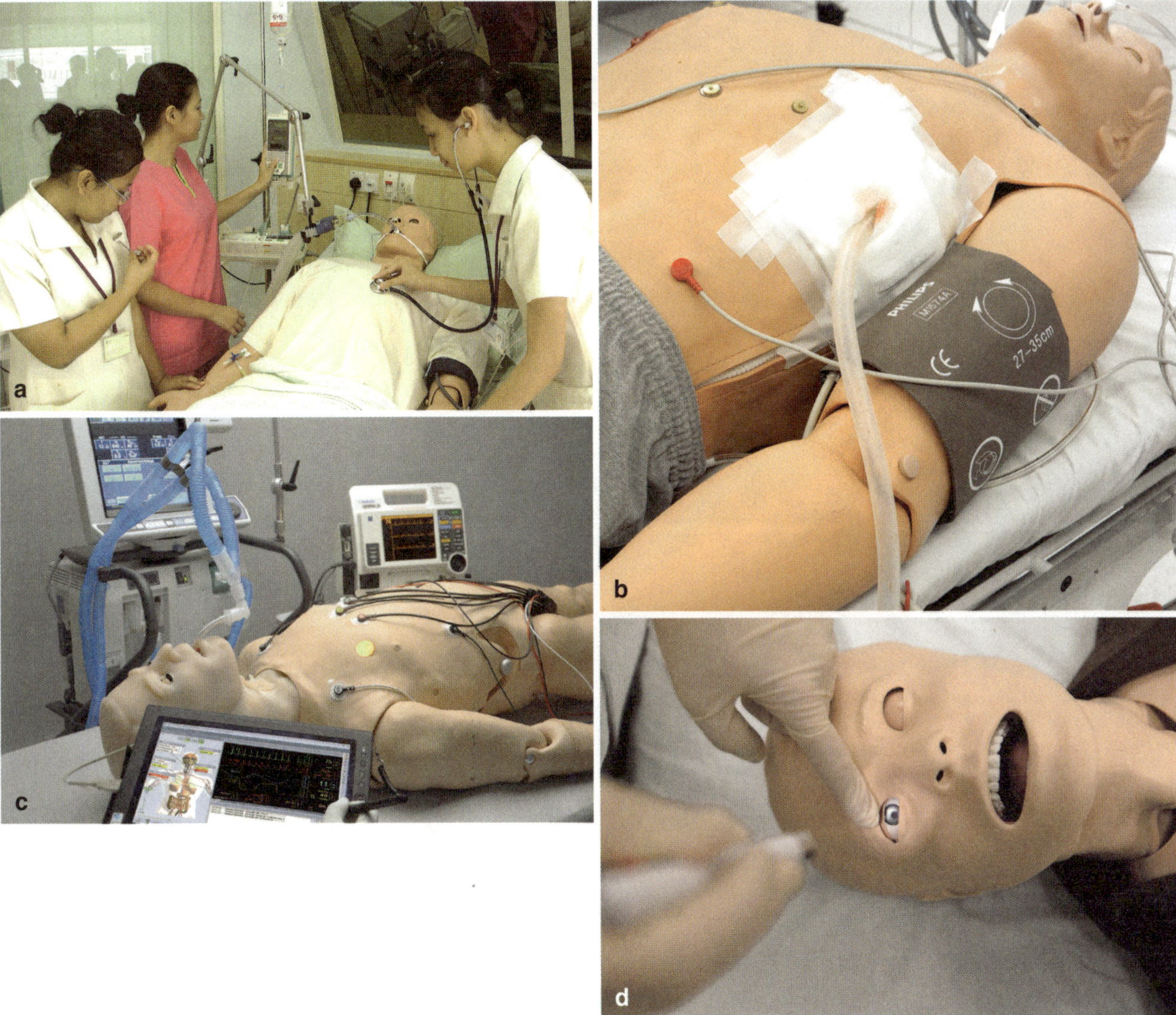

Fig. 29.7 (**a**) Nursing students practicing bedside ICU care using CAE METI HPS (Photo courtesy of CAE Healthcare ©2012 CAE Healthcare). (**b**) Chest tube management using the HPS (Photo courtesy of CAE Healthcare ©2012 CAE Healthcare). (**c**) Ventilator care using a Gaumard mannequin (Photo courtesy of Gaumard® Scientific 2012. All rights reserved). (**d**) Use of Sim Man 3G to teach neurologic assessment (Photo courtesy of Laerdal Medical. All rights reserved)

been restricted, in some hospitals, for caring for certain patients such as pediatric and critical care patients. Other schools must send students to facilities over 100 miles away to get these specialized experiences.

The complexity of today's acute and chronically ill patients is astounding compared to years past (Fig. 29.7a–d). Advances in technology, medications, and treatments have been shown to keep people alive longer and with more serious illnesses and disease processes. Often, the patients who are available to be assigned to students are just too ill for those students' level of care provision and capability. The student may need to understand advanced pathophysiology and pharmacology that they have yet to learn. The basic foundations may not have been laid for the student to understand the rationales for the care they are expected to give. This has the potential to result in an unsafe situation for the patient and requires diligence by the faculty and staff nurse assigned to the patient.

These situations help to explain why faculty and employers are concerned about the "gap" in expectations. Faculty have reported that graduates are ready to begin practice at a generalist level, but the employers of those graduates report that their new hires are not ready to care for patients [6]. Various preceptor or internship programs have been put in place, but it is not enough and educators and employers continue to work together to close this gap.

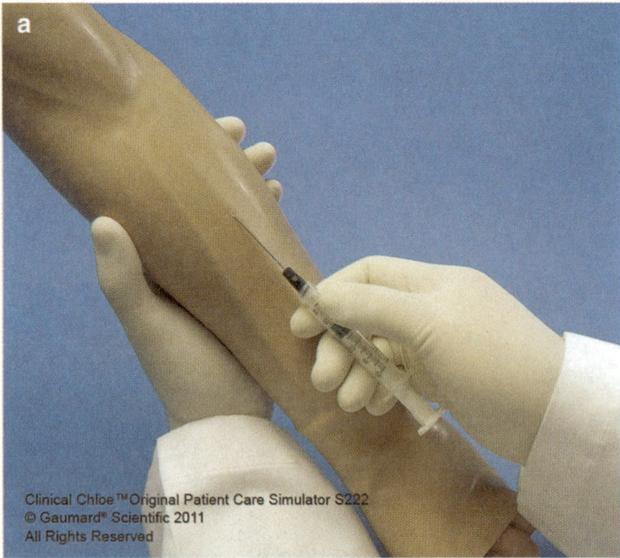

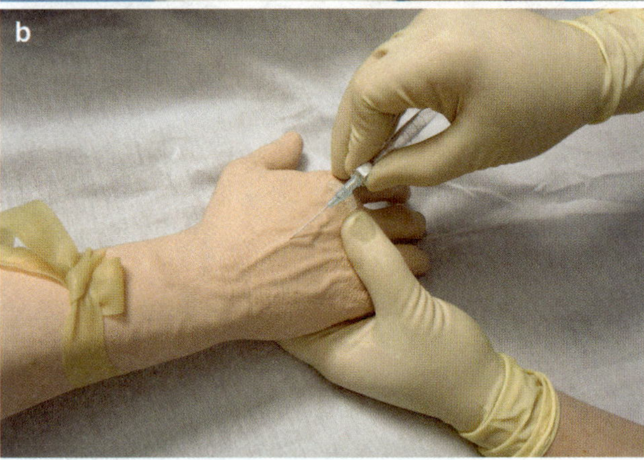

Fig. 29.8 (**a**) Gaumard IV training arm of Chloe™ Original Patient Care Simulator (Photo courtesy of Gaumard® Scientific 2012. All rights reserved) and (**b**) Laerdal IV training arm (Photo courtesy of Laerdal Medical. All rights reserved)

Practicing Nurses

Practicing nurses have many problems similar to the student nurses. Hospitals with IV teams have a core set of nurses who become masters at initiating IV therapy, but this may result in the remainder of the nurses losing that skill (Fig. 29.8a–b).

Similar results can happen when code teams manage all crises, as it is often heard and observed that the floor nurses "didn't know what to do before the team arrived" [7]. Nurses need to be able to quickly identify deterioration in the high-risk, low-volume patient, but without repetition, the ability to recognize problems diminishes [8] and it becomes less likely that the patient's problem will be caught in time.

The limitations identified in both the educational and practice environments make it clear that the use of patient simulation to educate students and nurses is one way to overcome these major issues and concerns.

Facilitating Learning with Simulation

The previous discussion lends insight into the challenges of nursing education and the difficulties to assure adequate preparation and repetition before actual clinical encounters. Repetition is critical and hones one's ability to recognize and mange clinical situations faster [9]. These conditions can be recreated in the simulated environment and can provide repetition and the opportunity for additional patient management experiences. Here we will review the simulation technologies and the application for nursing education.

There are several types of simulation that are used in nursing education to help students understand how to care for patients that they may, or may not, encounter in the traditional clinical environment. These types of simulation range from low fidelity to high fidelity, dependent upon the type of equipment used and the way it is used by the facilitator. The higher the fidelity, the more realistic the simulation encounter.

Screen-Based Simulation

Web-Based Simulators

Second Life® (SL) is an interactive virtual web-based environment (Chap. 14) that uses avatar technology to portray patients and colleagues. This virtual environment has been used for almost a decade to teach college courses in areas as diverse as art to architecture. Medical conferences have been held in this realm as well [10]. However, comparatively little has been accomplished using this environment to teach nursing students or practicing nurses. Primary uses for SL include role-playing, collaboration, real-time interaction between students and faculty, and alternative environment for simulations [11]. Aebersold et al. [10] suggest that the virtual world of SL is an excellent environment in which to explore dangerous scenarios or those that may be difficult to simulate realistically. One drawback mentioned was the low fidelity and resolution of graphics in SL. The use of SL by a college also requires purchase of an "island" or parcel of land that can be password protected, so only students of a particular course or program could have access to specific areas. Within SL, objects such as furniture, books, and buildings need to be created by the user, requiring time to learn and develop. In Rogers' [12] study of undergraduate nursing students learning in SL for the first time, he reported that participants were comfortable in the virtual environment, had little difficulty navigating the environment, and used trial and error methods when necessary.

Computer-Based Simulators

Another type of simulation used in nursing education is computer-based simulation. These simulations are conducted

Table 29.1 Methods to promote the holistic care of the simulated patient

Domain	Props	Patient situation	Learner response
Psychosocial	"Mother" at bedside	50-year-old man with ulcerative colitis; mother makes all decisions and answers all questions	Does the learner recognize the relationship as dysfunctional? Does the learner attempt to include the patient in all decision-making?
Spiritual	Religious icon or book at bedside	75-year-old female who has received a poor prognosis	Does the learner recognize the need to ask if spiritual advisor (minister, etc.) should be contacted?
Sociocultural	Purse on bedside stand	20-year-old female who is being discharged with several prescriptions	Does the learner consider the financial impact of the prescriptions and seek to understand if the patient can afford to fill them?
Developmental	Place a picture frame at the bedside of a young family with three to four children	45-year-old construction worker who experienced a myocardial infarction	Does the learner realize that the patient will likely not be able to return to his job? Do they understand the financial implications?
	Young mother	14-year-old female who just delivered a normal newborn	Do learners judge the patient?

through interactive multimedia programs that can be accessed on a computer. There is typically audio and video, graphics, and teaching questions and prompts. A scenario occurs in real time, and the learner is expected to manage the patient by using nursing judgment or interventions. Feedback is provided through the program if an incorrect decision is made [13]. Bonnetain et al. [13] studied the impact of learning with computer-based simulation on medical students and found that this was a good adjunct for mannequin simulation. Strengths of this type of simulation are that the programs tend to be easy to access and can be accessed as often as desired, increase knowledge and facilitate critical thinking, pace is set by learner, and low cost. Weaknesses are lack of physical interaction, less realistic, and it is not experiential learning [14].

Standardized Patients (SP)

Standardized patients (SP) (see Chap. 13) are actors trained to consistently portray a patient with a specific condition or concern when interacting with healthcare students [15]. These actors have been used since 1963, with varying degrees of acceptance. Considered high fidelity, SPs are now commonly used in medical and nursing schools, particularly during objective structured clinical examination (OSCE). The use of the SP helps to maintain consistency in each student's exam; however, there continue to be questions regarding reliability, validity, objectivity, and feasibility of this method of testing [16]. Lack of evidence has led some to challenge whether the use of the OSCE with SP is better than other methods of assessment, particularly because it is expensive and requires significant resources. Standardized patients must be recruited, trained, evaluated, and paid for their service. These costs can be substantial.

Although these examples of simulated learning methodologies are used to varying degrees in programs throughout the world, little research has been conducted to determine their impact on learning and whether there is demonstrated transference to the actual clinical practice.

Mannequin-Based Simulation

Benefits of Learning with High-Fidelity Patient Simulation

Mannequin-based (Chap. 15) SCEs are created in a manner that allows for impact on the psychomotor, cognitive, and affective domains. Psychomotor skills can be readily assessed during care of the simulated patient. As learners work together in small teams, they typically talk about how to manage the patient's care and often make decisions with input from the team. As a result of their discussions, the facilitator can observe their communication and problem-solving abilities. The cognitive skills, such as attention, memory, logic, and reasoning, can be observed and evaluated. The affective domain, one that is hard to impact by traditional teaching methods such as lecture, can be impacted by how the SCE is developed.

Creating situations that challenge the values, motivation, and attitudes of the learner will impact the affective domain. In simulation, facilitators can create challenges in the psychosocial, spiritual, sociocultural, and developmental domains of holistic patient care. These challenges are easily created and inexpensive to implement. It is important for nurses to understand that patient care is about more than the physiological care of the patient. Ways to promote holistic patient care are outlined in Table 29.1.

Facilitators can create experiences in which the learners care for patients that are not readily available to them in the traditional clinical site or are considered "low-volume, high-risk" patients. These types of patients will vary from facility to facility, but can be determined through consultation with

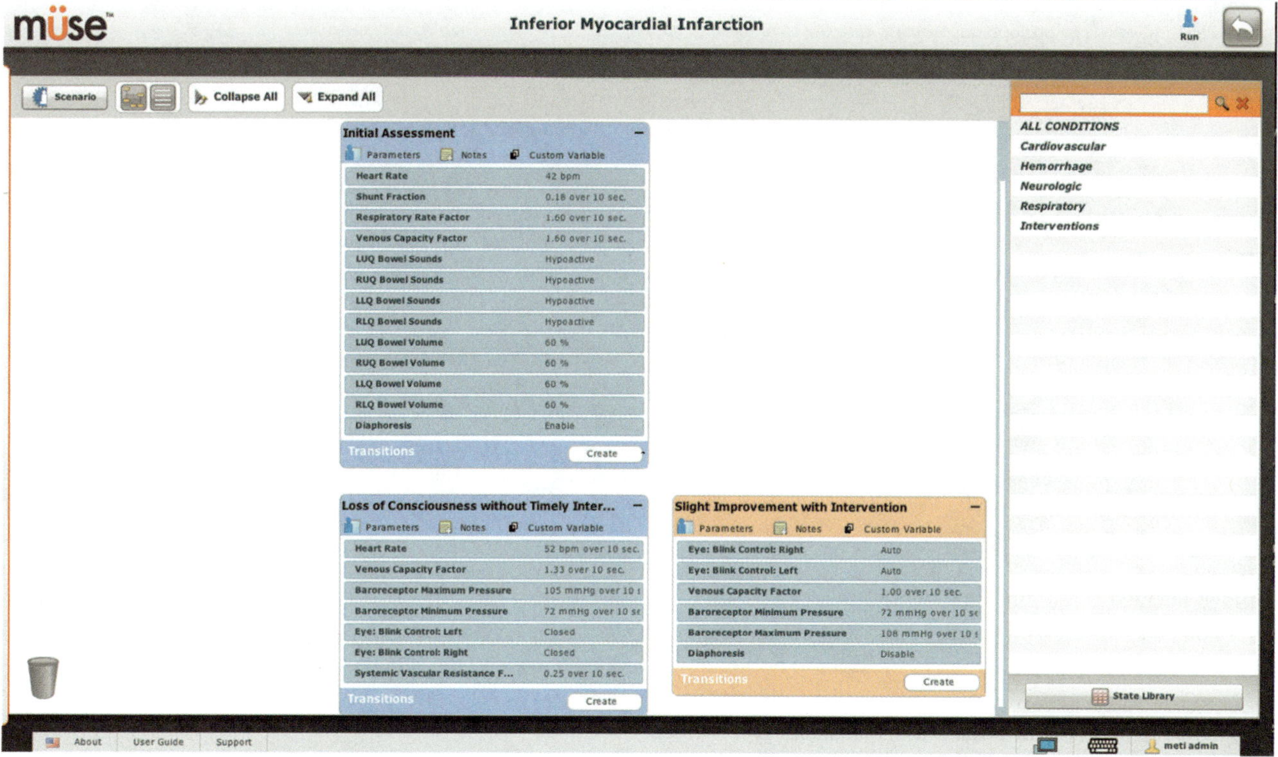

Fig. 29.9 Screenshot of preprogrammed scenario using CAE Muse interface (Photo courtesy of CAE Healthcare ©2012 CAE Healthcare)

the quality management department. Simulated patients can also be created to ensure that learners care for the most common types of patients they will care for. Data to determine this type of patient can be obtained from the clinical facility. Using information gleaned from The Joint Commission and other resources, facilitators can create simulated clinical experiences that address common errors identified through the root cause analysis procedure.

Another benefit of learning with patient simulation is that the learner, no matter the experience as a student or practitioner, is the nurse who can make decisions without having to seek input from the faculty or charge nurse. This allows the critical thinking process to play out so that learners can use their clinical judgment to provide care based on their own knowledge and understanding of the condition being simulated. Care decisions can be allowed to play out, whether right or wrong, so that learners can see the impact of their decisions on their patient's outcomes. The debriefing process helps the learner to better understand the decisions they made and the resulting outcomes.

During the SCE, learners have the opportunity to work in small teams while collaborating with their peers. Simulations for nurses and nursing students occur over varying lengths of time, typically from 20 min to 2 h. During this time, the learners practice organizational and prioritization skills while caring for the patient. This is done in a "safe" environment; however, many experts question the use of the term safe. While no harm comes to real patients and the simulation environment is considered a confidential space in which to learn, the learner must still perform in front of others and face the results of incorrect decisions. Additionally, if the learners are being evaluated, the safe environment ceases to exist for them. Caution should be used when describing the simulation environment as safe to ensure that learners understand this correctly.

Another benefit of the simulated environment is the ability to learn about ancillary devices that are necessary for safe patient care. An example of this is the electronic health record (EHR). There are several EHR products that have been designed specifically for use with simulation. As with hospital documentation systems, the products have different features. It has become increasingly important for faculty to ensure that they teach the principles of electronic documentation of patient care, which is the same as paper documentation. The specifics of a documentation platform will be learned during job orientation. This underscores the need for EHR use when caring for simulated patients. Practice implementing accurate, timely, and organized patient health information will help the student learn how to document, especially when opportunities in the traditional clinical environment are becoming limited.

Lastly, a benefit of using simulation lies in creating the ability to evaluate competency. Simulators can be programmed so that the exact same situation can play out for each learner (Fig. 29.9).

Audiovisual systems have improved so that facilitators can mark the recording at any time that they want to review

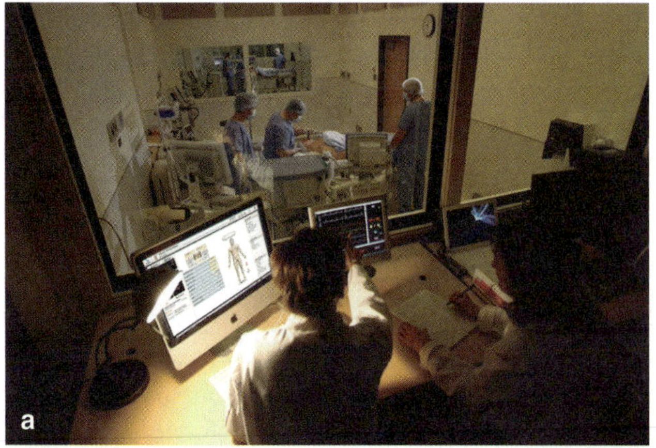

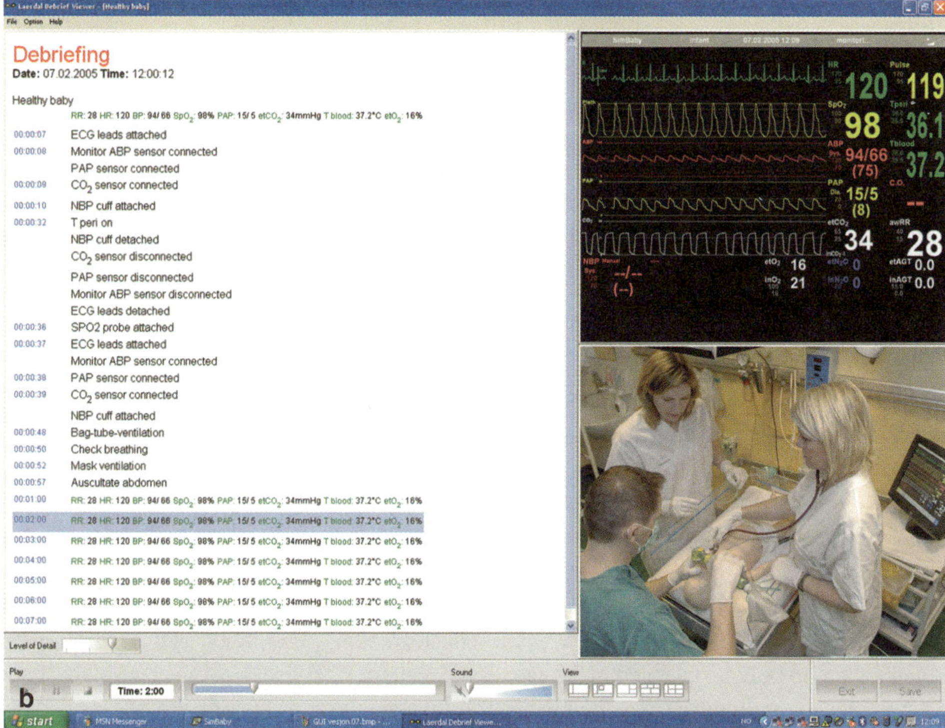

Fig. 29.10 (**a**) Observation of simulation scenario using CAE Learning Space (Photo courtesy of CAE Healthcare ©2012 CAE Healthcare) and (**b**) Laerdal SimBaby Feedback Screenshot (Photo courtesy of Laerdal Medical. All rights reserved)

and can also zoom in to see what the learner is doing (Fig. 29.10a–b).

Various checklists have been developed for use in competency evaluation, but it continues to be challenging to identify tools with established reliability and validity. Available tools have been identified and discussed by Kardong-Edgren et al. [17].

Challenges of Learning with High-Fidelity Patient Simulation

Several challenges inhibit the use of patient simulation for nursing including cost, human resources, and learning the technology. The challenges related to cost appear to be decreasing over time as the cost of the technology itself decreases. This phenomenon, which is unique to technology, occurs as smaller parts become available to do things that used to require larger parts and less complicated ways are identified to manage the technology. Compare the first computer available for a person's home to the abilities of the current smart phone, as an example. In addition, simulation is no longer viewed as a fad, but as a teaching strategy that is necessary. As such, grant money and donations have become focused to this area of education. Simulation laboratories and centers are often seen now as a point of status, and prospective students consider simulation availability when determining their college of choice.

Unfortunately, many colleges now have simulators, but they remain underused. When funding is obtained for equipment purchases, the need for faculty development is put aside or not understood. There is a steep learning curve for the technology itself but also for how to facilitate this type of learning. Initially, it was common to add simulation to the responsibilities of the skills lab coordinator, leading to the use of the simulator as another task trainer, in many cases. Over time, it has become clear that facilitating learning with simulation is a skill in its own right. Time and resources must be dedicated to this purpose for optimal learning to take place.

Faculty has also been leery of the technology. Simulators can be overwhelming in their complexity, are run by computer models that are not always understood, and require basic troubleshooting knowledge. Additionally, if audiovisual systems are used, these too must be learned so that they can be used concurrently with the simulator. The person running the simulator is often the voice of the patient, cueing the students, and may, in fact, also be the faculty facilitator of the SCE. Having all these various responsibilities can be overwhelming for the faculty who has not received adequate training.

Lastly, faculty must remember that this is a new way of learning for the students as well. Although they have grown up in a world of computers, they have continued to learn by lecture in most high schools. If they are expected to learn with the use of simulators, they must be oriented to the simulator, the environment, and the expectations prior to the SCE.

Integration of Simulation into the Nursing Curriculum

It is important to integrate simulation into the nursing curriculum at all levels. Some colleges use task trainers for lower-level students, reserving the high-fidelity simulators for upper-level students; however, the use of various types of simulators should always be based on the learning objectives for the experience. All levels of learners can benefit from high-fidelity learning experiences, no matter the level of simulator. The fidelity, or realism, of the experience draws the learner in, helping them to become engaged in the care of the patient.

A novice to expert approach is commonly used when integrating simulation throughout the curriculum, as it allows the students to build on previous experiences. Learners should have been exposed to the material being covered during the SCE, so it is important for the facilitator to be aware of what was covered in the curriculum. Expectations for preparation by the learner correspond to what their expectations are in the traditional clinical environment. In many colleges, simulation is considered a clinical experience, and therefore, the expectations of the learner should be the same in simulation as they are on the actual clinical wards. Examples of the integration of simulation into a nursing curriculum are provided in Table 29.2. These examples can be created using any type of simulation, virtual, screen based, or mannequin based, and used with any level of student or practitioner; the choice is dependent upon learning objectives and available resources.

As a result of integration of simulation throughout the curriculum, facilitators have the opportunity to observe learners for growth—or lack thereof. Being able to observe the learners in a controlled environment provides a way to evaluate learning that is not possible in the traditional clinical environment where students are spread out across an entire nursing unit or where the faculty may be responsible for students that are learning on several different patient care units. Having the students in the controlled simulation environment also allows for students to be assigned roles that they may be weak in, providing another learning opportunity tailored to their needs.

During the integration attempts, it is important for leadership to support the effort both financially and by their presence and verbal or written support. This will help to bring along faculty who may be more reluctant. An identified faculty champion, most commonly the simulation coordinator or facilitator, will also help to move faculty along as they demonstrate enthusiasm, a "can-do" attitude, and the willingness to help others learn more about simulation.

Creation of simulated clinical experiences is a very time-consuming endeavor, especially if they need to be programmed as well. Each of the major simulator vendors has a package of scenarios that have already been written and programmed. These scenarios are evidence based, built on learning objectives, provide information as to how to run the scenario, and were created by experts in simulation education. These scenarios can all be tailored to meet specific needs of the purchasing program and can save an immense amount of time, allowing quicker integration.

Table 29.2 Simulation across the nursing curriculum

Courses	Example
Fundamentals/skills	Urinary catheter insertion without urine return; student must evaluate for cause, such as tubing kink, dehydration, acute renal failure, chronic renal failure
Assessment	Hypertension, asthma; identify abnormals but may not have yet learned how to treat; tie in pathophysiology
Acute med/surg	Postoperative complications: deep vein thrombosis, hemorrhage, ileus
Chronic med/surg	Diabetes, coronary artery disease, chronic obstructive pulmonary disease
Mental health	Overdose, drug abuse, dysfunctional family dynamics
Obstetrics	Normal/abnormal delivery, postpartum hemorrhage, drug-addicted baby
Pediatrics	Dehydration, diabetic ketoacidosis, child abuse
Critical care	Pulmonary embolism, acute respiratory failure, trauma
Community health	Homeless patient, victim of violence, sexually transmitted disease

Table 29.3 Use of simulation in the hospital environment

Type of nursing/healthcare provider	Simulation experience
Neurological	Used in orientation program: assessment of a patient with a spinal cord injury, cardiovascular accident with and without indications for thrombolytics, acute head injury
Orthopedic	Post-op deep vein thrombosis followed by pulmonary embolism
ICU/CCU	Abdominal injury from car accident, internal bleeding requiring insertion of pulmonary artery catheter
Respiratory therapy	Individual competencies for managing respiratory emergencies
Helicopter service	Chronic obstructive pulmonary disease patient who requires intubation
Operating room	Malignant hyperthermia, sedation
ACLS	Implementation of ACLS following completion of courses
PACU	Unexpected cardiopulmonary arrest
NICU	Identification of deterioration and preparation for transport
Progressive	Management of cardiac drugs and drips
Rehab physical therapists	Moving a patient on a ventilator with an assortment of tubes and lines
RehabCare nurses	Management of patient on a ventilator

Use of Simulation in the Hospital Environment for Nurses

As mentioned earlier, simulation has been slower to enter the hospital environment, although it is quickly becoming more common now, likely as a result of the push for safer patient care. The benefits of using simulation in the hospital environment are to expose nurses to patient situations they might not often see, to practice using new equipment, and to evaluate competencies. The challenges are the same as those in the educational environment: time to learn and human resources. As the value of simulation continues to be shown in the literature, more hospitals are providing experiences for their new graduates and existing staff. Many have also incorporated simulation into their internship and/or orientation programs as well as into annual competency evaluations.

While nursing schools typically house their simulator(s) in a specific location where they stay all the time, hospitals more frequently will take the simulator to their staff. This overcomes the challenges of pulling staff away from their primary responsibilities of patient care. This *in situ* training is not without its challenges as the equipment and supplies must be gathered and relocated; surprise is often a factor as code scenarios are a favorite to run *in situ*, and Table 29.3 shows how simulation can be used for many different types of hospital nurses.

Nursing Assessment

Conducting assessment in the simulation environment is a controversial topic within the nursing education community. Many faculties have taken the philosophical approach that the simulation environment is to be one of learning in which formative assessment is completed, often during the debriefing process. The nature of simulation activities lends itself well to this formative assessment, as students receive immediate feedback from the simulator based on their decisions when providing care. Others promote the use of simulation when conducting high-stakes testing for the same reason—the simulator will react based on correct and incorrect choices that are made. However, caution must be taken when embarking on high-stakes testing, as consistency must be maintained between facilitators assuring that all students receive the same experience. This is inherently a challenge as simulation is considered a learner-driven activity and those learners do not always respond the same. These same cautions must be taken with practicing nurses, particularly if employment decisions are being made as a result of performance in simulation.

Research Needs and Opportunities

As a result of research supported by the National League for Nursing and Laerdal, Jeffries [18] published the first framework to support the creation and use of simulation: The Nursing Education Simulation Framework. This framework identified the concepts of (1) teacher, (2) student, and (3) educational practices and showed how those concepts had an impact on the simulation design characteristics and outcomes. The simulation design characteristics (objectives, fidelity, problem-solving, student support, and debriefing) also impact the outcomes (learning, skill performance, learner satisfaction, critical thinking, and self-confidence). This framework provides the support for researchers to conduct studies on any of these concepts and the role they play on other areas of simulation development. This framework is currently undergoing rigorous literature review to determine if any of the concepts in the framework need to be further developed. For example, the teacher is now commonly called facilitator.

There are variables that impact the teacher (demographics) and student (program, level, age) that can be further studied to see what that impact is and how it affects the learning outcomes. The lack of consistency with how simulation is facilitated and with how nurses are educated leads to numerous challenges when studying the outcomes of simulation. There are several efforts underway to assist in this area. The use of evidence-based scenarios, with sufficient information provided, allows for replication and standardization of experiences. The International Nursing Association for Clinical Simulation and Learning Board of Directors [19] published *Standards of Best Practice: Simulation* in an effort to help facilitators meet learning needs. The National Council of State Boards of Nursing is currently conducting a multisite, national, longitudinal study using standardized scenarios to help answer the question of how much simulation can replace clinical.

Additional research needs to be undertaken to determine the impact that learning with simulation has on patient safety and outcomes. There are studies completed that show a correlation; however, more need to be completed. Once research can solidly connect learning with simulation to better patient outcomes, then simulation will become the gold standard that it already is in the aviation field.

Conclusion

While simulation was slow to enter the arena of nursing education and practice, it has grown tremendously over the past few years. There are still challenges to full integration, such as cost, human resources, and training needs; however, the value is appreciated and the benefits are beginning to outweigh the challenges. It is vital that administrators and simulation enthusiasts continue to promote the effective use of simulation and provide the leadership to integrate this teaching methodology into the entire curriculum. Further research needs to be undertaken to identify the impact various conceptual areas have on learning outcomes as well as how learning with simulation impacts patient care and safety.

References

1. Kohn LT, Corrigan JM, Donaldson MS, editors. To err is human: building a safer health system. A report of the committee on quality of health care in America, Institute of Medicine. Washington: National Academy Press; 2000.
2. Page A, editor. Keeping patients safe: transforming the work environment of nurses. Board on Health Care Services. Washington: National Academies Press; 2003.
3. TeamStepps. National implementation. Agency for Healthcare Research and Quality (AHRQ). 2006. http://teamstepps.ahrq.gov/. Accessed on Oct 7, 2012.
4. Quality & Safety Education for Nurses. Robert Woods Johnson Foundation. 2005. http://www.qsen.org/overview.php. Accessed on Oct 25, 2012.
5. Benner P. From novice to expert: excellence and power in clinical nursing practice. Menlo Park: Addison-Wesley; 1984.
6. Ellis JR, Hartley CL. Nursing in today's world: trends, issues & management. 8th ed. New York: Lippincott Williams & Wilkins; 2004.
7. Leighton K, Scholl K. Simulated codes: understanding the response of undergraduate nursing students. Clin Simul Nurs. 2009;5(5): e187–94.
8. Gladwell M. Blink. New York: Little, Brown, & Company; 2005.
9. Wayne DB, Butter J, Siddall VJ, et al. Mastery learning of advanced cardiac life support skills by internal medicine residents. J Gen Intern Med. 2006;21(3):251–6. doi:10.1111/j.1525-1497.2006.00341.x.
10. Aebersold M, Tschannen D, Stephens M, et al. Second life! A new strategy in educating nursing students. Clin Simul Nurs. 2011. doi:10.1016/ j.ecns.2011.05.002. 8(9):e469–475.
11. Skiba DJ. Nursing education 2.0: a second look at second life. Nurs Educ Perspect. 2009;30(2):129–31.
12. Rogers L. Simulating clinical experience: exploring second life as a learning tool for nurse education. In: Same places, different spaces. Proceedings ascilite Auckland 2009. http://www.ascilite.org.au/conferences/auckland09/procs/rogers.pdf.
13. Bonnetain E, Boucheix JM, Hamet M, et al. Benefits of computer screen-based simulation in learning cardiac arrest procedures. Med Educ. 2010;44:716–22. doi:10.1111/j.1365-2923.2010.03708.x.
14. Li S. The role of simulation in nursing education: a regulatory perspective. National Council of State Boards of Nursing. Presented at AACN hot issues conference, Denver; 22 April 2007.
15. The INASCL Board of Directors. Standard I: terminology. Clin Simul Nurs. 2009;7(4S):s3–7. doi:10.1016/j.ecns.2011.05.005.
16. Wallace P. Following the threads of an innovation: the history of standardized patients in medical education. Caduceus. 1997;13(2):1–28.
17. Kardong-Edgren S, Adamson KA, Fitzgerald C. A review of currently published evaluation instruments for human patient simulation. Clin Simul Nurs. 2010;6(1):e25–35. doi:10.1016/jecns.2009.08.004.
18. Jeffries P. A framework for designing, implementing, and evaluating simulations used as teaching strategies in nursing. Nurs Educ Perspect. 2005;26:96–103.
19. INACSL Board of Directors. Standards of best practice: simulation. Clin Simul Nurs. 2011;7(6):e201–68.

Simulation in Obstetrics and Gynecology

30

Shad Deering and Tamika C. Auguste

Introduction

Simulation in obstetrics and gynecology is a critical resource that has and will continue to be used with ever-increasing frequency. While simulation-based education began in earnest in the field of anesthesiology, it has special significance in obstetrics and gynecology.

Obstetrics and gynecology is a unique specialty that requires a wide range of both clinical and operative surgical skills. While the general OB/GYN will see many routine medical issues similar to a family medicine provider, they are also required to be competent surgeons who also are experts in the management of pregnancy, labor, and delivery. Obstetricians must be equipped with the ability to manage two patients at the same time with the comprehension that interventions intended for the mother must be balanced with anticipated effects on the fetus. The sheer intellectual and technical breadth of the specialty combined with the emotions surrounding the event, that is, pregnancy and delivery, makes simulation training for the specialty of OB/GYN an imperative. Utilizing simulation to acquire and assess the surgical skills needed in gynecology as well as those routine and emergent procedures that occur on the labor and delivery floor is not only possible but necessary to ensure the best outcomes possible.

This chapter will be divided into two distinct sections, one that discusses the use of simulation for obstetrics and the other on the use for gynecology. There will be an emphasis not only what is currently being done but also the evidence for its effectiveness.

Obstetric Simulation

Background and History

While simulation training in obstetrics is often thought of as a relatively new field, its first use may actually predate written history. Archaeological records show that ancestors of the Siberian Mansai people created life-size leather birth models of women for rituals and teaching maneuvers to assist in birth [1]. In the eighteenth century, Madame du Coudray, who served as a midwife for the King of France, created a life-size leather birthing mannequin to educate women about childbirth management, and this impressively was reported to have resulted in reduced infant and maternal mortality [2]. However, it was not until the late 1990s and early 2000s that simulation training for obstetrics started to be evaluated in a scientific and systemic manner.

The need for simulation training in obstetrics is now recognized at both the national and international level. The American College of Obstetricians and Gynecologists (ACOG) and the Society for Maternal Fetal Medicine (SMFM) have both formed simulation committees to facilitate the incorporation of simulation into the field. In fact, AGOG has sponsored a hands-on obstetric emergencies simulation course every year since 2008.

Recently, a joint publication titled "Quality Patient Care in Labor and Delivery: A Call to Action" was endorsed by seven different societies including the American Academy

S. Deering, MD, LTC, MIL, USA, MEDCOM, MAMC (✉)
Department of Obstetrics/Gynecology,
Uniformed Services University of the Health Sciences,
Bethesda, MD, USA

Department of Obstetrics/Gynecology,
Madigan Army Medical Center,
Tacoma, WA, USA
e-mail: deering95@hotmail.com

T.C. Auguste, MD
Department of Obstetrics and Gynecology,
Georgetown University School of Medicine,
110 Irving Street NW, 58-18, Washington, DC 20010, USA

Department of OB/GYN Simulation,
Women's and Infants' Services,
Washington Hospital Center,
Washington, DC, USA
e-mail: tamika.c.auguste@medstar.net

A.I. Levine et al. (eds.), *The Comprehensive Textbook of Healthcare Simulation*,
DOI 10.1007/978-1-4614-5993-4_30, © Springer Science+Business Media New York 2013

of Family Physicians, American Academy of Pediatrics, the Association of Women's Health, Obstetric and Neonatal Nurses, American College of Nurse Midwives, the American College of Osteopathic Obstetricians and Gynecologists, ACOG, and SMFM [3]. In this publication, the consortium recommended that strategies be employed to ensure optimal care of obstetric patients to include drills, simulation exercises, and training in principles of crisis resource management (see Chap. 8).

Simulators are currently available for specific obstetric-related tasks such as episiotomy, amniocentesis, and vaginal and cesarean delivery and range from low- to high-fidelity female mannequins with the ability to hemorrhage and reproduce such medical emergencies as eclamptic seizures and cardiac arrest. A more comprehensive discussion of the actual simulators can be found in Chap. 15.

Evidence for and Current Usage in Training

Though new obstetric simulators are still being developed, there is now a reasonable body of literature available describing their use and utility. What follows in this section are examples of these obstetric simulations, a brief description of the simulators used, and the literature and outcomes associated with their use.

Amniocentesis

Amniocentesis is a relatively common procedure in obstetrics and is most often used for prenatal evaluation of fetal karyotype or determination of fetal lung maturity. Simulators for this procedure range from simple and inexpensive models made at the institution level (usually with gelatin mixtures or ultrasound gel and different targets inserted into ultrasound "phantoms" that allow for real-time scanning and procedures), to much higher-fidelity, commercially available, haptic-interface simulators [4–6].

Pittini et al. integrated a physical amniocentesis simulator with a standardized patient in order to assess both communication and technical skills related to the procedure [7]. In this study they assessed 30 trainees (including medical students, residents, and maternal fetal medicine fellows) and found significant improvement in both knowledge and technical performance after training. This study was important in that the authors attempted to evaluate communication and counseling and not just technical skills. Though there have been no studies yet that have evaluated whether or not better performance on an amniocentesis simulator translates to better outcomes with real patients, the commercial availability of relatively inexpensive models for a potentially morbid procedure makes training for this very reasonable.

Breech Vaginal Delivery

Breech vaginal delivery is no longer a routine procedure in obstetrics, especially now that the standard of care is to deliver a singleton breech by cesarean section. Therefore, current providers and recent graduates have significantly less experience in this type of delivery, yet there are still situations where patients present in advanced labor, and a breech vaginal delivery may be indicated.

The management for breech delivery can be simulated on a wide variety of obstetric birthing simulators, though not all models incorporate the delivery of a fetus with articulating joints. The latter would obviously be preferred since manipulating the baby can add fidelity and permit the practice of breech delivery maneuvers.

One article specifically evaluated the use of simulation training for breech vaginal delivery and reported on performance on a simulated breech vaginal delivery before and after training [8]. A total of 20 residents from two institutions completed the protocol and showed that after training, they had significantly higher scores for completion of critical delivery components ($p<0.05$) and that overall performance and safety of the delivery was also improved ($p=0.001$).

Maternal Cardiac Arrest

Care of a pregnant patient who experiences cardiac arrest is different since the team must take the unique physiology of pregnancy as well as the fetal status into account during the resuscitation. While it is possible to utilize male human patient simulators for these types of drills, for improved fidelity and the ability to monitor the fetal status, there are several high-fidelity full body birthing simulators available. There is a significant body of evidence in the literature suggesting the benefits of simulation and team training for improved code team performance and patient outcome, yet there is much less available data specific to pregnancy and the labor and delivery suite.

A recent article by Lipman et al. makes the case for the creation of an Obstetric Life Support program (OBLS) [9]. The authors discuss the similar nature of the neonatal resuscitation program (NRP) and explain how and why an OBLS course can be accomplished. One group studied the performance of multidisciplinary labor and delivery teams during maternal code events with a high-fidelity trainer [10]. They identified several common issues during these events such as poor communication with the pediatric resuscitation team, lack of leadership, and poor distribution of workload. Another group took this investigation a step further and attempted to determine if training could affect actual performance. Fisher et al. recruited 19 maternal fetal medicine staff to participate in a maternal arrest simulation program [11]. After training, they demonstrated significantly improved performance in both the time to initiate cardiopulmonary resuscitation and cesarean delivery during a simulated maternal code.

Cesarean Section

While often viewed as a routine procedure, a cesarean section is still a major abdominal operation and carries with it the potential for significant morbidity, especially when the patient has had previous abdominal surgery.

At present, simulators for this procedure are mostly limited to those made at the local institution level, though there is at least one simulation company (Gaumard Scientific, FL) that makes an abdominal cover for their birthing mannequin that contains simulated abdominal layers for a typical Pfannenstiel incision. New prototypes are also being built by others (examples of cesarean section simulator can be accessed at http://www.obgmanagement.com/pages.asp?id=6714 and http://www.savinglivesatbirth.net/summaries/43).

One study was performed that reported on the use of an intermediate-fidelity cesarean section simulator, created at the local level out of materials from a fabric store, for training new interns [12]. This group reported that the simulation exercises were effective in helping the interns define the steps of the procedure and in improving their overall comfort with assisting in performing the procedure.

Another recent publication used a high-fidelity birthing simulator and an abdominal model overlay to simulate a maternal cardiopulmonary arrest requiring the performance of a perimortem cesarean section [13]. In this trial, they randomized teams to encountering the cardiac arrest in either a delivery room or the operating room. They found that teams in the delivery room were more likely to deliver the fetus by perimortem cesarean section within the recommended 5-min time frame than the OR group (57% vs. 14%) during simulated drills.

Cordocentesis

During some pregnancies, there is a need to measure fetal hematocrit or platelet counts directly. This may require cordocentesis, where a needle is advanced into the fetal umbilical cord under direct ultrasound guidance. As the safety of this technical procedure is related to operator experience and the potential for serious complications is significant including fetal loss, this is an important area where simulation can have a major impact. To date, there are only a few publications related to the use of this type of simulator. One article, by Ville et al., describes a cordocentesis simulator in detail and also the training methods used to teach the procedure but failed to discuss evaluation of the efficacy of the training [14]. In another study from Thailand, a homemade cordocentesis simulator was used and a single trainee trained [15]. They then went on to describe outcomes from the first 50 cases that the trainee performed on actual patients and reported a 100% success rate during the procedures after training. While this is an interesting report, it is obviously limited by the inclusion of only a single trainee. At this time, there is one commercially available cordocentesis simulator for this type of training (Limbs & Things, UK).

Eclampsia

Eclampsia is an uncommon but significant obstetric emergency that involves generalized tonic-clonic seizures during pregnancy that is almost always associated with hypertension and proteinuria. Though the incidence of eclampsia is relatively low in the United States, the risk of both maternal and neonatal morbidity and mortality is significant when it does occur. Treatment of eclampsia involves supportive care during the seizure while managing hypertension, preventing aspiration, and administering medications (i.e., magnesium sulfate) to stop and prevent further seizures.

There are currently several options for simulators to address eclampsia. Some authors have used patient actors to play the part of a seizing pregnant patient, while others have simply stood behind the patient bed and physically shaken the mannequin to simulate the eclamptic seizure [16, 17]. One publication describes the creation of an external mechanism that made the maternal mannequin's head move in such a manner as to simulate a seizure [18]. Recently, new birthing simulators have been developed that include an internal seizure mechanism. This is the type of mannequin that is described in the multicenter implementation of an *in situ* obstetric emergency simulation training program [19].

Ellis et al. reported on the use of simulation training for eclampsia across six large hospitals in the UK [20]. A total of 140 participants were randomly assigned to 24 teams and assigned to simulation training either at a simulation center or at the hospital and with or without teamwork training. They found that after training, teams completed the basic tasks more quickly (55 s before vs. 27 s after, $p=0.012$) and that a magnesium sulfate loading dose was given much more often (92% of teams vs. 61% before training, $p=0.04$) and nearly 2 min earlier in simulated eclamptic seizure cases. There was no difference found between teams that trained in the simulation center or the hospital.

Episiotomy Repair

Although decreasing from 60.9% in 1979 to 24.5% in 2004, the rate of episiotomy during vaginal deliveries is still a very common procedure in modern obstetrics [21]. One study reported that almost 60% of OB/GYN residents surveyed reported receiving no formal education on episiotomy repair techniques [22]. Since poor repairs increase the risk for significant lacerations and complications during subsequent deliveries, it is important to be able to instruct trainees to safely perform this procedure. Fortunately, there are multiple models described in the literature and available commercially that can be used to do this. The locally made simulators range from a well-known beef tongue model to a "sponge perineum" that can be fabricated for very little money [23, 24].

In 2003, Nielsen et al. developed an objective structured assessment of technical skills (OSATS) and demonstrated that it was a reliable and valid measure of resident skill in the laboratory setting [25]. In their study, they also reported that 61% of the residents tested failed the assessment, further emphasizing the need for formal training opportunities. A more recent study by Uppal et al. reported on a similar evaluation of episiotomy repair skills of 40 OB/GYN residents from 13 different residency programs [26]. In their study, they found that participant level of training and prior experience had no effect on the pass rate and that, strikingly similar to Nielsen's results, the overall failure rate was 57.5%. Given the poor performance of residents over several different studies and the availability of validated training simulators and evaluation forms, incorporating episiotomy simulation into training programs is both important and feasible.

Operative Vaginal Delivery

In a recent article on operative vaginal delivery, a well-known expert stated that after didactic teaching on proper technique, the resident "…should then be assessed by both written examination and *formal simulation exercises* before allowing them to be primary operators on real patients" [27]. He went on to further say in the same article that "Simulation training can enhance residents' understanding of mechanical principles and should logically precede clinical work."

To date, models available for teaching these skills have been somewhat limited, as the ability to recreate the birth canal and delivery fetus with enough fidelity from material that will tolerate multiple procedures has been less than optimal. However, there are models that integrate the ability to provide feedback to trainees on both the correct angle used and the amount of force applied during the delivery.

Despite the limitations of current simulators, there is recognition that this type of training is needed. One report by Leslie et al. described connecting forceps to an isometric strength testing unit and demonstrated that residents could be taught the appropriate amount of force necessary during delivery and that they could reproduce this consistently after training [28]. Another very practical study by Dupuis et al. scored ten trainees on the accuracy of forceps blade placement utilizing a birthing simulator [29]. They found that the providers improved significantly with practice and estimated that approximately 35–45 placements were required to achieve 100% accuracy.

Postpartum Hemorrhage

With respect to postpartum hemorrhage, one of the leading causes of maternal mortality, the Joint Commission recommends that simulation exercises be run to "train staff in the [local] protocols, to refine local protocols, and to identify and fix systems problems that would prevent optimal care" [30]. In a similar manner, the UK Confidential Inquiries into maternal deaths also recommended that simulation drills and regular training for management of postpartum hemorrhage be conducted to reduce morbidity and mortality [31].

Specifically addressing simulation training for obstetric residents, Deering et al. reported on the performance of 40 residents from three different institutions during a simulated postpartum hemorrhage scenario [32]. They found that nearly half (47.5%) of the residents made some form of medication error during the exercise and that the level of experience was not a factor in their performance. This study emphasized the need for the type of training and education recommended by the national organizations discussed previously.

The ability to estimate blood loss also plays a key role in optimizing the management of postpartum hemorrhage. Two separate reports have been published addressing the estimation of blood loss using simulation. In a study by Maslovitz et al., they reviewed the performance of 50 obstetrical teams of physicians and nurses and evaluated their ability to estimate blood loss in an obstetric hemorrhage scenario [33]. They found that underestimating the degree of blood loss was common and that accuracy was only 50–60% for a hemorrhage of 3.5 l. A study by Bose et al. created 12 clinical simulation scenarios where estimation of blood loss was required [34]. Similar to the previously mentioned study, on evaluation of 103 physicians, midwives, nurses, and healthcare assistants, they found significant underestimation of blood loss as well.

Another study used simulation and recreated blood-soaked surgical sponges and under-buttocks drapes to determine if teaching providers what common surgical items look like with specified amounts of blood on them could improve their accuracy [35]. Assessment with simulated scenarios demonstrating different degrees of blood loss was done before and after this educational intervention on the visual estimation of blood loss (EBL). The group found that there was significant improvement and underestimation of EBL decreased from 62% to only 2% after training.

Spontaneous Vaginal Delivery

A vaginal delivery is one of the most common procedures done by medical students and residents in OB/GYN. It is usually straightforward, but it is difficult and awkward to try and teach the proper technique while the patient is pushing and the family is watching. Fortunately, there are several basic obstetric birthing simulators that work well to teach this. Examples of these can be seen in Chap. 15.

Uncomplicated Vaginal Deliveries

In a study of third year medical students, 56 were taught how to perform a vaginal delivery by lecture alone, while another group of 56 students were taught with a combination of lecture and simulation training [36]. At the end of their rotation, the students who participated in simulation training reported being more comfortable with their ability to perform a vaginal delivery and scored significantly higher on both their oral and written exams. Dayal et al. also examined the use of simulation to teach this skill to medical students [37]. After randomizing students to simulation training or standard didactics, the researchers observed performance of a simulated vaginal delivery at the beginning and end of their 6-week rotation. The simulation training group had higher overall delivery performance scores at both week 1 and week 5 after training, suggesting the ability to translate what they had learned in the lab into their practical demonstration.

Complicated Vaginal Deliveries

Shoulder Dystocia

The use of simulation to address outcomes in patients who experience a shoulder dystocia is probably the best studied area in obstetric simulation. Initial reports on the use of simulation to address shoulder dystocia training showed that a significant number of providers were not familiar with the common maneuvers required and that training could improve performance in a simulated shoulder dystocia scenario [38, 39]. Most important was the finding that a simulation training program could actually improve fetal outcomes. In 2006, Draycott et al. reported on the impact of the implementation of a shoulder dystocia simulation training program in the UK [40]. They reviewed all deliveries complicated by shoulder dystocia from the 4 years prior to the program and the 4 years after. While the incidence of shoulder dystocia was the same between the two time periods, the incidence of neonatal injury at birth after a shoulder dystocia was reduced nearly fourfold (9.3–2.3%; RR 0.25, CI 0.11–0.57). Similar findings were reproduced in the United States (10.1–2.6%, $p=0.03$) [41].

Simulation training has also been utilized in the evaluation of documentation after this common obstetric emergency, with multiple reports demonstrating significant gaps in documentation and that simulation training can help to improve documentation [42–44].

Umbilical Cord Prolapse

Upon diagnosis of umbilical cord prolapse, time is of the essence and an urgent cesarean section must be performed. This is a situation where the entire team must be involved, from the nurse or physician who makes the diagnosis to the anesthesia provider and pediatric support team that make the cesarean delivery and neonatal resuscitation possible. Simulation of this emergency is reproduced with almost any of the currently available birthing mannequins; the fetal umbilical cord is simply placed in the vagina in front of the presenting part. Including a fetal monitor to the simulation increases the fidelity since it allows for the trainer to create fetal heart rate abnormalities consistent with the cord compression often seen in this emergency.

A recent study from the UK reported on the implementation of a simulation training program for umbilical cord prolapse management at a large tertiary maternity unit [45]. They compared the diagnosis to delivery interval for all cord prolapse cases for the 6 years before and after simulation training. The group concluded that there was a significant decrease in the diagnosis to delivery interval from 25 to 14.5 min ($p<0.001$) and that the teams were much more likely to take the recommended actions to attempt to alleviate cord compression (34–82%, $p=0.003$). This landmark study was one of the first to demonstrate the benefits of simulation and team training on objective performance outcomes in obstetrics.

Teamwork Training

In the past, many attempts to improve patient outcomes in obstetrics were directed at the individual provider level with a focus on honing technical skills and increasing medical knowledge. However, it is now recognized that a majority of complications and morbidity actually result from ineffective teams rather than individual failures. A Sentinel Alert was issued by the Joint Commission in 2004 and reported that most cases of perinatal death and injury were caused by problems with an organization's culture and communication failures [46]. A year later, in 2005, another report stated that, despite increasing focus and awareness of the need to improve patient safety, there had not been a decrease in the death rate due to medical errors. They did note, however, that there were reductions in certain kinds of error-related deaths, including a 50% reduction in poor outcomes of preterm infants when labor and delivery staff had participated in team training [47]. (The basic principles of CRM are discussed in detail in Chap. 8.)

Teamwork training and assessment for obstetric residents demonstrated common significant communication and teamwork issues during emergencies including poor communication with the pediatric team, not assuming a leadership role, and poor workload distribution [10]. The use of mobile *in situ* simulation systems has been shown to be an effective method to train smaller hospitals and to identify and address latent safety threats on the actual labor and delivery unit [19, 48].

In 2010, a systemic review of simulation for multidisciplinary team training in obstetrics was published [49]. While 97 articles on the topic were identified, the authors chose to focus on eight that reported their outcomes of interest. They found that this type of training method was potentially effective in preventing errors and improving patient safety in acute obstetric emergencies but recommended that additional studies were needed. Since this publication, there was an article by Riley et al. that addressed the use of teamwork training with and without simulation training. In a 2011 study, Riley et al. chose to investigate three perinatal units at different hospitals [50]. At one hospital, there was no additional training, at another hospital they implemented TeamSTEPPS® training only, and at the third hospital, they conducted TeamSTEPPS® training that incorporated simulation training. Over a 3-year period, they measured the weighted adverse outcomes score (WAOS) and found no improvement in the first two hospitals but a 37% decrease in perinatal morbidity for the hospital that utilized teamwork and simulation training. While multiple confounders may have influenced these data, it is clear that simulation-based training may impact perinatal morbidity.

Art of Obstetric Simulation

Currently, there is an ongoing debate as to where obstetric simulation should be conducted, who should be involved, and how it can best be integrated for maximum benefit. The answers to these questions are important as we look at the future of simulation in this important area.

With regard to where obstetric simulation should be done, the answer, as with many things, is dependent on the goals of training. If the purpose of the training is to teach purely technical skills such as amniocentesis or forceps placement, then the ideal location may be a simulation center where the trainee is away from clinical distractions and has the complete attention of a mentor/instructor. However, if the goal is to practice teamwork or look at hospital systems issues (Chap. 10) that may affect patient care, then this training is almost certainly better done on the actual ward/unit itself (i.e., *in situ*) as it is impossible to recreate fully the physical location and systems in a center. An overview of this sort of training is outlined in Table 30.1. *In situ* simulation has been identified as an important component in the evaluation of newly constructed facilities [51]. In addition, having simulation capabilities available on the actual unit can allow for "just-in-time" training (i.e., warming up and reviewing the procedure just before performing it, similar to batting practice in baseball) for certain procedures such as amniocentesis or percutaneous umbilical blood sampling, which is something the authors have employed at their home institution.

In terms of who should be trained, there is growing evidence that the answer is the entire team, and not just the physicians. When reviewing programs that have demonstrated improvements in actual patient outcomes, Siassakos et al. noted that there were several common themes [52]. Key components of effective simulation training programs included the following:

1. Teamwork training combined with clinical training in a multidisciplinary format: There has been a shift in focus of training from working with just physicians. It is now recognized that communication issues are a leading cause of poor outcomes and that the entire team needs to be engaged in the effort.
2. Relevant, "in-house" training: Because of the difficulties getting complete teams together at simulation centers located outside of the hospital, many trained on their actual unit or at least in their hospital. This made multidisciplinary training possible and allowed for the identification of institution systems issues. Most importantly, these units worked to train almost 100% of their staff, and not just a select few.
3. Local solutions: The successful programs took national guidelines and then evaluated their own systems. They then created solutions that followed best practices and yet still worked within the capabilities of their institution.
4. Realistic training tools: With regard to simulators and training tools, the authors found that high fidelity and engagement of the learners was more important than having the most "high-tech" simulators available.
5. Institution-level incentives: Besides strong support from leadership, hospitals with effective programs often were offered financial incentives including significant discounts on their malpractice premiums.

Table 30.1 Location of obstetric simulation and efficacy

Location	Technical skills	Hospital systems issues	Teamwork/ Communication
In-situ/on ward	+	++	++
Simulation center	++	–	++

++ best fit, + possible, – not feasible

Gynecology Simulation

Background and History

Ancient Greece gave us the well-recognized apprenticeship model of training – *see one, do one, teach one*. This has been the mainstay of medical education, and especially surgical education, but has come under increased scrutiny in current times. This apprenticeship model is being recognized and identified as being outdated, inefficient, and potentially dangerous in the face of today's complicated surgical environments. There is also an increased awareness and appropriate intolerance of high error rates in healthcare. These issues are driving a mandate that alternative and safer methods of training be developed and implemented. Simulation has clearly emerged as part of the solution to this problem [53].

The concept of simulation is not novel in surgery. As early as 800 BC, Sushruta (one of two potential "fathers of surgery") recommended practicing on melons and wormed wood for training his students in surgery [54]. Many other sophisticated or high reliability organizations have used simulation technology for decades, and healthcare is only now trying to catch up. Aviation and nuclear energy for years have integrated simulation into both their education and quality improvement programs. The aviation industry has regularly scheduled assessments on flight simulators as an integral part of a pilot's maintenance of licensure and accreditation. Many of these simulators started out very simply, and this holds true in gynecologic surgery as well.

Early pioneers of simulation in healthcare like David Gaba (Chap. 2) introduced the modern era of simulation in healthcare by promoting mannequin training in the late 1980s [55]. It has only been within the last 15 years that disciplines like surgery and gynecology have embraced the concept of surgical simulation. Other pioneers in simulation have called for our specialty to move away from the subjective approach of assessing a trainee's skills and employ more objective metrics [56, 57]. It was also during this time that practice outside the operating room (OR) in either a simulated environment using box trainers or virtual reality was found to be more effective than traditional methods for developing operative skills [53, 58–60].

Simulation continued to develop and was growing as the landmark publication *To Err Is Human* became well known in 1999 [61]. The follow-up publication, *Crossing the Quality Chasm,* advocated the adoption of simulation training as a possible solution to the high error rates in healthcare [62]. After these publications, the promotions by leaders in the field, and the increasing evidence in the literature, simulation began to take hold as a serious contender as a method for learning surgical skills and especially in gynecology.

Gynecologic Simulators

A simulator can simply be an object, device, situation, or environment by which or in which a task or sequence of tasks can be realistically and effectively presented [63, 64]. Surgical simulators range from simple part-task trainers to sophisticated virtual reality simulators and from robotic simulators to standardized patients. In gynecology, many task trainers depict the pelvis and are used for specific procedures or skills like pelvic exams, intrauterine device (IUD) placement and removal, hysteroscopic resection, and urethral sling placement (Fig. 30.1).

When it comes to actual surgical procedures like laparoscopy, robotic surgery, or open gynecologic cases, the field of simulation has changed dramatically. For laparoscopic simulators, there are three basic types: (1) box trainers, (2) virtual reality, (3) hybrid simulators.

Box Trainers

As the name implies, box trainers consist of a box that mimics the abdominal cavity with different levels of realism. They are usually connected to a video camera that can project what the learner is doing in the box onto a video monitor. There are different training models that can be used with real laparoscopic instruments through trocars that are set in the lid or top of the box. A striking advantage to this form of simulation is that most people can fabricate their own box trainer using readily available inexpensive items such as a box, a light bulb, an inexpensive webcam, and a PC monitor. In addition, these are very portable and accessible on the ward or at home. The major drawbacks for this type of simulator include the inability to record the simulations, the lack of built-in assessment and feedback tools, and the lack of anatomic and haptic fidelity.

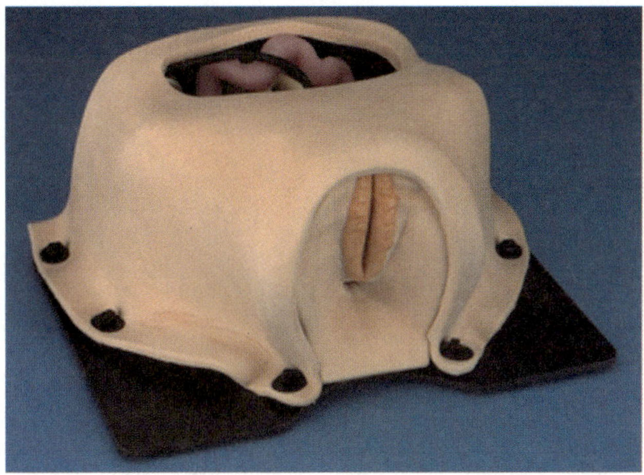

Fig. 30.1 Urethral sling procedure trainer. Limbs & Things, Savannah, GA (Photo courtesy of Limbs & Things ©2012 www.limbsandthings.com)

Virtual Reality (VR)

Virtual reality (VR) surgical simulators contain an array of electronic devices that function together to allow one to experience auditory and visual input in order to simulate a real setting or event. Most of the time these devices employ software running on a computer connected to a physical interface, like a handpiece [63]. The VR simulator can have different training tasks which mimic actions performed during surgery, with varying degrees of realism. A distinct advantage is that the computer will register and collect all movements and actions that are made, thus providing an excellent method of objective assessment and feedback for the trainee.

Historically speaking, VR simulation can be classified into four different generations of simulators. The *first generation* VR simulator was simple and based on the manipulation of abstract objects in a three-dimensional non-anatomical virtual space. These particular simulators were designed for the development of particular physical skills like visual-spatial perception, hand-eye coordination, and manual dexterity (Fig. 30.2). The *second generation* VR simulators introduced anatomical objects like the ovary or fallopian tube. This inherently made the experience

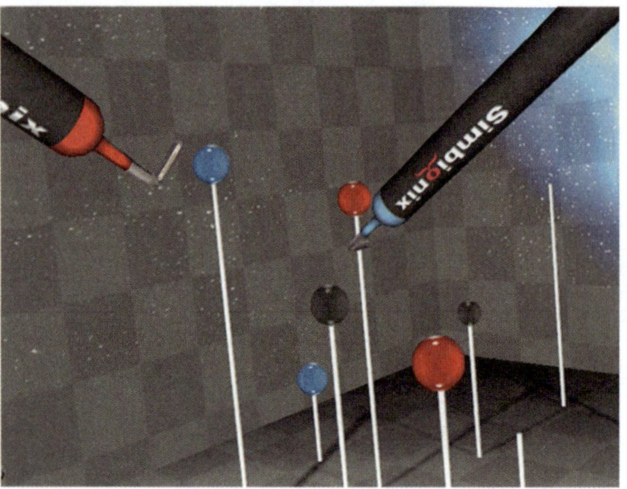

Fig. 30.2 Hand-eye coordination. LapMentor, Simbionix, Cleveland, OH (Used with permission from Simbionix, Cleveland, OH)

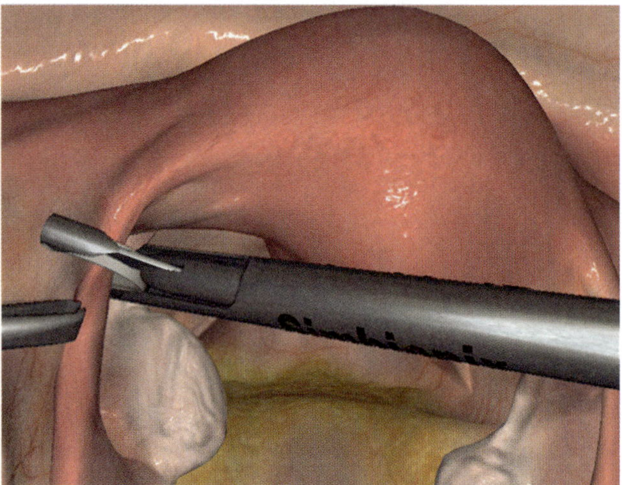

Fig. 30.3 Tubal sterilization, LapMentor, Simbionix, Cleveland, OH (Used with permission from Simbionix, Cleveland, OH)

more realistic (Fig. 30.3). The *third generation* VR simulators had more sophisticated software programs combined with an anatomically correct mannequin for very realistic training (Fig. 30.4). The *fourth generation* VR simulators include didactic teaching programs with prerecorded video examples. This generation often offers a combination of basic skills training like dexterity, hand-eye coordination, and instrument handling. This functionality incorporates a cognitive component of surgical anatomy, sequencing of operative procedures, and surgical decision making [63, 64]. The advantage to VR simulators lies in their realism and the potential to provide objective feedback based on the mechanism of the simulator. The distinct disadvantage to the VR simulator is their cost. These high-fidelity simulators can easily cost over $100,000, thereby limiting the number of institutions that can afford them.

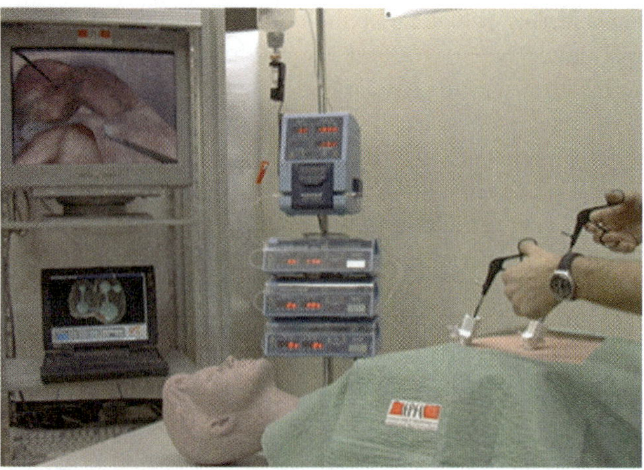

Fig. 30.4 VR simulator with high-fidelity mannequin

Hybrid Simulators

Hybrid simulators, as the name implies, are essentially a combination of a box trainer and a VR simulator and may be thought of as a computer-enhanced video box trainer [63]. The combination of VR imaging with real instruments and physical materials allows trainees to have the sensation of manipulating real physical objects. Some of these systems may also include computer-generated assessment and feedback (Fig. 30.5).

Robotic Surgery

Robotic laparoscopic surgery is the next frontier in gynecologic surgery and technology. While laparoscopic surgery has become fully integrated into the gynecology aspect of nearly all OB/GYN training programs, the future will have a heavy emphasis on robotic surgical training and techniques. Robotic technology in the OR offers minimally invasive surgery (MIS) options for many major surgical procedures. The robot is a combination of hardware and software programmed to communicate and interact with the environment. This technology markets itself as being different than the more traditional MIS method of laparoscopy (Fig. 30.6). In laparoscopy, the human eye perceives a two-dimensional view of the surgical site, while robotic equipment provides a three-dimensional view [65, 66]. Another difference is the ergonomics of conventional laparoscopy vs. the robot. In laparoscopy, the surgeon must stand while holding long instruments; with robotics the surgeons can sit while performing procedures [67]. Also, the robotic instruments provide significantly greater range of motion than traditional laparoscopic instruments, and the technology of the robot eliminates the "fulcrum effect" which in traditional laparoscopy forces surgeons to move their hands in the opposite direction of the instrument's tip [66]. Finally, another advantage of the robot is that it reduces any tremors the surgeon may have and allows the surgeon to select the scale of the

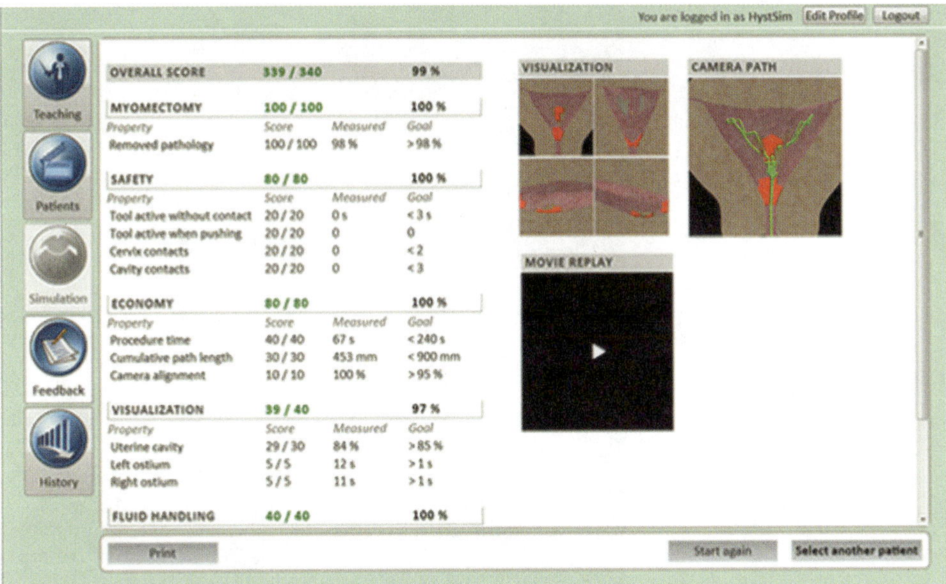

Fig. 30.5 VR simulator feedback, VirtaMed HystSim, Simbionix, Cleveland, OH (Used with permission from Simbionix, Cleveland, OH)

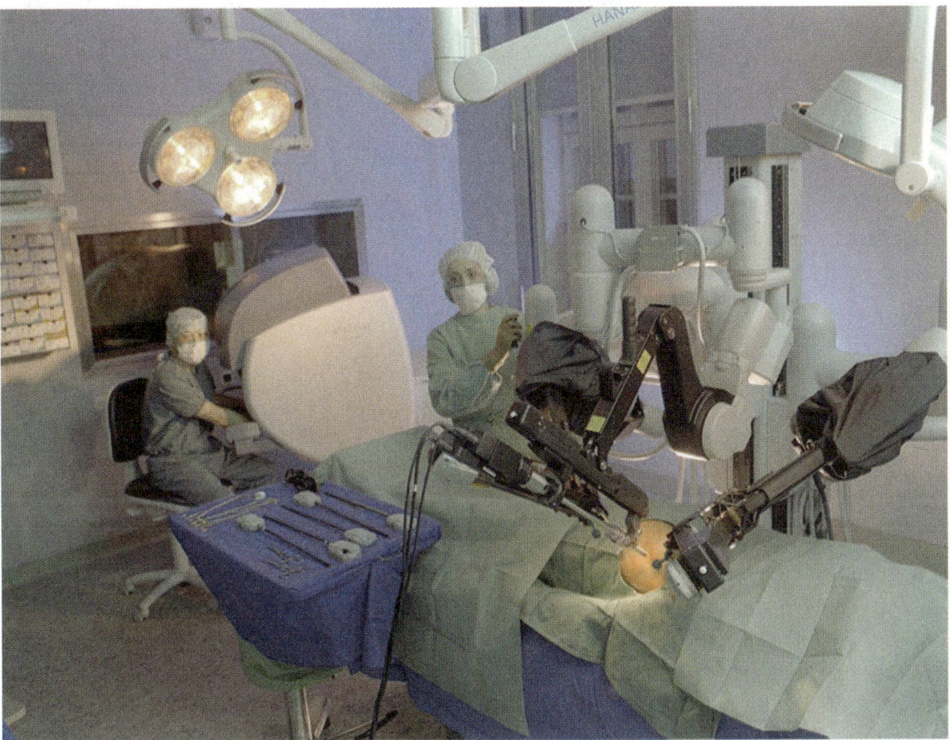

Fig. 30.6 Da Vinci robot. Intuitive Surgical, Sunnyvale, CA

ratio of the size of hand movements to the movement of the instrument tips [66, 68, 69].

While the da Vinci robotic surgery system offers several advantages in comparison to the traditional laparoscopic techniques, there are some disadvantages that limit its widespread use at all institutions. One of the main drawbacks of the robotic technology is the amount of time it is required for a surgeon to master its use. The next constraining factor is the cost of the device. The da Vinci robot costs well over $1 million, which makes it difficult for smaller hospitals to afford. Because of these factors, inexpensive simulation training methods are critical to decreasing learning time on the equipment.

Simulation for Gynecologic Procedures

While the traditional classroom setting cannot make up for actual hands-on operating time for a surgical trainee, the perceptual and psychomotor skills, which are of key importance for effective surgical technique, cannot be developed in lectures

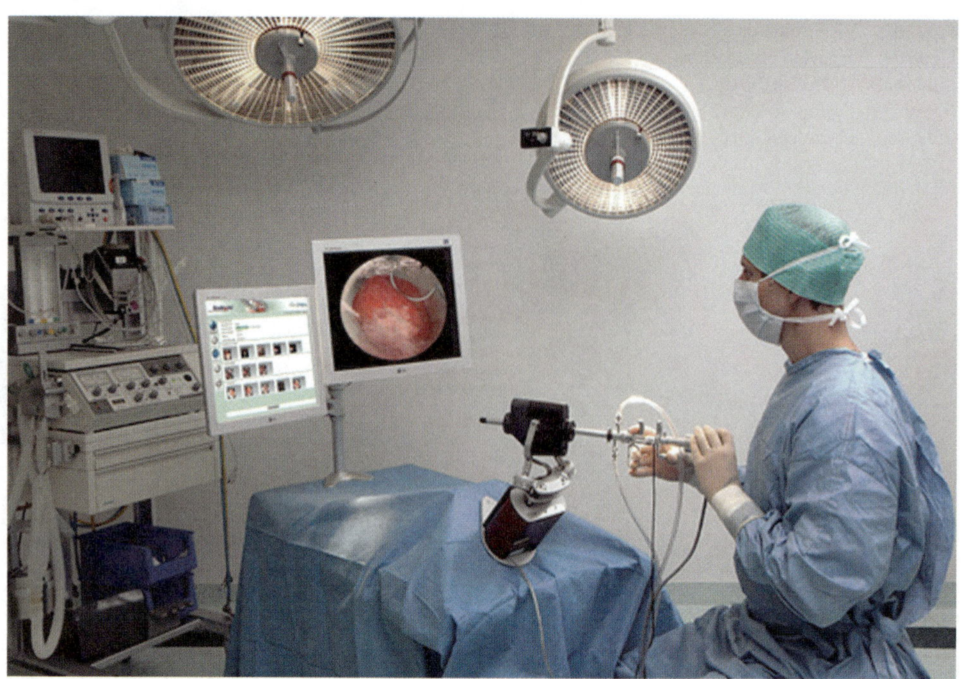

Fig. 30.7 Simbionix Hyst Sim (Used with permission from Simbionix, Cleveland, OH)

and seminars [70]. Simulation can provide additional learning opportunities in a way that can be self-directed and prepare the trainee for supervised training received in direct patient care [63]. Currently, there are simulators for gynecology that record the operator's performance and provide instant automated individualized feedback to its user. This feedback allows the trainee to monitor and refine their technique. The aim for trainees is to arrive at actual surgical procedures with better hand-eye coordination, greater familiarity of equipment, better efficiency in movement, and better knowledge of the surgical sequence [63]. The Simbionix Hyst sim and pelvic exam simulators help trainees acquire skills efficiently (Figs. 30.7 and 30.8).

Many institutions across the country are now developing and opening simulation centers to assist in the training of their students, residents, and physician staff. The centers may be discipline-specific or interdisciplinary. Many of these centers have sessions for training medical students, residents, nurses, and attending physicians individually and together in team training. Residency programs are also scheduling time with these centers to integrate simulation training into the curriculum. In institutions where there is no simulation center per se, departments can still use stand-alone task trainers and mannequins for training (Fig. 30.9a–c).

Simulation is also an excellent method for developing interdisciplinary team training in the operating room as well. A critical feature of any teamwork training program is a multidisciplinary approach. Multidisciplinary simulation-based training can be adapted to analyze team performance during a simulated gynecologic emergency. Many institutions are having their ORs adopt well-known and developed team training exercises using simulation to practice rare but catastrophic emergencies that could happen during actual surgical procedures. In these team training exercises, many of the gynecologic simulators such as a VR or box trainers are replaced with high-fidelity mannequins to simulate actual patients. At times a task trainer can be combined with a standardized patient actor to get a more realistic simulation. One report by Powers et al. examined OR teams during simulated surgeries and tasks that included trocar access and management of intra-abdominal hemorrhage utilizing a physical laparoscopic model and measured individual and overall team performance [71].

Evidence for and Current Usage in Training

When looking at simulators for adjuvant teaching modalities, it is critical that the simulator is able to differentiate between learners with different skill levels to determine whether there is any progress in learning or skill acquisition [53]. This is referred to as construct validity and is one of several levels of validation. Consistently showing the same measurement from the same skill levels is important and is termed reliability. The ultimate criteria for a simulator's value would be its predictive validity and transference to the actual OR, and this is the goal of all training programs.

In gynecology most studies have examined validation and transference in the use of box trainers or VR simulators. A study by Aggarwal et al. looked at one of the early commercially available laparoscopic VR simulators (LapSim®, Surgical Science Sweden, Göteborg, Sweden) and found that

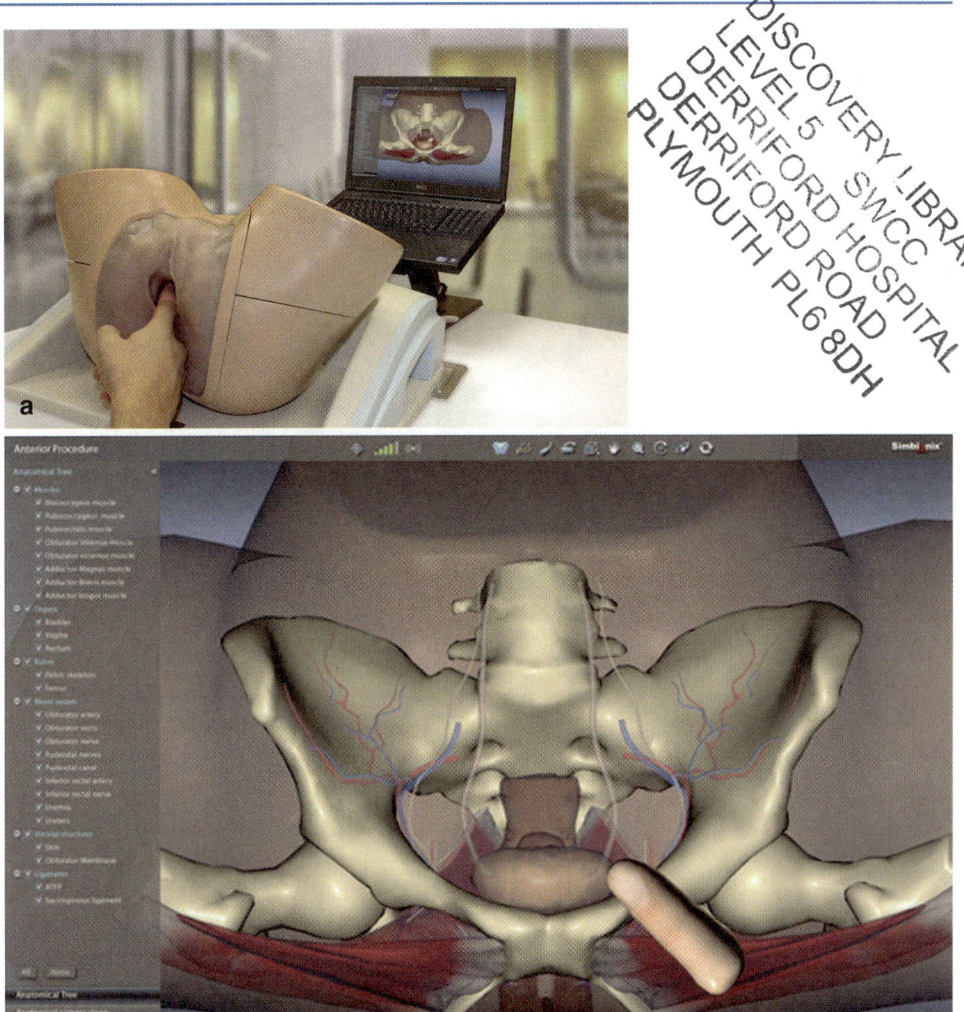

Fig. 30.8 (**a**) Simbionix pelvic trainer and (**b**) screen capture of trainee digit during pelvic palpation (Used with permission from Simbionix, Cleveland, OH)

intermediate and expert surgeons differed in their ability to complete a surgical module of salpingectomy for ectopic pregnancy [19]. This implied that the skills needed for VR are similar to those needed for real surgery, a good example of construct validity for this simulator [63, 72]. In the same study when novices and intermediate surgeons practiced on the VR simulator and improved their performance in the simulation laboratory, the result in the actual OR was a reduced median procedure time [72]. Another randomized controlled trial that compared VR simulation training was being added to clinical surgical training with traditional surgical training alone for salpingectomy and found a significantly shortened time in training to achieve competency in salpingectomy [73].

A recent Cochrane review of VR laparoscopic training in surgery has suggested that, in participants with limited laparoscopic experience, VR training results in a faster reduction in operating time, errors, and unnecessary movements than does standard laparoscopic training [74].

In the studies discussed, even though construct validity in realism and training was shown, it is still not clear whether the simulators used and/or the designed curriculum were appropriate predictors of clinical surgical ability. The predictive validity has yet to truly be shown in any well-designed study or trial. As educators and surgeons, it is essential to critically analyze the different components (i.e., blood loss, instrument path, or operating time) that make up some of the scores in these studies and see which are truly most important in real life [63].

Team Training in Gynecology

Simulation is clearly being used to teach technical skills, but by comparison, there has been relatively little work in the surgical simulation arena designed to teach or assess, interpersonal and communication skills and professionalism nontechnical skills [75]. Team training and simulation is not new

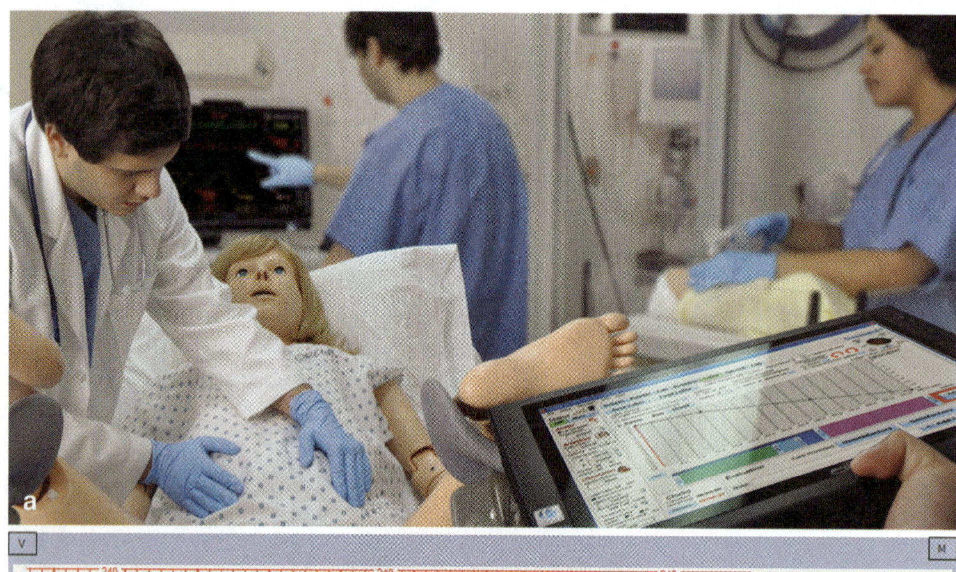

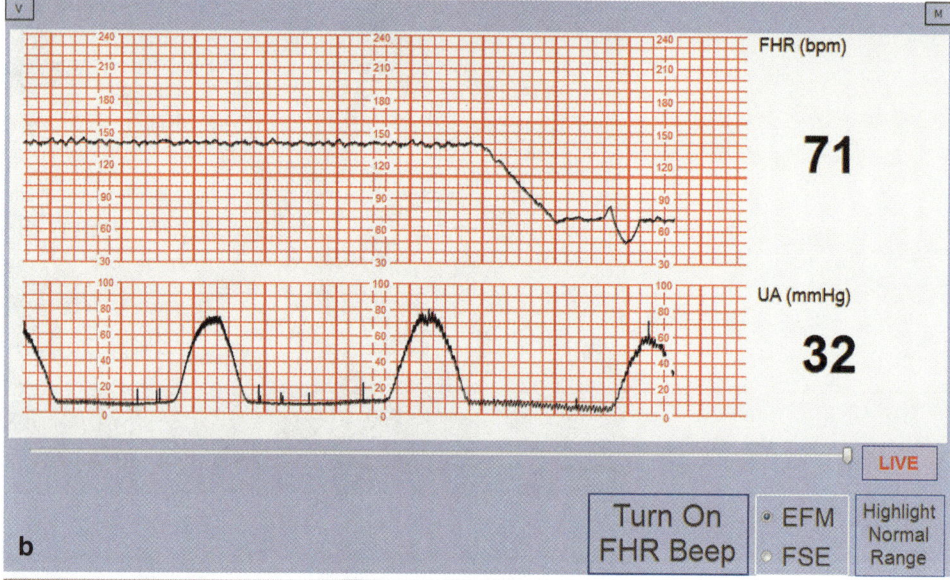

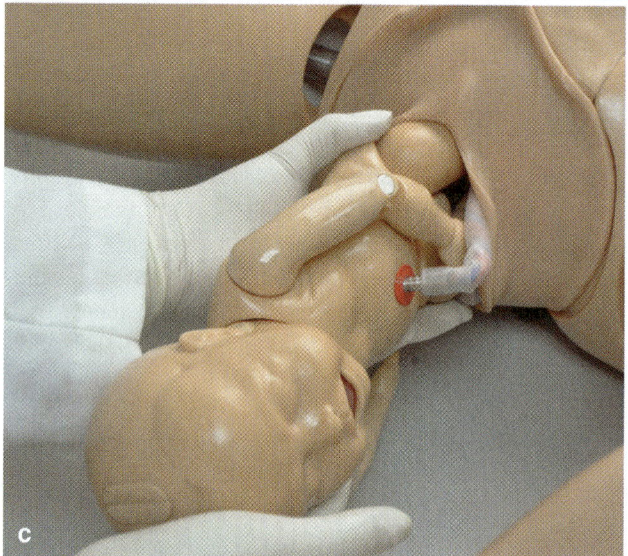

Fig. 30.9 (**a**) Multidisciplinary scenario of fetal distress (Photo courtesy of Gaumard), (**b**) simulated fetal heart tracing, and (**c**) delivery using Gaumard pregnancy simulator

in healthcare. There are many well-established programs across the United States; however, the overwhelming majority in our specialty focus on obstetrics not gynecology. In recent years, the Agency for Healthcare Research and Quality (AHRQ) has sponsored investigations in hopes of enhancing patient safety through team training simulations.

There are currently a few programs that are developing team training exercises in surgery. These include Kaiser Permanente's Highly Reliable Surgical Team (HRST) and the American College of Surgeons (ACS)/Association of Program Directors in Surgery (APDS) Surgical Skills Curriculum. The HRST and APDS Surgical Skills Curriculum are designed for different surgical specialties and are not specific for gynecology, though there is work to adapt them to the specialty. The ACS/APDS Surgical Skills Curriculum also includes team training that specifically aims to address nontechnical skills [76].

The (HRST) examines the relationship between their patient safety and highly reliable teams, and it is being shared with other institutions. For implementation, Kaiser collaborates with a hospital and begins with the identification and the training of project managers and a steering committee. After this, a safety survey is administered to all the staff, human factors training is provided, and metrics established. With the results of these parts, it is all integrated into the OR and includes items such as whiteboards, "glitch books," briefings, a surgical pause, routine debriefings, and regularly scheduled simulation training events. The required elements and the team training focus on teamwork and communication in the OR between all disciplines.

In recent studies, the ACS reported on their work to develop an objective scoring system for their surgical exercises. They have worked to determine construct validity of this objective scoring tool as well as other established rating tools for communication, teamwork, and workload [76]. Areas they examined included decision making, operating room communication, teamwork skills, and workload. The study focused on developing a de novo tool and applying other teamwork tools to the OR, and their findings did support construct validity for their tool [76]. The study also showed support from the participants in the form of favorable impressions of the developed module.

Although these reports represent initial efforts in the development of team training programs for surgery and specifically gynecology, properly validated rating tools to assess an individual's communication skill, specifically in the OR, are still lacking. The future of team training in the gynecology OR will begin with the development of these specific tools and then the proper design and evaluation of modules or scenarios to assess the communication and teamwork of participants.

The Art of Simulation in Gynecology

Currently, there is no national simulation curriculum in gynecology, but many different institutions are doing what they can to enrich the learning experience for their learners. As stated earlier in the chapter, many training programs have incorporated simulation training days for their residents. Most OB/GYN residents are being exposed to a variety of GYN simulation exercises during training. Many of these focus on specific skills. There are VR trainers for hysteroscopy (VirtaMed HystSim, Simbionix, Cleveland, OH) that have proven face and construct validity and are being used to introduce hysteroscopy and allow resident to practice particular skills like myomectomy and salpingectomy. Residents are also practicing laparoscopic skills on box trainers, and some are becoming certified in Fundamentals of Laparoscopic Surgery (FLS) and using task trainers to practice pelvic floor repairs.

GYN physicians in practice are also utilizing simulation modalities in their everyday practice. One of the most promising studies found that preoperative warm-up for 15–20 min with simple surgical exercises led to a substantial increase in surgical skill proficiency during follow-up tasks [77]. This is now translating to some surgeons practicing prior to laparoscopic surgeries on box trainers or VR trainers.

In addition, some residents and practicing physicians are taking the initiative and doing more independent training on box trainers to improve some of their basic or fundamental laparoscopic skills. Team training in gynecology is less prevalent but some institutions are using hybrid models or full mannequins in the ORs to practice a team's response to emergencies during gynecologic surgeries.

Future of Simulation in Gynecology

Implementation

Research on the effectiveness of simulation in gynecology is currently being done, and hopefully, it is only a matter of time before we, in gynecology, have the same evidence in support of simulation and team training that currently exists in obstetrics. For educators and trainers, there is a significant need for a clear plan to implement simulation into gynecologic training. Essential components of this plan must include (1) curriculum setting, (2) engagement, and (3) business planning [63].

Curriculum Setting/Design

A surgical skills curriculum needs to address multiple domains of learning: cognitive aspects (anatomy, instrument function, surgical steps), behavioral aspects (communication, composure, leadership), and technical proficiency (psychomotor skills and clinical experience) [63, 78]. A simulation curriculum in gynecology also needs to encompass all of these domains. Ideally, educators should collaborate to develop such a curriculum and then be able to have all trainees follow the same schedule. In order for a curriculum to be accepted nationally, there needs to be a predesigned template with guidance on use and basic equipment. As it stands now, there are some surgical societies or colleges that define requirements for skills training and are working on a predesigned curriculum for its members, but all hospitals or institutions are not necessarily obliged to implement these requirements in their training programs [79].

Engagement

It is important that educators and trainers find methods of engaging trainees. Self-motivation is a factor for the successful use of simulation training, but internal trainee motivation varies from person to person [80]. Understanding this basic principle and then developing methods to encourage and engage our trainees will be critical for the success of simulation training in gynecology. Trainees may still have the mindset of the Halstedian apprenticeship model of "see one, do one, teach one" and having a proctor present to "teach" them as the most effective way to learn, and not take the initiative to learn on their own [81]. Focus on independent practice on simulation modalities needs to be encouraged and fostered. One accepted method is to establish expectations of trainees to complete a standardized training module in simulation that is both introductory and procedural based, obtain proficiency in the simulation, and then test that proficiency before allowing them into the actual OR [73].

Business Planning

The expense of simulation training that encompasses simulators, physical space, technician time, and educator time is another common obstacle to implementation. The best method to approach the cost of simulation training is to balance it by the possibility of tangible financial savings [82, 83]. Evidence from obstetrics and other disciplines have shown improvement in patient safety and better outcomes. Simulation in gynecology may not only improve patient safety and provide women with better outcomes but also reduce health service costs by increasing clinical throughput [63, 84].

National Organizations

The American College of Obstetricians and Gynecologists (ACOG) has committed to simulation training and supports its utility across our discipline for students, residents, Junior Fellows, and Fellows. From the beginning, it was recognized that there was inconsistency in standards for simulation in our specialty. Because of this, the ACOG Education Division created a clinical simulation consortium that includes institutions from across the country with advanced OB/GYN simulation programs. The initial mission of this consortium was to develop and implement simulation-based curricula to assist residency programs to teach and improve residents' clinical performance. This curriculum is presently being standardized and validated across consortium members. Once completed, it will be made available to all residency programs in the USA. After this, the consortium will continue to work with ACOG on how to expand simulation training for the specialty.

Conclusion

Simulation training is a cornerstone for training all levels of providers in basic and advanced skills and emergencies in obstetrics and gynecology. It has application in the acquisition of technical skills as well as being a key part of effective teamwork training. As practitioners, educators, and trainees, we must become part of the ongoing programs of self-learning, assessment, and advancement if we are to remain relevant and current in our specialty. The field has grown exponentially in the past 10 years, and this will continue for the foreseeable future. It is an exciting time as evidence continues to be published that emphasizes the improved patient outcomes.

References

1. Macedonia CR, Gherman RB, Satin AJ. Simulation laboratories for training in obstetrics and gynecology. Obstet Gynecol. 2003;102:388–92.
2. Gelbart NR. The king's midwife: a history and mystery of Madame du Coudray. Berkeley: University of California Press; 1998. p. 16–7.
3. Quality patient care on labor and delivery: a call to action. Available at: http://www.acog.org/About_ACOG/ACOG_Departments/Patient_Safety_and_Quality_Improvement/~/media/F23BCE9264BF4F1681C1EB553DCA32F4.ashx. Accessed 29 Dec 2011.
4. Zubair I, Marcotte M, Weinstein L, Brost B. A novel amniocentesis model for learning stereotactic skills. Am J Obstet Gynecol. 2006;194(3):846–8.
5. Maher JE, Kleinman GE, Lile W, Tolaymat L, Steele D, Bernard J. The construction and utility of an amniocentesis trainer. Am J Obstet Gynecol. 1998;179(5):1225–7.
6. Duriez C, Lamy D, Chaillou C. A parallel manipulator as a haptic interface solution for amniocentesis simulation. In: IEEE international workshop on robot and human interactive communication, Bordeaux-Paris; 2001. pp. 176–81.
7. Pittini B, Oepkess D, Macrury K, Reznick R, Beyene J, Windrim R. Teaching invasive perinatal procedures: assessment of a high fidelity simulator-based curriculum. Ultrasound Obstet Gynecol. 2002;19:478–83.
8. Deering S, Brown J, Hodor J, Satin AJ. Simulation training and resident performance of singleton vaginal breech delivery. Obstet Gynecol. 2006;107(1):86–9.
9. Lipman SS, Daniels KI, Arafeh J, Halamek LP. The case for OBLS: a simulation-based obstetric life support program. Semin Perinat. 2011;35:74–9.
10. Daniels K, Lipman S, Harney K, Arafeh J, Druzin M. Use of simulation based team training for obstetric crises in resident education. Simul Healthcare. 2008;3:154–60.

11. Fisher N, Eisen LA, Bayya JV, et al. Improved performance of maternal-fetal medicine staff after maternal cardiac arrest simulation-based training. Am J Obstet Gynecol. 2011;205:239.e1–5.
12. Vellanki VS, Gillellamudi SB. Teaching surgical skills in obstetrics using a cesarean section simulator – bringing simulation to life. Adv Med Educ Pract. 2010;1:85–8.
13. Lipman S, Daniels K, Cohen SE, Carvalho B. Labor room setting compared with the operating room for simulated perimortem cesarean delivery: a randomized controlled trial. Obstet Gynecol. 2011;118:1090–4.
14. Ville Y, Cooper M, Revel A, Frydman R, Nicolaide KH. Development of a training model for ultrasound-guided invasive procedures in fetal medicine. Ultrasound Obstet Gynecol. 1995;5: 180–3.
15. Tongprasert F, Tongson T, Wanapirak C, Sirichotiyakul S, Piyamongkol W, Chanprapaph P. Experience of the first 50 cases of cordocentesis after training with model. J Med Assoc Thai. 2005;88(6):728–33.
16. Thompson S, Neal S, Clark V. Clinical risk management in obstetrics: eclampsia drills. BMJ. 2004;328:269–71.
17. Guise JM, Lowe NK, Deering S, Osterweil BS, O'Haire C, Irwin L, et al. Mobile in-situ obstetric emergency simulation and teamwork training to improve maternal-fetal safety in hospitals. Jt Comm J. 2010;36(10):443–53.
18. Daniels K, Parness AJ. Development and use of mechanical devices for simulation of seizure and hemorrhage in obstetrical team training. Simul Healthcare. 2008;3(1):42–6.
19. Deering SH, Rosen MA, Salas E, King HB. Building team and technical competency for obstetric emergencies: the Mobile Obstetric Emergencies Simulator (MOES) System. Simul Healthcare. 2009;4:166–73.
20. Ellis D, Crofts JF, Hunt LP, Read M, Fox R, James M. Hospital, simulation center, and teamwork training for eclampsia management: a randomized controlled trial. Obstet Gynecol. 2008;111:723–31.
21. Frankman EA, Wang L, Bunker CH, Lowder JL. Episiotomy in the United States: has anything changed? Am J Obstet Gynecol. 2009;200(5):573.e1–7. Epub 2009 Feb 24.
22. McLennan MT, Melick CF, Clancy SL, Artal R. Episiotomy and perineal repair. An evaluation of resident education and experience. J Reprod Med. 2002;47(12):1025–30.
23. Freeman J, Dobbie A. The "sponge perineum:" an innovative method of teaching fourth-degree obstetric perineal laceration repair to family medicine residents. Fam Med. 2006;38(8):542–4.
24. Woodman PJ, Nager CW. From the simple to the sublime: incorporating surgical models into your surgical curriculum. Obstet Gynecol Clin North Am. 2006;33:267–81.
25. Nielsen PE, Foglia LM, Mandel LS, Chow GE. Objective structured assessment of technical skills for episiotomy repair. Am J Obstet Gynecol. 2003;189:1257–60.
26. Uppal S, Hermanli O, Rowland J, Hernandez E, Dandolu V. Resident competency in obstetric anal sphincter laceration repair. Obstet Gynecol. 2010;115(2):305–9.
27. Yeomans ER. Operative vaginal delivery. Obstet Gynecol. 2010; 115(3):645–53.
28. Leslie KK, Dipasquale-Lehnerz P, Smith M. Obstetric forceps training using visual feedback and the isometric strength testing unit. Obstet Gynecol. 2005;105(2):377–82.
29. Dupuis O, Decullier E, Clerc J, et al. Does forceps training on a birth simulator allow obstetricians to improve forceps blade placement? Eur J Obstet Gynecol Reprod Biol. 2011;159(2):305–9.
30. Joint Commission. Preventing maternal death. Sentinel event alert. Jan 2010;(44):1–4.
31. Ge L. The Confidential Enquiry into Maternal and Child Health (CEMACH). Saving mothers' lives: reviewing maternal deaths to make motherhood safer – 2003-2005. The seventh report on confidential enquiries into maternal deaths in the United Kingdom. London: CEMACH; 2007.
32. Deering SH, Chinn M, Hodor J, Benedetti T, Mandel L, Goff B. Use of a postpartum hemorrhage simulator for instruction and evaluation of residents. J Graduate Med Educ. 2009;1(2):260–3.
33. Maslovitz S, Barkai G, Lessing JB, et al. Improved accuracy of postpartum blood loss estimation as assessed by simulation. Acta Obstet Gynecol Scand. 2008;87:929–34.
34. Bose P, Regan F, Paterson-Brown S. Improving the accuracy of estimated blood loss at obstetric haemorrhage using clinical reconstructions. BJOG. 2006;113:919–24.
35. Dildy GA, Paine AR, George NC, Velasco C. Estimated blood loss: can teaching significantly improve visual estimation? Obstet Gynecol. 2004;104(3):601–6.
36. Holmstrom SW, Downes K, Mayer JC, Learman LA. Simulation training in an obstetric clerkship. Obstet Gynecol. 2011;118(3): 649–54.
37. Dayal AK, Fisher N, Magrane D, Goffman D, Bernstein PS, Katz NT. Simulation training improves medical student's learning experiences when performing real vaginal deliveries. Simul Healthcare. 2009;4(3):155–9.
38. Deering S, Poggi S, Macedonia C, Gherman R, Satin AJ. Improving resident competency in the management of shoulder dystocia with simulation training. Obstet Gynecol. 2004;103(6):1224–8.
39. Crofts JF, Bartlett C, Ellis D, Hunt LP, Fox R, Draycott TJ. Training for shoulder dystocia: a trial of simulation using low-fidelity and high-fidelity mannequins. Obstet Gynecol. 2006;108(6):1477–85.
40. Draycott TJ, Crofts JF, Ash JP, Wilson LV, Yard E, Sibanda T, et al. Improving neonatal outcome through practical shoulder dystocia training. Obstet Gynecol. 2008;112(1):14–20.
41. Grobman WA, Miller D, Burke C, Hornbogen A, Tam K, Costello R. Outcomes associated with introduction of a shoulder dystocia protocol. Am J Obstet Gynecol. 2011;205(6):513–7.
42. Deering S, Poggi S, Hodor J, Macedonia C, Satin AJ. Evaluation of resident's delivery notes after a simulated shoulder dystocia. Obstet Gynecol. 2004;104:667–70.
43. Crofts JF, Bartlett C, Ellis D, et al. Documentation of simulated shoulder dystocia: accurate and complete? BJOG. 2008;115: 1303–3018.
44. Goffman D, Heo H, Chazotte C, Merkatz IR, Bernstein PS. Using simulation training to improve shoulder dystocia documentation. Obstet Gynecol. 2008;112:1284–7.
45. Siassakos D, Hasafa Z, Sibanda T, Fox R, Donald F, Winter C, et al. Retrospective cohort study of diagnosis-delivery interval with umbilical cord prolapse: the effect of team training. BJOG. 2009;116:1089–96.
46. Joint Commission on Accreditation of Healthcare Organizations. Sentinel event alert. Joint commission on accreditation of healthcare organizations. 2004;(30)
47. Leape LL, Berwick DM. Five years after to err is human: what have we learned? JAMA. 2005;293:2384–90.
48. Guise JM, Lowe NK, Deering S, et al. Mobile in situ obstetric emergency simulation and teamwork training to improve maternal-fetal safety in hospitals. Jt Comm J Qual Patient Saf. 2010;36(10): 443–53.
49. Merien AER, van de Ven J, Mol BW, Houterman S, Oie SG. Multidisciplinary team training in a simulation setting for acute obstetric emergencies. Am J Obstet Gynecol. 2010;115(5): 1021–31.
50. Riley W, Davis S, Miller K, Hansen H, Sainfort F, Sweet R. Didactic and simulation nontechnical skills team training to improve perinatal patient outcomes in a community hospital. Jt Comm J Qual Patient Saf. 2011;37(8):357–64.
51. Bender JG. In situ simulation for systems testing in newly constructed perinatal facilities. Semin Perinatol. 2011;35(2):80–3.
52. Siassakos D, Crofts JF, Winter C, Weiner CP, Draycott TJ. The active components of effective training in obstetric emergencies. BJOG. 2009;16:1028–32.

53. Smith M. Simulation and education in gynecologic surgery. Obstet Gynecol Clin North Am. 2011;38:733–40.
54. Sara FS, Parihar RS. Sushruta: the first plastic surgeon in 600 BC. Internet J Plast Surg. 2007;4:2.
55. Rosen KR. The history of medical simulation. J Crit Care. 2008;23:157–66.
56. Reznick RK. Teaching and testing technical skills. Am J Surg. 1993;3:358–61.
57. Darzi A, Smith S, Taffinder N. Assessing operative skill needs to become more objective. BMJ. 1999;318:887.
58. Rosser JC, Rosser LE, Savalgi RS. Skill acquisition and assessment for laparoscopic surgery. Arch Surg. 1997;132:200–4.
59. Scott PJ, Bergen PC, Rege RV, et al. Laparoscopic training on bench models; better and more cost effective than operating room experience? J Am Coll Surg. 2000;191:272–83.
60. Hyltander A, Liljegren E, Rhoden PH, et al. The transfer of basic skills learned in a laparoscopic simulator to the operating room. Surg Endosc. 2002;16:1324–8.
61. US Institute of Medicine; Committee on Quality of Health Care in America. To err is human: building a safer health system. Washington: National Academy Press; 1999.
62. US Institute of Medicine; Committee on Quality of Health Care in America. Crossing the quality chasm: a new health system for the 21st century. Washington: National Academy Press; 2001.
63. Burden C, Oestergaard J, Larsen CR. Integration of laparoscopic virtual-reality simulation into gynaecology training. BJOG. 2011;118 Suppl 3:5–10.
64. Larsen CR, Sorensen JL, Ottesen BS. Simulation training of laparoscopic skills in gynaecology. Ugeskr Laeger. 2006;168:2664–8.
65. Ballantyne GH, Moll F. The da Vinci telerobotic surgical system: the virtual operative field and the telepresence surgery. Surg Clinc North Am. 2003;83(6):1293–304.
66. Glickson J. Using simulation to train oncology surgeons: gynecologic oncologists practice OR's touch, feel and pressures. Bull Am Coll Surg. 2011;96(3):32–8.
67. Soni VK. Da Vinci robotic surgery: pros and cons. Health Liv. Available at: http://www.steadyhealth.com/articles/Da_Vinci_Robotic_Surgery_Pros_and_Cons_a1259.html. Accessed 19 Dec 2011.
68. Jacobsen C, Elli I, Hogan S. Robotic surgery update. Surg Endosc. 2004;18:1186–91.
69. Boehm DH, Detter C, Arnold MB, et al. Robotically assisted coronary bypass surgery with the ZEUS telemanipulator system. Semin Thor Card Surg. 2003;15(2):112–20.
70. Moorthy K, Munz Y, Sarker SK, Darzi A. Objective assessment of technical skills in surgery. BMJ. 2003;327:1032–7.
71. Powers K, Rehrig ST, Schwaitzberg SD, Callery MP, Jones DB. Seasoned surgeons assessed in a laparoscopic surgical crisis. J Gastrointest Surg. 2009;13:994–1003.
72. Aggarwal R, Tully A, Grantcharov T, et al. Virtual reality simulation training can improve technical skills during laparoscopic salpingectomy for ectopic pregnancy. BJOG. 2006;113:1382–7.
73. Larsen CR, Soerensen JL, Grantcharov TP, et al. Effect of virtual reality training on laparoscopic surgery: randomized controlled trial. BMJ. 2009;338:61802. doi:10.1136/bmj.b2074-20.
74. Gurusamy KS, Aggarwal R, Palanivelu L, Davidson BR. Virtual reality training for surgical trainees in laparoscopic surgery. Cochrane Database Sys Rev. 2009;(1):CD006575.
75. Arain NA, Hogg DC, Gala RB, et al. Construct and face validity of the American College of Surgeons/Association of Program Directors in Surgery laparoscopic troubleshooting team training exercises. Am J Surg. 2012;203(1):54–62.
76. Scott DJ. Laparoscopic troubleshooting module. In: Dunnington G, editor. American College of Surgeons (ACS)/Association of Program Directors in Surgery (APDS) surgical skills curriculum for residents phase III. 2008. Available from: http://www.facs.org/education/surgicalskills/html. Accessed: 11 Dec 2011.
77. Kahol K, Satava RM, Ferrara J, et al. Effect of short-term pretrial practice on surgical proficiency in simulated environments: a randomized trial of the "preoperative warm up" effect. J Am Coll Surg. 2009;208:255–68.
78. Seymour NE, Gallagher AG, Roman SA, et al. Virtual reality training improves operating room performance; results of a randomized, double-blinded study. Ann Surg. 2002;236:458–63.
79. Schreuder HW, Oei G, Maas M, et al. Implementation of simulation in surgical practice: minimally invasive surgery has taken the lead: the Dutch experience. Med Teach. 2011;33:105–15.
80. Van Dongen KW, van der Wal WA, Rinkes IH, et al. Virtual reality training for endoscopic surgery: voluntary or obligatory? Surg Endosc. 2008;22:664–7.
81. Auguste T, Henderson B, Loyd K. Protected proctored time on laparoscopic kits, does it help? Poster presentation APGO/CREOG annual meeting, March 2011, San Antonio.
82. Warren O, Kinross J, Paraskeva P, et al. Emergency laparoscopy-current best practice. World J Emerg Surg. 2006;31:1–24.
83. Kern K. Medico-legal perspectives on laparoscopic surgery. Current review of minimally invasive surgery. Philadelphia: Current Medicine; 1998. Chapter 21.
84. The productive operating theatre. Coventry: NHS Institute for Innovation and Improvement; 2009.

Simulation in Ophthalmology

31

Gina M. Rogers, Bonnie Henderson, and Thomas A. Oetting

Introduction

Simulation has been an important part of ophthalmic training for many years [1–3]. Generally, simulation-based training has focused on technical surgical training with much less emphasis on other aspects of ophthalmic competency such as exam skills, patient-physician communication, and professionalism. Simulation in ophthalmic surgical training is conventionally associated with "wet labs" which use cadaver or animal eyes. More recently, ophthalmic simulation has expanded to include cognitive simulation and sophisticated computer-based surgical simulators that are proving useful in ophthalmic training. Though a relatively young branch of medical simulation in the modern sense, ophthalmology is a fertile ground for innovation using simulators.

Like most complex tasks, ophthalmic surgery is associated with a significant learning curve. To this end, several studies have demonstrated that reduced complication rates can result from deliberate practice and clinical experience [4–7]. Randleman et al. found that complication rates were lower in a group of residents with 80 or more cases compared to those with fewer than 80 cases of cataract surgery experience [5]. Teus et al. showed that the first 28 cases with a type of refractive surgery were less safe than subsequent cases [6], and Bell et al. showed that higher volume surgeons had a lower complication rate than those performing fewer cases [7]. Perhaps simulation can be utilized to give novice trainees the equivalent experience necessary for improved patient outcomes while reducing patient risk during their preliminary training.

Ophthalmic surgery is complex and is therefore difficult to teach [8–10]. Most types of ophthalmic surgery are performed under magnification of some sort (e.g., loupe or operating microscope). There is a significant learning curve and period of adjustment of the user's eyes in this sort of surgery. Ophthalmology, compared to other divisions of surgery, poses additional difficulty to the trainee and trainer as the operative field is small and often only one set of hands can be operating at any given time. Additionally, ophthalmic surgery often requires the simultaneous use of all extremities to control various equipment (e.g., instruments in both hands, one foot on the microscope pedal, and one foot on the instrument pedal). In this chapter, we discuss the uses of and evidence for simulation in ophthalmology training from the traditional (i.e., wet lab simulation) to the modern (i.e., computer-based simulation). We also discuss potential ways in which these modalities can be employed to benefit trainees.

G.M. Rogers, MD (✉)
Department of Ophthalmology and Visual Sciences, University of Iowa Hospitals and Clinics, 200 Hawkins Drive, Iowa City, IA 52242, USA
e-mail: ginamrogers@gmail.com

B. Henderson, MD
Department of Ophthalmology, Harvard Medical School, Boston, MA, USA

Ophthalmic Consultants of Boston, 52 Second Avenue, Suite 2500, Waltham, MA 02451, USA
e-mail: bahenderson@eyeboston.com

T.A. Oetting, MS, MD
Department of Ophthalmology and Visual Sciences, University of Iowa Hospitals and Clinics, 200 Hawkins Drive, Iowa City, IA 52242, USA

Surgical Service Line, Department of Ophthalmology, Veterans Medical Center, UIHC-Ophthalmology, 200 Hawkins Drive, Iowa City, IA 52242, USA
e-mail: thomas-oetting@uiowa.edu

The Science of Ophthalmology Simulation

Wet Lab Simulation

Wet labs have been an important part of ophthalmic education for years [1–3, 11–14]. The wet lab is typically a simulation of the operating room that includes a microscope, instruments, and porcine cadaver or artificial eyes. As animal and cadaver eyes are used in these labs, they are typically not located in the actual operating room and the use of a separate set of instruments is required. In some programs the wet lab

A.I. Levine et al. (eds.), *The Comprehensive Textbook of Healthcare Simulation*, DOI 10.1007/978-1-4614-5993-4_31, © Springer Science+Business Media New York 2013

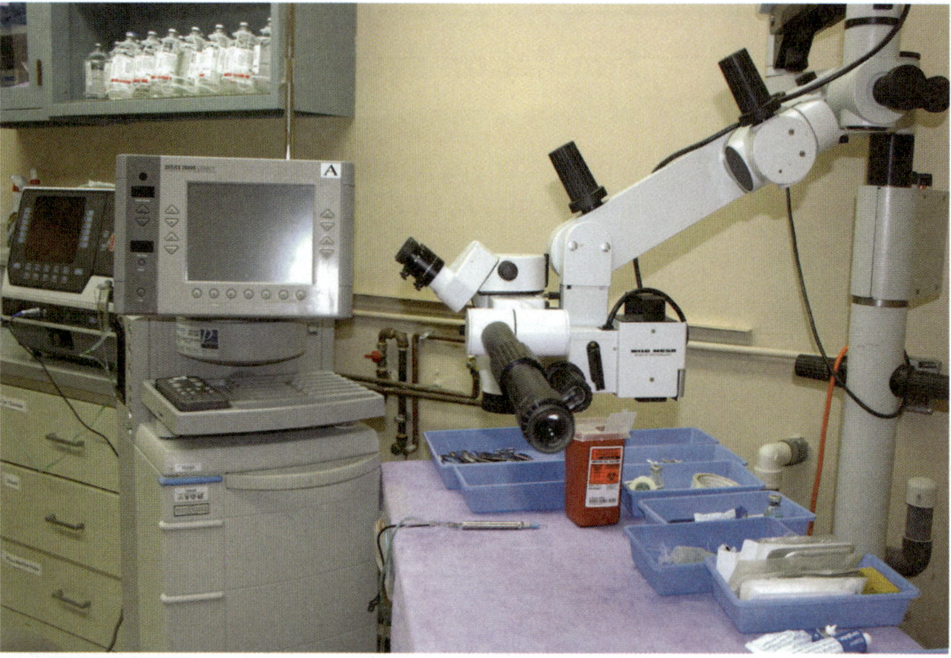

Fig. 31.1 Example of basic wet lab. This operating microscope has a second ocular for a second person to observe

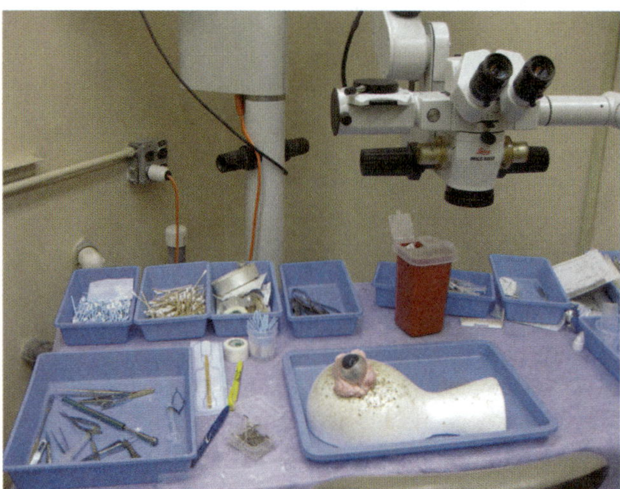

Fig. 31.2 View of wet lab setup with a porcine eye. It is evident that the porcine eye is much larger than the human eye

Table 31.1 Summary of First-Year Resident Iowa Wet Laboratory Curriculum

Objectives: During the first-year resident's rotation at a given center, the resident will have 5 half-day sessions in the wet laboratory under faculty supervision. Additional practice will be required and this is the responsibility of the resident. The resident is also required to read *Cataract Surgery for Greenhorns* by Oetting and *Phacodynamics* by Seibel prior to the first wet lab session:
1. Demonstrate fine motor and proprioception kills under the operating microscope. 2. Demonstrate proficiency in working in small surgical field alone and with an assistant. 3. Demonstrate knowledge of the various phacoemulsification machines and settings of each machine. 4. Demonstrate phacoemulsification machine and operating microscope pedal functions. 5. Demonstrate performance of five clear corneal and scleral incisions on animal eye. 6. Identify the steps of phacoemulsification. 7. Demonstrate the performance of the steps of phacoemulsification on animal eye. 8. Identify the various types of ophthalmic sutures. 9. Demonstrate placing corneal, scleral, conjunctival, and skin sutures.

is available at all times in dedicated labs, and in other programs the wet lab is set up a few times a year to allow practice. Similarly, curricula may or may not be well defined for the use of such labs [15] (see Figs. 31.1 and 31.2).

Lee et al. outlined the structured wet lab program developed at the University of Iowa [15]. In this program, a set of goals and objectives is established for trainees. This allows assessments tied to the objectives to ensure that the learner is ready for the next step. The program proposes a set of practical and didactic tests to ensure competence. This allows residents to learn skills at the appropriate time and provides a more reliable skill set prior to the resident's first real case in the operating room. One of the most important features and logistically challenging components of this program is having faculty available for significant portions of the wet lab training, which at best would occur during normal hours and not late at night or on weekends when faculty are less available (see Table 31.1).

Fisher outlined a structured skills "obstacle course" wet lab with specific stations to assess residents' skills on a variety of surgical tasks [16]. The "obstacle course" was designed to simulate three surgical procedures: (1) temporal artery biopsy and skin suturing, (2) muscle recession, and (3) phacoemulsification wound construction and suturing. All the procedures were performed in a wet lab using a pig foot and eye. The pig's foot was prepared for the temporal artery biopsy and skin suturing section by inserting a piece of red plastic tubing into the superficial facial to simulate the artery. At each station the resident was given a list detailing the required steps of the test and videotaped at each station. The videos were later reviewed by various experienced surgeons and given a score. The authors conclude that this wet lab obstacle course demonstrated development of an objective and standardized test of beginning surgical skills and established face and content validity for ophthalmic surgery [16].

Henderson et al. outlined the key components of an effective ophthalmic wet lab: setting up the physical space, establishing appropriate faculty and curriculum, obtaining the practice eye, stabilizing the eye, preparing the eye, and funding the wet lab [11]. Having a separate and dedicated space for the wet lab allows the trainee to practice when appropriate and when faculty and the resident are available. As mentioned above, a structured program is a key to a successful wet lab program [11, 15]. Practice eyes are sometimes expensive or hard to obtain. Typically, porcine eyes are used but grapes, sheep eyes, cadaver eyes, cadaver eyes with glued-on contact lenses, and plastic-fabricated eyes can be used for simulating the live human eye in the wet lab [15, 17–20]. Various techniques have been outlined to make the porcine eye behave more like the senile human eye, such as the application of fixative solutions and microwave energy [11]. Each of these techniques has its advantage in some capacity in attempting to simulate a human eye; however, no single technique or model is as good of a replacement as operating on a live, human eye. One of the most difficult issues of establishing a wet lab, however, is simply funding the lab which requires space, instruments, and most importantly faculty time. Still, few simulation modalities are as tried and true as the wet lab, and as such, this classic simulation has staying power.

Computer-Based Simulation

Advances in computer technology have led to increasingly sophisticated virtual reality simulators for surgical and procedural preparation. As outlined in this text, simulation training has been gaining popularity among many surgical subspecialties and in the education of teaching procedural tasks to nonsurgical residents. In ophthalmology, there are currently two commercially available ophthalmic simulators: PhacoVision® (Melerit Medical; http://www.meleritmedical.com/) and Eyesi® (VRmagic Holding AG; http://www.vrmagic.com/en/eyesi/) (Figs. 31.3, 31.4, 31.5, and 31.6). These devices are primarily aimed at cataract surgery; however, the initial versions of the Eyesi® simulator were designed to simulate vitreoretinal surgery [21–25]. Although both simulators have many similarities and functions, our discussion will focus on the Eyesi® simulator since it is the most widely studied device of the two [24, 26–29].

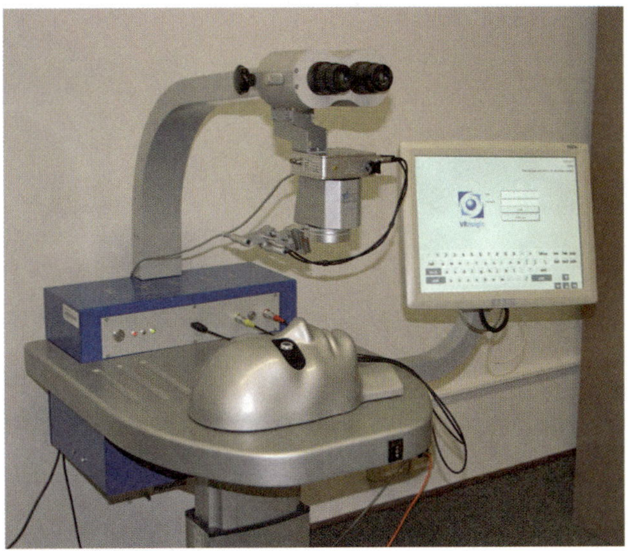

Fig. 31.3 The Eyesi® simulator. The system has oculars and operating scope model. The adjacent monitor will project the same view as the participant views through the ocular. There are two foot pedals designed in a similar fashion to the operating scope: foot pedal and the phacoemulsification machine pedal. The head can be positioned so that the operator can sit either temporally or superiorly

There are significant advantages in the use of virtual reality ophthalmologic simulators for training. The computer-based simulators such as the Eyesi® are cleaner than wet labs, allow for quick setup of simulation exercises, and do not require acquisition of practice eyes and facilities to support biological specimens. Trainees may position themselves at the simulator as they would be sitting in the operating room. A realistic microscope and instrument foot pedals as well as instruments for each hand are incorporated into the simulator. For the novice surgeon, positioning at the microscope, managing instrumentation, and maneuvering in the operative field simultaneously can present a major challenge. The simulation of using all extremities at once can be a very valuable experience especially if aided with faculty feedback (see Figs. 31.7 and 31.8).

Both computer simulation devices have a computerized eye model that includes a lens, iris, capsule, and cornea. The eye model is visible through the oculars, creating a stereo image to simulate the depth of the structures within the eye. The software senses the position of instruments and provides feedback or "grades" based on tissue handling and whether or not there was unintended damage of structures such as the cornea. The device provides an immediate numerical score on specific tasks (Capsulorhexis, Nucleofractis). Which can be used to track the progress of the trainee (see Figs. 31.9, 31.10, and 31.11).

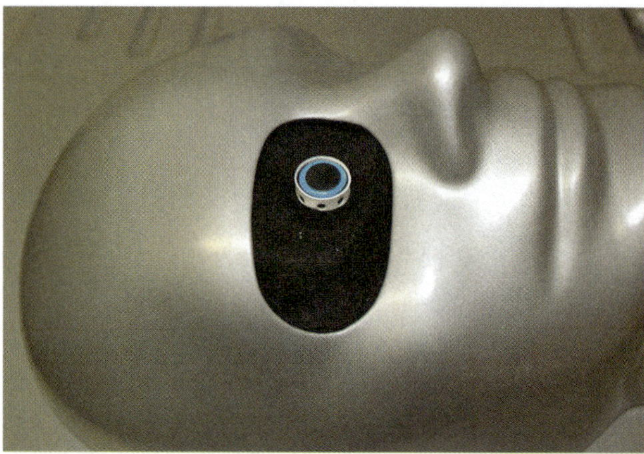

Fig. 31.4 The Eyesi® simulated patient and eye. Each of the ports on the outer aspect of the eye will allow for placement of one of the system's instruments

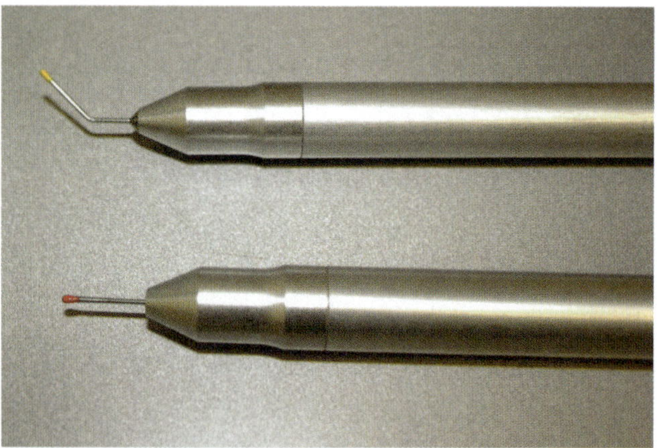

Fig. 31.5 Examples of the "handpieces" of the Eyesi® simulator. Once placed through one of the ports of the model eye, the instrument will appear as the needed instrument for the task i.e., capsulorhexis forceps, irrigation cannula, and phacoemulsification hand piece

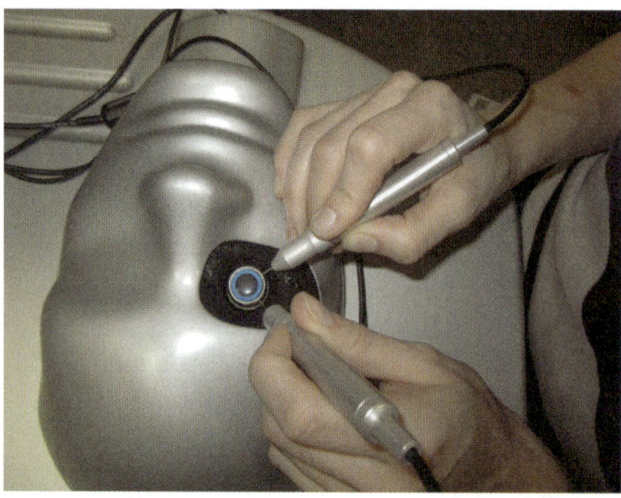

Fig. 31.6 The "handpieces" positioned within the simulated eye

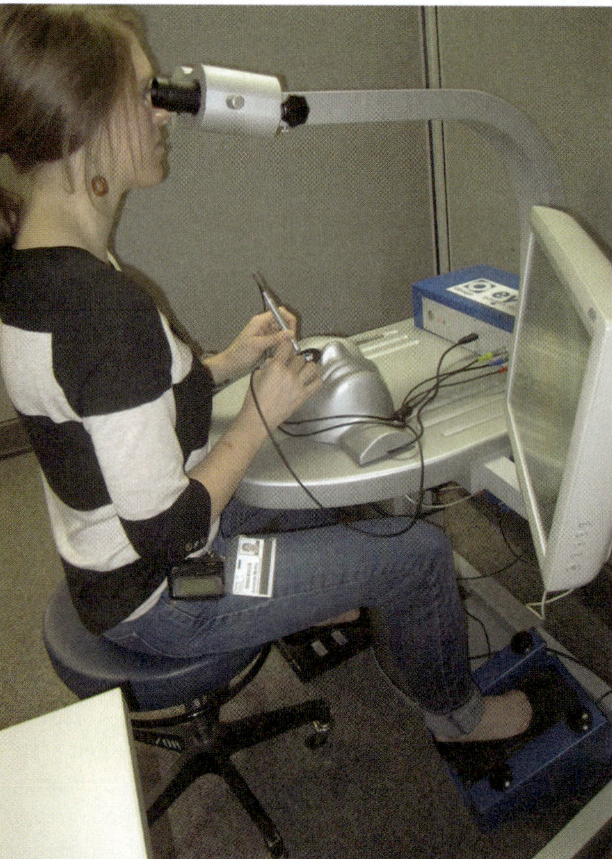

Fig. 31.7 Example of a trainee positioned at the Eyesi®. You can see that the trainee is positioned as if she was in the operating room: each foot upon the appropriate foot pedal, chair and ocular height adjusted to allow comfort, and hands positioned with instruments in the eye. There is a projected view of what the trainee is seeing/doing on the computer monitor alongside the trainee permitting someone else to observe

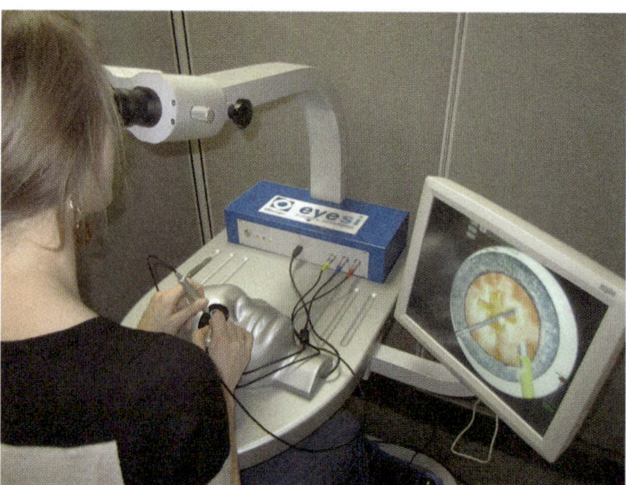

Fig. 31.8 Example of a trainee positioned at the Eyesi®

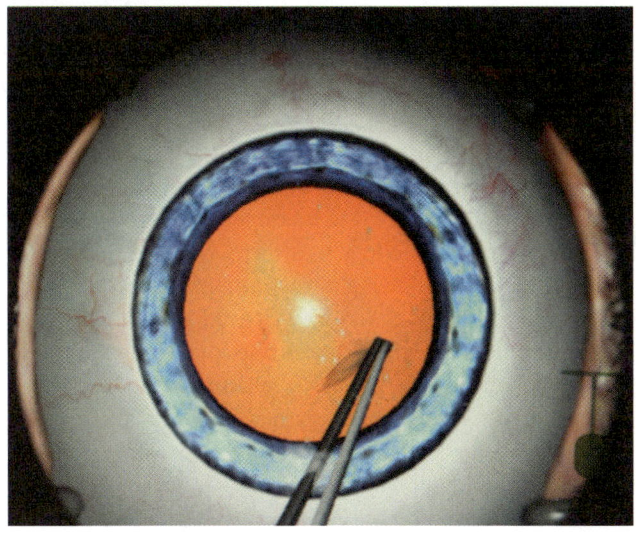

Fig. 31.9 Eyesi® simulation of creating a capsulorhexis

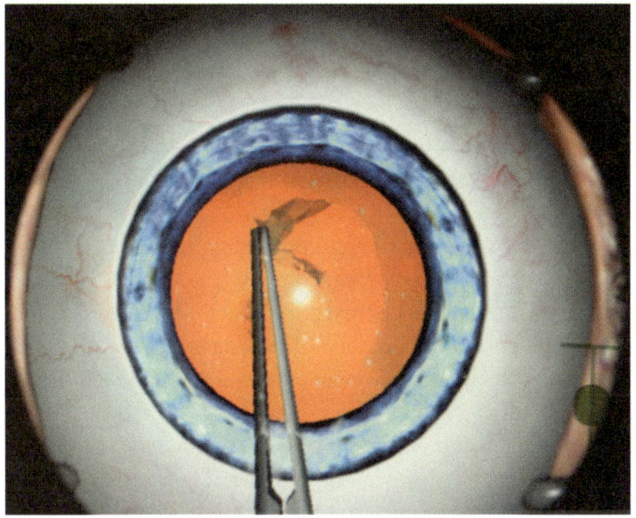

Fig. 31.10 Eyesi® simulation of creating a capsulorhexis

Advantages of Virtual Simulation

As outlined above, a wet lab offers a wide variety of opportunities for the trainee to practice surgical technique. However, setup for the wet lab often requires significant time and sometimes preparation of the tissue itself. This limits the ability to rapidly repeat a specific task, such as creating the capsulorhexis. With a wet lab, trainees may only be able to practice the capsulorhexis 2 or 3 times in an evening session before the biological eye is no longer usable to tissue disruption. With the Eyesi simulator, the resident can deliberately practice the capsulorhexis 100 times in an evening. The resident or faculty can set up technically difficult situations to allow for repeated practice which is not limited by setup time or delicate tissue disruption.

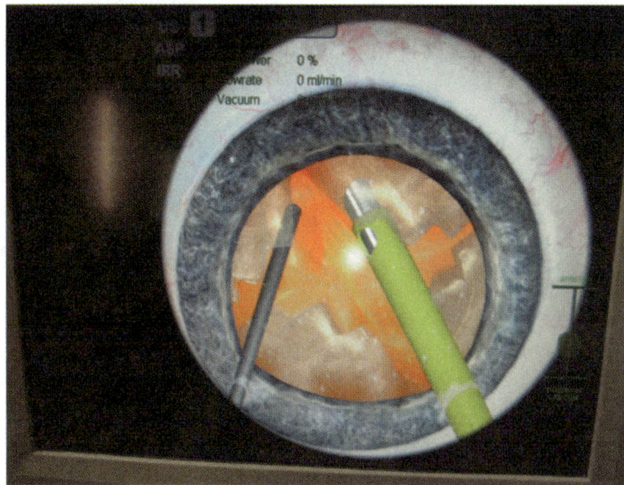

Fig. 31.11 Eyesi® simulation of nucleofractis

Another drawback to the wet lab is that for the training ophthalmic surgeon, feedback on performance is essential. A trainee can perform a given task repeatedly, but if they are executing the task improperly or stressing other tissues, then the practice of the improper technique is not beneficial. To ensure this does not occur, an experienced educator would need to be present observing and providing feedback to the trainee, which would require a significant amount of dedicated faculty time. While faculty presence is important in certain phases of computer simulation training, much can be done without faculty supervision after a set of exercises are established and real-time scoring is enabled. The simulators have software developed to "grade" the performance of trainees, and the trainee can indepedancy monitor their progress very easily and use this to train to competency.

The Evidence for Virtual Simulation

Several studies have demonstrated content and construct validity of the Eyesi® simulator. Mahr showed that the simulator's tremor and forceps module had validity [28]. Using the forceps module, experienced surgeons achieved statistically significant better total scores, with lower total task time and instrument-in-eye measurements than did novices. For the anti-tremor module, experienced surgeons also achieved statistically significant better total scores, with lower task time and instrument-in-eye time measurements than did novices. As such, the Eyesi simulator represents a very useful device with established validity.

One of the most difficult tasks for beginning cataract surgeon is creating the curvilinear capsulorhexis [8, 9]. In addition, an adequately sized continuous curvilinear capsulorhexis is critical to subsequent steps and long-term centration of the intraocular lens. Privett published a study which showed face validity for the Eyesi® simulator and the capsulorhexis portion of the procedure [30]. This study compared experienced surgeons to medical students on performance of the capsulorhexis on the Eyesi®. Experienced surgeons achieved statistically significant better scores in all parameters at the medium level, with better centering, less corneal injury, fewer spikes, less time operating without a red reflex, better roundness of the capsulorhexis, and less time completing tasks than novices. In general, all of the experienced surgeons that participated believed the simulator would be a useful training tool for beginning cataract surgeons (see Fig. 31.6).

A study conducted by the Department of Ophthalmology at the University of Tuebingen, Germany, compared performance in the wet lab between a control group and a group that had experience with the Eyesi® computer simulator [31]. Initially, the two groups were asked to perform the capsulorhexis in the wet lab. The group that was assigned to the virtual reality simulation then underwent training with two trials of the simulation modules. Both groups were then again asked to perform the capsulorhexis in the wet lab, and the group that was exposed to the virtual reality simulation showed statistically significant improvement in their median wet lab capsulorhexis overall performance score compared to controls. The capsulorhexis performance of virtual reality–trained students and residents were also more consistent with a lower standard deviation of scores compared to controls [31].

Senior residents find nucleofractis (i.e., breaking up and removing the nucleus of the cataractous lens) the most difficult step of the surgery [8]. A large portion of the difficulty in performing this task is that the novice surgeon is not accustomed to realizing the depth of the lens, successfully handling bimanual instrumentation, and manipulating nuclear fragments to safely remove the lens fragments. Belyea et al. found that residents who were exposed to the Eyesi® simulator were able to more quickly progress though the nucleofractis step of cataract surgery [27]. Belyea et al. reviewed 592 surgeries performed by residents in their program staffed by the same attending surgeon. Residents were divided into a simulator group and a non-simulator group based on the inclusion or absence of the eye-surgery simulator during their training period. They found a statistical between-group difference in mean phaco time, adjusted phaco time, and percentage phaco power. Regression analysis showed a significantly steeper slope of improvement in mean phaco time and power in the non-simulator group compared to the simulator group [27].

Interestingly, ophthalmic simulators have been used for a less traditional simulation studies. Waqar et al. studied the effect of fatigue on performance on the Eyesi® ophthalmic simulator [32]. Experienced surgeons received a standardized orientation and completed ten attempts on level-four forceps module of the Eyesi® simulator. To reduce the effect of the learning curve, a parameter "plateau" score was calculated for each surgeon (the average of their final four attempts). The surgeons then returned immediately after their scheduled surgery to complete ten more attempts on the same module, and similar parameters were recorded. The surgeons then repeated the module after a routine surgical day (197 min of operating time). The surgeon's simulator parameters were found to be improved, both total score and total time, concluding that there was no detrimental effect of fatigue following a routine operating room day. Park compared novice and experienced surgeons as they were exposed to a distracting exercise (performing arithmetic) while performing computer simulator modules [26]. Their study found that a distractive cognitive task reduced the ability of novice surgeons and expert surgeons to deal with that task, although their simulated surgical performance was not overtly compromised [26].

The continued advancement of computer technology and surgical simulators is exciting for ophthalmic surgeon educators as an adjunctive education tool. The ultimate role virtual reality will play in the evolution of ophthalmology surgical curriculum is still to be determined; it does appear that there are significant advantages to having this training opportunity.

The Art of Cognitive Simulation

Surgery involves coordination of cognitive and physical skills to successfully perform complex procedures. New residents are often overwhelmed during their first cases. Despite reading, watching videos, and observing surgical cases, they have not yet formed a complete mental map of each procedure including its major parts and all the small steps that comprise each part. They often do not understand the goal of each step or how the steps fit together. Their understanding can even be fragile; they are easily upset when a step does not go exactly as planned.

New residents often struggle to simply learn to make their hands (and sometimes feet) perform new, delicate maneuvers with a high cost of failure. This is aggravated by the fact that the preparatory activities are passive. Rather than learning these new physical skills through hands-on practice, until they are in the operating room, students mostly learn by reading or observation. This is somewhat akin to teaching someone to play baseball by having them spend months reading books about the game. Needless to say, this approach yields the expected results; residents who are performing surgery for the first time often lack the prerequisite cursor skills necessary to execute the simplest of procedural tasks.

Computer simulations enable us to eliminate the costs of failure while providing opportunities for practice in a way that helps residents develop more sophisticated and flexible knowledge bases. Simulation can be used to isolate the cognitive aspects of surgical tasks from the physical ones and, in

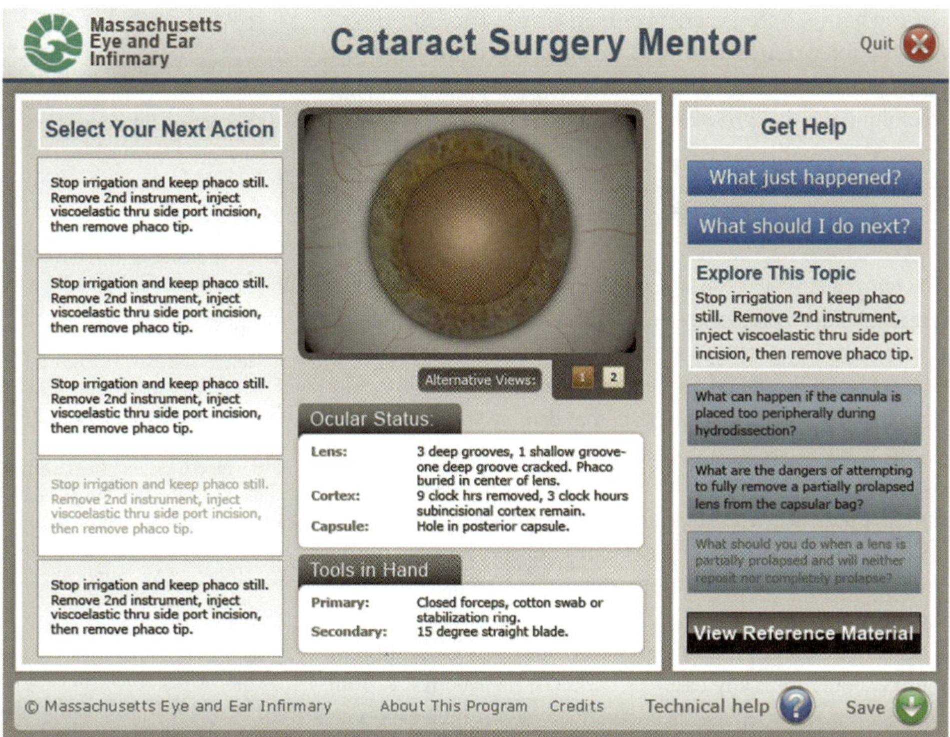

Fig. 31.12 Screen shot of the computer portion of the Massachusetts Eye and Ear Cataract Master®

doing so, reduce the cognitive load. For example, a simulation can enable students to practice just the cognitive aspects of a surgical procedure, having them make decisions about how the procedure should be executed without physically executing them. Unlike actual patients, simulated patients can be designed to focus students on the aspects of surgical procedures where errors and complications most commonly occur. By isolating the cognitive aspects of the task and facilitating practice within the safety of a simulation, the stress level, cognitive load, and time pressure on students can be more controlled. In addition, we can provide students with access to expert explanations addressing common errors and challenges.

A computer-based simulation program of cataract surgery designed to teach students the cognitive skills involved in the phacoemulsification procedure has been developed by the Massachusetts Eye and Ear Institute (MEEI) [33, 34]. This software which includes animation, video, and text is called the Massachusetts Eye and Ear Cataract Master® (Fig. 31.12). The software is based on an "immersive-story" curriculum. In brief, some of these principles are: (1) practice experience should be highly realistic, engaging students in the performance of authentic tasks in authentic roles and contexts, (2) students should be allowed to fail as they might in the real world since each such failure is a critical learning opportunity, and (3) at times of failure, students should get "just-in-time" feedback and support in the forms of stories and explanations from experts as well as through exposure to expert performance. This approach scaffolds learners by limiting the cognitive load they face when starting to learn cataract surgery. Learners can master the procedural sequences at a conceptual level but in a meaningful and memorable contextualized setting before having to worry about mastering them at a physical level.

The MEEI program is a learn-by-doing approach to teaching ophthalmology residents the cognitive skills involved in three approaches to phacoemulsification cataract surgery: scleral tunnel with divide and conquer, clear cornea with divide and conquer, and clear cornea with chopping techniques. The curriculum is designed to permit students to quickly recognize their misconceptions and knowledge gaps and then facilitate their expanded and revised understanding of cataract surgery. In addition to teaching the basics of cataract surgery, the curriculum places emphasis on a range of complications that can arise in cataract surgery and on areas where novices are most prone to potentially serious failures.

A cognitive simulation program can be used to facilitate reflection, since trainees will have a hands-on environment in which it is safe to review and revisit experiences they had in the OR. They can safely do things like play "what if?" games exploring the consequences of taking different approaches to a surgical procedure, possibly one they had just performed in the OR. Those trainees in need of remedial help and those with questions who might otherwise be embarrassed to ask would have a risk-free environment in which to learn.

While apprenticeship is the only proven method for learning to be a doctor, it still carries some of the risks suggested by the "have some to get some" paradox. There is a constant tension between the experiences learners need and the opportunities for practice available to them when they are not already highly skilled. Simulation technology will enable us to circumvent this problem.

Training Level-Specific Curriculum

The current apprentice system has served as the main mode of training surgeons for many years. With increasing demands to demonstrate competency of ophthalmic residents, new methods of teaching and training residents will continue to evolve. The University of Iowa published data that demonstrated improved senior resident surgical outcomes after an enhanced training curriculum was introduced to the junior resident's cataract training program [4]. The junior resident's first-year curriculum entails a structured wet lab with faculty supervision and "backing in" or performing the last portions of cataract surgery. The second-year curriculum has a "deliberate practice" rotation where the resident performs only the capsulorhexis portion of the procedure on many cases [4, 13]. The capsulorhexis from each case is recorded and the operative video is reviewed with faculty and the resident provided feedback. This innovative curriculum encompasses all of the simulation modalities discussed above, and resident feedback from this program has been very positive in their training experience.

Conclusion

We foresee that the purely apprenticeship model of teaching of the past will be replaced by a combination of apprenticeship and wet labs, computer and cognitive simulation, guided curriculums, and competency-based skills assessments [13, 14] in ophthalmology.

References

1. Lee AG, Carter KD. Managing the new mandate in resident education: a blueprint for translating a national mandate into local compliance. Ophthalmology. 2004;111:1807–12.
2. Oetting TA, Lee AG, Beaver HA, et al. Teaching and assessing surgical competency in ophthalmology training programs. Ophthalmic Surg Lasers Imaging. 2006;37:384–93.
3. Henderson BA, Ali R. Teaching and assessing competence in cataract surgery. Curr Opin Ophthalmol. 2007;18:27–31.
4. Rogers GM, Oetting TA, Lee AG, et al. Impact of a structured surgical curriculum on ophthalmic resident cataract surgery complication rates. J Cataract Refract Surg. 2009;35:1956–60.
5. Randleman JB, Wolfe JD, Woodward M, Lynn MJ, Cherwek DH, Srivastava SK. The resident surgeon phacoemulsification learning curve. Arch Ophthalmol. 2007;125:1215–9.
6. Teus MA, de Benito-Llopis L, Sánchez-Pina JM. Learning curve of laser-assisted subepithelial keratectomy: influence on visual and refractive results. J Cataract Refract Surg. 2007;33:1381–5.
7. Bell CM, Hatch WV, Cernat G, Urbach DR. Surgeon volumes and selected patient outcomes in cataract surgery: a population-based analysis. Ophthalmology. 2007;114:405–10. Epub 2006 Dec 14.
8. Dooley IJ, O'Brien PD. Subjective difficulty of each stage of phacoemulsification cataract surgery performed by basic surgical trainees. J Cataract Refract Surg. 2006;32:604–8.
9. Prakash G, Jhanji V, Sharma N, Gupta K, Titiyal JS, Vajpayee RB. Assessment of perceived difficulties by residents in performing routine steps in phacoemulsification surgery and in managing complications. Can J Ophthalmol. 2009;44:284–7.
10. Binenbaum G, Volpe NJ. Ophthalmology resident surgical competency: a national survey. Ophthalmology. 2006;113:1237–44. Epub 2006 May 24.
11. Henderson BA, Grimes KJ, Fintelmann RE, Oetting TA. Stepwise approach to establishing an ophthalmology wet laboratory. J Cataract Refract Surg. 2009;35:1121–8.
12. Oetting TA. Help ophthalmology residents achieve success: how to develop a comprehensive plan for evaluating surgical competency. Cataract Refract Surg Today. 2008;73–77.
13. Oetting TA. Teaching the capsulorhexis technique. Cataract Refract Surg Today. 2007;10:46–48.
14. Oetting TA. Surgical competency in residents. Curr Opin Ophthalmol. 2009;20:56–60.
15. Lee AG, Greenlee E, Oetting TA, et al. The Iowa ophthalmology wet laboratory curriculum for teaching and assessing cataract surgical competency. Ophthalmology. 2007;114:e21–6. Epub 2007 May 1.
16. Fisher JB, Binenbaum G, Tapino P, Volpe NJ. Development and face and content validity of an eye surgical skills assessment test for ophthalmology residents. Ophthalmology. 2006;113:2364–70.
17. Hashimoto C, Kurosaka D, Uetsuki Y. Teaching continuous curvilinear capsulorhexis using a postmortem pig eye with simulated cataract(2)(2). J Cataract Refract Surg. 2001;27:814–6.
18. Figueira EC, Wang LW, Brown TM, et al. The grape: an appropriate model for continuous curvilinear capsulorhexis. J Cataract Refract Surg. 2008;34:1610–1.
19. Lenart TD, McCannel CA, Baratz KH, Robertson DM. A contact lens as an artificial cornea for improved visualization during practice surgery on cadaver eyes. Arch Ophthalmol. 2003;121:16–9.
20. Rootman DS, Marcovich A. Utilizing eye bank eyes and keratoplasty techniques to teach phacoemulsification. Ophthalmic Surg Lasers. 1997;28:957–60.
21. Jonas JB, Rabethge S, Bender HJ. Computer-assisted training system for pars plana vitrectomy. Acta Ophthalmol Scand. 2003;81:600–4.
22. Wagner C, Schill M, Hennen M, et al. Virtual reality in ophthalmological education. Ophthalmologe. 2001;98:409–13.
23. Hikichi T, Yoshida A, Igarashi S, et al. Vitreous surgery simulator. Arch Ophthalmol. 2000;118:1679–81.
24. Rossi JV, Verma D, Fujii GY, et al. Virtual vitreoretinal surgical simulator as a training tool. Retina. 2004;24:231–6.
25. Grodin MH, Johnson TM, Acree JL, Glaser BM. Ophthalmic surgical training: a curriculum to enhance surgical simulation. Retina. 2008;28:1509–14.
26. Park J, Waqar S, Kersey T, Modi N, Ong C, Sleep T. Effect of distraction on simulated anterior segment surgical performance. J Cataract Refract Surg. 2011;37:1517–22.
27. Belyea DA, Brown SE, Rajjoub LZ. Influence of surgery simulator training on ophthalmology resident phacoemulsification performance. J Cataract Refract Surg. 2011;37:1756–61. Epub 2011 Aug 15.
28. Mahr MA, Hodge DO. Construct validity of anterior segment antitremor and forceps surgical simulator training modules: attending versus resident surgeon performance. J Cataract Refract Surg. 2008;34:980–5.
29. Webster R, Sassani J, Shenk R, et al. Simulating the continuous curvilinear capsulorhexis procedure during cataract surgery on the EYESI system. Stud Health Technol Inform. 2005;111:592–5.

30. Privett B, Greenlee E, Rogers G, Oetting TA. Construct validity of a surgical simulator as a valid model for capsulorhexis training. J Cataract Refract Surg. 2010;36:1835–8.
31. Feudner EM, Engel C, Neuhann IM, Petermeier K, Bartz-Schmidt KU, Szurman P. Virtual reality training improves wet-lab performance of capsulorhexis: results of a randomized, controlled study. Graefes Arch Clin Exp Ophthalmol. 2009;247:955–63.
32. Waqar S, Park J, Kersey TL, Modi N, Ong C, Sleep TJ. Assessment of fatigue in intraocular surgery: analysis using a virtual reality simulator. Graefes Arch Clin Exp Ophthalmol. 2011;249:77–81. Epub 2010 Oct 2.
33. Henderson BA, Neaman A, Kim BH, Loewenstein J. Virtual training tool. Ophthalmology. 2006;113:1058–9.
34. Henderson BA, Kim JY, Golnik KC, et al. Evaluation of the virtual mentor cataract training program. Ophthalmology. 2010;117:253–8.

Simulation in Orthopedic Surgery

32

Jay D. Mabrey, Kivanc Atesok, Kenneth Egol, Laith Jazrawi, and Gregory Hall

Introduction

Traditional orthopedic surgical education is rooted in the master-apprentice model in which residents are taught by senior staff using real patients [1]. While effective in the past, the rapid expansion of orthopedic procedures and significant changes in residency education have exposed important limitations. Complex operating room (OR) technologies and minimally invasive procedures are associated with steep learning curves [2], and resident work-hour restrictions, cost pressures, and patient safety measures are limiting trainees' exposure to real-time clinical material [3]. As a result, today's orthopedic trainees are challenged to acquire more complex and diverse surgical skills than their predecessors, but in less time [4]. Moreover, the actual requirements to complete a residency are rather broad. The Accreditation Council for Graduate Medical Education (ACGME) requires post-graduate-year two through five (PGY-2-5) residents to record their clinical experience in the ACGME Case Log System and only requires that the graduating resident log between 1,000 and 3,000 procedures [5]. Most importantly, it does not specify a specific number of total cases for proficiency at any given task. Unlike the majority of general surgery training programs that have had laparoscopic simulators available to their residents for several years, orthopedic training programs are only now being able to offer high-fidelity procedural simulators.

Once these residents are out in practice, it is just as critical for them to keep up their skill sets. Several studies have shown a positive correlation between the volume of cases performed by a surgeon and their outcomes including total shoulder [6], total hip [7], and total knee replacements [8].

As opportunities for learning through "on-the-job" training with "real" patients diminish, alternative training methods outside the OR environment are entering the curriculum [9, 10]. These include hands-on training in specially designed surgical skills laboratories, cadaver labs, synthetic bones and anatomical models, and computerized simulators. In this chapter we will explore the use of these educational devices for orthopedic education and assessment.

Surgical Skills Laboratories

Lab-based education aims to allow orthopedic residents to practice basic surgical skills in a risk-free, low-stress environment, affording them the opportunity to gain familiarity with techniques before they perform them on real patients in the OR [3]. Sonnadara et al. [3] demonstrated that an intensive surgical skills course can be highly effective at teaching and developing targeted basic surgical skills in first-year orthopedic residents. The authors compared a group of residents who were given a 30-day surgical skills laboratory ($n=6$) with a control group participating in standard residency training ($n=16$). There was no significant performance difference between the groups prior to the commencement of training using both the Objective Structured Assessment of Technical

J.D. Mabrey, MD, MBA (✉)
Department of Orthopaedics, Baylor University Medical Center, 3500 Gaston Ave., 6 Hoblitzelle, Dallas, TX 75246, USA
e-mail: jaym@baylorhealth.edu

K. Atesok, MD, MSc
Faculty of Medicine, Institute of Medical Science, University of Toronto, 28 Harrison Garden Blvd. Suite 301, Toronto, ON M2N 7B5, Canada
e-mail: kivanc.atesok@utoronto.ca

K. Egol, MD
Department of Orthopaedic Surgery, NYU Hospital for Joint Diseases, 301 E 17th St., New York, NY 10003, USA
e-mail: kenneth.egol@nyume.org

L. Jazrawi, MD
Division of Sports Medicine, Department of Orthopaedic Surgery, NYU Langone Medical Center Hospital for Joint Diseases, 301 E. 17th St., Suite 1402, New York, NY 10003, USA
e-mail: laith.jazrawi@nyumc.org

G. Hall, BA
Department of Orthopaedic Surgery, NYU Langone Medical Center Hospital for Joint Diseases, 301 E 17th, Rm. 1500, New York, NY 10003, USA
e-mail: gregory.hall@nyumc.org

A.I. Levine et al. (eds.), *The Comprehensive Textbook of Healthcare Simulation*, DOI 10.1007/978-1-4614-5993-4_32, © Springer Science+Business Media New York 2013

Skills (OSATS) standard checklist and global rating scale (GRS). OSATS is comprised of simulated surgical environments in which trainees receive instructions on the technical skills needed to accomplish surgical tasks under the direct observation of an expert. Examiners score candidates using two methods. The first is a task-specific checklist consisting of a set of specific surgical maneuvers that have been deemed essential elements of the procedure. The GRS includes specific surgical behaviors, such as respect for tissues, economy of motion, and appropriate use of assistants [10]. Residents in the intensive surgical skills course took half-day training sessions everyday in the morning, which included basic fracture fixation techniques, application of casts and splints, and familiarization with basic surgical instruments. These training sessions were followed by clinical duties during the afternoon similar to residents in the standard training group. Post-training scores were significantly better in the lab-trained group compared to standard residency group on both the OSATS checklists and GRS [3].

An example of the OSATS score sheet and GRS for carpal tunnel release has been reported by van Heest et al. (App) [11]. In this study of 28 orthopedic residents representing six levels of surgical training, using this tool significant differences were found between the year of training and the knowledge test score, global rating scale, and detailed checklist [11].

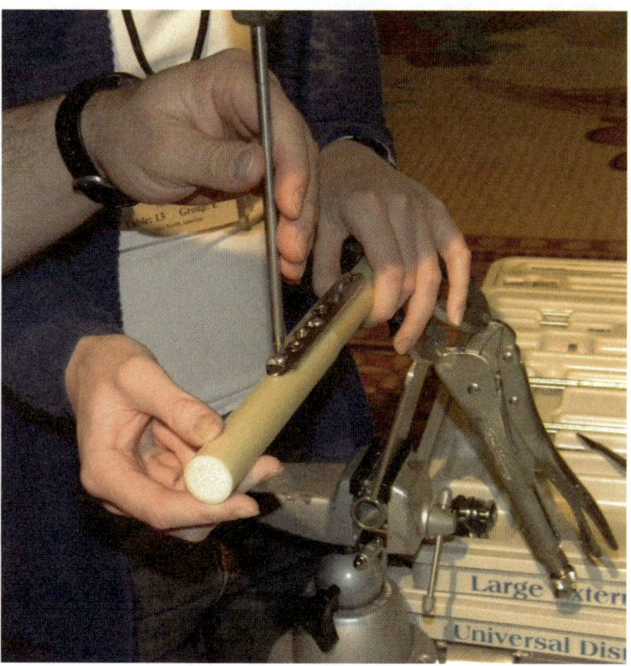

Fig. 32.1 Synthetic bone model in simulation lab

Cadaveric Models and Synthetic Bones

Cadaveric training has been part of surgical education as early as the sixteenth century [12]. Since then, it has remained the gold standard of surgical practice prior to operation on live patients [13]. The trainee is exposed to real anatomy with varying degrees of validity, depending upon whether the cadaver is fresh or embalmed. Disadvantages of this model include costs, difficulty in procurement, limited time frame of use, and the possibility of disease transmission.

Over the last few decades, synthetic or plastic bone models have been developed to replace cadaveric bones and serve as reproducible models to aid in the development of basic orthopedic surgical skills [14]. These models are consistent in size, shape, and density and can be modeled to nearly any form, no special storage techniques or ethics committee approval is required, and they are relatively inexpensive and reproducible in large numbers [15]. And while synthetic bones may lack "face validity" or a sense of realism [4], they still play a significant role in the training process (Fig. 32.1).

Fracture fixation is the most common application in cadaveric and synthetic bone skills training. Leong et al. [4] recruited 21 subjects to validate the use of three models of fracture fixation in the assessment of technical skills. The subjects were divided into three groups according to their experience in trauma procedures (novice, intermediate, and expert). Each subject was asked to perform three procedures: application of a dynamic compression plate on a cadaver porcine model, insertion of an un-reamed tibial intramedullary nail, and application of a forearm external fixator, the latter two on synthetic bone models. The primary outcome measures were the OSATS and GRS using video recordings of the procedures and motion analysis of the hand movements of the surgeons. Their results revealed significant differences among all three levels of expertise based on dynamic compression plate fixation of pre-fractured porcine tibia. External fixation of the pre-fractured synthetic ulna model did not differentiate among different expertise levels, and intramedullary nail insertion into a pre-fractured synthetic tibia model failed to differentiate between surgeons with intermediate and expert levels of expertise [4]. The authors noted: "This study has validated a low-cost, high-fidelity porcine dynamic compression plate model using video rating scores for skills assessment and movement analysis. It has also demonstrated that Synbone models for the application of an intramedullary nail and an external fixator are less sensitive and should be improved for further assessment of surgical skills in trauma" [4]. In the United States, the Orthopaedic Trauma Association (OTA – www.ota.org) and the AO Foundation a non profit organization of international surgeons specializing in the treatment of trauma and disorders of the musculoskeletal system lead the way for orthopedic trainees to gain experience at surgical simulation. During these courses, trainees become familiar with the various tools and implants utilized to repair common fractures. They learn

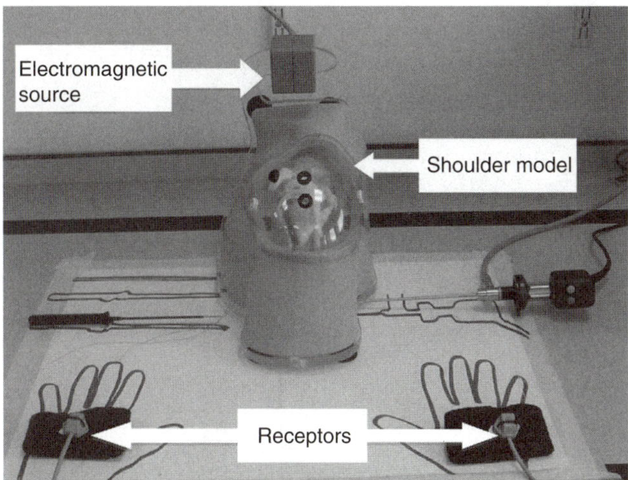

Fig. 32.2 The Alex Shoulder Professor benchtop simulator (Sawbones Europe, Malmö, Sweden) and the three-dimensional electromagnetic motion tracking system (PATRIOT; Polhemus, Colchester, Vermont) used to assess surgical performance (Howells et al. [17]. Used with permission from *Journal of Bone and Joint Surgery*)

reduction techniques as well as proper implant installation, drill technique, and screw placement.

Tuijthof and colleagues [16] developed the Practice Arthroscopic Surgical Skills for Perfect Operative Real-life Treatment (PASSPORT) training environment, a physical knee model that allows for realistic surgical actions. It includes standard portals, menisci that can be probed, and simulates problems such as bleeding and air bubbles. Medial and lateral springs enable application of varus and valgus stresses. Construct validity was assessed by testing 20 experienced arthroscopy surgeons (>50 knee arthroscopies per year) and 8 less-experienced residents in training (<20 arthroscopies per year). The experienced surgeons were significantly more efficient on PASSPORT than the residents, taking only 19.7 s on average to complete a specified set of tasks vs. the 55.2 s taken by the residents to complete the same tasks [16].

Howells et al. [17] using a laboratory-based shoulder simulator demonstrated that regular repetition of arthroscopic Bankhart repair was necessary to maintain optimum performance. Six fellowship-trained lower-extremity surgeons were trained to perform an arthroscopic Bankhart repair using the Alex Shoulder Professor simulator (Sawbones Europe, Malmö, Sweden) (Fig. 32.2). Having had no previous experience with Bankhart repair, these six surgeons demonstrated a learning curve as they improved significantly through their first 12 repetitions. The surgeons then returned to their respective lower-extremity practices and came back after 6 months to be tested again. The second set of results demonstrated that the surgeons had not retained any of their original improved technical skills; instead, they produced learning curves indistinguishable from the first set confirming loss of skill in performing Bankhart repair [17].

Computer Tools

Orthopedic surgery training requires knowledge and understanding of the three-dimensional (3D) anatomy of the skeleton and its spatial relation to other anatomical structures, encouraging the development of computer-based simulators aimed at residency training. Software simulation programs assist the trainee in conceptualizing complex fracture anatomy and allow them to carry out a given surgical procedure in a virtual 3D environment (Figs. 32.3a and b) [18]. Citak et al. [19] created standard acetabular fracture models in synthetic pelves and performed CT scans that were either registered with 3D planning software or used for conventional 2D paper planning. After the planning, the fractured pelvis model was submerged in a gel medium to simulate soft tissue resistance and to allow the fracture position to be maintained when the reduction was complete. The accuracy of the reduction was found to be significantly better following planning with virtual 3D software compared to the standard technique (Figs. 32.3c, d and e). Similar software with the ability of 3D image production and manipulation based on patient-specific CT data is also available for joint resurfacing arthroplasty or total joint replacement procedures to improve accuracy and shorten learning curves [20, 21].

Blyth et al. [22] studied a PC-based virtual reality training system designed to evaluate and improve a trainee's ability to accurately reduce and internally fix a hip fracture, using standard anteroposterior and lateral radiographs. The simulator software, with a download size of 4 MB, could be accessed over the Internet or run on a stand-alone computer. The software incorporated all relevant tasks of pinning a hip fracture, from positioning of the C-arm and fracture reduction to skin incision and placement of the sliding hip screw, plate, and cortical screws (Fig. 32.4a–e). Ten participants were included in the study with each performing six operative scenarios on the simulator. Results indicated that the simulator had good "face validity," providing a realistic view of the operating environment as well as testing problem-solving ability. The study was not comparative and conclusions were based on participants' subjective feelings with regard to potential advantages that the software might provide [22].

Although available for several years, rapid prototyping, or 3D printing, has dropped significantly in price, making it accessible to surgeons who wish to practice an upcoming surgical procedure on realistic plastic models generated from the patient's actual computerized tomography (CT) data [23].

Advances in computing processing and graphics cards now allow researchers to simulate complex injury mechanisms in real time. This is particularly useful in training in combat medicine. With body armor saving more and more lives, first

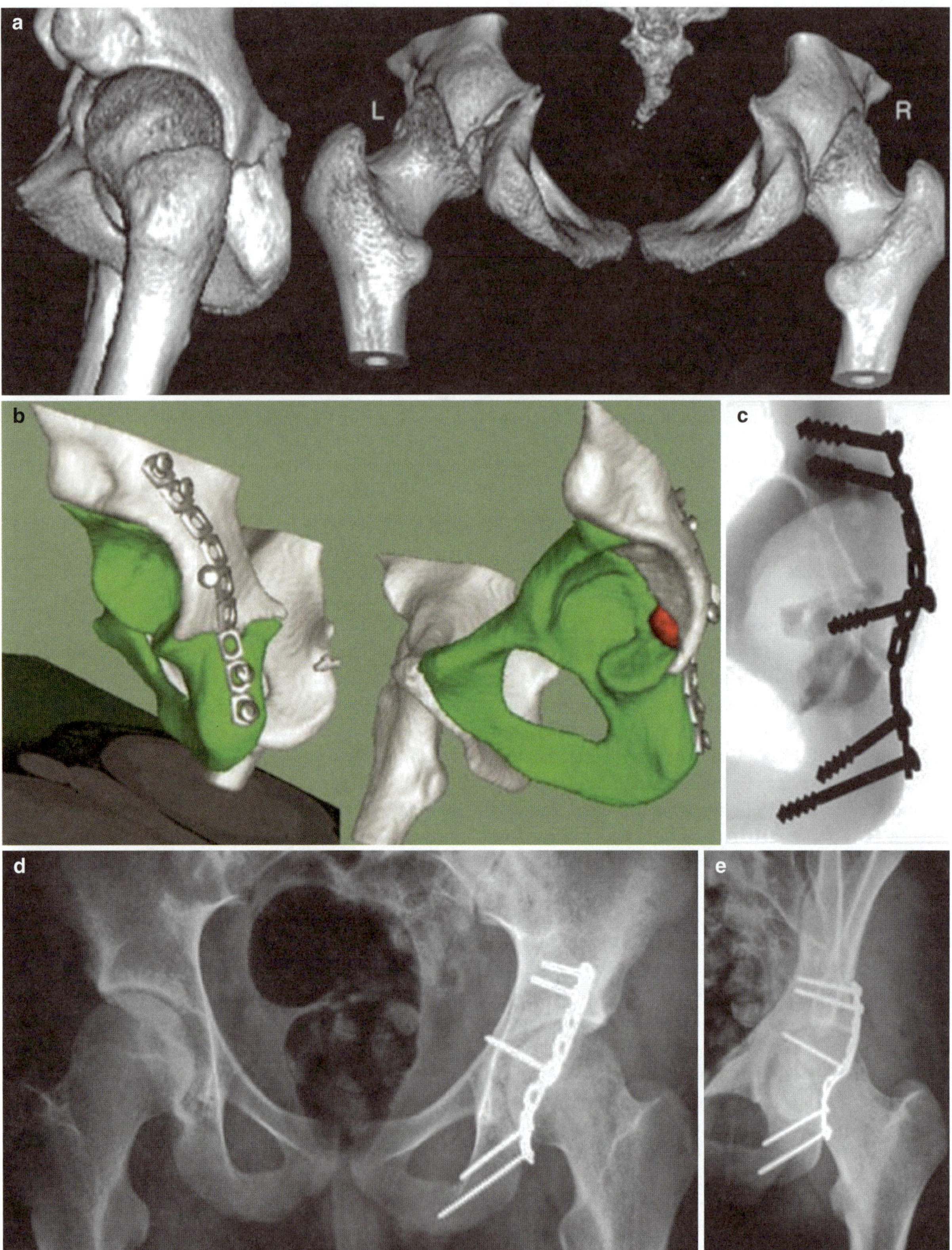

Fig. 32.3 (**a**) Lateral (*left*) and posteroanterior (*right*) three-dimensional (3D) computerized tomography (CT) reconstructions of a left acetabulum posterior wall fracture. (**b**) Virtual image of the fracture generated by the software based upon the preoperative CT images. The fracture fragments can be manipulated by the surgeon and reduced virtually after which the plate and the screws are applied. The fracture fragments are color-coded and the femur has been digitally subtracted for better visualization. (**c**) Rendering the bone translucent, as the surgeon would see it on fluoroscopy, created this virtual image. This enables better control of screw length and direction. (**d**, **e**) Actual postoperative radiographs of the pelvis and left hip. The final operative result is closely approximated by the preoperative virtual planning (© American Academy of Orthopaedic Surgeons. Reprinted from Atesok and Schemitsch [18], with permission)

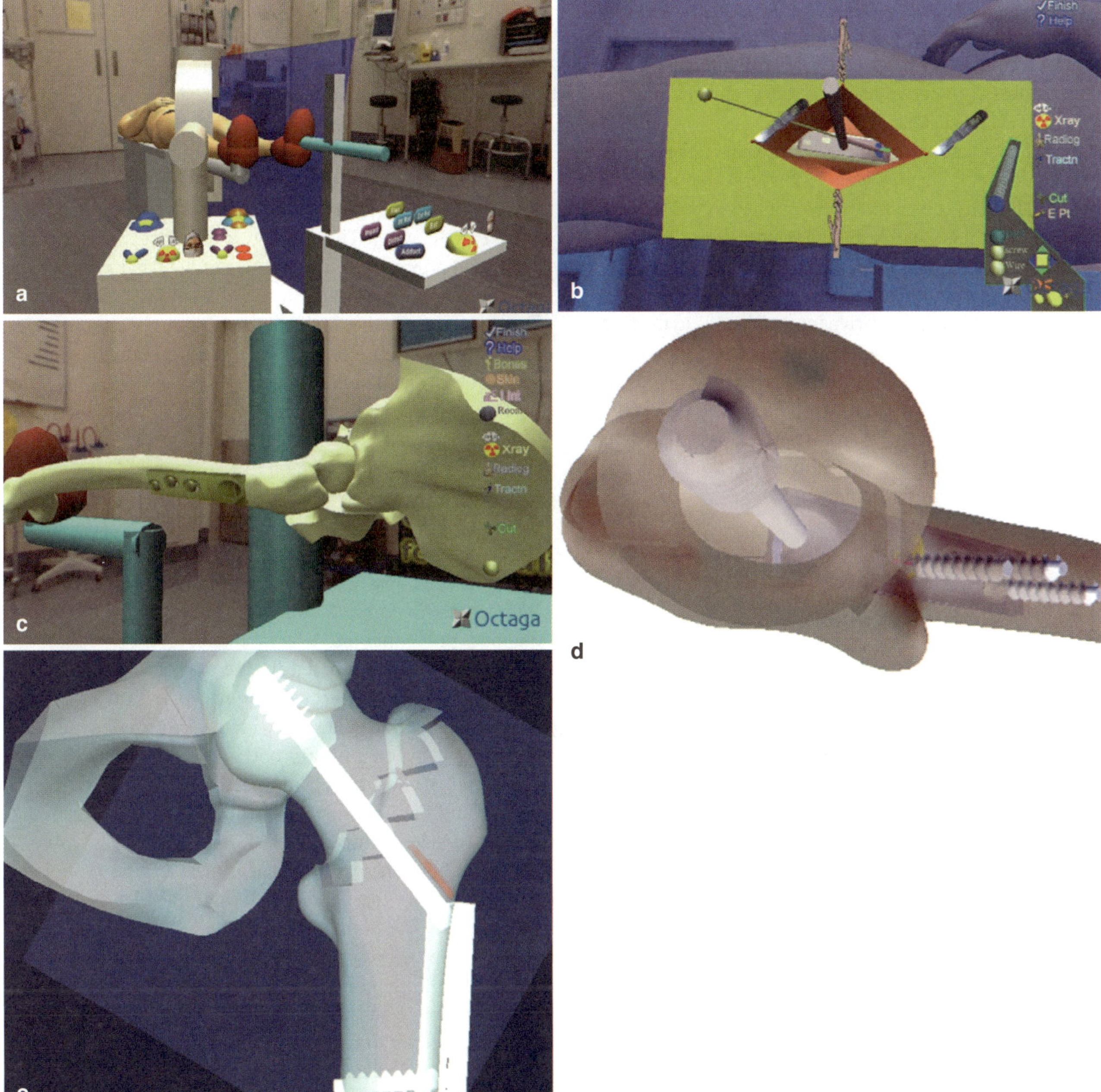

Fig. 32.4 Illustrations of a PC-based virtual reality training system for hip fracture fixation. (**a**) View of the virtual operating theater, showing the image intensifier and fracture table. (**b**) View of the virtual operative scene showing the skin incision, with the 135° guide plate visible on the femur. (**c**) Final reduction at the completion of the procedure with soft tissues removed. (**d**) Translucent femur demonstrating superiorly placed lag screw. (**e**) Virtual postoperative AP radiograph demonstrating fracture reduction and fixation placement (Reprinted from Blyth et al. [22], Copyright (2007), with permission from Elsevier)

responders and soldiers in the field are seeing a dramatic increase in extremity injuries including open fractures [24]. Reinig et al. [25] are developing a virtual environment for the United States Army to teach combat medics about thigh trauma. Using finite element modeling (FEM), the authors can predict and display how the femur and its surrounding soft tissues will respond to the application of various loads. The results are depicted as appropriate images on simulated radiographs, ultrasound, or computerized tomography. Thus, combat medics can practice ahead of time for the wide range of devastating injuries they will encounter in the field.

Haptics

A major complaint by trainees using early computer-based simulators has been the absence of physical feedback from the device. The introduction of haptics, or force feedback, to current orthopedic simulators gives the trainee a sense of shape and texture for the structure that they are working on. Haptics can produce either active feedback or passive feedback. In active haptic devices, devices such as the PHANTOM (Sensable Technologies, Inc., Woburn, MA) generate artificial mechanical resistance at the tip of the instrument being manipulated. However, some authors have noted that there is a lack of force applied to the shaft of the instrument being handled by the trainee [26]. This has led some researchers such as McCarthy et al. [26] to add passive haptic simulators that provide feedback along the shaft of a simulated arthroscopic instrument which adds to the realistic feel of the procedure. Vankipuram et al. [27] developed a simulation model which provides adequate haptic sensations for simulating drilling realistically. The authors suggested that simulated drilling with a virtual bone may improve trainees' basic skills and make a positive impact on their drilling tasks in real operating conditions.

Virtual Reality Simulators for Arthroscopy Training

Knee arthroscopy has increased 49% between 1996 and 2006 with 984,607 arthroscopes being performed in 2006 alone [28]. One might argue that this increase in numbers bodes well for the trainee; however, the majority of these arthroscopies are performed in free-standing ambulatory surgery centers, and most of those are not associated with training programs. Thus, there is an increasing demand for arthroscopy in the United States, yet orthopedic residency programs are faced with the challenge of providing sufficient training while restricting work hours. One survey of fifth-year, US orthopedic residents revealed that only 32% believed that their program devoted adequate time for training in arthroscopy in stark contrast to the 66% of program directors [29].

The Knee Arthroscopy Surgical Trainer (KAST) developed by the American Academy of Orthopaedic Surgeons' Task Force on Virtual Reality is designed to provide an intuitive and autonomous experience for the orthopedic resident [30]. KAST consists of a hardware component supported by proprietary software and a didactic component delivered on one of two monitors positioned in front of the trainee (Fig. 32.5a). The core of the hardware component is a pair of PHANTOM® haptic devices that recreate the feel of the arthroscope and the probe within the virtual knee (Fig. 32.5b). The workspace can be raised or lowered electronically to accommodate a wide range of statures, sitting or standing. To complete the feeling of performing a real arthroscopy, the trainee must manipulate a surrogate leg via flexion and extension of the knee and the application of varus and valgus forces. The simulator switches seamlessly between a right and a left knee, forcing the trainee to be ambidextrous with respect to the camera and probe.

The arthroscopic images, displayed on the right-hand monitor, are generated by a program that recreates three-dimensional models of the internal structures of the knee. These images are based on data from the Visible Human Project [31] or similar but higher-resolution cryosectioned data (Fig. 32.5d, e). These structures interact with the virtual probe and arthroscope, just as the cartilage and synovial lining of a real knee would interact. Techniques developed by Touch of Life Technologies alter the morphology, posture, and pathologies displayed from the data, giving a limitless supply of virtual patients [30].

The didactic component of KAST, known as the "Mentor," is displayed to the trainee on the left monitor (Fig. 32.5d). After logging on to KAST, the Mentor directs the trainee through a series of brief lessons demonstrating how to run the simulator. The Mentor program utilizes Hypertext Markup Language (HTML) to display text, audio, images, and video. In addition, the Mentor displays Interactive Anatomic Animations (IAA) utilizing texture-mapped polygonal models to render complex anatomic scenes that may be altered by the trainee's actions. After that, the trainee is instructed on how to perform a complete diagnostic sweep of the knee with the arthroscope only, followed by a sweep with a probe in the opposite hand. The Mentor continuously records all activity generated by the trainee and then provides sophisticated feedback concerning the trainee's progress.

Throughout the session, trainees must achieve proficiency while following the instructions from the Mentor program (Fig. 32.5d). The Mentor requires the trainee to score 100% on each step before proceeding to the next task. When they have successfully completed all required tasks, they do the entire procedure on their own and then one last time with the entire procedure timed. There is a "God's-eye view" of the outside of the knee that shows where the arthroscope and the probe are with respect to the knee anatomy to assist the trainee with triangulation (Fig. 32.5a). This view is not available once the trainee advances to the timed tasks. KAST will continue to evolve through software updates to include meniscal resection and ACL repair. KAST has been designed so that the same hardware can be used for simulation of shoulder arthroscopy [30].

The system is already up and running at several orthopedic residency training programs including the Durham Veterans' Hospital in North Carolina, the University of Michigan in Ann Arbor, the Pan Am Clinic in Winnipeg, Brooke Army Medical Center in San Antonio, Banner Health in Phoenix, and the University of Colorado at Denver [30].

Validity and Outcomes of Simulator-Based Arthroscopy Training

The major concerns with simulator-based arthroscopy training are the validity of the skills learned on the simulator and whether or not they can be transferred to the operating room. For many surgeons, VR surgical simulators represent little more than a means of evaluating a subject's dexterity and aptitude for video games [32]. Moreover, there is concern that most simulator systems provide training in psychomotor skills only and do not address the cognitive components of surgical competence (i.e., knowledge, decision making, and communication) [33].

Tuijthof et al. [34] evaluated two commercially available virtual reality knee simulators, the Insight ArthroVR arthroscopy simulator (GMV, Madrid, Spain) and the Knee Arthroscopy Surgical Trainer (Touch of Life Technologies, Aurora, CO, USA), with respect to construct validity (time to perform tasks) and face validity (realistic depiction of the procedure). Thirty-seven participants that were recruited from the authors' department consisting of three groups of increasing level of arthroscopic experience were evaluated:

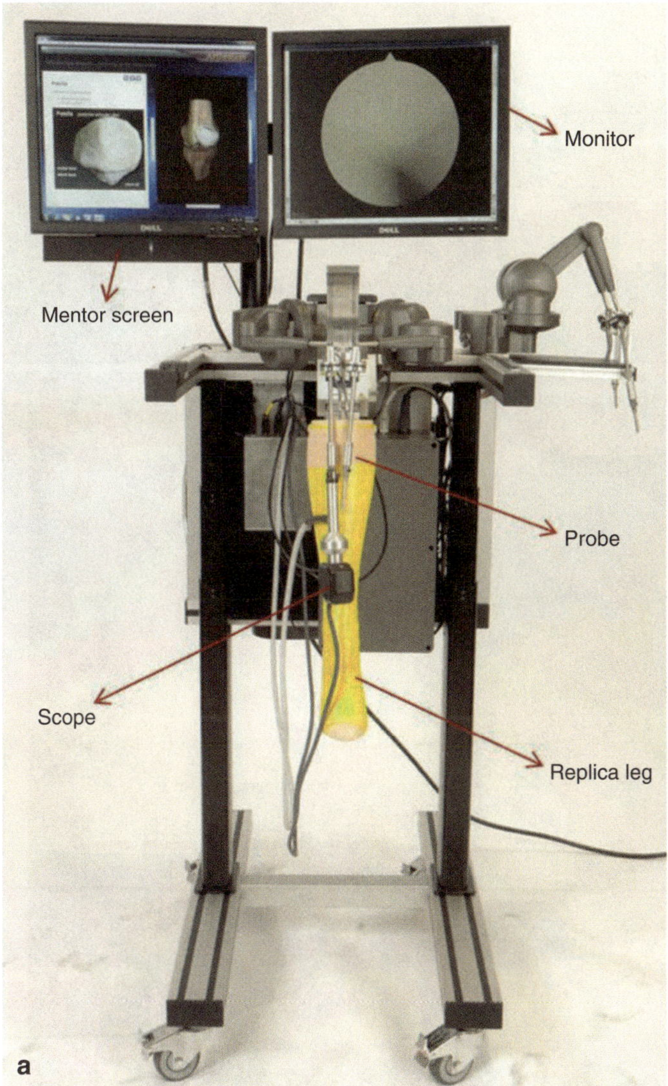

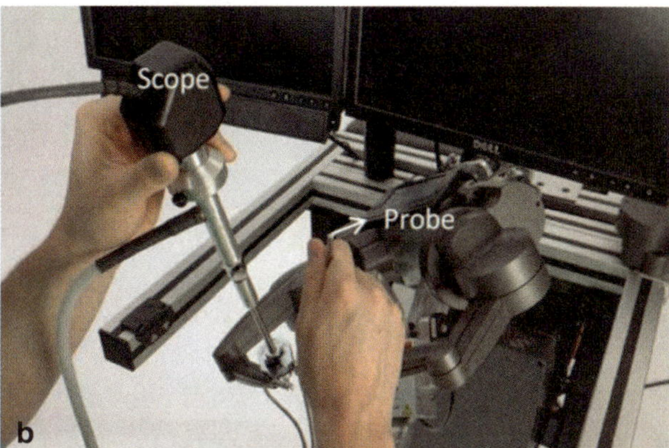

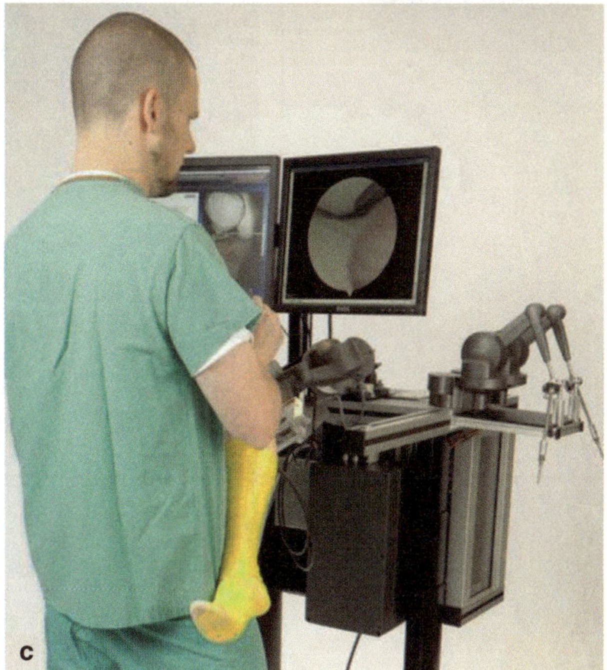

Fig. 32.5 (**a**) View of the Knee Arthroscopy Surgical Trainer (KAST). The Mentor screen (*left*) shows the instructions step by step with an animated view of each step. The arthroscopy monitor (*right*) displays the simulated procedure as in an actual arthroscopic procedure. (**b**) The scope and the probe are attached to separate PHANTOM haptic feedback devices. (**c**) The replica leg is used to apply varus and valgus stresses to the knee. Transducers built into the leg convey the information to the program, and the computer model responds appropriately. (**d**) The "Mentor" screen for KAST displays a set of instructions or tasks for the trainee on the left side and a "God's-eye" view on the right to help orient the trainee during the initial phases of instruction. Later, during timed tasks, the "God's-eye" view is not available. (**e**) The arthroscopy screen displays images as they would appear on a real monitor in the operating room

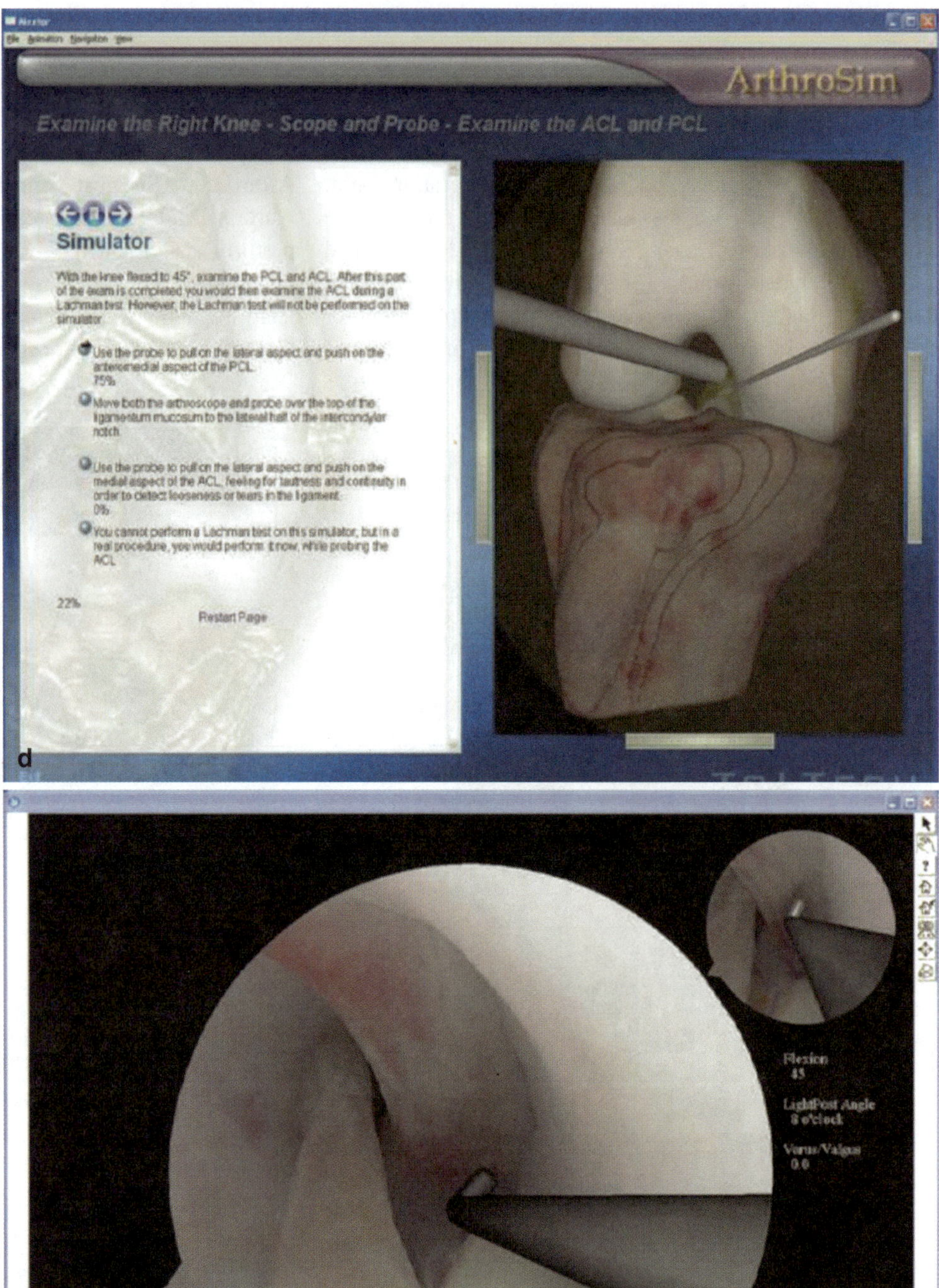

Fig. 32.5 (continued)

novices with zero cases, intermediates with up to 59 cases, and experts with 60 or more cases. The task to determine construct validity was designed to be replicated between the two simulators and consisted of probing nine anatomic landmarks from the anterolateral portal in knee simulation mode. Neither of the simulators were felt to demonstrate full construct validity as task times were similar among the three groups after only one or two repetitions [34]. The authors also reported observing face validity for both simulators but suggested that there was room for improvement. Both the intermediate and expert test subjects felt that the haptics felt unrealistic on both simulators [34]. It should be noted that both of the simulators tested rely upon active haptics provided by PHANTOM feedback devices.

McCarthy et al. [26] reported validation for the Sheffield Knee Arthroscopy Training System (SKATS) that uses only passive haptics provided by physical structures within the knee. Experienced surgeons performed significantly faster, located more pathologies, and demonstrated shorter arthroscope path lengths than a less-experienced group of subjects. Further studies are planned to investigate "skill transfer and training transfer" [26].

The virtual reality shoulder arthroscopy simulator introduced by Mentice (Mentice Corp, Gothenburg, Sweden) has been available for several years and has been a key component in validating virtual reality arthroscopic training. Gomoll et al. [9] studied the validity of simulator-based arthroscopy training by correlating the actual surgical experience with the performance on the simulator. Four groups of subjects with different levels of experience in arthroscopic procedures were compared based on their performance in a virtual reality simulator for shoulder arthroscopy. Their results revealed statistically significant differences across all groups (i.e., groups with more real experience in arthroscopic procedures performed better on the simulator) in all parameters of performance assessment such as time to completion of the module, the distance traveled with the tip of the probe compared with a computer-determined optimal distance, the average velocity of probe movement, and the number of probe collisions with tissues. Participants were also questioned on their prior experience with video games, and no significant difference was found on simulation performance between subjects with prior video game experience compared to those without. The authors stated that "This indicates that the skill set tested may be similar to the one developed in the operating room, thus suggesting its use as a potential tool for the future evaluation of surgical trainees" [9]. They then retested the trainees 3 years after their initial evaluation on an arthroscopy simulator and reported that individuals who had gained surgical experience in the interval between two identical arthroscopic simulation tests demonstrated substantially improved results on the simulator as well [35]. Pedowitz et al. [36] were among the first to demonstrate that the Mentice shoulder simulator could distinguish among medical students, orthopedic residents, and experienced faculty in terms of time of completion of task and in the efficiency with which they completed assigned tasks [36]. Similarly, Srivastava et al. [37] reported that experienced shoulder arthroscopists consistently performed better on the simulator than did surgeons in training or medical students.

More recently, Martin et al. [38] demonstrated a strong correlation between performance of basic arthroscopic tasks on the Insight Arthro VR shoulder simulator (Immersion, San Jose, California, USA) and performance of the same tasks in a cadaveric model. Their results provide further evidence supporting the validity of arthroscopic simulators as a beneficial educational tool in the assessment of performance in a surgical setting. Howells et al. [39] investigated the effects of lab-based simulator training on the ability of surgical trainees to perform diagnostic arthroscopy on real patients. A total of 20 junior orthopedic trainees were randomized to receive a standard protocol of arthroscopic simulator training ($n = 10$) or traditional training without simulation ($n = 10$). Participants were all within the first 2 years of training and had minimal experience of arthroscopy (i.e., assisted or observed <10 arthroscopies). Motion analysis method was used to track the improvements in performance of the trainees in the simulator group through the course of simulated training. Following 1 week of training, an experienced knee surgeon, who was blinded to groups, supervised all 20 trainees in the operating room while they were performing a diagnostic arthroscopy and assessed their performance using a standard checklist and an OSATS GRS. Motion analysis showed that the performance of all trainees in the simulator group improved significantly through subsequent training episodes at the end of training. Analysis of the performance in the operating room demonstrated that scores of the simulator group were significantly better according to standard checklist and global rating scores. The authors stated that "orthopaedic surgical trainees who have undergone a period of lab-based arthroscopic simulator training go on to demonstrate improved technical performance in the OR compared with an untrained group" [39].

Current data demonstrating the transfer validity of arthroscopic skills acquired through simulator-based training to the operating theater is limited. However, general opinion is that a standardized simulator training may allow orthopedic surgery residency programs to accelerate residents' acquisition of basic skills required in arthroscopy while minimizing the increased operative times and potential iatrogenic injury to patients that are associated with the learning of such skills during actual surgical procedures [39].

Practical and Future Applications

Perhaps the gold standard for orthopedic simulation is the OLC (Orthopaedic Learning Center) Education and Conference Center in Rosemont, Illinois. Operating on the first floor of the national headquarters of the American Academy of Orthopaedic Surgeons (AAOS), the OLC is a world-class bio-skills laboratory providing up to 20

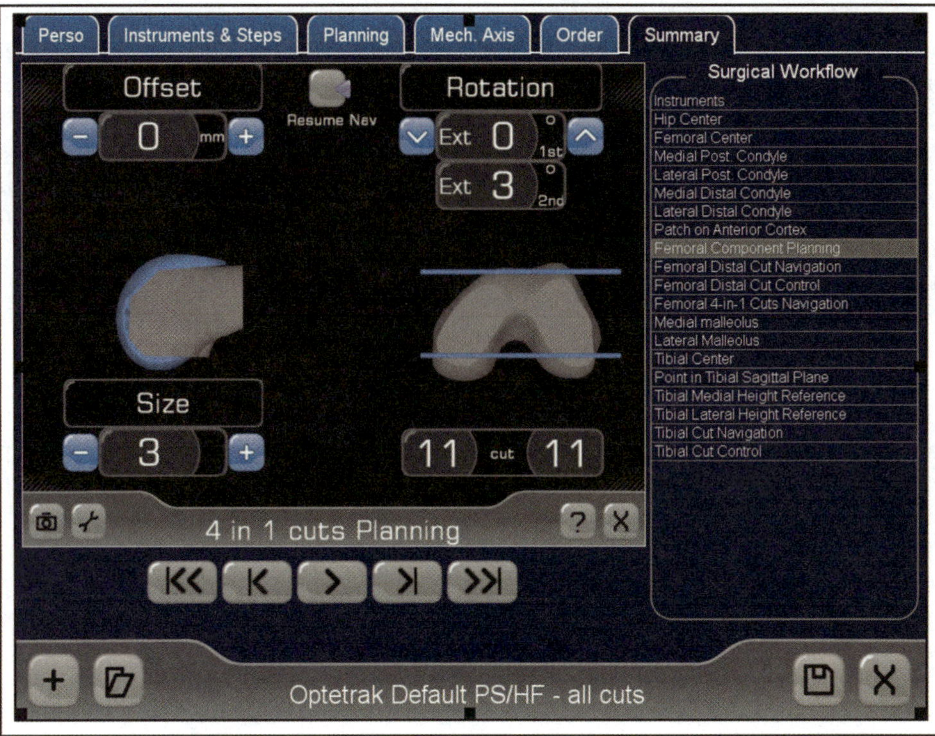

Fig. 32.6 Screen shot of computer-assisted surgery (CAS) system from Exactech, Gainesville, FL. The position and sizing of the implant is presented on the left of the screen, while the order of the surgical workflow is listed on the right with this step highlighted. Combined with traditional foam bone training, CAS may accelerate the learning curve for residents in training. Additional training of surgeons in practice may be enhanced by utilizing 3D printouts of femurs and tibias from actual patients with challenging deformities

workstations at a time for arthroscopy and total joint, spine, hand, foot, and trauma procedures. While primarily focusing on fresh cadavers as the main source of teaching material, there are plans to incorporate the KAST as an adjunct to arthroscopy training when it becomes more widely available.

One of the more innovative approaches in training orthopedic residents on how to perform total knee arthroplasty is the incorporation of computer-assisted surgery (CAS) tools such as BrainLAB into a traditional OSATS-style testing protocol [40]. Myden et al. developed a 3-day course that took junior orthopedic residents through a traditional OSATS skills test for total knee replacement (TKA) and then had the residents learn how to perform TKA on foam bones using computer-guided surgery [40]. Quantitatively, the junior residents participating in this combined program with just one standard TKA and two CAS TKAs improved as much as residents who had been trained with up to six TKAs on foam bones, suggesting that the use of the CAS system improved the residents' skills faster than the traditional method.

The advantage of CAS as an instructional tool for TKA is that it gives immediate feedback to the user in a very structured manner. Alignment of cutting blocks and components are readily displayed on the CAS screen (Fig. 32.6), and the entire procedure is presented in a stepwise fashion identical to the format used in the actual operating room.

The future of orthopedic simulation holds great promise, particularly with the advent of new motion-based game controllers such as the Wii Remote™ Plus from Nintendo® and the Xbox® Kinect™ from Microsoft®. It is not too hard to imagine individual companies developing their own web-based, motion-controlled surgical simulation programs that could be accessed through the Internet using a Kinect™ controller on an Xbox® 360 console purchased for less than $300 from Amazon.com®.

Conclusion

A variety of educational techniques are available to the orthopedic resident in training, ranging from simple Sawbones™ to complex virtual reality simulators. The degree to which these devices recreate actual orthopedic procedure varies with the tasks at hand. As with the other specialties in this book, the major hurdles toward integrating these techniques into the modern orthopedic curriculum are both cost and time. Costs for the high-end simulators will stabilize, but it is unlikely that they will reach the level of mass-produced video games and consoles, although McCarthy's group [26] is on track to develop a valid low-end knee simulator. Educators must make hospital administrators and medical school deans aware of the tremendous advantage in economics and safety of investing in simulator products that enable orthopedic trainees to enter the operating room for the first time with a preexisting skill set.

Appendix

TABLE E-1 Assessment of Operative Report Dictation (10 pts)

Use this form to review the Operative Report for Carpal Tunnel Syndrome Release.

1.	Preparation (consent/time out)	Yes ☐	No ☐
2.	Positioning/Prep of patient/arm	Yes ☐	No ☐
3.	Proper skin incision (describes landmarks)	Yes ☐	No ☐
4.	Proper dissection of tissue layers (skin, subcutaneous fat, palmar fascia, transverse carpal ligament)	Yes ☐	No ☐
5.	Proper identification and protection of structures at risk (palmar arch, branches of median nerve)	Yes ☐	No ☐
6.	Complete release of transverse carpal ligament (proximal and distal extent)	Yes ☐	No ☐
7.	Verification of integrity/condition of median nerve and recurrent motor branch	Yes ☐	No ☐
8.	Appropriate closure	Yes ☐	No ☐
9.	Demonstrates logical order of dictation	Yes ☐	No ☐
10.	Demonstrates efficient and concise description of the surgical procedure; completed within allotted time	Yes ☐	No ☐

TABLE E-2 Detailed Checklist - Carpal Tunnel Release Proctor Score Sheet*

Proctor Number: ____________________ Actual Start Time: ________________

Resident Number: ____________________ Actual Stop Time: ________________

Date: ________ Specimen #________

Checklist

Skin incision: _________

Yes	No	
☐	☐	Skin incision from wrist crease to Kaplan line, in line with radial aspect of ring finger- drawn appropriately
☐	☐	Holds knife perpendicular to tissue plane (incision is perpendicular to skin without flaps or skiving)
☐	☐	Applies appropriate pressure for skin penetration without multiple passes
☐	☐	Makes flaps with minimal tissue handling (minimal grasping, regrasping, tissue trauma, etc)

Layered dissection: ___________

Yes	No	
☐	☐	Incision is perpendicularly completed to the level of the palmar fascia
☐	☐	Proper use of tissue retractors for deeper dissection
☐	☐	Palmar fascia is incised perpendicular in the same plane through its length
☐	☐	Identifies distal border of transverse carpal ligament
☐	☐	Identifies and protects palmar arch at distal end of wound
☐	☐	Complete release of TCL

Transverse carpal ligament: ____

Yes	No	
☐	☐	TCL is incised on its ulnar border
☐	☐	TCL is incised perpendicular in the same plane through its length
☐	☐	Median nerve is visualized as decompressed through its distal extent
☐	☐	Median nerve is visualized as decompressed through its proximal extent
☐	☐	Recurrent motor branch is visualized as decompressed

Closure using 3 sutures: _____________

Yes	No	
☐	☐	Places suture following curve of needle AND passes needle through tissue with supination: pronates wrist to regrasp needle
☐	☐	Starts instrument tie with square throw AND subsequent throws are square to previous
☐	☐	Ties knot without tissue strangulation (appropriate skin tension)
☐	☐	Appropriate knot spacing

ADVERSE EVENTS

☐	☐	**Palmar arch injury**
☐	☐	**Guyon canal release**
☐	☐	**Median nerve or flexor tendon Injury**
☐	☐	**Other**

PASS/FAIL ASSESSMENT

☐ PASS ☐ FAIL

(*The detailed checklist was adapted from the task-specific checklist shown in: Reznick R, Regehr G, MacRae H, Martin J, McCulloch W. Testing technical skill via an innovative "bench station" examination. Am J Surg. 1997;173:226–30.)

TABLE E-3 Global Rating Scale of Operative Performance*

Resident Number_______; Proctor Number______:

Station Carpal Tunnel
To be completed by faculty observer

Please circle the number for each category, irrespective of the trainee's PGY level.

Instrument ID and Handling

1	2	3	4	5
Could not name instruments, selected wrong instrument(s); handled instruments inappropriately		Could name same, not all instruments; hesitated or changed mind in selecting instruments; handled them appropriately ***most*** of the time		Named all instruments; easily selected correct instruments; used them appropriately ***all*** of the time

Quality of Incision

1	2	3	4	5
Poor technique skin compromised, multiple passes		Moderately good technique skin roughly handled, difficulty with depth		Excellent technique single pass in one plane excellent depth

Quality of Suturing

1	2	3	4	5
Poor technique poor manual dexterity, uneven closure		Moderately good technique moderate dexterity, uneven spacing, acceptable closure		Excellent technique excellent dexterity excellent closure

Quality of Knots

1	2	3	4	5
Poor technique couldn't do all 3 ties, insecure knots		Moderately good technique some ties were done better than others, mostly secure knots		Excellent technique excellent execution of all 3 ties, very secure knots

Respect for Tissue

1	2	3	4	5
Frequently used unnecessay force, or caused damage on tissue		Careful handling of tissue but occasionally used damage		Very careful handling of tissues with minimal or no damage

Motion and Flow

1	2	3	4	5
Many unnecessary moves, frequent stops + starts, frequently grasped, regrasped tissue		Some unnecessary moves, reasonably efficient, smooth progression, occasional reprasing of tissue		Clear economy of movement easy flow /rhythm throughout, minimal regrasping of tissue

Score (6 -30): ________

(*Adapted from the Global Rating Scale of Operative Performance shown in: Reznick R, Regehr G, MacRae H, Martin J, McCulloch W. Testing technical skill via an innovative "bench station" examination. Am J Surg. 1997;173:226–30.)

References

1. Engels PT, de Gara C. Learning styles of medical students, general surgery residents, and general surgeons: implications for surgical education. BMC Med Educ. 2010;10:51.
2. Wang B, Lu G, Patel AA, Ren P, Cheng I. An evaluation of the learning curve for a complex surgical technique: the full endoscopic interlaminar approach for lumbar disc herniations. Spine J. 2011; 11(2):122–30.
3. Sonnadara RR, Van Vliet A, Safir O, et al. Orthopedic boot camp: examining the effectiveness of an intensive surgical skills course. Surgery. 2011;149(6):745–9.
4. Leong JJ, Leff DR, Das A, et al. Validation of orthopaedic bench models for trauma surgery. J Bone Joint Surg Br. 2008;90(7):958–65.
5. ACGME ACfGME. ACGME Program Requirements for Residency Education in Orthopaedic Surgery. 2012; Available at http://www.acgme.org/acWebsite/downloads/RRC_progReq/260_orthopaedic_surgery_07012012_TCC.pdf. Accessed 20 Feb 2012.
6. Jain N, Pietrobon R, Hocker S, Guller U, Shankar A, Higgins LD. The relationship between surgeon and hospital volume and outcomes for shoulder arthroplasty. J Bone Joint Surg Am. 2004;86- A(3):496–505.
7. Katz JN, Losina E, Barrett J, et al. Association between hospital and surgeon procedure volume and outcomes of total hip replacement in the United States medicare population. J Bone Joint Surg Am. 2001;83-A(11):1622–9.
8. Katz JN, Barrett J, Mahomed NN, Baron JA, Wright RJ, Losina E. Association between hospital and surgeon procedure volume and the outcomes of total knee replacement. J Bone Joint Surg Am. 2004;86-A(9):1909–16.
9. Gomoll AH, O'Toole RV, Czarnecki J, Warner JJ. Surgical experience correlates with performance on a virtual reality simulator for shoulder arthroscopy. Am J Sports Med. 2007;35(6):883–8.
10. Reznick RK, MacRae H. Teaching surgical skills – changes in the wind. N Engl J Med. 2006;355(25):2664–9.
11. Van Heest A, Putnam M, Agel J, Shanedling J, McPherson S, Schmitz C. Assessment of technical skills of orthopaedic surgery residents performing open carpal tunnel release surgery. J Bone Joint Surg Am. 2009;91(12):2811–7.
12. Ferrari G. Public anatomy lessons and the carnival: the anatomy theatre of Bologna. Past Present. 1987;117:50–106.
13. Holland JP, Waugh L, Horgan A, Paleri V, Deehan DJ. Cadaveric hands-on training for surgical specialties: is this back to the future for surgical skills development? J Surg Educ. 2011;68(2):110–6.
14. Schneider U, Heller R. Plastic Bone Used for Training Purposes by Surgeons. US Patent 4,106,219, filed November 19, 1976, and issued August 15, 1978.
15. Hausmann JT. Sawbones in biomechanical settings – a review. Osteo Trauma Care. 2006;14(4):259–64.
16. Tuijthof GJ, van Sterkenburg MN, Sierevelt IN, van Oldenrijk J, Van Dijk CN, Kerkhoffs GM. First validation of the PASSPORT training environment for arthroscopic skills. Knee Surg Sports Traumatol Arthrosc. 2010;18(2):218–24.
17. Howells NR, Auplish S, Hand GC, Gill HS, Carr AJ, Rees JL. Retention of arthroscopic shoulder skills learned with use of a simulator. Demonstration of a learning curve and loss of performance level after a time delay. J Bone Joint Surg Am. 2009;91(5):1207–13.
18. Atesok K, Schemitsch EH. Computer-assisted trauma surgery. J Am Acad Orthop Surg. 2010;18(5):247–58.
19. Citak M, Gardner MJ, Kendoff D, et al. Virtual 3D planning of acetabular fracture reduction. J Orthop Res. 2008;26(4):547–52.
20. Cobb JP, Kannan V, Dandachli W, Iranpour F, Brust KU, Hart AJ. Learning how to resurface cam-type femoral heads with acceptable accuracy and precision: the role of computed tomography-based navigation. J Bone Joint Surg Am. 2008;90 Suppl 3:57–64.
21. Gofton W, Dubrowski A, Tabloie F, Backstein D. The effect of computer navigation on trainee learning of surgical skills. J Bone Joint Surg Am. 2007;89(12):2819–27.
22. Blyth P, Stott NS, Anderson IA. A simulation-based training system for hip fracture fixation for use within the hospital environment. Injury. 2007;38(10):1197–203.
23. Brown GA, Firoozbakhsh K, DeCoster TA, Reyna Jr JR, Moneim M. Rapid prototyping: the future of trauma surgery? J Bone Joint Surg Am. 2003;85-A Suppl 4:49–55.
24. Owens BD, Kragh Jr JF, Macaitis J, Svoboda SJ, Wenke JC. Characterization of extremity wounds in Operation Iraqi Freedom and Operation Enduring Freedom. J Orthop Trauma. 2007; 21(4):254–7.
25. Reinig K, Lee C, Rubinstein D, Bagur M, Spitzer V. The United States military's thigh trauma simulator. Clin Orthop Relat Res. 2006;442:45–56.
26. McCarthy AD, Moody L, Waterworth AR, Bickerstaff DR. Passive haptics in a knee arthroscopy simulator: is it valid for core skills training? Clin Orthop Relat Res. 2006;442:13–20.
27. Vankipuram M, Kahol K, McLaren A, Panchanathan S. A virtual reality simulator for orthopedic basic skills: a design and validation study. J Biomed Inform. 2010;43(5):661–8.
28. Kim S, Bosque J, Meehan JP, Jamali A, Marder R. Increase in outpatient knee arthroscopy in the United States: a comparison of National Surveys of Ambulatory Surgery, 1996 and 2006. J Bone Joint Surg Am. 2011;93(11):994–1000.
29. Hall MP, Kaplan KM, Gorczynski CT, Zuckerman JD, Rosen JE. Assessment of arthroscopic training in U.S. orthopedic surgery residency programs – a resident self-assessment. Bull NYU Hosp Jt Dis. 2010;68(1):5–10.
30. Mabrey JD, Reinig KD, Cannon WD. Virtual reality in orthopaedics: is it a reality? Clin Orthop Relat Res. 2010;468(10):2586–91.
31. Ackerman MJ. The Visible Human Project: a resource for anatomical visualization. Stud Health Technol Inform. 1998;52(Pt 2):1030–2.
32. Rosser Jr JC, Lynch PJ, Cuddihy L, Gentile DA, Klonsky J, Merrell R. The impact of video games on training surgeons in the 21st century. Arch Surg. 2007;142(2):181–6; discusssion 186.
33. Grantcharov TP. Is virtual reality simulation an effective training method in surgery? Nat Clin Pract Gastroenterol Hepatol. 2008;5(5):232–3.
34. Tuijthof GJ, Visser P, Sierevelt IN, Van Dijk CN, Kerkhoffs GM. Does perception of usefulness of arthroscopic simulators differ with levels of experience? Clin Orthop Relat Res. 2011;469(6):1701–8.
35. Gomoll AH, Pappas G, Forsythe B, Warner JJ. Individual skill progression on a virtual reality simulator for shoulder arthroscopy: a 3-year follow-up study. Am J Sports Med. 2008;36(6):1139–42.
36. Pedowitz RA, Esch J, Snyder S. Evaluation of a virtual reality simulator for arthroscopy skills development. Arthroscopy. 2002; 18(6):E29.
37. Srivastava S, Youngblood PL, Rawn C, Hariri S, Heinrichs WL, Ladd AL. Initial evaluation of a shoulder arthroscopy simulator: establishing construct validity. J Shoulder Elbow Surg. 2004; 13(2):196–205.
38. Martin KD, Belmont PJ, Schoenfeld AJ, Todd M, Cameron KL, Owens BD. Arthroscopic basic task performance in shoulder simulator model correlates with similar task performance in cadavers. J Bone Joint Surg Am. 2011;93(21):e1271–5.
39. Howells NR, Gill HS, Carr AJ, Price AJ, Rees JL. Transferring simulated arthroscopic skills to the operating theatre: a randomised blinded study. J Bone Joint Surg Br. 2008;90(4):494–9.
40. Myden CA et al. Computer-assisted surgery simulations and directed practice of total knee arthroplasty: Educational benefits to the trainee. Comput Aided Surg. 2012;17(3):113–27.

Simulation in Otolaryngology

33

Ellen S. Deutsch and Luv R. Javia

Introduction

The myriad of simulators developed in otolaryngology broadly span the disciplines of otology, rhinology, airway, and head and neck surgery. Moreover, interpersonal, professional, and communication clinical skills can be honed using simulators. These distinct and individual simulators can be organized into curricula and delivered in various formats whether as weekly didactic curricula for residents and fellows or as aggregated, concentrated exposures in courses. Simulators in otolaryngology will continue to thrive, evolve, and play a greater, more vital role in the future education of residents and even skills improvement for experienced surgeons.

Otolaryngologists have approached simulation with a broad perspective and have developed or adapted a wide variety of simulators and types of simulation. Simulators in Otolaryngology range from simple, physical models to virtual electronic marvels and from low cost to high technology. Some of these simulators have been developed by otolaryngologists for specific Otolaryngologic purposes and some have been designed for other purposes but have been adopted or adapted for Otolaryngology. Based on identified learning objectives, otolaryngologists have incorporated these simulators into a spectrum of simulations which may address technical skills, medical management and judgment, communication, teamwork and leadership, and systems improvements. Otolaryngologists are also using simulation as a platform from which to develop and refine assessment methods and tools and to provide objective documentation of both technical and nontechnical skills.

As in other specialties, simulation can be used to develop, maintain, optimize, and test skills [1].

Simulation uniformly includes directed practice and debriefing, which are essential components of adult education [2]. Simulation allows learners to explore, make mistakes, and recover from mistakes without direct risk to patients. Simulation incorporated into a comprehensive curriculum provides learning opportunities based on the needs of learners rather than the needs of patients [3]. In some circumstances, using simulation-based education may be an ethical imperative [4]. Simulation provides essential tools which allow clinical educators to take advantage of the rapid pace of technologic advances, as well as helping manage the impact of resource limitations and ever-increasing societal expectations.

In parallel with other specialties, the issue of simulator and simulation fidelity, or realism, is also of major concern for otolaryngology. This characteristic relates to the entire simulation and encompasses more than the features of the simulator. Fidelity is not the same as the level of technology of a particular simulator, e.g., a low technology simulator may be high fidelity for a specific learning objective and vice versa. Fidelity is a complex combination of the physical and technologic characteristics of the simulator, the setting and circumstances in which the simulation occurs, and their relationship to the educational needs of the learner(s).

Within Otolaryngology, there are notable areas of expertise in developing simulators and simulations and in the development of tools and strategies to assess learning and competence. In this chapter we explore the diversity of simulators and simulation used in otolaryngology.

E.S. Deutsch, MD, FACS, FAAP (✉)
Department of Anesthesia and Critical Care,
Center for Simulation, Advanced Education, and Innovation,
The Children's Hospital of Philadelphia,
Room 8NW100, 3400 Civic Center Blvd.,
Philadelphia, PA, USA
e-mail: deutsches@email.chop.edu

L.R. Javia, MD
Department of Otorhinolaryngology/Head and Neck Surgery,
Perelman School of Medicine at the University of Pennsylvania,
Philadelphia, PA, USA

Department of Pediatric Otolaryngology,
Children's Hospital of Philadelphia,
34th Street and Civic Center Blvd., 1 Wood Building,
Philadelphia, PA 19104, USA
e-mail: javia@email.chop.edu

A.I. Levine et al. (eds.), *The Comprehensive Textbook of Healthcare Simulation*,
DOI 10.1007/978-1-4614-5993-4_33, © Springer Science+Business Media New York 2013

Overview of Simulation for Otolaryngology

There is a long, proud history of simulation in otolaryngology. Chevalier Jackson, who shaped modern bronchoesophagology, advocated practice and demonstrated his methods using simulation techniques almost a century ago. Films donated to the American Bronchoesophagological Association by his family show him demonstrating both bronchoscopic and open surgical procedures which can be viewed online (at http://abea.net) [5, 6].

Dissecting cadaveric temporal bones to learn both the anatomy and the techniques important for mastoid surgical procedures is a time-honored mainstay of otolaryngology residencies. Learners have long used cadavers, anesthetized animals, and other biologic tissue to improve their anatomic knowledge and surgical skills. Even experienced surgeons use various types of simulation to explore new technologies and to hone their skills as advances in imaging, surgical tools, surgical devices, and surgical procedures evolve.

A variety of simulators are described below, but they represent only the beginning of the process of developing a simulation. When seeking pure task training to develop technical skills, an isolated simulator may be optimal, and the opportunity to practice specific skills in a solitary manner is invaluable. If learning objectives addressing skills such as teamwork, communication, and leadership are sought, entire scenarios can be created, including case descriptions which incorporate the same content as a clinical encounter, providing opportunities for realistic, even interprofessional, diagnostic, and management interactions and interventions. To augment the realism and comprehensiveness of a simulation, use of actual surgical equipment, or relevant radiographic studies, or even a fog machine to simulate smoke may be warranted. Realism can also be augmented by conducting the simulation in a space designed to look like an operating room or a clinic or a patient care room – or the realism could be optimized by conducting the simulation "in situ," in a real operating room. Learners may also benefit from interacting with a "confederate" who role-plays another participant, a skilled "standardized patient" who is trained to represent specific conditions and provide feedback to the learner, or other learners in the setting of multidisciplinary or interprofessional simulations.

Otology Simulators

Cadaveric temporal bones used for dissection represent one of the oldest simulators that are used to train otologic surgery. Anatomic relationships within the temporal bone are complex and challenging. The ossicles, cochlea, vestibular labyrinth, and facial nerve, which control hearing, balance, and facial motion, are all very small structures which can be difficult to localize and identify but lay in close proximity within the surgical field. Dissection through the temporal bone is also used to provide access to the skull base. Cadaveric dissection sets the standard against which other methods must compare in order to gain general acceptance as valid training alternatives to live surgery [7]. However, infectious concerns and increasing difficulty procuring cadaveric temporal bones limit exposure of trainees to this type of simulator. These challenges to cadaveric temporal bone dissection have spawned interest in alternate otologic simulators.

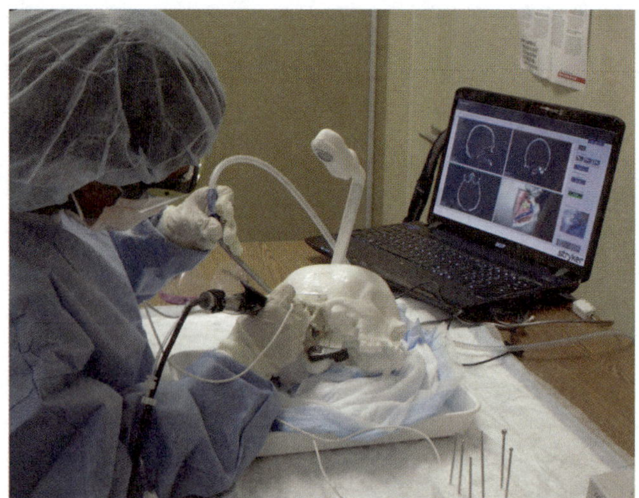

Fig. 33.1 Physical temporal bone simulator with electronic interface (Stryker, Kalamazoo, MI) providing metrics and image guidance

Several types of non-cadaveric temporal bone simulators have been developed. Some are actual physical models made out of artificial materials. The Pettigrew bone is made of plastic and incorporates colored structures to highlight relevant otologic anatomy [7, 8]. Recent 3D printing technology has further expanded the possibilities for this sort of simulator. This novel technology may someday allow us to print physical models based on actual patient pathology from radiographic imaging data already available. Furthermore, as this technology advances, it may allow us to improve upon the anatomic fidelity of currently available physical temporal bone models. Stryker (Kalamazoo, MI) markets a physical temporal bone composed of a bone-like material which can be drilled using standard tools but has an electronic interface including embedded electrodes and an image guidance system, both of which can provide feedback to trainees in real time as they drill (Fig. 33.1). The electrodes can ascertain when vital structures, such as the facial nerve, are damaged or violated and provide metric summaries for performance analysis.

Kuppersmith et al. were among the first proponents of the power of virtual reality simulators for otology training by otolaryngology trainees. They specifically discussed the development of an anatomically accurate virtual 3D environment whereby trainees could practice surgical skills with force, vibratory, and auditory feedback [9]. Several other groups have developed virtual reality (VR) temporal bone dissection simulators including Agus et al., the Ohio State VR simulator, the Stanford VR simulator, the VOXEL-MAN TempoSurg VR simulator (Fig. 33.2), the Visible Ear Surgery VR simulator, the CSIRO/Melbourne VR simulator, and the Karl Storz Surgical Cockpit ENT VR simulator [10–15].

Most of the VR simulators incorporate haptic and auditory feedback. Kerwin et al. reported on increasing the realism of VR temporal bone drilling by rendering fluid dynamics including bleeding effects, meniscus rendering, and refraction [16]. The neurosurgical literature also reports a VR simulator designed for transpetrous extended approaches [17]. Unfortunately, many of these simulators are prototypes and not commercially available for purchase.

Besides the challenges of development and production, there is also the burden upon the developers to undertake the great monetary and time investment of intensive validation. Wiet et al. have recently published a manuscript detailing the validation of the Ohio State VR temporal bone simulator at eight different institutions across the USA; practice on their VR simulator was found to be equivalent to practice on cadaveric temporal bones [18].

Similar to physical models with electronic interfaces, VR simulators allow unlimited opportunities for practice including some components of competency assessment and feedback without requiring the presence of an expert surgeon during each dissection. Time for dissection, identification and violation of key structures, and efficiency of movement can all be measured. Additionally, comparing VR temporal bone simulators to both cadaveric and physical models, there is not a physical limit as to the number of temporal bones available for dissection, mistakes can be "reversed," and the trainee does not have to discard a temporal bone to start over. Moreover, by comparing the "pixels" or areas of bone removed by a trainee to compiled data from expert dissections, one can score adequacy of dissection [12, 18]. Incorporation of these competency measurements into the simulator is an active area of research. As computer hardware and software technology advances, so to will the realism of current VR platforms. Some have proposed that during the early stages of training, three-dimensional models and virtual reality temporal bone simulators are more than adequate to meet trainees' needs…[and] the holistic benefits of cadaveric dissection would be better utilized once trainees have reached the "autonomous" stage [7].

Although there is a lot of interest and great potential for the use of technology-augmented simulators, several low technology otologic simulators also exist. Mathews et al. describe an incus and stapes footplate simulator for stapes prosthesis placement comprised of a disposable drinking cup, toothpicks, and a tongue depressor [19]. Similarly, Owa et al. describe another low-cost simulator for stapes prosthesis placement made out of ward-based materials [20].

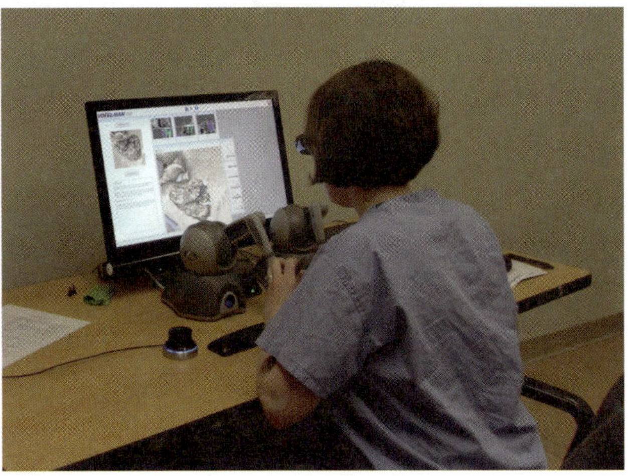

Fig. 33.2 Virtual reality temporal bone simulator (VOXEL-Man, Hamburg, Germany), providing auditory information, haptic interface, and metrics

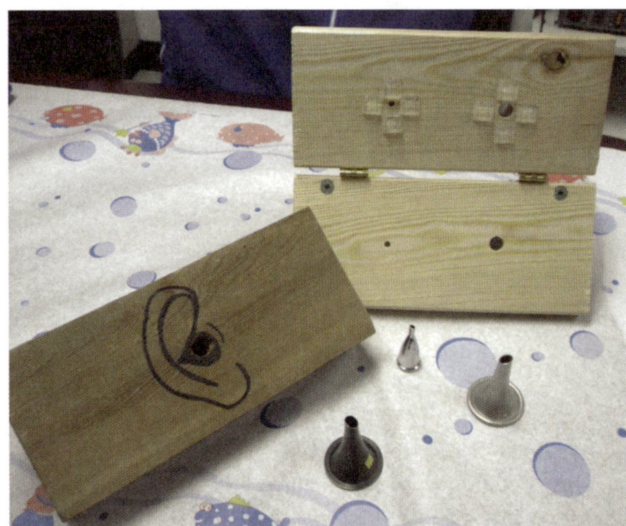

Fig. 33.3 Constructed otology simulator, for practicing myringotomy tube insertion and office-based procedures. A piece of plastic inserted between the wooden blocks functions as a tympanic membrane. Foreign bodies, or lotion to represent otorrhea, can be placed in the external ear canal. The narrower aperture represents a stenotic ear canal. Simulator developed by Steve Handler, MD

For the novice otolaryngologist, even myringotomy tube insertion, which typically includes the use of a microscope, is challenging and can be simulated. Several otolaryngologists have constructed simple models designed to allow beginners to practice hand-eye or hand-eye-microscope coordination (Fig. 33.3). Volsky et al. describe a physical anatomic model of a head with tympanic membrane cartridge components which fit inside the ear canal, allowing for repeated attempts at performing myringotomy and pressure equalization tube placement. Construct validity has been demonstrated for this simulator, as it has been shown to discriminate novice from non-novice users [21]. There are also virtual reality simulators for performing a myringotomy [22, 23].

Sinus Simulators

Rhinologic and sinus simulators have some characteristics which are similar to otology simulators, in that the underlying anatomic framework which the simulator replicates is bone, but there are also important differences. In contrast to the rigidity of much of the temporal bone, many of the bones in the nose and sinuses are thin and are manipulated or displaced (i.e., "outfractured") during surgical procedures, so it would be optimal to represent them as non-static structures. The delicate soft tissue interface within rhinosinus anatomy is also complex. Sinus simulator development has parallels with otology simulator development, in that both 3-dimensional and virtual models have been built.

The ES3 simulator, a virtual sinus simulator with an anatomic, haptic interface, has been extensively studied by Weghorst, Rudman, Edmond, Fried, and several coauthors, and is one of the most comprehensively validated extant simulators [1]. Learning exercises with this simulator include both nonanatomic skills (e.g., using a surgical orientation, but manipulating abstract shapes) and specific anatomic exercises, such as middle turbinate medialization and uncinectomy [1]. Additional virtual simulators include the Nasal Endoscopy Simulator [24, 25], the Voxel Man SinuSurg [26], and a simulator described by Caversaccio et al. [27]. Most of the virtual sinus simulators include haptic feedback and an anatomic interface; and most are in the prototype phase. Caversaccio et al. found no improvement in actual procedures on patients [27]. Edmond suggested and Fried et al. documented improved operative technique and performance during actual surgery related to training with the ES3 simulator [1, 28].

Several physical rhinosinus models have been developed [29–31]. Leung et al. describe both a physical and cadaveric model which can be used for both nonanatomic and anatomic skill training [32]. Malekzadeh et al. have developed and validated a low cost, low technology gelatin model which is semi-anatomic (Fig. 33.4) [33].

An epistaxis simulator can be constructed from material generally available in simulation centers and is useful for novices who are learning how to utilize a headlight as well as how to construct and apply nasal packing (Fig. 33.5) [34]. Thin tubing inserted through the back of the mannequin's head and into its nose allows simulated blood to flow until the learner inserts packing materials or an epistaxis control device to staunch the bleeding. Both anterior and posterior nasal packs can be inserted.

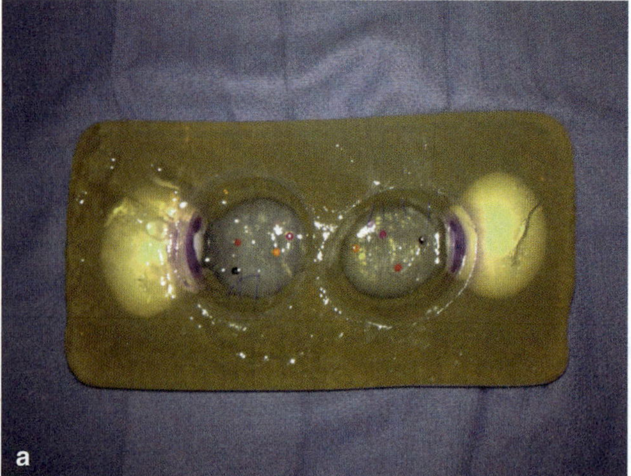

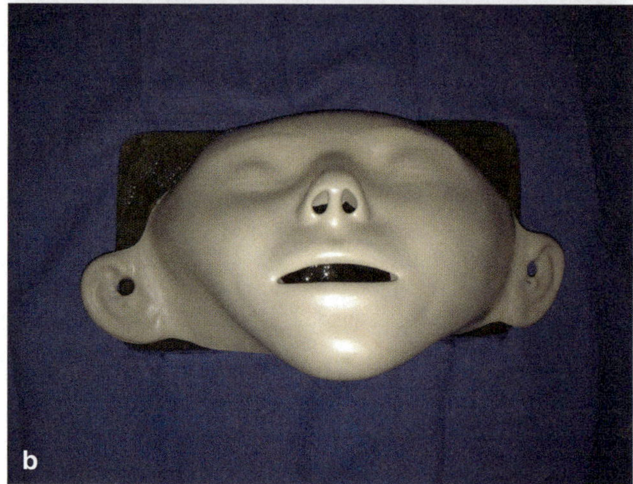

Fig. 33.4 Sinus surgery model constructed from gelatin and other items. The gelatin model (**a**) is placed behind the mannequin face (**b**). Entering the maxillary sinuses releases the contents of the raw eggs, which can be suctioned. Simulator developed by, and photos courtesy of, Sonya Malekzadeh, MD

Airway Simulators

Although all surgical procedures require skill and involve risk for patients, airway work exemplifies the challenges which make simulation valuable to the otolaryngologist, the anesthesiologist, and their patients. For example, a typical resident would be expected to manage between 0.2 and 3.9 cases of foreign body aspiration per year, depending on their training location [35]. Traditionally, simulation used to learn these techniques occurred in an animal laboratory. Currently the management of aspirated foreign bodies can also be practiced by inserting a foreign body into a variety of full body mannequins, and this exercise can be repeated as many times as desired (Fig. 33.6) [36].

In general, the mannequins' airway characteristics are not identical to those of humans, but they are sufficiently representative, particularly for novices who are also learning how to manipulate the appropriate instruments. When a physical

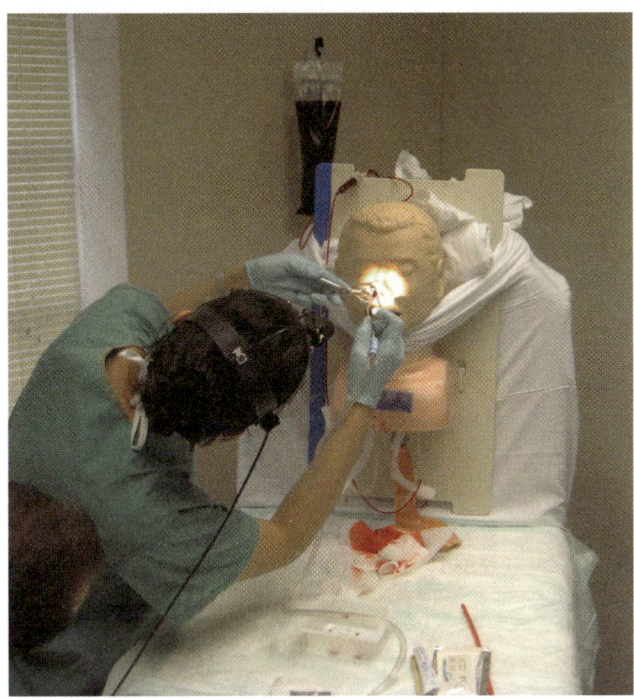

Fig. 33.5 Epistaxis model. Faculty controls the flow of "blood" through the tubing inserting from the back of the head into the nasal cavity

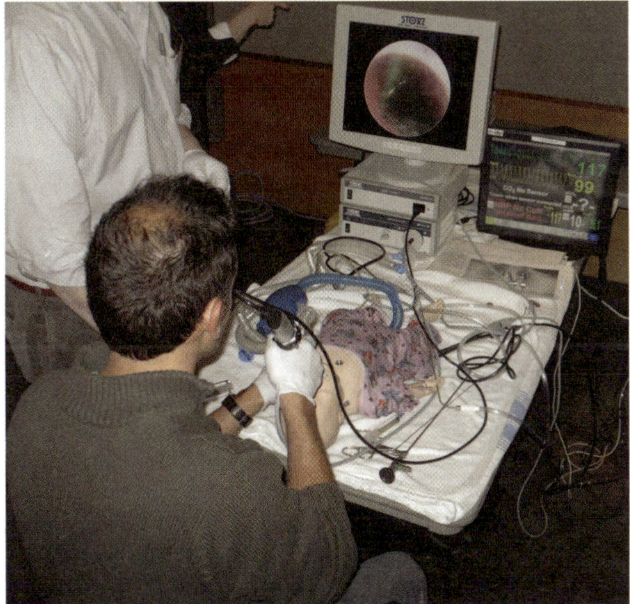

Fig. 33.6 Resident removing an "aspirated" foreign body from a high-technology infant simulator (SimBaby, Laerdal, Wappinger Falls, NY) in an "ad hoc" simulation setting during an Airway Foreign Body Course. Note the image from the bronchoscope on the endoscopy monitor, and the vital signs monitor displaying physiologic data; the pulse oximeter also provides audible information. If the mannequin is not adequately ventilated, the pulse oximetry reading will decrease; if the endoscopist does not adequately coordinate with the "anesthesiologist," the mannequin will demonstrate laryngospasm

model with representative laryngeal, tracheal and endobronchial anatomy is used (whether low or high technology), airway anatomy can be learned using actual equipment, such as laryngoscopes, rigid telescopes or fiberoptic bronchoscopes. Howells et al found that students who had trained on a simulator were able to develop intubation skills in actual patients more quickly and safely than those without simulator training [37]. Rowe and Cohen demonstrated improved skills during bronchoscopy on real patients after residents trained on a VR bronchoscopy simulator [38]. Jabbour et al. are developing fabricated organosilicate airway complexes which provide additional anatomic fidelity [39].

After the learner manages basic instrument manipulation skills, the complexity of the simulation can be increased to represent a more comprehensive experience, including reviewing radiographs prior to performing the procedure, planning and coordinating with the anesthesiologist, etc. If a high-technology mannequin is used, additional conditions and characteristics can be modeled, such as oxygen desaturation, asymmetric chest wall expansion, and laryngospasm.

Burns et al. have adapted a model which takes advantage of the small caliber vascular network present in the chorioallantoic membrane of chicken eggs, providing a responsive biologic platform for laser and microlaryngeal procedures [40, 41]. Several models have been developed for simulating tonsillectomy; most attempt to replicate the challenge of accessing distant structures (e.g., the tonsils in the oropharynx) through a relatively narrow aperture in a very representative fashion [42, 43].

Head and Neck Simulators

Recent advances in Head and Neck Surgery with Transoral Robotic Surgery has created a new need for training both new and experienced otolaryngologists in these novel techniques. This has spawned the creation of robotic skill training simulators including *da Vinci Skills Simulator* (Intuitive Surgical, Sunnyvale, CA); and Robotic Surgical Simulator (Simulated Surgical Systems, Williamsville, NY) for robot-assisted surgical procedures. The *da Vinci Skills Simulator* is a training device that integrates into an existing surgeon's console and includes abstract and anatomic virtual reality exercises that can be projected to the trainee through the binocular optics (Fig. 33.7). A simulator can also be created with the robotic arms and the surgeon's console. Physical task training exercises can also be performed using the actual robotic instrumentation. The virtual reality exercises have all the aforementioned advantages of virtual reality simulators, including the ability to repeat exercises, the ability to practice skills without the need of an attendant experienced surgeon, and the ability to compile data regarding competency assessment, such as time to completion of tasks, instrument collisions, and movement efficiency, with real-time feedback.

Despite these recent advances, not all head and neck simulators require expensive or complex technology. Simulators valuable in training head and neck techniques of local flaps

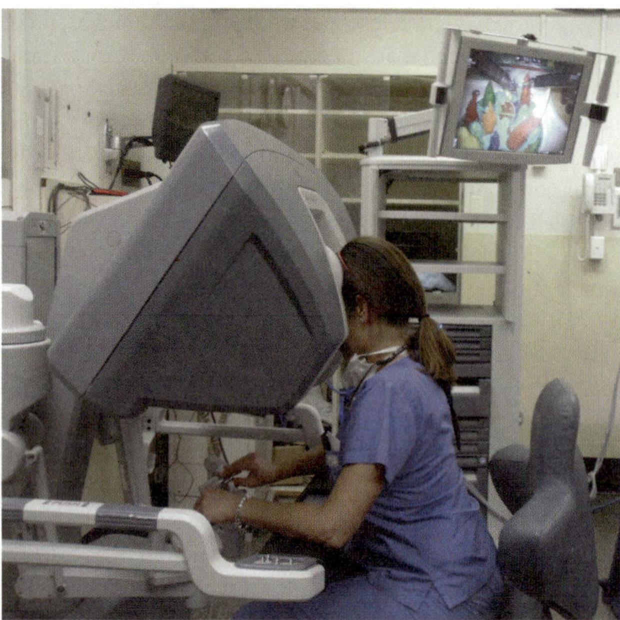

Fig. 33.7 Learner at a robotic console (da Vinci, Intuitive, Sunnyvale, CA), demonstrating practice of robotic manipulation skills with nonanatomic tasks

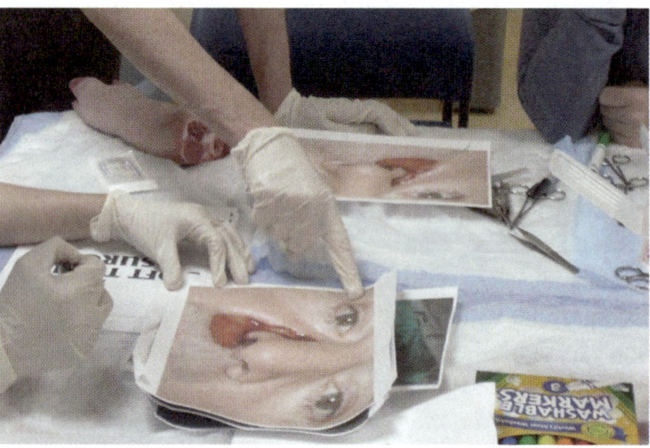

Fig. 33.8 Participants design local rotation and advancement flaps on photographs of lesions and then execute the flaps on biologic tissue (pigs' feet)

include the traditional use of pig's feet and photographs. Local rotation and advancement flaps can be marked out and planned on pictures of patients with actual lesions in various anatomic regions. Trainees can then go a step further and actually practice executing these local flaps using pigs' feet, surgical instrumentation, and suturing techniques (Fig. 33.8) [44].

Microvascular anastomosis is another skill set with an available simulator. Biomet (Warsaw, Indiana) has a kit which is a physical task trainer with a delicate synthetic vessel that must be anastomosed with appropriate suture (Fig. 33.9). Following the completion of the anastomosis, the trainee can inject simulated blood through the vessel to check for leaks. Trainees ideally should wear surgical loupes or use surgical microscopes to increase the realism of the simulation.

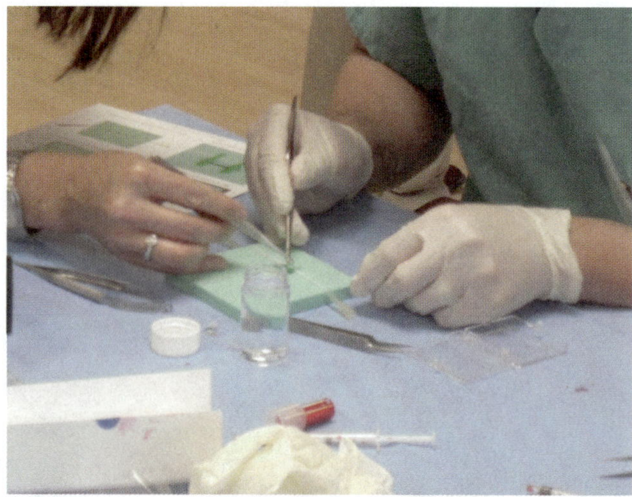

Fig. 33.9 Task trainer for practicing microvascular anastomosis (Biomet, Warsaw, IN)

Plating courses sponsored by organizations such as the AO Foundation (Davos, Switzerland) or plating manufacturers such as Synthes (West Chester, PA) or Stryker (Kalamazoo, MI) can provide hands-on training with physical task trainers in which craniofacial plates can be affixed to simulated skulls to practice treating various craniofacial fractures. This allows the trainees to become familiar with not only the plating technology and instrumentation but also the techniques of facial fracture repair prior to performing on real patients.

Cricothyroidotomy simulators are abundant and varied in their characteristics. They range from full body, high-tech mannequins with the capability of simulating a "can't ventilate, can't intubate" scenario requiring cricothyroidotomy or tracheotomy to physical task trainers which can be constructed more economically. Liu et al. have created a virtual simulator with haptic feedback [45] which employs a Phantom haptic interface device (SensAble Technologies, Wilmington, MA) and can simulate cervical landmark identification, incision with a scalpel blade with bleeding and resistance as the scalpel goes through skin, and the resistance of inserting an airway into the trachea. Physical task trainers can be constructed from mannequins (without using the high-fidelity capabilities) [46–48], corrugated tubing [48], cadaveric tissue, a porcine airway model [49], sheep trachea model [50], and converted/recycled mannequin heads [51] to name a few. Some would argue that there is a role for high-fidelity mannequins that these low-fidelity options are not able to fulfill.

John et al. examined the role of stress by comparing the time to perform a cricothyroidotomy on a physical task trainer in a classroom setting to a "medium-fidelity" simulator incorporated in a "can't intubate, can't ventilate" scenario including pharyngeal edema, laryngospasm, and restricted neck extension as well as a vital signs display in a simulated

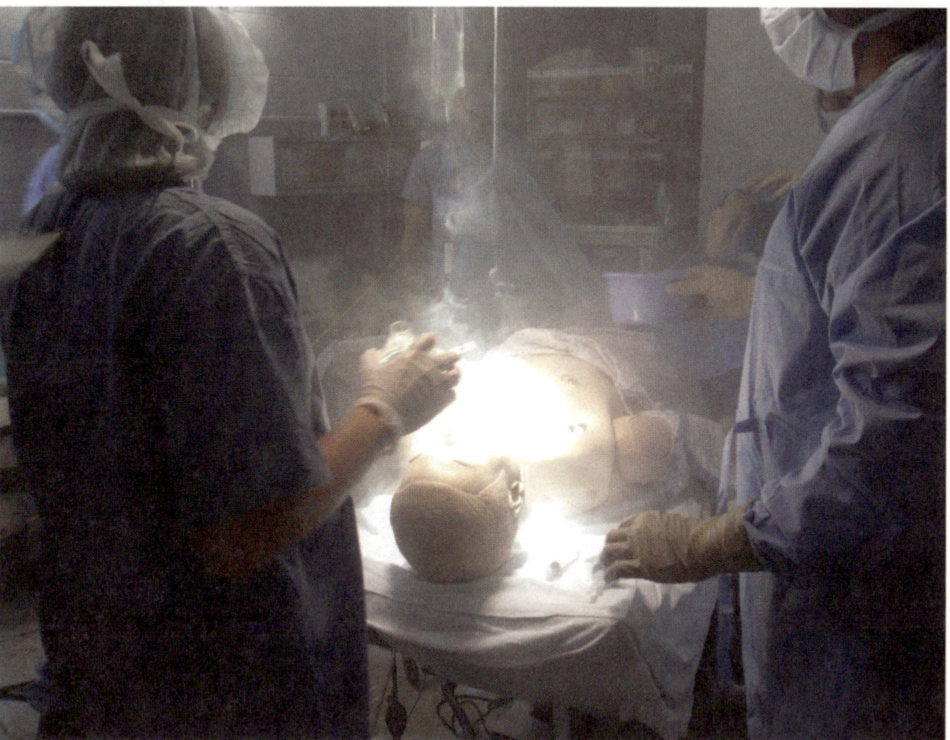

Fig. 33.10 Simulated operating room fire during simulated tonsillectomy involving both Otolaryngology residents and student registered nurse anesthetists. Simulation designed by Kelly Malloy, MD, James Kearney, MD and Maria Magros, CRNA, MS, MSN

operating room setting [47]. Seventy-seven percent of tested anesthesiologists in this randomized crossover study took longer with the medium-fidelity simulator as compared to the physical task trainer suggesting that stress and time pressures in real-life scenarios may affect the performance of cricothyroidotomy. From a strictly skills acquisition perspective, Friedman et al. suggest in their study that a simple inexpensive model constructed from corrugated tubing achieved the same effect on objectively rated skill acquisition as did an expensive high-fidelity simulator [48].

Interpersonal and Professional Clinical Skills Simulation

Besides simulating surgical skills, simulations can be designed to help learners acquire or hone communication skills, including obtaining informed consent, and delivering "bad news" (which includes any sort of information which is unpleasant or uncomfortable for the person receiving the information). The most advanced of these simulations employ "standardized patients," who are professionals trained not only to interact with the learner but also to evaluate and provide feedback to the learner. Less rigorous methods to simulate a "delivering bad news" situation include using faculty, or even other learners, to role-play as a reluctant patient, an anxious family member, or even a difficult faculty member who must be awakened in the middle of the night with unpleasant information [52].

Opportunities to practice leadership as well as difficult discussions can be built into simulations addressing a variety of crises, including "can't intubate, can't ventilate" airway obstruction emergencies, airway fires, and hemorrhage (Fig. 33.10). The difficult discussions can focus on working with another healthcare provider with strongly different management opinions or disclosure of an adverse event to a patient or family member. The participant group can range from single-discipline to interprofessional combinations, and the setting can range from participants sitting in chairs in a circle to a high-technology in situ or even immersive environment. A typical simulation would involve an otolaryngologist coordinating with an anesthesiologist and one or more nurses to optimize team functions including communication, while managing a mannequin with foreign body aspiration.

Practical Implementation of Simulation in Otolaryngology

A series of simulations, based on gap or needs analyses, can be organized into curricula and delivered in various formats. Simulations can be interspersed into the weekly didactic curricula for residents and fellows, replacing specific standard lectures or can be aggregated into concentrated exposures.

For example, the Airway Foreign Body Endoscopy course given at the Children's Hospital of Philadelphia includes an animal laboratory, an interactive, case-based decision-making session, and an ad hoc simulation laboratory incorporating

Table 33.1 Components of the Airway Foreign Body Endoscopy course; a 1-day course designed for novice Otolaryngology Residents and Pediatric Surgery Fellows; developed by Ian N. Jacobs, MD; Ellen S. Deutsch, MD; and Karen B. Zur, MD and held at the Children's Hospital of Philadelphia

Topic or skill	Components
Basic understanding of foreign body aspiration, anesthesia, anatomy, instruments and related topics	Keynote address, plus 4 brief related lectures
Removal of various aspirated foreign bodies from an animal model	Animal laboratory
Removal of aspirated foreign bodies from a high-technology mannequin, including complications such as laryngospasm	High-technology infant mannequin
Delivering bad news	Role-playing difficult conversations, facilitated by faculty
Virtual bronchoscopy	Virtual reality bronchoscopy simulator
Foreign body aspiration case-based decision making	Powerpoint-based presentation of a case of foreign body aspiration, requiring a series of decisions as the patient progresses from presentation in the Emergency Department through complications in the operating room, utilizing an audience response system to stimulate discussion

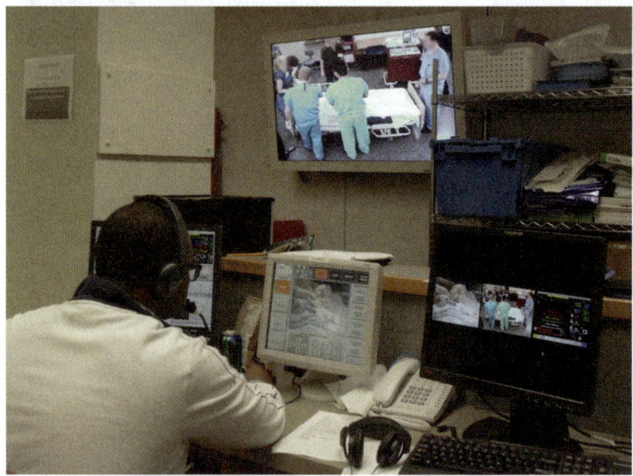

Fig. 33.11 Control area for complex scenario, involving multiple participants managing a surgical complication in a high-technology mannequin (Photograph taken at the Penn Medicine Clinical Simulation Center, Philadelphia, PA, during the 2012 ORL Rising Chief Boot Camp)

high-technology full body simulators used for foreign body removal, a virtual reality simulator used to explore endobronchial anatomy, and a "delivering bad news" role-playing session designed to help residents prepare for "difficult" conversations (Table 33.1). The course is given over one intensive day, which starts with a few brief lectures and then the residents rotate through each of the stations.

Both an "Otolaryngology (ORL) Emergencies Boot Camp" for junior ORL residents and an "ORL Rising Chief boot camp" are also single intensive days, designed to provide progressive experience in isolated skills, then more complex tasks, and finally procedures and management requiring teamwork and communication as well as technical skills. For example, in the ORL Emergencies Boot Camp, residents perform skills such as intubation and then more complex tasks, such as anterior and posterior nasal packing to manage epistaxis, and then participate in "complex scenarios" in which a small group of residents collaborates to diagnose and manage an expanding neck hematoma in a high-technology mannequin [53]. In the ORL Rising Chief Boot Camp, residents begin by participating in skills such as designing and performing local flaps on pigs' feet, then practice with robots and both virtual and physical temporal bone simulators, and finally collaborate to manage an airway emergency in a high-technology mannequin, which includes interacting with a "confederate" role-playing an uncooperative consultant (Fig. 33.11).

Challenges and Opportunities in Otolaryngology Simulation

Challenges for simulation in general include the potential for discrepant modeling, a plateau effect, lack of skill translation, and the rapid evolution of technology, making comparisons difficult. Simulation is often more valuable for novices, but this will likely change as simulators improve over time, and when using them to model the anatomy of specific patients to practice specific procedures becomes easier.

There are also challenges for simulation specific to otolaryngology. Although Otolaryngology shares the need to learn and finesse interpersonal and professional skills with all medical specialties, and many surgical skills, such as suturing the surfaces of organs, with other surgical specialties, we also have unique learning and practice requirements. Many of our procedures require indirect manipulation of tissue; we use instruments to access structures which we cannot reach manually and work at the far end of narrow tunnels from entryways with narrow apertures. In these circumstances, the impact of edema and hemorrhage are magnified, but these complications are not yet well modeled by most simulators. Endoscopic removal of endobronchial foreign bodies in children provides a challenging example. Additionally, many of our procedures are accomplished on extraordinarily small structures, such as the ossicles within the temporal bone.

Simulation has been used to test the reliability of an objective Operative Competency Assessment Tool developed by Ishman and colleagues [54, 55]. This type of tool may be useful for competency-based accreditation which will likely be required in the future by regulatory organizations such as the Accreditation Council for Graduate Medical Education (ACGME). With some creativity, simulation can be used in partial fulfillment of all of the current ACGME competency requirements [56]. The relatively small numbers of residents and fellows per year in training programs makes collaboration essential for meaningful validation, although it should not be presumed that research should be limited to otolaryngologists still in training.

Otolaryngology simulation extends beyond training endeavors. Roy and Smith used biologic tissue as a model to evaluate the impact of varying oxygen concentrations and surgical instruments on the risk of initiating an operating room fire within a cavity [57].

Looking forward, the American Academy of Otolaryngology – Head and Neck Surgery has established an Otolaryngology Surgical Simulation Task Force which is evaluating the current state of the art of simulation, providing information about simulation to academy membership, nurturing collaborations and making recommendations for applications and future directions for simulation in Otolaryngology.

Conclusions

Simulators have long been used in otolaryngology, but educational and technologic advances create the opportunities, and resource limitations and societal expectations create the need to use them more broadly. Otolaryngologists have risen to this challenge and developed or adapted simulators for otolaryngology which include low and high-technology models, physical and virtual models, inexpensive and expensive models, home-made and commercial models, live humans, cadavers, anesthetized animals, and biologic tissue which can be purchased at the grocery store. The diversity of options are complementary [52], allowing selection of the most appropriate simulator for specific learning objectives. These simulators are then incorporated into simulations which address technical and medical skills, as well as safety, teamwork, and communication. Several specific simulators have achieved face, content, and construct validity, [1, 18, 58] and specific simulators have also been demonstrated to improve skills in simulated settings and even operational performance in actual patient care [1, 12, 18, 37, 38]. Simulation is revolutionizing surgical training for learners at all career stages. The complexity and importance of expertise in otolaryngology provides many opportunities to expand and shape simulation to benefit our patients. The field of otolaryngology simulation, built on deep roots, is vibrant and thriving.

References

1. Fried MP, Sadoughi B, Gibber MJ, et al. From virtual reality to the operating room: the endoscopic sinus surgery simulator experiment. Otolaryngol Head Neck Surg. 2010;142(2):202–7.
2. Ericsson KA. Deliberate practice and acquisition of expert performance: a general overview. Acad Emerg Med. 2008;15(11): 988–94.
3. Kneebone RL. Practice, rehearsal, and performance: an approach for simulation-based surgical and procedure training. JAMA. 2009;302(12):1336–8.
4. Ziv A, Wolpe PR, Small SD, Glick S. Simulation-based medical education: an ethical imperative. Acad Med. 2003;78(8):783–8.
5. History: Jackson speaks. 2012. http://abea.net/about/historical/jacksonspeaks/index.html. Accessed 26 Apr 2012.
6. History: Jackson tracheotomy. 2012. http://abea.net/about/historical/jacksontracheotomy/index.html. Accessed 20 May 2012.
7. George AP, De R. Review of temporal bone dissection teaching: how it was, is and will be. J Laryngol Otol. 2010;124(2):119–25.
8. Varadarajan V, Verma R, Auccott W. The portable temporal bone lab – a useful training adjunct for the ENT trainee. Clin Otolaryngol. 2010;35(5):449–50.
9. Kuppersmith RB, Johnston R, Jones SB, Jenkins HA. Virtual reality surgical simulation and otolaryngology. Arch Otolaryngol Head Neck Surg. 1996;122(12):1297–8.
10. Agus M, Giachetti A, Gobbetti E, et al. Mastoidectomy simulation with combined visual and haptic feedback. Stud Health Technol Inform. 2002;85:17–23.
11. Wiet GJ, Stredney D, Sessanna D, Bryan JA, Bradley Welling D, Schmalbrock P. Virtual temporal bone dissection: an interactive surgical simulator. Otolaryngol Head Neck Surg. 2002;127(1):79–83.
12. Sewell C, Morris D, Blevins NH, et al. Providing metrics and performance feedback in a surgical simulator. Comput Aided Surg. 2008;13(2):63–81.
13. Pflesser B, Petersik A, Tiede U, Hohne KH, Leuwer R. Volume cutting for virtual petrous bone surgery. Comput Aided Surg. 2002;7(2):74–83.
14. Trier P, Noe KO, Sorensen MS, Mosegaard J. The visible ear surgery simulator. Stud Health Technol Inform. 2008;132:523–5.
15. Hutchins M, O'Leary S, Stevenson D, Gunn C, Krumpholz A. A networked haptic virtual environment for teaching temporal bone surgery. Stud Health Technol Inform. 2005;111:204–7.
16. Kerwin T, Shen HW, Stredney D. Enhancing realism of wet surfaces in temporal bone surgical simulation. IEEE Trans Vis Comput Graph. 2009;15(5):747–58.
17. Bernardo A, Preul MC, Zabramski JM, Spetzler RF. A three-dimensional interactive virtual dissection model to simulate transpetrous surgical avenues. Neurosurgery. 2003;52(3):499–505.
18. Wiet GJ, Stredney D, Kerwin T, et al. Virtual temporal bone dissection system: OSU virtual temporal bone system: development and testing. Laryngoscope. 2012;122 Suppl 1:S1–12.
19. Mathews SB, Hetzler DG, Hilsinger Jr RL. Incus and stapes footplate simulator. Laryngoscope. 1997;107(12 I):1614–6.
20. Owa AO, Gbejuade HO, Giddings C. A middle-ear simulator for practicing prosthesis placement for otosclerosis surgery using ward-based materials. J Laryngol Otol. 2003;117(6):490–2.
21. Volsky PG, Hughley BB, Peirce SM, Kesser BW. Construct validity of a simulator for myringotomy with ventilation tube insertion. Otolaryngol Head Neck Surg. 2009;141(5):603; 608.e1.
22. Sowerby LJ, Rehal G, Husein M, Doyle PC, Agrawal S, Ladak HM. Development and face validity testing of a three-dimensional myringotomy simulator with haptic feedback. J Otolaryngol Head Neck Surg. 2010;39(2):122–9.
23. Wheeler B, Doyle PC, Chandarana S, Agrawal S, Husein M, Ladak HM. Interactive computer-based simulator for training in blade navigation and targeting in myringotomy. Comput Methods Programs Biomed. 2010;98(2):130–9.
24. Bockholt U, Ecke U, Muller W, Voss G. Realtime simulation of tissue deformation for the nasal endoscopy simulator (NES). Stud Health Technol Inform. 1999;62:74–5.
25. Ecke U, Klimek L, Muller W, Ziegler R, Mann W. Virtual reality: preparation and execution of sinus surgery. Comput Aided Surg. 1998;3(1):45–50.

26. Tolsdorff B, Pommert A, Hohne KH, et al. Virtual reality: a new paranasal sinus surgery simulator. Laryngoscope. 2010;120(2): 420–6.
27. Caversaccio M, Eichenberger A, Hausler R. Virtual simulator as a training tool for endonasal surgery. Am J Rhinol. 2003;17(5): 283–90.
28. Edmond Jr CV. Impact of the endoscopic sinus surgical simulator on operating room performance. Laryngoscope. 2002;112(7I): 1148–58.
29. Ossowski KL, Rhee DC, Rubinstein EN, Ferguson BJ. Efficacy of sinonasal simulator in teaching endoscopic nasal skills. Laryngoscope. 2008;118(8):1482–5.
30. Nogueira Junior JF, Cruz DN. Real models and virtual simulators in otolaryngology: review of literature. Rev Bras Otorrinolaringol (Engl Ed). 2010;76(1):129–35.
31. Stamm A, Nogueira JF, Lyra M. Feasibility of balloon dilatation in endoscopic sinus surgery simulator. Otolaryngol Head Neck Surg. 2009;140(3):320–3.
32. Leung RM, Leung J, Vescan A, Dubrowski A, Witterick I. Construct validation of a low-fidelity endoscopic sinus surgery simulator. Am J Rhinol. 2008;22(6):642–8.
33. Steehler MK, Pfisterer MJ, Na H, Hesham HN, Pehlivanova M, Malekzadeh S. Face, content, and construct validity of a low-cost sinus surgery task trainer. Otolaryngol Head Neck Surg. 2012; 146(3):504–9.
34. Pettineo CM, Vozenilek JA, Kharasch M, Wang E, Aitchison P. Epistaxis simulator. Simul Healthc. 2008;3(4):239–41.
35. Shah RK, Patel A, Lander L, Choi SS. Management of foreign bodies obstructing the airway in children. Arch Otolaryngol Head Neck Surg. 2010;136(4):373–9.
36. Deutsch ES. High-fidelity patient simulation manikins to facilitate aerodigestive endoscopy training. Arch Otolaryngol Head Neck Surg. 2008;134(6):625–9.
37. Howells TH, Emery FM, Twentyman JE. Endotracheal intubation training using a simulator. An evaluation of the Laerdal adult intubation model in the teaching of endotracheal intubation. Br J Anaesth. 1973;45(4):400–2.
38. Rowe R, Cohen RA. An evaluation of a virtual reality airway simulator. Anesth Analg. 2002;95(1):62–6.
39. Jabbour N, Reihsen T, Sweet RM, Sidman JD. Psychomotor skills training in pediatric airway endoscopy simulation. Otolaryngol Head Neck Surg. 2011;145(1):43–50.
40. Burns JA, Kobler JB, Heaton JT, Anderson RR, Zeitels SM. Predicting clinical efficacy of photoangiolytic and cutting/ablating lasers using the chick chorioallantoic membrane model: implications for endoscopic voice surgery. Laryngoscope. 2008;118(6): 1109–24.
41. Higbie E, Howitt B. The behavior of the virus of equine encephalomyelitis on the chorioallantoic membrane of the developing chick. J Bacteriol. 1935;29(4):399–408.
42. Street I, Beech T, Jennings C. The Birmingham trainer: a simulator for ligating the lower tonsillar pole. Clin Otolaryngol. 2006; 31(1):79.
43. Ross SK, Jaiswal V, Thomas S. Re: Yorick's skull model for tonsillectomy tie training. Clin Otolaryngol. 2008;33(6):630.
44. Cook T, editor. Basic soft tissue surgery. Washington: American Academy of Facial Plastic and Rconstructive Surgery; 1982.
45. Liu A, Bhasin Y, Bowyer M. A haptic-enabled simulator for cricothyroidotomy. Stud Health Technol Inform. 2005;111:308–13.
46. King PH, Blanks ST, Rummel DM, Patterson D. Simulator training in anesthesiology: an answer? Biomed Instrum Technol. 1996;30(4): 341–5.
47. John B, Suri I, Hillermann C, Mendonca C. Comparison of cricothyroidotomy on manikin vs. simulator: a randomised cross-over study. Anaesthesia. 2007;62(10):1029–32.
48. Friedman Z, You-Ten KE, Bould MD, Naik V. Teaching lifesaving procedures: the impact of model fidelity on acquisition and transfer of cricothyrotomy skills to performance on cadavers. Anesth Analg. 2008;107(5):1663–9.
49. Murphy C, Rooney S, Maharaj C, Laffey J, Harte B. A comparison of three cuffed emergency percutaneous cricothyroidotomy devices with surgical cricothyroidotomy performed by experienced anaesthesiologists. Eur J Anaesthesiol. 2009;26:220.
50. Pettineo CM, Vozenilek JA, Wang E, Flaherty J, Kharasch M, Aitchison P. Simulated emergency department procedures with minimal monetary investment cricothyrotomy simulator. Simul Healthc. 2009;4(1):60–4.
51. Ryzynski A. Airway part-task trainer: how to be green and budget lean. Can J Anesth. 2010;57:S22.
52. Deutsch ES, Christenson T, Curry J, Hossain J, Zur K, Jacobs I. Multimodality education for airway endoscopy skill development. Ann Otol Rhinol Laryngol. 2009;118(2):81–6.
53. Malekzadeh S, Malloy KM, Chu EE, Tompkins J, Battista A, Deutsch ES. ORL emergencies boot camp: using simulation to onboard residents. Laryngoscope. 2011;121(10):2114–21.
54. Ishman SL, Brown DJ, Boss EF, et al. Development and pilot testing of an operative competency assessment tool for pediatric direct laryngoscopy and rigid bronchoscopy. Laryngoscope. 2010; 120(11):2294–300.
55. Ishman SL, Benke JR, Johnson K, et al. Blinded evaluation of interrater reliability of an operative competency assessment tool for direct laryngoscopy and rigid bronchoscopy. Arch Otolaryngol Head Neck Surg. 2012 Sep 17:1–7. doi:10.1001/2013.Jamaoto.115.
56. ACGME general competencies. http://www.acgme.org/outcome/comp/GeneralCompetenciesStandards21307.pdf. Accessed 10 June 2011.
57. Roy S, Smith LP. What does it take to start an oropharyngeal fire? Oxygen requirements to start fires in the operating room. Int J Pediatr Otorhinolaryngol. 2011;75(2):227–30.
58. Schout BMA, Hendrikx AJM, Scherpbier AJJA, Bemelmans BLH. Update on training models in endourology: a qualitative systematic review of the literature between January 1980 and April 2008. Eur Urol. 2008;54(6):1247–61.

Simulation in Pain and Palliative Care

34

Yury Khelemsky and Jason Epstein

Introduction

Pain medicine and palliative care are diverse and challenging fields with overlapping disciplines that include anesthesiology, physical medicine and rehabilitation, neurology, psychiatry, and geriatrics. In order to achieve a high degree of fidelity in simulating the complex multidisciplinary fields of pain medicine and palliative care, simulation curricula must encompass technical and nontechnical skills utilizing standardized patients, procedure-based part-task trainers, as well as rare occurrence management on full human patient simulators. This chapter will review the state of simulation-based education in pain medicine and palliative care, outline future directions, and present an example of complex multimodal simulation that addresses the needs of trainees and practicing physicians in these fields.

Simulation Modalities

Provider Interaction: Standardized Patients and Virtual Reality

Provider interaction with patients, family members, caretakers, and other healthcare practitioners is an integral part of pain medicine and palliative care practices. These interactions, which may include the delivery of bad news, provision of emotional support, discussion of end-of-life care (i.e. DNR orders, etc.) integration of evidence-based medicine into recommendations, evaluation of management and total suffering, and titration of analgesics, among others can be simulated with the use of standardized patients (SP) or computer-based virtual reality (VR) programs [1–5]. Unfortunately, simulation is rarely integrated into the training of physicians who must provide difficult news—in one survey only 13% of respondents experienced it during their training. The same study noted that simulation training may help physicians feel prepared for difficult conversations and that ongoing experience was strongly associated with comfort level [6].

Y. Khelemsky, MD (✉)
Department of Anesthesiology,
Icahn School of Medicine at Mount Sinai, New York, NY, USA

Department of Anesthesiology,
The Mount Sinai Medical Center, New York, NY, USA
e-mail: yury.khelemsky@gmail.com

J. Epstein, MD
Department of Anesthesiology,
Icahn School of Medicine at Mount Sinai, New York, NY, USA
e-mail: jhe2001@med.cornell.edu

Standardized Patients (SP)

Both standardized patients and standardized patient families have been used in palliative care education and have been found to be valuable at improving and assessing the provision of palliative care [1, 7–13]. Standardized patient families have been employed to educate gerontological nurse practitioner students about the needs of patients and their families during the end-of-life period [1]. A simulation designed to elicit the ability of ICU physicians to initiate palliative care was found not only to be a high-fidelity tool but highlighted a significant variability in treatment decisions [6]. In another ICU-based study, an Objective Structured Clinical Examination (OSCE) was developed to assess the ability of surgical residents to lead an end-of-life discussion and to disclose an iatrogenic complication. This pilot OSCE was found to provide residents with a positive learning experience and valid formative feedback; however, as is the case with all SP simulations, a review of the tapes revealed a need for greater standardization of the actor's roles [7].

The use of standardized patients was useful in training pediatric residents to communicate bad news and understand the emotions that they and the parents may experience [9]. A multi-professional communication skills program that relied on standardized patients to explore the challenges of communicating with cancer patients and their families appeared to be effective in providing a meaningful learning

A.I. Levine et al. (eds.), *The Comprehensive Textbook of Healthcare Simulation*,
DOI 10.1007/978-1-4614-5993-4_34, © Springer Science+Business Media New York 2013

experience [8]. In order to address the longitudinal nature of patient-provider interactions in palliative care, an extended standardized patient scenario (ESPS) was developed, which was presented over several sessions, depicting various points in the patient's disease progression [10]. While the use of SPs in pain medicine has not been described, as a field it readily lends itself to the application of above strategies, as well as those from other closely related disciplines [14–16].

Virtual Reality (VR)

Computer-based patient simulation offers an effective means of providing simulation training to large numbers of individuals. Avatar (a virtual reality patient)-mediated training has several advantages over SPs, such as superior standardization, breadth of simulated personalities and pathologies, ease of scheduling, and decreased expense [2, 17]. A recent study using avatars found that participants responded favorably to this educational modality and had improved self-efficacy in delivering bad news [2]. Other research indicates that computer-based simulation is useful as a teaching tool for residents treating malignancy related pain—improving the residents' abilities to rapidly initiate analgesia, measure pain scores at appropriate intervals, and titrate long acting agents, resulting in a significant reduction of pain scores [18]. Interestingly, strategies of using VR not only for provider education in palliative care but as a therapeutic modality for patients in end-of-life care have been proposed [12, 19, 20]. Use of VR in Pain Medicine has not been described, but it is clear that improvement of provider competence in pharmacologic, behavioral, social, and interpersonal aspects of patient care is critical to successful multidisciplinary management of pain and suffering [15, 21].

Future Directions

There are multiple interpersonal interaction scenarios in palliative care and pain medicine to which standardized patients and VR technologies may be readily applied. For example, new patient interviews that would prompt the trainee to elicit certain history and physical exam findings, order appropriate diagnostic workup, as well as tailor a treatment regimen. Scenarios that involve dealing with aberrant drug behavior would hone a practitioner's skills in identifying and managing at-risk individuals. Additionally, simulated interactions with other members of the treatment team, such as referring physicians, could develop a trainee's ability to clearly and effectively communicate, a cornerstone of providing efficient comprehensive care in a multidisciplinary environment. As with all simulation, these exercises would be useful in both education and assessment of practitioners and should be designed with level of training in mind. Basic scenarios may be introduced early in training, with more complex scenarios reserved for fellowship training, board certification or recertification.

As this chapter is being written, the authors are designing a comprehensive simulation-based pain medicine curriculum for the American Society of Anesthesiologists (ASA) Maintenance of Certification in Anesthesiology for Subspecialties (MOCA-SUBS) Program. Part IV of this program, Practice Performance Assessment and Improvement (PPAI), requires that physicians participate in a simulation course at an ASA-endorsed center (see Chaps. 17 and 48) during each 10-year accreditation cycle [22]. SPs, VR, as well as modalities discussed later in this chapter such as part-task trainers, and full-scale mannequin simulations are being employed to craft a multimodality high-fidelity, self-assessment, and learning tool for current practitioners in the field of pain medicine.

Procedure-Based Simulators

Current Technology

Strict procedural skills fall under the domain of pain medicine more so than of palliative care. Multiple studies have shown that simulation is effective in teaching procedural skills in the fields of general surgery, robotic surgery, urology, otorhinolaryngology, neurosurgery, medicine, anesthesiology, pain medicine, among others [23–31]. However, few studies have been designed to show direct improvements in clinical outcomes from the use of simulation for training [31].

Procedures may be simulated with the aid of live human models, cadavers, animal models, part-task trainers, and VR—each modality possessing inherent benefits and limitations. While live human models offer the highest fidelity to teach gross and radiographic anatomy and are extensively used in simulation of ultrasound-guided regional anesthesia and pain medicine procedures, the actual procedure itself cannot be performed for obvious reasons. Use of live animal models for procedural simulation is very limited due to ethical considerations and cost but can offer high fidelity. Part-task trainers, such as those produced by Blue Phantom™, for simulation of spinal/epidural and ultrasound-guided peripheral nerve blocks offer high fidelity in procedural performance, but studies detailing their impact on trainees do not exist (Figs. 34.1 and 34.2). Furthermore, a study comparing simulated placement of an epidural catheter in a high- vs. low-fidelity model revealed no differences in the Manual Skill Checklist or Global Rating Scale scores between the two modalities [32]. Haptic actuators for simulation of epidural anesthesia and other needle insertion procedures have been described but are not currently commercially available [33].

Virtual reality procedural simulators combine haptics (tactile feedback technology) with images of either gross and/or

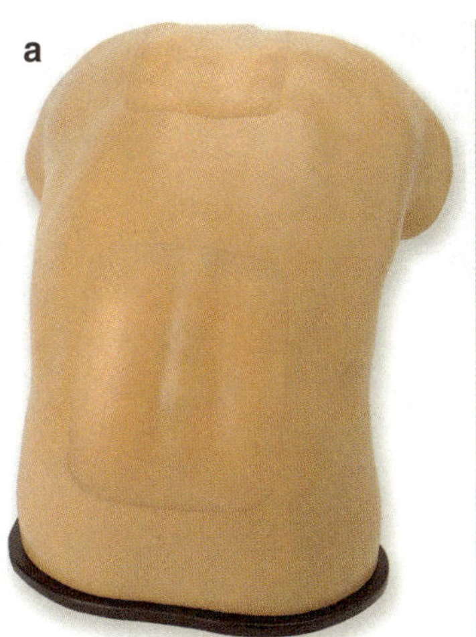

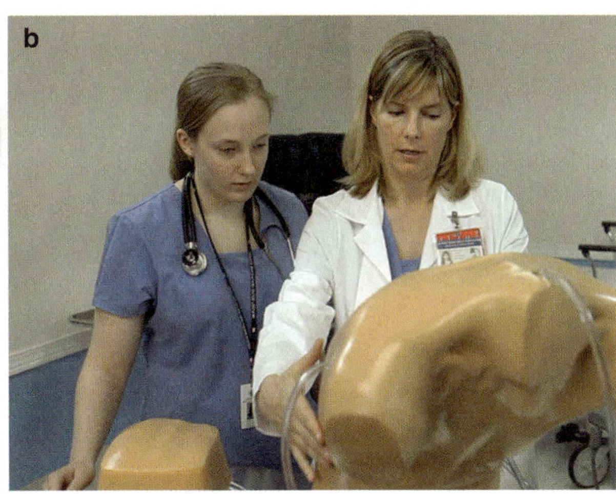

Fig. 34.1 Lumbar/thoracic epidural/spinal placement simulator (**a**) Simulator with back insert in place (**b**) Teaching epidural placement with the simulator (Reproduced with permission from Blue Phantom™, Redmond, VA)

imaging (i.e., ultrasound) derived anatomy. One such device is the Common Platform Medical Skills Trainer (CPMST) from Touch of Life Technologies (Fig. 34.3). Images of gross anatomy derived from the Visible Human Dataset (detailed dataset of cross-sectional photographs of the human body) and of corresponding ultrasound anatomy are coupled with haptic devices, allowing for an immersive, high-fidelity environment for performing ultrasound-guided nerve blocks.

Another VR device is Medical Simulation Corporation's (MSC) SimSuite® neurostimulation simulator (Fig. 34.4). This technology offers healthcare providers an environment in which to advance their skills in spinal cord stimulation (SCS) from needle insertion to manipulation of leads to mapping for optimal pain management. Simulation features include virtual fluoroscopy for 3D tracking of needle, C-arm manipulation with lateral views, tactile feedback, needle and lead navigation and manipulation, programmable complications, suture skill practice, mapping to optimize pain management for a variety of patient presentations, and patient interaction.

In addition to allowing practitioners to hone their procedural skills in a risk-free environment, these simulators are portable, allowing for on-site education. Unfortunately, there are no studies detailing outcomes of provider training with either of these simulation platforms.

Future Directions

Most pain medicine procedures are minimally invasive image guided in nature—a combination that readily lends itself to procedural simulation. For example, the CPMST or SimSuite could be expanded to allow for ultrasound, fluoroscopically, or CT-guided procedures such as celiac plexus block, stellate ganglion block, vertebral augmentation, spinals/epidurals, cervical medial branch blocks, and multiple other minimally invasive pain medicine procedures. Synthetic anatomically driven part-task trainers, like those used for peripheral ultrasound-guided blocks, can also be adapted for pain specific procedural simulation.

Rare and Critical Occurrence Management

High-fidelity mannequin simulation of rare and critical events has been well described in multiple medical disciplines; however, little work has been done in the fields of Palliative Care and Pain Medicine [31, 34–38]. An implementation of a simulation program for palliative care providers at the Montagu Clinical Simulation Center in the UK has been described [39]. Scenarios, which were jointly written by staff from several hospitals included anaphylaxis, collapse of a relative, hypercalcemia, spinal cord compression, hemorrhage, an end-of-life event, finding an overdosed patient, and a relative wishing to reverse a "do not resuscitate" directive immediately post cardiac arrest. Elements of crisis avoidance and resource management were integrated into the debriefing process. Participants in this 1-day program reported increased confidence in the management of rare events, greater awareness of the need to plan for such events, consolidation of existing knowledge, appreciation for being able to communicate with colleagues away from situational pressures, and a high sense of personal achievement associated with completing a psychologically demanding educational event. This program provides a good framework for the creation of other Palliative Care simulation curricula.

Application of full-scale mannequin simulation specifically to pain medicine has not been described, although a report has linked a case of successful resuscitation of bupivacaine-induced cardiac arrest to recent simulation training [40]. As previously discussed, the authors are currently creating a MOCA-SUBS Pain Medicine Simulation Curriculum. In addition to the mannequins, the multimodality simulations will include SPs and VR and address topics like anaphylaxis (to IV contrast or local anesthetics), seizure (e.g., IV injection of local anesthetic complicating stellate ganglion block or IV phenol complicating celiac plexus block), respiratory arrest (inadvertent while refilling an intrathecal pump), torsades de points (secondary to methadone

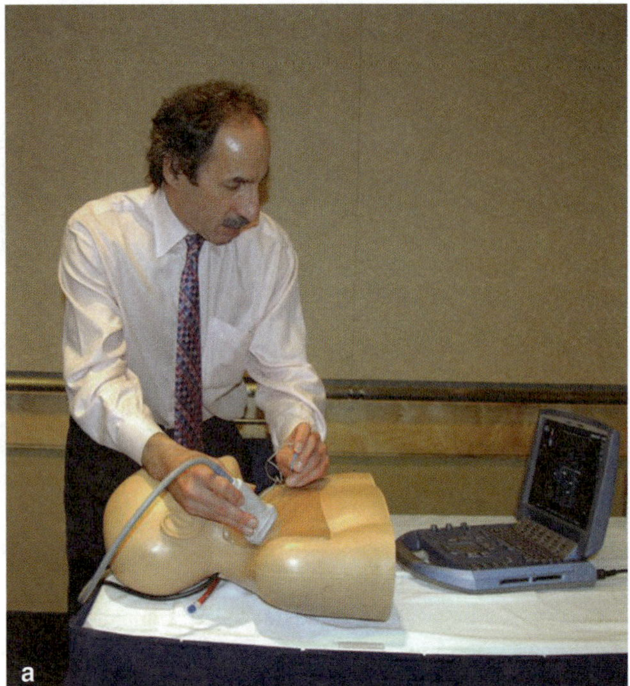

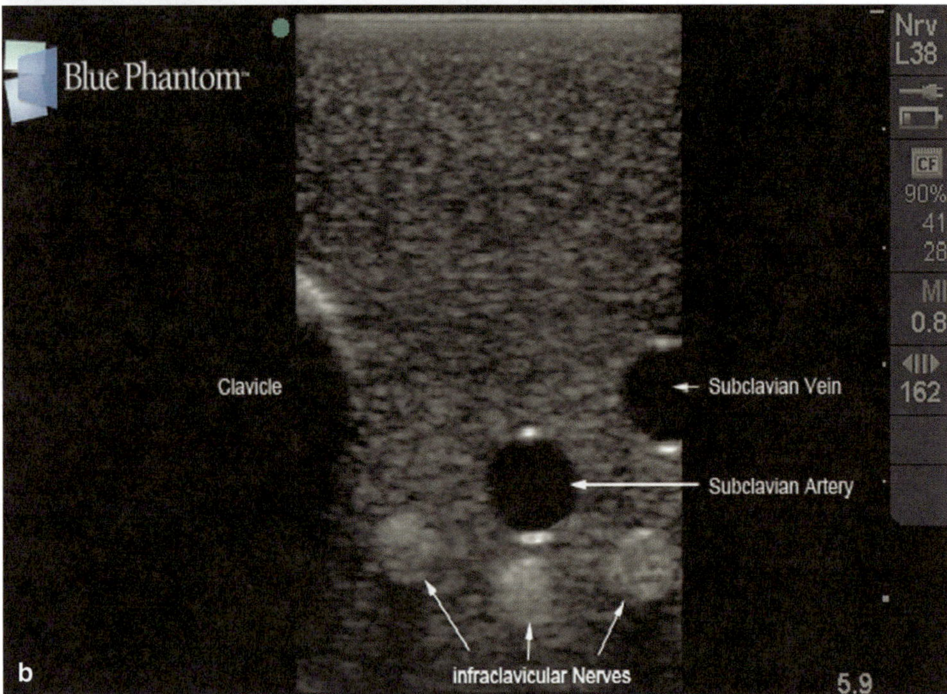

Fig. 34.2 (a) "Ultrasound Andy," the original Blue Phantom™ head-neck-upper torso ultrasound-guided regional anesthesia and central venous access model. (b) Ultrasound image of "Ultrasound Andy's" infraclavicular brachial plexus (Reproduced with permission from Blue Phantom ™, Redmond, VA)

toxicity), serotonin syndrome (drug-drug interaction between opioids and tricyclic antidepressants), hypertensive emergencies (during cervical epidural steroid injection), pneumothorax (after paravertebral or intercostal nerve block) and hypotension (due to sympathectomy post celiac plexus block), among others. These simulations will be multimodal, incorporating rare and critical occurrence management simulation, SPs/VR, and procedure simulation in order to enhance their fidelity [22].

Proposed Multimodal Curriculum

The following example, comprised of four stages, is a comprehensive simulation of the management of a 62-year-old male with intractable pain secondary to pancreatic adenocarcinoma presenting for celiac plexus block (Table 34.1).

In the initial stage, the practitioner will interact with a simulated patient (either SP or VR) to perform an assessment and decide if a celiac plexus block is an appropriate

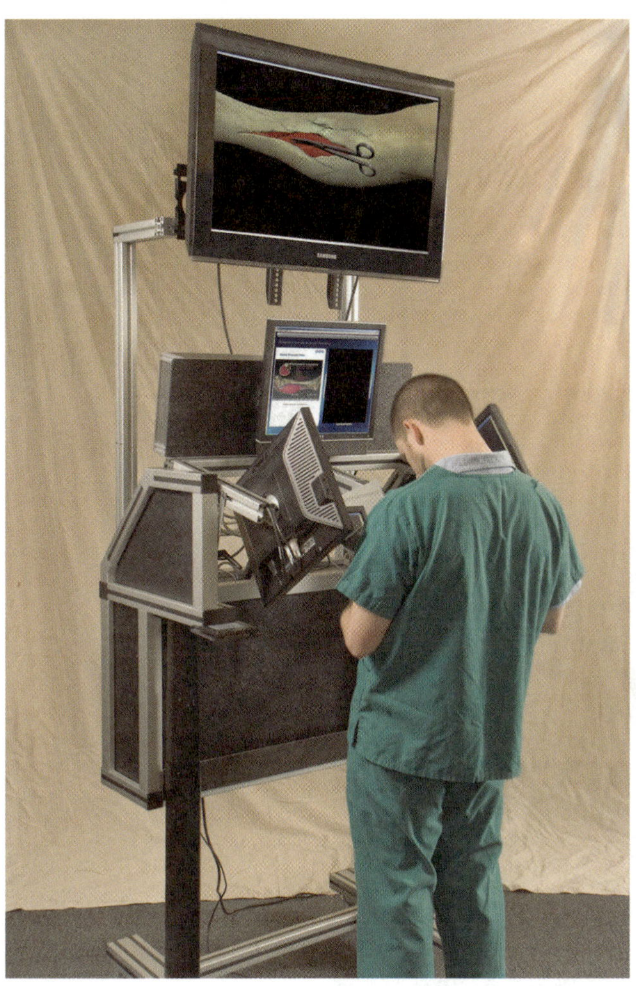

Fig. 34.3 Common Platform Medical Skills Trainer (CPMST) (Courtesy of Touch of Life Technologies, Aurora, CO)

intervention. If so, a thorough explanation of the procedure must be provided and consent obtained.

During the second stage of the simulation the practitioner will move to a part-task device where s/he will perform a simulated CT or fluoroscopically guided celiac plexus block. Upon completion of the block the practitioner would have to diagnose that the patient is experiencing local anesthetic toxicity (LAST).

For the third stage of the simulation, a full-scale mannequin simulator will be used to replicate the complication, and the practitioner will proceed to initiate management and activate a help system.

In the final stage of the simulation, the practitioner would return to a standardized patient/s (SP or VR) in order to brief the patient's family on the procedure, complication, and a proposed pain management plan.

Conclusion

By combining multiple simulator technologies into a suite of simulations, educators can present a comprehensive, engaging experience to introduce and reinforce key concepts and procedural tasks salient to pain and palliative care practitioners. Alternatively, the simulator suite approach allows facilitators to design a thorough assessment of the breadth of a practitioner's skill set for evaluative purposes. While some of the technologies described in this chapter are still under development, pain and palliative care practitioners involved in simulation can use this generalized multimodal approach with available equipment to create valuable education and evaluation tools.

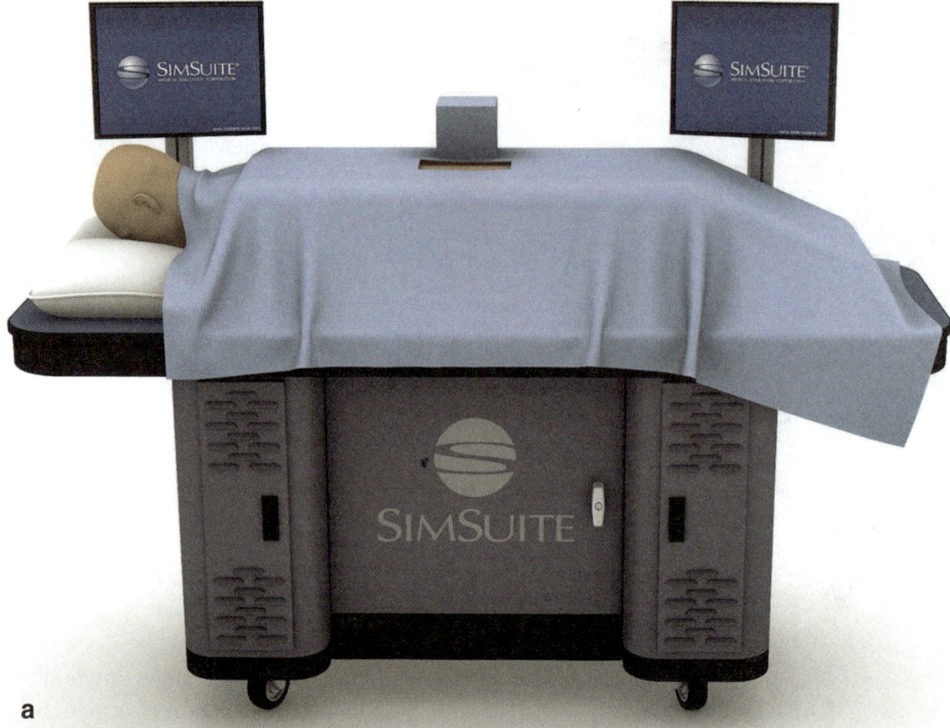

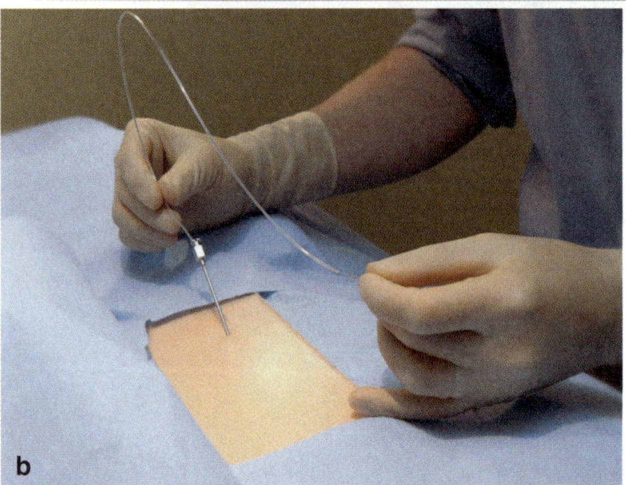

Fig 34.4 (**a**) SimSuite® Neurostimulation Simulator. (**b**) Practitioner advancing a spinal cord stimulator lead. SimSuite® Neurostimulation Simulator (Courtesy of Medical Simulation Corporation, Denver, CO)

Table 34.1 Four stages of a proposed multimodal simulation in pain medicine

1. Patient interview and consent
2. Performance of celiac plexus block
3. Management of post-procedure complication
4. Discussion with family/patient

References

1. Shawler C. Palliative and end-of-life care: using a standardized patient family for gerontological nurse practitioner students. Nurs Educ Perspect. 2011;32(3):168–72.
2. Andrade AD, Bagri A, Zaw K, Roos BA, Ruiz JG. Avatar-mediated training in the delivery of bad news in a virtual world. J Palliat Med. 2010;3(12):1415–9.
3. Freer JP, Zinnerstrom KL. The palliative medicine extended standardized patient scenario: a preliminary report. J Palliat Med. 2001;4(1):49–56.
4. Oyama H. Virtual reality for the palliative care of cancer. Stud Health Technol Inform. 1997;44:8794.
5. Waisel DB, Simon R, Truog RD, Baboolal H, Raemer DB. Anesthesiologist management of perioperative do-not-resuscitate orders: a simulation-based experiment. Simul Healthc. 2009;4(2):70–6.
6. Kersun L, Gyi L, Morrison WE. Training in difficult conversations: a national survey of pediatrichematology-oncology and pediatric critical care physicians. J Palliat Med. 2009;12(6):507–8.
7. Barnato AE, Hsu HE, Bryce CL, Lave JR, et al. Using simulation to isolate physician variation in intensive care unit admission decision making for critically ill elders with end-stage cancer: a pilot feasibility study. Crit Care Med. 2008;36(12):3156–63.
8. Chipman JG, Beilman GJ, Schmitz CC, Seatter SC. Development and pilot testing of an OSCE for difficult conversations in surgical intensive care. J Surg Educ. 2007;64(2):79–87.

9. Donovan T, Hutchison T, Kelly A. Using simulated patients in a multiprofessional communications skills programme: reflections from the programme facilitators. Eur J Cancer Care. 2003;12(2):123–8.
10. Serwint JR. The use of standardized patients in pediatric residency training in palliative care: anatomy of a standardized patient case scenario. J Palliat Med. 2002;1:146–53.
11. Finlay IG, Stott NC, Kinnersley P. The assessment of communication skills in palliative medicine: a comparison of the scores of examiners and simulated patients. Med Educ. 1995;29(6):424–9.
12. Faulkner A. Using simulators to aid the teaching of communication skills in cancer and palliative care. Patient Educ Couns. 1994; 23(2):125–9.
13. Pratt SD. Recent trends in simulation for obstetric anesthesia. Curr Opin Anaesthesiol. 2012;25(3):271–6.
14. Cooper JB, Singer SJ, Hayes J, Sales M, et al. Design and evaluation of simulation scenarios for a program introducing patient safety, teamwork, safety leadership, and simulation to healthcare leaders and managers. Simul Healthc. 2011;6(4):231–8.
15. McNaughton N, Ravitz P, Wadell A, Hodges BD. Psychiatric education and simulation: a review of the literature. Can J Psychiatry. 2008;53(2):85–93.
16. Cantrell MJ, Deloney LA. Integration of standardized patients into simulation. Anesthesiol Clin. 2007;25(2):377–83.
17. López V, Eisman EM, Castro JL. A tool for training primary health care medical students: the virtual simulated patient. In: 2008 20th IEEE international conference on tools with artificial intelligence. Dayton; 2008. p. 194–201.
18. Harting B, Hasler S, Abrams R, Odwazny R, McNutt R. Computer-based simulation as a teaching tool for residents treating patients with cancer-related pain crises. Qual Manag Health Care. 2008; 17(3):192–9.
19. Oyama H. Virtual reality for palliative medicine. Stud Health Technol Inform. 1998;58:140–50.
20. Gershon J, Zimand E, Lemos R, Rothbaum BO, Hodges L. Use of virtual reality as a distractor for painful procedures in a patient with pediatric cancer: a case study. Cyberpsychol Behav. 2003;6(6): 657–61.
21. Augarten A, Zaslansky R, Matok Pharm I, Minuskin T, et al. The impact of educational intervention programs on pain management in a pediatric emergency department. Biomed Pharmacother. 2006; 60(7):299–302.
22. http://www.theaba.org/pdf/MOCA-SUBS-LAUNCH.pdf. Accessed on 4/3/12.
23. Sachdeva AK, Buyske J, Dunnington GL, Sanfey HA, et al. A new paradigm for surgical procedural training. Curr Probl Surg. 2011; 48(12):854–968.
24. Schreuder HW, Wolswijk R, Zweemer RP, Schijven MP, et al. Training and learning robotic surgery, time for a more structured approach: a systematic review. BJOG. 2012;119(2):137–49.
25. Nestel D, Groom J, Eikeland-Husebø S, O'Donnell JM. Simulation for learning and teaching procedural skills: the state of the science. Simul Healthc. 2011;6(Suppl):10–3.
26. Ahmed K, Jawad M, Abboudi M, Gavazzi A, et al. Effectiveness of procedural simulation in urology: a systematic review. J Urol. 2011;186(1):26–34.
27. Clifton N, Klingmann C, Khalil H. Teaching otolaryngology skills through simulation. Eur Arch Otorhinolaryngol. 2011;268(7): 949–53.
28. Malone HR, Syed ON, Downes MS, D'Ambrosio AL, et al. Simulation in neurosurgery: a review of computer-based simulation environments and their surgical applications. Neurosurgery. 2010; 67(4):1105–16.
29. Castanelli DJ. The rise of simulation in technical skills teaching and the implications for training novices in anaesthesia. Anaesth Intensive Care. 2009;37(6):903–10.
30. Bould MD, Crabtree NA, Naik VN. Assessment of procedural skills in anaesthesia. Br J Anaesth. 2009;103(4):472–83.
31. Okuda Y, Bryson EO, DeMaria Jr S, Jacobson L, et al. The utility of simulation in medical education: what is the evidence? Mt Sinai J Med. 2009;76(4):330–43.
32. Friedman Z, Siddiqui N, Katznelson R, Devito I, et al. Clinical impact of epidural anesthesia simulation on short- and long-term learning curve: high-versus low fidelity model training. Reg Anesth Pain Med. 2009;34(3):229–32.
33. Magill JC, Byl MF, Hinds MF, Agassounon W, et al. A novel actuator for simulation of epidural anesthesia and other needle insertion procedures. Simul Healthc. 2010;5(3):179–84.
34. Houben KW, van den Hombergh CL, Stalmeijer RE, Scherpbier AJ, et al. New training strategies for anaesthesia residents. Curr Opin Anaesthesiol. 2011;24(6):682–6.
35. Murray DJ. Current trends in simulation training in anesthesia: a review. Minerva Anestesiol. 2011;77(5):528–33.
36. Yager PH, Lok J, Klig JE. Advances in simulation for pediatric critical care and emergency medicine. Curr Opin Pediatr. 2011; 23(3):293–7.
37. Weinberg ER, Auerbach MA, Shah NB. The use of simulation for pediatric training and assessment. Curr Opin Pediatr. 2009;21(3): 282–7.
38. McLaughlin S, Fitch MT, Goyal DG, Hayden E, et al. Simulation in graduate medical education 2008: a review for emergency medicine. Acad Emerg Med. 2008;15(11):1117–29.
39. Pease N. High fidelity clinical simulation in cancer and palliative care. In: Foyle L, Hostad J, editors. Innovations in cancer and palliative care education. Oxon: Radcliffe Publishing Ltd; 2007. Chapter 1.
40. Smith HM, Jacob AK, Segura LG, Dilger JA, et al. Simulation education in anesthesia training: a case report of successful resuscitation of bupivacaine-induced cardiac arrest linked to recent simulation training. Anesth Analg. 2008;106(5):1581–4.

Simulation in Pediatrics

35

Vincent Grant, Jon Duff, Farhan Bhanji, and Adam Cheng

Introduction

Resuscitation of pediatric patients is complex and can prove challenging even for experienced healthcare providers. Survival following pediatric cardiac arrest remains poor in both the in- and out-of-hospital settings [1, 2]. Fortunately pediatric cardiac arrests occur infrequently [3]. This likely relates to the predominant nature of pediatric cardiac arrests, where early recognition of respiratory compromise or shock with appropriate, rapid intervention can prevent the progression to cardiac arrest [4, 5]. Training programs to educate healthcare providers (HCPs) on early recognition and initial management of acutely ill pediatric patients, along with continuous quality improvement measures to ensure appropriate systems, and delivery of care should be fundamental concepts in caring for pediatric patients.

The American Academy of Pediatrics Committee on Pediatric Emergency Medicine noted concerns regarding the variability of training and the lack of pediatric experience of HCPs providing emergency care for pediatric patients [6]. Additionally, a survey of emergency medicine residency program directors found that there was variable and insufficient exposure to acutely ill pediatric patients for their trainees—yet despite this limited pediatric acute care training, most residents were expected to care for acutely ill pediatric patients once in practice [7]. It is therefore no surprise that, while a significant majority of practicing emergency medicine physicians felt their residency completely prepared them to manage adult cardiac arrest (76%) and trauma resuscitation (60%), only a quarter of the survey respondents felt completely prepared to manage pediatric cardiac arrest or trauma following residency [8]. Similarly, in a large pediatrics training program, only about a third of senior residents had ever led a resuscitation with only one-sixth of all residents ever discharging a defibrillator on an actual patient [9]. Advanced resuscitation courses can be helpful to learn resuscitation skills, but these skills typically deteriorate within months, particularly when there is not adequate clinical experience [10, 11].

Simulation-based educational programs are particularly suited to address some of the challenges in training HCPs to care for sick children. Adults learn best when they are actively engaged in the process, both cognitively and emotionally [12, 13]. Simulation allows for experiential learning that may not be possible in the clinical setting [14]. The process of learning by "doing," reflecting on the performance to define the performance gaps and how to address them helps incorporate the lessons learned into future practice. Fundamental to this learning is the process of debriefing, where a "safe" and supportive environment is created to allow for the open and honest communication of experiences and thoughts of team members [13]. Without this facilitated reflection process,

V. Grant, MD, FRCPC (✉) • A. Cheng, MD, FRCPC, FAAP
Section of Emergency Medicine,
Department of Paediatrics, University of Calgary,
Calgary, AB, Canada

KidSIM Pediatric Simulation Program,
Alberta Children's Hospital,
2888 Shaganappi Trail NW, Calgary, AB T3B 6A8, Canada
e-mail: vincent.grant@albertahealthservices.ca;
chenger@me.com

J. Duff, MD, FRCPC
Division of Critical Care, Department of Pediatrics,
University of Alberta, Edmonton, AB, Canada

Edmonton Clinic Health Academy (ECHA),
11405 87 Avenue, Edmonton, AB T6G 1C9, Canada
e-mail: jon.duff@albertahealthservices.ca

F. Bhanji, MD, FRCPC, MSc, FAHA
Department of Pediatrics, Richard and Sylvia Cruess Faculty Scholar
in Medical Education, McGill University,
Montreal, QC, Canada

Divisions of Pediatric Emergency Medicine and Pediatric Critical Care,
Montreal Children's Hospital,
Montreal, QC, Canada
e-mail: farhan.bhanji@mcgill.ca

A.I. Levine et al. (eds.), *The Comprehensive Textbook of Healthcare Simulation*,
DOI 10.1007/978-1-4614-5993-4_35,

improvements in future performance may be limited or actually not occur at all [15, 16]. Simulation allows learners to appropriately debrief performance following a controlled resuscitation event, something that is not often possible for the limited pediatric resuscitations that do occur in the (sometimes chaotic) clinical environment [17]. While clearly the relevance and emotional impact of a real resuscitation make it an ideal learning opportunity, their relative rarity and the inability to optimally debrief the event (or sometimes debrief at all) preclude using clinical training exclusively.

Simulation-based education also allows for continuous quality improvement in pediatric acute care when the frequency of true resuscitation events remains low. It is well accepted that medical error accounts for a large number of hospital-related deaths [18]. What may not be as well recognized is that children are at particular risk of these errors, with drug dosing errors being the most frequent issue, particularly in the acute care setting [19, 20]. Traditional educational programs have not successfully addressed the issue [21]. Simulation provides opportunity for deliberate practice, a more effective method of instruction than traditional clinical education that may help correct/prevent errors [22, 23]. Simulation sessions also allow teams (or larger "systems") to practice in order to identify potential problems that can subsequently be addressed—problems that would not be identified in clinical practice until they actually cause harm! This could include the identification of specific knowledge gaps of team members [24, 25], teamwork issues that can be addressed with subsequent (re)training or even organizational issues when in situ simulation is utilized (e.g., the identification of a malfunctioning defibrillators or inadequate or improper sizes of available equipment) [26–28].

While the focus of simulation-based education in pediatrics is frequently on acute life-threatening events or teamwork/crisis resource management, simulation can be useful in a variety of other domains such as the training of procedural or surgical skills [29] competence, the development of communication skills or in more novel methods such as helping the participant develop their own teaching skills. In this chapter we will address the use of simulation for education and assessment in pediatrics.

The "Science" of Pediatric Simulation

Best Evidence of Impact

Simulation-based education is not meant to replace training in the pediatric clinical environment but rather to complement it and is gaining momentum as a method to educate healthcare providers for a myriad of reasons. These include, but are not limited to: the unpredictable clinical environment where important case presentations may present infrequently; a growing patient safety culture that does not allow (sometimes unqualified) learners to practice on patients; and reduced work hours of medical trainees limiting clinical experience and continuity of care [30].

Kirkpatrick's classic work outlined levels of training evaluation: learner reaction (i.e., how much they liked it), learning transfer (i.e., did it result in improved performance in the clinical environment), and results (i.e., did it improve patient outcomes) [31]. Similarly, McGaghie suggests a classification system that evaluates learning outcomes in the controlled educational laboratory (T1), transfer to patient care practice (T2), and ultimately to improved patient outcomes (T3) [32]. Unfortunately, relatively few published articles on education for clinical practitioners focus on patient outcome, the highest level of impact from training [33].

The literature in simulation-based education is evolving rapidly with important new articles published almost monthly. The evidence of increased learner satisfaction and actual learning is relatively common with learners demonstrating a preference for simulation over traditional learning formats [34–37]. Recent publications also suggest that healthcare providers improve their confidence in their resuscitation skills with increased opportunities for simulation-based training and that confidence correlates better with their mock code experience than the number of real codes they attended [17, 38, 39]. This may relate in part to the more active roles and the consistency of debriefing that they receive in the simulation environment. Self-efficacy, or belief in one's capability to organize and execute the course of action required to achieve desired outcomes [40], is poor amongst frontline physicians caring for sick pediatric patients [41, 42]. Increased self-efficacy in a task has been associated with an increase in subsequent performance of that behavior. Therefore, resuscitation education programs should aim not only to improve performance but also the self-efficacy of the learners, as even those who are knowledgeable and skilled in resuscitation may not apply lifesaving interventions if they do not believe in their ability [43, 44].

The evidence for pediatric simulation affecting clinical performance and patient outcomes is beginning to appear in the medical literature. A recent randomized control trial demonstrated residents learning lumbar punctures (LP) with simulation-based deliberate practice were more successful on their next LP attempt on actual patients—an important outcome from a child's or parent's perspective [29]. For observed and evaluated intubations in the Pediatric Intensive Care setting, teams performed better if at least two of the team members had undergone simulation training [45]. Finally, in a landmark study, Andreatta and colleagues demonstrated dramatically improved patient survival from cardiac arrest after introducing a formal simulation-based mock code program. The outcomes of patients at their particular institution improved from a survival of rate of 33% to a dramatic 56%. Particularly striking from this study was the notion that

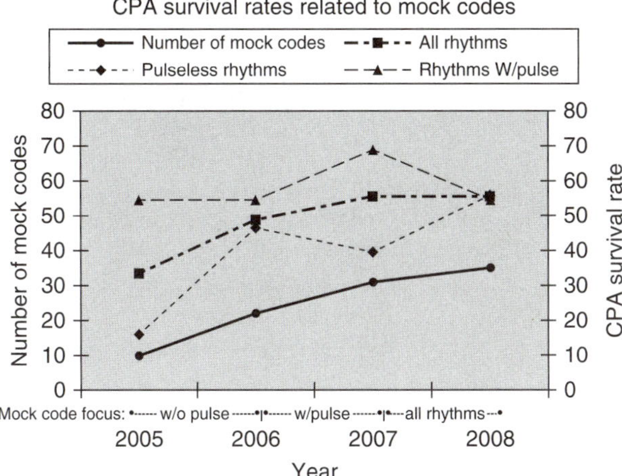

Fig. 35.1 Real pediatric survival rates (*right scale*) related to the number of mock codes (*left scale*). *CPA* cardiopulmonary arrest (Reprinted with permission from Andreatta et al. [46])

cardiac arrest survival correlated to the number of simulation sessions conducted in that particular year—and that the specific type of rhythms focused on within the mock code program (e.g., pulseless or with a pulse) showed the greatest improvements in clinical outcomes for the years they were focused on in the mock code program (Fig. 35.1) [46].

Discipline-Specific Curricula

General and In-Patient Pediatrics

Pediatric training programs have struggled to provide adequate exposure to acute care cases and opportunities for advanced procedural skills for residents in training. Traditional "mock code" programs with static mannequins lacked realism and relied heavily on the instructor to provide timely feedback during the scenario. Over the years, educators have recognized the benefits of simulation and how a higher level of environmental and physical realism can enhance the learning outcomes for trainees of all levels. Simulation allows participants to practice in an environment that closely mimics real life, thus allowing learners to be fully immersed and engaged in the learning experience [47].

Recently, leaders in pediatric resuscitation education have incorporated more simulation-based education into both the Neonatal Resuscitation Program (NRP) and the Pediatric Advanced Life Support (PALS) course. The use of increased realism and debriefing in this context will provide pediatric healthcare providers the foundation of knowledge and skills necessary to look after acutely ill children. The growth of simulation around the world has also lead to the genesis of novel simulation curricula that have been integrated into preexisting pediatric curricula. These curricula have been developed to enhance three primary skill sets: cognitive skills (content knowledge), technical skills, and crisis resource management.

Pediatric simulation educators recently developed a curriculum which integrated modular, training year-specific simulation courses with a longitudinal just-in-time mock code program. The program was developed based on a thorough needs assessment, which included a comprehensive review of Royal College of Physicians and Surgeons of Canada (RCPSC) and Accreditation Council for Graduate Medical Education (ACGME) objectives for pediatric residency training. Three year-specific simulation-based courses were then developed and implemented which were run once a year for residents in years 1, 2, and 3 of pediatric residency training. These 1-day courses included a mix of learning formats—including lecture, high-realism simulation, debriefing, and small group discussions. Table 35.1 outlines the curriculum content for each year-specific course [48].

In addition to the modular, year-specific courses, the curriculum included longitudinal in situ just-in-time mock codes using high-realism simulation in an interprofessional setting. The topic of the mock code was determined by selecting the sickest patient on the clinical teaching unit, and simulating their status should they deteriorate. This approach allowed the residents (and the entire HCP team) to be prepared for a potential deterioration of that patient, familiarized them to the equipment for resuscitation, and provided them the opportunity to practice in a multidisciplinary team-based environment. The use of pediatric mock codes is reviewed further in section "Pediatric Critical Care Medicine".

Pediatric Emergency Medicine

There has been a significant implementation of simulation-based learning in pediatric emergency medicine (PEM) training. Adler et al. described the implementation of a 1-day, six-case simulation-based pediatric emergency medicine curriculum and concluded that focused, frequent, and effortful instructional interventions are necessary to achieve substantial performance improvements [49]. A longitudinal approach to the integration of simulation into the PEM curriculum was taken by Cheng et al. who developed a package of 43 different acute care scenarios that were delivered over 2 years of PEM training, packaged as 12 different core and subspecialty modules. Each module, consisting of three or four simulation cases, was designed to be delivered over 3–4 h, with learning targeted at a specific theme or specialty. Knowledge, technical skills, and behavioral skills were discussed and reviewed after each simulation with a 30–40-min facilitated debriefing session. Although trainee performance and patient outcomes were not measured after the implementation of the curriculum, those PEM residents participating in the training reported very high satisfaction ratings for this method of acute care education. Table 35.2 provides an

Table 35.1 Pediatric simulation curriculum outline

Longitudinal just-in-time mock codes		
Realistic, multidisciplinary response to acute deterioration of patients		
Year-1 course	*Year-2 course*	*Year-3 course*
Critical first 5 min	Complex medical management	Crisis resource management
Knowledge	*Knowledge*	*Knowledge*
Respiratory failure	Rapid sequence intubation	Leadership
Shock	Inotropic support	Communication
Seizures	Postarrest management	Resource management
		Situational awareness
Skills	*Skills*	*Skills*
Bag-valve-mask ventilation	RSI and intubation	Code team leader role
IV fluid setup and administration	Intraosseous needle insertion	Post-resuscitation debriefing
Chest compressions		
Simulation cases	*Simulation cases*	*Simulation cases*
Hypovolemic shock	Status asthmaticus	Status asthmaticus
Bronchiolitis	Septic shock	Septic shock
Anaphylaxis	Status epilepticus	Status epilepticus
Status asthmaticus	Cardiogenic shock	Cardiogenic shock
Trauma		
Aspiration pneumonia		
Status epilepticus		

This information was originally published in Sam et al. [48, pp. e16–20]. Reprinted by permission
Abbreviations: *IV* intravenous, *RSI* Rapid Sequence Intubation

Table 35.2 Pediatric emergency medicine curriculum outline: scenario list by modules

Year 1	*Core modules*	*Total of 23 scenarios*
	Respiratory emergencies	Status asthmaticus, aspiration pneumonia, upper airway obstruction, acute chest syndrome
	Cardiac emergencies	Supraventricular tachycardia, unstable ventricular tachycardia, ventricular fibrillation, PEA/asystole
	Shock	Septic shock, hypovolemic shock, anaphylactic shock, cardiogenic shock
	Blunt trauma	Abdominal trauma, major head injury, orthopedic trauma, thoracic trauma
	Environmental emergencies	Near drowning/hypothermia, electrical injury, smoke inhalation/carbon monoxide poisoning
	Infant/neonatal emergencies	Nonaccidental injury, bronchiolitis, congenital diaphragmatic hernia, congenital heart disease
Year 2	*Subspecialty modules*	*Total of 20 scenarios*
	Toxicology emergencies	Sympathomimetic, anticholinergic, cholinergic and opioid toxidromes
	Endocrinological emergencies	Diabetic ketoacidsosis, adrenal crisis, thyroid storm
	Oncological emergencies	Mediastinal mass, hyperleukocytosis/stroke, tumor lysis syndrome
	Nephrological emergencies	Hypertensive emergency, acute renal failure/hyperkalemia, hyponatremia
	Neurological emergencies	Status epilepticus, coma/depressed level of consciousness, combative/encephalopathy
	Penetrating trauma	Thoracic trauma, neck trauma, spinal cord trauma, abdominal trauma

Adapted with permission from Cheng et al. [50]

overview of the curriculum, along with a description of the cases in each module [50]. Other centers have used simulation to improve the performance of pediatric trauma teams noting improved subsequent performance in the simulated scenarios [35].

Neonatal Intensive Care

Simulation-based training is gaining momentum in neonatal intensive care units (NICU) across the world. Although neonatal resuscitation is common, neonates requiring aggressive resuscitation at birth are rare. This low-frequency but potentially high-risk event lends itself well to simulation-based training [51]. The traditional NRP program improves cognitive and technical skills but gaps in behavioral skills and other areas have been identified [52–56] and knowledge retention is poor [57]. Simulation is now tightly integrated into the NRP curriculum [58].

Research to determine the impact of simulation-based education on neonatal resuscitation is accumulating. Two studies have explored the use of a single high-fidelity simulation session compared to either low-fidelity simulation or self-study and found no difference in multiple choice examination scores post-learning though the high-fidelity groups did require less prompting during simulated resuscitations [59, 60]. These studies are limited by the use of a single simulation session and only cognitive knowledge as the outcome variable. More frequent simulation sessions may be required to improve knowledge transfer [61].

Simulation is also being developed and used in novel methods for neonatal intensive care. It has been studied as a "booster" to previous NRP training to remote communities to prevent knowledge decay [62]. A group consortium has formed to develop a "living text book" and "living world" for neonatal nurse practitioner education [63]. Simulation is also being used as part of a larger initiative to improve communication in the labor and delivery environment and during end-of-life care [64, 65].

Research evaluating the impact of neonatal simulation on patient outcome is limited to date. One study in neonatal airway management taught to pediatric residents using a single session revealed that although the learners demonstrated improved skills on a neonatal mannequin, a benefit in actual clinical performance was not found (although the study was likely underpowered for this outcome) [66]. In a landmark study, Draycott et al. developed an annual simulation-based training intervention for obstetrical and neonatal teams [67]. Their intervention decreased the incidence of newborn hypoxic-ischemic encephalopathy from 27.3 to 13.6 per 10,000 births over a 5-year period, demonstrating the potential benefit of simulation-based training on actual patient outcomes. Future neonatal simulation studies need to continue to evaluate changes in actual clinical performance.

Pediatric Critical Care Medicine

The challenges that exist in the neonatal intensive care environment are mirrored in the pediatric intensive care unit (PICU). In a recent survey of 76 pediatric residents, it was clear that although many of them were involved in the resuscitation of an acutely ill child, they were not adequately trained to respond, especially in basic life support and the use of a defibrillator [9]. These gaps were noted again in a simulator-based study evaluating the performance of pediatric residents during a resuscitation and in airway management [68]. Given these studies one could consider it unethical to solely rely on clinical experience to educate our trainees in pediatric resuscitation.

A number of simulation-based curricula have been developed and studied in pediatric critical care. Nishisaki and colleagues developed a multi-institutional "boot camp" for PICU fellows [69]. Learners participated in whole and small group discussions, task training, and high-fidelity simulation sessions covering airway management, vascular access, sepsis, resuscitation, traumatic brain injury, and delivering bad news. In the latter half of the course, each simulation session was followed by a debriefing session and then a second simulation scenario similar to the first to allow for deliberate

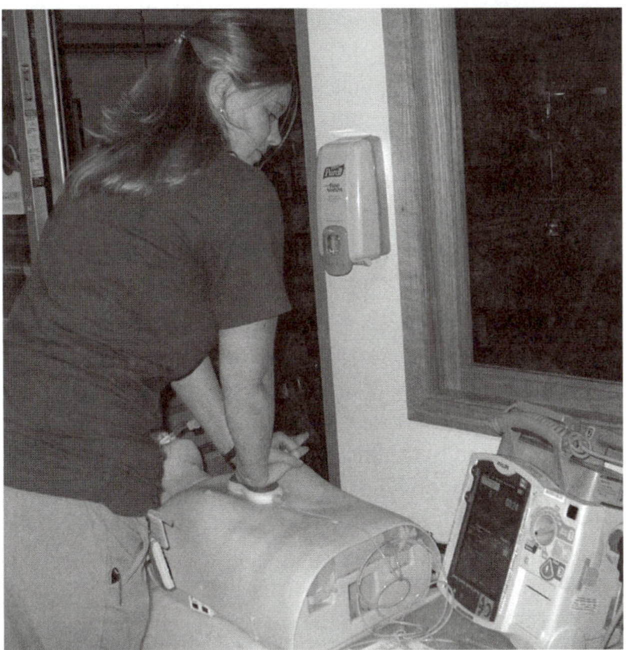

Fig. 35.2 "Rolling Refresher" CPR skill training using "just-in-time" and "just-in-place" simulation (Reprinted from Niles et al. [71]. Copyright 2009, with permission from Elsevier

practice. On a follow-up survey, participants reported increased perceived confidence and competence following the training. The use of the "train-to-success" strategy significantly improved the learners' perception of the training effectiveness.

Education provided just prior to a clinical event may be more effective than standard courses. A "just-in-time" simulator-based refresher training on airway management in the PICU was developed and clinical outcomes assessed [70]. Although this approach had no effect on first-time intubation success rate by pediatric residents, there was increased resident participation as the initial laryngoscopist with no concomitant increase in adverse events when compared to historical controls. Such training may make senior PICU staff more comfortable in allowing junior trainees to perform tasks in the PICU. A similar study examined frequent just-in-time simulator training in CPR (Fig. 35.2). It was well received by staff and those that were refreshed ≥2/month demonstrated significantly shorter time to effective CPR on subsequent mannequin assessment [71]. Subsequent studies demonstrated that instructor-led mannequin-based CPR booster sessions of pediatric ward staff could improve CPR skill acquisition rates and maintain retention of CPR skills [72, 73]. The use of frequent simulation-based updates may be a useful method for providers to maintain their skills in dealing with rare events, such as pediatric intubation and cardiac arrest.

In order to increase availability of simulation in critical care, in situ simulation is becoming more prevalent, either permanently located in the PICU, or mobile systems, useable virtually anywhere [74, 75]. One popular use of this technique is mock codes in which resuscitation teams are called to surprise simulations [76]. These exercises can identify learning needs or systemic latent errors that need to be addressed [26, 77]. Niebauer et al. found a very high incidence of hyperventilation by healthcare providers during mock resuscitations with a mean ventilation rate of 40.6 breaths per minute, a problem which has recently been confirmed in the clinical environment [78, 79]. Hunt and colleagues found that there were deviations from standardized basic life support protocols in 75% of resuscitations [28]. These programs have the potential of a large clinical impact as demonstrated by Andreatta's study discussed previously.

Pediatric transport is another domain using simulation-based training. Although research in this area to date is limited, the development of untethered portable pediatric mannequins allows simulation-based training to be done in multiple environments including elevators, ambulances, and helicopters.

As cardiac intensive care develops as a separate subspecialty of pediatric critical care, simulation has also been incorporated there as an educational technique. Several studies have demonstrated increased learner self-confidence in resuscitation following simulation training [39, 80]. Pye and colleagues used simulation to introduce parental presence during resuscitation to their cardiac ICU staff [81].

In addition to more traditional simulations, cardiac-specific interventions have been studied. An echocardiography trainer for identification of various pediatric congenital heart defects has been developed, and though some technical challenges remain, it was felt to be realistic and useful [82]. Lo and colleagues have developed a reusable chest opening task trainer and have shown improvement in team skills with serial simulations of urgent sternal opening in a decompensating postoperative patient [83].

Simulation-based training has also been used in extracorporeal life support and continuous renal replacement therapy (CRRT). Lopez-Herce and colleagues used a multimodal educational intervention including high-fidelity simulation, didactic lectures, and task training with both CRRT and peritoneal dialysis machines. Their intervention improved cognitive measures and performance by learners as demonstrated by MCQ and simulated performance assessment [84]. Conventional pediatric mannequins have also been modified to interact with extracorporeal membrane oxygenation (ECMO) circuits [85]. Simulation-based training with these modified simulators has improved performance in the simulated environment as well as some modest improvements in the clinical environments [86, 87].

Pediatric Surgery and Pediatric Anesthesia

Another domain adopting simulation as an educational tool is pediatric surgery. It has been used to develop cognitive and behavioral skills as well as more specific surgical task training. Various task trainers using physical models and virtual reality have been developed to allow surgical trainees to develop competence in such procedures such as bronchoscopy, gynecological examinations, cleft lip repair, and laparoscopic surgery [88–92]. Patient-specific anatomy can also be created in a task trainer to allow practice prior to complex surgeries, such as repair of congenital heart conditions [93]. However, widespread adoption for task training has been somewhat limited by the relative lack of pediatric-specific mannequins and a recent survey of pediatric surgical trainees and program directors noted that currently available simulators may not be adequate to improve their skills [94]. More work is required to create more realistic surgical task trainers. In a recent survey of pediatric surgical trainees and their program directors, although 86.2% of respondents felt that simulation-based minimally invasive surgery training improves training efficiency, only 31.1% actually felt that current simulators had actually improved their skills [94]. In the adult population, the use of simulator-based minimally invasive surgery training did reduce error rates in the clinical environment [95].

Simulation has also been used to improve surgical team communication. Auguste reported using simulation to prepare surgical teams for a hospital's first EXIT procedure for a baby with hypoplastic left heart syndrome [96]. Surgical handover is another area where errors are common and simulation is being used to train residents in strategies to improve the quality of handover [97].

Although simulation has been used prominently in adult anesthesia pediatric data is limited [98, 99]. Howard-Quijano et al. used simulation to evaluate the ability of pediatric anesthesia trainees to manage intraoperative cardiac arrest [100]. Shavit and colleagues assessed a simulation-based sedation course that they developed and noted that simulation-trained physicians demonstrated improved performance in actual patient sedations [101]. However, more research is clearly needed.

Adolescent Medicine/Psychiatry

A final area where the use of simulation has been adopted as an important educational tool is in the area of adolescent medicine. In particular, issues pertaining to the assessment of mental health have been explored and measured. The simulation used in this group is exclusively standardized patients (SP). Some programs have even started to train and use actual adolescents in the role of SP. The use of actual adolescents as SP has been evaluated positively by students interacting with adolescents in this role [102]. However, authors warn that the adolescents must be chosen carefully and trained well [103].

In general, using standardized patients to practice interviewing and counseling skills has a positive effect on students.

These students have been shown to score significantly higher on both measures of knowledge and clinical skills [104]. Additionally, the use of standardized patients has been evaluated in both medical students and residents who have been trained in programs that supplemented traditional mental health teaching with simulated interactions with a standardized patient in the role of an adolescent with mental health issues. Several studies have shown positive effects in the areas of knowledge, clinical skills, confidence, and interpersonal skills. These positive effects have been shown in the mental health areas of major depressive disorders and suicide risk assessment [105, 106]. The future of simulation in this patient group will focus on other mental health conditions. More research is needed into the factors that improve the selection and training of adolescents to play the role of SP.

Team Training in Pediatrics

As specialized teams deliver increasing amounts of pediatric care, the importance of teamwork is receiving increased attention. Greater evidence is becoming available on the widespread prevalence of human factor errors during pediatric resuscitations [26, 28] and the importance of good teamwork skills in improving resuscitation team performance [54]. These skills are not explicitly taught in standard training programs. An alert from the Joint Commission for the Accreditation of Healthcare Organizations (JCAHO) noted that of 47 cases of neonatal mortality or severe morbidity reviewed, ineffective team dynamics played a role in almost 75% of them [107]. The Commission recommended that all healthcare organizations provide team training, clinical drills, and debriefings to evaluate team performance and identify gaps. Simulation-based training provides an opportunity to provide this education [108] and has been recommended by the International Liaison Committee on Resuscitation [109].

To date, there is little data on the use of team training in pediatrics. Gilfoyle and colleagues developed a workshop with a plenary session followed by simulation sessions to teach teamwork skills to pediatric residents [42]. They demonstrated that residents had improved teamwork skills both following the initial training and in a 6-month follow-up when compared to a control group. A similar improvement in collaboration between physicians and nurses was noted after multidisciplinary simulation sessions in another study [110].

A more recent study randomized participants into three groups: standard NRP, standard NRP plus 2 h of team training or high-fidelity NRP with team training [111]. As expected, participants receiving team training demonstrated more team skills, and this improvement was maintained at 6-month follow-up. However, team training with low-fidelity simulation did not improve teamwork skills as compared to control suggesting the value of fidelity in simulation-based training. Riley and colleagues developed a perinatal team training intervention based on the Team STEPPS® program developed by the Agency for Healthcare Research and Quality [112]. A didactic-only and simulation plus didactic education program was compared to control in this small cluster randomized trial. The simulation-based cluster had a 37% reduction in neonatal adverse outcomes. No improvement was noted in the didactic-only group when compared to control. These studies demonstrate that team training can improve patient outcomes, but didactic training alone is not enough.

Assessment Tools in Pediatrics

Many evaluation tools have been developed for use in simulation-based education. These assessment tools have been developed to evaluate clinical performance, leadership skills, and teamwork skills. Several assessment tools to evaluate crisis resource management (both team and leader performance) were recently reviewed in the literature [113]. However, until recently, very few of these tools have been developed or validated in pediatrics. Table 35.3 summarizes a variety of assessment tools developed in pediatrics.

The "Art" of Pediatric Simulation

There is no area of simulation where artful creativity is better expressed than in the area of pediatrics. The unique elements of caring for pediatric patients and their families present unique opportunities to apply simulation in very novel ways. The following section reviews some of the very unique and novel ways that simulation has been used in pediatrics. We also present innovative collaborations and networks that have been developed for the provision and assessment of simulation-based education. Finally, we present some of the unique challenges and barriers to providing pediatric simulation education.

Barriers and Challenges

Pediatric simulation education programs face a barrier unique to other areas of simulation: the diverse range of sizes of pediatric patients. From preterm infants, to toddlers, to school-aged children, and finally to adolescents, the significant range of patient sizes creates a potential problem for simulation educators in terms of maintaining contextual realism. This problem exists across the whole spectrum of simulation, from standardized patients through to high-fidelity patient mannequins. Many programs have successfully

Table 35.3 Pediatric assessment tools

Author	Focus of assessment	Environment where studied/validated	Scale used	Psychometrics measured/reported
Donoghue et al. [114]	Clinical skills	Pediatric residents performing PALS scenarios	3-point scale	Interrater reliability (IRR); $r=0.82$ Score variance attributable to rater: 1.4%
Lockyer et al. [115]	Clinical skills	Students taking an NRP course	3-point scale	Internal consistency; $\alpha = 0.70$
van der Heide et al. [116]	Clinical skills	Resident adherence to NRP guidelines	Weighted scoring system	IRR; $r=0.77$
Ishman et al. [117]	Technical skills	Resident performance with pediatric direct laryngoscopy/rigid bronchoscopy	5-point scale (two checklists: surgical checklist and global assessment of surgical performance)	IRR; intraclass coefficient=0.49 for surgical checklist and=0.70 for global assessment Internal consistency; $\alpha = 0.97$
Brett-Fleegler et al. [118]	Hybrid (clinical/leadership skills)	Pediatric residents	Dichotomous (Yes/No)	IRR; intraclass coefficient=0.8
Grant et al. [119]	Leadership (2 subscales: leadership/communication skills and knowledge and clinical skills)	Pediatric residents leading PALS-based resuscitations	4-point scale	Internal consistency; $\alpha = 0.82$ Generalizability coefficient=0.76 (acceptable for testing purposes)
Reid et al. [120]	Team assessment	Pediatric "experts" vs pediatric residents	3-point scale	IRR; intraclass coefficient=0.81 Good discrimination: "expert" 84% vs residents 66%
Anderson et al. [121]	Team assessment	Neonatal resuscitation providers	5-point scale	Internal consistency; $\alpha = 0.83–0.92$
Anderson et al. [122, 123]	Team Assessment	Multiple pediatric providers	5-point scale	IRR; intraclass coefficient=0.97–0.98 Internal consistency; $\alpha = 0.97$
Sigalet et al. [124]	Team Assessment	Undergraduate students from medicine, nursing, and respiratory therapy	5-point scale with defined anchors	IRR; intraclass coefficient=0.87–0.91 Internal consistency; $\alpha = 0.90$

Table 35.4 Summary of pediatric simulation mannequins

Vendor	High-fidelity mannequin	Age ranges represented
Laerdal	SimNewB™	Premature infant
	SimBaby™	Infants (<1 year)
	SimJunior™	5–9 year olds
	SimMan®	Adult (surrogate for adolescent)
CAE/METI	BabySIM®	Infants/young toddler (<2 years)
	PediaSIM®	5–9 year olds
	iStan®/HPS®/ECS®	Adult (surrogate for adolescent)
Gaumard	Premie HAL®	Premature infant
	Newborn HAL®	Infants (<1 year)
	Pediatric HAL® One Year	1–3 year olds
	Pediatric HAL® Five Year	5–9 year olds
	HAL®/Susie®	Adult (surrogate for adolescent)

integrated adolescent standardized patients into their training and evaluation (OSCEs), while fewer have incorporated school-aged children. The younger the child, the more difficult it is for them to be truly standardized making it impossible to use young children and toddlers as standardized patients. In terms of mannequin-based simulation, and in particular high-fidelity patient mannequins, mannequin vendors have responded to the problem of a diverse patient population by creating different versions of mannequins to represent different sizes of patients required within pediatric simulation. Although a detailed discussion of the pediatric mannequins can be formed in chapter 15, Table 35.4 provides a summary of the main mannequin vendors with their high-fidelity pediatric versions.

One of the most significant barriers to new and growing pediatric simulation programs is the initial cost of purchasing enough simulators to span the age ranges desired. Most adult-based simulation programs will often choose one model of simulator that they find useful and use that in their center. The advantage of this is that facilitators and educators only have to learn one mannequin platform. In pediatrics, a program that wants to cover all available ages would have be proficient with at least two mannequin platforms, which can be very stressful for program staff, facilitators, and educators.

Additionally, not all pediatric mannequins are created equal. Mannequin vendors have not equally assigned the same level of fidelity to each of their mannequins, meaning that some of the mannequins are better used for certain scenario types than others, further compounding the issue raised above. For example, some mannequins are better at simulating patients with a changing level of consciousness, simply because they have automatic eye opening and closing versus other mannequins who do not. Some mannequins recreate a seizure better than others, while others recreate respiratory distress better. Other examples of variability include pupillary changes and reaction to light, ability to obtain a reasonable seal with positive pressure ventilation using a bag and mask, chest compressibility, number and distribution of speakers for chest sounds, number of pulses and variable filling, among others. These are important issues to consider when deciding on the types of scenarios and the right mannequin to match the objectives to maintain the best contextual realism. Finally, there are a number of features missing from the current generation of pediatric mannequins that may become available in the future. The first is a real time streaming voice that is age appropriate. Currently, most mannequins only have "canned" phrases that the mannequin is able to say in an age appropriate voice. However, in order to most appropriately interact with the healthcare team working with the mannequin, a real time streaming voice is essential. This ability currently exists in the mannequins; however, there is no voice changing ability inherent in the software of the mannequins to change the voice from that of the adult simulation facilitator to a more appropriate pediatric one. It is anticipated that this would become a routine feature of pediatric mannequins in the future.

The other clinical finding likely to be of significant use to pediatric simulation educators would be the ability to more accurately portray cardiopulmonary perfusion. It would be extremely useful to have both peripheral pulses that could move through a range of filling and not just dichotomous or trichotomous choices. The incorporation of both central and peripheral capillary refill as a routine feature of the mannequins would also be extremely valuable to the educators and learners.

Although there remain significant barriers for pediatric simulation educators to overcome, many instructors have introduced clever scenario designs to overcome the challenges. This includes the use of clinical photographs or video to show capillary refill time, increased work of breathing, patient rashes, patient mentation, and seizure activity amongst others. Educators have used confederates to provide the "history" and some of the "clinical findings," particularly for scenarios involving infants and young children. Clearly these limitations have emphasized the importance of the "art" of pediatric simulation education delivery.

Novel Uses of Simulation

"Confederate" Parents and Family Members

One of the more unique aspects of pediatric healthcare is dealing with a group of patients that may not be able to communicate directly with the healthcare team. This is primarily the case in young infants and toddlers. Similarly, it can create challenges with the contextual realism of pediatric simulation scenarios as the team may not be able to elicit important information from the simulated patient (depending on age). As in real life, the presence of a parent becomes essential. There are many simulation programs that are successfully incorporating confederates acting in the role of a parent.

Although having a parent is important for enhancing the contextual realism of pediatric simulation scenarios, the parent role can also be used as a potential distracter for the team. Parent(s) can portray different emotions, including fear and anger, as well as repeatedly asking questions or trying to interfere with the communication flow in teams. Objectives and debriefing of such scenarios may include the appropriate communication of the team and the distracting parent.

In terms of the background and training for confederates acting as parents, some programs have incorporated trained actor SPs. Although likely the most realistic, this is also the most expensive of the options. Other programs have used cheaper alternatives, including offering comprehensive training to lay people who are either program staff or volunteers to effectively portray family members in scenarios (Marc Auerbach MD, written communication December 2011; Louis Halamek MD, written communication December 2011).

Difficult Conversations

A number of pediatric simulation programs have also incorporated the parent role as the primary element where the mannequin is used more like a "prop." For instance, this may be done for the purpose of breaking bad news to families such as revealing a difficult diagnosis or prognosis or to facilitate difficult conversations such as those surrounding cases of nonaccidental trauma (child abuse), disclosure of medical error, or even discussions around end-of-life care and organ donation. Using confederates as parents in these scenarios can be a powerful way of meeting objectives in those challenging areas particularly when real-world clinical experiences present so infrequently (Vinay Nadkarni MD, written communication, December 2011; Louis Halamek MD, written communication, December 2011; Kathy Tobler MD, written communication, December 2011; Vincent J. Grant, MD, written communication, December 2011).

End-of-Life Scenarios

In a similar vein, pediatric simulation with the addition of a confederate parent has been used to re-create difficult situations at the end of life. These not only include the difficult conversations highlighted above, but the re-creation of the clinical findings of a patient near the end of life allow for powerful experience for the appropriate learning group (Vinay Nadkarni MD, written communication, December 2011).

Teaching Parents and Families via Simulation

One of the more unique opportunities being explored at present is the possibility of using high-fidelity simulation to enhance the teaching of parents and other caregivers of patients with known medical needs (Fig. 35.3). In some ways, this has been occurring for decades with the way that cardiopulmonary resuscitation has been taught, but some simulation programs have started to include high-fidelity

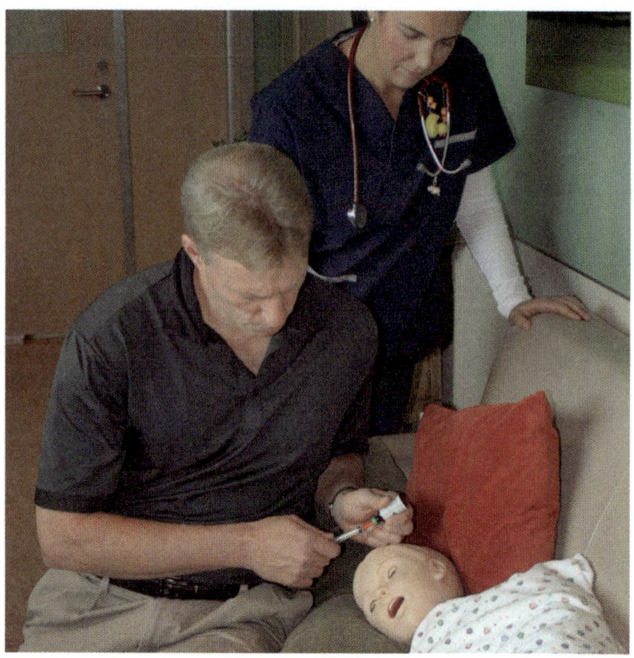

Fig. 35.3 Teaching a father to administer a rescue medication to his seizing child using a simulation mannequin (©KidSIM™ Pediatric Simulation Program, Alberta Children's Hospital/University of Calgary 2012. Reproduced with permission)

simulation specifically to provide instruction, feedback, and practice in the specific area of management. Multiple institutions are currently exploring the feasibility and outcome of using simulation-based education with families for seizure management and rescue medication administration in patients with intractable epilepsy and atypical febrile seizures, anaphylaxis, apnea spells, home supplemental oxygen, and tracheostomy care. In fact, simulation-based education may now be included into the discharge planning process for patients with complex medical needs (Vincent J. Grant MD, written communication, December 2011; David Grant MD, written communication, December 2011; Farhan Bhanji, written communication, January 2012)

Outreach Education

Up to 95% of pediatric emergency department visits occur outside of pediatric tertiary care centers and underscores the need for pediatric acute care training in those environments. Rural and remote care providers feel very uncomfortable and lack confidence in their ability to look after ill or injured children. This leads to a significant degree of stress when faced with these challenging situations. Simulation-based experiential learning may have a particular role in those environments. This training can be provided at the major teaching center or through Pediatric Simulation Outreach Programs that provide training in the local environment. It makes intuitive sense that training teams in their own environment, with their own clinical equipment and with their usual team members allows for a richer learning environment where issues of system, team process, and individual knowledge can be improved. It is not uncommon that the barriers to performance in this environment are related to room and equipment-specific issues related to the care of pediatric patients, which once addressed, lead the teams to greater rates of success (Vincent J. Grant MD, written communication, December 2011). Other novel applications of distance education include a distance telesimulation program between the Children's Hospital of Philadelphia and programs in Japan where facilitators in Philadelphia are able to lead debriefing on scenarios occurring in real time across the world (Vinay Nadkarni MD, written communication, December 2011).

Other Novel Uses of Simulation in Pediatrics

- Mannequin modifications to accommodate the placement of umbilical arterial/venous catheters wiring for ECMO/ECLS circuits (Jon Duff MD, written communication, January 2012)
- Multidisciplinary in situ simulation involving patient aggression and restraint (Marc Auerbach, written communication, December 2011)
- Using eye tracking software to differentiate novice from expert bedside caregivers based upon eye tracking (Marino Festa MD, written communication, January 2012)
- Extramural deliveries with parking attendants in parkade (following a real event) (Marc Auerbach MD, written communication, December 2011)
- Simulation around rare surgical events: fetal surgery and separation of conjoint twins (Vinay Nadkarni MD, written communication, December 2011)
- Debriefing for hospital administration—comprehensive training program to prepare hospital administrators and other leaders to effectively interact with staff and debrief critical incidents as well as routine events (Louis Halamek MD, written communication, December 2011)
- Child abduction scenario—multiday exercise where faculty first try to obtain access to hospital uniforms over a course of days prior to the event, then on the day of the abduction the event is declared as soon as a confederate gains unchallenged access to a ward (David Grant MD, written communication, December 2011)

Innovative Collaboration

The rapid growth of simulation-based education in pediatrics has lead to the genesis of several innovative collaborations, all with the common vision of enhancing the application of simulation to improve the healthcare outcomes of infants and children. The Canadian Pediatric Simulation Network (CPSN) is an interprofessional network of pediatric simulation educators in Canada who have met annually since 2007 [125]. The network's goal is to foster the growth of simulation by promoting effective networking amongst simulation educators in Canada. Over the past 4 years, this network has been successful at implementing a number of projects such as a national crisis resource management course and provides a good example of how combined expertise in simulation can be effective in achieving projects at the national level.

Two different pediatric simulation research networks have evolved in the past 5 years. The Examining Pediatric Resuscitation Education using Simulation and Scripting (EXPRESS) Collaborative and the Patient Outcomes In Simulation Education (POISE) Network have both successfully conducted multicenter, simulation-based research trials by bringing together simulation research experts from across North America. Led by experts in pediatric acute care and simulation, the EXPRESS collaborative's primary aim is to improve the delivery of medical care to critically ill children by answering important research questions pertaining to pediatric resuscitation, education and simulation [126]. The first EXPRESS project involved the development of a debriefing script for pediatric advanced life support (PALS) instructors, which ultimately led to the inclusion of a debriefing tool in the 2011 PALS instructor materials [127]. The POISE network members have collaborated in the development of educational interventions related to infant lumbar puncture and neonatal intubation procedures. Along with the implementation and testing of simulation-based training and assessments, POISE has established a community of simulation educators by offering monthly webinar sessions and educational content on its website (Marc Auerbach MD, written communication, December 2011). In January 2012, recognizing their common goals and vision, the EXPRESS collaborative and POISE network formally merged to form the largest simulation research and education network in the world: the International Network in Simulation-based Pediatric Innovation, Research, and Education (INSPIRE) (Vinay Nadkarni MD, written communication, December 2011). This new network will continue the work previously done by EXPRESS and POISE and also aims to invite collaboration from educators and researchers from all parts of the world to advance the field of pediatric simulation.

In 2010, the International Pediatric Simulation Society (IPSS) was born, dedicated to pediatric, perinatal, and associated healthcare providers and organizations who use simulation-based education to improve care and safety for children. IPSS will promote and support multidisciplinary simulation-based education, training, and research among all pediatric subspecialties focused on the unique nature and needs of caring for the pediatric and perinatal patient, including advocacy for simulation internationally by addressing issues such as technology, funding, legislation, and public policy (www.ipedsim.com, accessed Dec 21, 2010).

The "Future" of Pediatric Simulation

The success of innovation and collaboration within pediatric simulation education has already set the field in a positive direction heading into the future. However, educators in this

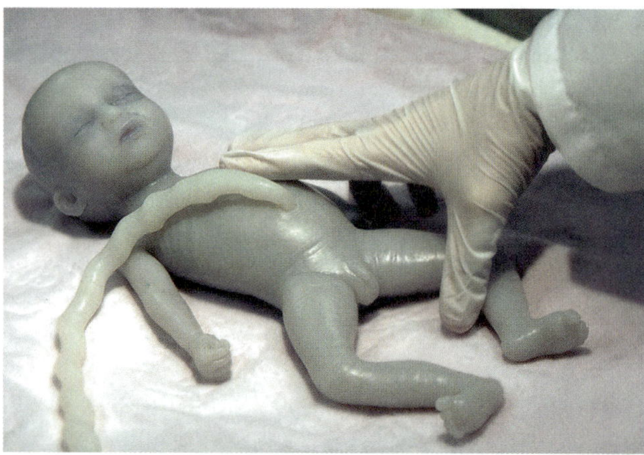

Fig. 35.4 Limbs and Things' fetal demise simulator (Photo courtesy of Limbs & Things ©2012 www.limbsandthings.com)

domain must continue to push the envelope in five important areas (that are not exclusive to pediatric simulation) where a greater amount of academic understanding is required.

The first and foremost is the assessment of simulation-based education on actual patient outcomes. Simulation will benefit in its reputation, acceptance, and funding sources when it can link training to improved patient outcomes. Although this is extremely challenging based on the logistics of viewing or reviewing actual patient events when they are rare in pediatrics, it is of utmost importance that simulation academics begin to make these linkages.

The second is the incorporation of simulation into high-stakes examinations. Simulation has, to date, focused primarily on training and formative assessment with issues of successful completion of rotations, licensing, and revalidation left aside. Some effort now has the be placed on the use of simulation to assess competence in order to both ensure appropriate qualifications of healthcare providers and as a tool to "drive" student/practitioner learning to the relevant learning outcomes (e.g., as compared to written tests that may guide learning in other directions). In order for this paradigm shift to occur there needs to be a development of valid assessment tools to assess the relevant competence. There has been some work introducing simulation into this environment, and if simulation is the best method to educate in some areas of our healthcare curriculum, than it might also be the best way of assessing competence in these same areas. Further work needs to be done into the development of valid assessment tools to measure competence in areas that have been shown to be better taught using this education technique.

The third area is a better understanding of the ways we have been assisting learners to reflect on their experiences. The learning from simulation-based education is highly reliant on the quality of this reflection and the learner's ability to understand new concepts from it. Only recently have educators began to look at the quality of debriefing and to develop tools to better understand its basic elements. The development

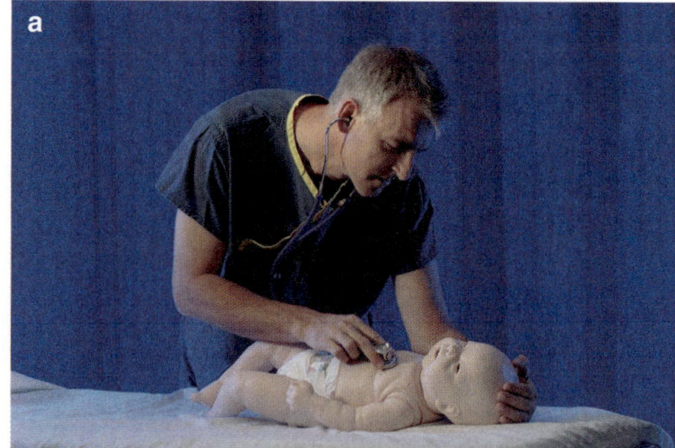

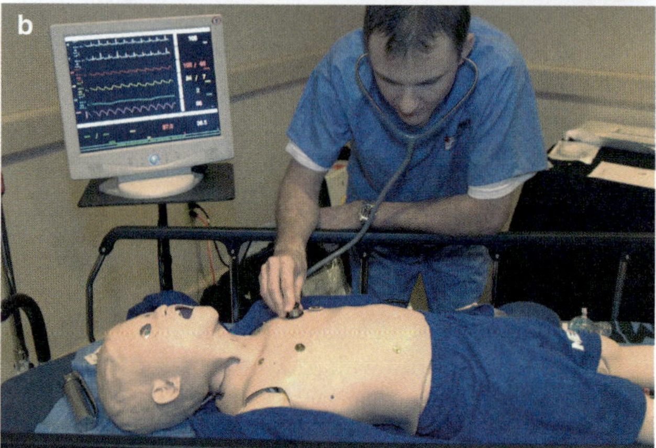

Fig. 35.5 (**a**) CAE BabySim and (**b**) CAE Pediasim (Photo courtesy of CAE Healthcare ©2012 CAE Healthcare)

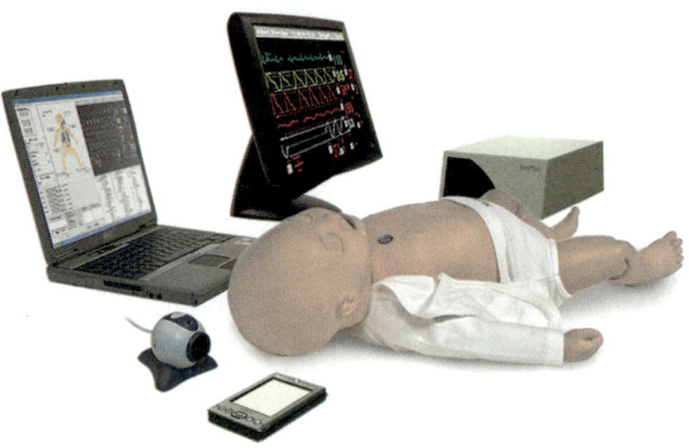

Fig. 35.6 Laerdal SimBaby (Photo used courtesy of Laerdal)

of these tools should lead to better benchmarks on what quality debriefing looks like and how to ensure it exists universally throughout the world of simulation.

The fourth is the need to increase the amount of realism in scenario delivery, including creatively maximizing the realism of the teaching environment, as well as continuing to push mannequin vendors to further improve their mannequins. Several of the currently available simulators are shown in Figs. 35.4, 35.5, 35.6, 35.7, and 35.8. These and other simulators will be necessary for the fidelity of pediatric simulation to progress.

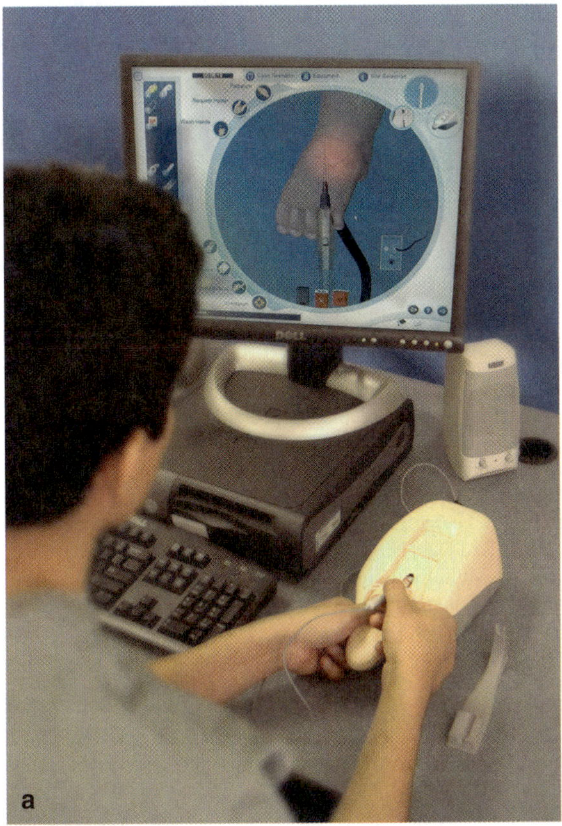

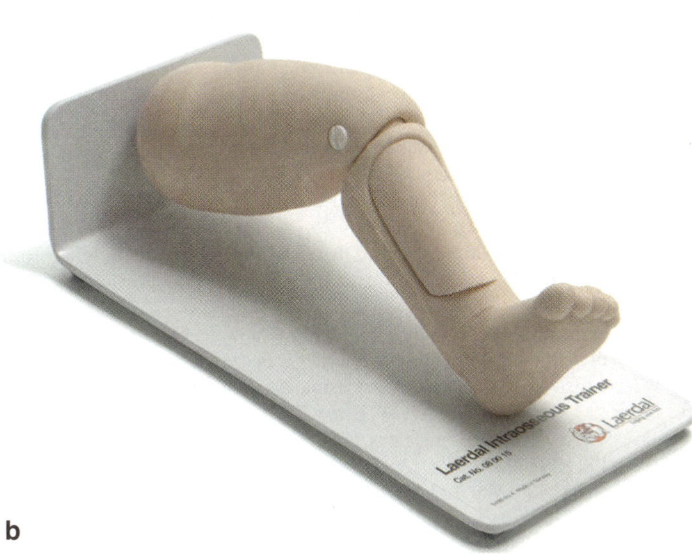

Fig. 35.7 (**a**, **b**) Laerdal Infant IV and intraosseous trainers (Photo used courtesy of Laerdal)

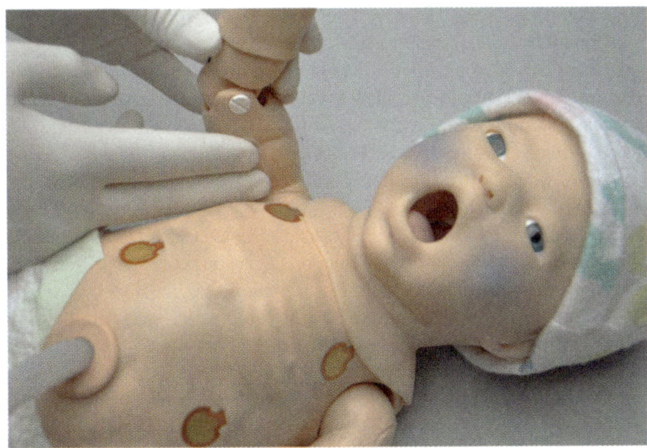

Fig. 35.8 Gaumard Baby simulator with cyanosis (Photo used courtesy of Gaumard)

Conclusion

The pediatric collaborations identified earlier in the chapter need to be fostered and continue to grow. Only in working together with educators from across our individual countries and the entire world will we be able to face the challenges listed above and to answer the important questions that will ultimately lead to better patient outcome, as well as to continue to keep pediatric simulation at the "cutting edge" of simulation-based delivery and outcomes.

References

1. Nadkarni VM, Larkin GL, Peberdy MA, Carey SM, Kaye W, Mancini ME, et al. First documented rhythm and clinical outcome from in-hospital cardiac arrest among children and adults. JAMA. 2006;295:50–7.
2. Donoghue AJ, Nadkarni V, Berg RA, Osmond MH, Wells G, Nesbitt L, et al. Out-of-hospital pediatric cardiac arrest: an epidemiologic review and assessment of current knowledge. Ann Emerg Med. 2005;46:512–22.
3. Tibballs J, Kinney S. A prospective study of outcome of in-patient paediatric cardiopulmonary arrest. Resuscitation. 2006;71:310–8.
4. Kleinman ME, de Caen AR, Chameides L, Atkins DL, Berg RA, Berg MD, et al. On behalf of the Pediatric Basic and Advanced Life Support Chapter Collaborators. Part 10: Pediatric Basic and Advanced Life Support: 2010 International Consensus on Cardiopulmonary Resuscitation and Emergency Cardiovascular Care Science With Treatment Recommendations Circulation. 2010;122:S466–515.
5. Cheng A, Bhanji F. A case-based update: 2010 paediatric basic and advanced life-support guidelines. Paediatr Child Health. 2011;16:295–7.
6. American Academy of Pediatrics, Committee on Pediatric Emergency Medicine. Access to pediatric emergency medical care. Pediatrics. 2000;105:647–9.
7. Tamariz VP, Fuchs S, Baren JM, Pollack ES, Kim J, Seidel JS. Pediatric emergency medicine education in emergency medicine training programs. Acad Emerg Med. 2000;7:774–8.

8. Langhan M, Keshavarz R, Richardson LD. How comfortable are emergency physicians with pediatric patients. J Emerg Med. 2004;26:465–9.
9. Hunt EA, Patel S, Vera K, Shaffner DH, Pronovost PJ. Survey of pediatric resident experiences with resuscitation training and attendance at actual cardiopulmonary arrests. Pediatr Crit Care Med. 2009;10:96–105.
10. Bhanji F, Mancini ME, Sinz E, Rodgers DL, McNeil MA, Hoadley TA, et al. Part 16: education, implementation, and teams: 2010 American Heart Association Guidelines for Cardiopulmonary Resuscitation and Emergency Cardiovascular Care. Circulation. 2010;122:S920–33.
11. Ali J, Howard M, Williams J. Is attrition of advanced trauma life support acquired skills affected by trauma patient volume? Am J Surg. 2002;183:142–5.
12. Halamek LP. Teaching versus learning and the role of simulation-based training in pediatrics. J Pediatr. 2007;151:329–30.
13. Fanning RM, Gaba DM. The role of debriefing in simulation-based learning. Simul Healthc. 2007;2:115–25.
14. Kolb D, Fry R. Towards an applied theory of experiential learning. In: Cooper C, editor. Theories of group processes. London: John Wiley; 1975.
15. Savoldelli GL, Naik VN, Park J, Joo HS, Chow R, Hamstra SJ. Value of debriefing during simulated crisis management: oral versus video-assisted oral feedback. Anesthesiology. 2006;105:279–85.
16. Marteau TM, Wynne G, Kaye W, Evans TR. Resuscitation: experience without feedback increases confidence but not skill. BMJ. 1990;300:849–50.
17. van Schaik SM, Von Kohorn I, O'Sullivan P. Pediatric resident confidence in resuscitation skills relates to mock code experience. Clin Pediatr. 2008;47:777–83.
18. Kohn L, Corrigan J, Donaldson M. To err is human: building a safer health system. Washington, D.C.: National Academy Press; 2000.
19. Kaushal R, Bates DW, Landrigan C, McKenna KJ, Clapp MD, Federico F, et al. Medication errors and adverse drug events in pediatric inpatients. JAMA. 2001;285:2114–20.
20. Kozer E, Scolnik D, Macpherson A, Keays T, Shi K, Luk T, et al. Variables associated with medication errors in pediatric emergency medicine. Pediatrics. 2002;110:737–42.
21. Kozer E, Scolnik D, Macpherson A, Rauchwerger D, Koren G. The effect of a short tutorial on the incidence of prescribing errors in pediatric emergency care. Can J Clin Pharmacol. 2006;13:e285–91.
22. Ericsson KA. Deliberate practice and the acquisition and maintenance of expert performance in medicine and related domains. Acad Med. 2004;79:S70–81.
23. McGaghie WC, Issenberg SB, Cohen ER, Barsuk JH, Wayne DB. Does simulation-based medical education with deliberate practice yield better results than traditional clinical education? A meta-analytic comparative review of the evidence. Acad Med. 2011;86:706–11.
24. Spanos SL, Patterson M. An unexpected diagnosis: simulation reveals unanticipated deficiencies in resident physician dysrhythmia knowledge. Simul Healthc. 2010;5:21.
25. Shilkofski NA, Nelson KL, Hunt EA. Recognition and treatment of unstable supraventricular tachycardia by pediatric residents in a simulation scenario. Simul Healthc. 2008;3:4–9.
26. Garden AL, Mills SA, Wilson R, Watt P, Griffin JM, Gannon S, et al. In situ simulation training for paediatric cardiorespiratory arrest: initial observations and identification of latent errors. Anaesth Intensive Care. 2010;38:1038–42.
27. Hunt EA, Hohenhaus SM, Luo X, Frush KS. Simulation of pediatric trauma stabilization in 35 North Carolina emergency departments: identification of targets for performance improvement. Pediatrics. 2006;117:641–8.
28. Hunt EA, Walker AR, Shaffner DH, Miller MR, Pronovost PJ. Simulation of in-hospital pediatric medical emergencies and cardiopulmonary arrests: highlighting the importance of the first 5 minutes. Pediatrics. 2008;121:e34–43.
29. Kessler DO, Auerbach M, Pusic M, Tunik MG, Foltin JC. A randomized trial of simulation-based deliberate practice for infant lumbar puncture skills. Simul Healthc. 2011;6:197–203.
30. Okuda Y, Bryson EO, DeMaria Jr S, Jacobson L, Quinones J, Shen B, et al. The utility of simulation in medical education: what is the evidence? Mt Sinai J Med. 2009;76:330–43.
31. Kirkpatrick DL. Evaluating training programs: the four levels. San Francisco: Berrett-Koehler; 1994.
32. McGaghie WC. Medical education research as translational science. Sci Transl Med. 2010;2:19cm8.
33. Belfield C, Thomas H, Bullock A, Eynon R, Wall D. Measuring effectiveness for best evidence medical education: a discussion. Med Teach. 2001;23:164–70.
34. Donoghue AJ, Durbin DR, Nadel FM, Stryjewski GR, Kost SI, Nadkarni VM. Effect of high-fidelity simulation on Pediatric Advanced Life Support training in pediatric house staff: a randomized trial. Pediatr Emerg Care. 2009;25:139–44.
35. Hunt EA, Heine M, Hohenhaus SM, Luo X, Frush KS. Simulated pediatric trauma team management: assessment of an educational intervention. Pediatr Emerg Care. 2007;23:796–804.
36. Falcone Jr RA, Daugherty M, Schweer L, Patterson M, Brown RL, Garcia VF. Multidisciplinary pediatric trauma team training using high-fidelity trauma simulation. J Pediatr Surg. 2008;43:1065–71.
37. Binstadt ES, Walls RM, White BA, Nadel ES, Takayesu JK, Barker TD, et al. A comprehensive medical simulation education curriculum for emergency medicine residents. Ann Emerg Med. 2007;49: 495–504.
38. Mikrogianakis A, Osmond MH, Nuth JE, Shephard A, Gaboury I, Jabbour M. Evaluation of a multidisciplinary pediatric mock trauma code educational initiative: a pilot study. J Trauma. 2008;64:761–7.
39. Allan CK, Thiagarajan RR, Beke D, Imprescia A, Kappus LJ, Garden A, et al. Simulation-based training delivered directly to the pediatric cardiac intensive care unit engenders preparedness, comfort, and decreased anxiety among multidisciplinary resuscitation teams. J Thorac Cardiovasc Surg. 2010;140:646–52.
40. Bandura A. Self-efficacy: the exercise of control. New York: W.H. Freeman and Company; 1997.
41. Grant EC, Marczinski CA, Menon K. Using pediatric advanced life support in pediatric residency training: does the curriculum need resuscitation? Pediatr Crit Care Med. 2007;8:433–9.
42. Gilfoyle E, Gottesman R, Razack S. Development of a leadership skills workshop in paediatric advanced resuscitation. Med Teach. 2007;29:e276–83.
43. Turner NM, Dierselhuis MP, Draaisma JM, ten Cate OT. The effect of the Advanced Paediatric Life Support course on perceived self-efficacy and use of resuscitation skills. Resuscitation. 2007;73:430–6.
44. Maibach EW, Schieber RA, Carroll MF. Self-efficacy in pediatric resuscitation: implications for education and performance. Pediatrics. 1996;97:94–9.
45. Nishisaki A, Nguyen J, Colborn S, Watson C, Niles D, Hales R, et al. Evaluation of multidisciplinary simulation training on clinical performance and team behavior during tracheal intubation procedures in a pediatric intensive care unit. Pediatr Crit Care Med. 2011;12:406–14.
46. Andreatta P, Saxton E, Thompson M, Annich G. Simulation-based mock codes significantly correlate with improved pediatric patient cardiopulmonary arrest survival rates. Pediatr Crit Care Med. 2011;12:33–8.
47. Cheng A, Duff J, Grant E, Kissoon N, Grant V. Simulation in pediatrics: an educational revolution. Paediatr Child Health. 2007;12:465–8.
48. Sam J, Pierse M, Al-Qahtani Q, Cheng A. Implementation and evaluation of a simulation curriculum for pediatric residency programs including just in time in-situ mock codes. Pediatr Child Health. 2012;17:1–5.
49. Adler M, Vozenilek J, Trainor J, et al. Development and evaluation of a simulation-based pediatric emergency medicine curriculum. Acad Med. 2009;84:935–41.

50. Cheng A, Goldman R, AbuAish M, Kissoon N. Integration and evaluation of a simulation-based acute care curriculum into a pediatric emergency medicine fellowship training program. Pediatr Emerg Care. 2010;26:475–80.
51. Halamek LP. The simulated delivery-room environment as the future modality for acquiring and maintaining skills in fetal and neonatal resuscitation. Semin Fetal Neonatal Med. 2008;13:448–53.
52. Carbine DN, Finer NN, Knodel E, Rich W. Video recording as a means of evaluating neonatal resuscitation performance. Pediatrics. 2000;106:654–8.
53. Anderson JM, Warren JB. Using simulation to enhance the acquisition and retention of clinical skills in neonatology. Semin Perinatol. 2011;35:59–67.
54. Rovamo L, Mattila MM, Andersson S, Rosenberg P. Assessment of newborn resuscitation skills of physicians with a simulator manikin. Arch Dis Child Fetal Neonatal Ed. 2011;96:F383–9.
55. Thomas EJ, Sexton JB, Lasky RE, Helmreich RL, Crandell DS, Tyson J. Teamwork and quality during neonatal care in the delivery room. J Perinatol. 2006;26:163–9.
56. Bismilla Z, Finan E, McNamara PJ, LeBlanc V, Jefferies A, Whyte H. Failure of pediatric and neonatal trainees to meet Canadian Neonatal Resuscitation Program standards for neonatal intubation. J Perinatol. 2010;30:182–7.
57. Kaczorowski J, Levitt C, Hammond M, Outerbridge E, Grad R, Rothman A, et al. Retention of neonatal resuscitation skills and knowledge: a randomized controlled trial. Fam Med. 1998;30:705–11.
58. Arnold J. The Neonatal Resuscitation Program comes of age. J Pediatr. 2011;159:357–8.
59. Campbell DM, Barozzino T, Farrugia M, Sgro M. High-fidelity simulation in neonatal resuscitation. Paediatr Child Health. 2009;14:19–23.
60. Cavaleiro AP, Guimaraes H, Calheiros F. Training neonatal skills with simulators? Acta Paediatr. 2009;98:636–9.
61. Sawyer T, Sierocka-Castaneda A, Chan D, Berg B, Lustik M, Thompson M. Deliberate practice using simulation improves neonatal resuscitation performance. Simul Healthc. 2011;6:327–36.
62. Curran VR, Aziz K, O'Young S, Bessell C. Evaluation of the effect of a computerized training simulator (ANAKIN) on the retention of neonatal resuscitation skills. Teach Learn Med. 2004; 16:157–64.
63. LeFlore J, Thomas PE, Zielke MA, Buus-Frank ME, McFadden BE, Sansoucie DA. Educating neonatal nurse practitioners in the 21st century. J Perinat Neonatal Nurs. 2011;25:200–5.
64. Ohlinger J, Kantak A, Lavin Jr JP, Fofah O, Hagen E, Suresh G, et al. Evaluation and development of potentially better practices for perinatal and neonatal communication and collaboration. Pediatrics. 2006;118:S147–52.
65. Armentrout D, Cates LA. Informing parents about the actual or impending death of their infant in a newborn intensive care unit. J Perinat Neonatal Nurs. 2011;25:261–7.
66. Finan E, Bismilla Z, Campbell C, Leblanc V, Jefferies A, Whyte HE. Improved procedural performance following a simulation training session may not be transferable to the clinical environment. J Perinatol. 2012;32(7):539–44. doi:10.1038/jp.2011.141.
67. Draycott T, Sibanda T, Owen L, Akande V, Winter C, Reading S, et al. Does training in obstetric emergencies improve neonatal outcome? BJOG. 2006;113:177–82.
68. Hunt EA, Vera K, Diener-West M, Haggerty JA, Nelson KL, Shaffner DH, et al. Delays and errors in cardiopulmonary resuscitation and defibrillation by pediatric residents during simulated cardiopulmonary arrests. Resuscitation. 2009;80:819–25.
69. Nishisaki A, Hales R, Biagas K, Cheifetz I, Corriveau C, Garber N, et al. A multi-institutional high-fidelity simulation "boot camp" orientation and training program for first year pediatric critical care fellows. Pediatr Crit Care Med. 2009;10:157–62.
70. Nishisaki A, Donoghue AJ, Colborn S, Watson C, Meyer A, Brown 3rd CA, et al. Effect of just-in-time simulation training on tracheal intubation procedure safety in pediatric intensive care unit. Anesthesiology. 2010;113:214–23.
71. Niles D, Sutton RM, Donoghue A, Kalsi MS, Roberts S, Boyle L, et al. "Rolling Refreshers": a novel approach to maintain CPR psychomotor skill competence. Resuscitation. 2009;80:909–12.
72. Sutton RM, Niles D, Meaney PA, Aplenc R, French B, Abella BS, et al. Low-dose, high-frequency CPR training improves skill retention of in-hospital pediatric providers. Pediatrics. 2011;128:e145–51.
73. Sutton RM, Niles D, Meaney PA, Aplenc R, French B, Abella BS, et al. "Booster" training: evaluation of instructor-led bedside cardiopulmonary resuscitation skill training and automated corrective feedback to improve cardiopulmonary resuscitation compliance of Pediatric Basic Life Support providers during simulated cardiac arrest. Pediatr Crit Care Med. 2011;12:e116–21.
74. Weinstock PH, Kappus LJ, Kleinman ME, Grenier B, Hickey P, Burns JP. Toward a new paradigm in hospital-based pediatric education: the development of an onsite simulator program. Pediatr Crit Care Med. 2005;6:635–41.
75. Weinstock PH, Kappus LJ, Garden A, Burns JP. Simulation at the point-of-care: reduced-cost, in situ training via a mobile cart. Pediatr Crit Care Med. 2009;10:176–81.
76. Palmisano JM, Akingbola OA, Moler FW, Custer JR. Simulated pediatric cardiopulmonary resuscitation: initial events and response times of a hospital arrest team. Respir Care. 1994;39:725–9.
77. Brooks-Buza H, Fernandez R, Stenger JP. The use of in situ simulation to evaluate teamwork and system organization during a pediatric dental clinic emergency. Simul Healthc. 2011;6:101–8.
78. Niebauer JM, White ML, Zinkan JL, Youngblood AQ, Tofil NM. Hyperventilation in pediatric resuscitation: performance in simulated pediatric medical emergencies. Pediatrics. 2011;128:e1195–200.
79. McInnes AD, Sutton RM, Orioles A, Nishisaki A, Niles D, Abella BS, et al. The first quantitative report of ventilation rate during in-hospital resuscitation of older children and adolescents. Resuscitation. 2011;82:1025–9.
80. Kane J, Pye S, Jones A. Effectiveness of a Simulation-Based Educational Program in a pediatric cardiac intensive care unit. J Pediatr Nurs. 2011;26(4):287–94.
81. Pye S, Kane J, Jones A. Parental presence during pediatric resuscitation: the use of simulation training for cardiac intensive care nurses. J Spec Pediatr Nurs. 2010;15:172–5.
82. Weidenbach M, Razek V, Wild F, Khambadkone S, Berlage T, Janousek J, et al. Simulation of congenital heart defects: a novel way of training in echocardiography. Heart. 2009;95:636–41.
83. Lo TY, Morrison R, Atkins K, Reynolds F. Effective performance of a new post-operative cardiac resuscitation simulation training scheme in Paediatric Intensive Care Unit. Intensive Care Med. 2009;35:725–9.
84. Lopez-Herce J, Ferrero L, Mencia S, Anton M, Rodriguez-Nunez A, Rey C, et al. Teaching and training acute renal replacement therapy in children. Nephrol Dial Transplant. 2012;27(5):1807–11.
85. Anderson JM, Boyle KB, Murphy AA, Yaeger KA, LeFlore J, Halamek LP. Simulating extracorporeal membrane oxygenation emergencies to improve human performance. Part I: methodologic and technologic innovations. Simul Healthc. 2006;1:220–7.
86. Anderson JM, Murphy AA, Boyle KB, Yaeger KA, Halamek LP. Simulating extracorporeal membrane oxygenation emergencies to improve human performance. Part II: assessment of technical and behavioral skills. Simul Healthc. 2006;1:228–32.
87. Burton KS, Pendergrass TL, Byczkowski TL, Taylor RG, Moyer MR, Falcone RA, et al. Impact of simulation-based extracorporeal membrane oxygenation training in the simulation laboratory and clinical environment. Simul Healthc. 2011;6:284–91.
88. Brydges R, Farhat WA, El-Hout Y, Dubrowski A. Pediatric urology training: performance-based assessment using the fundamentals of laparoscopic surgery. J Surg Res. 2010;161:240–5.
89. Schendel S, Montgomery K, Sorokin A, Lionetti G. A surgical simulator for planning and performing repair of cleft lips. J Craniomaxillofac Surg. 2005;33:223–8.

90. Loveless MB, Finkenzeller D, Ibrahim S, Satin AJ. A simulation program for teaching obstetrics and gynecology residents the pediatric gynecology examination and procedures. J Pediatr Adolesc Gynecol. 2011;24:127–36.
91. Hamilton JM, Kahol K, Vankipuram M, Ashby A, Notrica DM, Ferrara JJ. Toward effective pediatric minimally invasive surgical simulation. J Pediatr Surg. 2011;46:138–44.
92. Deutsch ES. High-fidelity patient simulation manikins to facilitate aerodigestive endoscopy training. Arch Otolaryngol Head Neck Surg. 2008;134:625–9.
93. Shiraishi I, Yamagishi M, Hamaoka K, Fukuzawa M, Yagihara T. Simulative operation on congenital heart disease using rubber-like urethane stereolithographic biomodels based on 3D datasets of multislice computed tomography. Eur J Cardiothorac Surg. 2010;37:302–6.
94. Lasko D, Zamakhshary M, Gerstle JT. Perception and use of minimal access surgery simulators in pediatric surgery training programs. J Pediatr Surg. 2009;44:1009–12.
95. Zendejas B, Cook DA, Bingener J, Huebner M, Dunn WF, Sarr MG, et al. Simulation-based mastery learning improves patient outcomes in laparoscopic inguinal hernia repair: a randomized controlled trial. Ann Surg. 2011;254:502–9.
96. Auguste TC, Boswick JA, Loyd MK, Battista A. The simulation of an ex utero intrapartum procedure to extracorporeal membrane oxygenation. J Pediatr Surg. 2011;46:395–8.
97. Chen JG, Mistry KP, Wright MC, Turner DA. Postoperative handoff communication: a simulation-based training method. Simul Healthc. 2010;5:242–7.
98. Gozal D, Gozal Y. Pediatric sedation/anesthesia outside the operating room. Curr Opin Anaesthesiol. 2008;21:494–8.
99. Cravero JP, Havidich JE. Pediatric sedation – evolution and revolution. Paediatr Anaesth. 2011;21:800–9.
100. Howard-Quijano KJ, Stiegler MA, Huang YM, Canales C, Steadman RH. Anesthesiology residents' performance of pediatric resuscitation during a simulated hyperkalemic cardiac arrest. Anesthesiology. 2010;112:993–7.
101. Shavit I, Keidan I, Hoffmann Y, Mishuk L, Rubin O, Ziv A, et al. Enhancing patient safety during pediatric sedation: the impact of simulation-based training of nonanesthesiologists. Arch Pediatr Adolesc Med. 2007;161:740–3.
102. Bokken L, Van Dalen J, Scherpbier A, Van der Vleuten C, Rethans J-J. Lessons learned from an adolescent simulated patient educational program: five years of experience. Med Teach. 2009;31: 605–12.
103. Blake K. Sex, drugs and rock and roll – teaching with adolescent standardized patients. Med Teach. 2009;31:571–3.
104. Feddock CA, Hoellein AR, Griffith CH, Wilson JF, Lineberry MJ, Haist SA. Enhancing knowledge and clinical skills through an adolescent medicine workshop. Arch Pediatr Adolesc Med. 2009;163:256–60.
105. Lewy C, Sells CW, Gilhooly J, McKelvey R. Adolescent depression: evaluating pediatric residents' knowledge, confidence, and interpersonal skills using standardized patients. Acad Psychiatry. 2009;33:389–93.
106. Fallucco EM, Hanson MD, Glowinski AL. Teaching pediatric residents to assess adolescent suicide risk with a standardized patient module. Pediatrics. 2010;125:953–9.
107. Sentinel Event Alert: Preventing infant death and injury during delivery. The Joint Commission for the Accreditation of Healthcare Organizations. 2004. http://www.jointcommission.org/sentinel_event_alert_issue_30_preventing_infant_death_and_injury_during_delivery/. Accessed 19 Dec 2011.
108. Halamek LP, Kaegi DM, Gaba DM, Sowb YA, Smith BC, Smith BE, et al. Time for a new paradigm in pediatric medical education: teaching neonatal resuscitation in a simulated delivery room environment. Pediatrics. 2000;106:E45.
109. Perlman JM, Wyllie J, Kattwinkel J, Atkins DL, Chameides L, Goldsmith JP, et al. Neonatal Resuscitation Chapter Collaborators. Part 11: Neonatal resuscitation: 2010 International Consensus on Cardiopulmonary Resuscitation and Emergency Cardiovascular Care Science With Treatment Recommendations. Circulation. 2010;122:S516–38.
110. Messmer PR. Enhancing nurse-physician collaboration using pediatric simulation. J Contin Educ Nurs. 2008;39:319–27.
111. Thomas EJ, Williams AL, Reichman EF, Lasky RE, Crandell S, Taggart WR. Team training in the neonatal resuscitation program for interns: teamwork and quality of resuscitations. Pediatrics. 2010;125:539–46.
112. Riley W, Davis S, Miller K, Hansen H, Sainfort F, Sweet R. Didactic and simulation nontechnical skills team training to improve perinatal patient outcomes in a community hospital. Jt Comm J Qual Patient Saf. 2011;37:357–64.
113. Cheng A, Donoghue A, Gilfoyle E, Eppich W. Simulation-based crisis resource management training for pediatric critical care medicine: a review for instructors. Pediatr Crit Care Med. 2012;13(2):197–203.
114. Donoghue A, Nishisakia A, Sutton R, Hales R, Boulet J. Reliability and validity of a scoring instrument for clinical performance during Pediatric Advanced Life Support simulation scenarios. Resuscitation. 2010;81:331–6.
115. Lockyer J, Singhal N, Fidler H, Weiner G, Aziz K, Curran V. The development and testing of a performance checklist to assess neonatal resuscitation megacode skill. Pediatrics. 2006;118:e1739–44.
116. van der Heide PA, van Toledo-Eppinga L, van der Heide M, van der Lee JH. Assessment of neonatal resuscitation skills: a reliable and valid scoring system. Resuscitation. 2006;71:212–21.
117. Ishman SL, Brown DJ, Boss EF, Skinner ML, Tunkel DE, Stavinoha R, et al. Development and pilot testing of an operative competency assessment tool for pediatric direct laryngoscopy and rigid bronchoscopy. Laryngoscope. 2010;120:2294–300.
118. Brett-Fleegler MB, Vinci RJ, Weiner DL, Harris SK, Shih M-C, Kleinman ME. A simulator-based tool that assesses pediatric resident resuscitation competency. Pediatrics. 2008;121:e597–603.
119. Grant EC, Grant VJ, Bhanji F, Cheng A, Duff JP, Lockyer JM. The development and assessment of an evaluation tool for pediatric resident competence in leading simulated pediatric resuscitations. Resuscitation. 2012;83(7):887–93. doi:10.1016/j.resuscitation.2012.01.015.
120. Reid J, Stone K, Brown J, Caglar D, Kobayashi A, Lewis-Newby M, et al. The Simulation Team Assessment Tool (STAT): development, reliability and validation. Resuscitation. 2012;83(7):879–86.
121. Anderson JM, Yaeger K, Halamek LP, Murphy A. Evaluation of behavior in the delivery room: validation of a scoring tool. Simul Healthc. 2006;1:138.
122. LeFlore J, Anderson JM, Cheng A, Boyle KB, Leonard DT, Corbin L, et al. Development and reliability of a behavioral scoring tool for simulated pediatric resuscitation: a report from the EXPRESS Pediatric Research Collaborative. Simul Healthc. 2009;4:304.
123. Anderson JM, LeFlore J, Cheng A, Boyle KB, Leonard DT, Corbin L, et al. Validation of a behavioral scoring tool for simulated pediatric resuscitation: A report from the EXPRESS Pediatric Research Collaborative. Simul Healthc. 2009;4:305.
124. Sigalet E, Donnon T, Grant V. Assessment of undergraduate health professional team performance: the development of the KidSIM Teamwork Performance Scale. Simul Healthc. 2011;6:382.
125. Grant V, Cheng A. The Canadian Pediatric Simulation Network: a report from the second national meeting in September 2009. Simul Healthc. 2010;5:355–8.
126. Cheng A, Hunt E, Donoghue A, Nelson K, LeFlore J, Anderson J, et al. EXPRESS – Examining Pediatric Resuscitation Education using Simulation and Scripting: the birth of an international pediatric simulation research collaborative – From concept to reality. Simul Healthc. 2011;6:34–41.
127. Cheng A, Rodgers D, Van Der Jagt E, Eppich W, O'Donnell J, for the American Heart Association Pediatric Subcommittee. Evolution of the Pediatric Advanced Life Support course: Enhanced learning with a new debriefing tool and Web-based module for Pediatric Advanced Life Support instructors. Pediatr Crit Care Med. 2012;13:589–95.

Simulation in Psychiatry

36

Elizabeth Goldfarb and Tristan Gorrindo

Abbreviations

CSAT	Computer simulation assessment tool
DSM-IV	Diagnostic and Statistical Manual of Mental Disorders IV
MSE	Mental status examination
OSCE	Objective Structured Clinical Examination
PTSD	Posttraumatic stress disorder
SP	Standardized or simulated patient
USMLE Step 2CS	United States Medical Licensing Examination Step 2: Clinical Skills
VR	Virtual reality

DOC: WHAT BRINGS YOU HERE MR. SAUNDERS?
COMPUTER: WELL MY WIFE WANTED ME TO COME.
DOC: YES.
COMPUTER: IT'S NOT MY IDEA THAT'S FOR SURE. SHE TOLD ME I OUGHT TO SEE A PSYCHIATRIST. SHE SAID.........SHE SAID SHE WAS GOING TO LEAVE IF I DIDN'T GO.
DOC: HOW DO YOU FEEL ABOUT SEEING A PSYCHIATRIST?
COMPUTER: YOU KNOW WHAT I THINK ABOUT PSYCHIATRISTS. I THINK THEY ARE THE BIGGEST BUNCH OF PHONIES THERE EVER WAS.
DOC: WHAT MAKES YOU THINK THAT?
COMPUTER: I DIDN'T COME HERE TO DISCUSS PSYCHIATRISTS.

~ *Excerpt from Starkweather and colleagues 1967* [1]

E. Goldfarb, BA (✉)
Department of Psychology,
New York University, New York, NY, USA
e-mail: goldfe01@nyu.edu

T. Gorrindo, MD
Division of Postgraduate Medical Education,
Massachusetts General Hospital, Boston, MA, USA

Department of Psychiatry,
Massachusetts General Hospital, Boston, MA, USA
e-mail: tristan.gorrindo@mgh.harvard.edu

Introduction

The above dialogue shows a programmed patient responding to a human interviewer. While this conversation is clearly not going well, one of the advantages to using simulation in mental health education is that trainees can learn to be more effective clinicians at no risk to real patients or themselves. The practice of providing care for mental illness necessitates experiential learning [2] and assessment. While simulation has only been used in mental health education for the past few decades, it has quickly become indispensable. Simulation enhances exposure to a variety of patients and to a range of psychopathologies [3]. This is particularly advantageous with regard to high-risk patients and highly volatile psychopathologies, situations that pose safety risks for trainees and patients [4]. Further, as these high-risk situations occur infrequently in most clinical practices, it is critical that trainees have the opportunity to practice before they arise [5].

Current Use in Mental Health Education

The uses of simulation in mental health education can be broken down into two broad categories: *teaching clinical skills* and *assessment*.

Teaching Clinical Skills

In mental health education, simulation has been used to teach clinical skills at various levels of training, including medical students [6–11], residents [12, 13], nursing students [14–18], nurses [19], and experienced therapists [4, 20]. Techniques include the use of human SPs[1] and mannequins, as well as virtual tools (for details, see Table 36.1).

[1] Before continuing, it is important to clarify terminology related to "SPs." The "patients" used in high-fidelity simulation are variously referred to as "simulated" and "standardized." As discussed by Brenner,

A.I. Levine et al. (eds.), *The Comprehensive Textbook of Healthcare Simulation*,
DOI 10.1007/978-1-4614-5993-4_36, © Springer Science+Business Media New York 2013

Table 36.1 Simulation techniques used to train mental health skills

How are these skills taught?
A variety of techniques have been used as interventions to teach skills in mental health education:
SPs [3, 6–10, 12, 13, 16, 21]
Mannequins [14, 15, 22, 23]
Virtual patients [24]
Virtual reality [4, 25]
Computers [1, 26, 27] and Internet [28]
Audiotapes/MP3s [5, 17, 18, 20]

In psychiatry, the process of teaching clinical skills is well suited to simulations [4, 13]. The unpredictability of when learning occurs, the constraints on service delivery as determined by reimbursement sources, the complexity of skills required, the nature of the population receiving therapy, and the time lag before trainees receive feedback create serious difficulties in teaching psychiatric skills [13]. This time lag is especially problematic for teaching new skills, as supervision does not always occur during clinical encounters [4]. Within the guild tradition of psychiatry training, trainees often see patients without the direct observation of a supervising clinician as it is felt that the negative comments made by a supervisor during an encounter with a real patient may make the trainee feel chastened. Subsequently, the patient may feel embarrassed, uncomfortable, and potentially uncared for as the focus shifts to the trainee [10]. Even when patients have agreed to participate in treatment with a supervisor in the session, some may cancel abruptly or not appear for a training session, perhaps as a result of their diagnoses [29].

Simulation helps to address these challenges. As Beutler and Harwood point out, "Specifically, contemporary technology offers a means for instituting training procedures that (a) are standardized, (b) maintain a realistic and reliable portrayal of the training stimuli, (c) allow immediate feedback on skill development, (d) can provide corrective feedback for therapist arousal of defense or anxiety, (e) are safe for both patient and therapist, and (f) are cost efficient to deliver" [4]. There are also logistical challenges associated with the evolving field of mental health. While psychiatry has become a mostly ambulatory practice with brief inpatient stays, medical student clerkships in psychiatry still occur on the inpatient unit, making simulations vital opportunities for trainees to practice outpatient, emergency room, and consult liaison-based clinical skills [10, 21].

A broad array of clinical skills in psychiatry is conducive to simulation training. As early as 1987, a text-based computer tool was developed for trainees to select different assessments, diagnoses, and treatments for a virtual patient. Afterward, the trainees could compare their selections to the ideal decisions, based on expert opinions, for the patient [26]. The initial interview is a critical skill for mental health clinicians in all professions, providing an opportunity for assessment of symptoms and determination of care.

Simulations have been used extensively to train in interviewing skills. As Gay and colleagues note, "simulated-patient interview provides a unique opportunity to put educational needs before patient care issues" [10]. Simulations target different areas of this process, including interpersonal skills [6, 9, 16, 30] and the establishment of rapport under time constraints [31]. Others aim to train in specific interviewing styles [12], recognition of specific diagnostic categories [11], working with difficult patients [30], and discerning latent verbal and nonverbal cues [32]. For more specific descriptions of interviewing skills targeted in simulation training, please see Table 36.2 [6, 9–12, 16, 27, 30–32].

Of particular interest in psychiatry is the teaching of the mental status examination (MSE) [7–9]. Often considered the equivalent of a physical examination for psychiatry, MSE training has incorporated simulation by having a large group of medical students observe a lecturer perform an MSE on a SP [7] and having groups of medical students conduct MSEs on SPs simulating various mental health diagnoses [8]. Overall, students liked both approaches, with 93.9% of the lecture group responding that using an SP was a useful tool to teach the MSE [7] and 98% of the students conducting group interviews reporting that they enjoyed the session and learned from it [8].

On a systems level, simulation using SPs has been used to train mental health teams and improve leadership skills in designing treatment plans. As part of a larger initiative to improve interdisciplinary teamwork and patient care, participants viewed videotapes of an SP being interviewed by a clinician. They also had access to "mock" charts, intake assessment information, admitting notes, and results of laboratory tests. The overall helpfulness of these simulated treatment planning sessions were rated as "good" or "excellent" by almost 75% of participants [33]. In another novel treatment team activity, a virtual online case unfolded in real time over the course of a week, facilitating an electronic-based discussion between students and faculty [34].

Teaching clinicians to be empathic is another unique application for simulation [17, 18, 20, 35, 36]. It is known that stereotyping of and bias against individuals with mental illnesses can hinder a clinician's ability to respond empathetically [17]. This is especially problematic as mental

---

these terms have different connotations, where simulated implies a step below the real patient experience and standardized suggests something superior to the inconsistencies of real patients [3]. In another commentary, McNaughton identifies simulated patients as healthy people who have been carefully coached, whereas standardized patients are individuals trained to portray their own problems (or individuals without a disease trained to portray a specific patient's problems) in a consistent manner [21]. Both terms are used throughout the literature, sometimes referring to trained actors and other times to mental health experts who portray patients. We will use "SP" to refer to the full range of human standardized and simulated patients.

Table 36.2 Use of simulation to train interviewing skills

Simulation technique	Interviewing skills	Citation
SP	Distinguishing between diagnoses in complex mental health presentations	[10]
SP	Interpersonal effectiveness for range of psychopathologies	[6]
SP	"Exploratory" interviewing, as opposed to a more directive series of history-taking questions	[12]
SP	Case-based goals including: Eliciting a history Determining concurrent challenges Demonstrating interviewing strategies to make the patient comfortable Identifying necessary diagnostic procedures Obtaining helpful background information	[16]
SP	Interpersonal skills Eliciting complete history Conducting mental status examination Making differential diagnosis Developing comprehensive treatment plan	[9]
SP	Therapeutic communication Working with patients who accuse provider of stealing/lying to them Diffusing patient's agitation Caring for patients who feel sense of entitlement to specific care	[30]
SP	Using patient-centered communication techniques Building rapport during short interview Detecting mental health issues during Post-Deployment Health Reassessment	[31]
SP	Beginning to pick up latent meaning of verbal messages Beginning to pick up nonverbal messages Understanding the effect of the patient on the therapist and vice versa Conducting sensitive initial psychotherapeutic interview	[32]
Virtual patient	Interviewing techniques Knowledge of signs and symptoms of conduct disorder	[11]
Computer program	Questioning process Attitude (convergent, ambiguous, divergent)	[27]

health clinicians learn to use their empathic response to a patient as part of the diagnostic process [3]. As psychotic symptoms are often stereotyped and stigmatized, several interventions have focused on exposing participants to simulated hallucinations, often based on the hallucinations of real patients. Techniques include using MP3 players to play audio recordings [20], participating in elaborate role-plays where participants have different perceptions of a situation [37], and even the construction of a virtual hospital ward in the commercial virtual world system *Second Life* [25]. Such interventions have been used with mental health professionals [20], nursing students [17, 18], undergraduates [35], correctional officers [36], and the general public [25].

Simulation also provides the opportunity to foster skills that, while important for mental health education, are not specific to the profession. These include critical thinking, communication [14, 22], decision-making [19], self-efficacy, confidence, cultural competency [19, 28], clinical reasoning [23], and general interviewing skills [21]. Conversely, techniques such as virtual reality (VR) have been used to train professionals in other disciplines who are entering mental health settings [19].

Assessment

Simulation is particularly suited to assess competencies that necessitate a clinician-patient interaction [38] and are difficult to observe or interpret consistently within a clinical setting. This is often the case in mental health, which features sensitive or private conversations and varied clinical presentations that would be difficult to compare across learners [39]. Simulations can be used for *formative* (low-stakes) assessments for which trainees receive feedback and remediation, as well as *summative* (high-stakes) assessments that determine competencies and lead to certification or licensing [21, 39]. As with any testing modality, simulations need to be designed with clear outcomes that distinguish between low, medium, and high performers [39].

For similar ethical reasons to those discussed for interventions in mental health, there are advantages to using simulation rather than real patients for *formative* assessment to test the effectiveness of an educational intervention. This is particularly important for studies that want to compare competence in a trained group to an untrained control group. While the total number of simulations used in mental health is limited, SPs have been used to assess whether interventions teaching cognitive behavioral therapy improved social worker [40] and general practitioner [41] competence in using these skills. Both studies videotaped the SP encounters and rated them using the Cognitive Therapy Scale, finding in both cases that the intervention group performed significantly better than the control group. SPs have also been used to assess pediatric resident's use of *Diagnostic and Statistical Manual of Mental Disorders IV* (DSM-IV) criteria to diagnose adolescent depression [42]. Outcomes of training in relevant skills, such as assessment of contextual factors [43], have also been ascertained using SPs. Performance with an SP during the Objective Structured Clinical Examination (OSCE) has been used as an outcome measure, examining the effect of communication skills training [44] as well as the completion of a psychiatry clerkship [45]. In both studies, the group that had participated in the intervention performed significantly better with SPs than the group that had not.

There are several challenges inherent in using real patients for assessment of trainees. First, a sample of real patients is not always representative, and presentations cannot be selected systematically. As a result, trainees may not see enough patients during an exam to provide a fair assessment of their skills. Additionally, there are concerns that chronically mentally ill patients may not have the capacity to consent to participation [12, 46]. By providing greater consistency in level of difficulty and type of patient response, simulation can fill the assessment requirements of (1) stability of competence over time for the same trainee and (2) fairness and consistency across different SPs [46, 47]. In general, simulation is superior to "role-playing" for assessment. Conflicts of interest and breaches of confidentiality can occur when a student portrays a patient for another student during a high-stakes examination [21].

Summative performance assessments are required at many levels of mental health training. One performance assessment paradigm that frequently uses simulation is the OSCE, reviewed in depth by McNaughton and colleagues (see also Chap. 13) [21]. OSCEs are used at multiple levels of mental health education, most notably as part of the United States Medical Licensing Examination Step 2: Clinical Skills (USMLE Step 2CS) exam which has been designed to assess competence in various clinical encounters [46]. These exams typically contain "stations" in which trainees interact with SPs, some of which focus on mental health condition [21]. Examination benchmarks focus on students' abilities to detect nuances of communication as well as interpersonal cues [38]. Some focus on a specific competency, such as assessing and managing suicide risk [48].

In some cases, the SPs provide ratings that constitute a component of a trainee's score on the assessment [39]. Some researchers indicate that SPs have the greatest reliability when rating more than 30 items [39]. One study found SPs' ratings of trainee performance of a psychiatric interview to correlate with clinical evaluators' assessments of these videotaped interactions, as well as with trainees' performance on a written differential diagnosis and mental health treatment plan [49]. Another found only moderate agreement between SPs and physician examiners regarding trainee communication skills [50]. This discrepancy has led some to caution against using SPs to assess complex interpersonal skills, particularly empathy [3].

In addition to OSCEs, SPs have been used to assess other competence in clinical mental health skills. For example, to assess the competence of mental health and addiction workers in the technique of motivational interviewing, one study videotaped interactions with SPs [47]. This technique was shown to have good test-retest reliability, as participants' performance scores stayed constant when they interacted with SPs weeks apart. In addition, SPs have been trained to simulate depression, enabling them to visit doctors' offices incognito to provide an assessment of doctors' diagnosis and management of depression [51, 52].

While SPs are frequently used to perform in or score assessments, virtual techniques have been used as well [53–56]. A web-based platform designed for psychiatry, the computer simulation assessment tool (CSAT) (Fig. 36.1), allows trainees to act as clinicians in a clinical encounter with a virtual SP, in a manner similar to that described by Srinivasan and colleagues [39]. After choosing an action, participants are directed to a video clip. The website also features branching capabilities based on the trainee actions. At the end of the simulation, the CSAT tool provides immediate targeted remediation based on the trainee's performance during the encounter. This tool has been used to assess psychiatry residents' competency in obtaining informed consent to initiate medication treatment for a patient with depression [53]. Virtual patients have also been used to assess competency in determining a differential diagnosis [54]. Another virtual technique, known as the objective structured video exam (OSVE), involves trainees watching a video vignette of an interview and completing an answer sheet detailing their observations, knowledge, and recommendations regarding key communication skills [55, 56]. OSVEs have been used with trainees at varying levels of education, including undergraduates [57], first-year medical students [55], and third-year medical students [56], and for diverse processes, including to gauge the effectiveness of communication skills training [57] or as part of a training curriculum [56]. Unlike the OSCE, the OSVE is designed to elucidate "covert cognitive scripts underlying overt communication behavior" [56]. While several different video vignettes were used, inter-rater reliability was high [55–57] and one study found high correlation with examiner ratings of trainees' performance in the OSCE (though not with standardized patient ratings of trainees' OSCE performance) [55].

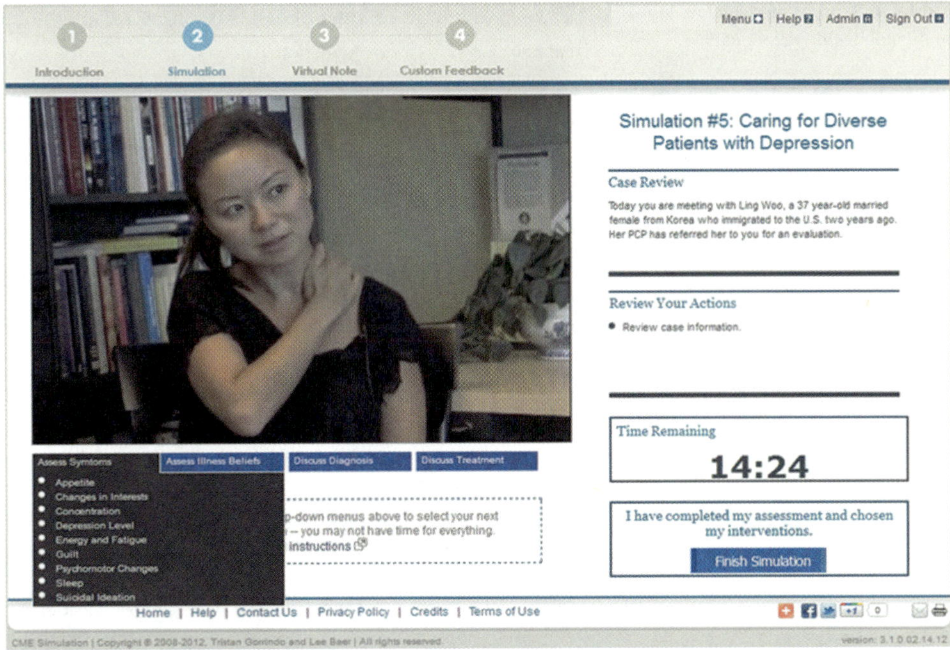

Fig. 36.1 Screenshot of computer simulation assessment tool (CSAT)

Other Applications of Simulation in Mental Health

Therapeutic Simulation for Mental Health Patient Care

Unlike other fields of medicine, simulation in mental health has been used extensively with patients, both as a treatment modality and a tool for diagnosis and assessment (see Table 36.3 for summary). Knowledge of these applications is particularly informative for educators who may wish to alter or build upon existing patient care modalities for later use as training tools.

Treatment and Skill Building

VR has been used in mental health treatment since the 1990s, often as a tool for exposure therapy [86]. The use of VR to augment exposure therapy is ideal for disorders that interfere seriously with the normal functioning of a patient's life (fear of dogs); are more expensive, unsafe, or impossible to use in vivo exposure (fear of flying, heights, or driving) [87, 88]; and are time sensitive [63]. Further, knowing that the simulation can be paused during a session may make the treatment less aversive, increasing the number of patients seeking treatment and decreasing attrition rates [87].

To date, VR has been used as an exposure tool for fears of flying (see Fig. 36.2) [64, 65], driving [67, 68], and spiders, as well as addiction [58], social phobia, posttraumatic stress disorder (PTSD) [66, 69–76], and other forms of anxiety [61–63]. For example, exposing patients with fear of heights to a series of virtual environments including a virtual glass elevator, an outdoor balcony, and a footbridge helped patients decrease their anxiety using exposure-response prevention techniques [63]. VR exposure has been used for PTSD [66] both with civilian [69] and military populations [70–76]. With PTSD, in vivo exposure is often impossible, and patients may have difficulty imagining, visualizing, or describing the traumatic experience [63]. Follow-up studies suggest that this type of virtual exposure has sustained long-term positive effects [87].

Simulation has provided the opportunity for mental health patients to practice and learn specific skills. VR has been used to simulate environments such as virtual cafes and virtual supermarkets for patients with autism, enabling them to practice social skills. These patients learn to use the VR equipment quickly and have shown performance improvements both within the VR environment and in real life. Advantages to VR for this training include the removal of confusing or competing stimuli, the ability to manipulate time (the clinician can pause the simulation to discuss important points), and the ability to allow subjects to learn while playing. In some cases, the clinician can also be an avatar in the virtual environment [89]. VR has also been used to facilitate social skills training for patients with schizophrenia [80]. One particular social skill, the job interview, is critical for patients with severe mental illness who wish to return to the workforce. Preliminary data from a job interview simulation study suggest that patients found the tool easy to use, realistic, and helpful [79]. VR has also been used to teach fire and street safety to children with fetal alcohol syndrome and autism spectrum disorder [78]. The program *Second Life* has been used to provide experiential learning to patients regarding their illness and facilitate group sessions in which patients

Table 36.3 Uses of virtual reality in mental health patient care

Use in patient care	Clinical area	Focus	Citations[a]
Treatment	Addiction		[58]
	Anorexia		[59, 60]
	Anxiety		[61[b], 62[b], 63]
	Anxiety	Flying	[64, 65]
	Anxiety, PTSD		[66]
	Phobia	Driving	[67, 68]
	PTSD	Civilian	[69]
	PTSD	Active duty military	[70–72]
	PTSD	Military	[73–76]
Skill training	Autism	Social skills	[77]
	Autism, fetal alcohol syndrome	Safety skills	[78]
	Psychiatric	Job interview	[79]
	Schizophrenia	Social skills	[80]
Assessment	Depression	Spatial memory	[81]
	Psychiatric	Cognitive performance	[24]
	Mentally disordered offenders	Risk assessment	[82]
	Schizophrenia	Medication management	[83]
	Schizophrenia	Diagnosis	[84]
	Schizophrenia	Driving	[85]

[a]These citations are not meant to be comprehensive
[b]Indicates meta-analysis

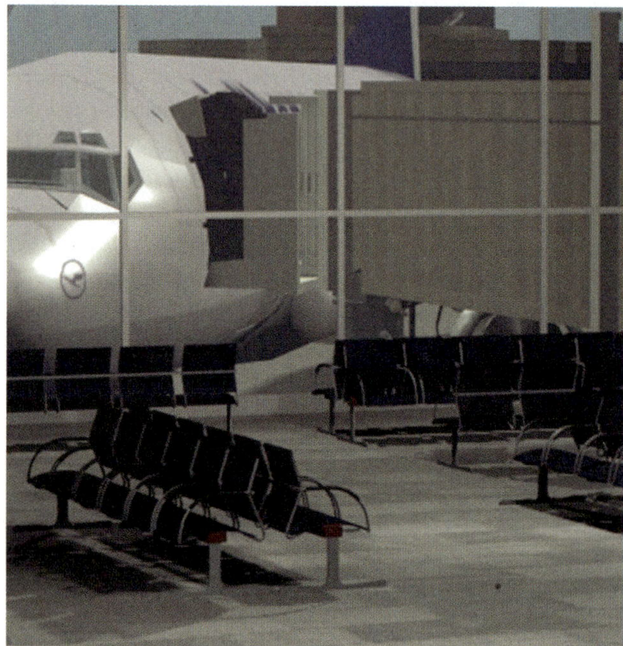

Fig. 36.2 Virtual environment used in exposure therapy for fear of flying

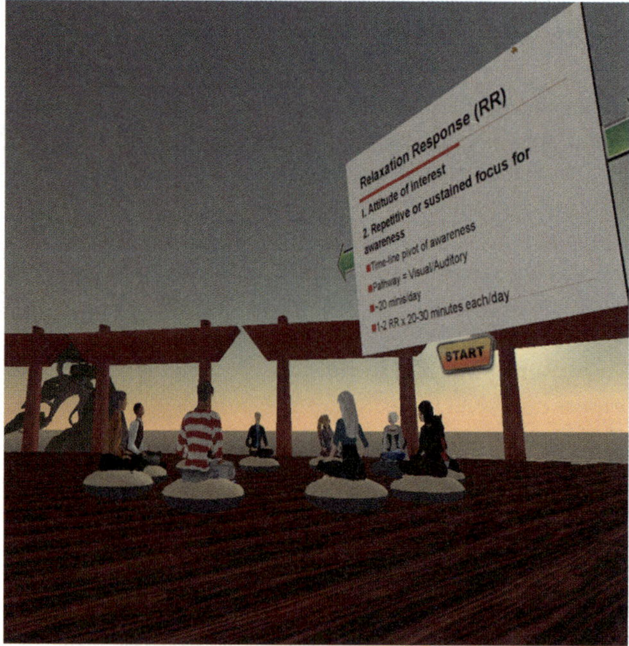

Fig. 36.3 Training patients in relaxation techniques using Second Life

learn psychology-based skills such as the relaxation response (Fig. 36.3) [90].

While most uses of simulation for treatment and skill building directly involve a clinician, simulation has also been used to form peer-run virtual support groups for patients with mental illnesses [91]. In another example, virtual clinicians (referred to as embodied conversational agents) complete daily check-ins with patients. Data from the check-ins, including the patient's mood state and patient adherence, are then referred back to the real-world treatment team [91].

Assessment and Diagnosis

In addition to treatment and skill building, simulation has aided in the assessment of patients with mental health disorders. One group developed a 15-min virtual reality cognitive performance assessment test, which demonstrated good convergent and discriminant validity when compared with a traditional (1.5-h) neuropsychological test battery [24]. Using a virtual town (a surrogate for spatial memory), investigators could distinguish between patients with depression and controls, a level of sensitivity not found in a neuropsychological test battery [81]. Based on performance profiles in a virtual maze (a surrogate for working memory), investigators were able to distinguish between patients with schizophrenia and controls [84]. In another study of patients with schizophrenia, adherence to a simulated medication regimen in a virtual apartment had significant agreement with a validated measure of medication management skills [83].

Simulation is also beginning to find use in forensic psychiatry. A computer-based simulation tool has been used with mentally disordered offenders who committed violent crimes, enabling them to choose actions and observe the consequences of those actions (Fig. 36.4). While it is currently in the pilot phase, it holds potential as a risk assessment tool [82].

Simulation in Mental Health Research

Within the mental health field, simulation has become a powerful research tool. It has provided the opportunity to deepen understanding of mental health disorders as well as the clinicians who treat them.

A great deal of VR research with mental health patients has focused on addiction disorders and the concept of cue reactivity [92–99]. Using VR for this type of research allows patients to be exposed to more complex stimuli, creating a more realistic substance use environment and creating opportunities for future use in treatment [92]. VR techniques have also been used in tandem with functional neuroimaging to determine areas of differential activation associated with cue reactivity within these immersive environments [98].

Simulation can provide the opportunity to evaluate adaptive and functional abilities in diagnostic domains beyond addiction. One study assessed the driving ability of patients with schizophrenia prior to discharge from inpatient treatment, finding overall poor performance as well as significant differences based on treatment type [85]. Another study assessed spatial learning performance in patients with schizophrenia using a virtual 8-arm radial maze [100]. Finally, VR has been used as an outcome measure to assess the effectiveness of treatment interventions for patients with social phobia [101].

A simulation research tool has been used for patients with mental health diagnoses as well as prescribing healthcare providers. This web-based tool (called "reverse" simulation as it shows a standardized doctor instead of a standardized patient) shows a doctor obtaining informed consent to start a patient on a psychoactive medication. Participants then evaluate and reflect on the doctor's performance. By disseminating this to patients, healthcare providers, and lay caregivers, the goal of the project is to collaboratively enhance best practice standards for informed consent within psychiatry [102].

There have been several uses of simulation in research of clinician behaviors. As far back as 1972, one paper describes the process by which a heuristic computer program was developed to simulate psychiatrists' judgment and decision-making processes, a program that showed good agreement with real clinicians' assessments [103]. In another study, psychology students trained as SPs (referred to as "pseudopatients") simulated mental health conditions so that they were admitted to inpatient treatment. Their observations provided insight into systems and personnel-level issues within psychiatric hospitals [104].

Introduction
Scenario
History
Notes
Exit
If you were Anders, what would you do now?
I would sit down in the kitchen and wait for mum to come out of the bathroom
I would sit down outside the bathroom and plan for revenge
I would scream to mum that she has to open the door
I would knock on the door and ask mum to hurry up
I would kick and hit the door
I would break something that belong to mum
I would sit down outside the bathroom and wait for mum to come out and then hit her
I would take an axe and break the bathroom door

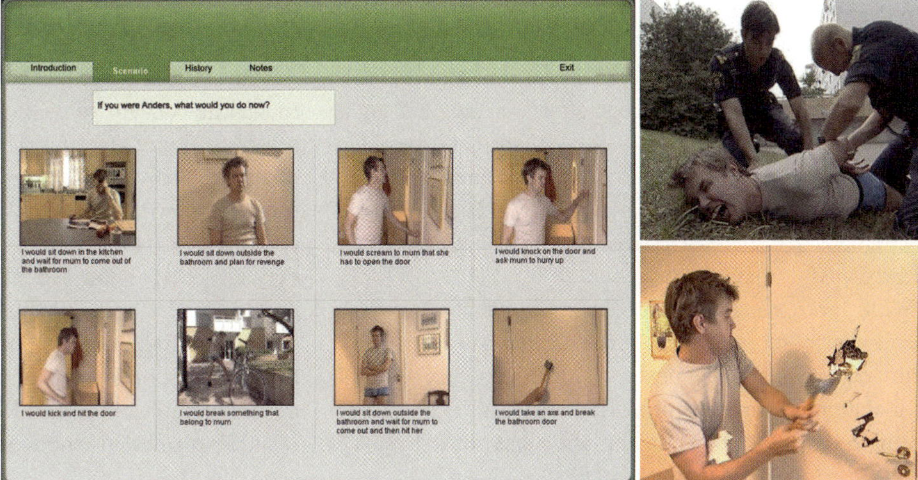

Fig. 36.4 Screenshot of computer-based simulation used with mentally disordered offenders

The Art of Mental Health Simulation

The design and implementation of simulation in psychiatry requires special considerations. Unlike many medical simulations which focus on the acquisition of procedural skills, mental health simulations often examine the interaction between patient and clinician. As such, particular attention to case design, patient selection, and verbal and nonverbal communication is warranted.

Rethinking Clinical Encounters: The Art of Writing a Good SP Case

Developing a clinical case can be simultaneously the most challenging and the most rewarding aspect of simulation. While portraying a psychologically complex patient is a challenge for the SP, it is also the clinician educator's responsibility to write a good case and to train the SP thoroughly [21]. One group estimated that it took 20 h to write the case and select and train the actor [8]. Some groups begin with an established case, such as one from the DSM Casebook [105] or one published in the literature [49].

However the case is designed, it is critical that it adheres to the learning objectives for the activity. For example, when designing a simulation for assessment, Srinivasan and colleagues recommend that educators ask what specifically they want to assess, how reliable and valid the assessment mechanisms are, and what outcomes are expected from the assessment [39]. Brown cautions that educators must identify and prioritize areas of the curriculum amenable to simulation. Simply focusing on an activity that lends itself to active engagement is not sufficient; due to the time and resources spent on designing a case, simulations should relate to essential learning outcomes that are best taught through simulation. For psychiatric nursing, recommended competencies include therapeutic communication, crisis management, interdisciplinary collaboration, and technical skills (e.g., medication administration, use of diagnostic tools) [5]. In their paper, Srinivasan and colleagues present a table including a "skills to be assessed" section that shows practical considerations associated with assessing specific clinical skills [39]. For example, if "communication" is the skill to be assessed, they point out the limitations of current natural language processing technology, strongly recommending that real people be used for assessment. With "self-assessment," they emphasize the necessity of developing feedback mechanisms.

With appropriate learning objectives in hand, writing the clinical case can be an educational activity in itself. Starkweather and colleagues note that the process of building a computer program for a clinical simulation "force[s] assumptions into the open. Implicit ideas must be made explicit and contingencies must be foreseen which, in the course of normal work, are seldom thought about in advance" [1]. Bellman and colleagues presented the simulation of a psychiatric interview as a mathematical process, in which there are different probabilities of the patient responding in certain ways based upon rapport with the therapist [27]. Naylor and Gianturco go so far as to define simulation as "A numerical technique for conducting experiments on certain types of mathematical and logical models describing the behavior of a system (or some component thereof) on a digital computer over extended periods of real time" [106].

Challenges in Mental Health Simulation

> A simulation need only be 'good enough' to reliably evoke the behavior to be assessed
>
> ~ *Yudkowsky, 2002* [46]

While Yudkowsky's statement is accurate, making a simulation "good enough" for applications in mental health is a delicate process. Despite the ethical and practical advantages of using non-patients, there are difficulties inherent in using such non-patients to portray mental health problems, which are well reviewed by Brenner [3]. Understanding these challenges also provides insight into dimensions necessary for simulation in mental health contexts.

In an educational context, the validity of mental health simulation has its limitations. The first area of tension is with regard to the subject's objectives during an examination and interview. While an SP portraying a mental health patient wants to evoke an emotional response, the goals of real patients tend to be more conflicted. In some cases, they may feel divided about what symptoms they want their clinician to know, and other times, they may resist knowing themselves. Further, there is a tension in real clinical encounters between a clinician's desire to deeply understand the patient's symptoms and the patient's desire for treatment to alleviate those symptoms. This pressure may not be felt when interacting with an SP.

Another challenge using non-patients in psychiatry relates to a particular type of mental health presentation, that of dissembling or malingering. There is a necessary suspension of disbelief when working with non-patients; in most cases, trainees know that these individuals do not actually have the condition that they are simulating. However, this makes it very difficult for non-patients to accurately simulate a condition in which a patient is lying [3].

As discussed earlier, one role for simulation in mental health education is to enhance empathy. However, this is one of the areas in which mental health simulation is complicated. If an SP evokes an emotional reaction, this could be due to their effective performance rather than the clinician's empathy [3]. Trainees and faculty have also reported difficulty developing empathy with SPs [29].

When using SPs in any branch of medical education, there is the question of whether someone can realistically portray a condition that he/she has not experienced [21]. In one study, investigators bypassed this issue by recruiting SPs from a theater group composed of individuals with former substance misuse problems [47], but this is not feasible for most mental health presentations. There is debate over whether roles should be based on SPs' previous real-life experiences, even if they have never met criteria for a psychiatric diagnosis. Some consider this necessary to producing a realistic simulation, while others think that this undermines the safety of the SP encounter [105]. Of course, part of the ethical advantage of using SPs is that they are not truly suffering from the conditions portrayed [105]. Keltner and colleagues consider actors trained in Constantin Stanislavski's *method acting* to be ideal, as they display honest emotion and "are trained never to use any trauma from their own past to induce an emotional episode," which can be harmful to the actor and difficult to repeat [107]. Other studies do not indicate a preference of acting style [108]. Research currently being conducted in Australia and Switzerland is focusing on the question of the neurological validity of actors' portrayals [109, 110]. Researchers have shown some evidence that *method* actors can activate specific brain regions when simulating emotional states [109]. Even when conditions are portrayed realistically, there is concern about variability between performances with regard to affect and responses to open-ended questions [21].

In addition to the educational concerns, there are considerations involved when using SPs to portray patients with mental health conditions. In a survey by McNaughton and colleagues, SPs with an average of 5 years of experience "unanimously considered [psychiatry roles] more exhausting, both physically and mentally [than non-psychiatry roles]. A huge amount of concentration and emotional investment is required to simulate these roles" [108]. SPs also reported that portraying highly affective psychiatric roles repeatedly in an OSCE setting had negative impacts extending beyond the time of the performance, with some SPs continuing to experience the psychiatric symptoms of their simulated character.

There are strategies that can be employed to mitigate these adverse effects, both before and after the simulation activity. When careful selection criteria—involving the completion of standardized measures to rule out psychopathology and an employment interview—were completed, adolescents portraying SPs in a psychiatry OSCE were found to experience far more benefits than risks [111]. Sufficient training is necessary, especially if the SP is providing feedback to the trainee [46]. For all SP roles, adequate time for rehearsal, as well as encouragement and feedback from mental health experts, is important [107]. Varying degrees of role instruction have been used, including providing the purpose of the interview and asking the SPs to enter with a real or pretend problem [32], providing a brief one-paragraph identity [12], and providing physical description, social history, medical history, and family history, as well as specific directions for affect, behaviors, body language, and mental processes [16]. The more "hands-off" approaches tend to be used with veteran SPs. Debriefing and de-"role"-ing are also critical parts of the process [21]. Many SPs plan their strategies for transitioning from the roles into their normal lives [112], such as removing makeup or engaging in a social activity [108]. With careful planning, SPs report many more benefits than negative effects of the experience. The process is often described as educational [108], both with regard to understanding mental health patients and the clinical process. In fact, performing as an SP may reduce stigma toward mental health patients [112, 113].

While VR avoids some issues with human simulation by creating an adequate, consistent, fair, and believable portrayal, this medium is currently limited in mental health applications with regard to presenting social environments and complex interactions [4]. Production standards are also high, as users expect interfaces similar in quality to commercially available videogames and animated movies [39]. Cybersickness is a concern that could limit the use of VR with mental health patient populations [63, 87, 89, 114]. Further, it is not yet clear what factors make for successful VR treatment (e.g., demographic and personality characteristics) or how many sessions is sufficient for a patient to gain therapeutic benefit [87].

Integrated mannequins, which can incorporate realistic high-acuity events such as epilepsy [23] and can have interactivity, verbal functions, and physiological parameters [23], also come with challenges. Problems include difficulty reproducing clinical scenarios, accounting for equally acceptable treatment choices, prioritizing necessary actions, sampling enough behavior, funding the high cost associated with development, and simulating realistic emotions [39], as well as limitations in simulating nonverbal communication, the latter two of which are especially critical for simulation in mental health education [5].

Future Directions

As the use of simulation in mental health is comparatively new, there are many exciting future applications. Within education, a critical next step will be to clarify whether clinician's performance in a simulation is a true surrogate for their performance in a real clinical encounter. This will open up a wide range of applications, including as a robust outcome measure for an educational intervention, such as performance improvement continuing medical education programs. Using a "secret-shopper" paradigm, some have suggested that it would also be useful to have incognito SPs visit doctors' offices simulating psychiatric diagnoses in addition to depression [51]. Srinivasan and colleagues suggest several other next steps, including using virtual worlds in which trainees could create avatars to interact in clinical settings, in which trainees could play the role of a patient, clinician, or family member. They suggest that scenarios with mannequins could "include management of critical side-effects of antipsychotic drugs, exploration of team dynamics in psychiatric emergencies, and management of suicidal patients and their families" [39]. McGarry and colleagues suggest that, with improved verbal function in mannequins, they can be used to train clinicians in narrative therapy [23].

One unexpected finding suggests a new use for simulation in mental health education. Hall and colleagues found that performance during interviews with SPs identified students having difficulty early in their clerkship. This poor performance was determined by observing faculty and by checklists filled out by SPs, specifically regarding interpersonal and communication skills. They suggest that "the simulation course format was uniquely able to reveal concerns in students' interactions with patients that needed attention" [6]. This type of performance simulation could provide a documented needs assessment and help inform future educational interventions at multiple stages of training. While it is clear that simulations need to be thoughtfully implemented for learning objectives that require experiential learning, future research should clarify how and when to best incorporate simulation into a mental health training curriculum.

With regard to patient care, clinicians hope to expand the use of simulation to identify and treat a broader range of psychiatric disorders. For example, with a diagnosis like schizophrenia, VR could function as a component of cognitive behavioral therapy, serve as a platform for exposure to persecutory fears, and teach skills to cope with symptoms as they occur [114]. Building on previous studies using VR to study cue reactivity in patients with substance abuse disorders, there is also interest in using VR for assessment and treatment of patients with eating disorders [92]. In another example, clinicians are hoping to use VR for assessment and treatment of obsessive-compulsive disorder, both as an exposure tool (as has been used for other anxiety disorders) and as a way to precisely measure performance in a customized and controlled environment [115] Finally, given children and adolescents' enthusiasm for virtual experiences, clinicians are interested in exploring more uses of simulation that are specific to assessing and treating symptoms in this demographic [116].

There are many new directions for research in mental health using simulation. The expansion of the "reverse" simulation model to multiple diagnostic categories will help elicit the essential elements of the informed consent process in psychiatry. Freeman suggests many potential uses for VR (simulating a social environment) in the study of psychotic disorders, including determining behavioral and physiological correlates of symptoms, identifying individual factors that predict threatening interpretations of others, and examining whether environmental elements increase the likelihood of particular symptoms [114].

Conclusion

The future for simulation in psychiatry will advance considerably in the coming years as technology enables simulation to adequately reproduce the complexities of human interactions, particularly the portrayal of mental health symptoms. However, technology will never replace the usefulness of SPs for the basic training and assessment of mental health professionals. The unique needs of psychiatry compel the field of medical simulation to adapt and develop new tools which will shape simulation throughout healthcare.

References

1. Starkweather JA, Kamp M, Monto A. Psychiatric interview simulation by computer. Methods Inf Med. 1967;6:15–23.
2. Crider MC, McNiesh SG. Integrating a professional apprenticeship model with psychiatric clinical simulation. J Psychosoc Nurs Ment Health Serv. 2011;49:42–9.
3. Brenner AM. Uses and limitations of simulated patients in psychiatric education. Acad Psychiatry. 2009;33:8.
4. Beutler LE, Harwood TM. Virtual reality in psychotherapy training. J Clin Psychol. 2004;60:317–30.
5. Brown JF. Applications of simulation technology in psychiatric mental health nursing education. J Psychiatr Ment Health Nurs. 2008;15:638–44.
6. Hall MJ, Adamo G, McCurry L, et al. Use of standardized patients to enhance a psychiatry clerkship. Acad Med. 2004;79:28–31.
7. Birndorf CA, Kaye ME. Teaching the mental status examination to medical students by using a standardized patient in a large group setting. Acad Psychiatry. 2002;26:180–3.
8. Rubenstein R, Niccolini R, Zara J. The use of live simulation in teaching the mental status examination to medical students. J Med Educ. 1979;54:663–5.
9. Bennett AJ, Arnold LM, Welge JA. Use of standardized patients during a psychiatry clerkship. Acad Psychiatry. 2006;30:185–90.
10. Gay TL, Himle JA, Riba MB. Enhanced ambulatory experience for the clerkship: curriculum innovation at the University of Michigan. Acad Psychiatry. 2002;26:90–5.
11. Parsons TD, Kenny P, Ntuen CA, et al. Objective structured clinical interview training using a virtual human patient. Stud Health Technol Inform. 2008;132:357–62.
12. Lewis JM. On the use of standardized patients. Acad Psychiatry. 2002;26:193–6.
13. Coyle B, Miller M, McGowen KR. Using standardized patients to teach and learn psychotherapy. Acad Med. 1998;73:591–2.
14. Kameg K, Howard VM, Clochesy J, Mitchell AM, Suresky JM. The impact of high fidelity human simulation on self-efficacy of communication skills. Issues Ment Health Nurs. 2010;31:315–23.
15. Morrison AM, Catanzaro AM. High-fidelity simulation and emergency preparedness. Public Health Nurs. 2010;27:164–73.

16. Shawler C. Standardized patients: a creative teaching strategy for psychiatric-mental health nurse practitioner students. J Nurs Educ. 2008;47:528–31.
17. Dearing KS, Steadman S. Enhancing intellectual empathy: the lived experience of voice simulation. Perspect Psychiatr Care. 2009;45: 173–82.
18. Hamilton Wilson JE, Azzopardi W, Sager S, et al. A narrative study of the experiences of student nurses who have participated in the Hearing Voices that are Distressing simulation. Int J Nurs Educ Scholarsh. 2009;6:Article 19.
19. Guise V, Chambers M, Valimaki M. What can virtual patient simulation offer mental health nursing education? J Psychiatr Ment Health Nurs. 2012;19(5):410–8.
20. Goulter N. Simulation in mental health education. Aust Nurs J. 2011;19:41.
21. McNaughton N, Ravitz P, Wadell A, Hodges BD. Psychiatric education and simulation: a review of the literature. Can J Psychiatry. 2008;53:85–93.
22. Sleeper JA, Thompson C. The use of hi fidelity simulation to enhance nursing students' therapeutic communication skills. Int J Nurs Educ Scholarsh. 2008;5:Article 42.
23. McGarry D, Cashin A, Fowler C. "Coming ready or not" high fidelity human patient simulation in child and adolescent psychiatric nursing education: Diffusion of Innovation. Nurse Educ Today. 2011;31(7):655–9.
24. Parsons TD, Silva TM, Pair J, Rizzo AA. Virtual environment for assessment of neurocognitive functioning: virtual reality cognitive performance assessment test. Stud Health Technol Inform. 2008; 132:351–6.
25. Yellowlees PM, Cook JN. Education about hallucinations using an internet virtual reality system: a qualitative survey. Acad Psychiatry. 2006;30:534–9.
26. Lambert ME. A computer simulation for behavior therapy training. J Behav Ther Exp Psychiatry. 1987;18:245–8.
27. Bellman R, Friend MB, Kurland L. Simulation of the initial psychiatric interview. Behav Sci. 1966;11:389–99.
28. Smith BD, Silk K. Cultural competence clinic: an online, interactive, simulation for working effectively with Arab American Muslim patients. Acad Psychiatry. 2011;35:312–6.
29. Krahn LE, Bostwick JM, Sutor B, Olsen MW. The challenge of empathy: a pilot study of the use of standardized patients to teach introductory psychopathology to medical students. Acad Psychiatry. 2002;26:26–30.
30. Grant JS, Keltner NL, Eagerton G. Simulation to enhance care of patients with psychiatric and behavioral issues: use in clinical settings. J Psychosoc Nurs Ment Health Serv. 2011;49: 43–9.
31. Training addresses returning service members' mental health needs. 2011. Available at http://news.vanderbilt.edu/2011/12/returning-soldiers-mental-health/. Accessed 8 Feb 2012.
32. Klamen DL, Yudkowsky R. Using standardized patients for formative feedback in an introduction to psychotherapy course. Acad Psychiatry. 2002;26:168–72.
33. Fichtner CG, Stout CE, Dove H, Lardon CS. Psychiatric leadership and the clinical team: simulated in vivo treatment planning performance as teamwork proxy and learning laboratory. Adm Policy Ment Health. 2000;27:313–37.
34. Hilty DM, Alverson DC, Alpert JE, et al. Virtual reality, telemedicine, web and data processing innovations in medical and psychiatric education and clinical care. Acad Psychiatry. 2006;30: 528–33.
35. Brown SA. Implementing a brief hallucination simulation as a mental illness stigma reduction strategy. Community Ment Health J. 2009;46:500–4.
36. Ando S, Clement S, Barley EA, Thornicroft G. The simulation of hallucinations to reduce the stigma of schizophrenia: a systematic review. Schizophr Res. 2011;133:8–16.
37. Ballon BC, Silver I, Fidler D. Headspace theater: an innovative method for experiential learning of psychiatric symptomatology using modified role-playing and improvisational theater techniques. Acad Psychiatry. 2007;31:380–7.
38. Vaidya NA. Psychiatry clerkship Objective Structured Clinical Examination is here to stay. Acad Psychiatry. 2008;32:177–9.
39. Srinivasan M, Hwang JC, West D, Yellowlees PM. Assessment of clinical skills using simulator technologies. Acad Psychiatry. 2006; 30:505–15.
40. Armstrong G, Blashki G, Joubert L, et al. An evaluation of the effect of an educational intervention for Australian social workers on competence in delivering brief cognitive behavioural strategies: a randomised controlled trial. BMC Health Serv Res. 2010; 10:304.
41. Blashki GA, Piterman L, Meadows GN, et al. Impact of an educational intervention on general practitioners' skills in cognitive behavioural strategies: a randomised controlled trial. Med J Aust. 2008;188:S129–32.
42. Lewy C, Sells CW, Gilhooly J, McKelvey R. Adolescent depression: evaluating pediatric residents' knowledge, confidence, and interpersonal skills using standardized patients. Acad Psychiatry. 2009;33:389–93.
43. Schwartz A, Weiner SJ, Harris IB, Binns-Calvey A. An educational intervention for contextualizing patient care and medical students' abilities to probe for contextual issues in simulated patients. JAMA. 2010;304:1191–7.
44. Yedidia MJ, Gillespie CC, Kachur E, et al. Effect of communications training on medical student performance. JAMA. 2003;290: 1157–65.
45. Goisman RM, Levin RM, Krupat E, Pelletier SR, Alpert JE. Psychiatric OSCE performance of students with and without a previous core psychiatry clerkship. Acad Psychiatry. 2010;34:141–4.
46. Yudkowsky R. Should we use standardized patients instead of real patients for high-stakes exams in psychiatry? Acad Psychiatry. 2002;26:187–92.
47. Bennett GA, Roberts HA, Vaughan TE, Gibbins JA, Rouse L. Evaluating a method of assessing competence in Motivational Interviewing: a study using simulated patients in the United Kingdom. Addict Behav. 2007;32:69–79.
48. Hung EK, Binder RL, Fordwood SR, Hall SE, Cramer RJ, McNiel DE. A method for evaluating competency in assessment and management of suicide risk. Acad Psychiatry. 2012;36:23–8.
49. McLay RN, Rodenhauser P, Anderson DS, Stanton ML, Markert RJ. Simulating a full-length psychiatric interview with a complex patient: an OSCE for medical students. Acad Psychiatry. 2002; 26:162–7.
50. Whelan P, Church L, Kadry K. Using standardized patients' marks in scoring postgraduate psychiatry OSCEs. Acad Psychiatry. 2009; 33:319–22.
51. Shirazi M, Sadeghi M, Emami A, et al. Training and validation of standardized patients for unannounced assessment of physicians' management of depression. Acad Psychiatry. 2011;35:382–7.
52. Carney PA, Dietrich AJ, Eliassen MS, Owen M, Badger LW. Recognizing and managing depression in primary care: a standardized patient study. J Fam Pract. 1999;48:965–72.
53. Gorrindo T, Baer L, Sanders KM, et al. Web-based simulation in psychiatry residency training: a pilot study. Acad Psychiatry. 2011; 35:232–7.
54. Williams K, Wryobeck J, Edinger W, McGrady A, Fors U, Zary N. Assessment of competencies by use of virtual patient technology. Acad Psychiatry. 2011;35:328–30.
55. Humphris GM, Kaney S. The Objective Structured Video Exam for assessment of communication skills. Med Educ. 2000;34:939–45.
56. Hulsman RL, Mollema ED, Oort FJ, Hoos AM, de Haes JC. Using standardized video cases for assessment of medical communication skills: reliability of an objective structured video examination by computer. Patient Educ Couns. 2006;60:24–31.

57. Baribeau DA, Mukovozov I, Sabljic T, Eva KW, Delottinville CB. Using an objective structured video exam to identify differential understanding of aspects of communication skills. Med Teach. 2012;34:e242–50.
58. Girard B, Turcotte V, Bouchard S. Crushing virtual cigarettes reduces tobacco addiction and treatment discontinuation. Cyberpsychol Behav. 2009;12:477–83.
59. Cardi V, Krug I, Perpina C, Mataix-Cols D, Roncero M, Treasure J. The use of a nonimmersive virtual reality programme in anorexia nervosa: a single case-report. Eur Eat Disord Rev. 2012;20:240–5.
60. Riva G, Bacchetta M, Baruffi M, Rinaldi S, Molinari E. Virtual reality based experiential cognitive treatment of anorexia nervosa. J Behav Ther Exp Psychiatry. 1999;30:221–30.
61. Opris D, Pintea S, Garcia-Palacios A, Botella C, Szamoskozi S, David D. Virtual reality exposure therapy in anxiety disorders: a quantitative meta-analysis. Depress Anxiety. 2012;29(2):85–93.
62. Powers MB, Emmelkamp PM. Virtual reality exposure therapy for anxiety disorders: a meta-analysis. J Anxiety Disord. 2008;22: 561–9.
63. Rothbaum BO, Hodges LF. The use of virtual reality exposure in the treatment of anxiety disorders. Behav Modif. 1999;23:507–25.
64. Wiederhold BK, Jang DP, Gevirtz RG, Kim SI, Kim IY, Wiederhold MD. The treatment of fear of flying: a controlled study of imaginal and virtual reality graded exposure therapy. IEEE Trans Inf Technol Biomed. 2002;6:218–23.
65. Rothbaum BO, Anderson P, Zimand E, Hodges L, Lang D, Wilson J. Virtual reality exposure therapy and standard (in vivo) exposure therapy in the treatment of fear of flying. Behav Ther. 2006; 37:80–90.
66. Gerardi M, Cukor J, Difede J, Rizzo A, Rothbaum BO. Virtual reality exposure therapy for post-traumatic stress disorder and other anxiety disorders. Curr Psychiatry Rep. 2010;12:298–305.
67. Wald J, Taylor S. Preliminary research on the efficacy of virtual reality exposure therapy to treat driving phobia. Cyberpsychol Behav. 2003;6:459–65.
68. Wiederhold BK, Wiederhold MD. Virtual reality treatment of post-traumatic stress disorder due to motor vehicle accident. Cyberpsychol Behav Soc Netw. 2010;13:21–7.
69. Difede J, Cukor J, Jayasinghe N, et al. Virtual reality exposure therapy for the treatment of posttraumatic stress disorder following September 11, 2001. J Clin Psychiatry. 2007;68:1639–47.
70. McLay RN, Wood DP, Webb-Murphy JA, et al. A randomized, controlled trial of virtual reality-graded exposure therapy for post-traumatic stress disorder in active duty service members with combat-related post-traumatic stress disorder. Cyberpsychol Behav Soc Netw. 2011;14:223–9.
71. Reger GM, Gahm GA. Virtual reality exposure therapy for active duty soldiers. J Clin Psychol. 2008;64:940–6.
72. Reger GM, Holloway KM, Candy C, et al. Effectiveness of virtual reality exposure therapy for active duty soldiers in a military mental health clinic. J Trauma Stress. 2011;24:93–6.
73. Rizzo AS, Difede J, Rothbaum BO, et al. Development and early evaluation of the Virtual Iraq/Afghanistan exposure therapy system for combat-related PTSD. Ann N Y Acad Sci. 2010;1208:114–25.
74. Rothbaum BO, Hodges LF, Ready D, Graap K, Alarcon RD. Virtual reality exposure therapy for Vietnam veterans with posttraumatic stress disorder. J Clin Psychiatry. 2001;62:617–22.
75. Rothbaum BO, Rizzo AS, Difede J. Virtual reality exposure therapy for combat-related posttraumatic stress disorder. Ann N Y Acad Sci. 2010;1208:126–32.
76. Wood DP, Murphy J, McLay R, et al. Cost effectiveness of virtual reality graded exposure therapy with physiological monitoring for the treatment of combat related post traumatic stress disorder. Stud Health Technol Inform. 2009;144:223–9.
77. Lahiri U, Warren Z, Sarkar N. Design of a gaze-sensitive virtual social interactive system for children with autism. IEEE Trans Neural Syst Rehabil Eng. 2011;19:443–52.
78. Strickland DC, McAllister D, Coles CD, Osborne S. An evolution of virtual reality training designs for children with autism and fetal alcohol spectrum disorders. Top Lang Disord. 2007;27: 226–41.
79. Bell MD, Weinstein A. Simulated job interview skill training for people with psychiatric disability: feasibility and tolerability of virtual reality training. Schizophr Bull. 2011;37 Suppl 2:S91–7.
80. Park KM, Ku J, Choi SH, et al. A virtual reality application in role-plays of social skills training for schizophrenia: a randomized, controlled trial. Psychiatry Res. 2011;189:166–72.
81. Gould NF, Holmes MK, Fantie BD, et al. Performance on a virtual reality spatial memory navigation task in depressed patients. Am J Psychiatry. 2007;164:516–9.
82. Wijk L, Edelbring S, Svensson AK, Karlgren K, Kristiansson M, Fors U. A pilot for a computer-based simulation system for risk estimation and treatment of mentally disordered offenders. Inform Health Soc Care. 2009;34:106–15.
83. Kurtz MM, Baker E, Pearlson GD, Astur RS. A virtual reality apartment as a measure of medication management skills in patients with schizophrenia: a pilot study. Schizophr Bull. 2007;33: 1162–70.
84. Sorkin A, Weinshall D, Modai I, Peled A. Improving the accuracy of the diagnosis of schizophrenia by means of virtual reality. Am J Psychiatry. 2006;163:512–20.
85. Brunnauer A, Laux G, Zwick S. Driving simulator performance and psychomotor functions of schizophrenic patients treated with antipsychotics. Eur Arch Psychiatry Clin Neurosci. 2009;259:483–9.
86. Foa EB, Kozak MJ. Emotional processing of fear: exposure to corrective information. Psychol Bull. 1986;99:20–35.
87. Gregg L, Tarrier N. Virtual reality in mental health. Soc Psychiatry Psychiatr Epidemiol. 2007;42:343–54.
88. Glantz K, Durlach NI, Barnett RC, Aviles WA. Virtual reality (VR) and psychotherapy: opportunities and challenges. Presence (Camb). 1997;6:87–105.
89. Bellani M, Fornasari L, Chittaro L, Brambilla P. Virtual reality in autism: state of the art. Epidemiol Psychiatr Sci. 2011;20:235–8.
90. Watson AJ, Grant RW, Bello H, Hoch DB. Brave new worlds: how virtual environments can augment traditional care in the management of diabetes. J Diabetes Sci Technol. 2008;2:697–702.
91. Gorrindo T, Groves JE. Computer simulation and virtual reality in the diagnosis and treatment of psychiatric disorders. Acad Psychiatry. 2009;33:413–7.
92. Bordnick PS, Carter BL, Traylor AC. What virtual reality research in addictions can tell us about the future of obesity assessment and treatment. J Diabetes Sci Technol. 2011;5:265–71.
93. Bordnick PS, Copp HL, Traylor A, et al. Reactivity to cannabis cues in virtual reality environments. J Psychoactive Drugs. 2009;41: 105–12.
94. Paris MM, Carter BL, Traylor AC, et al. Cue reactivity in virtual reality: the role of context. Addict Behav. 2011;36:696–9.
95. Traylor AC, Bordnick PS, Carter BL. Using virtual reality to assess young adult smokers' attention to cues. Cyberpsychol Behav. 2009; 12:373–8.
96. Kuntze MF, Stoermer R, Mager R, Roessler A, Mueller-Spahn F, Bullinger AH. Immersive virtual environments in cue exposure. Cyberpsychol Behav. 2001;4:497–501.
97. Saladin ME, Brady KT, Graap K, Rothbaum BO. A preliminary report on the use of virtual reality technology to elicit craving and cue reactivity in cocaine dependent individuals. Addict Behav. 2006;31:1881–94.
98. Lee JH, Lim Y, Wiederhold BK, Graham SJ. A functional magnetic resonance imaging (FMRI) study of cue-induced smoking craving in virtual environments. Appl Psychophysiol Biofeedback. 2005;30:195–204.
99. Culbertson C, Nicolas S, Zaharovits I, et al. Methamphetamine craving induced in an online virtual reality environment. Pharmacol Biochem Behav. 2010;96:454–60.

100. Spieker EA, Astur RS, West JT, Griego JA, Rowland LM. Spatial memory deficits in a virtual reality eight-arm radial maze in schizophrenia. Schizophr Res. 2012;135(1–3):84–9.
101. Donahue CB, Kushner MG, Thuras PD, Murphy TG, Van Demark JB, Adson DE. Effect of quetiapine vs. placebo on response to two virtual public speaking exposures in individuals with social phobia. J Anxiety Disord. 2009;23:362–8.
102. Goldfarb E, Fromson JA, Gorrindo T, Birnbaum RJ. Enhancing informed consent best practices: Gaining patient, family, and provider perspectives using reverse simulation. J Med Ethics. 2012; 38:546–51.
103. Beenen F, van Frankenhuysen JH, Veldkamp JG. The construction of a descriptive diagnostic system in psychiatry: first experiences with a computer simulation. Behav Sci. 1972;17: 278–87.
104. Winkler RC. Research into mental health practice using pseudopatients. Med J Aust. 1974;2:399–403.
105. Taylor JS. The moral aesthetics of simulated suffering in standardized patient performances. Cult Med Psychiatry. 2011;35: 134–62.
106. Naylor TH, Gianturco DT. Computer simulation in psychiatry. Arch Gen Psychiatry. 1966;15:293–300.
107. Keltner NL, Grant JS, McLernon D. Use of actors as standardized psychiatric patients. J Psychosoc Nurs Ment Health Serv. 2011; 49:34–40.
108. McNaughton N, Tiberius R, Hodges B. Effects of portraying psychologically and emotionally complex standardized patient roles. Teach Learn Med. 1999;11:135–41.
109. Inside the brain of a human emotion machine. The Daily Telegraph, 2001. Available at http://www.jeffstanden.net/fmri%201.pdf. Accessed 16 Dec 2011.
110. Institute for the performing arts and film: Authenticity of emotion. 2008. Available at http://ipf.zhdk.ch/english/research/current-research-projects/authenticity-of-emotion. Accessed 16 Dec 2011.
111. Hanson M, Tiberius R, Hodges B, et al. Adolescent standardized patients: method of selection and assessment of benefits and risks. Teach Learn Med. 2002;14:104–13.
112. Woodward CA, Gliva-McConvey G. The effect of simulating on standardized patients. Acad Med. 1995;70:418–20.
113. Hanson MD, Johnson S, Niec A, et al. Does mental illness stigma contribute to adolescent standardized patients' discomfort with simulations of mental illness and adverse psychosocial experiences? Acad Psychiatry. 2008;32:98–103.
114. Freeman D. Studying and treating schizophrenia using virtual reality: a new paradigm. Schizophr Bull. 2008;34:605–10.
115. Kim K, Kim CH, Kim SY, Roh D, Kim SI. Virtual reality for obsessive-compulsive disorder: past and the future. Psychiatry Investig. 2009;6:115–21.
116. Emmelkamp PM. Effectiveness of cybertherapy in mental health: a critical appraisal. Stud Health Technol Inform. 2011;167:3–8.

37 Simulation in Pulmonary and Critical Care Medicine

Adam D. Peets and Najib T. Ayas

Introduction

In fast-paced specialties such as pulmonary and critical care medicine, healthcare professionals are called upon to manage highly unstable patients and must make rapid decisions, perform invasive procedures, and communicate effectively within a team environment to provide optimal patient care. In the past, these professionals would achieve competency in performing each of these tasks after years of clinical experience with patients. However, in the last 20 years, there has been a significant paradigm shift in the way we teach these skills. For numerous reasons including technological advances, the patient safety movement, and efforts to optimize educational experiences of medical trainees, simulation-based training has now taken on a leading role in this domain.

This chapter will focus on both the science and the art of simulation-based training within pulmonary and critical care medicine. First we will review different ways in which simulation is being used within these specialties and the evidence supporting these practices, and subsequently we will describe some practical principles to optimize its use. Our goal is to provide the reader with an overview of the current state of the art and science of simulation in these specialties so that they may then decide how best to integrate simulation technology into their own practice.

A.D. Peets, MD, MSc (Med Ed) (✉)
Department of Critical Care Medicine,
University of British Columbia,
Rm 239 Comox Building, 1081 Burrard St,
Vancouver, BC V6Z 1Y6, Canada
e-mail: apeets@providencehealth.bc.ca

N.T. Ayas, MD, MPH
Department of Medicine, University of British Columbia,
Room 224 Comox Building, 1081 Burrard Street,
Vancouver, BC, Canada
e-mail: nayas@providencehealth.bc.ca

The Evidence Base for Simulation in Critical Care

Medical Knowledge

Simulation has been successfully used to help teach a wide variety of content areas within pulmonary and critical care medicine including early goal-directed therapy for severe sepsis and septic shock, respiratory failure, mechanical ventilation, and shock [1, 2]. It has been found to be at least equivalent, if not superior, to lecture, small group sessions, and problem-based learning (PBL) [3–7]. For example, 31 4th-year medical students were randomly assigned to either PBL or simulator sessions in order to learn the concepts of acute dyspnea and abdominal pain [3]. Students trained with simulation had an incremental increase in final test scores that was significantly higher than those who had undergone PBL sessions (25% increase vs. 8%, $p<0.04$). Although it may require a significant investment of time and money, simulation can be a very effective method for teaching content knowledge to trainees within pulmonary and critical care medicine.

Technical Skills

Practitioners within pulmonary and critical care medicine must be competent to perform a wide variety of procedures, some of which they may encounter infrequently. A growing body of literature suggests simulation, with its ability to provide opportunities for deliberate practice, may be an effective way to teach and maintain these technical skills.

Airway Management

While numerous investigations involving simulation training for airway management have been undertaken in the anesthesia and emergency medicine realms [8, 9], there are surprisingly few investigations specific to the critical care environment (see Fig. 37.1).

A.I. Levine et al. (eds.), *The Comprehensive Textbook of Healthcare Simulation*,
DOI 10.1007/978-1-4614-5993-4_37, © Springer Science+Business Media New York 2013

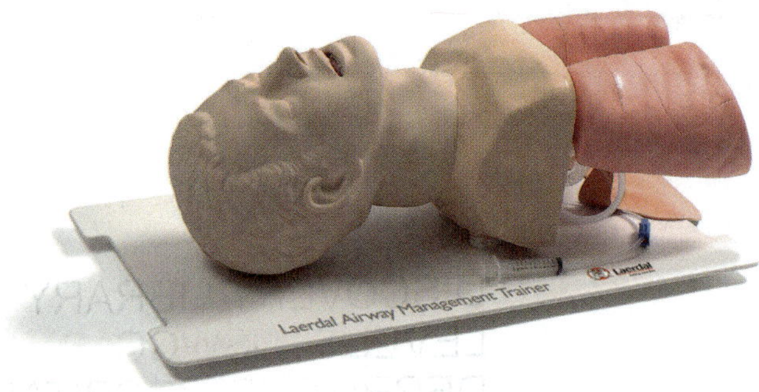

Fig. 37.1 Part-Task trainer to help teach endotracheal intubation (Used with permission of Laerdal)

Dr. Mayo and colleagues have published a series of studies investigating the use of simulation as part of a training program for initial airway management skills (i.e., bag-mask ventilation and preparation for intubation). They found that both interns and senior residents can effectively learn to perform these skills by participating in a 30-min session that utilizes deliberate practice with a high-fidelity human patient simulator and comprehensive debriefing [10, 11]. Interestingly, the outcomes for interns taking these sessions were similar whether the session was taught by attending physicians or by house staff, which included postgraduate year 2 or 3 residents completing ICU rotations, chief residents, or pulmonary fellows [12]. This supports the notion that content expertise is not necessarily a prerequisite for instructors of simulation sessions and highlights the importance of providing trainees with the opportunity to simply practice a procedure in a hands-on fashion. Importantly, this group also found that participants continued to use the skills they learned in the session when performing initial airway management with real patients, suggesting that skills taught through simulation are potentially transferrable to and sustainable in the clinical environment [10].

Only one study in the critical care setting has described the potential impact of simulation training on endotracheal intubation (ETI) [13]. As part of an intensive quality improvement initiative for ETI at their center, Mayo and colleagues trained pulmonary/critical care fellows on the technique of endotracheal intubation and the process of team leadership. Over a period of 3 years, they were able to demonstrate that trainees had complication rates similar to those previously reported in the anesthesia literature and deemed the quality improvement process to be a success. Given the high risk of potential complications associated with out-of-operating-room emergency ETIs [14] and the specific skillset required to manage these situations, further investigations to delineate the role that simulation has in optimizing performance should be undertaken.

Central Venous Catheterization

Central venous catheters (CVC) are frequently required in the critical care environment [15]. However, insertion of these catheters is not without risk [16]. While the use of ultrasound guidance for venous cannulation has led to a reduction in the complication rate, training with simulation provides promise for further improvements in the safety profile of this invasive procedure [17].

A recent meta-analysis found that simulation-based training for CVC insertion was associated with high learner satisfaction, improved learner confidence in their ability to perform the procedure, and better ability to actually perform the procedure on a mannequin [17]. Additionally, there is preliminary evidence to suggest that simulation training for CVCs could have a "snowball effect." To illustrate, Barsuk et al. found that after training 1 year of residents to perform CVC with high-fidelity mannequins, junior residents in each of two subsequent years had improved skills at baseline compared to those who came before them [18]. On a baseline assessment of their ability to insert internal jugular catheters, junior residents' scores went from 46.7% in 2007 to 55.7% in 2008 and 70.8% in 2009 ($P < .001$). The authors hypothesized an increase in the quantity and/or the quality of bedside CVC teaching that each successive year of junior residents received from senior residents could be responsible and that this unforeseen side effect could have significant benefits for medical trainees and the healthcare system alike. As discussed in more detail in the "Patient Outcomes" section, there is also evidence to suggest that simulation training for CVCs can lead to improvements in relevant patient outcomes.

Cardiac Life Support

The use of simulation is now considered standard practice when teaching basic or advanced cardiac life support [19–21]. While the majority of the evidence suggests learning cardiac life support with simulation improves future performance on mannequins [22–25] and potentially even positively impacts patient outcomes [26–30], other studies have not found this to be the case [31]. Further complicating matters are the inconsistent results of studies evaluating the impact of mannequin fidelity on relevant outcomes, with some showing improved outcomes with high-fidelity mannequins [22–25, 32–34] and others showing no difference between low- or high-fidelity mannequins [30, 34–36]. Given the available evidence, international guidelines currently recommend simulators be used when training individuals to perform cardiac life support and that either high- or low-fidelity mannequins may be used [20].

Extracorporeal Support

The use of extracorporeal support to sustain critically ill patients is increasing [37]. However, given the complex nature of the technology involved and the potential for catastrophic consequences should technical emergencies arise, there is a need to determine how best to educate ICU

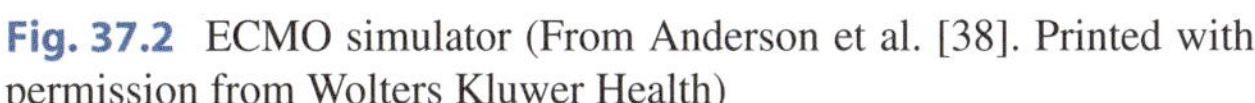

Fig. 37.2 ECMO simulator (From Anderson et al. [38]. Printed with permission from Wolters Kluwer Health)

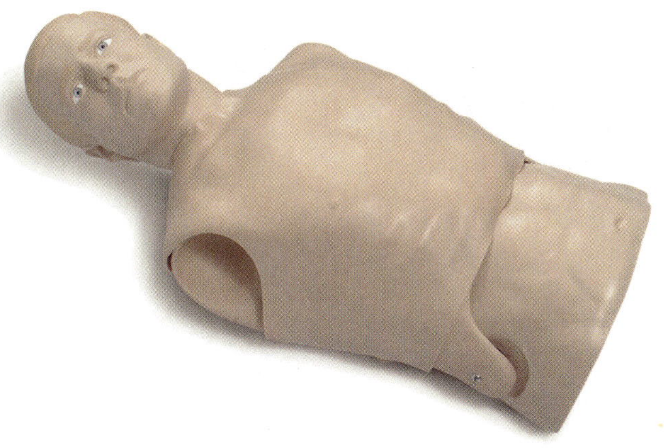

Fig. 37.3 Mannequin for chest tube insertion (Used with permission of Laerdal)

personnel in using and troubleshooting bedside extracorporeal support. One approach described by Anderson et al. involved developing an educational intervention that included a high-fidelity simulator modified to accept an extracorporeal circuit [38] (Fig. 37.2). They subsequently demonstrated that participants not only had the subjective belief that the simulator was superior to traditional extracorporeal membrane oxygenation (ECMO) training but that there was also an objective improvement in their technical and behavioral skills following the session [38, 39]. However, a more recent trial failed to demonstrate an improvement in participants' ECMO-related technical skills after a simulation session, regardless of whether they were being assessed in a simulated or true clinical environment [40]. While there is certainly face validity to use simulation to teach the technical skills associated with ECMO, further investigations need to be undertaken to provide guidance on its optimal use.

Bronchoscopy

The first description of a high-fidelity computer-based bronchoscopy simulator was published in 1999 [41]. and was followed shortly thereafter by two studies demonstrating that pulmonary and critical care medicine fellows who trained using the simulator had dramatically accelerated learning curves than those trained in the traditional fashion [42, 43]. More recently, perhaps reflecting the growth of interventional pulmonary medicine as a distinct subspecialty, there has been a rapid increase in the number of investigations published [44].

In general, these studies have found that simulation is an effective and efficient way for trainees to acquire bronchoscopy skills. For example, Moorthy et al. found that after five attempts on a virtual reality bronchoscopy simulator, novices were performing at an equivalent level of proficiency on the simulator as bronchoscopists who had performed between 200 and 1,000 bronchoscopies on real patients [45]. Additionally, Wahidi et al. found that pulmonary fellows who received simulator training demonstrated the same level of competency after 20 real bronchoscopies as traditionally trained fellows achieved after 50 bronchoscopies [46]. There is even evidence to suggest that the technical skills learned over a short period of time on a bronchoscopy simulator are transferrable to situations involving real patients. Blum et al. demonstrated that interns trained on a simulator required less assistance and were more thorough when performing bronchoscopy on real patients in the operating room than those interns who had not received training [47].

While the majority of studies have used high-fidelity virtual reality simulators, a wide assortment of lower-fidelity models is also available [44]. The high-fidelity virtual reality simulators have been found to be preferable for learning simple bronchoscopy, but for invasive procedures like transbronchial needle aspiration, low-fidelity models such as those made from plastic or animals are felt to be better at recreating the feel of true human anatomy [48, 49]. Simulators have also been used to help teach other tasks such as chest tube insertion and endobronchial ultrasound (Fig. 37.3).

Other Procedures

The discussion above has focused on a number of procedures that are regularly performed within the domains of pulmonary and critical care medicine. We have not included other potentially relevant procedures because either the role of simulation in teaching that skill has not been rigorously evaluated (e.g., thoracentesis) or extensive evaluations have taken place primarily within other specialties (e.g., endotracheal intubation within the field of anesthesiology). For the latter category, excellent reviews of the relevant evidence can be found in other chapters in this book (chap 17).

Maintenance of Skill

While individuals trained with simulation-based medical education can rapidly achieve a high level of technical competency

Table. 37.1 Summary of the impact of simulation-based training compared to traditional education (From McGaghie et al. [54]. Printed with permission from Wolters Kluwer Health)

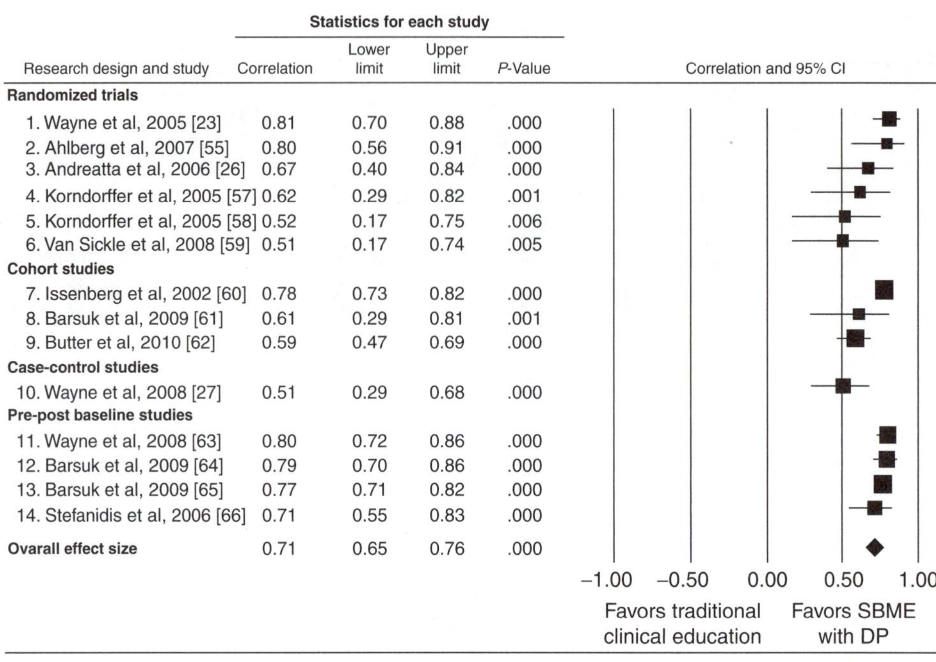

Research design and study	Statistics for each study: Correlation	Lower limit	Upper limit	*P*-Value
Randomized trials				
1. Wayne et al, 2005 [23]	0.81	0.70	0.88	.000
2. Ahlberg et al, 2007 [55]	0.80	0.56	0.91	.000
3. Andreatta et al, 2006 [26]	0.67	0.40	0.84	.000
4. Korndorffer et al, 2005 [57]	0.62	0.29	0.82	.001
5. Korndorffer et al, 2005 [58]	0.52	0.17	0.75	.006
6. Van Sickle et al, 2008 [59]	0.51	0.17	0.74	.005
Cohort studies				
7. Issenberg et al, 2002 [60]	0.78	0.73	0.82	.000
8. Barsuk et al, 2009 [61]	0.61	0.29	0.81	.001
9. Butter et al, 2010 [62]	0.59	0.47	0.69	.000
Case-control studies				
10. Wayne et al, 2008 [27]	0.51	0.29	0.68	.000
Pre-post baseline studies				
11. Wayne et al, 2008 [63]	0.80	0.72	0.86	.000
12. Barsuk et al, 2009 [64]	0.79	0.70	0.86	.000
13. Barsuk et al, 2009 [65]	0.77	0.71	0.82	.000
14. Stefanidis et al, 2006 [66]	0.71	0.55	0.83	.000
Ovarall effect size	0.71	0.65	0.76	.000

SBME simulation based medical education, *DP* deliberate practice

[27, 46, 50], studies have also shown that these skills may be lost rapidly if not reinforced on a regular basis. Smith et al. randomized 53 residents to be trained to perform CVC insertion with either traditional training throughout their ICU rotation or traditional training plus a one-time simulator session just prior to their ICU rotation [51]. While the residents who were trained with simulators had an initial significant improvement in their performance, 3 months later, their performance had deteriorated and was no different than those residents who had undergone traditional training. The authors hypothesized that because residents did not have the opportunity to practice the skills they had acquired during the simulation (on average, they each inserted less than two CVCs over the course of an entire rotation), they lost any gains that had been made. Similarly, Roy et al. found a significant deterioration in the ability of pediatric residents to appropriately manage life-threatening events from 4 to 8 months after their initial training session, leading the authors to raise the issue of whether more frequent training should be mandated to ensure practitioners maintain competency in this critical skill [52].

While there is some evidence to suggest that certain skills, such as those that rely on algorithms (ACLS management) or motor memory (procedural skills), may be more resistant to decay [53], the higher-order skills mentioned above, such as clinical reasoning, are at higher risk to be lost without ongoing reinforcement [52].

Summary for Technical Skills

The results above are consistent with a recent meta-analysis that demonstrated simulation-based educational sessions were superior to traditional clinical education for teaching technical skills, with a large effect size of 0.71 (95% CI 0.65–0.76; $p<0.001$, see Table. 37.1) [54]. In addition, the demonstration of accelerated learning curves when simulators are used to teach procedural skills [67] when combined with the potential decline in these skills over time without deliberate practice [51, 52] suggests that simulation could play an important role in pulmonary and critical care medicine not only for acquiring competency but also for maintaining that competency over the course of a career.

Communication

Effective verbal communication within the healthcare team and between the healthcare team and patients and their families is a crucial component of providing optimal patient care [68]. In particular, in the fast-paced ICU setting, ineffective communication has been shown to be an important risk factor for adverse events [69, 70]. Therefore, it is extremely important to provide healthcare practitioners opportunities to achieve and maintain competency with respect to communication skills.

Simulation-based medical education has been shown to be an effective method not only for novice learners to acquire fundamental communication skills for family meetings in the critical care setting [71] but also for experienced practitioners and teams to refine their existing skills [72, 73]. For example, 40 cardiac arrest teams from a number of different hospitals were found to have significant improvements in leadership, team coordination, and verbalizing situational information after a day-long educational session that involved simulation-based learning of crisis resource management skills [72]. De Vita et al. also demonstrated a significant improvement in crisis resource management skills after medical emergency team (MET) members underwent simulation training [73].

Recently, there has also been increasing interest in exploring the effectiveness of communication between healthcare providers. In particular, the issue of handover, or transfer of patient information from one healthcare provider to another, has been garnering more attention. Each time a handover occurs, important information may be lost [74]. As the number of consecutive hours physicians are able to work continues to decrease, there is an obligatory increase in the number of handovers of patient information that must occur. Therefore, there has been interest in improving the quality of this process in order to minimize the impact of discontinuity of care on patient outcomes [75, 76].

Within the critical care environment, simulation has been used to improve the effectiveness of communication and information transfer during nursing handover at shift change [77]. When compared to baseline, nurses were significantly more effective in communicating key pieces of information like demographics and physiologic data after completing a workshop. The effectiveness of simulation to teach and assess physicians' communication skills specifically during handover has been used in other specialties [78] but, to our knowledge, has not yet happened in pulmonary or critical care medicine. Given the potential negative impact of discontinuity of care on patients, providing individuals the opportunities to learn these skills, especially within the safe environment made possible with simulation training, should be an educational priority.

Patient Safety

An argument for the development of a simulation-based curriculum that focuses on patient safety and crisis resource management in the ICU has previously been proposed by Fox-Robichaud and Nimmo [79]. After acknowledging the groundbreaking work that anesthesiologists have made by integrating crisis resource management training in their field, the authors highlight a number of differences in the critical care environment, including shared decision-making and managing multiple critically ill patients simultaneously, that justify modifying the "tried and true" methods to achieve additional ICU-specific competencies. There are now numerous examples of simulation-based initiatives that have been developed to improve patient safety within the critical care environment.

For example, mock codes conducted throughout a hospital have been used not only to improve how the cardiac arrest team functions but can also be used to help optimize logistics at a systems level (see Chap. 10). Villamaria et al. describe the use of mock codes not only to help orient the code blue team to a new hospital but also to troubleshoot the building in order to improve patient safety [80]. After conducting 12 mock codes in different areas of the hospital, they identified issues such as locked doors, inadequate phone access, and suboptimal crash cart placement, all of which were subsequently addressed prior to any actual patient harm as a consequence of these system deficiencies.

Another example of simulation being used to improve patient safety comes from Ford and colleagues [81]. When compared to didactic sessions, nurses who received training with simulation-based sessions had significantly less medication administration errors.

Additionally, Burton et al. used a high-fidelity simulator to provide nurses and respiratory therapists the opportunity to undertake deliberate practice of technical and nontechnical skills related to ECMO [40]. Over the course of the study, significant improvements were seen in participants' knowledge and attitudes toward safety and their ability to work effectively as a team. Clearly, simulation shows promise as an educational technique for teaching the principles of this important construct to healthcare professionals.

Patient Outcomes

There is increasing evidence that structured simulation-based education that targets mastery learning through deliberate practice can positively impact patient outcomes [82, 83]. Within the fields of pulmonary and critical care medicine, there are a number of studies that provide indirect evidence of this relationship. Examples include improved adherence to ACLS protocols during actual code events [27], decreased number of needle passes during central line insertion [64], and a reduction in the incidence of catheter-related bloodstream infections (CRBSI) [84]. While this last example led to a significant cost savings of over $700,000 per year [85], the impact that the decrease in CRBSI had on direct patient outcomes such as length of stay or mortality was not reported.

One recent study in the critical care environment provides more direct evidence that a positive relationship between simulation-based medical education and patient outcomes may exist. Over a 4-year period, Andreatta et al. conducted an increasing number of simulated codes with debriefings as part of an educational initiative for residents and code team members at one hospital [26]. They found a significant increase in the number of patients who survived code blues, rising from a baseline of 33–56% after the fourth year of implementation. While there were a number of limitations with the design of the study including lack of information regarding individual resident performance and some important details of the codes themselves, this still provides a strong signal that simulation-based medical education has the potential to improve patient outcomes.

Importantly, the vast majority of the relevant studies in this area have compared simulation-based medical education to no intervention [82]. Therefore, results need to be interpreted with this in mind and future studies designed to provide a realistic comparison of educational techniques.

Assessment and Evaluation

As medical education moves toward a competency-based framework [86], simulation is poised to take on a greater role in assessment and evaluation because of its ability to assess what medical professionals' actually do, rather than simply what they say they would do [87]. This may be particularly important within the specialties of pulmonary and critical care medicine as many of the required core competencies, including technical skills, ability to communicate, and team-based care, are extremely difficult to assess with written exams or other traditional methods of assessment [79].

For example, the creation of reliable and valid checklists now allows for objective assessments to take place for technical skills such as endotracheal intubation [88], advanced cardiac life support protocols [23], central venous catheter insertion [89] and bronchoscopy [90], communication skills [91], and complex patient management skills [92–95]. While simulation has been used almost exclusively for formative assessments within the specialties of pulmonary and critical care medicine, given the rapid advances being made in simulation technology and development of assessment tools with rigorous psychometric properties, it may now be ready for use in high-stakes certifying examinations at a national level, much like it has in other specialties [96, 97].

Within a competency-based training framework, simulation assessments at regular intervals could provide useful information to both program directors and trainees. For example, Wahidi et al. found that pulmonary trainees demonstrated significant interindividual variation in their skill level despite having performed the same number of bronchoscopies [46]. Therefore, information from these assessments could be used to create and periodically modify a more personalized schedule of learning experiences for each trainee over the course of their residency based on their specific needs. Once a physician has completed their training, simulation could also be used as a tool to assess maintenance of competency over time, identify areas for remediation, or to assess to what degree a disability or impairment impacts clinical performance [98].

In addition to evaluating the performances of individuals, simulation can be used to assess teams or systems. Marsch et al. used a high-fidelity human patient simulator to assess the quality of care provided during mock cardiac arrests in the intensive care unit [99]. They found that there were significant gaps in quality of care, such as delays in initiation and subsequent suboptimal quantity of CPR provided, and that there was lack of creation of an effective team environment. This powerful information was subsequently used to create initiatives to improve patient care.

With its ability to consistently recreate scenarios in a standard fashion, simulation has the potential to play an important role in formative, summative, and certifying assessments of individual medical professionals, teams, and systems within the specialties of pulmonary and critical care medicine.

Overall Comment on the State of the Science

In general, simulation has been shown to be at least equivalent, if not superior in performance to traditional methods of education [82]. While the evidence base for simulation continues to grow at a rapid pace, there remain significant gaps in our knowledge that we need to fill in order to best guide exactly when, how, and for what simulation should be used in the specialties of pulmonary and critical care medicine.

The Art of Critical Care Simulation

Much like in other areas of medicine, when evidence is still in evolution, relying on experience and best judgment to make decisions is the next best option. Based on the experiences of others and our own, in this section we outline a number of key issues that warrant consideration when aiming for a successful simulation experience within pulmonary and critical care medicine, they include places, people, pedagogy, and practicality.

Places

Traditionally, large stand-alone simulation centers have been constructed in an attempt to centralize both technical and human resources. While these centers still play an important role in conducting large-scale scheduled simulation endeavors, in recent years there has been a movement toward the use of in situ simulation within critical care medicine because of a number of potential advantages [100]. First, learning in the same environment in which that knowledge or skillset will later be used has previously been demonstrated to improve learning outcomes [101, 102] and even potentially contribute to improved patient outcomes [26].

Second, in situ simulation provides tremendous flexibility. Similar to anesthesia and the surgical specialties, some aspects of pulmonary and critical care medicine occur within a defined environment and therefore lend themselves nicely to training in simulation laboratories. However, because

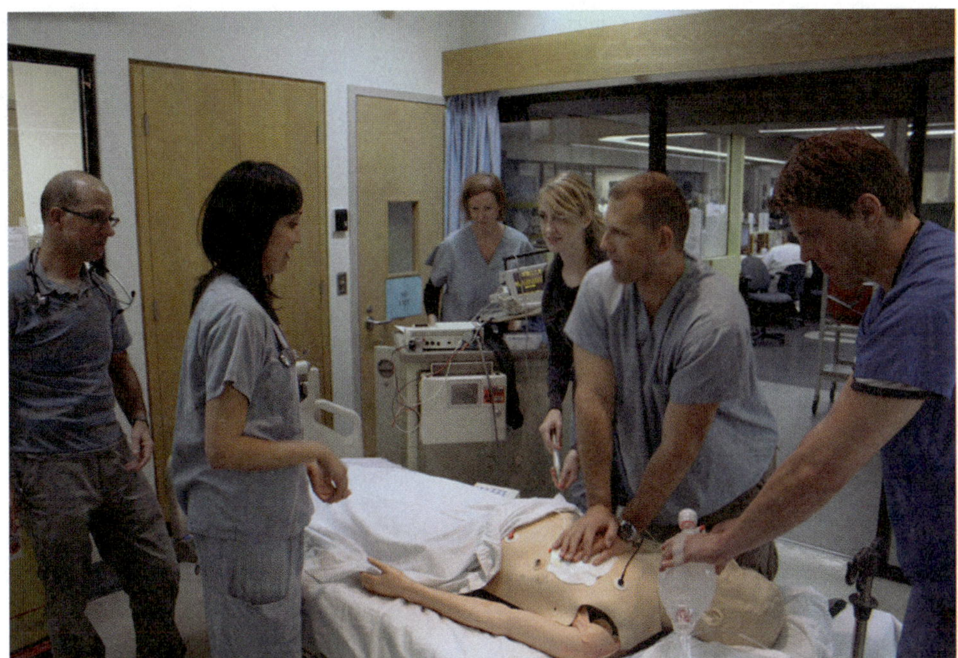

Fig. 37.4 In situ setting for simulation at St. Paul's Hospital

other aspects, like cardiac arrests or medical emergency team calls, can occur in any part of the hospital, a simulation laboratory may not be able to accurately replicate the environment. Using in situ simulation, mock cardiac arrests can be performed in any location (hallway, staircase, outside the hospital, etc.) at any time of day or night based on what is needed to achieve the specific learning objectives.

Third, compared to off-site simulation centers, accessibility is dramatically improved; as a result, trainees are more likely to receive simulation-based training when the simulator is readily available [103]. Finally, while the cost to purchase the current generation of portable high-fidelity human patient simulator is still significant, it is significantly less than those required to procure, renovate, and maintain dedicated simulation laboratory space [104]. Given all of these reasons, we have been increasingly using in situ simulation in our ICUs in recent years (Fig. 37.4).

People

The first group of "people" involved in simulation are the learners. Within the critical care environment in particular, it is important to be cognizant of the wide variety of learners that may be participating. There are not only medical trainees from numerous specialties and at various stages of training but also learners from many other disciplines including nursing, respiratory therapy, pharmacy, social work, and physiotherapy that could be involved in simulation on a daily basis. Additionally, a multitude of other specialties or healthcare services from outside the ICU might be appropriate to be included in sessions. Since a "one-size-fits-all" approach to simulation will not lead to optimal learning outcomes, identifying the various groups and engaging them to determine their learning needs is a worthwhile endeavor.

The second group of "people" are the facilitators and educators involved in making the simulation actually happen. Ideally, a committee of dedicated and enthusiastic individuals with representatives from each of the disciplines listed above should be assembled. They should receive appropriate training, including topics such as curriculum design and evaluation, case development, and debriefing techniques. In addition, ensuring appropriate remuneration and nonmonetary recognition for their efforts is extremely important in order to ensure sustainability of the program. Also, when the simulation involves multiple disciplines, we have found it useful to have a facilitator from each of those disciplines present to provide face validity and content expertise if needed.

It goes without saying that having an individual who takes on the role of "champion" is crucial for developing and sustaining a simulation program. Since there are always more priorities in a healthcare system than there is money or human resources to support, having an enthusiastic and effective leader to ensure that simulation is seen as a valuable priority is extremely important.

Pedagogy

Our approach to any educational session involves three steps: plan, teach, and review.

Table 37.2 Sample content from a pulmonary and critical care medicine simulation curriculum for learners at different stages of training

	Knowledge domains	Procedural skills	Process skills
Medical students	Cardiac arrest Shock Acute respiratory failure Acid–base derangements Hyperkalemia	CPR ACLS protocols Bag-mask ventilation Intubation using laryngoscope CVC insertion Thoracentesis Paracentesis	Introduction to communicating in an emergency situation
Residents	In addition to knowledge listed above: Physiologic basis for resuscitation Coma/seizure Hypertensive emergencies Multisystem trauma	In addition to skills listed above: Intubation using simple airway adjuncts Chest tube insertion Ultrasound for CVC insertion Transvenous pacemaker	Basic crisis resource management skills
Fellows	In addition to knowledge listed above: Toxidromes Severe respiratory failure Refractory shock Transportation medicine Obstetrical emergencies	In addition to skills listed above: Advanced airway adjuncts (fiber-optic, surgical airway, etc.) Bronchoscopy Advanced ventilation strategies ECMO management	Advanced crisis resource management skills Advanced communication skills (families, interprofessional conflict, etc.)

CPR cardiopulmonary resuscitation, *ACLS* advanced cardiac life support, *CVC* central venous catheter, *ECMO* extracorporeal membrane oxygenation

Plan

There are three steps to planning simulation sessions that we have found useful. First is to plan how and when simulation will be used within the context of an entire educational curriculum. Without a systematic approach, there may be a tendency to focus solely on content that can be taught with simulation and, in the process, miss other important topics, or try to use simulation to teach everything, when in fact different teaching modalities would be more effective for some content areas (see Table 37.2). Second, once the learning objectives that will be most effectively met using simulation have been identified, the specific details for each session, such as case scripting, location, props, and scheduling, can be planned.

The third step is planning for spontaneous sessions. Occasionally, clinical service demands are such that an unscheduled simulation session can occur. We have found these to be extremely high yield because the sessions can be used to cover content areas or skills that the learners have identified as being immediately relevant. For example, if a debriefing session following a real cardiac arrest identified a number of areas for opportunities, the team could immediately practice by using the simulator to recreate the same situation. Although planning for this type of session is challenging, steps such as developing a library of cases, training most if not all faculty members to use simulation technology and having a basic approach to simulation sessions that both the learners and facilitators are familiar with can greatly enhance their effectiveness and the likelihood that they will occur.

Teach

Based on the learning objectives within your curriculum, simulation can be used to teach a wide variety of content knowledge and skills as outlined above in the Science section. However, we find it most useful to facilitate learning skills that are more difficult to acquire when using traditional instructional modalities. For example, we focus less on content knowledge that can be acquired from books or didactic sessions and more on technical skills, communication skills, and leadership skills (see Table 37.3). In our institution, the physician membership of the cardiac arrest team changes every 4 weeks as residents complete their rotations. As a result, we have found simulation to be an invaluable resource to orient new residents and provide opportunities for deliberate practice in patient and team management skills.

While important learning gains can be made by simply participating in a simulation session, in our experience the most effective learning occurs during debriefing when feedback is provided and teaching points are highlighted. Based on the learning objectives of the case, we target a maximum of three teaching points for each debriefing; we otherwise find that learners get overloaded and fail to retain key information. Having well-trained and experienced facilitators who can identify these relevant teaching points, create a safe atmosphere, engage learners, and provide honest and constructive feedback is crucial to the success of the session.

We feel that all specialists in pulmonary and critical care medicine should have the opportunity to acquire this skillset and so have incorporated this teaching into our fellowship

Table 37.3 Sample scenario: code blue communication

Difficulty:
Easy
Target:
Junior ICU resident
Objectives:
1. Demonstrate appropriate management of a cardiac arrest according to current ACLS guidelines (pulseless VT)
2. Demonstrate the ability to effectively communicate with members of the multidisciplinary healthcare team during a crisis situation when limited information is initially available (should include evidence of data gathering, active listening, clear communication of orders, and thought processes)
Setting:
Intensive care unit
Props:
Mannequin, already intubated
BMV unit
IV, central line, saline bags, stocked arrest cart
Cast:
1–2 residents (one will be the code team leader)
2 bedside nurses (can give meds, history, assist in CPR)
2 respiratory therapists (can provide assistance with airway, assist in CPR)
Overview:
The resident team is called to the bedside of a 78-year-old patient in the ICU who was admitted last night. The only information that they will be given is a brief synopsis that the post-call resident gave during handover this morning. (*Severe community-acquired pneumonia, required intubation, broad-spectrum antibiotics started, started to improve hemodynamically, and from an oxygenation perspective post-intubation*). Further details are available only from the nurses and respiratory therapists at the bedside during the scenario
Upon arrival, the residents will find the patient in pulseless ventricular tachycardia. Details of the events leading up to the arrest (past history of CAD with NSTEMI 2 weeks ago and over past hour increasing tachycardia and increasing norepinephrine infusion with sudden decompensation into VT 1 min ago) can be obtained from the nurses and RTs if asked
Performance evaluation:
Code blue communication checklist

VT ventricular tachycardia, *BMV* bag-mask ventilation, *NSTEMI* non st elevation myocardic infraction, *RT* respiratory therapist

program. In different academic sessions throughout their training, fellows learn about the basics of simulation, scenario creation, and techniques for teaching, debriefing, and providing feedback. They have the opportunity to observe faculty facilitators during sessions with more junior residents and subsequently facilitate these sessions themselves with direct observation and feedback from faculty.

In addition to its role as an instructional modality, we have found simulation very useful for assessing our critical care medicine fellows' progression over the course of their 2-year training in areas such as content knowledge, communication skills, crisis resource management, and procedural skills. The results are used in a formative fashion to create and revise their personal learning plan on an ongoing basis.

Review

Following every simulation session, it is important to review positive aspects and identify opportunities for improvement based on the input of all participants and by undertaking a process of self-reflection. In general, we have found written anonymous feedback to be an effective means to obtain honest and constructive comments from participants, although not all choose to complete it and those that do often leave little in the way of detailed information. However, if a team has been working together with the same facilitator for a number of sessions, they may be able to develop a level of trust that enables feedback to be given verbally; in our experience, this usually provides the most meaningful suggestions for change.

Self-reflecting on the session, the facilitator's personal performance and the feedback that others provided can be a particularly challenging thing to do, especially when the session has not gone well. However, it is an important way to improve as a facilitator and can provide valuable feedback for improving the sessions and curriculum.

It is also important that review be undertaken at a systems level and that feedback be used to help guide curriculum renewal on a regular basis.

Practicality

We believe that this is one of the most important aspects of a successful simulation program in pulmonary and critical care medicine and applies to each of the three other key issues described above. For example, simulation should be easily accessible, easy to use, and have reasonable initial and ongoing costs. The learning objectives and the simulation experience need to be flexible, seen as relevant by each participant, and enjoyable for both participants and facilitators.

In our opinion, practicality should receive a higher priority than fidelity. We find it much more practical to use lower-fidelity simulators that are stored in the ICU than to have to go off-site to use a higher-fidelity model. We have also found that it is the facilitators rather than the fidelity of a mannequin that can make or break a session. Financially, if we had to choose between buying a new simulator or investing in our facilitators, we would choose the latter every time.

While these are just a few of many potential examples, the important point is recognizing the impact that practicality can have on the sustainability of a successful simulation program.

Conclusion

Despite the gaps in available evidence, the use of simulation-based training in the specialties of pulmonary and critical care medicine is almost certain to continue to increase given the current patient safety climate and the face validity that it has as an educational technique. The important task ahead of us will be determining how best to combine this exciting technology with existing instructional techniques in order to optimize the learning of current and future healthcare professionals.

References

1. Nguyen HB, Daniel-Underwood L, Van Ginkel C, et al. An educational course including medical simulation for early goal-directed therapy and the severe sepsis resuscitation bundle: an evaluation for medical student training. Resuscitation. 2009;80:674–9.
2. Schroedl CJ, Corbridge TC, Cohen ER, et al. Use of simulation-based education to improve resident learning and patient care in the medical intensive care unit: a randomized trial. J Crit Care. 2012;27(2):219.e7–13. doi:10.1016/j.jcrc.2011.08.006.
3. Steadman RH, Coates WC, Huang YM, et al. Simulation-based training is superior to problem-based earning for the acquisition of critical assessment and management skills. Crit Care Med. 2006; 34:151–7.
4. Ten Eyck RP. Improved medical student satisfaction and test performance with a simulation-based emergency medicine curriculum: a randomized controlled trial. Ann Emerg Med. 2009;54:684–91.
5. Cant RP, Cooper SJ. Simulation-based learning in nurse education: systematic review. J Adv Nurs. 2010;66:3–15.
6. Murphy PW, Engle K, Jorns LJ, Herrington CP, Lindsey LM. Comparison of PBL and simulation educational methods for the acquisition of medical knowledge. Respir Care Educ Annu. 2009; 18:31–7.
7. McCoy CE, Menchine M, Anderson C, Kollen R, Langdorf MI, Lotfipour S. Prospective randomized crossover study of simulation vs. didactics for teaching medical students the assessment and management of critically ill patients. J Emerg Med. 2011;40(4):448–55.
8. Goldmann K, Ferson DZ. Education and training in airway management. Best Pract Res Clin Anaesthesiol. 2005;19:717–32.
9. Wang EE, Quinones J, Fitch MT, et al. Developing technical expertise in emergency medicine – the role of simulation in procedural skill acquisition. Acad Emerg Med. 2008;15:1046–57.
10. Mayo PH, Hackney JE, Mueck JT, Ribaudo V, Schneider RF. Achieving house staff competence in emergency airway management: Results of a teaching program using a computerized patient simulator. Crit Care Med. 2004;32:2422–7.
11. Kory PD, Eisen LA, Adachi M, Ribaudo VA, Rosenthal ME, Mayo PH. Initial airway management skills of senior residents: simulation training compared with traditional training. Chest. 2007;132: 1927–31.
12. Rosenthal ME, Adachi M, Ribaudo V, Mueck JT, Schneider RF, Mayo PH. Achieving housestaff competence in emergency airway management using scenario based simulation training: comparison of attending vs housestaff trainers. Chest. 2006;129:1453–8.
13. Mayo PH, Hegde A, Eisen LA, Kory P, Doelken P. A program to improve the quality of emergency endotracheal intubation. J Intensive Care Med. 2011;26:50–6.
14. Griesdale DEG, Bosma TL, Kurth T, Isac G, Chittock DR. Complications of endotracheal intubation in the critically ill. Intensive Care Med. 2008;34:1835–42.
15. Berthiaume LR, Peets AD, Schmidt U, et al. Time series analysis of use patterns for common invasive technologies in critically ill patients. J Crit Care. 2009;24:471.e9–471.e14.
16. McGee DC, Gould MK. Preventing complications of central venous catheterization. N Engl J Med. 2003;348:1123–33.
17. Ma IWY, Brindle ME, Ronksley PE, Lorenzetti DL, Sauve RS, Ghali WA. Use of simulation-based education to improve outcomes of central venous catheterization: a systematic review and meta-analysis. Acad Med. 2011;86:1137–47.
18. Barsuk JH, Cohen ER, Feinglass J, McGaghie WC, Wayne DB. Unexpected collateral effects of simulation-based medical education. Acad Med. 2011;86:1513–7.
19. Bhanji B, Mancini ME, Sinz E, et al. Part 16: education, implementation, and teams: 2010 American Heart Association Guidelines for Cardiopulmonary Resuscitation and Emergency Cardiovascular Care. Circulation. 2010;122 suppl 3:S920–33.
20. Soar J, Monsieurs KG, Ballance JH, et al. European Resuscitation Council guidelines for resuscitation 2010 Section 9. Principles of education in resuscitation. Resuscitation. 2010;81(10):1434–44.
21. Perkins GD. Simulation in resuscitation training. Resuscitation. 2007;73:202–11.
22. Owen H, Mugford B, Follows V, Plummer JL. Comparison of three simulation-based training methods for management of medical emergencies. Resuscitation. 2006;71:204–11.
23. Wayne DB, Butter J, Siddall VJ, et al. Simulation-based training of internal medicine residents in advanced cardiac life support protocols: a randomized trial. Teach Learn Med. 2005;17:210–6.
24. Ali J, Cohen RJ, Gana TJ, Al-Bedah KF. Effect of the Advanced Trauma Life Support program on medical students' performance in simulated trauma patient management. J Trauma. 1998;44:588–91.
25. Hunt EA, Vera K, Diener-West M, et al. Delays and errors in cardiopulmonary resuscitation and defibrillation by pediatric residents during simulated cardiopulmonary arrests. Resuscitation. 2009;80:819–25.
26. Andreatta P, Saxton E, Thompson M, Annich G. Simulation-based mock codes significantly correlate with improved pediatric patient cardiopulmonary arrest survival rates. Pediatr Crit Care Med. 2011; 12:33–8.
27. Wayne DB, Didwania A, Feinglass J, Fudala MJ, Barsuk JH, McGaghie WC. Simulation-based education improves quality of care during cardiac arrest team responses at an academic teaching hospital: a case–control study. Chest. 2008;133:56–61.
28. Pottle A, Brant S. Does resuscitation training affect outcome from cardiac arrest? Accid Emerg Nurs. 2000;8:46–51.
29. Schneider T, Mauer D, Diehl P, Eberle B, Dick W. Does standardized mega- code training improve the quality of pre-hospital

advanced cardiac life support (ACLS)? Resuscitation. 1995; 29:129–34.

30. Birnbaum ML, Robinson NE, Kuska BM, Stone HL, Fryback DG, Rose JH. Effect of advanced cardiac life-support training in rural, community hospitals. Crit Care Med. 1994;22:741–9.
31. Miotto HC, Couto BR, Goulart EM, Amaral CF, Moreira Mda C. Advanced cardiac life support courses: live actors do not improve training results compared with conventional mannequins. Resuscitation. 2008;76:244–8.
32. Donoghue AJ, Durbin DR, Nadel FM, Stryjewski GR, Kost SI, Nadkarni VM. Effect of high-fidelity simulation on Pediatric Advanced Life Support training in pediatric housestaff: a randomized trial. Pediatr Emerg Care. 2009;25:139–44.
33. Campbell DM, Barozzino T, Farrugia M, Sgro M. High-fidelity simulation in neonatal resuscitation. Paediatr Childs Health. 2009; 14:19–23.
34. Rodgers D, Securro SJ, Pauley R. The effect of high-fidelity simulation on educational outcomes in an advanced cardiovascular life support course. Simul Healthc. 2009;4:200–6.
35. Schwartz LR, Fernandez R, Kouyoumjian SR, Jones KA, Compton S. A randomized comparison trial of case-based learning versus human patient simulation in medical student education. Acad Emerg Med. 2007;14:130–7.
36. Hoadley TA. Learning advanced cardiac life support: a comparison study of the effects of low- and high-fidelity simulation. Nurs Educ Perspect. 2009;30:91–5.
37. Brodie D, Bacchetta M. Extracorporeal membrane oxygenation for ARDS in adults. N Engl J Med. 2011;365:1905–14.
38. Anderson JM, Boyle KB, Murphy AA, Yaeger KA, LeFlore J, Halamek LP. Simulating extracorporeal membrane oxygenation emergencies to improve human performance. Part I: methodologic and technologic innovations. Simul Healthc. 2006;1:220–7.
39. Anderson JM, Murphy AA, Boyle KB, Yaeger KA, Halamek LP. Simulating extracorporeal membrane oxygenation emergencies to improve human performance. Part II: assessment of technical and behavioral skills. Simul Healthc. 2006;1:228–32.
40. Burton KS, Pendergrass TL, Byczkowski TL, Taylor RG, Moyer MR, Falcone RA, et al. Impact of simulation-based extracorporeal membrane oxygenation training in the simulation laboratory and clinical environment. Simul Healthc. 2011;6:284–91.
41. Bro-Nielsen M, Tasto JL, Cunningham R, Merril GL. PreOp endoscopic simulator: a PC-based immersive training system for bronchoscopy. Stud Health Technol Inform. 1999;62:76–82.
42. Colt HG, Crawford SW, Galbraith O. Virtual reality bronchoscopy simulation: a revolution in procedural training. Chest. 2001;120: 1333–9.
43. Ost D, De Rosiers A, Britt EJ, Fein AM, Lesser ML, Mehta AC. Assessment of a bronchoscopy simulator. Am J Respir Crit Care Med. 2001;164:2248–55.
44. Stather DR, Lamb CR, Tremblay A. Simulation in flexible bronchoscopy and endobronchial ultrasound: a review. J Bronchol Intervent Pulmonol. 2011;18:247–56.
45. Moorthy K, Smith S, Brown T, Bann S, Darzi A. Evaluation of virtual reality bronchoscopy as a learning and assessment tool. Respiration. 2003;70:195–9.
46. Wahidi MM, Silvestri GA, Coakley RD, et al. A prospective multicenter study of competency metrics and educational interventions in the learning of bronchoscopy among new pulmonary fellows. Chest. 2010;137:1040–9.
47. Blum MG, Powers TW, Sundaresan S. Bronchoscopy simulator effectively prepares junior residents to competently perform basic clinical bronchoscopy. Ann Thorac Surg. 2004;78:287–91.
48. Davoudi M, Wahidi MM, Rohani NZ, Colt HG. Comparative effectiveness of low- and high-fidelity bronchoscopy simulation for training in conventional transbronchial needle aspiration and user preferences. Respiration. 2010;80:327–34.
49. Konge L, Arendrup H, von Buchwald C, Ringsted C. Virtual reality simulation of basic pulmonary procedures. J Bronchol Intervent Pulmonol. 2011;18:38–41.
50. Holcomb JB, Dumire RD, Crommett JW. Evaluation of trauma team performance using an advanced human patient simulator for resuscitation training. J Trauma. 2002;52:1078–86.
51. Smith CC, Huang GC, Newman LR, et al. Simulation training and its effect on long-term resident performance in central venous catheterization. Simul Healthc. 2010;5:146–51.
52. Roy KM, Miller MP, Schmidt K, Sagy M. Pediatric residents experience a significant decline in their response capabilities to simulated life-threatening events as their training frequency in cardiopulmonary resuscitation decreases. Pediatr Crit Care Med. 2011;12:e141–4.
53. Wayne DB, Siddall VJ, Butter J, et al. A longitudinal study of internal medicine residents' retention of advanced cardiac life support skills. Acad Med. 2006;81:S9–12.
54. McGaghie WC, Issenberg SB, Cohen ER, Barsuk JH, Wayne DB. Does simulation-based medical education with deliberate practice yield better results than traditional clinical education? A meta-analytic comparative review of the evidence. Acad Med. 2011;86:706–11.
55. Ahlberg G, Enochsson L, Gallagher AG, Hedman L, Hogman C, McClusky DA, et al. Proficiency-based virtual reality training significantly reduces the error rate for residents during their first 10 laparoscopic cholecystectomies. Am J Surg. 2007;193:797–804.
56. Andreatta PB, Woodrum DT, Birkmeyer JD, Yellamanchilli RK, Doherty GM, Gauger PG, et al. Laparoscopic skills are improved with LapMentor training: Results of a randomized, double-blinded study. Ann Surg. 2006;243:854–63.
57. Korndorffer JR, Dunne JB, Sierra R, Stefanidis D, Touchard CL, Scott DJ. Simulator training for laparoscopic suturing using performance goals translates to the operating room. J Am Coll Surg. 2005;201:23–9.
58. Korndorffer JR, Hayes DJ, Dunne JB, Sierra R, Touchard CL, Markert RJ, et al. Development and transferability of a cost-effective laparoscopic camera navigation simulator. Surg Endosc. 2005; 19:161–7.
59. Van Sickle KR, Bitter EM, Baghai M, Goldenberg AE, Huang IP, Gallagher AG, et al. Prospective, randomized, double-blind trial of curriculum-based training for intracorporeal suturing and knot tying. J Am Coll Surg. 2008;207:560–8.
60. Issenberg SB, McGaghie WC, Gordon DL, Symes S, Petrusa ER, Hart IR, et al. Effectiveness of a cardiology review course for internal medicine residents using simulation technology and deliberate practice. Teach Learn Med. 2002;14:223–8.
61. Barsuk JH, Ahya SN, Cohen ER, McGaghie WC, Wayne DB. Mastery learning of temporary hemodialysis catheter insertion by nephrology fellows using simulation technology and deliberate practice. Am J Kidney Dis. 2009;53:A14–7.
62. Butter J, McGaghie WC, Cohen ER, Kaye M, Wayne DB. Simulation-based mastery learning improves cardiac auscultation skills in medical students. J Gen Intern Med. 2010;25:780–5.
63. Wayne DB, Barsuk JH, O'Leary KO, Fudala MJ, McGaghie WC. Mastery learning of thoracentesis skills by internal medicine residents using simulation technology and deliberate practice. J Hosp Med. 2008;3:48–54.
64. Barsuk JH, McGaghie WC, Cohen ER, Balachandran JS, Wayne DB. Use of simulation-based mastery learning to improve the quality of central venous catheter placement in a medical intensive care unit. J Hosp Med. 2009;4:397–403.
65. Barsuk JH, McGaghie WC, Cohen ER, O'Leary KS, Wayne DB. Simulation-based mastery learning reduces complications during central venous catheter insertion in a medical intensive care unit. Crit Care Med. 2009;37:2697–701.
66. Stefanidis D, Sierra R, Korndorffer JR, Dunne JB, Markley S, Touchard CL, et al. Intensive continuing medical education course

training on simulators results in proficiency in laparoscopic suturing. Am J Surg. 2006;191:23–7.
67. Kruglikova I, Grantcharov TP, Drewes AM, Funch-Jensen P. Assessment of early learning curves among nurses and physicians using a high-fidelity virtual-reality colonoscopy simulator. Surg Endosc. 2010;24:366–70.
68. Leonard M, Graham S, Bonacum D. The human factor: the critical importance of effective teamwork and communication in providing safe care. Qual Saf Health Care. 2004;13:85–90.
69. Wright D, Mackenzie SJ, Buchan I, Cairns CS, Price LE. Critical incidents in the intensive therapy unit. Lancet. 1991;338:676–8.
70. Reader TW, Flin R, Cuthbertson BH. Communication skills and error in the intensive care unit. Curr Opin Crit Care. 2007;13:732–6.
71. Lorin S, Rho L, Wisnivesky JP, Nierman DM. Improving medical student intensive care unit communication skills: a novel educational initiative using standardized family members. Crit Care Med. 2006;34:2386–91.
72. Frengley RW, Weller JM, Torrie J, et al. The effect of a simulation-based training intervention on the performance of established critical care unit teams. Crit Care Med. 2011;39:2605–11.
73. De Vita MA, Schaefer J, Lutz J, Dongilli T, Wang H. Improving medical crisis team performance. Crit Care Med. 2004;32:S61–5.
74. Horwitz LI, Moin T, Krumholz HM, Wang L, Bradley EH. Consequences of inadequate signout for patient care. Arch Intern Med. 2008;168:1755–60.
75. Riesenberg LA, Leitzsch J, Massucci JL, et al. Residents' and attending physicians' handoffs: a systematic review of the literature. Acad Med. 2009;84:1775–87.
76. Gordon M, Findley R. Educational interventions to improve handover in health care: a systematic review. Med Educ. 2011;45:1081–9.
77. Berkenstadt H, Haviv Y, Tuval A, et al. Improving handoff communications in critical care: utilizing simulation-based training toward process improvement in managing patient risk. Chest. 2008;134:158–62.
78. Farnan JM, Paro JAM, Rodriguez RM, et al. Hand-off education and evaluation: piloting the observed simulated hand-off experience (OSHE). J Gen Intern Med. 2010;25:129–34.
79. Fox-Robichaud AE, Nimmo GR. Education and simulation techniques for improving reliability of care. Curr Opin Crit Car. 2007;13:737–41.
80. Villamaria FJ, Pliego JF, Wehbe-Janek H, et al. Using simulation to orient code blue teams to a new hospital facility. Simul Healthc. 2008;3:209–16.
81. Ford DG, Seybert AL, Smithburger PL, Kobulinsky LR, Samosky JT, Kane-Gill SL. Impact of simulation-based learning on medication error rates in critically ill patients. Intensive Care Med. 2010;36:1526–31.
82. Cook DA, Hatala R, Brydges R, et al. Technology-enhanced simulation for health professions education: a systematic review and meta-analysis. JAMA. 2011;306:978–88.
83. McGaghie WC, Draycott TJ, Dunn WF, Lopez CM, Stefanidis D. Evaluating the impact of simulation on translational patient outcomes. Simul Healthc. 2011;6:S42–7.
84. Barsuk JH, Cohen ER, Feinglass J, McGaghie WC, Wayne DB. Use of simulation-based education to reduce catheter-related bloodstream infections. Arch Intern Med. 2009;169:1420–3.
85. Cohen ER, Feinglass J, Barsuk JH, et al. Cost savings from reduced catheter-related bloodstream infection after simulation-based education for residents in a medical intensive care unit. Simul Healthc. 2010;5:98–102.
86. Frank JR, Snell LS, Cate OT, et al. Competency-based medical education: theory to practice. Med Teach. 2010;32:638–45.
87. Holmboe E, Rizzolo MA, Sachdeva AK, Rosenberg M, Ziv A. Simulation-based assessment and the regulation of healthcare professionals. Simul Healthc. 2011;6:S58–62.
88. Nishisaki A, Nguyen J, Colborn S, et al. Evaluation of multidisciplinary simulation training on clinical performance and team behavior during tracheal intubation procedures in a pediatric intensive care unit. Pediatr Crit Care Med. 2011;12:406–14.
89. Dong Y, Suri HS, Cook DA, et al. Simulation-based objective assessment discerns clinical proficiency in central line placement: a construct validation. Chest. 2010;137:1050–6.
90. Davoudi M, Osann K, Colt HG. Validation of two instruments to assess technical bronchoscopic skill using virtual reality simulation. Respiration. 2008;76:92–101.
91. Schmitz CC, Chipman JG, Luxenberg MG, Beilman GJ. Professionalism and communication in the intensive care unit: reliability and validity of a simulated family conference. Simul Healthc. 2008;3:224–38.
92. Kim J, Neilipovitz D, Cardinal P, Chiu M, Clinch J. A pilot study using high-fidelity simulation to formally evaluate performance in the resuscitation of critically ill patients: The University of Ottawa Critical Care Medicine, High-Fidelity Simulation, and Crisis Resource Management I Study. Crit Care Med. 2006;34:2167–74.
93. Kim J, Neilipovitz D, Cardinal P, Chiu M. A comparison of global rating scale and checklist scores in the validation of an evaluation tool to assess performance in the resuscitation of critically ill patients during simulated emergencies. Simul Healthc. 2009;4:6–16.
94. Malec JF, Torsher LC, Dunn WF, et al. The Mayo high performance teamwork scale: reliability and validity for evaluating key crew resource management skills. Simul Healthc. 2007;2:4–10.
95. Ottestad E, Boulet JR, Lighthall GK. Evaluating the management of septic shock using patient simulation. Crit Care Med. 2007;35:769–75.
96. Hatala R, Kassen BO, Nishikawa J, Cole G, Issenberg SB. Incorporating simulation technology in a Canadian Internal Medicine specialty examination: a descriptive report. Acad Med. 2005;80:554–6.
97. Berkenstadt H, Ziv A, Gafni N, Sidi A. The validation process of incorporating simulation-based accreditation into the anesthesiology Israeli national board exams. Isr Med Assoc J. 2006;8:728–33.
98. Sharpe R, Koval V, Ronco JJ, et al. The impact of prolonged continuous wakefulness on resident clinical performance in the intensive care unit: a patient simulator study. Crit Care Med. 2010;38:766–70.
99. Marsch SCU, Tschan F, Semmer N, Spychiger M, Breuer M, Hunziker PR. Performance of first responders in simulated cardiac arrests. Crit Care Med. 2005;33:963–7.
100. Yager PH, Lok J, Klig JE. Advances in simulation for pediatric critical care and emergency medicine. Curr Opin Pediatr. 2011; 23:293–7.
101. Smith SM, Vela E. Environmental context-dependent memory: a review and meta-analysis. Psychon Bull Rev. 2001;8:203–20.
102. Godden DR, Baddeley AD. Context-dependent memory in two natural environments: on land and underwater. Br J Psychol. 1975; 66:325–31.
103. Weinstock PH, Kappus LJ, Kleinman ME, et al. Toward a new paradigm in hospital-based pediatric education: the development of an onsite simulator program. Pediatr Crit Care Med. 2005;6:635–41.
104. Weinstock PH, Kappus LJ, Garden A, Burns JP. Simulation at the point of care: reduced-cost, in situ training via a mobile cart. Pediatr Crit Care Med. 2009;10:176–82.

38 Simulation in Radiology: Diagnostic Techniques

Alexander Towbin

Introduction

Radiology has evolved to become essentially two distinct but closely related fields: diagnostic and interventional radiology. The use of simulation is therefore diverse in its nature when applied to radiology. In this chapter, we present the role of simulation in diagnostic radiology, which includes not only its role for practitioner training but its role as an education tool for our patients as they prepare to undergo potentially frightening procedures. Simulation has been utilized in very novel ways for these purposes, and we believe much of this material will be of interest to the reader and may provide others with potential beneficial applications to a variety of other specialties. In the following chapter (Chap. 39), the role of simulation in interventional radiology is presented. Given the nature of invasive radiology and its grounding as a procedure-centric specialty, simulation in this field is more similar to other interventional fields and has shown great promise.

Simulators in diagnostic radiology are an interesting dichotomy. Surprisingly there is perhaps no specialty that uses simulators as much as radiology (i.e., case-based lectures, online modules, and phantoms to calibrate modalities); yet, if you ask most radiologists, they will tell you that they never use simulation. When thinking of simulators in radiology, it helps to consider them from three points of view: directly helping the patient, directly helping the imaging technology, and directly helping the radiologist. In this chapter, we present the point of view and the evidence for the use of simulation in each. We also have embedded practical applications for simulation for these three arenas.

A. Towbin, MD
Department of Radiology,
Cincinnati Children's Hospital Medical Center,
3333 Burnet Ave, ML 3051,
Cincinnati, OH 45229, USA
e-mail: alexander.towbin@cchmc.org

Simulators in Radiology: Preparing the Patient

In radiology, high-quality imaging is often required to make a diagnosis or evaluate an abnormality. In order to obtain high-quality, diagnostic images, radiologists must rely on their patient's cooperation and ability to follow specific instructions. Simulators are used to help prepare patients for examinations prior to imaging. This is most prevalent in pediatric radiology where simulators are widely utilized to help children understand the processes and procedures they will undergo as part of the examination. In this setting, simulators can be placed into three broad categories: demonstration, practice, and play therapy. In reality, however, all three methods are often used in combination.

Demonstration is perhaps the simplest method of simulation. The patient is shown the machines and equipment with which they will be interacting during the procedure. This demonstration can vary widely depending on the study that is being demonstrated.

MRI is an ideal procedure for demonstration as the long scan times, relatively small scanner bore, and loud noises make it at times a difficult study for patients to undergo without sedation. Mock scanners (scale or full-size models of the clinical scanners) have been used to prepare children for the experience of undergoing MRI (Fig. 38.1) [1–6]. While this practice is not widespread, in hospitals that provide this experience, the patient is able to take a tour of the radiology department and see a life-sized scanner. While in the practice scanning room, MRI sounds can be played over speakers in the room or via headphones to prepare the patient for the noises they will hear during scanning.

Several studies have been performed evaluating the utility of mock MRI in preparing children for MRI and evaluating its effect on the need for anesthesia [1, 2]. In the largest study, a mock MRI program was able to reduce the need for sedation by almost 17% in patients aged 3–8 years old [1]. It is likely that such programs would benefit patients with anxiety, claustrophobia, or other limitations when undergoing MRI.

A.I. Levine et al. (eds.), *The Comprehensive Textbook of Healthcare Simulation*,
DOI 10.1007/978-1-4614-5993-4_38, © Springer Science+Business Media New York 2013

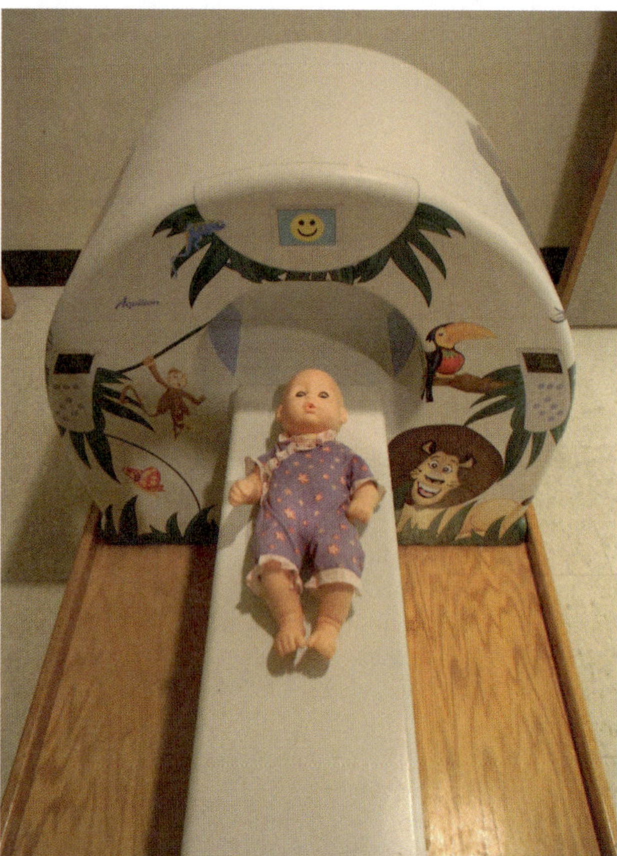

Fig. 38.1 Mock CT scanner. The scanner is a 1:10 size scale model of the clinical scanner. The small size allows children to prepare for the actual scan by placing a doll or stuffed animal on the table and moving it through the gantry

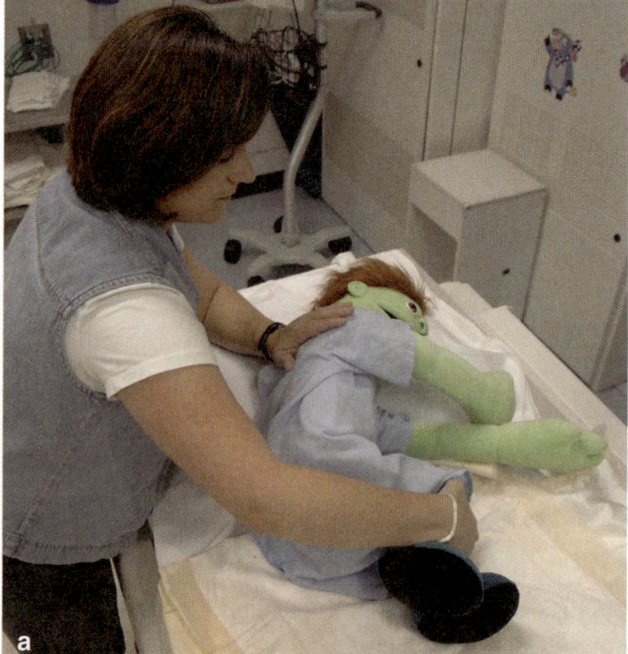

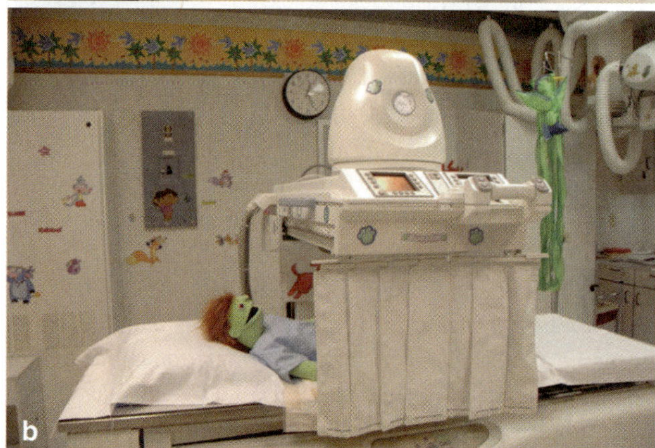

Fig. 38.2 (a) Dolls can be used to help prepare children for different examinations. In fluoroscopy, child life specialists can demonstrate correct positioning for a contrast enema using a doll. (b) Dolls can also be used to show children how the machines works

Fluoroscopy is another modality where demonstration is often used. The fluoroscopic environment is often frightening to patients as they are forced to lie down on a hard table in a dark room while a large camera comes down close to their body. The group of medical personnel standing over them performing the study can also be intimidating. Because of the way the test is performed, the patient is rarely sedated; yet, they are subject to invasive and sometimes painful procedures. Demonstration cannot completely prepare a child for this scenario, but it can help them to understand what will happen during the study.

Child life specialists are an invaluable resource in helping children prepare for fluoroscopic procedures in an age-appropriate manner. Before the study is performed, the child life specialist welcomes the child and brings him or her to the fluoroscopy suite. Once there, the child life specialist shows the patient the fluoroscopy machine and how it works. Patients are allowed to touch the machine and the table. Then, the child life specialist explains the procedure to the patient using a picture book where a doll is shown to be the patient. Depending on the child and his or her level of understanding and anxiety, the child life specialist can then demonstrate what the child will experience by using the doll (Fig. 38.2). The child is able to feel all tubes or catheters that will be used during the procedure so that he or she is better prepared once the radiologist enters the room.

Practice is another method that is used extensively to help simulate the procedure and help the patient prepare for an exam. An example of practice is in preparing patients for MR elastography (MRE). In this procedure, the patient undergoes an MRI while a 7-in. plastic speaker, called the passive driver, is placed on the patient. The passive driver is connected via pneumatic tubing to the active driver, an audio subwoofer, in the MRI control room. In order to prepare patients for the vibration sensation that they will feel during scanning, child life specialists use a vibrating passive driver

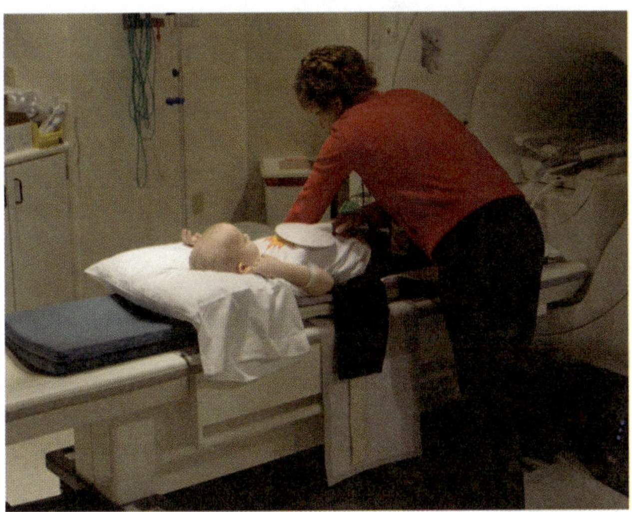

Fig. 38.3 In order to obtain high-quality images, it helps to prepare patients for unexpected or unusual sensations. In MR elastography, child life specialists prepare children for the vibrations they will feel by placing the passive driver on the abdomen prior to scanning

simulator on the child prior to the MRE (Fig. 38.3). The prescan simulation helps prepare patients for the sensation they will feel during scanning and helps to reduce patient anxiety and sudden movements at the start of the actual MRE sequence.

Practice is often coupled with demonstration in an attempt to prepare patients for a procedure. What is practiced often depends on the invasiveness of the procedure. In noninvasive procedures, patients are able to experience a large portion of what they will undergo in a nonthreatening and staged approach.

Using a full-scale mock MRI as an example, the following procedure has been described as a method to help prepare children for scanning [1]. First, the child and his or her caregiver are assessed for their level of anxiety. The responses then help to guide the remainder of education, practice, and demonstration. The child life specialist then uses age and developmentally appropriate methods to teach the patient about the procedure. This education can involve picture books, videos, listening to sounds recorded from the MR scanner, and demonstration with dolls. Finally, the patient is able to lie in the mock scanner, lie in a radiofrequency coil, and practice lying still. They are able to pick the music they would like to listen to or the movie that they would like to watch during scanning. In this scenario, they are able to simulate the entire scanning process prior to the scan itself.

In more invasive procedures such as a voiding cystourethrogram (VCUG) or contrast enema, it is not possible to practice the most difficult portions of the procedure. For these procedures, the child life specialist demonstrates the procedure through picture books or demonstration on dolls. The child is then placed on the fluoroscopy table where they are able to practice relaxation techniques and the positions in

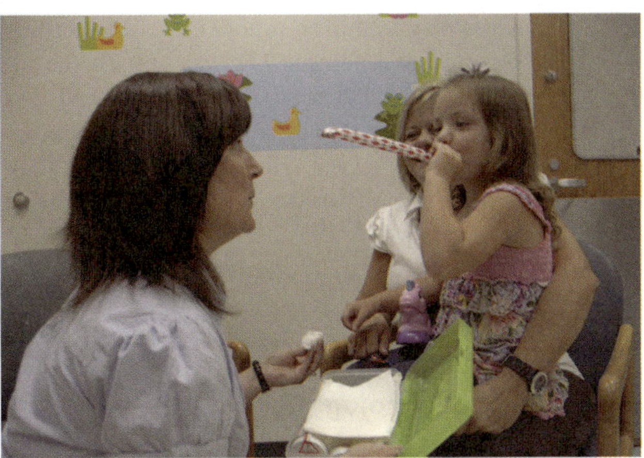

Fig. 38.4 Child life specialists use age-appropriate tools such as party blowers or bubbles to help children learn deep-breathing techniques for relaxation prior to undergoing a painful or anxiety-provoking procedure

which they will be placed. Child life specialists use age-appropriate tools such as party blowers or bubbles not only to perform deep breathing during painful portions of the procedure but also as a means of distraction and play (Fig. 38.4). Prior to the procedure, children practice these techniques while on the fluoroscopy table to simulate as much of the procedure as possible.

The final technique of simulation used in patient preparation in pediatric radiology is play therapy. This is perhaps the most immersive technique in that children are able to become more comfortable with the procedure by simulating the examination through play. One of the benefits of play therapy is that a child life specialist can observe the child and identify their specific anxieties. They are then able to target education and relaxation techniques directly to this portion of the examination.

In preparation for CT or MRI, play therapy can be used as another method to reduce anxiety. Scale model scanners have been developed so that a doll or stuffed animal can undergo the scan (Fig. 38.1). The child is able to place his or her doll on the model scanner and push it through the machine. While they are playing, children will often explain the procedure from their point of view to their doll. Child life specialists are able to use this play to help explain specific parts of the examination to the child.

Play is often a large part of practice as well. For example, when practicing deep breathing with party blowers, child life specialists can turn the deep-breathing technique into a game. Instead of just blowing through the party blower, the children can aim for their parents or a technologist's nose (Fig. 38.4). This can turn an anxiety-provoking scenario into a game where everyone in the room is laughing.

While demonstration, practice, and play therapy often help to prepare children for a procedure, the material used must be appropriate for the child. At least one study has suggested that these techniques may lead to an overall increase in anxiety. This study showed that in children 7–12 years of age, the preparatory material used led to increased questioning and anxiety by the child [7]. It is possible that the anxiety provoked in this study is an anomaly related to the techniques used as several other studies have shown that demonstration, practice, and play can be used to decrease anxiety and the need for sedation during a procedure [1–3, 6].

Simulators in Radiology: Preparing the Imaging Technology

Simulators are most extensively used in radiology to help test and calibrate the imaging modalities. Every radiology department uses phantoms as part of its check on quality control and quality assurance for each modality. Each test acts as a check on the performance or internal consistency of the machine with key outcomes related to image quality, sensitivity of the machine in detecting subtle lesions, the radiation output of the machine, or the reproducibility of findings. The type of phantom used varies depending on the machine that is being tested and the feature being evaluated. Phantoms are commonly used in radiography, CT, MRI, and nuclear medicine. Because each modality employs a number of different tests, many of which require an understanding of the physics of that specific modality, only a few tests on select modalities are described here. The modalities selected for this chapter are the focus of active research or are thought to be good examples of phantoms used to test the modality.

With the rapid increase in the use of CT for diagnosing and managing a wide variety of conditions, there has been considerable research performed to develop methods to increase image quality while at the same time decreasing the radiation dose to the patient [8]. Because each CT scan delivers radiation to the patient, it is impractical and unethical to perform this testing on patients. Two main methods have been developed to evaluate the radiation dose delivered by a certain study: phantom-based studies and computer simulation.

Phantoms can vary in complexity and sophistication depending on the measured variable. For CT, the simplest phantom is a water phantom [9]. This type of phantom is created by filling a structure with water. The water phantom works on the principal that water has a defined CT density (0 Hounsfield units). Any variation from this is the image noise. As the radiation used to acquire the image is decreased, the noise increases. The water phantom can thus be used to measure image noise.

Test phantoms can vary considerably. One type of phantom called a "performance phantom" allows various cylinders of different densities to be inserted into the phantom. This is also used to detect image noise as well as the reproducibility of measurements [10]. Low-contrast phantoms are used to assess the sensitivity of nodule detection. In these phantoms, there are multiple cylinders of varying diameter. Each cylinder has a density slightly higher than water. These phantoms work on the principal that as noise increases, the lesions will become more and more difficult to identify. Linearity phantoms are used to ensure that a known element has a specific density on CT (Fig. 38.5). In this phantom, there are multiple pins, each containing a known density. The pins are placed in a cylinder that has water density. The phantom is scanned and

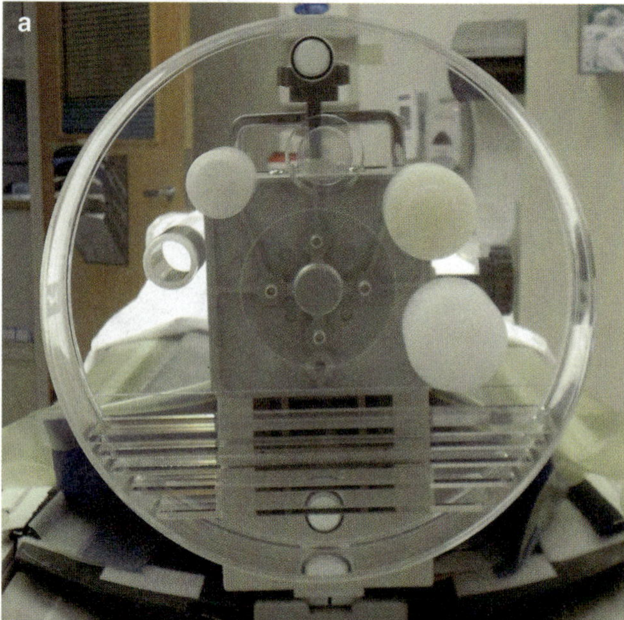

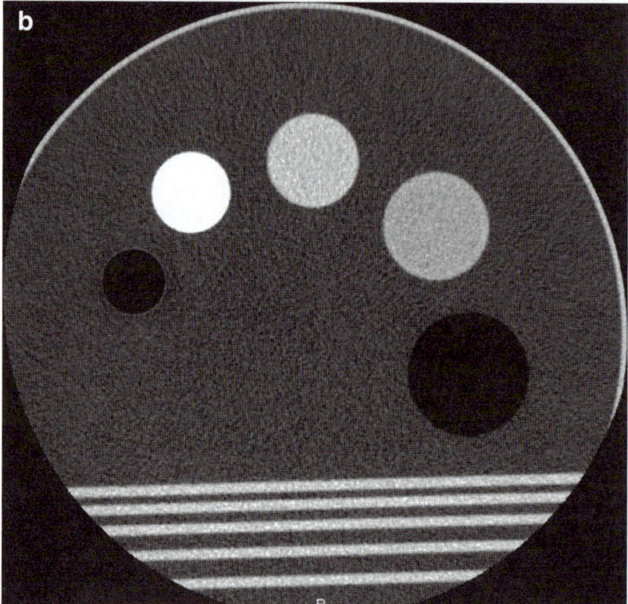

Fig. 38.5 (**a**) Photograph and (**b**) CT of a linearity phantom. Phantoms are used in every radiology department to help calibrate the modalities. Linearity phantoms are used for CT to ensure that the density of the structures meets a known standard

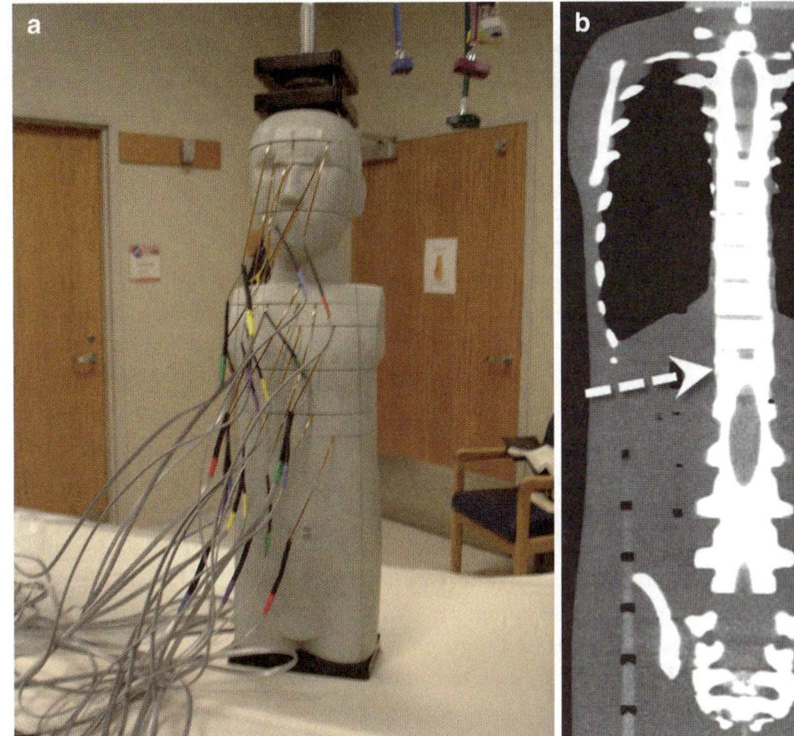

Fig. 38.6 (**a**) Anthropomorphic phantoms can vary in complexity depending on their purpose. The anthropomorphic phantom in this photograph has multiple leads attached to it in order to measure the radiation dose at different locations. (**b**) CT image of the same phantom shows soft tissue (*arrow*), bone (*dashed arrow*), and air-filled structures (*arrow head*), similar to a patient

the density of each element is measured and plotted to ensure the accuracy of the CT numbers.

The most advanced phantom is the anthropomorphic phantom (Fig. 38.6). Anthropomorphic phantoms can be constructed in various shapes and sizes to simulate the differences between males and females or patients of different sizes and ages. Even though these phantoms are designed to simulate the human body in shape and internal appearance, they can vary considerably. Some anthropomorphic phantoms are designed for a specific application such as lung nodule detection [11], while others are used to evaluate the whole body [10, 12–14].

The majority of the current research performed using anthropomorphic phantoms involves the calculation of radiation dose [12–14]. Anthropomorphic phantoms are useful for dose calculations because they take differences in body contour and different tissue interactions into account [14]. High-quality anthropomorphic phantoms will include all major internal organs. Phantoms used for dose calculations have multiple holes within them so that dosimeters can be placed within the phantom and organ doses can be measured. Using anthropomorphic phantoms in this manner allows for a standard method of calculating dose that is reproducible across different machines and differing technologies.

Some of the newest phantoms are entirely computerized. High-quality computerized phantoms help to address the main shortcoming of anthropomorphic phantoms, namely, the cost associated with fabricating the number of phantoms required to simulate the large range of patient sizes, clinical needs, and physiologic motion [8]. Computerized phantoms are therefore incredibly useful in "characterizing, evaluating, and optimizing CT imaging systems and image processing and reconstruction methods" [8]. The biggest disadvantage of computerized phantoms is that there is no physical object to scan; thus, the actual dose cannot be measured.

There are two main types of computerized phantoms: voxelized and mathematical [8]. Voxelized phantoms are based on patient data obtained from CT or MRI and appear very lifelike. They are useful in evaluating specific organs and image quality; however, their main disadvantage is that to simulate motion or anatomic variation, interpolation must be used, introducing error [8]. Mathematical phantoms use geometric shapes to construct organs. Because the shapes are predefined, they are easily manipulated to account for anatomic variation and motion. The major limitation of mathematical phantoms is the simplistic equations on which they are based. This limits exact modeling of human physiology [8]. As computers become more powerful, hybrid phantoms have been created that are based on patient imaging data and use more complex mathematical models to define the internal structures [8].

Because all modern radiologic imaging is digital, the images acquired as part of a clinical scan can be used for further simulation to evaluate the effect that changing imaging parameters has on image quality [15, 16]. Several hybrid studies have been performed where simulated noise has been added to clinical scans as a way to produce scans with noise equivalent to reducing dose. This method allows researchers to perform large-scale studies evaluating the effect reduced dose has on image quality and diagnostic accuracy [15]. The benefit of this data is that new imaging techniques can be evaluated and tested while the patient is imaged based on the current clinical standard.

Although not used to the same degree as CT, simulators have been created to optimize image quality for radiographs [17–19]. These simulators work on principles similar to those of CT simulators. Simulated images are created either through computer modeling, manipulating clinical images, or imaging phantoms of varying complexity.

Simulators in Radiology: Preparing the Radiologist

Simulators designed for radiologists are most akin to simulators in other fields of medicine. These simulators can be placed into two broad categories: those used to teach image interpretation and those used to teach a specific technique or procedure.

Diagnostic Simulators

Diagnostic radiology is ideally suited for simulation. All of the imaging and information related to its interpretation are digital. This makes reproduction of any imaging study for simulator use simple and likely effective as long as true representations are provided. Digital images allow creators of radiology simulators to create unique workflows for image interpretation such as creating digital "hotspots" to identify abnormalities. Further, radiologists are used to working in a digital environment so that a simulated environment can look and feel exactly like the real production environment, simply by the presentation of digital material.

Despite the relative ease with which simulation can be used in this field, simulation in diagnostic radiology has lagged behind other medical specialties. Most simulation is designed to teach a specific skill or technique. In radiology, diagnostic interpretation involves complex pattern recognition of a heterogeneous group of studies, involving multiple modalities and encompassing multiple body parts. Basic radiology interpretation involves creating a search pattern and methodically using this pattern every time to identify differences from the imagined standard (i.e., "normal") for the imaged body part. The complexity of creating such a system to teach image interpretation is beyond the scope of most applications.

One could argue that another reason for the lag is that although simulation is used in radiology, it has not progressed into the digital era. Radiology education has traditionally included case conferences where the trainee is asked to interpret an unknown case in front of his or her peers. This type of education plays an important role in radiology because it allows a large group of trainees to see rare cases that may not be encountered during their training. Case conferences allow the educator to identify key pertinent positive and negative findings based on the discussion by the trainee. This type of simulation is helpful in that other trainees can observe the process their peers use to form a differential diagnosis. The disadvantage of this method is that only one trainee can actively participate at a time. This unknown case format has been transmitted into the digital era via cases of the day or week on popular radiology websites such as the American College of Radiology's *Case in Point* (http://www.acr.org/HomePageCategories/CaseInPoint.aspx), AuntMinnie.com's *Case of the Day* (http://www.auntminnie.com), and the Society of Pediatric Radiology's *Case of the Week* (http://www.pedrad.org).

Perhaps the main reason simulators have not been widely developed for diagnostic radiology is the lack of a perceived need. The impetus of most medical simulators is patient safety, particularly in relationship to resident and fellow training. In diagnostic radiology, the trainees are almost always supervised. This is particularly true for the junior-most residents where their case load is limited both in volume and complexity. For residents, every study is overread by a staff radiologist before the final report is released. During the overread process, trainees are instructed on findings that they missed or overinterpreted. At many institutions, the only time unsupervised preliminary image interpretations are released to the hospital is overnight. Radiology residents must have 1 year of radiology training before they are allowed to take unsupervised call. Even with this regulation, many hospitals have instituted 24-h faculty coverage, making unsupervised image interpretation almost nonexistent.

Given that unsupervised overnight time potentially represents the biggest risk to patient safety in diagnostic radiology, several simulators have been created to help prepare residents for this overnight call [20–28]. These simulators have ranged in complexity in their included cases, included modalities, file format of the digital image, and method of interpretation.

The first digital image simulators focused on specific indications or types of studies to teach one skill such as identifying intracranial hemorrhage on CT of the head or buckle fractures in pediatric patients (Fig. 38.7) [25, 26, 29]. With these simulators, the user was asked to answer one question, namely, is a specific abnormality present or is the study normal? In constructing the simulators, diagnostic images were converted from their native Digital Imaging and Communications in Medicine (DICOM) format to a JPEG formatted image via a screen capture. Digital hotspots were then added so that the user could click on any potential area

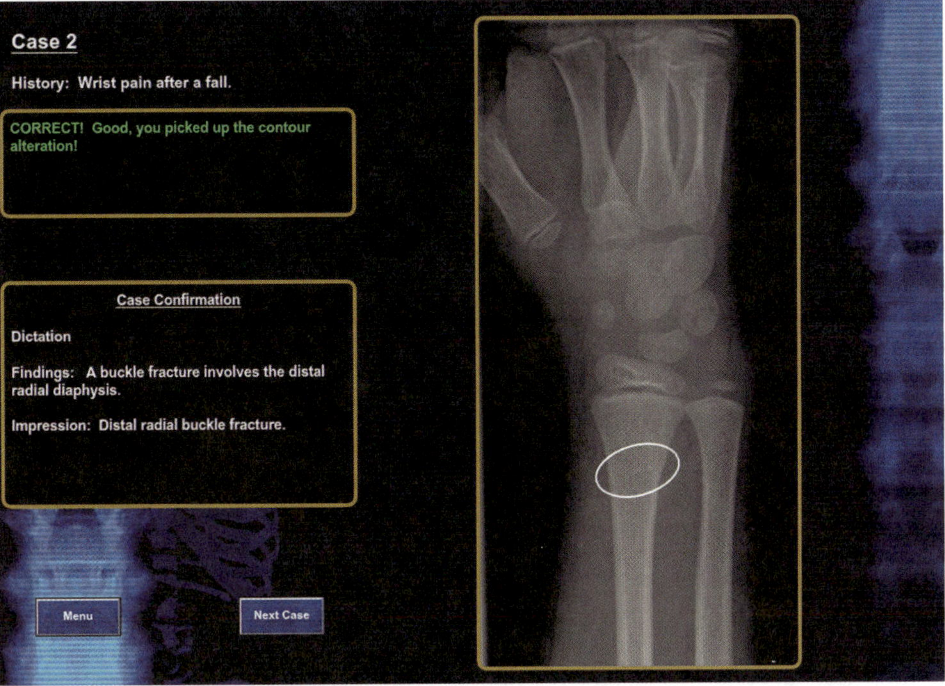

Fig. 38.7 Several indication-specific simulators have been developed. These simulators typically function in a web-based environment where the user clicks on a digital hotspot (*oval*) that contains the finding

of abnormality. Using a pretest and posttest, this type of simulator was shown to be effective in teaching trainees to make a specific finding [25, 26]. There have been no studies evaluating the user's actual clinical performance before and after using this simulator.

There were several advantages to this type of focused simulator. First, the simulator was easy to use and required little training. Second, the user was able to see a large number of challenging cases in a small amount of time. Finally, because users received instantaneous feedback on what they missed, they learned as the simulation module progressed.

Even though these focused simulators were effective, there were several disadvantages that limited their adaptation. First, there are a limited number of diagnoses that have subtle imaging findings yet occur with a high-enough frequency to warrant inclusion into a simulator. Second, even though radiologists work in a digital environment, they are used to DICOM images. Modern picture archiving and communication systems (PACS) allow the user to magnify images, window/level, make measurements, and even provide sharpening algorithms to improve edge detection. Without these tools, the focused simulators are not truly able to mimic a radiologist's work environment. Third, focused simulators often used one or several images, not the entire data set. The trainees knew that if an abnormality was present, it would be on the provided image. While this helps the trainee identify subtle findings on the image and can help with the search pattern, it does not mimic the current practice in radiology where a radiologist must scroll through a large volume of images to make a diagnosis. Finally, the creation of focused simulators was often seen to be too time intensive for the indications where they worked best. Most medical simulators are used to help teach clinicians how to manage rare or particularly dangerous indications. The indications that work best in focused radiology simulators are neither rare nor dangerous.

As the next generation of diagnostic simulators was created, the components of an ideal simulator were discussed [22]. First, it is thought that the simulator should mimic the appearance and functionality of the clinical PACS in use in the radiologist's normal environment. This would allow the radiologist to use the tools required to make a diagnosis in an environment similar to everyday practice. Second, the simulator should accept fully anonymized DICOM data sets. Having the data in a DICOM format would allow radiologists to use the clinical tools with which they are familiar, such as window/level and measurement tools. Perhaps the most significant advantage of having the entire imaging data set is that it allows the radiologist to simulate clinical practice closely by evaluating every image and every sequence for pertinent positive and pertinent negative findings. The third feature of an ideal simulator is easy case entry. For simulators to enjoy widespread use, administrators must be able to add cases quickly with limited interaction. Finally, the ideal simulator should provide both immediate and long-term feedback so that users can assess their progress at every step of their training.

At least one simulator has been created that employs these principles [21, 22]; however, this simulator only works in one environment, at one hospital, for one purpose, and is not commercially available. The simulator was designed using hypertext markup language (HTML) and interfaced to the PACS via an open application programming interface, a feature unique to the Philips iSite PACS (Philips; Best, The Netherlands). While there were features unique to the simulator (such as the worklist, the method of entering the interpretation, and the feedback mechanism), the overall process of image viewing was identical to the clinical practice.

For the most part, diagnostic radiology simulators have not progressed beyond this point. There are several reasons for this failure. Perhaps the main reason that simulators have not been developed is that they cannot meet the first component of an ideal simulator: that they mimic the appearance and functionality of the clinical PACS. Because there are a large number of PACS vendors, it is not possible to create a simulator that will suit every user base.

Even with this limitation, it is possible to create a simulator using a local PACS. The easiest way to do this is to use the test PACS environment (if available) to house each diagnostic study. If the test PACS is used, many of the features of an ideal radiology simulator can be realized: The environment closely mimics the production system, fully anonymized DICOM data sets can be imported to the test environment, and finally, pushing DICOM images between the production and test environments is easy and can be performed by a PACS administrator.

Even though this process works to transfer and view images, there are several limitations. User access to the test PACS environment is often limited; some institutions are limited by the number of user logins that can be assigned to the test PACS. If this limitation exists, the production PACS can be used as a repository for anonymized data sets. This functionality is possible only if the number used as the unique identifier for each study can be manipulated so that two instances of the same study can live in the production environment. While this method has been used at some institutions [30], it may not be an acceptable solution at other locations.

Another major limitation of using the test PACS environment as a simulator is that there is no easy way for users to enter their interpretations. If the test PACS is used, the simplest method of case interpretation is to either allow the user to dictate their interpretation using a digital recorder or to ask the user to write or type their impression. In either scenario, the process is not entirely the same as their standard clinical practice.

The final limitation of using the test PACS as a simulator is that there is no way to provide immediate or long-term feedback to the user. If the interpretation is written down or dictated, a third party must grade the responses. While this method of adjudication can be useful for certain purposes, it does not allow trainees to work independently while tracking their progress.

Simulation for the Practicing Radiologist

There are many potential uses of simulators in radiology besides on-call preparation [22]. Perhaps the use with the biggest potential is in postresidency training. For faculty radiologists, it is often difficult to master a new technique such as MR elastography or effectively read studies with new contrast agents such as hepatocyte-specific contrast agents or blood pool agents. Simulators allow radiologists to read a large volume of cases in a short period of time, gaining the knowledge it would otherwise take months to learn on their clinical service.

Simulators could also be used as part of a continuing medical education program. For example, a course could offer a simulator as a way to augment lectures on a certain topic. The attendees would then be able to use their newfound knowledge to interpret challenging cases and thus solidify their understanding of a new concept. This type of active learning is much more effective than the passive learning employed in typical didactic lectures. Through their strong industry ties, the American College of Radiology (ACR) has been able to create an education center that uses this type of learning. The ACR Classroom has several features to optimize learning including a large volume of educational cases, a small student to faculty ratio, and individual PACS workstations for each learner with their PACS viewer of choice. In addition to providing training, course attendees receive a certificate of completion which can be used to certify competency in certain types of exams such as cardiac CT and CT colonography. While their education center is seen as a model of radiology education, it suffers from a lack of portability (i.e., the cases and simulation cannot be brought home for continued practice).

Simulation for Assessment and Testing

Simulation can also be used as a testing tool. While this concept is standard with simulators in scenarios such as CPR training, it is thus far foreign in radiology. Current testing for maintenance of certification or certificates of added qualification is computer based; however, the exams rely on static images of a specific abnormality and focus on the examinee's ability to make a diagnosis. While this is helpful, it does not truly test the entire process of what makes a good radiologist, namely, the ability to identify findings, recognize pertinent positive and negative findings, form a differential diagnosis, and communicate the results to the ordering health care provider. Simulator-based testing would allow the certifying board to test these skill sets.

In addition to board examinations, simulators could also be used in testing trainees. Through prerotation tests and postrotation tests, radiology residency programs could prove that their trainees had gained competency in certain fields. Competency-based tests could also be used to prove readiness for call or even be a requirement for graduation from a training program. Once validated, this type of testing would allow training programs to have more objective data proving that their graduates are ready to care for patients independently.

Procedural Simulators

The procedural-based simulators used in radiology are more typical of simulators used in other fields of medicine. This class of simulators helps to teach the user a specific task or technique in a safe environment removed from patients. Procedural simulators vary in complexity from the simplest simulators created using typical household objects to the most complex simulators created with advanced computer interfaces and anthropomorphic models. The simulators discussed below are separated by modality.

Ultrasound

Ultrasound simulators have been used for two main purposes: teaching scanning technique and teaching ultrasound-guided interventions. One use of simulators that teach scanning technique is to help prepare junior-level residents to be on call [28]. Ultrasound makes up a large percentage of cases ordered from the emergency department because of its availability, safety, and wide range of indications [28]. While at some hospitals trainees only need to know the basics of scanning in order to be able to troubleshoot difficult cases after hours, at other hospitals the trainee is responsible for both performing and interpreting after-hour scans. In order for a scan to be diagnostic, the sonographer must be able to locate and optimize the organ or abnormality of interest, obtain images in standard planes, provide appropriate measurements, and, if needed, use advanced functionality such as Doppler waveforms. In addition to being able to master all of these skills, the trainee must be able to complete the scan in a timely fashion.

Even though trainees must master the skills of scanning before being able to scan patients independently, it is difficult for them to gain this experience. Modern sonography departments are busy, and rapid patient throughput does not allow time for deliberate training [28]. Because of these limitations, simulator-based training is required. Traditionally, trainees have turned to each other, taking turns at being a mock patient while they let their classmates practice scanning. While this allows the user to get familiar with the machine and certain body parts, it does not allow the user to practice scans such as transvaginal sonography or scrotal ultrasound. To address this concern and to allow for a more standardized education, ultrasound simulators have been developed and are commercially available [28]. These simulators function as stand-alone machines where the sonographer scans a mannequin yet is able to provide real-time ultrasound images. Modules can be purchased to focus on specific body parts such as the abdomen, the breast, or female pelvis. Each module allows the user to scan abnormal patients and practice performing and interpreting the study.

Other ultrasound simulators have been developed to teach users how to scan a small patient population for a specific indication such as craniosynostosis in infants [31]. This type of simulator has typically been used to teach a new technique to users already familiar with ultrasound. The first step in creating an indication-specific simulator is to create a model/phantom for the disease process. Creating a model often requires lots of trial and error; however, several principles should be kept in mind.

There are several features of an ideal phantom for ultrasound [32]. First, the model should have a similar size and shape to the body part being scanned. This allows the user to practice their technique accurately. Second, the phantom should have similar acoustic properties to the desired organ or pathology. Many ultrasound phantoms can be constructed using common household items. Care must be made so that the constructed phantom looks similar to the organ in real life. This again helps the user prepare for the patient scenario. Next, the ideal model would be cheap and easy to produce and be reusable and reproducible. If a simulator program is to be effective, the phantom must be similar each time it is used so that the training experience is standardized. Finally, targets must be distinguishable from surrounding medium and must not corrode with time. If the phantom will be used to test an intervention such as a biopsy, it should be clear to the user when contact has been made with the target.

Ultrasound is commonly used for image-guided biopsies as it has many advantages compared to other imaging modalities [32]. The chief advantage of ultrasound is that it allows for real-time imaging while the procedure is being performed. This allows the interventionalist to watch the needle at all times during the procedure. Because the ultrasound probe is relatively small, patients can often be positioned in a way that is both comfortable and provides an adequate window to the organ or pathology. The final advantage of ultrasound over other types of image guidance is the lack of ionizing radiation.

Even though there are many advantages of ultrasound, its use can be limited due to the skill required to perform ultrasound-guided interventions. Some operators, particularly trainees, find it difficult to control the ultrasound probe with one hand and the needle or biopsy gun with the other hand. Ultrasound simulators have been used to help users gain this skill in a safe environment.

Many simulators have been developed for ultrasound-guided interventions; this chapter will focus on simulators developed for the breast and kidney [32–42]. Simulators for breast ultrasound are typically used to help users learn breast biopsy. While commercial simulators that model the human breast exist [Blue Phantom, http://www.bluephantom.com/product/Breast-Biopsy-Ultrasound-Training-Model.aspx?cid=438; CIRS, http://www.cirsinc.com/products/modality/76/needle-breast-biopsy-phantom-with-amorphous-lesions/; Kyoto Kagaku, http://www.kyotokagaku.com/

products/detail03/us-6.html], many institutions prefer creating their own phantoms using natural materials, such as chicken or turkey breasts, or manufactured materials such as gelatin.

Commercial phantoms have several disadvantages that make them less useful than homemade phantoms [33]. First, the consistency of commercial phantoms is often different than the human breast, and the shape is more dome-shaped compared to the breast in a supine patient. Second, the echotexture is uniform, making the needle easy to identify. While this may be an advantage for early trainees, it differs compared to the experience of working with a real breast. Finally, commercial phantoms are often expensive compared to the low cost of the homemade phantoms.

The homemade breast phantoms often employ fruits or vegetables to simulate lesions [33, 35–37]. Targets that can mimic solid lesions include grapes, peas, potatoes, and olives. Strawberries can be particularly useful as the seeds can help to mimic a calcified lesion [36]. Cysts can be simulated by filling a latex glove with water and tying off the fingers [36, 37]. By simulating different types of lesions, the user is able to practice different techniques such as biopsy and cyst aspiration in the same setting.

Simulators for renal ultrasound have focused on performing renal biopsy and placement of nephrostomy tubes [39–42]. Similar to the breast, commercial renal phantoms are available [Blue Phantom, http://www.bluephantom.com/product/Replacement-kidneys-for-renal-biopsy-ultrasound-training-model.aspx?cid=545; CIRS, http://www.cirsinc.com/products/modality/81/kidney-training-phantom/]; however, many institutions prefer homemade phantoms due to cost. Homemade phantoms can again be biologic or manufactured. Biologic phantoms have been described using the kidneys of recently slaughtered pigs inserted in either a chicken breast or gelatin [40, 41]. The advantage of these phantoms is that the kidneys match the appearance and consistency of the human kidney. The biggest disadvantage of the biologic phantoms is they do not last long before they must be disposed and they pose risks inherent to biologic systems. Manufactured phantoms may avoid the disadvantages of biologic phantoms; however, they are time-consuming to produce, may not look and feel like a human kidney, and, depending on their construction, may not allow the user to perform the range of interventions possible with a biologic phantom.

Fluoroscopy

Most fluoroscopy simulators have been created for interventional radiology and will be discussed in Chap. 38. Only a few simulators have been developed that mimic procedures typically performed in fluoroscopy [43, 44]. Each of these simulators was designed to teach a specific skill.

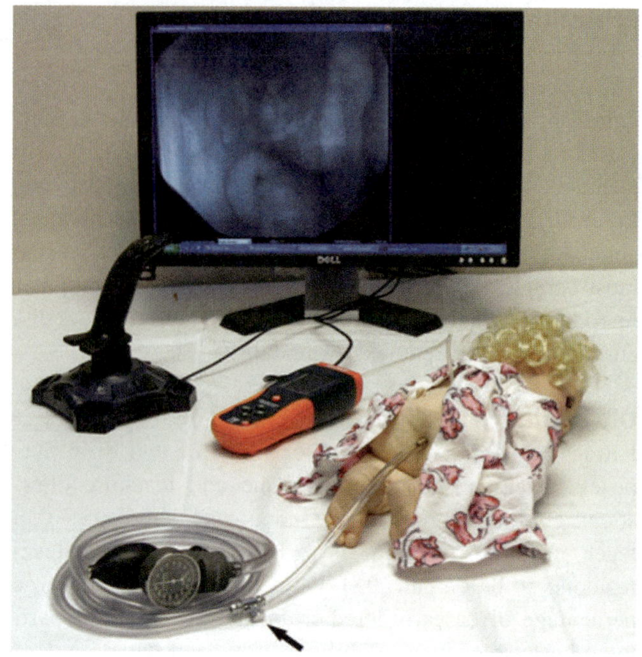

Fig. 38.8 Photograph of a simulator created for practicing intussusception reduction. Plastic tubing with the external release valve (*arrow*) connects the aneroid gauge and bulb insufflator to the cylinder within the doll. Additional tubing extends from the doll to a pressure sensor and is transmitted via USB cable to a computer. The computer displays simulated images taken during an intussusception reduction (Reprinted from Stein-Wexler et al. [43], with permission from Springer)

Intussusception is a relatively common cause of an acute abdomen in children between 6 months and 2 years of age. It is unique in that it is treated with an air or fluid contrast reduction under fluoroscopy. While it is relatively common, more than 40% of radiology residents have little or no experience in treating the disorder [43]. Because fluoroscopic reduction of intussusception can be the definitive treatment, the radiologist must be proficient at performing the procedure. In order to teach trainees this skill as well as how to deal with rare complications, a simulator was developed in one department using a doll and computer interface (Fig. 38.8). This simulator allowed faculty radiologists to teach trainees the technique required to reduce an intussusception without placing a patient at risk. There have been no studies comparing the clinical performance of trainees who have used the simulator versus trainees who did not use the simulator.

The intussusception simulator was designed to teach trainees a technique that is performed infrequently and carries a risk of bowel perforation that, while rare, can be catastrophic. The simulator that was created for gastrojejunal tube placement was designed for different reasons [44]. This procedure is very common and has rare, treatable risks yet is technically demanding. The goal of this simulator is to help trainees become proficient in the technique before they are

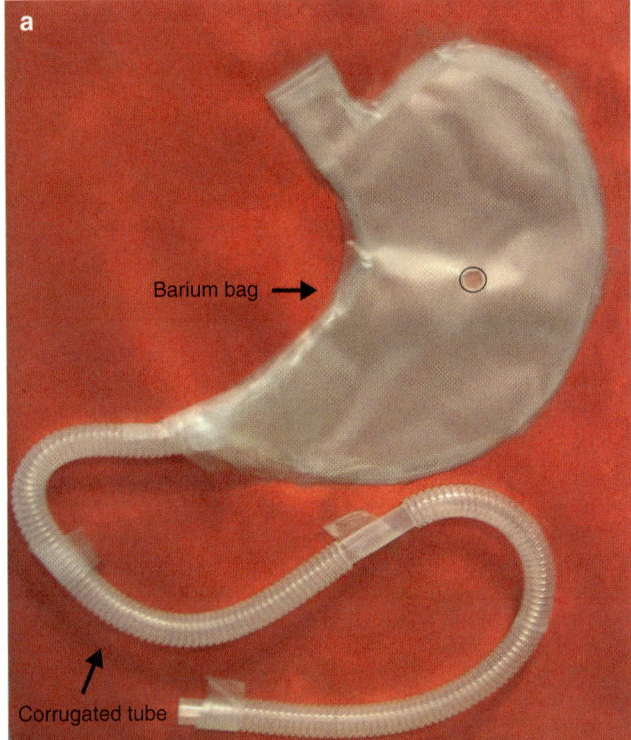

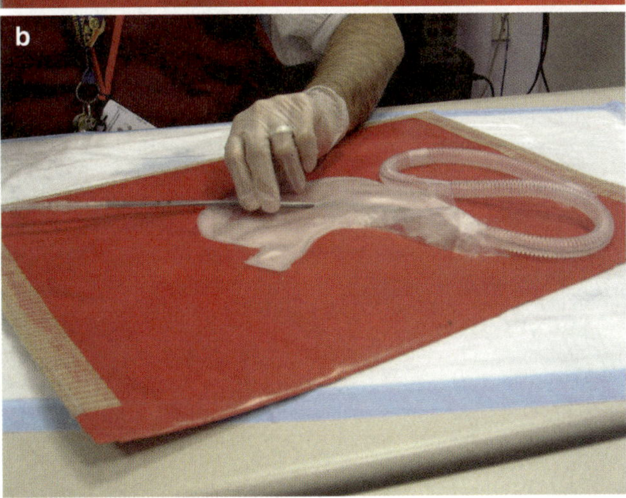

Fig. 38.9 (a) A simulator for placement of a gastrojejunostomy tube was constructed using a barium enema bag cut into the shape of stomach and a translucent corrugated tube bent to simulate the course of duodenum. (b) Image showing a radiology resident practicing placing a gastrojejunostomy tube using the simulator (Images courtesy of Ray Sze, MD)

care for patients to reduce the use of excessive fluoroscopy time. This type of simulator provides an environment where users can repeatedly practice new techniques (Fig. 38.9).

Interventional Radiology

Interventional radiology (IR) involves minimally invasive procedures that require specialized fine motor and visuospatial endovascular skills using imaging (e.g., X-ray fluoroscopy, ultrasound) to guide the manipulation of needles, wires, and catheters in vascular and organ systems. Because of the high level of manual dexterity required to perform procedures, IR is ideally suited for the use of simulator-based training. Several simulators have been developed for this purpose. They are described in detail in Chap. 39.

Conclusion

The current trend in medicine is to move away from the traditional models of learning and toward a more objective/structured approach to education and performance evaluation. This trend is mirrored in radiology where simulators are being used to help prepare patients, test and calibrate imaging modalities, and train radiologists. While the use of simulators in training radiologists has lagged behind other specialties, simulators used for other purposes (such as calibrating modalities) are a part of the standard practice of every radiology department. It is likely that with work-hour restrictions and fewer patient encounters, trainees will have greater exposure to simulation as time goes by, as will practicing radiologists through certification processes and CME.

References

1. Carter AJ, Greer ML, Gray SE, Ware RS. Mock MRI: reducing the need for anaesthesia in children. Pediatr Radiol. 2010;40:1368–74.
2. Hallowell LM, Stewart SE, de Amorim E, Silva CT, Ditchfield MR. Reviewing the process of preparing children for MRI. Pediatr Radiol. 2008;38:271–9.
3. Rosenberg DR, Sweeney JA, Gillen JS, Kim J, Varanelli MJ, O'Hearn KM, et al. Magnetic resonance imaging of children without sedation: preparation with simulation. J Am Acad Child Adolesc Psychiatry. 1997;36:853–9.
4. Pressdee D, May L, Eastman E, Grier D. The use of play therapy in the preparation of children undergoing MR imaging. Clin Radiol. 1997;52:945–7.
5. Edwards AD, Arthurs OJ. Paediatric MRI under sedation: is it necessary? What is the evidence for the alternatives? Pediatr Radiol. 2011;41:1353–64.
6. de Bie HM, Boersma M, Wattjes MP, Adriaanse S, Vermeulen RJ, Oostrom KJ, et al. Preparing children with a mock scanner training protocol results in high quality structural and functional MRI scans. Eur J Pediatr. 2010;169:1079–85.
7. Hartman JH, Bena J, McIntyre S, Albert NM. Does a photo diary decrease stress and anxiety in children undergoing magnetic resonance imaging? A randomized, controlled study. J Radiol Nurs. 2009;28:122–8.
8. Segars WP, Mahesh M, Beck TJ, Frey EC, Tsui BM. Realistic CT simulation using the 4D XCAT phantom. Med Phys. 2008;35:3800–8.
9. Frush DP, Slack CC, Hollingsworth CL, Bisset GS, Donnelly LF, Hsieh J, et al. Computer-simulated radiation dose reduction for abdominal multidetector CT of pediatric patients. AJR Am J Roentgenol. 2002;179:1107–13.
10. Joemai RM, Geleijns J, Veldkamp WJ. Development and validation of a low dose simulator for computed tomography. Eur Radiol. 2010;20:958–66.

11. Hanai K, Horiuchi T, Sekiguchi J, Muramatsu Y, Kakinuma R, Moriyama N, et al. Computer-simulation technique for low dose computed tomographic screening. J Comput Assist Tomogr. 2006;30:955–61.
12. Kim S, Yoshizumi TT, Frush DP, Toncheva G, Yin FF. Radiation dose from cone beam CT in a pediatric phantom: risk estimation of cancer incidence. AJR Am J Roentgenol. 2010;194:186–90.
13. Yoshizumi TT, Goodman PC, Frush DP, Nguyen G, Toncheva G, Sarder M, et al. Validation of metal oxide semiconductor field effect transistor technology for organ dose assessment during CT: comparison with thermoluminescent dosimetry. AJR Am J Roentgenol. 2007;188:1332–6.
14. Hurwitz LM, Yoshizumi TT, Goodman PC, Frush DP, Nguyen G, Toncheva G, et al. Effective dose determination using an anthropomorphic phantom and metal oxide semiconductor field effect transistor technology for clinical adult body multidetector array computed tomography protocols. J Comput Assist Tomogr. 2007;31:544–9.
15. Britten AJ, Crotty M, Kiremidjian H, Grundy A, Adam EJ. The addition of computer simulated noise to investigate radiation dose and image quality in images with spatial correlation of statistical noise: an example application to X-ray CT of the brain. Br J Radiol. 2004;77:323–8.
16. Fefferman NR, Bomsztyk E, Yim AM, Rivera R, Amodio JB, Pinkney LP, et al. Appendicitis in children: low-dose CT with a phantom-based simulation technique – initial observations. Radiology. 2005;237:641–6.
17. Winslow M, Xu XG, Yazici B. Development of a simulator for radiographic image optimization. Comput Methods Programs Biomed. 2005;78:179–90.
18. Fanti V, Marzeddu R, Massazza G, Randaccio P, Brunetti A, Golosio B. A Simulator for X-ray images. Radiat Prot Dosimetry. 2005;114:350–4.
19. Veldkamp WJ, Kroft LJ, van Delft JP, Geleijns J. A technique for simulating the effect of dose reduction on image quality in digital chest radiography. J Digit Imaging. 2009;22:114–25.
20. Desser TS. Simulation-based training: the next revolution in radiology education? J Am Coll Radiol. 2007;4:816–24.
21. Towbin AJ, Paterson B, Chang PJ. A computer-based radiology simulator as a learning tool to help prepare first-year residents for being on call. Acad Radiol. 2007;14:1271–83.
22. Towbin AJ, Paterson BE, Chang PJ. Computer-based simulator for radiology: an educational tool. Radiographics. 2008;28:309–16.
23. Ganguli S, Pedrosa I, Yam CS, Appignani B, Siewert B, Kressel HY. Part I: preparing first-year radiology residents and assessing their readiness for on-call responsibilities. Acad Radiol. 2006;13: 764–9.
24. Yam CS, Kruskal J, Pedrosa I, Kressel H. Part II: preparing and assessing first-year radiology resident on-call readiness technical implementation. Acad Radiol. 2006;13:770–3.
25. Halsted MJ, Perry LA, Perry DJ, Benton C. Development of an interactive model for teaching emergency pediatric radiography: preliminary report. J Am Coll Radiol. 2005;2:701–3.
26. Halsted MJ, Guluzian JK, Little IG, Perry LA, Perry D, Benton C. Development of a new instructional tool to increase the diagnostic accuracy of radiology residents interpreting emergency pediatric neuroradiology studies. J Am Coll Radiol. 2006;3(11):893–4.
27. Halsted MJ, Guluzian JK, Perry LA, Little IG, Benton C. What is normal? A clinically useful reference collection of pediatric radiology cases created within a PACS. J Am Coll Radiol. 2005;2: 189–92.
28. Monsky WL, Levine D, Mehta TS, Kane RA, Ziv A, Kennedy B, et al. Using a sonographic simulator to assess residents before overnight call. AJR Am J Roentgenol. 2002;178:35–9.
29. LoRusso AP, Bassignani MJ, Harvey JA. Enhanced teaching of screening mammography using an electronic format. Acad Radiol. 2006;13:782–8.
30. Gutmark R, Halsted MJ, Perry L, Gold G. Use of computer databases to reduce radiograph reading errors. J Am Coll Radiol. 2007;4:65–8.
31. Ngo AV, Sze RW, Parisi MT, Sidhu M, Paladin AM, Weinberger E, et al. Cranial suture simulator for ultrasound diagnosis of craniosynostosis. Pediatr Radiol. 2004;34:535–40.
32. Nicholson RA, Crofton M. Training phantom for ultrasound guided biopsy. Br J Radiol. 1997;70:192–4.
33. Harvey JA, Moran RE, Hamer MM, DeAngelis GA, Omary RA. Evaluation of a turkey-breast phantom for teaching freehand, US-guided core-needle breast biopsy. Acad Radiol. 1997;4:565–9.
34. Vidal FP, Villard PF, Holbrey R, John NW, Bello F, Bulpitt A, et al. Developing an immersive ultrasound guided needle puncture simulator. Stud Health Technol Inform. 2009;142:398–400.
35. Hassard MK, McCurdy LI, Williams JC, Downey DB. Training module to teach ultrasound-guided breast biopsy skills to residents improves accuracy. Can Assoc Radiol J. 2003;54:155–9.
36. Morehouse H, Thaker HP, Persaud C. Addition of Metamucil to gelatin for a realistic breast biopsy phantom. J Ultrasound Med. 2007;26:1123–6.
37. Meng K, Lipson JA. Utilizing a PACS-integrated ultrasound-guided breast biopsy simulation exercise to reinforce the ACR practice guideline for ultrasound-guided percutaneous breast interventional procedures during radiology residency. Acad Radiol. 2011;18: 1324–8.
38. Phal PM, Brooks DM, Wolfe R. Sonographically guided biopsy of focal lesions: a comparison of freehand and probe-guided techniques using a phantom. AJR Am J Roentgenol. 2005;184:1652–6.
39. Rock BG, Leonard AP, Freeman SJ. A training simulator for ultrasound-guided percutaneous nephrostomy insertion. Br J Radiol. 2010;83:612–4.
40. Strohmaier WL, Giese A. Ex vivo training model for percutaneous renal surgery. Urol Res. 2005;33:191–3.
41. Hammond L, Ketchum J, Schwartz BF. A new approach to urology training: a laboratory model for percutaneous nephrolithotomy. J Urol. 2004;172:1950–2.
42. John BS, Rowland D, Patel U, Pilcher J, Anson K, Nassiri D. Evaluation of the accuracy of 3-dimensional ultrasonography of the kidney using an in vitro renal model. J Ultrasound Med. 2009; 28:155–62.
43. Stein-Wexler R, Sanchez T, Roper GE, Wexler AS, Arieli RP, Ho C, et al. An interactive teaching device simulating intussusception reduction. Pediatr Radiol. 2010;40:1810–5.
44. Hayeri MR, Sze R. An easily constructed simulator facilitates training of radiologists in gastrojejunal tube insertion. Pediatr Radiol. 2010;40:1138–9.

Simulation in Radiology: Endovascular and Interventional Techniques

39

Amrita Kumar and Derek Gould

Introduction

Interventional radiology (IR) and specialties performing endovascular procedures (e.g., vascular surgery, invasive cardiology and cardiothoracic surgery, and neurosurgery) involve minimally invasive procedures that require specialized fine motor and visual-spatial endovascular skills using imaging (e.g., X-ray fluoroscopy, ultrasound) to guide the manipulation of needles, wires, and catheters in vascular and organ systems. Even today, training of complex and core IR skills largely uses a traditional master-apprenticeship model in the fashion of Halstead and Hippocrates, where invasive medical procedures are learned and practiced on patients, albeit with supervision by a senior "master." Although it is time tested and has worked successfully for years, there are many disadvantages associated with this traditional method of training since it can be inefficient, unpredictable, and expensive [1, 2].

As is the case with healthcare in general, there are many influences that have driven the development of simulation within IR [3]. Work hour limits in the USA and Europe limit in-hospital work of trainees, therefore reducing the time and case mix available to train. The popularity of interventional training impacts on the available case mix, which may vary between centers, and inevitably limits exposure to rare and adverse events. Other drawbacks include time and cost of a mentor's supervision, lack of transparency, and the inevitable added risks to patients.

One of the main drivers toward simulation-based education has been a strong emphasis toward patient safety. Reports such as "To err is human" by the Institute of Medicine [4] highlighted for the first time to the public, medical professionals and the government, the realities, and consequences of medical errors. This report stated that 44,000–98,000 patients may die per annum as a result of medical errors in the USA alone and that this is the eighth leading cause of death, exceeding motor vehicle accidents. More than half of these errors were thought to be preventable, and the report specifically recommended reduction of error by using simulation methods to improve the effectiveness of training and patient safety. This has led to patient safety and medical errors being high on the medical and political agendas.

Simulation has been used for some time in other, risk-averse industries such as aviation and the military, introducing environments to train and assess complex and hazardous tasks in safety where the real-world experience is both costly and dangerous. The technical demands of medical tasks similarly require specific cognitive and perceptual-motor skills for success and safety. There are risks of an inexperienced medical trainee learning such skills in an apprenticeship model, and these risks may be reduced through "pre-patient training" that uses medical simulation technologies to improve safety for patients [5].

Benefits of Simulation for IR

The benefits of introducing simulation into a training curriculum for IR include an opportunity to gain experience in an environment free from risk to patients, to learn from mistakes, to rehearse complex cases, and to obtain objective assessments free from bias. A broad range of simulation

A. Kumar, MD, BSc, MBBS, MSc, FRCR (✉)
Department of Medical Imaging,
Royal Liverpool University Hospital, Liverpool, UK

Department of Imaging,
University College Hospital London, London, UK
e-mail: amritasinha@doctors.org.uk

D. Gould, MB, ChB, FRCP, FRCR
Department of Medical Imaging,
Royal Liverpool University Hospital, Liverpool, UK

Department of Radiology,
Royal Liverpool University NHS Trust, Liverpool, UK

Faculty of Medicine,
University of Liverpool, Prescot Street, Liverpool L7 8XP, UK
e-mail: dgould@liv.ac.uk

A.I. Levine et al. (eds.), *The Comprehensive Textbook of Healthcare Simulation*,
DOI 10.1007/978-1-4614-5993-4_39, © Springer Science+Business Media New York 2013

methods include scenarios using actors, trainers, and complete teams; fixed and homemade models; animals and cadavers; augmented reality and virtual environments; and hybrid simulations using a combination of technologies, methods, and arrangements for context. None of these methods fully replicates the "gold standard" fidelity (faithfulness of replication) of the patient, and thus, each method has limitations, including fragility and a lack of variability of fixed models, cost, lack of suitable anatomy and pathology, ethics and political issues of using animals, and hardware challenges for computer simulations. However, simulation can nonetheless replicate key procedural steps and even the complete tasks to a sufficient level of fidelity and content that, once validated, can be used to learn skills that transfer to performance in patients.

While simulator models themselves can be costly to manufacture, simulations can be cost-effectively aligned to a range of specialty groups with common training objectives. This might apply to IR skills that are a focus of interest to related specialties such as endovascular access and procedures in cardiology or vascular surgery. Such simulations have been developed by academic centers in the UK using virtual reality, where the core skills of interpreting 2D X-ray or ultrasound images are reproduced in a simulator in the same way as they are viewed in real-life procedures. These virtual reality (VR) models have been developed using content (visual and tactile) developed from in-depth procedural knowledge with the aim of realistically simulating a patient; such an approach has groundbreaking training potential.

Achieving High-Fidelity IR Simulation

A well-developed simulator should mimic the real-world task, performing the critical actions in real time and allowing the observer to suspend their belief [6]. It should provide appropriate content (what we can actually see, feel, and/or do in the simulation) and fidelity (faithfulness of reproduction) for the key components of the task so that consistent and uniform skills can be learned and assessed.

To attain correct content that realistically reflects the real-world task, developers need to draw upon the in-depth procedural knowledge of subject matter experts (SME) to form a clear understanding of the processes involved in achieving the desired training objectives in the curriculum. The ultimate aim is for the participant to believe in the realism of the artificial field that they are immersed in within the simulated environment. Ideally they should experience the same apprehensions and concerns in the virtual patient, as they would in the real-life setting.

Role of Task Analysis in Development

For this to occur, key steps in a simulation are first identified by a team of human factors experts using task analysis (TA) which acts as the basis of simulator development. Without this there would be little hope to mirror the real-world task or provide effective training.

Although TA techniques have played an important role in the development of training for the last 100 years and formed much of the health and safety legislation currently in operation [7], they are still in their infancy as tools within healthcare. The emergence of TA techniques has started to be used as an educational resource within the medical community, in the development of IR simulators [8] and surgical training [9].

TA originally focused on observable behaviors that complete a given task. However, to fully understand and appreciate complex procedural tasks, a more detailed mapping of operators' thought processes has to be undertaken in the form of hierarchical and cognitive TA. This includes discussions, interviews, and, perhaps, video-recording and observing procedures performed by SMEs. The detailed procedural documentation obtained covers all, or many of the key steps of the procedures and forms the basis of a technical blueprint for simulator model development. Computer-based simulations bring the added benefit of objective assessment of trainee performance, to identify safe completion of a training objective within the target curriculum and allow proficiency-based training. Task analysis also provides the essential data to inform development of relevant metrics that assess safety and correct completion of the specified training objective. The simulator model's metrics which are technical tools, created by computer scientists and supported by SMEs' identification of critical performance steps (CPS) from the TA, using a questionnaire tailored to the task. CPS not only generate a simulator's metrics and assessment report, but can provide evidence for observer-based assessment checklists and global scoring systems.

It can be seen that TA provides essential data for a simulator model's content and development, to create an illusion of the real-world process [10]. The ability to use metrics that have been objectively derived from TA meets a requirement for credibility of the simulator, particularly where there may be consideration of use for credentialing and revalidation purposes. In this way, the TA process defines all aspects of the simulator, how it seems to an observer, its internal algorithms, its operational scope, and what it can assess [8]. All stages of simulator development should be conducted in close collaboration with the credentialing organization and its training curriculum.

Validation

Validation determines the authenticity of the simulation and the relevance of any metrics. An appropriate level of validity is required to ensure fitness for the purpose of training and assessment, before being formally used within a curriculum [11]. To be effective, a simulation should be an accurate representation of the real-world system that would normally be used for a given training objective. Hence validation starts with building the right simulation model for the task to be trained, where development is informed by a detailed task analysis from its inception.

Although validation is new to surgery, it has been well developed in psychology and behavioral sciences. A valid instrument's assessment tools correctly measure procedure steps that are important to safe completion of the training objective (construct validity) and train skills that transfer to actual procedures in patients in the clinical environment (transfer of training) [12]. Validation is usually achieved through the calibration of the model to actual system behavior using the discrepancies between the two, and the insights gained, to improve the model. For medical simulation this process is formed by SME review of the content and appearances of the simulation, feeding discrepancies back to developers until the accuracy of a model's content is judged to be acceptable (content validity).

Once the steps of a simulation are correctly replicated (content validity), and the simulation and its context appear realistic to an operator (face validity), there is a need to demonstrate transfer of training, and that these skills are retained over time (skills maintenance). For predictive validity, the simulation's assessment should predict future competence in patients as confirmed in a subsequent clinical study. Lastly, concurrent validity correlates the new method with a gold standard such that the performance of experts can be distinguished from that of novices during the same time frame.

Although the transfer of skills has been shown for simulations of laparoscopic surgery [13], colonoscopy [14], and anesthesia [15], very few simulations in radiology have been successfully validated to show improvement in technical skills in patients. Some evidence is now being collected for interventional and endovascular procedures [8, 16].

Procedural Simulations in Interventional Radiology

Procedural simulators are of particular interest in IR. Computer-based simulations, in particular, provide IR trainees the chance to learn and be assessed while performing interventional tasks in a safe environment. Integrated computer hardware, interface devices, and custom software provide some realistic tactile sensation and force feedback to enable the user to react in accordance with near real-world visual cues in an on-screen display [17]. Such training may be well suited to IR techniques as it enables trainees to learn basic wire and catheter handling skills, with the promise of allowing experts an opportunity for procedural rehearsal and skills maintenance. It provides procedural simulation with real-time interactions; two-dimensional (and sometimes three-dimensional) graphic displays of angiographic anatomy; mechanical interfaces using real guidewires, sheaths, and catheters that provide some degree of haptic feedback; and modeling of physiologic and pharmacologic responses [18].

Simulators have been incorporated into training programs for physicians learning vascular interventions such as carotid artery stenting (CAS), iliac and renal artery stenting, and visceral procedures such as nephrostomy drainage, ultrasound targeted liver biopsy, and inferior vena cava filter placements.

Endovascular Simulators

Mentice VIST™ (Vascular Intervention Simulation Trainer; Gothenburg, Sweden) claims to be a high-fidelity endovascular simulator that provides realistic hands-on training for angiographic and interventional procedures. The simulator comprises a mechanical haptics interface unit housed within a plastic mannequin cover, a high-performance desktop computer, and two display screens. Modified instruments are inserted through an access port into the haptics device that imparts tactile sensation and force feedback. The physician is able to select appropriate endovascular tools and perform interventional procedures guided by visual cues from the simulated fluoroscopic screen. The performance is measured using assessment parameters such as contrast fluid used, total procedure time, fluoroscopy time, and some clinical parameters (endovascular tools used, stent placement accuracy). A procedure report is provided automatically for each session. At the same time, the construct validity of such a simulation might be enhanced by using evidence-based metrics [12].

The cases available on this simulator include comprehensive modules on cerebral, carotid, coronary, renal, and iliac/SFA angiography, including stenting and coiling. The various modules are claimed to facilitate the development of equipment handling skills and clinical decision-making abilities by providing multiple access options and a variety of patient scenarios, thus challenging the learner's procedural capabilities.

Multiple validation studies proving face and construct validity have been carried out on the VIST, but two important studies have shown that this high-fidelity simulator equates to an effective training and assessment model, with transfer of training being shown in vivo [16, 19]. This has even led to the production of a portable version of the simulator, VIST-C™.

The Simbionix AngioMentor™ Ultimate (Simbionix, Cleveland, OH) is another endovascular trainer that has a similar range of arterial procedures to the VIST including the use of haptics technology. This simulator offers greater emphasis on patient monitoring with a comprehensive drug panel, vital signs and ECG monitoring, drug administration, and response to physiological disturbances (Fig. 39.1).

Even though research has not been performed confirming that the training users receive on this simulator is able to be transferred to real patients, research has confirmed that the AngioMentor can reliably discriminate between different levels of experience when performing a percutaneous endovascular carotid stenting procedure, thus demonstrating construct validity [20]. This has led to two further device versions including the AngioMentor Express (portable version) and the AngioMentor Express dual access (for use in challenging endovascular procedures that require two access sites in the same intervention).

The Simsuite SIMANTHA® (Medical Simulation Corporation, Denver, CO) is a larger, high-fidelity simulator system incorporating situations with multiple events, immediate feedback, and high sensory load, with up to six interactive screens to facilitate multidisciplinary team training. This system also includes response to patient physiology features,

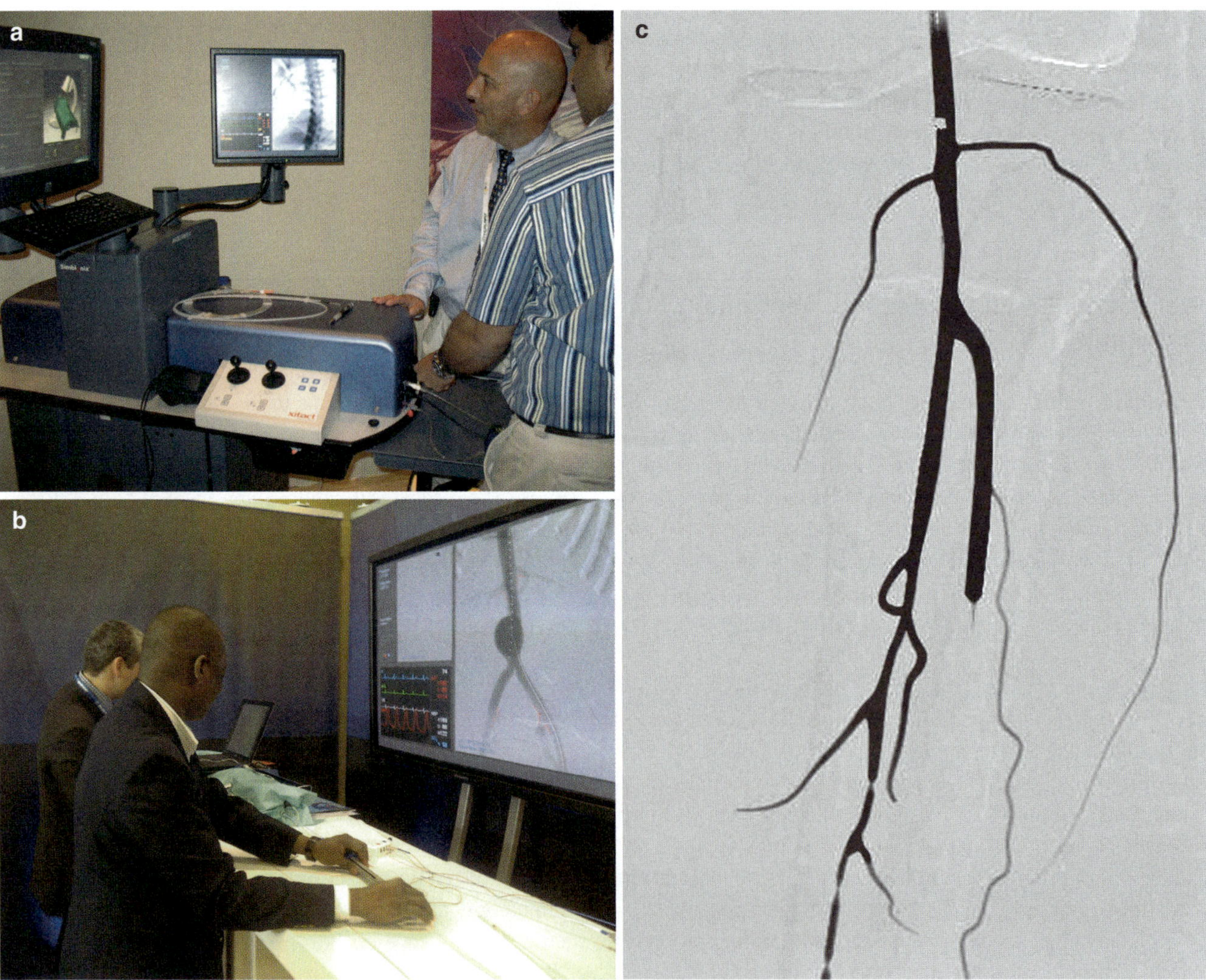

Fig. 39.1 Simbionix AngioMentor: (**a**) AngioMentor workstation, (**b**) workstation with projected image (note physiologic data inlay), (**c**) virtual angiographic image, (**d**) CT image corresponding to fluoroscopic views of abdominal aortic aneurysm, and (**e**) vascular segmentation workstation showing aortic pathology and corresponding CT images (Photos used courtesy of Simbionix)

Fig. 39.1 (continued)

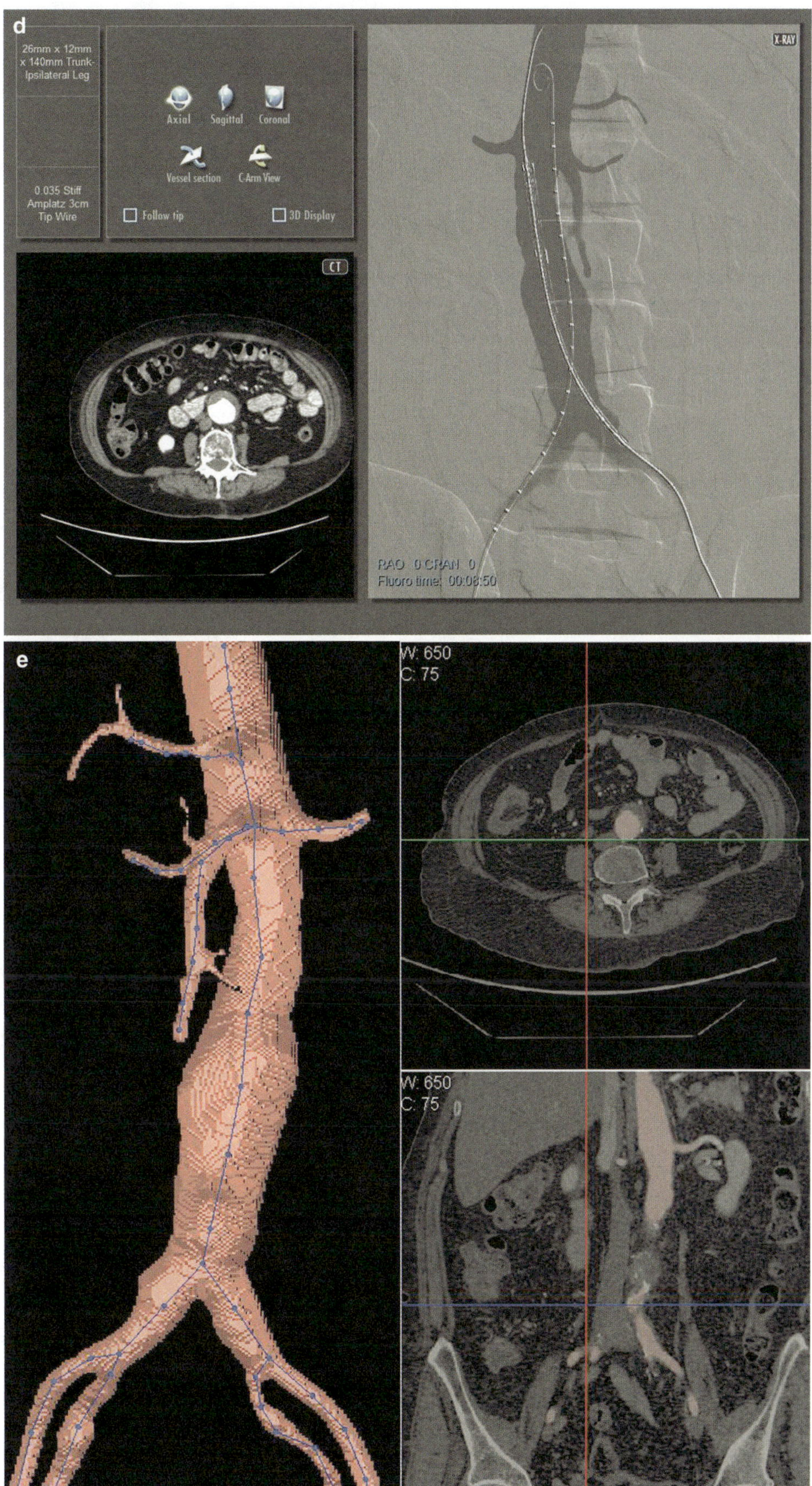

as well as covering the procedural and skills training of the entire process of care.

A study performed using this simulator showed significant improvement in the technical skills of nine residents over a 3-day period following simulator-based training [21]. The residents significantly improved in three categories, including total procedure time (decreased 54%), volume of contrast (decreased 44%), and fluoroscopy time (decreased 48%) in repeated simulation-based testing.

The CathLabVR™ (CAE, Montreal, Quebec) also boasts peripheral arterial, carotid, renal, and coronary simulation modules with metrics-based assessment. To date no significant transfer of training study has been carried out with this simulator. There has, however, been evidence for construct validity for cardiac lead placement, which differentiated procedural efficiency (less time in procedure and in fluoroscopy and better tissue visualization by X-ray) among three cohorts according to their experience level [22] (Fig. 39.2).

The latest endovascular simulator that has shown transfer of training is the ImaGINe-Seldinger, developed by the Craive Collaboration in the United Kingdom [23]. This high-fidelity VR simulator consists of two workstations that simulate, separately, the needle insertion and guidewire/catheter exchange steps of the Seldinger technique, together allowing practice of all the steps of this task. ImaGINe-Seldinger incorporates 23 critical procedure steps based on an exhaustive task analyses that allows for more thorough performance assessment and feedback. The multicenter validation study showed that the simulator exhibited face and construct

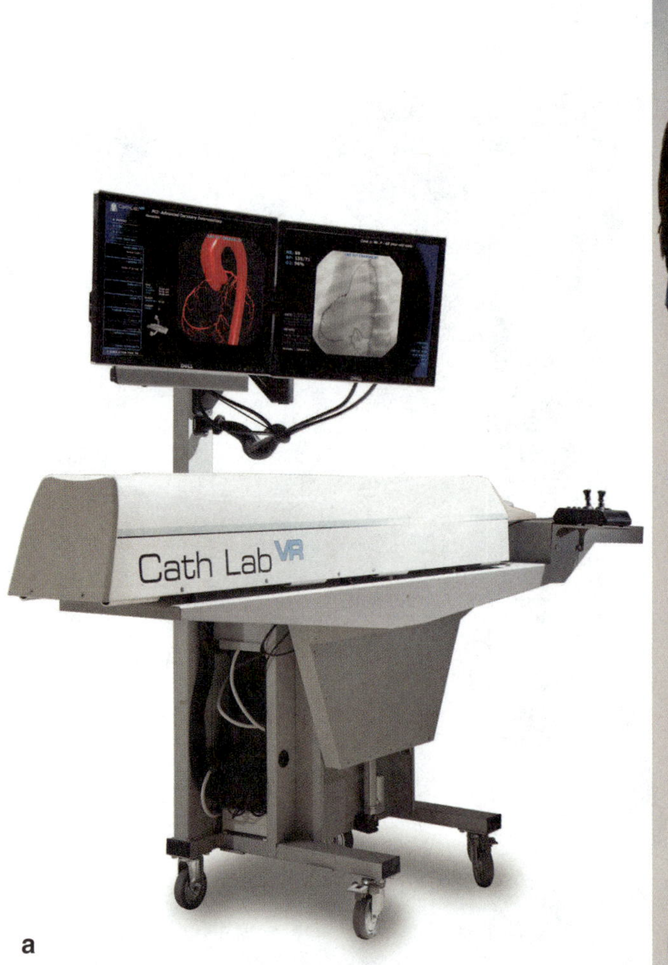

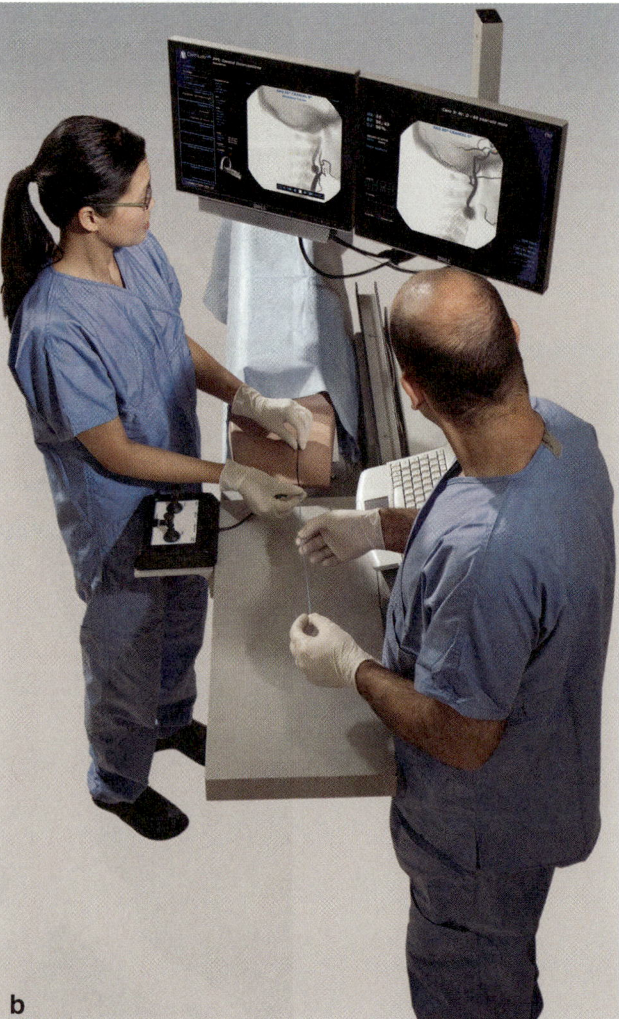

Fig. 39.2 CAE Cath Lab VR: (**a**) Cath Lab VR workstation, (**b**) participants performing cerebral angiogram, and (**c**) screen shot of coronary and aortic angiogram (Photos courtesy of CAE Healthcare ©2012 CAE Healthcare)

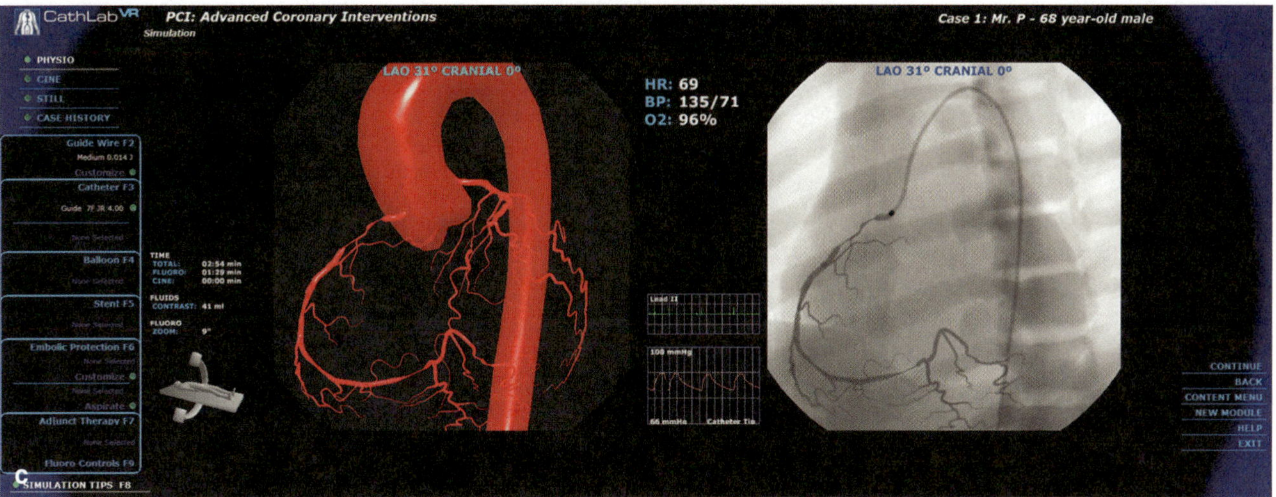

Fig. 39.2 (continued)

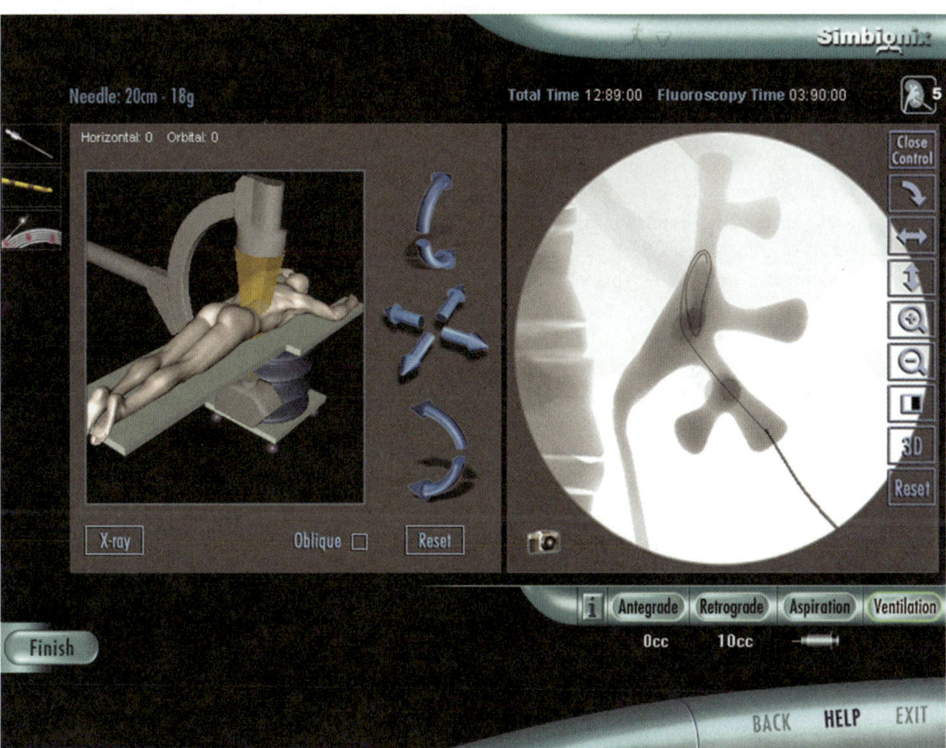

Fig. 39.3 Simbionix Perc Mentor screen shot (Photo used courtesy of Simbionix)

validity, as well as transfer of training; a simulator-trained cohort received significantly higher mean performance ratings than a control group on subsequent patient procedures [23]. This collaboration has gone on to develop the ImaGINe-S simulator for liver biopsy and nephrostomy procedures, showing construct validity with more experienced participants consistently receiving better performance scores on all 19 of the simulator model's performance metrics [8]. In Fig. 39.3, we present a screenshot from the Simbionix percutaneous nephrostomy simulator (Perc Mentor).

Conclusion

The current trend in interventional radiology is to move away from the traditional models of learning and towards a more objective/structured approach to performance evaluation. The presence of face, content, and construct validity will normally indicate an effective training and assessment tool, but this cannot be automatically assumed. There is a need for objective, transfer of training studies to fully sanction the use of a simulation as a training and assessment tool. As has been discussed, there is now evidence to support informed adoption of simulation-based skills training into a range of medical specialities [24]. In interventional radiology, evidence is now accumulating for simulations to commence use within the IR curriculum (see Table 39.1). As a result, it can be seen that medical simulation is here to stay, being best employed to prepare learners for real patient contact.

Table 39.1 Recommendations for adopting simulation into IR curriculum

1. Define target curriculum.
2. Subject matter experts identified by credentialing organization in that curriculum.
3. SMEs identify simulation appropriate curriculum training objectives and content and Critical Performance Steps (CPS).
4. Identify relevant existing simulations that could meet the requirements of content and CPS: (i) Content must be correctly replicated with appropriate fidelity (ii) Metrics must reflect and be specific for CPS for construct validity
5. Require simulator model manufacturers to provide a though specification, including detailed system architecture, intended target curriculum, how and by whom content and metrics were identified and developed, outcomes of any validation studies.
6. Assess candidate simulations, their specifications, and any prior validation studies.
7. Implementation. Where a minimum of content and face validity is present, a simulation can be considered for curriculum training. For assessments, construct validity must be present.
8. Infrastructure including funding bodies present, rationalize cost, accommodation, monitor training outcomes, and validate in curriculum.
9. Collaborate with local and national simulation networks and organizations, e.g., SIR simulation task force, Philadelphia simulation center, Crossroads Institute.

References

1. Bridges M, Diamond DL. The financial impact of teaching surgical residents in the operating room. Am J Surg. 1999;177:28–32.
2. Salim A, Teixeira PG, Chan L, Oncel D, Inaba K, Brown C, et al. Impact of the 80-hour workweek on patient care at a level I trauma center. Arch Surg. 2007;142:708–12.
3. Bradley P. The history of simulation in medical education and possible future directions. Med Educ. 2006;40:254–62.
4. Kohn LT, Corrigan JM, Donaldson MS, editors. To err is human: building a safer health system. Washington, D.C.: National Academy Press; 1999.
5. Grantcharov T, Reznick R. Teaching procedural skills. BMJ. 2008;336(7653):1129–31.
6. Gould DA, Chalmers N, Johnson SJ, Kilkenny C, White MD, Bech B, et al. Simulation: moving from technology challenge to human factors success. Cardiovasc Intervent Radiol. 2012;35(3):445–53.
7. Militello LG, Hutton RJ. Applied cognitive task analysis (ACTA): a practitioner's toolkit for understanding cognitive task demands. Ergonomics. 1998;41(11):1618–41.
8. Johnson SJ, Hunt CM, Woolnough HM, Crawshaw M, Kilkenny C, Gould DA, et al. Virtual reality, ultrasound-guided liver biopsy simulator: development and performance discrimination. Br J Radiol. 2012;85(1013):555–61.
9. Grunwald T, Clark D, Fisher SS, McLaughlin M, Narayanan S, Piepol D. Using cognitive task analysis to facilitate collaboration in development of simulator to accelerate surgical training. Stud Health Technol Inform. 2004;98:114–20.
10. Bech B, Lönn L, Falkenberg M, Bartholdy NJ, Räder SB, Schroeder TV, et al. Construct validity and reliability of structured assessment of endoVascular expertise in a simulated setting. Eur J Vasc Endovasc Surg. 2011;42(4):539–48.
11. Smith S, Wan A, Taffinder N, Read S, Emery R, Darzi A. Early experience and validation work with Procedicus VA – the Prosolvia virtual reality shoulder arthroscopy trainer. Stud Health Technol Inform. 1999;62:337–43.
12. Gould DA, Kessel DO, Healey AE, Johnson SJ, Lewandowski WE. Simulators in catheter-based interventional radiology: training or computer games? Clin Radiol. 2006;61:556–61.
13. Seymour NE, Gallagher AG, Roman SA, O'Brien MK, Bansal VK, Andersen DK, et al. Virtual reality training improves operating room performance: results of a randomized, double-blinded study. Ann Surg. 2002;236:458–63.
14. Sedlack RE, Kolars JC. Computer simulator training enhances the competency of gastroenterology fellows at colonoscopy: results of a pilot study. Am J Gastroenterol. 2004;99:33–7.
15. Rowe R, Cohen RA. An evaluation of a virtual reality airway simulator. Anesth Analg. 2002;95:62–6.
16. Chaer RA, Derubertis BG, Lin SC, Bush HL, Karwowski JK, Birk D, et al. Simulation improves resident performance in catheter-based intervention: results of a randomized, controlled study. Ann Surg. 2006;244:343–52.
17. Dawson S. Procedural simulation: a primer. J Vasc Interv Radiol. 2006;17:205–13.
18. Dawson DL. Training in carotid artery stenting: do carotid simulation systems really help? Vascular. 2006;14:256–63.
19. Berry M, Lystig T, Beard J, Klingestierna H, Reznick R, Lönn L. Porcine transfer study: virtual reality simulator training compared with porcine training in endovascular novices. Cardiovasc Intervent Radiol. 2007;30:455–61.
20. Weis G, Devaud J, Ramee S, Reisman M, Stone G, Gray W. The use of interventional cardiovascular simulation to evaluate operator performance: The Carotid Assessment of Operator Performance by the Simbionix Carotid StEnting Simulator Study (ASSESS). Simul Healthc. 2007;2:81.
21. Dawson DL, Meyer J, Lee ES, Pevec WC. Training with simulation improves residents' endovascular procedure skills. J Vasc Surg. 2007;45:149–54.
22. Wong T, Darzi A, Foale R, Schilling RJ. Virtual reality permanent pacing: Validation of a novel computerized permanent pacemaker implantation simulator. J Am Coll Cardiol. 2001;37(Suppl A):493A–4.
23. Johnson SJ, Guediri SM, Kilkenny C, Clough PJ. Development and validation of a virtual reality simulator: human factors input to interventional radiology training. Hum Factors. 2011;53(6):612–25.
24. Cleave-Hogg D, Morgan P. Experiential learning in an anaesthesia simulation centre: analysis of students' comments. Med Teach. 2002;24(1):23–6.

Simulation in Basic Science Education

40

Staci Leisman, Kenneth Gilpin, and Basil Hanss

Introduction

Simulation is now ubiquitous in medical education. Throughout the continuum of learning, opportunities have arisen for further integration of this teaching technique, and educators have, for the most part, embraced this evolution fully. While the clinical portion of medical education lends itself well to the use of simulation, the basic science years are also an area where simulation may address many educational challenges and demands. In this chapter, we will discuss some of the key tenets of medical education from which simulation has emerged. We will Presents some potential uses for Simulation, in the preclinical years. Finaly we will also take a brief diversion and dicuss some of the challenges with a specific focus on hemodynamic modeling for physiology instruction.

A History of Changes in Medical Education

Since the influential Flexner Report in 1910, the standard framework for American medical education has been two preclinical years of basic science education, followed by 2 years of clinical, apprentice-based teaching in a hospital setting [1]. Flexner realized that after a comprehensive study of basic science, future physicians would need to learn how to apply that knowledge to care for patients. To address this, he advocated for additional clinical years in which students would train underskilled clinicians, integrating basic science knowledge with the realities of patient care. He believed that the best teachers would be physician-scientists skilled in investigation, research, and patient care and that students would benefit from having the same teachers throughout their medical education. By World War I, all medical schools had adopted his recommendations [2], and the basic framework for medical education that Flexner promoted has remained more or less intact to the present.

Since Flexner's time, however, the medical education landscape has changed dramatically. Recent advances in learning theory have posited that adults learn best when facts and concepts are presented in the appropriate context [3], yet students continue to have most of their preclinical education presented in large lecture hall formats. As science itself becomes ever more specific, there are fewer clinician-scientists who can devote equal attention to both their bench work and clinical work, as research is no longer primarily based on the direct observation of patients, but rather on molecular mechanisms and models [4]. This results in medical students spending their preclinical years learning basic science from full-time scientists, to be later instructed by junior and senior clinicians during their clinical clerkships. Unfortunately, these same clinicians often have time constraints preventing them from optimally teaching basic science during the clerkships [5]. Simultaneously, major changes to healthcare and science financing have evolved, such that medical schools and teaching hospitals derive significant funding from governmental sources. This puts a substantial burden on scientists to publish, and for clinicians to see patients, which also constrains their educational efforts [4]. Medical residents, another prime source of teaching to medical students, increasingly are being subject to work-hour restrictions, further limiting the available time for teaching students on clerkships. Finally, due to pressures from managed care organizations, patients are frequently discharged once they achieve clinical stability, which limits

S. Leisman, MD (✉) • B. Hanss, PhD
Department of Medicine, Icahn School of Medicine at Mount Sinai, One Gustave Levy Place, Box 1243, New York, NY 10029, USA
e-mail: staci.leisman@mssm.edu; basil.hanss@mssm.edu

K. Gilpin, MD, ChB, FRCA
Department of Anaesthesia, Cambridge University, Cambridge, UK

Anaesthetic Department, Cambridge University Hospital, 15 High Street, Little Eversden, Cambridge, UK
e-mail: kenneth.gilpin@nhs.net

A.I. Levine et al. (eds.), *The Comprehensive Textbook of Healthcare Simulation*,
DOI 10.1007/978-1-4614-5993-4_40,

Fig. 40.1 Changes in physician culture (Reprinted from Morrison et al. [12], with permission from Wiley)

Changes in Physician Culture between the 1910 Flexner Report and 2010

The 20th century physician	The 21st century physician
• Accumulate knowledge	• Acquire and use knowledge
• Individual scholarly work	• Interdisciplinary research teams
• Autonomous	• Collaborative
• Cooperative	• Share accountability
• Individual achievement	• Interdisciplinary teams
• Solo experts (physician-centered)	• Coordination of care (patient-centered)

students' time to see cases from start to finish [6] and decreases the variety of the cases seen [7]. Thus, medical students may not be exposed to optimal levels of basic science and clinical integration during their clerkships. Simulation, starting in the preclinical years, is a rational way to have students overcome these potential deficits.

Changes in the Medical Education Landscape Since Flexner's Report

As the medical landscape has changed—increased specialization, an explosion in mechanistic knowledge and available treatments, changes in payment models, and the prominence of other members of the medical team—so too have the requirements of the physician. In contrast to the long-standing paradigm of a solo generalist physician treating every problem, in today's medical practice, no one physician is able to master the enormous complexity of medical knowledge and treatments, and so patients now see a multitude of specialists. The healthcare team has expanded from a physician and nurse, to include dietitians, social workers, case managers, nurse practitioners, physician assistants, and medical specialists from various areas. It is no surprise then that team training is increasingly being recognized as a key feature to prevent medical errors [7] and to ensure optimal care for the patient [8] (Fig. 40.1).

To help address this, medical education has naturally evolved over the past 40 years—first, with the focus on small group, case-based learning and second, with the introduction to clinical medicine occurring earlier in the students' education. Beginning in 1969 at McMaster University in Ontario [9], case-based learning and small group formats began to permeate modern medical schools. By 2003, 70% of all US medical schools reported using problem-based learning (PBL) in the preclinical years [10]. Problem-based learning was designed to integrate basic and clinical sciences and represented a fundamental shift from lecture-based learning. The hallmark of PBL is small student-led teams, working together and applying basic science principles to help solve a clinically based case. Problem-based learning is thought to improve retention by focusing students on larger scientific principles, fostering independent learning, expanding teaching methodology, and allowing learning to occur in a more realistic setting [11]. Additionally, problem-based learning teaches students skills critical to working as a team; in order for students to best manage the case, they must communicate well, work together, and teach and learn from one another [12]. It has been suggested that prior to the emphasis of case-based learning, mastery of basic science was presented as an end unto itself, instead of emphasizing its importance and application to the practice of clinical medicine. In case-based learning, students understand why basic science instruction is relevant for their future as physicians [9]; however, despite its benefit, schools primarily used PBL to complement formal, more traditional teaching, with only 6% of programs in 2003 using PBL for more than half of their instruction [10].

Schools also began to experiment by introducing clinical experiences upon entry into medical school, rather than waiting until the later clinical years. In the 1990s, medical history and physical exam skills were still taught in a classroom—a setting devoid of patient encounters. Schools experimented with making these tasks more realistic by allowing students to practice their history and physical exam skills on real or standardized patients. Students were given opportunities to use these skills early in their medical education and to integrate them with other courses; surveys revealed that students responded favorably to those changes [13].

Flexner Revisited

Acknowledging both the changes in medical education, the shifting culture of the physician, as well as the changes in healthcare and science, multiple groups revisited the Flexner Report at its centenary and used that opportunity to issue new guidelines for medical education [2, 5]. The International Association of Medical Science Educators (IAMSE) surveyed leaders in medical education, including the national organizations of multiple basic science specialties. The consensus of the various groups was that basic science studies should be early and throughout the 4 years of medical school to improve knowledge retention. They advocated for increased integration of the basic and clinical sciences, with an emphasis on feedback and mastery of knowledge, rather than having basic sciences front loaded into the medical school curriculum. In one suggested approach, which they termed "ICE" (Ideas, Connections, and Extensions), students are first introduced to an *idea*, they then *connect* that idea with other teachings to place it within a contextual framework, and finally they *extend* the teaching by applying it to real-life examples. One of the suggested methods to improve the basic science and clinical integration is via the use of simulators [5].

The Carnegie Foundation, who commissioned the original Flexner Report, also chose to review the state of medical education at the 100-year anniversary of Flexner's seminal work. Central themes in the commission's recommendations were the need to make the learning process more learner centric, the "integration of formal knowledge and clinical experience, and the development of habits of inquiry and improvement" [2] (Fig. 40.2). Many of their recommendations, including connecting formal teaching to clinical experiences, providing challenging problems and giving students the ability to participate in authentic care, and incorporating teamwork into the curriculum, are well suited to simulation. Simulation lends itself to integration of basic science and clinical work and promotes both teamwork and scientific inquiry by engaging learners in challenging problems and giving them tools with which to participate.

Simulation Is Widely Practiced in Medical Schools

Medical simulation is most often associated with clinical education; indeed, the earliest examples of medical simulation involved obstetric mannequins, and mannequins designed to teach airway and resuscitation, which have existed since the 1950s [14, 15]. In the intervening years, the field of simulation has seen vast improvements in the fidelity and accuracy of these models, and its use has become widespread in medical education. A 2010 survey of 90 medical schools by the AAMC showed that 84 and 91% of respondents used simulation in the 1st year and 2nd year courses, respectively. Per the survey, the most common courses in which simulation was employed were Clinical Skills, Introduction to Clinical Medicine, and Physical Diagnosis, suggesting that while simulation use is widespread in the preclinical years, it is still predominantly being used to enhance clinical medicine experiences rather than for basic science education (Fig. 40.3). Less than half of the schools surveyed used simulation in nonclinical subjects such as anatomy, pharmacology, and physiology [6].

To some degree, simulation in preclinical education is not a new concept. Anatomy courses, in which students dissect cadavers to learn the relationships between physical structures, have been a part of medical education for centuries. Physiology and pharmacology courses have long employed animal labs to simulate the physiologic responses to pharmacologic and physiologic intervention. These animal labs are particularly useful for augmenting lecture material by demonstrating core physiologic concepts, such as cardiac and pulmonary function, and the physiologic responses to perturbations to homeostasis. Students must generate hypotheses, manipulate variables, and observe and record their effects; the labs allow participants to integrate core concepts and appreciate the interrelatedness and unpredictability of live bodies [16]. Animal labs are not without their limitations—they are expensive and time-consuming, employ an animal surrogate to teach about the human body, and are fraught with ethical considerations. They present a large amount of data quickly, requiring students to focus on numerous variables simultaneously [16]. Should students miss a critical feature of the experiment, it is difficult to go back and redo that portion. There are a finite number of interventions (such as drugs) that can be performed per session—and if a mistake is made, the organ cannot be "reset." There are limitations on the measurements, which can be performed on an organ—especially within the economic constraints of the student laboratory. Due to changing cultural attitudes towards vivisection, some students have difficulty focusing on the goals of the experiment [16], whereas others have found that a large majority of students exposed to a dog laboratory found it to reinforce lecture material, despite approximately 20% of students reporting discomfort in using dogs to demonstrate pharmacologic concepts [17]. As technologic capabilities have expanded, high fidelity and computer simulators seemed ideal replacements for these animal labs.

Simulation in Preclinical Years

Simulation for clinical education, both in clerkship training, residency, and postresidency, has been extensively studied, with the earliest published report from 1969 [18]. A recent meta-analysis, spanning 20 years of data, showed that simulation-based medical education with clinical practice was superior to traditional medical education for acquisition of skills that ranged from laparoscopy and central venous catheter insertion to advanced ACLS and cardiac auscultation [19]. As the equipment and expertise have become more widespread among medical school and training programs and faculty have become adept at their use, it is no surprise that they have moved into the preclinical years.

Problematically, research on simulation in the preclinical years is sparse and typically consists of reports from one center. A 2007 conference on Educational Research rated simulation the highest priority for educational research (out of 11 possible options) [20]. One key item discussed by

Theme	The Carnegie Report of 2010 — Challenges	Recommendations
Standardization and individualization	• Medical education is:	• Standardize learning outcomes through assessment of competencies
	○ Not outcomes based	• Individualize learning process, allow opportunity to progress within and across levels when competencies are achieved
	○ Inflexible	• Offer elective programs to support the development of skills for inquiry and improvement
	○ Overly long	
	○ Not learner-centered	
Integration	• Poor connections between formal knowledge and experiential learning	• Connect formal knowledge to clinical experience, including early clinical immersion and adequate opportunities for more advanced learners to reflect and study
	• Fragmented understanding of patient experience	• Integrate basic, clinical, and social sciences
	• Poorly understood nonclinical and civic roles of physicians	• Engage learners at all levels with a more comprehensive perspective on patients' experience of illness and care, including more longitudinal connections with patients
	• Inadequate attention to the skills required for effective team care in a complex health care system	• Provide opportunities for learners to experience the broader professional roles of physicians
		• Incorporate interprofessional education and teamwork in the curriculum
Habits of injury and improvement	• Focused on mastering today's skills and knowledge without also promoting knowledge-building and an enduring commitment to excellence	• Prepare learners to attain both routine and adaptive forms of expertise
	• Limited and often pro forma engagement in scientific inquiry and improvement exercises	• Engage learners in challenging problems and allow them to participate authentically in inquiry, innovation, and improvement of care
	• Inadequate attention to patient populations, health promotion, and practice-based learning and improvement	• Engage learners in initiatives focused on population health, quality improvement, and patient safety
	• Insufficient opportunity to participate in the management and improvement of the health care systems within which they learn and work	• Locate clinical education in settings where quality patient care is delivered, not just in university teaching hospitals
Identity formation	• Lack of clarity and focus on professional values	• Provide formal ethics instruction, storytelling, and symbols (honor codes, pledges, and white coat ceremonies)
	• Failure to assess, acknowledge, and advance professional behaviors	• Address the underlying messages expressed in the hidden curriculum and strive to align the espoused and enacted values of the clinical environment
	• Inadequate expectations for progressively higher levels of professional commitments	• Offer feedback, reflective opportunities, and assessment on professionalism, in the context of longitudinal mentoring and advising
	• Erosion of professional values because of pace and commercial nature of health care	• Promote relationships with faculty who simultaneously support learners and hold them to high standards
		• Create collaborative learning environments committed to excellence and continuous improvement

Fig. 40.2 The Carnegie Report of 2010 (Reprinted from Irby et al. [2], with permission from Wolters Kluwer)

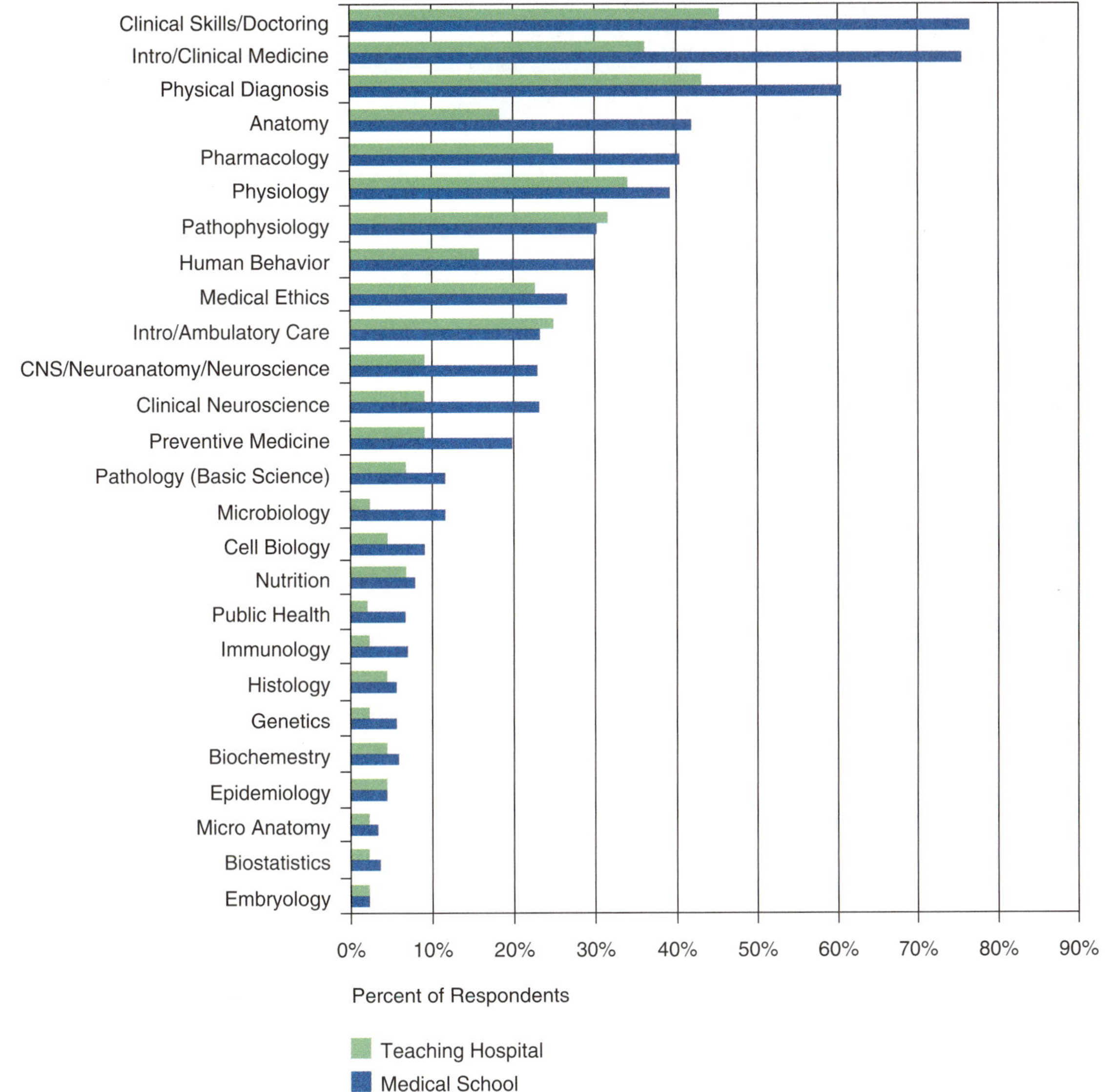

Fig. 40.3 Use of simulation in medical education. From AAMC Survey, September 2011 (©2011 Association of American Medical Colleges. All rights reserved. Reproduced with permission)

researchers is the need for simulation use to be integrated throughout the medical school curriculum, so that students are able to develop expertise over time [21] and benefit from repetitive practice [7]. While these statements refer to task-based simulation, it can be inferred that by introducing simulation earlier, students can develop more general simulation skills: teamwork, facility with mannequins and computers, and familiarity with terms and devices. Students' reflections on their first encounters with patients reveal them to be anxious and insecure—fearful of all there is to remember, a belief that they have insufficient knowledge and skills and guilt over using patients for "practice" [22]. Using simulated patient encounters, even if their primary role is to cement and supplement basic science concepts, may relieve some of that anxiety. A major challenge to integrating simulation more fully into the preclinical years is well-designed, well-validated simulators and simulations that educators will accept as a suitable replacement or function to enhance existing practices and educational activities.

Using Computer Simulation to Teach Basic Science

There are some benefits of using computer models to teach basic science:

1. *Original experiments can be recreated more easily*—Classic experiments, such as the original experimental

work by Starling [23], are relatively easy to construct and provide the opportunity for students to follow the same path of discovery.

2. *Some measurements or interventions are easier to demonstrate with simulation than in vivo*—Pulmonary venous pressure or ventricular volume is technically very difficult to determine due to the constraints of measurement within a living organism. Measuring cell membrane voltages is difficult due to the sensitivity of equipment to ambient noise and is realistically impossible during a busy lab class. These phenomena are relatively easy to demonstrate with simulation as no environmental noise is present in the simulated screen-based environment.
3. *More interventions can be performed within a given time*—The rapidity which a simulation model can be loaded and "prepared" allows multiple experiments on a theme within a given learning session. This is especially true for more complex interventions. A single experiment can be performed several times with each sequence measuring different variables in quick succession.
4. *A simulation can be reset*—Animal organs have a limited lifespan *ex vivo*, and any experimental error is likely to necessitate a fresh preparation. The ease with which a computer simulation can be restarted gives the educator more flexibility to allow students to commit mistakes and take the results to their conclusion.
5. *Virtual organs can be studied in situ*—Studying the heart or lungs as isolated organs belies the fact that their function depends on their environment (in these examples, the vascular system). Giving epinephrine to an isolated heart would increase the heart rate and force of contraction. However, giving epinephrine to a heart *in situ* would also increase the afterload (which in turn affects the heart work, coronary perfusion, and cardiac output) and has an effect of contracting plasma volume and thereby increasing the preload as well.
6. *Entirely virtual systems can be low cost*—Although designing the computer program can be expensive, the marginal cost is thereafter very small as the program can be shared globally. This is in contrast to vivisection, with high marginal and running costs which can be shared via teleconference only partially if at all.

Best Practices in Preclinical Simulation

Whereas simulation in clinical years, especially simulation related to acquisition of procedural skills, has been studied extensively, simulation in preclinical education has not. Most published data has been on individual schools' experience with simulation and/or small, single-center pilot studies, and the published literature includes data on computer- and mannequin-based simulation. However, there have been similar themes that run across these accounts and provide a useful framework for discussion of simulation in basic science education.

Complement of Lecture-Based Material

In all reports, the simulator is used to enhance, rather than teach, the primary material. The simulated cases should be designed to enhance course objectives and goals [24]. Typically, simulators require the consolidation of knowledge gained from the lecture hall, independent study, and real-life experiences of the students, who have had limited experience with clinical medicine. Because the goal is not to treat and cure the patient, but to explore and expand upon basic science foundations, students should be encouraged to suggest and use drugs/interventions that may not exist or be optimal treatment but are physiologically and/or pharmacologically plausible [24]. For example, if the simulated patient was exhibiting bradycardia, students could elect to give atropine (a medication that opposes vagal action), epinephrine (a beta-agonist), or say "we should give a drug that would oppose the vagus nerve." Simulation is also best served when it is integrated carefully into the curriculum, allowing students to contextualize the scientific material which they have been presented [25]. Much like simulation cannot replace clinical experience, simulation should not replace traditional basic science education. It requires thoughtful placement into the curriculum, serving to enhance and exemplify teaching, but not be the primary learning modality, and is optimal when it is a mandatory, not optional, activity [7].

Expert Instructor, Defined Group Size, and Defined Timeline

Most reports indicate that simulation groups function best with 1–2 expert instructors, who can both provide accurate and physiologically sound responses to student intervention and have expertise in the working of the software [24, 25]. Having experts assist with simulation also allows prompt recognition, and correction, of any inaccuracies within the simulator and ensures that students do not leave the simulation session with misconceptions about the normal physiologic and/or pharmacologic responses [25]. The cases should be managed exclusively by the students, with instructor observing closely and interjecting only to guide (but not rescue) the students should they become stuck or suggest an inappropriate intervention [24]. Groups should be small enough so that all students can participate and be engaged and large enough to obligate students to work as a team. Team training is increasingly recognized as a critical skill in caring of patients, as medical students will eventually be required to work with other physicians, nurses, social workers, and other allied health professionals [7, 12], and by introducing team training early into the medical school curriculum, students will develop tools for successful teamwork. Additionally, research has shown that when students are required to teach each other, and use data to solve problems, they learn more than when they are listening to lecture or are reviewing notes [12] and that students working in collaborative settings demonstrate more enthusiasm for collaborative approaches compared to students working in lecture-based settings [13]. However, care should be taken to avoid a too large a group, because when groups become too large, students are not able to participate as well and may not be able to observe relevant changes [26]. We generally limit our mannequin-based simulation groups to ten or less.

Deliberate Practice and Individualized Learning

The educational literature increasingly recognizes that for optimal performance to occur, certain criteria of deliberate practice must be met, including repetitive performance of the skill (including cognitive skills) and skills assessment with specific feedback [7]. Deliberate practice has been validated in clinical skills such as bedside cardiology, advanced cardiac life support, surgical skills, and invasive procedures [19]. Data on the use of deliberate practice in learning and integrating basic science knowledge are lacking, but studies have shown that students perform better on examinations when the test items are designed as clinical vignettes, suggesting that retention is improved when students are required to use basic science in a clinical context rather than as isolated facts [5]. Active participation by learners allows them to focus on the core concepts that they need to master and proceed at a pace that best suits them [7]. To further promote individualized learning, some centers have implemented "simulator on demand" sessions that allow students to reserve time with the simulator and trained facilitators and explore topics which they have found difficult [25].

Debriefing

High-quality simulation requires scheduled and thorough debriefing by a clinician or other expert teacher [15]. In a 2005 systematic review of best practices in medical education simulation, almost half of the papers reviewed listed feedback as the most critical feature of simulation [7]. The teacher's role is to integrate the features of the case with the objectives of the course, assist the students in reflecting on their experience in caring for their "patient" [24], and compare and contrast the methods of treatment employed by the students. The facilitator also guides preclinical students in the subtleties of the language and syntax of patient care—discussing the chief complaint of the patient, the ways in which students form and test hypotheses, and conclusions they draw from the signs and symptoms the patient demonstrates. In this way, the students are better prepared with an organizational foundation for their clinical years [24]. Feedback is essential to medical simulation and one of the most challenging for preceptors to master. A study comparing oral, videotape assisted, and no debriefing found that oral and videotape-assisted feedback were equally successful in improving nontechnical skills (teamwork, task management, situation awareness, and decision making) but that participants who had not received feedback had no improvement on a posttest [27]. Successful feedback can be videotaped, oral, or built into the simulator [7], but should include 12 evidence-based best practices, which have been adapted by McGaghie to simulation feedback (Table 40.1).

Table 40.1 Evidence-based best practices in simulation feedback

Debriefs must be diagnostic
Ensure that the facilitators create a supportive learning environment for debriefs
Encourage team leaders and team members to be attentive of teamwork processes during performance episodes
Educate team leaders on the art and science of leading team debriefs
Ensure that team members feel comfortable during debriefs
Focus on a few critical performance issues during the debriefing process
Describe specific teamwork interactions and processes that were involved in the team's performance
Support feedback with objective indicators of performance
Provide outcome feedback later and less frequently than process feedback
Provide both individual- and team-oriented feedback, but know when each is most appropriate
Shorten the delay between task performance and feedback as much as possible
Record conclusions made and goals set during the debrief to facilitate feedback during future debriefs

Data from McGaghie et al. [21], with permission from Wiley

The difficulty in providing feedback that meets best practices is that it is labor, resource, and time intensive. Facilitators need to be trained in administering simulation and providing feedback; because simulation is often done in small group settings, multiple facilitators are required.

Students Appreciate and Value Their Simulation Experiences

Overall, students rate simulation experiences very highly, believing them worthwhile and recommended for future courses and other students (Table 40.2).

Numerous studies, across multiple centers and fields of study, show students believe that simulators enhance and

Table 40.2 Student rating of simulation experiences

Study author and date	Was simulation experience: Worthwhile?	Recommend for future years/ other courses (% who agreed)
Zvara, 2001 [29]	95%—worthwhile 85%—contributed to understanding	92%
Samsel, 1994 [17]	4.78 out of 5 5 = very useful	4.89 out of 5 5 = highly recommended
Tan, 2002 [27]	94.5%	96%
Rodriguez-Barbaro, 2008 [30]	81%	NA
Gordon, 2006 [31]	90%	90%
Heitz, 2009 [32]	97%	NA

improve their knowledge of physiology [6] and allow them to more easily grasp concepts [26] and see realistic changes [26]. Students and teachers who have used computer modeling to simulate renal and cardiovascular physiology have reported improved integration and understanding of physiologic processes and assisted in conceptualizing "whole-body homeostasis" when combined with traditional lecture-based learning [28]. When computer simulation has been applied to neurophysiology to demonstrate membrane potentials, a large majority of students believed that the program increased their understanding [29]. While such self-efficacy data represent "soft" outcomes on the surface, having students believe in their own education is a major challenge to educators in many fields. Almost universally, simulation improves student confidence in themselves and in the instruction they received. That alone can be a victory for educators.

Simulators' Impact on Learning Is Less Clear

While numerous studies have indicated students *believe* that simulation improves their understanding of scientific concepts, the data on their effectiveness as a learning tool is mixed when compared to traditional learning formats [18, 26, 29–32]. Some researchers have found improvements in immediate and long-term testing [30, 33], and others have found that students who were exposed to simulation were better at making measurements, but scored equally in their understanding of neurophysiologic events [31]. Students exposed to a large-group autonomic nervous system simulation were able to recall data presented during the simulator, but were not able to apply that data to a different clinical scenario [29]. In other reports, after exposure to a simulator, students and teachers felt that the students could be overwhelmed by the large amount of data received and had difficulty in determining the relevant data [28] and that changes occurred too quickly for students to appreciate the key points to be learned [26]. Other data, from non-simulation literature, have shown that when students are given a basic science mechanistic explanation of diseases, students' retention of the disease's clinical features is improved [34]. Cook, in a comprehensive review and meta-analysis from 2011, found that simulation was associated with large gains in knowledge outcomes compared to pre-intervention or no-intervention controls, but noted that there was large variation among studies and some studies that reported negative findings [32]. Overall, there is a clear need for more research into the effectiveness in simulation on learning basic science concepts, especially given its costs.

Limitations of Simulation

Cost

Compared to a lecture format—in which one needs an auditorium with basic audiovisual equipment—running simulators can be extremely expensive. Schools must meet the capital cost of purchasing simulation equipment and budget for the recurrent cost of repairs, support, and upgrades. Medical schools on average dedicate 33 rooms for simulation, with an average 6,400 square feet, although those numbers include space dedicated for standardized patient exams. In 2009, the annual operating budgets for simulation centers was not consistent, but about half of the schools had an annual budget of less than $500,000 [6] (Fig. 40.4). The majority of the funding for medical school simulation-related expenses comes directly from the medical school [6].

However, as simulation becomes more prevalent in residency and clinical programs, it is possible for the preclinical students to borrow the simulators and faculty that exist for other purposes. For simulation which is entirely virtual, there is the potential to save money as computer software has a low marginal cost and requires no excessive space to be housed, and as technology advances, the cost of simulators

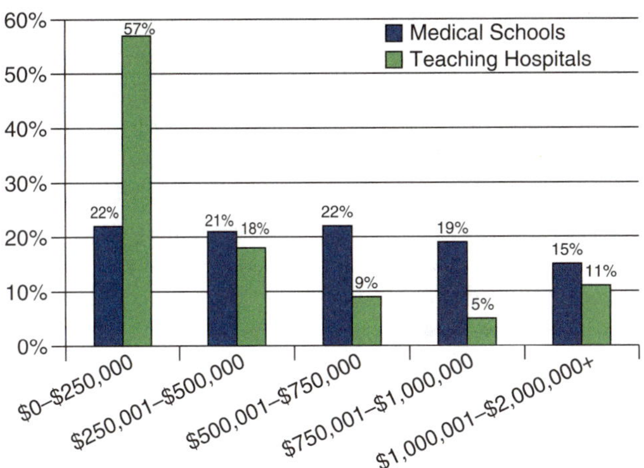

Fig. 40.4 Operating budgets for simulation centers. From AAMC Survey of Simulation in Medical Schools, September 2011 (©2011 Association of American Medical Colleges. All rights reserved. Reproduced with permission)

has also fallen [6]. Some have suggested adapting existing teaching cases to the simulator, obviating the need to develop entirely original cases for simulator use [35].

Trained Personnel

Personnel must be trained in equipment use and troubleshooting, with the median number of dedicated, full-time equivalent personnel reported by respondents in 2010 to be 5 (including administrators, curriculum authors, technicians, facilitators, and directors) [6]. As mentioned above, for immersive model-driven simulation, facilitators/educators must have a sound knowledge of physiology. Representative teaching cases must be written and programmed thoughtfully, with input from the simulation staff and the course directors of the subjects being integrated. These new time demands are occurring simultaneously with rising clinical and research productivity demands, which can limit the available time for teaching [2]. Finding adequate numbers of faculty required to run simulations and debrief afterwards can be challenging. Some data have suggested that residents can be trained as experts [36] (see Chapter 41, The Clinical Educator Track for Medical Students and Residents, which discusses a successful strategy used in the Department of Anesthesiology at Icahn School of Medicine at Mount Sinai) or that students can learn in larger group formats or via teleconference [29, 36], although these scenarios may not be ideal for all educational scenarios.

Clinicians have billing requirements, and scientists are pushed to write and obtain grants; incentives need to be given when pulling them away from traditional "money-making" activities. Medical education funding has been a noted challenge. One strategy that has been promoted by the University of Washington is to formalize agreements between departmental chairs and the simulation center, in which departmental chairs fund and ensure protected time for interested faculty's efforts in the simulation center, in exchange for access to the simulation center and the establishment of a dedicated faculty member to teach that department's trainees. They also advocate teaching portfolios to be used when considering academic promotion and have found that these strategies have resulted in 95% retention of their faculty pool [37].

Limited Time

Because medical schools have a limited amount of time in which to teach students, any expansions of the curriculum inevitably result in decreases in time for other components. Medical school curricula have undergone numerous modifications over the years, in response to biomedical discoveries, new technologies, and curricular mandates by governing bodies [5], yet still remain a 4-year endeavor. Research is still needed to determine the optimal way to structure the preclinical education, in order to make it as efficacious and efficient as possible.

Logistical Challenges

In order to keep groups small, schools must either have numerous simulators running simultaneously (which can be cost, space and faculty prohibitive) or sequentially, which can be time prohibitive. Frequently, other groups—clerkship students, residents in many departments, other allied health personnel, and continuing education courses—also require use of the simulator. In order to run smoothly, dedicated schedulers and support personnel are crucial [25].

Practical Implementation: Icahn School of Medicine at Mount Sinai

The simulation team from the Department of Anesthesiology at the Mount Sinai Medical Center has been conducting simulator-based physiology labs for Icahn School of Medicine at Mount Sinai (MSSM) since 1996. The current course covers the cardiovascular, respiratory, and autonomic nervous systems over 3 weeks and has been mostly unchanged since 1999. Prior to this time, truncated simulations were performed.

The simulation-based physiology lab series is an integral mandatory component of the first-year physiology course at the MSSM. Students participate in three different 2-h simulation-based laboratories taught by a team of 2–3 anesthesiologists (residents and attendings) in groups of 7–10 students per session. The first lab covers cardiovascular physiology, the second covers respiratory physiology, and the final session is a trauma scenario/autonomic nervous system lesson. During these fundamental laboratories, the simulator serves as a means to demonstrate normal and deranged physiology. In the final session, students apply principles of basic cardiovascular and pulmonary physiology to idealize oxygen tissue delivery in order to successfully resuscitate a simulated hypotensive trauma patient.

Full environment simulation (FES) is staged for each session using a CAE/METI Human Patient Simulator. The HPS has full drug recognition capabilities, and monitoring data are displayed on a large 50-in. plasma cell with Smart Board overlay capability (SMART Technologies Inc.). The overlay affords the ability to operate any Windows-based (Microsoft Corporation) program from the plasma cell or write directly on the screen via a blackboard function. The facilitators rapidly change the display between physiologic data and blackboard in order to review key physiologic concepts as the scenarios unfold. The experience is Socratic, and the students are expected to apply physiologic concepts learned in the classroom in order to interpret clinically relevant patient care issues. Each scenario is stopped and started as needed to discuss the application of classroom knowledge to the clinical situation and to allow participants time to develop diagnostic and therapeutic plans.

It is crucial that the lecture material precede simulation for these participants. Therefore, it is critical that the physiology course directors and the simulation course directors work closely together to organize and schedule both didactic and simulation curriculum in sequence. On one occasion, this was not the case, and much of the simulation session devolved into a didactic exercise so that the students could learn fundamental cardiovascular equations. This situation was less than ideal.

Integrated Cardiovascular Physiology Laboratory

The labs begin similarly. The students are asked not to take notes and to immerse themselves fully in the environment. The cardiovascular lab begins with the evaluation of an unconscious person in the field where a discussion is conducted regarding the sort of cardiovascular information a clinician can gather with one finger (i.e., heart rate, rhythm, estimate of blood pressure). The patient is then moved to the emergency room where the students choose monitors to more closely evaluate the cardiovascular system, ultimately leading to a patient with a full invasive set of monitors including an ECG, a noninvasive blood pressure cuff, an arterial line, a pulmonary artery catheter, and a transesophageal echocardiogram. All the while, monitor placement, data interpretation, indications, contraindications, risks, and benefits are discussed for each monitor. Once the pulmonary artery catheter is floated, several experiments are conducted, and the students must predict the impact of a change in heart rate on cardiac output and stroke volume. During the lab the students encounter various conditions resulting in a destabilized cardiovascular system requiring them to intervene with pharmacologic agents (atropine and lidocaine), cardioversion, and vagal maneuvers. The students appreciate how understanding cardiac physiology guides their therapeutic intervention and helps them idealize cardiac function. In a separate session run simultaneously in another classroom remote from the simulation laboratories, the students learn about transesophageal echocardiography with an emphasis on form and function to demonstrate the kinds of information one can gather from this modality.

Integrated Pulmonary Physiology Laboratory

The respiratory lab follows the path of a molecule of oxygen from the atmosphere into the bloodstream and onto a red blood cell. The patient is an asthmatic in acute bronchospasm, and he deteriorates during the scenario until he ultimately requires mechanical ventilation. Blood gases are drawn and their values discussed. Participants discuss salient equations and physiologic principles related to oxygenation and ventilation including shunt, dead space, and the relevance of the alveolar gas equation and learn about the monitoring and therapeutic modalities available for this system (e.g., pulse oximetry, capnography, oxygen delivery systems, bronchodilators, ventilators).

Integrated Autonomic Nervous System Laboratory

The third lab introduces the students to a trauma patient who comes to the emergency room hypotensive and tachycardic after a motor vehicle accident. The students use what they learned from labs one and two to resuscitate the patient and monitor, evaluate, and idealize both the cardiovascular and pulmonary systems to improve oxygen delivery to tissues. The students also learn new clinical skills such as the primary and secondary survey in order to apply what they learned in the classroom and prior labs to care for a patient in shock of unknown origin. Despite fluid and blood transfusion, the patient is persistently hypotensive, and the students are required to develop a differential diagnosis including hemorrhage, tension pneumothorax, cardiac tamponade, embolic disease, transfusion reaction, and anaphylaxis. These labs have been consistently rated among the highest exercises by the first year class and have been very rewarding for the anesthesiologists involved in the course. In a manuscript currently in press, the team found that not only were the labs well received, but they actually improved students' perceptions towards anesthesiologists as these were the course facilitators. In addition, students rated their likelihood to choose anesthesiology as a career option as higher after attending the course [38].

Conclusions

Simulation provides preclinical students the ability to integrate basic science teachings in a clinically relevant way and allows students to experiment, question, and explore scientific theories in a safe and focused manner. Simulation, if done carefully and thoughtfully, allows students to practice without risk to the patient [4, 25, 33] and may improve retention of basic science facts [26, 29, 30, 32, 33]. Research in preclinical use of simulation is sparse, but general principles of effective and prompt feedback, thoughtful integration with the basic science curriculum, and individualized learning are associated with better outcomes. Simulation use is limited by its cost, need for trained personnel, the need for peer-reviewed models, and the realization that the models for simulation are constrained by our limited understanding of the physiological processes that underpin them.

Appendix: Design Paradigms in Physiologic Model Construction

Introduction

Understanding the programming paradigms behind simulation physiologic modeling may prove beneficial to basic and clinical scientist considering creating simulation-based educational exercises or preparing simulation-based scenarios for their basic science curriculum. In this section we offer a unique insight into the development of physiologic modeling so educators can best understand the strengths and limitations of existing simulation as they apply this new technology to their curriculum.

"Static Data vs. Synthetic"

Broadly speaking there are two approaches to designing a physiological model, each of which introduces specific constraints about how the model can then be used. A classification of simulators along these lines has been proposed by Cumin and Merry [1]. However, most commercial simulators are built using combinations of these two strategies and cannot be easily categorized.

"Static Data" Approach

In a "static data" paradigm, real physiological data is stored and directly displayed to the student without any attempt to recreate the underlying mechanism. Any interaction with the model directs the student to a different set of static data. An example would be an ECG, stored in the simulator as an image, or a set of coordinates. If the user then gave a high dose of potassium to the simulated patient, the simulator would be directed to show a second static ECG demonstrating the effects of hyperkalemia. This method allows the supervisor to easily control the simulation directly (and sometimes called "script control" [1]).

There are two significant advantages to modeling a physiological system in this way. The first is that static data models are simpler (and therefore cheaper) to construct. The second is that because real experimental data is used directly, no assumptions about the static accuracy of the model need to be made. For applications where visual fidelity is paramount, such as the current echocardiography simulators (CAE ViMedix, Heartworks), static data models are easy to make visually convincing.

One direct consequence of using a static data set is that the model is then confined to adjusting its output discretely, due to the instant transition from one data source to another. This is apparent in ECG simulators where the displayed waveform can abruptly change from one archetypal pattern to another.

Another consequence is that the interactivity of the model is limited by the size of the dataset. When a simulator can have more than one interaction, in combination this leads to a geometric increase in possible outputs and therefore dataset size. In the example above, if the student has the option to give a lower dose of potassium to the simulator, a third ECG showing the effects of less-pronounced hyperkalemia would need to be displayed (and therefore, created and programmed into the simulator). If the simulator were equipped to have the student give another drug—such as calcium—then the total amount of ECGs in the databank would have to be doubled (ECGs demonstrating normokalemia, mild hyperkalemia, and severe hyperkalemia, with and without hypercalcemia). This geometric increase in total output options serves as a limitation to interactivity and therefore the scope of "top-down" simulation (Table 40.3).

Table 40.3 Static data paradigm: If there are five states for potassium, calcium, and heart rate and each combination is valid, then a total of 5 × 5 × 5 = 125 different ECG images will need to be created

Variable	Possible state
Potassium	Severe and mild hypokalemia Severe and mild hyperkalemia Normokalemia
Calcium	Severe and mild hypocalcemia Severe and mild hypercalcemia Normocalcemia
Heart rate	Very slow Slow Normal Fast Very fast

Reprinted from Holubarsch et al. [2], with permission from Wolters Kluwer

"Synthetic" Approach

The "Synthetic" paradigm is more complex, but potentially of higher fidelity compared to the "static data" approach. In this method, the designer attempts to create a mathematical representation of the structure and function of human physiology. This is referred to by some as "model-driven simulation" [1]. It involves simplification and *abstraction* of the real physical system (which is often irresolvable complex). The more abstract the mathematical model, the less its structure represents the real physiological process it intends to imitate. Taken to extremes, this produces a "black box" model, where the output is produced from the input with no mechanistic assumptions at all. Classical three-compartment pharmacokinetic models are an example of this. In order to recreate the above ECG example in a synthetic model, the programmer could attempt to create an electrical model of the heart which produces the ECG voltage. To do so, they could program multiple "myocytes" which depolarize and repolarize in response to physiologic stimuli (e.g., serum electrolyte levels, parasympathetic and sympathetic stimulation, and ischemia). In addition to the challenges of converting these electrical, physiological, hormonal, and other stimuli to programming language, these models require prior elucidation of the body's underlying physiologic mechanisms. It is this architectural complexity—rather than lack of computing power—which has slowed the adoption of "synthetic" modeling in simulation.

As a general rule, models with fewer interactions are easier to build in a "static data" pattern. However, as the number of desired interactions increases (especially in combination), it can become easier to attempt to create a synthetic model.

Synthetic models solve the discrete output and interactivity problems of static data models, allowing much more complex simulation scenarios. There is no absolute limit on the degree of model complexity save the difficulty in constructing the underlying model architecture, but their applicability is affected by problems which fundamentally limit model construction.

Real Physiological and Pathological Processes Have Not Been Fully Elucidated

In aviation simulation, the mechanics that determine the aircraft behavior are largely described and are underlined by physical laws expressed as mathematical equations. In contrast, most biological simulated conditions rely on a complex causal web of mechanisms with incompletely understood relationships. Real patients also exhibit phenotypic variation, which obscures these mechanisms and can in itself be challenging to simulate. This is explored further in the example below.

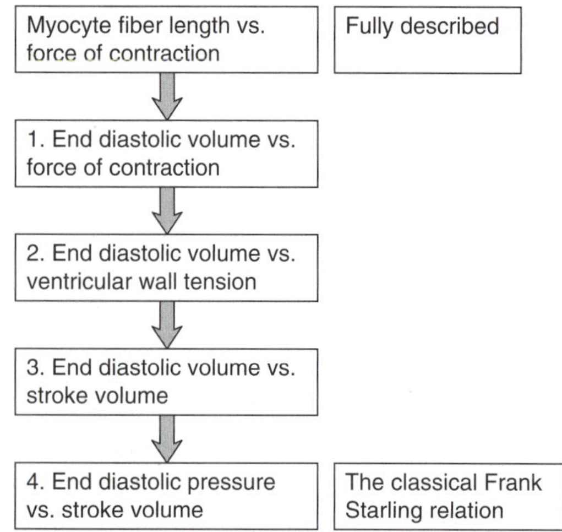

Fig. 40.5 The mechanisms which allow us to follow the genesis of the Frank Starling curve from the force of contraction of a myocyte according to its length to the change in SV of a heart according to its EDP have not been fully described. This means that an empirical model of this mechanism cannot be constructed

Modeling the Frank Starling Curve

We have a good understanding of the relationship between myocyte fiber length and force of contraction (FOC) for a myocyte, and we also have a wealth of experimental data to support the classical Frank-Starling relation of end-diastolic pressure (EDP) and stroke volume. We also know that the myocyte length/FOC relation is the prime underlying cause of the Frank-Starling relation. However, in order to create a model, we need to construct a set of mathematical relations that quantify the etiological progression from one to the other. Figure 40.5 shows an attempt to do this, with comments on the four arbitrary steps below:

1. Firstly, the relation between myocyte fiber length and end-diastolic volume (EDV) is (probably irresolvable) complex as the muscle fibers exist in multiple orientations and the heart cannot be reduced to a geometric shape.
2. Subsequently, the translation from myocyte tension to ventricular wall tension also depends upon the mechanical advantage of each fiber—which is also related to the orientation.
3. Modeling the stroke volume from the ventricular wall tension depends largely on the effect of the vascular system on the afterload and preload of the heart *in situ* and how this might affect the fluid dynamics of blood ejection.
4. Converting from ventricular volume to pressure equates to compliance. Experimental data exists to support this, although in an *in vivo* heart compliance changes actively and is energy dependent (i.e., diastolic dysfunction).

This example shows a typical pattern in trying to model biological systems. Supporting experimental data exists in isolation, but cannot be joined to form a coherent description of how a system works. Overarching all of this is the tremendous phenotypic variation between different individuals, frustrating attempts to identify mathematical patterns.

Mathematical Limitations Prevent the Accurate Description of Human Physiology in a Model

Many physiological processes require significant computing resources to solve. Additionally, and in contrast to pharmaceutical and research modeling, the mathematical solutions need to run in real time and on low-powered devices. It is worth mentioning that some problems offer no mathematical solution at all [3, 4] which means that human physiology will *never* be accurately modeled in its entirety.

Consequences of Synthetic Model-Driven Simulation

Patient Parameters Have to Be Set Indirectly via Their Causal Parameters

When changing a value such as blood pressure in a pure "static data" simulation, the value is entered directly by the supervisor and is then displayed to the student. However, in a "synthetic" simulation, the model needs to know the underlying cause of the hypotension in order to recreate it. In this example, blood pressure is a function of the cardiac output and the systemic vascular resistance, and the supervisor would need to choose which one of those variables to alter. If the supervisor reduces the cardiac output, then the model would need to know whether this was due to a reduction in heart rate or stroke volume (Fig. 40.6). This etiological progression continues until the *fundamental* parameters are reached—which are parameters which do not depend on any other for their value and can safely be changed. This also marks the limit of the model architecture, and as the model construction deepens, the supervisor is required to manipulate ever more fundamental parameters, which in turn requires a deeper knowledge of physiology and the model behavior. In an environment where most simulation is performed by technicians these problems may serve as a limit to synthetic model complexity.

Patient Parameters Cannot Be Predicted

Many physiological processes cannot be solved arithmetically and need to be approximated by induction. Consequently, the output of the model cannot be predicted from its starting position (i.e., the output is reached by induction). Returning to the example above, the future effect on the blood pressure of reducing the vagal tone cannot be precisely quantified. If the supervisor wanted to reduce the blood pressure by a defined amount or achieve an exact value (e.g., precisely

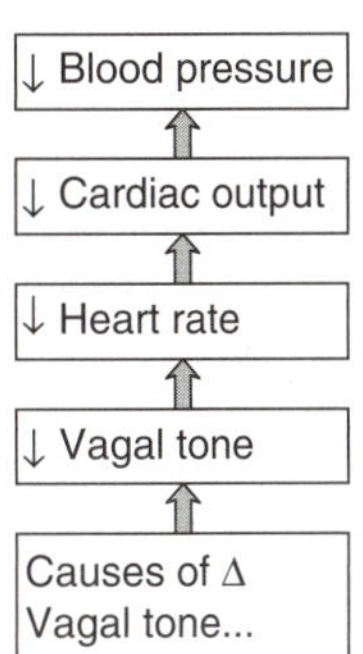

Fig. 40.6 Reducing the blood pressure of a "bottom-up" simulation by increasing the vagal tone. The blood pressure cannot be changed directly as it is controlled by the model

120/80 mmHg), this would be very difficult to implement, and programming solutions add considerably to the model complexity.

Validating Physiological Models

There is an abundance of published data on the role of simulators in the educational process and their value as a learning tool [5–8]. In contrast there is almost no information regarding the accuracy of the physiological models that drive these systems, although it is noted that there are no agreed standards for simulation accuracy [9]. There is an explicit risk that an inaccurate simulation model could cause *negative learning* in the student. Although this concept has not been explored in medical simulation, there is a documented case in aviation where a pilot used a maneuver that he learned in a simulator which resulted in a crash when used in a real aircraft [10].

Validating the *fixed* output of a "static data" model is possible, as published data can be used directly, with reliance on peer review of the supporting paper. In a "synthetic" model, the author has to use published data indirectly, together with peer opinion and personal experience, to construct the model. This interpretation potentially adds another source of error.

Another problem with validating synthetic models is that they often simulate physiological extremes where there is a paucity of supportive published data of any type. The designer is then reduced to relying on an informal review of the model behavior by his peers. This is *de facto* practice in resuscitation simulation and is compounded by the lack of feedback channels the supervisors can use when trying to report inaccurate model behavior to the manufacturer.

The difficulty in validating the dynamic response of a synthetic model should be contrasted with that of a static data model. In a synthetic model the dynamic response to an intervention (such as a drug) can be validated, and the limitations openly defined. In a static data model, the response to this intervention is provided manually by the supervisor, who has to interpret both the student's actions and the likely behavior of the virtual patient. The

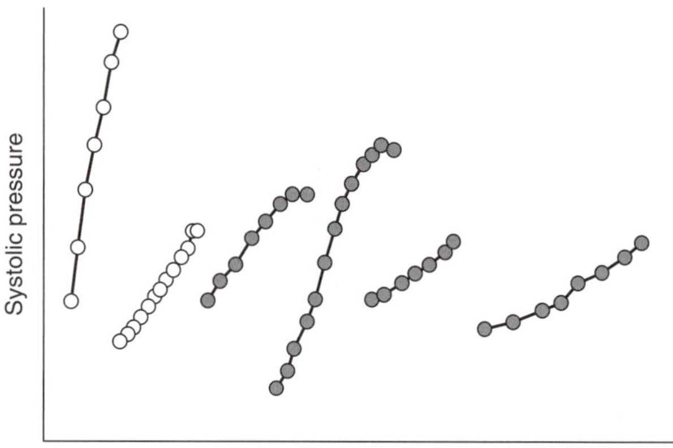

Fig. 40.7 A wide variation in shape and amplitude of Frank Starling curves is seen when comparing isolated hearts (here normal hearts are open symbols; dilated cardiomyopathic hearts are closed). This produces a broad target when attempting to recreate them artificially

supervisor's actions (and therefore the accuracy of the simulation) will vary depending on the individual concerned and cannot be quantified. In a "static data" model then, the source of the risk of inaccuracy and negative learning moves from the model to the supervisor.

The problem of validity is mitigated (or at least obscured) to some extent by the large phenotypic variation in the human population. Because of this, physiologists accept a very broad definition of what would be a normal response, and the model output can fall anywhere within these limits and still be considered acceptable (Fig. 40.7).

An elegant solution is to build this population variability into the model itself. This has already been attempted to a limited degree with some immersive simulators allowing the simulation director to choose the type of patient (e.g., young or old) for the simulation scenario. This digital representation of phenotypic variation will hopefully be replaced by analogue models in the future, but this will open a new layer of modeling which will also need to be validated.

There is a joint responsibility between the manufacturers and the medical community to transparently validate the physiological models that drive simulators and explicitly quantify their limitations. However, the onus is on all supervisors who run interactive simulations to be aware of the inaccuracies of the simulator (be it the physical manikin or physiological model) and how these might cause negative learning.

References

1. Cumin D, Merry AF. Simulators for use in anaesthesia. Anaesthesia. 2007;62(2):151–62.
2. Holubarsch C et al. Existence of the Frank-Starling mechanism in the failing human heart: investigations on the organ, tissue, and sarcomere levels. Circulation. 1996;94(4):683–9.
3. Berger R. Memoirs of the American Mathematical Society The Undecidability of the Domino Problem. vol. 66. Providence: American Mathematical Society; 1966.
4. Wang H. Proving theorems by pattern recognition – II. At&T Tech J. 1961;40(1):1–41.
5. Draycott T, Sibanda T, Owen L, et al. Does training in obstetric emergencies improve neonatal outcome? Bjog-Int J Obstet Gy. 2006;113(2):177–82.
6. Good ML. Patient simulation for training basic and advanced clinical skills. Med Educ. 2003;37:14–21.
7. Maran NJ, Glavin RJ. Low- to high-fidelity simulation – a continuum of medical education? Med Educ. 2003;37:22–28.
8. Wong AK. Full scale computer simulators in anesthesia training and evaluation. Can J Anaesth. 2004;51(5):455–64.
9. Cumin D, Merry AF, Weller JM. Standards for simulation. Anaesthesia. 2008;63(12):1281–4.
10. Airbus SAS. Submission to the National Transportation Safety Board for the American Airlines Flight 587 Accident Investigation. 2001. http://usread.com/flight587/Airbus_submission.pdf Accessed on 2001..

References

1. Flexner A, Carnegie Foundation for the Advancement of Teaching, Pritchett HS. Medical education in the United States and Canada; a report to the Carnegie Foundation for the Advancement of Teaching. New York City; 1910.
2. Irby DM, Cooke M, O'Brien BC. Calls for reform of medical education by the Carnegie Foundation for the Advancement of Teaching: 1910 and 2010. Acad Med. 2010;85(2):220–7.
3. Bransford J, Brown AL, Cocking RR, National Research Council (U.S.). Committee on Developments in the Science of Learning. How people learn : brain, mind, experience, and school. Washington, D.C.: National Academy Press; 1999.
4. Cooke M, Irby DM, Sullivan W, Ludmerer KM. American medical education 100 years after the Flexner report. N Engl J Med. 2006;355(13):1339–44.
5. Finnerty EP, Chauvin S, Bonaminio G, Andrews M, Carroll RG, Pangaro LN. Flexner revisited: the role and value of the basic sciences in medical education. Acad Med. 2010;85(2):349–55.
6. Passiment M, Sacks H, Huang G. Medical Simulation in Medical Education: Results of an AAMC Study. American Association of Medical Colleges. Sept 2001.
7. Issenberg SB, McGaghie WC, Petrusa ER, Lee Gordon D, Scalese RJ. Features and uses of high-fidelity medical simulations that lead to effective learning: a BEME systematic review. Med Teach. 2005;27(1):10–28.
8. Kirch DG. Commentary: the Flexnerian Legacy in the 21st century. Acad Med. 2010;85(2):190–2.
9. Sweeney G. The challenge for basic science education in problem-based medical curricula. Clin Invest Med. 1999;22(1):15–22.
10. Kinkade S. A snapshot of the status of problem-based learning in U. S. medical schools, 2003–04. Acad Med. 2005;80(3):300–1.
11. Azer SA, Eizenberg N. Do we need dissection in an integrated problem-based learning medical course? Perceptions of first- and second-year students. Surg Radiol Anat. 2007;29(2):173–80.
12. Morrison G, Goldfarb S, Lanken PN. Team training of medical students in the 21st century: would Flexner approve? Acad Med. 2010;85(2):254–9.
13. Curry RH, Makoul G. An active-learning approach to basic clinical skills. Acad Med. 1996;71(1):41–4.
14. Bradley P. The history of simulation in medical education and possible future directions. Med Educ. 2006;40(3):254–62.

15. Okuda Y, Bryson EO, DeMaria Jr S, et al. The utility of simulation in medical education: what is the evidence? Mt Sinai J Med. 2009;76(4):330–43.
16. Samsel RW, Schmidt GA, Hall JB, Wood LD, Shroff SG, Schumacker PT. Cardiovascular physiology teaching: computer simulations vs. animal demonstrations. Am J Physiol. 1994;266(6 Pt 3):S36–46.
17. Willis LR, Besch Jr HR. Effect of experience on medical students' attitudes toward animal laboratories in pharmacology education. Acad Med. 1995;70(1):67–9.
18. Steinberg M, Cook DA, Gilbert M, et al. Towards targeted screening for acute HIV infections in British Columbia. J Int AIDS Soc. 2011;14:39.
19. McGaghie WC, Issenberg SB, Cohen ER, Barsuk JH, Wayne DB. Does simulation-based medical education with deliberate practice yield better results than traditional clinical education? A meta-analytic comparative review of the evidence. Acad Med. 2011;86(6):706–11.
20. Fincher RM, White CB, Huang G, Schwartzstein R. Toward hypothesis-driven medical education research: task force report from the Millennium Conference 2007 on educational research. Acad Med. 2010;85(5):821–8.
21. McGaghie WC, Issenberg SB, Petrusa ER, Scalese RJ. A critical review of simulation-based medical education research: 2003–2009. Med Educ. 2010;44(1):50–63.
22. Pitkala KH, Mantyranta T. Feelings related to first patient experiences in medical school. A qualitative study on students' personal portfolios. Patient Educ Couns. 2004;54(2):171–7.
23. Patterson SW, Starling EH. On the mechanical factors which determine the output of the ventricles. J Physiol. 1914;48(5):357–79.
24. Oriol NE, Hayden EM, Joyal-Mowschenson J, Muret-Wagstaff S, Faux R, Gordon JA. Using immersive healthcare simulation for physiology education: initial experience in high school, college, and graduate school curricula. Adv Physiol Educ. 2011;35(3):252–9.
25. Gordon JA, Hayden EM, Ahmed RA, Pawlowski JB, Khoury KN, Oriol NE. Early bedside care during preclinical medical education: can technology-enhanced patient simulation advance the Flexnerian ideal? Acad Med. 2010;85(2):370–7.
26. Tan GM, Ti LK, Suresh S, Ho BS, Lee TL. Teaching first-year medical students physiology: does the human patient simulator allow for more effective teaching? Singapore Med J. 2002;43(5):238–42.
27. Savoldelli GL, Naik VN, Park J, Joo HS, Chow R, Hamstra SJ. Value of debriefing during simulated crisis management: oral versus video-assisted oral feedback. Anesthesiology. 2006;105(2):279–85.
28. Rodriguez-Barbero A, Lopez-Novoa JM. Teaching integrative physiology using the quantitative circulatory physiology model and case discussion method: evaluation of the learning experience. Adv Physiol Educ. 2008;32(4):304–11.
29. Heitz C, Brown A, Johnson JE, Fitch MT. Large group high-fidelity simulation enhances medical student learning. Med Teach. 2009;31(5):e206–10.
30. Gordon JA, Brown DF, Armstrong EG. Can a simulated critical care encounter accelerate basic science learning among preclinical medical students? A pilot study. Simul Healthc. 2006;1 Spec no:13–7.
31. McGrath P, Kucera R, Smith W. Computer simulation of introductory neurophysiology. Adv Physiol Educ. 2003;27(1–4):120–9.
32. Cook DA, Hatala R, Brydges R, et al. Technology-enhanced simulation for health professions education: a systematic review and meta-analysis. JAMA. 2011;306(9):978–88.
33. Halm BM, Lee MT, Franke AA. Improving toxicology knowledge in preclinical medical students using high-fidelity patient simulators. Hawaii Med J. 2011;70(6):112–5.
34. Woods NN, Brooks LR, Norman GR. It all make sense: biomedical knowledge, causal connections and memory in the novice diagnostician. Adv Health Sci Educ Theory Pract. 2007;12(4):405–15.
35. Gordon JA, Oriol NE, Cooper JB. Bringing good teaching cases "to life": a simulator-based medical education service. Acad Med. 2004;79(1):23–7.
36. Cooper JB, Barron D, Blum R, et al. Video teleconferencing with realistic simulation for medical education. J Clin Anesth. 2000;12(3):256–61.
37. Kim S, Ross B, Wright A, et al. Halting the revolving door of faculty turnover: recruiting and retaining clinician educators in an academic medical simulation center. Simul Healthc. 2011;6(3):168–75.
38. DeMaria Jr S, Bryson EO, Bodian C, et al. The influence of simulation-based physiology labs taught by anesthesiologists on the attitudes of first-year medical students towards anesthesiology. Middle East J Anesthesiol. 2011;21(3):347–53.

Part IV

Professional Development in Simulation

The Clinical Educator Track for Medical Students and Residents

41

Alan J. Sim, Bryan P. Mahoney, Daniel Katz, Rajesh Reddy, and Andrew Goldberg

Introduction

Every physician must be equipped with the skills requisite to that of an educator. The physician's ability to teach effectively and communicate information to others is tested constantly through numerous interactions with patients, medical students, residents, and fellow practitioners, usually under a variety of circumstances. This role as "teacher" begins as a student in one's clinical years of medical school and continues to develop further during one's postgraduate training. Such an integral skill set, however, is not innate; rather, it must be learned and frequently improved upon. It is clear that competency in education or the ability to educate others effectively should be incorporated into any physician-training program. The recognition of this necessity has led to the formal integration of education training into the paradigm of physician education. The American Council for Graduate Medical Education (ACGME) common program requirements for residency training state: *Residents are expected to develop skills and habits to be able to participate in the education of patients, families, students, residents, and other health professionals* [1], while the Liaison Committee on Medical Education (LCME) mandates: Residents must be *prepared for their roles as teachers and evaluators of medical students* [2].

While the benefits of resident-as-teacher and educator mentoring programs have been well documented [3], the utilization of a simulation education program as the site for the development of faculty and medical educators has not been explored. This chapter will review the history and literature on resident and medical student educator mentoring, citing the benefits, differing modes of implementation, and integration of models for adult learning while identifying the role for simulation in regards to the mentoring of medical educators.

A.J. Sim, MD (✉) • D. Katz, MD
Department of Anesthesiology,
Icahn School of Medicine at Mount Sinai, New York, NY, USA
e-mail: alan.sim@mountsinai.org; daniel.katz@mountsinai.org

B.P. Mahoney, MD
Department of Anesthesiology,
Ohio State Wexner Medical Center, Ohio, USA
e-mail: mahoney.181@usa.edu

R. Reddy, MD
Department of Anesthesiology,
Icahn School of Medicine at Mount Sinai,
215 E. 95th St., Apt. 6L, New York, NY 10128, USA
e-mail: raj.reddy@mountsinai.org

A. Goldberg, MD
Department of Anesthesiology,
Icahn School of Medicine at Mount Sinai,
1249 Park Ave., Apt. 14E, New York, NY, USA
e-mail: andrew.goldberg@mountsinai.org

Resident and Medical Student Education Training: A Brief History

The term "doctor" is etymologically derived from the Latin word *docere*, "to show, teach, cause to know," and therefore carries within its meaning a presumption of competency and excellence in education. Given such a longstanding reputation of a physician's role as educator, it is somewhat surprising to see only a recent focus on educator training in residency programs. Formal resident-as-teacher curricula emerged within a very small number of residency training programs in the 1970s [4, 5]. Initially, only anecdotal evidence on a program-by-program basis was available. The majority of these programs illustrated that using peers as teachers was cost-effective [6], non-inferior to using attending physicians as teachers, and most importantly, due to the closeness of age and perspective in the medical field, peer educators allowed the teacher to put himself in the shoes of his student and thus be an empathetic educator [6]. This allows for unique and highly effective educational methods. Peer educators can draw from their familiarity of being a student and use it to overcome difficulties, barriers, frustrations, and fears experienced by the student inherent to the expectations of learning a vast array of material in a short amount of time [6, 7].

A.I. Levine et al. (eds.), *The Comprehensive Textbook of Healthcare Simulation*,
DOI 10.1007/978-1-4614-5993-4_41, © Springer Science+Business Media New York 2013

In light of these benefits, using peers as teachers was a promising initiative in the evolution of graduate medical education. However, it was observed that without proper instruction regarding the skill set necessary to become a teacher, peer teaching would never reach its full potential. Although there exists a level of expectation that all physicians have an *a priori* ability to teach, this is simply not true. Physicians, like any other teacher, must be properly trained in the skills required to pass on and communicate knowledge effectively and succinctly. As residency programs started to appreciate this fact, the number of formal teaching skills improvement programs (TSIPs) increased. By the early 1990s, roughly 20% of residency programs offered TSIPs [8]. As the number of these programs increased, so did the support of their worth. Programs noticed that TSIPs could increase a resident educator's ability to teach effectively [9, 10], promote self-confidence [11, 12], hone perceived clinical knowledge [3, 13], and stimulate interest to pursue careers in academic medical centers [14, 15]. Most importantly, these programs reiterated that peers were not only non-inferior to their attending counterparts [16] but also potentially superior educators due not only to their unique perspective but also to their distinctive understanding and experiential "mastery" of the material they attempted to teach [17, 18]. By 2001, approximately half of all residency programs in the USA offered some formal training in teaching skills [19]. Other studies illustrated that in addition to residents being powerful and effective educators, medical students themselves can also be used as a valuable pool of teachers.

Programs designed to develop medical students as teachers (MED-SATS) have been reported as early as the 1970s, describing senior medical students teaching medical history taking and demonstrating skills in physical diagnosis to junior students [6, 7]. Since this time, there have been multiple descriptions of MED-SATS in peer tutoring [20, 21], teaching basic life support and cardiopulmonary resuscitation [22], instruction in the basic sciences, and moderating case-based learning sessions [23]. Many of these programs are designed with the specific goal of providing experience and instruction in teaching skills [24, 25]. The overriding theory is that early education of medical students on their expected roles as physician educators will improve their abilities to teach, broaden their educational skill set, and motivate them to pursue careers in academia [15].

Currently, it is widely accepted that programs that teach both residents and medical students how to teach are beneficial to medical education. Younger students find it helpful to have peers as teachers [24], while senior students and residents find the experience to be rewarding, useful in improving educational skills, and often request or desire more opportunities to teach. In the next section of this chapter, we describe how the simulation environment provides the ideal setting for the development of student as educator.

Simulation as a Tool for Clinical Educator Development

Mannequin-based simulation has been used for medical education since its inception in the early 1960s. During the last 50 years, its use has become more pervasive as a teaching tool. As a result, simulation centers established within medical institutions for undergraduate and graduate medical education have become virtually ubiquitous (see Fig. 41.1). The

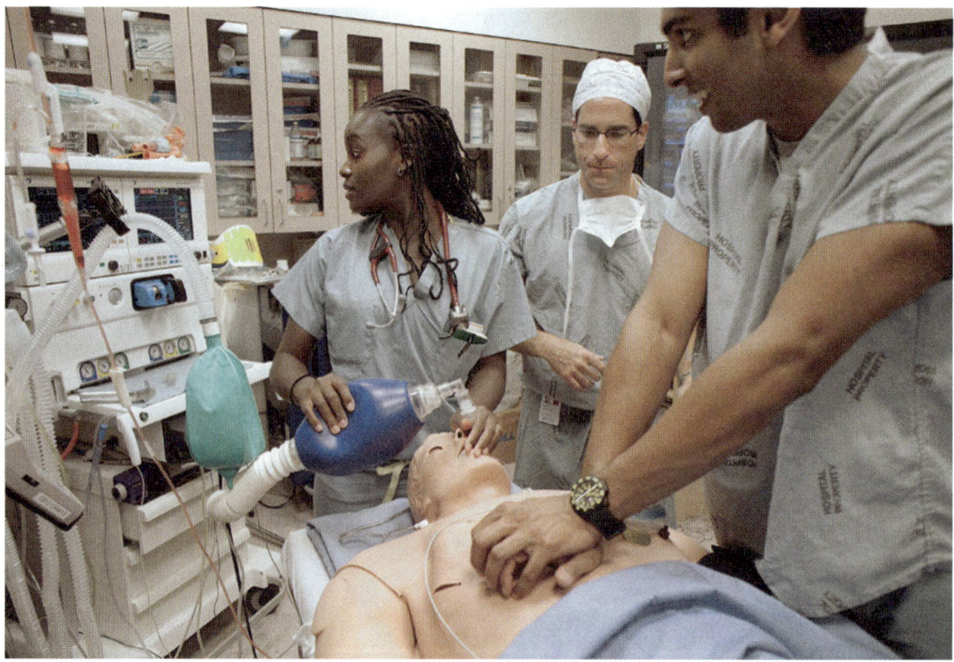

Fig. 41.1 Mannequin-based simulation exercise

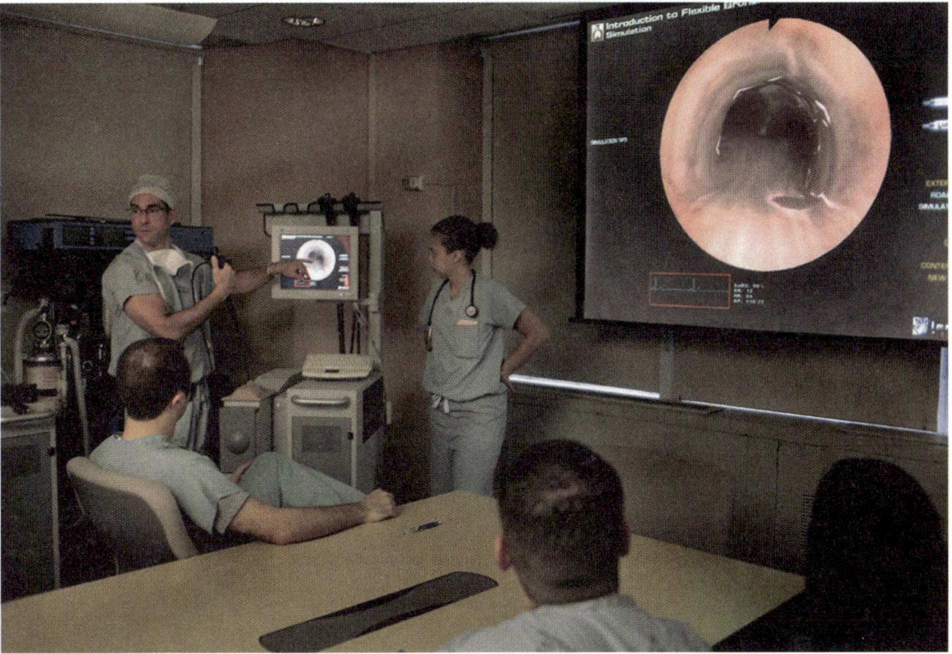

Fig. 41.2 Small-group simulation exercise

benefits and utilization of simulation as a resource to teach learners are discussed in great detail throughout this book. These tools and the simulated environment also prove to be a powerful and nearly limitless workshop for potential educators to create, test, and refine their educational methods. Many of the pedagogical principles that apply to clinical educators can be employed within the forum of the human simulator and its environment for medical students and residents.

Diverse Audience Exposure

Simulation offers many unique advantages for novice educators to perfect teaching skills and curricula design development in a safe, controlled, and manipulatable setting. Being a virtual classroom, the simulated environment presents a vast array of options, in terms of audience composition and class size. Course material, teaching style, and therefore simulations can be tailored to a variety of audiences, giving the student educator the ability to perform, test, and master their curricula on novice-level learners, such as high school or premedical students before attempting to teach to more experienced learners.

Class Size Options

The ability to control class size is also another significant advantage of the simulated environment. Teaching in front of a full lecture hall can be daunting even for a seasoned educator, but it is incredibly anxiety provoking and intimidating for the novice. While some simulation-based scenarios will be done on a "grand" scale, involving multiple locations, advanced telecommunications, and large conference rooms, the majority of simulations can be done more intimately with small groups. Controlling class size in the simulated environment allows novice educators the ability to gain experience and confidence with a manageable number of students (see Fig. 41.2).

Feedback and Mentorship

The "hands on," small group aspect of simulation-based teaching also permits frequent and immediate feedback opportunities for student and educator alike. The environment affords a unique opportunity for the novice educator to be observed and mentored from more seasoned student educators and faculty. The idea of a tiered system of mentorship is an integral component of the student-as-teacher model and creates a "farm team" of educators and mentors, who start as novice educators, gain experience and skills, and become education mentors to more junior teachers (described in more detail below). Teaching in this nonintimidating environment is a perfect proving ground for young educators to experiment, build self-confidence, acquire and reinforce knowledge, and continually improve based on immediate student and mentor feedback.

Experiential Curricular Design

Creating experiential courses conducted in a simulated environment facilitates curricular development and improves teaching skills for the student educator. The simulation classroom enables the student educator to create scenarios drawn

Table 41.1 Anesthetic planning scenario based on a residents' personal experience

State	Patient status	Learner objectives	Operator notes/teaching points/triggers
1. Baseline	Patient is anxious, asks for meds to relax him	*Learner actions*: Will identify self to team and locate appropriate patient history. Attach monitors, reassure patient	*Operator*: Baseline healthy patient loaded in sinus tach *Teaching points*: Appropriate history obtained, decide whether or not to proceed with the plan decided on *Trigger*: Participant applies monitors to patient
2. Pre-sedation	Patient found to be tachycardic with normal blood pressure upon placement of monitors	*Learner actions*: Recognize sinus tachycardia, cause is anxiety and let them treat as they want	*Operator*: Change to sinus rhythm with sedation. *Teaching points*: Recognition of anxiety *Trigger*: Surgeon asks if he can start
3. Sedation	Patient becomes profoundly agitated and moves around	*Learner actions*: Manages the MAC case by giving more sedation, may try narcotics or hypnotics	*Operator*: Patient becomes apneic temporarily but recovers, have them manipulate the airway to ensure patency *Teaching points*: Recognition of sedation. Diagnose why the patient continues to respond to stimuli *Trigger*: Patient calms temporarily
4. Intra-Op	Patient is comfortable, but upon manipulation of the hernia beings to move around and groan. Surgeon complains. Entice them to give more sedation	*Learner actions*: Recognize level of sedation inadequate, respond to surgeon the definition of MAC. Often more sedation given	*Operator*: Upon further sedation patient becomes completely apneic and unresponsive. Desaturation ensues *Teaching points*: Recognition of inadequate anesthesia, realization of poor technique for this case *Trigger*: Patient begins to desaturate, remains unarousable, becomes difficult to ventilate
5. Intubation	Patient remains in extremis, airway management needed. Convert to general anesthesia with an ET tube	*Learner actions*: Rescue the airway via intubation, mechanical ventilation. Alter anesthetic drugs or levels appropriately. Treat pain	*Operator*: Patient recovers from respiratory insult. Once tube in place surgeon is happy with conditions, asks for relaxation *Teaching points*: Ability to rescue the airway. Explain the quick desaturation. Discover how they painted themselves into a corner *Trigger*: Successful patient management
6. Emergence and recovery	Procedure ends, patient emerges, gets extubated	*Learner actions*: Proper emergence. Decide need for reversal. After extubation gives proper sign out	*Operator*: Patient emerges well, surgeon happy procedure is done, normal PACU sign out *Teaching points*: Decision of extubation, proper PACU sign out
7. Debriefing	Patient now awake	*Learner actions*: Self-assessment of performance initiated. Completion of debriefing with demonstration of understanding of diagnosis and management of blunt trauma and hypotension	*Operator*: Administer standardized debriefing. *Teaching points*: Discuss MAC vs. general, need for airway management and back-up plan. Proper consent process. Feedback regarding strengths and weaknesses in simulation completion. Allow for revisit of simulation immediately to apply recently acquired feedback. *Trigger*: Completion of debriefing

from their own patient encounters during their training. Experiential curricular development offers student educators exceptional familiarity with a subject. This "ownership" of material imparts a level of confidence and knowledge of the curriculum that will result in a more confident and knowledgeable educator compared to counterparts who may not have had the same experience. This unique perspective gives student educators the ability to recreate their own experiences and impart particular emotions, people, events, and decision trees that were encountered in real life. As student educators and residents progress through their training, they can continue to make and reinforce connections between real-life experience and their simulation curriculum. Eventually, through multiple iterations and mastery of an experiential simulation, the student educator gains more confidence with the creation of novel simulation-based experimental scenarios. This creativity is fostered, and new simulations are designed with basic principles learned from prior successful simulations and enhanced by knowledge gained as they progress through their medical and educator training (see Table 41.1). Upon completion of their training, the student educator is expected to acquire a broad educational repertoire. Not only should they have amassed a collection of simulations and the comfort to teach to a variety of audiences, but should finish training having honed the skills to develop spontaneous novel scenarios that addresses future educational needs.

Dynamic Education

The creation of a simulation scenario, whether experiential or by spontaneous design, requires a student educator to research

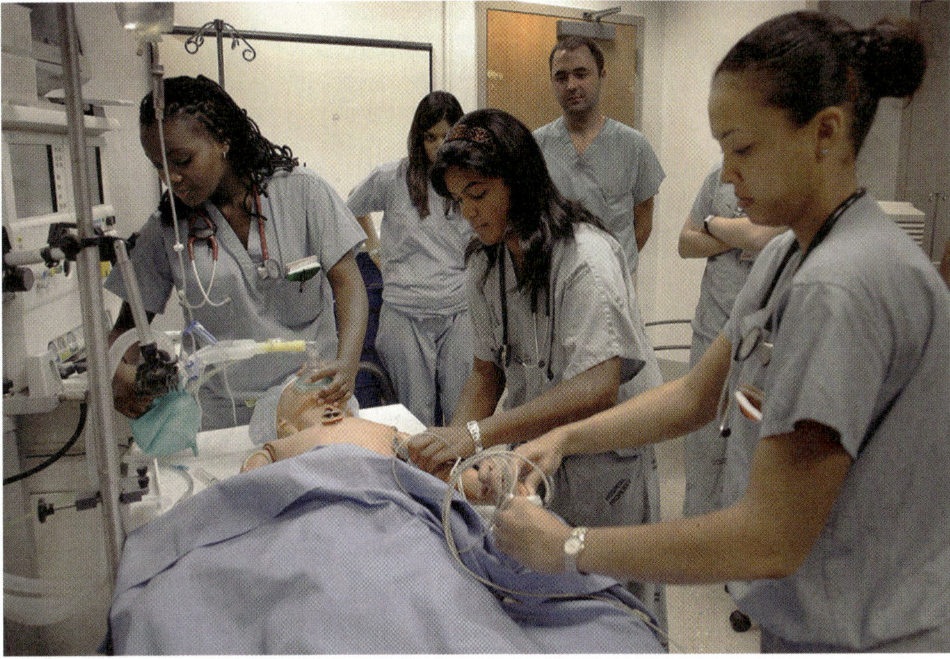

Fig. 41.3 Full-scale simulation involving three clinical educators of varying experience creating a fully immersive teaching environment

a given topic and master a set of information, much like any other didactic exercise. Most didactics follow a linear path, an outline is given, information is communicated, and the lesson plan follows accordingly. The major difference is that due to the immersive and sometimes unpredictable environment the simulator provides, like the actual clinical environment, the student educator must be a *dynamic educator*, prepared to deal with unexpected questions, technical errors, and unanticipated decision trees the learners may provide throughout the scenario. For example, a drug error may occur, an "impossible airway" may prove easy, or an intervention may be performed for which the simulation educator was not prepared. Though this presents the student educator with significant challenges, it does not halt the process of education for both the teacher and the student, rather it forces the teacher to be resourceful, think quickly, and be versatile. It also mandates that the educator must plan ahead for possible pitfalls. As one garners more experience with a given scenario, more unforeseen events occur, and the educator gains a greater mastery of a subject or given simulation. By learning to anticipate unanticipated questions, and by making adjustments, they solidify previously existing knowledge, build self-confidence, and learn to communicate information effectively. The educator can also learn to better control what is taught, reach greater understanding by their students, and learn to influence their audience to "follow the script" and reduce the amount of unexpected questions and actions. Therefore, the rich and dynamic simulated teaching environment can serve to reinforce educator knowledge, increase self-confidence, and hone their teaching skill set. All of these are vital aspects to growing educators who are enthusiastic about teaching and maximizing the education of those being taught.

The "Farm Team" Approach to Mentorship

As stated before, simulator-trained educators have the ability to teach multiple audiences; create innovative, immersive, and adaptive simulations that refine their medical knowledge; and provide excellent feedback through practiced communication. Of all the benefits described, perhaps the most valuable benefit to simulator-trained educators is the formation of relationships between medical students, residents, and faculty resulting in a unique, incredibly rewarding, and effective mentoring system. Instillation of young educators at the level of student or resident places them in a system that repeatedly reinforces itself. Residents learning to educate are positioned to mentor students whom themselves are also learning to educate. For example, creating a robust simulated operating room environment often calls for multiple educators, some may be tasked with running the simulation software, others portraying patients or surgeons, and others involved in the initiation of inciting events (see Fig. 41.3). These educators may be of different levels of training, ranging from attending physician to student. Through their participation in the simulated scenario, all student educators gain knowledge in experience in simulation and educational training by their observation of those around them and execution of their assigned roles within the simulated scenario. This mentorship allows for sharing of teaching experiences between more senior educators and junior educators, ultimately creating a "farm team" model. Within this system, junior educators are trained and mentored by senior educators, eventually taking over increasingly greater teaching responsibilities and administrative duties as they progress through their residency. Ultimately, upon completion of their

Table 41.2 Sample medical student simulation elective timetable

Goals and objectives	Week 1	Week 2	Week 3	Week 4
Educational skill building	Observe prescheduled sessions	Assist senior clinical staff in scheduled simulations	Assist senior clinical staff in running your specific scenario	Perform your scenario and didactic session with minimal senior clinician input
Simulation design and execution	Learn basic simulator function and design	Design clinical simulation scenario	"Drive" your scenario during live sessions	Finalize your scenario
	Pick a unique clinical simulation scenario based on experience	Test simulation and concurrent didactic session	Modify your scenario based on feedback	Submit to clerkship coordinator for formal evaluation

training, these educators can transition easily from residents to faculty with the proper tools for a career in academia and simulation-based training. What follows is our institutional model for a "Clinical Educator Track" within an anesthesiology residency program utilizing simulation-based educational training.

The Clinical Educator Track and Simulation-Based Elective for Medical Students

Our program has an initial formal mentorship program for fourth-year medical students interested in clinical educator careers. Medical students join our program during a unique one-month elective in anesthesiology simulation and learn to educate in the simulated environment. Under the guidance of attending-level faculty and senior residents within our anesthesiology program, the students learn to develop their own curriculum by observing and helping teach during existing simulator-based sessions. The students learn to be effective communicators for a variety of student audiences and learn to create their own immersive simulations and case-based scenarios for junior level and premedical learners. Depending on the events scheduled for the month in which they are enrolled, they also attend simulation-based courses conducted for various audiences (e.g., community service programs with middle school students or CME courses for attending-level staff). In these courses they assume various roles while learning a good deal with "over the shoulder" observation to learn how to run scenarios. In addition to obtaining skills in curricular development with the human simulator, the student educators learn to appreciate and respect the needs and abilities of the students they teach.

By the end of their month, students are expected to have designed and taught one novel simulation scenario to third-year medical students on their 1-week anesthesia clerkship. This scenario is created under the guidance of resident and/or attending faculty supervision and is observed by one of the simulation faculty to assist the student with running the scenario, debriefing the students, and to order to provide feedback to the elective student educator (see Table 41.2).

The Clinical Educator Track for Residents

Our program recruits many of these students into our anesthesiology residency program who then continue as resident educators. Also, many of our residents become interested in teaching and ask to be involved in simulation-based education after they are exposed to their clinical anesthesia (CA)-1 anesthesia boot camp—a series of simulations over a 7-week period. CA-1 residents with an interest in medical education are recruited from our residency program to join our "Clinical Educator Track" (CET) and participate in our department's simulation-based educator program for community service and teaching of medical students, residents, and occasionally retraining physicians. The residents first participate in an advanced simulator elective and are taught to develop and conduct both didactic and simulator-based educational activities. As a component of their residency responsibilities, these residents learn to be effective educators for a variety of audiences, organize and conduct the didactic curriculum for our third-year anesthesia clerkship, teach in our simulator-based physiology labs, help conduct simulator-based courses for residents and retraining attending-level physicians, and participate in extensive community service teaching which includes underprivileged students from local elementary and middle and high schools. In addition, the residents participate in regional, national, and international meetings helping faculty conduct simulation-based workshops (see Fig. 41.4).

Initially, junior residents are encouraged to observe senior resident educators during didactic and simulator-based educational sessions. Further training on the simulator is performed in conjunction with the simulation educational fellow and attending faculty to help residents develop their own

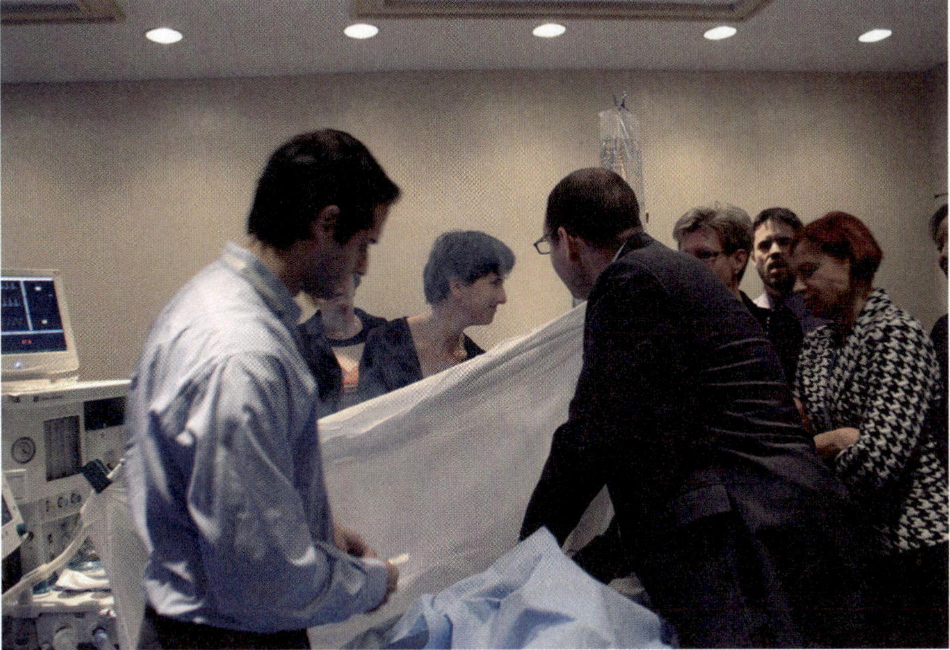

Fig. 41.4 Attending and resident clinical educators simulate an airway fire at a national meeting

curriculum while they also help teach during existing simulator-based sessions. The residents learn to be effective communicators for a variety of student audiences and also learn to develop successful simulations and educational modules through participation in existing educational sessions. Residents are strongly encouraged to develop their own unique and innovative didactic and simulator-based curriculum in an open-ended model where they have no specific requirements for a scenario type or setting but are expected to develop and use a repertoire of scenarios for the various audiences they encounter, (e.g., designing a scenario that is fun and represents an innovative way to orient new medical students to the department) (see Table 41.3). With a large complement of resident educators (roughly 3–5 per year), the result is a large breadth and wide variety of lessons. Many of the residents find it a rewarding experience which allows them to create an educational portfolio for those continuing in a career in academic medicine.

Our residents are given the opportunity to teach in conjunction with their clinical responsibilities by signing up to work a financially compensated pre or post-call educational day. Residents must be Accreditation Council of Graduate Medical Education (ACGME) work-hour compliant and cannot violate the work-hour restrictions placed by the ACGME. Since the call schedule and resident rotation schedule vary from month to month, it is ideal to have a large complement of residents to fulfill the department's educational goals. An online, internet-based calendar has been set up for residents to sign up for education days (see Table 41.4). This calendar is available to the resident education coordinators (CA3 residents experienced with teaching) and the rest of the residents to avoid scheduling conflicts. Dates are then communicated to the program director and medical students to maintain logistical organization.

The goals and objectives for the CET is that residents learn curricula development, curricula assessment, simulation programming, and simulation-based teaching modalities over the course of their 3-year training (see Table 41.5). They are encouraged to keep track of their educational experiences, and methods are provided by which they receive feedback from medical students in order to better hone their skills and further develop new educational exercises.

Residents conduct simulation-based educational activities throughout the year including:

1. Community service education for underprivileged students
2. Premed and humanities and medicine curriculum
3. Integrated simulation-based physiology labs for first-year medical student
   (a) Pulmonary physiology
   (b) Cardiovascular physiology
   (c) The autonomic nervous system
4. Anesthesia curriculum for third-year medical student clerks
5. Curriculum for fourth-year students participating in a simulation or basic anesthesiology elective
6. Introduction to internship for PGY-1 anesthesiology residents

Table 41.3 Innovative orientation curriculum designed by a resident clinical educator

Lesson Title: Workroom Scavenger Hunt	
Teacher: Jason H Epstein, MD **Date**: 17 January 2012 **Students**: Visiting MS4 students	
Lesson objectives	**Key points**
Students will be able to find the GP3, Ann6, and Ann7 anesthesia workrooms Students will be able to describe the categories of equipment to be found in the anesthesia workrooms Students will be able to describe the differences between standard, anode, RAE, and blue line tubes Students will have fun	Anesthesia workrooms can be a confusing, complicated place to be Support staff are key members of the anesthesia team Introduce them to one of the anesthesia techs if possible
Assessment tools Scavenger Hunt (see below)	
What/When	**How**
Opening hook/connection to prior knowledge (15 min)	Welcome to MSSM. Ask who has gotten lost so far Give them a scenario of having an unexpected difficult airway in your room and being asked to quickly grab a fiber-optic scope and a 6.0 ETT. Imagine the challenge of even finding the workroom and then how to get the equipment
Workroom tour (30 min)	Visit the three workrooms: Ann7/Ann6/GP3 West Review equipment as follows: Ann7: Airway and regional (ENT/GU cases) Ann6: IVs and fluids (Peds/ambulatory cases) GP3: Drugs
Workroom scavenger hunt (30 min)	Divide into three groups Each group is given the scavenger hunt form below and is assigned to a different workroom Ensure each group has someone with a smartphone to take pictures. Take a picture of the things on the scavenger hunt items labeled [1]. Encourage taking pictures otherwise you will have lots of stuff to return to the workrooms at the end of the day Give them 20 min to meet back on KCC8 conference room
Scavenger hunt review (20 min)	Review answers Score liberally (note that some of the questions have more than one correct answer) Give out candy – winning group gets to pick first
Department connection (10 min)	Make sure you get something from the workroom for your cases tomorrow
Materials and attachments Scavenger hunt ×4 Candy!	

7. Introduction to anesthesiology for CA-1 anesthesiology residents
8. Simulation-based PALS for CA-2 residents
9. Airway assessment and management for critical-care fellows
10. Simulation workshops at the New York State Society of Anesthesiologist (NYSSA) Postgraduate Assembly (PGA)
11. Simulation for the thoracic workshop at the American Society of Anesthesiologists (ASA) annual meeting
12. Regional training level-specific simulation-based seminar for anesthesiology residents (milestones, outcomes, and competencies for anesthesiology residents [MOCAR])
13. Departmental educational meetings (The New York Review, Clinical updates in Anesthesiology, Surgery and Perioperative Medicine)

Table 41.4 Sample teaching schedule based on resident call schedule

Date	Name	Session	Location
Mon Oct 31 9–11AM	Silverman (Post 2A)	MS4 orientation	KCC 8-04
Tue Nov 2 2–4PM	Reddy (Pre-OB)	MS4 (OB and Epidurals)	KCC 8-04
Wed Nov 2 1–3PM	Blasius (Pre TL)	MS4 (human patient simulation)	Sim Lab
Thurs Nov 3 2–4PM	Hernandez (Post-long)	MS4 (intro to workroom)	KCC 8-58
Fri Nov 4 1:30–3:30PM	Ezziddin (Pre-OB)	MS4 (intro to Peds)	KCC 8-04
Fri Nov 4 9AM–1PM	Reddy (DAS)	CA-1 FLOAT	KCC 8-04
Wed Nov 9 3–5PM	Hofer (Post-long)	MS4 (induction)	Meet on KCC8
Thu Nov 13 2–4PM	Epstein (Pre-OB)	CA-0	Sim Lab
Fri Nov 11 9AM–1PM	Reddy (DAS)	CA-1 FLOAT	KCC 8-04
Fri Nov 11 9AM–3PM	Katz (Post-OB)	CA-1 SIM LAB	KCC 8-04
Mon Nov 14 1–3PM	Epstein (Pre-TL)	MS4	KCC 8-04
Wed Nov 16 1–3PM	Afonso (Pre-Elm)	MS4	Meet on KCC8
Thu Nov 17 1–3PM	Blasius (Pre-TL)	CA-0	Sim Lab
Thu Nov 17 1–3PM	Hofer (Pre-OB)	MS4 (Thoracic)	Meet on KCC8
Fri Nov 18 9AM–1PM	TBD	CA-1 FLOAT	KCC 8-04
Mon Nov 21 9–11AM	Ezzidin (Post-OB)	MS3 Orientation	TBD
Tue Nov 22 2–4PM	Blasius (Pre-2B)	MS3 (intro to anesthesia)	Sim Lab
Tue Nov 29 1–3PM	Afonso (Pre-Elm)	MS4 (intro to workroom)	KCC 8-04

Table 41.5 Sample clinical educator responsibility flow chart

Clinical education responsibilities	CA-1	CA-2	CA-3
Community service education for high school students	Teach	Supervise	Supervise
Premed education	Teach	Supervise	Supervise
MS1 physiology labs	Observe/act	Drive/teach	Teach
MS3 anesthesiology clerkship	Teach	Teach	Supervise
MS4 anesthesiology elective	Drive/teach	Teach	Teach
PGY1 Introduction to internship	Observe/act	Observe/act/drive	Teach
CA-1 "boot camp"	N/A	Observe/act/drive	Drive/teach
CA-2 PALS exercise	Observe	N/A	Teach

The Advanced Clinical Educator Track for Residents

The Advanced Clinical Educator Track (ACET) is a unique 2–4-month concentrated rotation for CA-3 residents engaged in simulation-based education throughout their training who have demonstrated an interest and an aptitude as resident educators. This advanced track gives CA-3 residents the opportunity to further hone their skills by receiving more consistent formal mentorship with advanced training in simulation-based education and assessment during dedicated nonclinical time. In addition, they are given administrative responsibilities and are expected to help schedule, organize, and staff the various educational programs run by our department and the other clinical educators. Known as Resident Education Coordinators, these residents are CA-3s who have been involved in the Clinical Educator Track and wish to pursue an academic career. Their responsibilities include the organization and conduct of the third-year medical student clerkship in anesthesiology, creating a dynamic and viable curriculum, and assisting in "faculty" development by keeping track of feedback for resident educators and offering constructive criticism (see Fig. 41.5). They also learn simulation-based research design and complete an grant an IRB application. CA-3 ACET residents are encouraged to participate in educational research projects and assist during local and national meetings. It is the goal of our program to provide residents upon completion of the Advanced Clinical Educator Track all the tools and skills necessary for an academic career whereby they are excellent clinician educators and clinician scientists. Over the last 7 years 92% (11 of 12) of the ACET residents have pursued careers in academics as simulation experts.

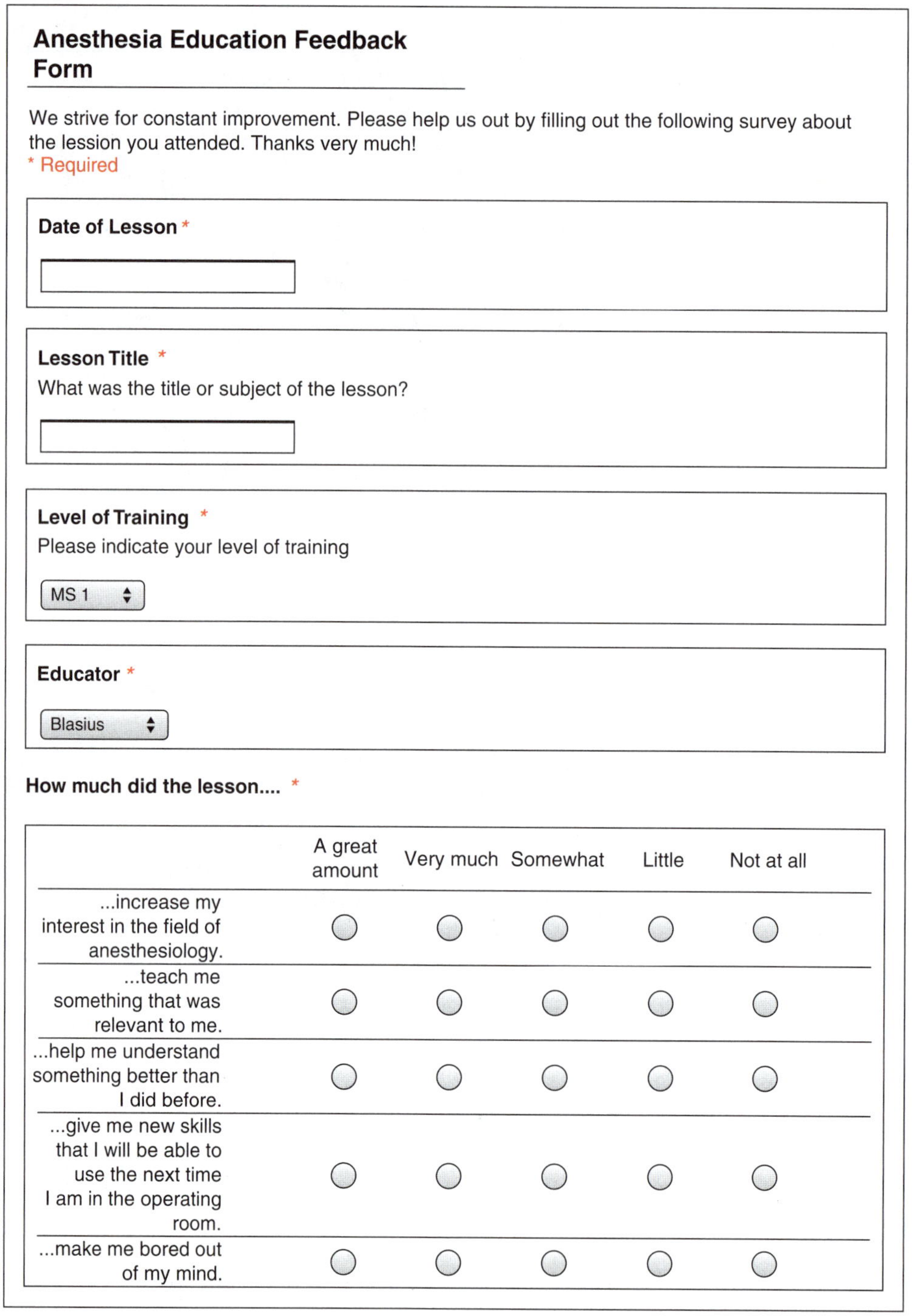

Fig. 41.5 Sample online feedback form

Anesthesia Education Feedback Form

We strive for constant improvement. Please help us out by filling out the following survey about the lession you attended. Thanks very much!
* Required

Date of Lesson *

Lesson Title *
What was the title or subject of the lesson?

Level of Training *
Please indicate your level of training

MS 1

Educator *

Blasius

How much did the lesson.... *

	A great amount	Very much	Somewhat	Little	Not at all
...increase my interest in the field of anesthesiology.	○	○	○	○	○
...teach me something that was relevant to me.	○	○	○	○	○
...help me understand something better than I did before.	○	○	○	○	○
...give me new skills that I will be able to use the next time I am in the operating room.	○	○	○	○	○
...make me bored out of my mind.	○	○	○	○	○

Conclusion

The study of medicine and training of a physician in many ways retains its origins as a relationship between a master and an apprentice. Like many trades, medicine is an amalgamation of skills that are best transmitted by members of that profession. The guild structure of trade expertise – apprentice, journeyman, and master – reflects our modern-day student, resident, and attending physician phases which reflect movement toward independence. Residents, like journeymen, represent the mid-level trainee of our profession, able to teach, yet still in want of further training. Clearly, simulation has already changed the way we as physicians educate our students. Combined with the idea that teaching and learning for physicians must always go hand in hand, simulation has the potential to change the way we as physicians train our teachers and provides creative and novel pathways to reach true masters of medicine and medical education.

References

1. Accreditation Council for Graduate Medical Education (ACGME) Common Program. 2011. ACGME Web site. Available at: http://www.acgme.org/acWebsite/navPages/nav_PDcoord.asp. Accessed 2 Mar 2012.
2. Standards for Accreditation of Medical Education Programs leading to the M.D. degree. 2010. Liason Committee on Medical Education Web Site. Available at: http://www.lcme.org/standard.htm. Accessed 2 Mar 2012.
3. Busari JO, Scherpbier AJ. Why residents should teach: a literature review. J Postgrad Med. 2004;50:205–10.
4. Meleca CB. A house staff training program to improve clinical teaching. Annu Conf Res Med Educ. 1977;16:332–3.
5. Meleca CB, Schimpfhauser FT, Witteman JK, Sachs LA. Clinical instruction in medicine: a national survey. J Med Educ. 1983;58:395–403.
6. Barnes HV, Albanese M, Schroeder J, Reiter S. Senior medical students teaching the basic skills of history and physical examination. Acad Med. 1978;53:432–4.
7. Flax J, Garrard J. Students teaching students: a model for medical education. Acad Med. 1974;49:380–3.
8. Bing-You RG, Tooker J. Teaching skills improvement programmes in US internal medicine residencies. Med Educ. 1993;27:259–65.
9. Edwards JC, Kissling GE, PlauchÉ WC, Marier RL. Evaluation of a teaching skills improvement programme for residents. Med Educ. 1988;22:514–7.
10. Julian KA, O'Sullivan PS, Vener MH, Wamsley MA. Teaching residents to teach: the impact of a multi-disciplinary longitudinal curriculum to improve teaching skills. Med Educ Online. 2007; 12:1–6.
11. Jewett LS, Greenberg LW, Goldberg RM. Teaching residents how to teach: a one-year study. J Med Educ. 1982;57:361–6.
12. Greenberg LW, Goldberg RM, Jewett LS. Teaching in the clinical setting: factors influencing residents' perceptions, confidence and behaviour. Med Educ. 1984;18:360–5.
13. Wamsley MA, Julian KA, Wipf JE. A literature review of "resident-as-teacher" curricula: do teaching courses make a difference? J Gen Intern Med. 2004;19:574–81.
14. Martins AR, Arbuckle MR, Rojas AA, Cabaniss DL. Growing teachers: using electives to teach senior residents how to teach. Acad Psychiatry. 2010;34:291–3.
15. Amarosa JMH, Mellman LA, Graham MJ. Medical students as teachers: how preclinical teaching opportunities can create an early awareness of the role of physician as teacher. Med Teach. 2011;33:137–44.
16. Haist SA, Wilson JF, Fosson SE, Brigham NL. Are fourth-year medical students effective teachers of the physical examination to first-year medical students? J Gen Intern Med. 1997;12:177–81.
17. Escovitz ES. Using senior students as clinical skills teaching assistants. Acad Med. 1990;65:733–4.
18. Solomon P, Crowe J. Perceptions of student peer tutors in a PBL program. Med Teach. 2001;23:181–6.
19. Morrison EH, Friedland JA, Boker J, Rucker L, Hollingshead J, Murata P. Residents-as-teachers training in US residency programs and offices of graduate medical education. Acad Med. 2001;76:S1–4.
20. Schaffer JL, Wile MZ, Griggs RC. Students teaching students: a medical school peer tutorial programme. Med Educ. 1990;24:336–43.
21. Krych AJ, March CN, Bryan RE, Peake BJ, Pawlina W, Carmichael SW. Reciprocal peer teaching: students teaching students in the gross anatomy laboratory. Clin Anat. 2005;18:296–301.
22. Mowbray A, McCulloch JD, Conn AG, Spence AA. Teaching of cardiopulmonary resuscitation by medical students. Med Educ. 1987;21:285–7.
23. Johansen ML, Martenson DF, Bircher J. Students as tutors in problem-based learning: does it work? Med Educ. 1992;26:163–5.
24. Blatt B, Greenberg L. A multi-level assessment of a program to teach medical students to teach. Adv Health Sci Educ. 2007;12:7–18.
25. Pasquinelli LM, Greenberg LW. A review of medical school programs that train medical students as teachers. Teach Learn Med. 2008;20:73–81.

Fellowship Training in Simulation

42

Emily M. Hayden and James A. Gordon

Introduction

A fellowship program in the health professions typically implies clinical subspecialty training, often approved by the Accreditation Council for Graduate Medical Education (ACGME) or other institutional regulatory bodies. In addition, mentored research training programs, often sponsored by governmental agencies, foundations, or individual specialty societies, have supported fellowship training for faculty development in the health sciences. Academic expertise in the learning sciences also requires an intensive period of dedicated study and support; however, opportunities for dedicated fellowship study in medical education generally [1–3], and simulation in particular, are comparatively limited. Based on experience with simulation fellows over nearly a decade [4, 5], we describe here a model for fellowship training designed to foster expertise and leadership in the growing field of medical simulation. Typically offered as a 1–2-year program of professional development, the fellowship is designed to extend focused training beyond individual faculty development courses and continuing medical education programs, offering an advanced career pathway in the field. This chapter will explore simulation fellowships using a curricular development framework described in Kern's Curriculum Development for Medical Educators [6] (Table 42.1); this approach is intended to provide both theoretical and organizational structure for discussion.

E.M. Hayden, MD, MHPE (✉) • J.A. Gordon, MD, MPA
MGH Learning Laboratory,
Division of Medical Simulation,
Department of Emergency Medicine,
Massachusetts General Hospital,
Boston, MA, USA

Gilbert Program in Medical Simulation,
Harvard Medical School,
Boston, MA, USA
e-mail: emhayden@partners.org; jgordon3@partners.org

Table 42.1 Kern's Curriculum Development Framework for Medical Educators [6]

Problem identification and general needs assessment
Needs assessment of targeted learners
Goals and objectives
Educational strategies
Implementation
Evaluation and feedback

Problem Identification and General Needs Assessment

Early general and specialty medical education fellowships were developed to augment teaching skills, create communities of educators, and develop educational leaders at a time of growing interest in medical education scholarship [2]. Similarly, health services research fellowships, sponsored by groups like the Robert Wood Johnson Foundation, also offered academic, methodologic, and leadership training in order to help selected clinicians better understand nonmedical disciplines essential to health care. Today, the rapidly increasing interest in simulation [7, 8] has driven a new demand for specialty leaders. These individuals need the training to lead, develop, teach, and evaluate the kind of simulation-based initiatives which promise wide-ranging impact on health care quality and safety. While medical students and residents interested in staying in academia increasingly view simulation as a viable career pathway, they need a support infrastructure to develop and sustain education-based careers. Fellowship work can help trainees efficiently acquire needed skills by providing an intensive period of time, focus, and support.

A.I. Levine et al. (eds.), *The Comprehensive Textbook of Healthcare Simulation*,
DOI 10.1007/978-1-4614-5993-4_42, © Springer Science+Business Media New York 2013

Table 42.2 Potential objectives for simulation fellowship

By the end of the simulation fellowship, all fellows should have the skills to:
1. Describe historical and current theoretical and scientific foundations of simulation-based medical education
2. Conceive, develop, and run simulation-based training and assessment modules
3. Help create, administer, and evaluate new simulation programs, centers, and technology
4. Critically appraise and/or conduct simulation-based medical education research

Needs Assessment of Targeted Learners

Most current simulation fellowships are focused on physician trainees who have just completed residency training. These individuals are more likely to have experienced simulation in their prior training but typically have limited training in the theory, style, administration, and science of simulation-based education. Potential fellows can identify a range of focus areas during a simulation fellowship, including clinical teaching, medical education research, leadership and administration, and biomechanical engineering. Some institutions have chosen to combine medical education and simulation fellowships into a unified whole, complementing those shared competencies (i.e., teaching methodology, competency assessment, curriculum development, program evaluation, organizational structure, and educational scholarship) with more simulation-specific skills like technology-enhanced case development, scenario implementation, and debriefing strategies.

Goals and Objectives

The primary goal of simulation fellowship programs is to create experts and leaders in the field of healthcare simulation by providing dedicated experience and mentored training in simulation-based medical education. A sample list of objectives is listed in Table 42.2.

Other objectives are at the discretion of the fellowship director and fellow, such as those focusing on specific projects tailored to the fellows' goals and the local environment. Fellowship program objectives should adapt with changing institutional or fellow needs.

Educational Strategies

The strategies employed for any fellowship should reflect the local environment in terms of objectives, resources, and faculty. It is more efficient to make use of existing courses and infrastructure, such as master's degree coursework or certificate programs, and established faculty development workshops. It is helpful if the simulation fellows can join an existing cohort of research and education trainees in other disciplines to learn from one another, share research ideas, and participate in collective "works-in-progress" presentation and feedback sessions.

Educational strategies should map to the objectives of the program. The sample objectives from Table 42.2 are recounted below with example strategies matched to each item:

1. *Describe the historical and current theoretical and scientific foundations of simulation-based medical education*:
   - Attend local faculty lectures and participate in community discussion.
   - Engage in guided readings and/or journal club.
   - Attend regional and national simulation/medical education meetings/exhibits.
   - Participate in graduate-level coursework and continuing education offerings.
2. *Conceive, develop, and run simulation-based training and assessment modules* (in addition to the above):
   - Engage in a longitudinal teaching practicum (supervised practical teaching experience).
   - Learn and practice how to operate and teach with all simulation equipment.
   - Observe both novice and master simulation instructors.
   - Encourage direct observation of one's own instruction and solicit peer feedback.
   - Assume leadership in selected course design, administration, and evaluation.
   - Participate in reflective practice
3. *Help create, administer, and evaluate new simulation programs, centers, and technology (in addition to* the above):
   - Attend local simulation operations, planning, and leadership meetings.
   - Attend faculty development and leadership workshops (locally and nationally).
   - Assume leadership for a programmatic component of the local teaching unit.
   - Assist in evaluation of new equipment and financing.
   - Participate in the hiring and human resources process for new fellows and staff.
4. *Critically appraise and/or conduct simulation-based medical education research* (in addition to the above):
   - Completion of an IRB/Human subjects review application.
   - Write and submit scholarly abstract(s) for peer review and presentation.

- Design, implement, and complete a scholarly project through to manuscript.
- Participate in peer review of others' work (formal or informal).

Implementation

The implementation of a fellowship program will be driven by the local environment and resources. This section will be a general discussion of simulation fellowship program implementation, with framework adapted from Kern's curricular development model [6], including a discussion of resources, support, administration, barriers, and introduction of the curriculum.

While not required for the academic training component of the fellowship, clinicians need a venue to maintain their clinical skill during the fellowship period. This clinical component complements the simulation fellowship work and is typically arranged in collaboration with the relevant clinical department of the base institution. However, some fellows may arrange clinical work independently, as long as it fits within the structure and time demands of the fellowship curriculum. Under special arrangement, some fellows, particularly international research physicians, will be eligible only for nonclinical fellowship experience.

Identification of Resources

Resources required for any fellowship program revolve around discussion of applicants, faculty, time, facilities, and funding considerations.

Fellow Applicants

Fellowship training in medical simulation is applicable across specialties, but a broad clinical background is helpful in serving the diverse constituencies of most simulation programs. Selection criteria and clinical responsibilities will vary by institution. Those programs that facilitate clinical placement will interview and select applicants for both clinical and fellowship work.

Faculty

Faculty can be drawn from both within and outside the institution, guided by the fellowship director, who typically serves as a primary mentor. Often the local simulation center director is also the simulation fellowship director, which provides important synergy and programmatic context for the fellow. Clinical mentorship is provided by the relevant departmental leadership and practice group.

Time

Typical allocation of time for fellowship duties (vs. clinical/other non-simulation-related work) ranges from 50 to 80% academic "protected" time for new skill acquisition. For clinicians, this often translates to 1–2+ days of clinical work a week, complementing 3–4 days reserved for fellowship work. Those fellowships that do not arrange clinical placement typically allow fellows to moonlight; however, clinical work beyond the time allocations noted risks detracting from the fellowship training itself. The fellowship time is often the only dedicated period an individual will have for several years to build a solid foundation for an academic career.

Fellowship programs are usually 1–2 years in length. Typically a 1-year simulation fellowship program will allow a fellow to survey the different types of simulation available and learn to teach in these environments. Given all of the concurrent responsibilities of a new fellow/faculty member (e.g., transitioning to new clinical role often in a new healthcare system), some fellows choose not to develop an independent research project during the first year, focusing instead on simulation teaching and course administration. A 2-year fellowship allows the fellow to spend more time on scholarship in simulation, and those so inclined can opt for a second year to focus on academic and research development. A sample template of a 1-year fellowship is shown in Table 42.3; this template is used locally for the fellowship based at Massachusetts General Hospital but is designed to be accessible and available as a joint fellowship structure in collaboration with other institutions (i.e., all formal coursework can be done by distance or in short on-site bursts in Boston; all teaching and programmatic experience is conducted at the home institution/simulation center).

Facilities

A simulation center sponsoring a simulation fellowship should be able to host a wide variety of simulation technologies and teaching approaches, offering experience both in the laboratory and in situ within a clinical/hospital setting. A fellow should also have a dedicated work space which can be provided by the simulation laboratory or within an affiliated clinical department.

Table 42.3 Template of a 1-year simulation fellowship

July	Orientation to the simulation laboratory, hospital, clinical department, and medical/nursing school Help with simulation-based orientation activities for new hospital trainees and house staff
August	Mentored teaching in simulation-based orientation activities for new medical/nursing students
September	Mentored teaching in simulation activities (simulation laboratory and in situ)
October	Attend the 1-week Institute for Medical Simulation Comprehensive Workshop (Center for Medical Simulation, Boston, MA) [9, 10] Mentored teaching in simulation activities (simulation laboratory and in situ)
November	Supervised simulation teaching (simulation laboratory and in situ)
December	Supervised simulation teaching (simulation laboratory and in situ)
January	Attend 2-week winter session for the Harvard Macy Institute's Program for Educators in the Health Professions (Harvard Medical School and Graduate School of Education, Boston, MA) [11, 12] Attend the Society for Simulation in Healthcare's International Meeting on Simulation in Healthcare
February	Start academic teaching practicum through the MGH Institute of Health Professions (a graduate school founded by Massachusetts General Hospital). This semester-long activity can be done by distance for nonlocal fellows. In combination with the Institute for Medical Simulation and Harvard Macy Institute course offerings (above), completion of this practicum qualifies the fellow for the graduate school's Certificate of Teaching and Learning with a Concentration in Healthcare Simulation Lead simulation teaching activities (simulation laboratory and in situ)
March	Lead simulation teaching activities (simulation laboratory and in situ) Continue teaching practicum course
April	Lead simulation teaching activities (simulation laboratory and in situ) Continue teaching practicum course
May	Attend 1-week spring session of the Harvard Macy Institute's Program for Educators in the Health Professions Lead simulation teaching activities (simulation laboratory and in situ) Complete teaching practicum course and earn graduate-school level Teaching and Learning Certificate
June	Lead simulation teaching activities (simulation laboratory and in situ)

During the year fellows are also required to attend weekly simulation laboratory operations meetings and a monthly simulation education and research forum; individual scholarly work is planned in collaboration with program faculty and extended to a second year focus (often with initiation or extension of Master's degree coursework) for those fellows wishing to concentrate on educational research

Funding

The number of fellowship positions offered may be determined by a variety of factors, including availability and structure of funding, teaching volume, faculty oversight, and clinical placement opportunities. For example, some programs can accommodate two fellows per year, while others will accommodate one every other year based on a 2-year fellowship cycle.

Funding of the fellowship is also dependent on the local environment. One common option is to have the fellow work a reduced/part-time clinical load at the attending salary rate. This is often estimated at between 20 and 50%, or 1–2+ clinical days, with the caveat that more clinical time translates to more income but less focus available for fellowship work. To mitigate, additional stipend funds can be added to prioritize funding for the simulation fellowship work. That stipend can come from multiple sources, whether from the simulation center funds, grant work, or other institutional/departmental allocations. The size of that stipend will vary by program and funding source and depends on availability and/or desirability of clinical practice as part of an integrated fellowship model.

While some institutions choose to segregate clinical appointments from academic fellowship roles (i.e., a fellow in medical simulation can also work as an attending physician in their area of board preparation/certification), others do not. This precludes a salary model supported by clinical work. Extending the academic stipend model above, another option is to pay the fellow the corresponding postgraduate trainee salary rate which would be supported by dedicated academic fellowship funds. For example, if the fellow has just completed a 4-year residency, they would now be considered a PGY-5 and paid the corresponding institutionally approved salary rate.

Obtaining Support

Internal support of all stakeholders for the fellowship needs to be gathered to ensure a successful program. These stakeholders include fellows, clinical department leadership, graduate medical leadership, and simulation faculty. While simulation/education fellowships by their very nature are not ACGME eligible, many institutions will have an oversight and "accreditation" pathway for nonclinical fellowships that is very helpful in establishing and maintaining a simulation training program.

Administration

While some fellowships will be highly structured, others will be more flexible. In alignment with the principles of adult learning that focuses on making the learning relevant to the learner, some fellows will manage their own learning throughout the fellowship. A simulation director will always guide the fellow and advise which activities would be higher yield than others; but in the more flexible model, the fellowship period is inherently time for discovery learning. The administrative structure of the fellowship is typically straightforward with the simulation center director often also serving as the fellowship director and mentor, and affiliated simulation community providing faculty support. As the fellow gains experience, they may assume supervised administrative and leadership roles within the group.

Anticipating Barriers

Taking steps to prevent obstacles will lessen foreseeable barriers to the program. Support of the simulation center, respective clinical departments, and hospital are crucial. An internal (institutional) application process for fellowships can be very helpful in gathering feedback and support. Those fellows who integrate clinical work into the fellowship will need the same level of clinical supervision and mentorship as any new faculty member and must be allocated the same level of support.

Introducing the Curriculum

For new programs, one common approach is to introduce the curriculum and pilot the first year with an internal candidate. This allows the fellowship to have an initial incumbent that is known and familiar with local culture and practice and can take maximum advantage of existing resources; this individual can also provide critical insight into institution-specific opportunities and challenges as the program expands.

Evaluation and Feedback

A robust program with a systematic approach incorporates thoughtful assessment of the fellow and faculty, as well as evaluation of the program.

Assessment

The fellow should receive formative feedback as often as possible throughout their training. This feedback can be from the fellowship director, faculty, simulation technicians, and simulation participants. Summative assessment likely would be in the form of 6-month or yearly evaluation forms that are completed by the fellowship director and faculty. The fellow should be advised to start a teaching portfolio to keep track of their instructional assessments/evaluations. Meetings should be planned every 6 months for discussion of the fellow's progress.

Program Evaluation

Multiple sources of fellowship program evaluation can be employed. The most immediate sources of evaluative information are from evaluation forms that fellows and faculty complete. Tracking the fellows' scholarship, awards, leadership positions, and promotions both during and after fellowship is also helpful in gauging the impact of fellowship work.

Conclusion

As the field of medical simulation grows, there is increasing demand for experts and leaders in the field. Simulation fellowships are one venue for intensive training and faculty development for a focused academic career. As more simulation fellowships and associated training opportunities are offered in the USA and abroad, a well-trained community of simulation leaders will increasingly be available to help guide and sustain the field.

References

1. Gruppen L, Simpson D, Searle N, Robins L, Irby D, Mullan P. Educational fellowship programs: common themes and overarching issues. Acad Med. 2006;81:990–4.
2. Searle N, Hatem C, Perkowski L, Wilkerson L. Why invest in an educational fellowship program? Acad Med. 2006;81:936–40.
3. Hatem C, Lown B, Newman L. The Academic Health Center Coming of Age: helping faculty become better teachers and agents of educational change. Acad Med. 2006;81:941–4.
4. Gordon J, Oriol N, Cooper J. Bringing good teaching cases "to life": a simulator-based medical education service. Acad Med. 2004;79:23–7.
5. Gordon JA. As accessible as a book on a library shelf: the imperative of routine simulation in modern healthcare. Chest. 2012;141(1):12–6.
6. Kern D, Thomas P, Howard D, Bass E. Curriculum Development for Medical Education: a six-step approach. Baltimore: The Johns Hopkins University Press; 1998.
7. Okuda Y, Bond W, Bonfante G, et al. National growth in simulation training within emergency medicine residency programs, 2003–2008. Acad Emerg Med. 2008;15:1113–6.
8. Fernandez R, Wang E, Vozenilek J, et al. Simulation Center Accreditation and Programmatic Benchmarks: a review for emergency medicine. Acad Emerg Med. 2010;17:1093–103.

9. Rudolph J, Simon R, Raemer D, Eppich W. Debriefing as formative assessment: closing performance gaps in medical education. Acad Emerg Med. 2008;15:1010–6.
10. Gordon J, Cooper J, Simon R, Raemer D. The Institute for Medical Simulation: a new resource for medical educators worldwide [abstract]. Anesthesiol Analg. 2005;101:S22.
11. Armstrong E, Doyle J, Bennett N. Transformative professional development of physicians as educators: assessment of a model. Acad Med. 2003;78:702–8.
12. Armstrong E, Barison S. Using an outcomes-logic-model approach to evaluate a faculty development program for medical educators. Acad Med. 2006;81:483–8.

Specialized Courses in Simulation

43

Deborah Navedo and Robert Simon

Introduction

The purpose of all simulations is to gain insight – insight about the nature of disease progression, about the efficacy of interventions or treatments, or even insight about one's own assumptions, decisions, or performance gaps – and to reflect on teamwork, decision making, and communication. The art and science of creating such learning environments in the health professions has evolved. Explicit learning outcomes include a spectrum of competencies from the demonstration of skills and compliance with algorithms and protocols to effective participation in an interprofessional team to provide comprehensive care in various settings [1].

For even seasoned educators, managing such an array of learning experiences requires special preparation in the form of faculty development or formal education in specialized "simulationist" courses. These courses go beyond the introductory level of faculty development that can be offered in single-session courses. Some of the courses are more immersive and comprehensive than others, exploring pedagogical principles such as adult and experiential learning to create evidence-based learning environments and providing methods to contribute knowledge to the field through systematic research. Most of the latter courses are emerging within institutions of higher education and offer credit and possibly academic credentials or degrees.

Previous chapters focused on formal education training for medical students, residents and fellows. This chapter offers an overview of the increasing value placed on educational competencies of simulation instructors for the practicing healthcare provider. We will review a sampling of currently available specialized courses and describe future directions in faculty development for simulation-based education.

Calls for Educational Reform Toward Simulation-Based Learning

There has been an increasing call for health profession education reform include the need for evidence-based teaching techniques rather than relying on clinical expertise alone [2–4]. Traditionally, healthcare providers lacked formal training in education. Although it was assumed that practitioners would naturally be effective educators, this is not generally the case. The Accreditation Council for Graduate Medical Education (ACGME) has emphasized the importance of communication and teaching and requires all training programs to create an environment that fosters students as educators [5]. As is the case in clinical practice, the adage, see one, do one, teach one, is no longer valid when one is discussing teaching skills. In addition clinical instruction had been based on teaching cases used by veteran faculty. As grant funded simulation centers started appearing in the past decade, these cases were often recreated with mannequin simulators. Simulation sessions were focused on programming the mannequins to mirror the physiology of the clinical cases. Clinical expertise is not entirely sufficient to claim competence in this new and unique environment. Simulation-based educational experiences tend to be stressful for participants, complex for instructors, and have an emotional component for learners. They are focused on changing learner behaviors, including fostering reflective practitioners, and require that participants be debriefed. This requirement for debriefing is not only an educationally sound

D. Navedo, PhD, CPNP, CNE (✉)
Center for Interprofessional Studies and Innovation,
MGH Institute of Health Professions,
Charlestown Navy Yard, 36 First Ave.,
Boston, MA 02129-4557, USA

MGH Learning Laboratory,
Massachusetts General Hospital, Boston, MA, USA
e-mail: dnavedo@mghihp.edu

R. Simon, EdD
Department of Anesthesia,
Harvard Medical School, Boston, MA, USA

Center for Medical Simulation,
100 First Ave, Building 39, 4th Floor, Charlestown, MA 02129, USA
e-mail: rsimon2@partners.org

A.I. Levine et al. (eds.), *The Comprehensive Textbook of Healthcare Simulation*,
DOI 10.1007/978-1-4614-5993-4_43, © Springer Science+Business Media New York 2013

practice (see Chaps. 6 and 7) but also has an ethical component, i.e., unlike the clinical environment wherein patients are subject to many forces beyond the control of the educator. Instructors using simulation purposely put learners in difficult events and thus have a moral obligation to do their best to leave the learner well-informed about what happened and emotionally sound. These considerations and others have resulted in current demand for the infusion of educational expertise to improve educational efficacy in simulation environments [6].

Beginning with a shifting focus away from the technology (i.e., technical aspects of the simulator and complementing equipment), toward the techniques (pedagogy, learning theory) [1], desired learning outcomes have been defined with increasing complexity from successful completion of tasks or skills to effective performance within an interprofessional team. Due to the need to thoughtfully create such complex learning environments and to ensure that effective learning occurs in this new and powerful setting, specialized courses are being developed and provided for faculty development.

In 2005, Pamela Jeffries described a framework for implementing and assessing simulation within nursing education. She called for additional research to substantiate the prerequisite educator competencies for this growing teaching modality [7]. On the occasion of the 100th anniversary of the Flexner Report [8] and the Goldmark Report [9], which called for a scientific basis and approach to medical and nursing education, various studies were conducted to gauge the current progress in these fields. Two recent manuscripts, from the Lancet commission and the Carnegie Foundation, resulted in calls for further reform in healthcare education.

The Lancet commissioned report, *Health professionals for a new century: transforming education to strengthen health systems in an interdependent world* [4], identified problems requiring a redesign of the professional health education system. The report goes on to say that simulation-based education may be one potential solution to the problems. Identified barriers to effective healthcare included (1) a mismatch of competencies to patient needs, (2) inconsistent teamwork skills, (3) too narrow a focus on technical skills without broader contextual understanding, and (4) the tendency of the various professions to act in isolation from each other, risking communication and continuity errors.

Similarly, the Carnegie Foundation for the Advancement of Teaching reports on nursing and physician education called for improved pedagogy, which could be increased through the use of simulation as a complementary teaching strategy. Specifically, the report *Educating Nurses: A Call for Radical Transformation* [2] called for a radical rethinking about how to better integrate classroom teaching with clinical practice. Also, the report *Educating Physicians: A Call for Reform of Medical School and Residency* [3] called for incorporating early clinical experiences into medical education and offering more opportunities for medical students to train in teams with nursing and other health profession students.

In summary, emerging literature is calling for efficient integration of clinical experiences early in the educational process that is more interprofessional and team-base focused. Simulation-based education offers consistent clinical learning experiences without increasing patient risk and, if managed correctly, offers a psychologically safe and supportive learning environment for the trainees. Creating such learning environments requires a specialized skill set. Therefore, the need for infusion of improved and broadened educator skills is needed to optimize simulation-based learning. This need is creating a demand for specialized courses in simulation-based education in the context of the health professions.

Toward Standardized Educator Competencies

Expert clinicians are not by default expert educators. Educator competencies include a range of skills such as the ability to identify cognitive, psychomotor, and affective learning outcomes; knowing how to effectively teach different materials to different types of learners; and understanding how learners learn are not innate skills. These competencies need to be practiced and coached, just like any other professional training program, to result in knowledgeable and effective educators. Very few health profession schools provide their clinicians with a structured curriculum on learning theory and practices such as learning in an experiential context, designing courses and curricula, teaching techniques, learning outcome assessment, program assessment, and improvement. Moreover, very few health profession schools' clinical curricula provide information and insight into human factors, teamwork, organizational behavior, and social psychology. The knowledge of these concepts is vital for instructors so they are capable of teaching these important behavioral aspects of clinical care to their learners.

Existing programs to educate health professions faculty have mostly been oriented to single discipline and single specialty training. There are a significant number of master's level programs in nursing education and a growing number of physician or specialty-specific programs for physician educators. Each has developed their own program outcomes, but there is a paucity of coordinated literature describing the competencies of health profession educators in general, thus leaving little guidance for the simulation-based educator. As recently as 2006, published program development strategies for increasing simulation-based education did not include consideration for faculty development needs [10], but instead focused on curriculum development and organizational infrastructure including equipment acquisition.

Some organizations have begun efforts to define educator expectations with varying degrees of specificity. While some organizations defined the role of the educator as extrinsic and often not as content expert [11], other organizations have begun moving toward increasing the professional development for the existing clinician faculty in the areas of educator competency [12, 13].

Two interprofessional efforts underway are from the Society for Simulation in Healthcare (SSH) and the US Veteran's Administration (VA). The SSH has started a process of certifying simulation instructors [14]. Other organizations have been cooperating with the effort including the Australian Society for Simulation in Healthcare, the Association for Standardized Patient Educators, the International Nursing Association for Clinical Simulation and Learning and the Society in Europe for Simulation Applied to Medicine. The general topical areas are consistent with the simulation-based educator competencies described by the VA [15], on their SimLEARN Web page under the heading "General Competencies for SimInstructors." The areas include (1) program administration, (2) instructional skills, (3) technical skills for the simulation equipment, (4) curriculum planning and session design, and (5) assessment of learning and evaluation of program effectiveness. As these simulation-based instructor competencies are vetted, published, and validated, professional development activities for instructors, be it conference sessions, multiday CME courses, or formalized graduate programs in academia, may begin to align their curricula with these competencies.

Specialized Instructor Courses for Simulation-Based Teaching and Learning

Recently there has been an emergence of specialized simulation-based educator courses that aim to integrate evidence-based teaching practices into the simulated cases. Some are multiday faculty development or continuing education (CE) courses within existing simulation centers, while others are emerging as formal courses in institutions of higher education such as certificate programs or even concentrations in degrees programs. In this chapter we review only the multiday courses and graduate-level courses. [See Chap. 44 for descriptions of single-session offerings from SSH, INACSL, SESAM, etc.]

Examples of existing multiday CE programs for faculty development and instructor training can be seen in those offered by active simulation centers, often as part of their ongoing faculty development offerings. Typically, these programs are on-site, intensive experiences with established and well-defined learning outcomes (see Table 43.1). Most offer

Table 43.1 Sample multiday continuing education instructor courses

Name of course	Location	Collaborating simulation center	Approx. length
Institute for Medical Simulation (IMS): Comprehensive Instructor Course	Boston, MA	Center for Medical Simulation (CMS)	5 days
Improving Simulation Instructional Methods (ISIM)	Pittsburg, PA	Winter Institute for Simulation Education and Research (WISER)	3 days
Train the Trainer	Bristol, UK	Bristol Medical Simulation Center	2 days
International Workshop	Tel Hashomer, Israel	Israel Center for Medical Simulation (MSR)	5 days
Instructor Training Course	Sydney, Australia	Sydney Clinical Skills and Simulation Center	2 days
Center for Immersive and Simulation-Based Learning (CISL) Instructor Course	Stanford, CA	Center for Immersive and Simulation-based Learning (CISL) Stamford Medical School	2.5 days
Certificate in Simulation	Philadelphia, PA	Drexel College of Nursing and Health Professions	5 days
Australian Simulation Educators and Technician Trainers (AusSETT)	Rotating locations within Australia	Monash University (lead), The University of Melbourne, Edith Cowan University, Flinders University, The University of Queensland and Queensland Health	3 days
Coordinated Approach to Simulation Training (CAST)	East Bentleigh VIC, Australia	Southern Health Simulation Center, Monash Medical Center	5 days
Instructor Development: Simulation-Based Education Design and Debriefing	Rochester, MN	Mayo Clinic	3 days
Certificate in Simulation	Philadelphia	Center for Interdisciplinary Clinical Simulation and Practice, Drexel University College of Nursing and Health Professionals	5 days
The Basic EuSim Simulation Instructor Course and the Advanced EuSim Simulation Instructor Course	Copenhagen, Tuebingen, Bilthoven, London	Danish Institute for Medical Simulation (DIMS), Center for Patient Safety and Simulation (TuPASS), BARTS and The London NHS Trust	3 days
Keystones of Healthcare Simulation Certificate	Toronto, Canada	SIM-One, Ontario Simulation Network, University of Toronto and Waters Family Simulation Center	Three multiday courses and presentation at conference required

Table 43.2 Graduate certificate programs

Name of certificate	Institution of higher education	Collaborating simulation center	Credit requirements	Format	Practicum required	Comments
Certificate in Simulation Education	BryanLGH College of Health Sciences	(own)	9 credits	Online	No	
Teaching and Learning Certificate with Concentration in Healthcare Simulation	MGH Institute of Health Professions	Center for Medical Simulation	9 credits	Hybrid–online theory course, on-site instructor course, and practicum	Yes, (50 h hands-on)	
Graduate Certificate in Clinical Simulation	Monash University	(own)	24 credit points		Yes	1 year part-time
Postgraduate Certificate in Medical Simulation	University of Bedfordshire and Hertfordshire Medical School	London Deanery and Butterfield Park Simulation Center	Various based on level	Hybrid–online modules with on-site intensives	Four contact days per term	Two units over two terms required

Table 43.3 Degree programs specializing in simulation-based education

Institution	Degree	Simulation concentration requirements	Length (credits)	Collaborating center
New York College of Osteopathic Medicine of New York Institute of Technology	Master of Science in Medical/Health Care Simulation	Common focus throughout the program	Part-time (44 credits)	NYCOM/NYIT's Institute For Clinical Competence
Vanderbilt School of Medicine	Master of Health Professions Education	2 semester hours (available as elective)	2 years (36 h)	Center for Experiential Learning (CELA)
MGH Institute of Health Professions	Master of Science in Health Professions Education	6 semester credits (available as concentration)	1 year full time or 2–4 years part-time (33 credits)	Center for Medical Simulation (CMS).
London Deanery and the Institute of Education of the University of London	MA in Technology and Simulation in Clinical Practice	Common focus throughout the program	1 year full time, or 2–4 years part-time	

overviews in teaching and learning theory, introduction to simulation-based learning, orientation to the equipment, debriefing fundamentals, and management of common problems and offer hands-on opportunities to practice.

Significantly, many of the centers have developed distinct principles and philosophies around creating learning environments (such as psychological safely), unique debriefing approaches, and professional development pathways leading to further opportunities for instructor development. Each has access to faculty from within or from affiliated institutions. Selection of the appropriate course should be based on matching these characteristics with the participant's needs.

For those instructors and faculty who aspire a deeper understanding of the practice and scholarship of simulation-based education, there are graduate-level courses resulting in certificates and master's degrees, with specific focuses on simulation-based education. Although many schools of education allow student projects in the context of health professions and even simulation-based education, only recently are master's degrees being offered with explicit concentrations or emphasis available in healthcare simulation.

A few accredited institutions of higher education are now offering graduate-level credit and certificates of advanced studies in simulation-based education. A few examples of such programs that are situated in graduate schools are found in Table 43.2.

Some of the courses are completely or predominantly online while other courses are on-site intensives. Some certificate programs require a mentored practicum, while others do not. Finally, many instructors and faculty are seeking to formalize their study of education by pursing a master's level program in health professions education, where they can study the effective use of simulation-based teaching. A few such programs are now emerging (see Table 43.3).

Some of these programs are designed to pipeline or progress from center-based intensive experiential-based instructor training courses to articulate into master's degree requirements. Again, a thoughtful assessment of possible career paths will help a participant choose between programs by taking into account the various access points and potential for further study. Examples of articulated programs that are designed to encourage progression include the London

Deanery/University of London program and the Massachusetts General Hospital Institute of Health Professions program in Boston. Both programs explicitly articulate from graduate-level certificate courses, often in the form of several days intensive and immersive training, which count toward future master's degree requirements.

Such articulation programs are possible where a regional collaboration has been formed between centers for professional development offering specialized courses and institutions of higher education. As with any degree program in higher education, a formal application and admissions process would be required for the degreed program. As most certificate program enrollees are not ready to commit to a master's degree program during certificate requirement completion, a separate application process for matriculation into the degree program would be required. Most master's degree programs are based on education degree models, so the curricula include courses beyond the practical aspects of simulation-based teaching such as the fundamentals of adult learning, research methods in education, technology in education, learning outcome assessment, course and program design and evaluation, leadership and organizational change, and scholarly writing. Master's programs in medical education or nursing education have seen steadily increasing enrollments over the past decades; however, the infusion of simulation as a concentration or focus has been considered innovative and is relatively new in the USA as evidenced by the very few programs that explicitly offer such a focus.

Future Directions

There is broad recognition that educational expertise is a requisite skill to run simulation-based learning activities and that clinical expertise alone is no longer sufficient. Additionally, simulation is likely to become increasingly central in both prelicensure [16] and postlicensure programs, driving the need for concurrent improvement in instructor competencies on all levels. Continued development of collaborations and partnerships between clinical simulation centers and formal health professions educator programs to increase the quality of educational outcomes through education and research is now an imperative. The field of simulation-based interprofessional education is also ripe for intensified collaboration with other fields such as cognitive and social sciences, organizational behavior, human factors, aviation, games, education, aviation, and the military. As evidence-based teaching continues to develop, continuing innovations should be tied closely to outcomes assessment and scholarship of teaching and learning.

Conclusion

As specialized courses for instructor training grow in number, increased vigilance toward defining educator competencies will be required in order to promote incorporation of best practices in simulation education. Most importantly, an increased demand for evidence-based teaching and learning practices should drive progress toward future innovations in simulation-based education and support for research. Funding of such educational initiatives should be prioritized as the scholarship of teaching and learning is focused on the critical task of program development and evaluation.

References

1. Gaba D. The future vision of simulation in health care. Qual Saf Health Care. 2004;13 Suppl 1:i2–10.
2. Carnegie Foundation for the Advancement of Teaching. Educating nurses: a call for radical transformation. San Francisco: Jossey-Bass; 2010.
3. Carnegie Foundation for the Advancement of Teaching. Educating physicians: a call for reform of medical schools and residency. San Francisco: Jossey-Bass; 2010.
4. Frenk J et al. Health professionals for a new century: transforming education to strengthen health systems in an interdependent world. Lancet. 2010;10:1–35.
5. Accreditation Council for Graduate Medical Education. ACGME Competencies. Available from: acgme.org/acwebsite/home/home.asp. Cited 22 June 2012.
6. Boulet J et al. Reliability and validity of a simulation-based acute care skills assessment for medical students and residents. Anesthesiology. 2003;99(6):1270–80.
7. Jeffries P. A frame work for designing, implementing, and evaluating simulations used as teaching strategies in nursing. Nurs Educ Perspect. 2005;26(2):96–103.
8. Carnegie Foundation for the Advancement of Teaching. Medical Education in the United States and Canada. Stanford; 1910.
9. Rawnsley MM. The Goldmark report: midpoint in nursing history. Nurs Outlook. 1973;21(6):380–3.
10. Gould D. SIR/RSNA/CIRSE joint medical simulation task force strategic plan executive summary. J Vasc Interv Radiol. 2007;18:953–5.
11. Passiment M, Sacks H, Huang G. Medical simulation in medical education: results of an AAMC Survey. https://www.aamc.org/download/259760/data/medicalsimulationinmedicaleducationanaamcsurvey.pdf. 2011.
12. Jackson BS. Nursing faculty qualifications and roles. The National Council of State Boards of Nursing. https://www.ncsbn.org/Final_08_Faculty_Qual_Report.pdf. 2008.
13. Jeffries PR. Getting in S.T.E.P. with simulations: simulations take educator preparation. Nurs Educ Perspect. 2008;29(2):70–3.
14. Society for Simulation in Healthcare. Certification standards and elements. https://ssih.org/uploads/static_pages/PDFs/Certification/CHSE%20Standards.pdf. 2012.
15. SimLEARN: How to be a Simulation Instructor. Available from: http://www.simlearn.va.gov/SIMLEARN/RSRC_9-How_to_be_a_Simulation_Instructor.asp. Cited 22 June 2012.
16. Nehring W. U.S. boards of nursing and the use of high-fidelity patient simulators in nursing education. J Prof Nurs. 2008;24(2):109–17.

Continuing Education in Simulation

44

Ronald Levy, Kathryn Adams, and Wanda Goranson

Introduction

Every healthcare professional has an ethical obligation to maintain competency and provide the best evidence-based care available [1–3]. Healthcare professionals do not discontinue their education at the end of their formal training, but frequently renew their proficiencies throughout their careers, learning and updating cognitive knowledge, psychomotor skills, and teamwork techniques. This chapter will review continuing education accreditation and oversight, examine the necessary criteria for CE development, and present available simulation-based CE opportunities. Specifically, the content development process used for the Society for Simulation in Healthcare's (SSH) International Meeting on Simulation in Healthcare (IMSH) will be highlighted as an example of the processes and considerations involved in developing healthcare CE offerings.

Continuing Education Accreditation

The purpose of continuing education is to advance the knowledge and skills of professionals delivering care. Educational programs are offered on many topics, but not all educational programs qualify for continuing education credits. In order to receive CE credit, the activity/program must meet strict standards set forth by various accrediting organizations. Most healthcare disciplines have an accrediting organization (Table 44.1) that oversees continuing education. Accrediting organizations seek to assure the public that healthcare education is independent, free from commercial bias, based on valid content, and effective in improving the quality and safety of patient care [1, 2].

Accreditation Council for Continuing Medical Education (ACCME)

The ACCME, founded in 1981, is a nonprofit corporation based in Chicago, Illinois [1]. The ACCME accreditation system provides accreditation to US institutions that offer continuing medical education (CME) to physicians and other healthcare professionals. The mission of the ACCME is "the identification, development, and promotion of quality continuing medical education utilized by physicians in their maintenance of competence and incorporation of new knowledge to improve quality medical care for patients and their communities" [1].

Participation in accredited CME assists physicians in meeting the requirements for maintaining licensure, maintaining board certification specialties, credentialing, sustaining membership in professional societies, and upholding other professional privileges. State medical boards vary in the specific number of CME hours required for license renewal. While some states have no CME requirements for license renewal, others require up to 50 credits per year [4]. Approximately 700 organizations are ACCME-accredited as CME providers, including medical schools, nonprofit physician organizations, healthcare delivery systems, publishing and education companies, government and military organizations, and insurance and managed-care companies. Approximately 23 million

R. Levy, MD, DABA (✉)
Patient Simulation Center,
Departments of Anesthesiology/Neuroscience and Cell Biology,
University of Texas Medical Branch at Galveston,
Galveston, TX, USA
e-mail: rslevy@utmb.edu

K. Adams, BS
Department of Continuing Education,
Society for Simulation in Healthcare, Minneapolis, MN, USA
e-mail: kadams@ssih.org

W. Goranson, MSN, RN-BC
Department of Clinical Professional Development,
Iowa Health – Des Moines, 1200 Pleasant Street,
Des Moines, IA 50309, USA
e-mail: goransws@ihs.org

A.I. Levine et al. (eds.), *The Comprehensive Textbook of Healthcare Simulation*,
DOI 10.1007/978-1-4614-5993-4_44, © Springer Science+Business Media New York 2013

healthcare professionals attend more than 125,000 ACCME activities/programs annually [1].

The American Nurses Credentialing Center (ANCC)

The ANCC is the nation's leader in accreditation of continuing nursing education and provides standards to ensure quality programs. The mission of the American Nurses Credentialing Center is "to promote excellence in nursing and healthcare globally through credentialing programs" [2]. ANCC has both accredited providers, which are organizations that provide their own continuing education activities, and accredited approvers, which are organizations that approve continuing education activities for nonaccredited organizations. Nursing CE requirements for license renewal also varies by state.

Table 44.1 Accreditation agencies

Profession	Accrediting CE organization
Physicians	Accreditation Council for Continuing Medical Education (ACCME)
Nurses	American Nurses Credentialing Center (ANCC)
Pharmacists	Accreditation Council for Pharmacy Education (ACPE)
Respiratory care	American Association of Respiratory Care (AARC)
Paramedics/emergency medical services (EMS) personnel	Continuing Education Coordinating Board for Emergency Medical Services (CECBEMS)

Accreditation Council for Pharmacy Education (ACPE)

The ACPE establishes the standards for the education of pharmacists [3]. In 1975, the ACPE started accreditation for continuing pharmacy education. The Board of Directors of the ACPE is chosen from the American Association of Colleges of Pharmacy, the American Pharmacist Association, the National Association of Boards of Pharmacy, and the American Council on Education. A list of ACPE accredited providers can be found on the ACPE website (https://www.acpe-accredit.org).

Joint Accreditation

These three organizations, the ACCME, ANCC, and ACPE, have collaborated to develop a joint accreditation opportunity for providers, granting a Provider of Interprofessional Continuing Education designation to qualifying entities. Organizations that retain this accreditation may also offer continuing education credit for physicians, nurses, or pharmacists separately.

Steps in Planning Simulation-Based CE Activities

The planning steps for providing continuing education are similar across most of the healthcare disciplines.

1. Assess learner needs and professional practice gaps. Learner needs are assessed by various methods, including surveys of the target audience, self-recognition through pretesting, clinical quality indicators, focus groups, and literature and regulatory review, just to name a few. A practice gap will exist when new evidence or guidelines are released that require learners to update their knowledge [5].
2. Identify the learner population. The learner's stage of professional development and area of specialty will define the scope and content of the CE activity [5]. Some activities are designed for a single discipline, while others are developed with an interprofessional focus.
3. Create a planning committee. The planning committee should consist of the following: a planner from each discipline represented within the learner population, an education specialist, a content expert, and a member of the target audience. If ANCC credits are being offered, a nurse planner must also participate in planning the CE content [2].
4. Identify learning objectives for the activity. The planning committee will develop overall goals for the educational program as well as specific objectives that address identified learner gaps. Each individual activity will have specific learning objectives containing an action component, a subject component, and a measurable outcome.
5. Develop a budget. A budget, developed early in the process, will guide the planning committee on how much can be spent on faculty, printing, audiovisual needs, room fees, etc. Also, if expected revenue is intended to cover expenses, a budget will assist in setting registration fees.
6. Develop activity content and corresponding learning formats. Content for the educational activity is developed under the direction of the planning committee.

The planning committee is charged with developing targeted and effective content to provide interventions for identified learner gaps. Content can be developed in a number of ways, but it is always under the guidance of needs-based assessment findings. Instructional strategies, delivery methods, learner feedback mechanisms, and the learning resources/modalities are all components of the content development process.

7. Select facilitator/faculty. The course director and faculty are instrumental in developing the specific learning objectives, cases, prerequisites, and evaluation methods for the learning activity. Thus, the selected faculty participants should be content experts specific to the discipline and knowledgeable of the overall goals of the learning activity.
8. Resolve potential conflicts of interest. Disclosures of financial interest should be obtained from all activity planners and presenters to identify existing financial, professional, or personal relationships with entities producing healthcare or simulation-related goods and services. Those relationships must then be assessed to determine if the potential exists for commercial bias in the educational activity [6].
9. Create the evaluation methods. The planning committee and faculty will plan, design, and review evaluation tools and methods. Most CE activities use an evaluation survey, or "happy sheet," to capture the reaction of the learners which is the lowest of Kirkpatrick's levels of evidence [7]. Faculties are encouraged to find ways to evaluate learner changes in knowledge and behavior. Knowledge acquisition can be measured by pre- and posttests of participants, as well as through observations. Behavior changes are more difficult to measure because the desired changes typically occur over time.
10. Apply for CE credit through an accredited approver. If an organization is not accredited, but wishes to provide continuing education activities, CEUs can be obtained through an application process to an accredited approver. A list of accredited approvers can generally be found on each accrediting organization's website [1–3]. When applying for CE through an accredited approver, the lead planner for the educational activity is required to complete an application process and provide supporting documentation, fees, and post-activity documents. The sponsoring organization can choose to offer CE credits for one or multiple disciplines. If applying for ANCC credits, a lead nurse planner must be identified.
11. Promote and advertise the activity. After the activity is planned and the CE credits are approved, promotion of the program occurs. A cost-effective way to promote the CE activity is through emails to target audience members and on Internet websites.
12. Implement activity logistics. The planning committee develops and implements the infrastructure for the entire educational activity. The logistical implementation of the learning activity is often assisted by meeting coordinators and event professionals proficient in handling educational activity management.
13. Maintain activity records. Providing comprehensive reports about the learning activity process is essential in order to precisely detail all undertakings/actions associated with the activity. Thorough records include planning committee minutes, communication regarding content development and learner assessment, faculty disclosure statements, documentation of resolutions to identified faculty conflicts of interest, industry support documentation of any financial or in-kind support given to the educational program, certificates of attendance, participant and faculty listings, financial documentation, and final course promotional materials.

Providers of Continuing Education in Healthcare Simulation

Listed below are some of the major national and international interdisciplinary organizations that provide continuing education in simulation.

Society for Simulation in Healthcare (SSH)

The Society for Simulation in Healthcare (SSH) is the world's largest professional organization representing the field of healthcare simulation. The society is multidisciplinary, representing all fields and specialties in healthcare.

The society first convened in 1995 and 1996 in Rochester, NY, as a group of anesthesia educators interested in simulation. The society officially came into existence in 1998 and 1999 at a joint conference with the Society for Technology in Anesthesia (STA). Known as the International Meeting on Medical Simulation (IMMS), early organizers broadened the scope of the conference to include other medical specialties and healthcare providers. At the time, the meeting was small with between 100 and 250 participants. The IMMS continued as part of STA for several more years, and participation steadily increased. It became evident to leaders that a critical mass had been reached and the time had come to establish an independent society. The Society for Simulation in Healthcare was officially established in 2004.

The society annually hosts the largest international gathering of simulation educators and researchers at its International Meeting on Simulation in Healthcare (IMSH). The annual offering in 2012 broke attendance records with over 3,100 participants registered from 37 different countries.

The CE program designed for IMSH offers a comprehensive selection of continuing education courses for healthcare simulation administrators, managers, educators, researchers, and simulation technicians. Over 300 individual courses are offered throughout the 5-day meeting. Each of these individual learning activities is designed using the ACCME and ANCC criterion for the development of continuing education activities. Continuing education units (CEUs) are awarded after learner participation has concluded.

There are various learning formats offered at IMSH. The plenary sessions showcase leaders in healthcare simulation, as well as inspirational and innovative speakers who are on the cutting edge in related disciplines. Didactic lectures, expert panels, round table discussions, and hands-on workshops offer venues to accommodate varied learning styles. At IMSH are the immersive courses, in which faculty and learners re-create simulated learning environments, design and develop curriculum and delivery methods, train faculty, and perform various assessment techniques.

International Nursing Association of Clinical Simulation and Learning (INACSL)

The International Nursing Association of Clinical Simulation and Learning (INACSL) represents nurses working to promote research and evidence-based practice standards in clinical simulation methods and learning environments. The annual conference of INACSL is a forum for nurse educators, researchers, nurse managers, and staff development professionals. A wide variety of course offerings provide a comprehensive curriculum in simulation education, research, practice, and administration [8].

International Pediatric Simulation Society (IPSS)

The International Pediatric Simulation Society (IPSS) is an international, multidisciplinary organization dedicated to the practice and advancement of simulation-based education used in all subspecialties involved in the care of pediatric patients. The IPSS annual meeting, the International Simulation Symposia and Workshops (IPSSW), is the world's largest gathering of professionals working in pediatric and perinatal simulation. The IPSSW held its first meeting in 2008 in Stockholm, Sweden, and, like other meetings in simulation, has since experienced a rapid growth in attendance [9].

Society in Europe for Simulation Applied to Medicine (SESAM)

This multidisciplinary membership organization, formed in 1994 [10], encourages and supports the use of simulation in training and research. SESAM, primarily developed in Europe, includes members from all over the world. The organization includes members from a diverse spectrum of healthcare professionals including physicians and nurses from several specialties, technicians, engineers, psychologists, physicists, and biologists.

Association for Standardized Patient Educators (ASPE)

ASPE, formed in 1991, is the international organization for professionals in the field of simulated and standardized patient (SP) methodology. ASPE dedicates time and research to the advancement of SP research and related scholarly activities and works to establish and regulate standards of improved practice in patient-centered care [11].

Specialty Organizations Providing Simulation-Based CE

There are other organizations that offer simulation as a component of their continuing education content, some of which are briefly described below. This list is by no means inclusive, but it is designed to give the reader an idea of the breadth of simulation opportunities available in the medical community.

Society for Education in Anesthesia (SEA)

The SEA is a nonprofit educational organization for anesthesiologists who strive to enhance their abilities and scholarly endeavors in the field of education. Biannual meetings routinely include workshops and presentations focused on simulation.

American Society of Anesthesiologists (ASA) and the Post Graduate Assembly of the New York State Society for Anesthesiology (PGA)

These organizations, which comprise the largest annual meetings for anesthesiologists, offer workshops and immersive courses utilizing simulation.

Society of American Gastrointestinal and Endoscopic Surgeons (SAGES)

This society, dedicated to training gastrointestinal and endoscopic surgeons, offers a wide variety of simulation-based courses focused on the mastery of laparoscopic surgical techniques.

National League for Nursing

The NLN is dedicated to excellence in education for nursing leaders and educators. Several sessions at the NLN Annual Summit showcase the use of simulation in nursing education.

Private Providers of Simulation-Based Continuing Education

In addition to these national and international organizations, there are numerous opportunities to obtain CE credit from simulation centers around the country that offer courses specifically for the simulation educator. Not all centers offer a comprehensive menu, and it may require investigation to find courses on specific topics. Examples of several available course topics are generically described below.

Difficult Airway Management

These courses generally run 1–2 days and emphasize the skills required to operate various airway adjuncts. Most of these courses utilize task trainers, but some include full-body mannequins and incorporate scenario-based training opportunities.

Maintenance of Certification in Anesthesiology (MOCA)

This 6- to 8-h course is offered by ASA-endorsed simulation programs (Simulation Education Network) (see Chap. 48) for anesthesiologists required to complete a simulation experience as part of the MOC. The course highlights the management of complex anesthetic situations and crisis resource management.

Instructor and/or Debriefing Training

These courses prepare educators to develop, manage, teach, and assess the healthcare simulation program. Topics generally include behavior theory, adult learning concepts/methodologies, debriefing theories and strategies, program administration, program assessment, and program evaluation (see Chap. 43).

International Meeting on Simulation in Healthcare: A CE Exemplar

Planning for the Society for Simulation in Healthcare's Annual International Meeting on Simulation in Healthcare (IMSH) begins 18 months prior to the actual date of the conference. Nearly 200 volunteers and staff work to plan the most comprehensive international simulation continuing education conference in the world.

The first priority is to select the date and location. Historically, IMSH has been held in warm US cities, as the meeting always occurs in January.

The SSH Board of Directors selects three chairpersons to lead the IMSH Planning Committee after considering a slate of candidates recommended by previous planning committees and society leadership. Currently, there are three planning committee chairpersons: one physician, one nurse, and at least one ad hoc society member. Since the SSH has an international focus, at least one chairperson must reside outside of the USA. Early selection of these chairpersons allows time for mentoring and orienting the chairpersons to the IMSH planning process. Both outgoing and incoming chairs meet at the conclusion of IMSH to begin the planning for the next year. The IMSH chairs conduct weekly conference calls and hold several face-to-face meetings throughout the year. Meetings also include society staff members, as well as a member from the SSH Meeting Oversight Committee. A liaison from the SSH Education Committee and the SSH Research Committee is also assigned to assist in the planning process. The SSH Office of Continuing Education guides the planning process throughout the year.

Annually, the SSH Education Committee conducts a needs assessment for members regarding their educational requests/preferences by sending an electronic survey to all members of SSH. The Education Committee also summarizes the IMSH evaluations from the previous annual meeting. Faculty members who receive high ratings and positive comments will be encouraged to submit course proposals for the next meeting. Since meeting participants have options on which sessions to attend, those sessions with high attendance numbers are also considered to be effective and valuable. Other member needs are identified by noting common themes on the Society Listserv, recently published SSH journal articles, and by the identification of quality issues arising in the healthcare field. The Special Interest Groups (SIGs) of SSH are also involved in this process to assure that medical specialty needs are represented at the meeting (Table 44.2).

All needs assessment data is summarized and forwarded to the IMSH Planning Committee. The summary report includes an itemized list of the major curriculum categories that should be used to organize the content and the relative percentages of basic to advanced content that should be included in the report. The report becomes a blueprint for the final educational program. Content for IMSH is organized as

Table 44.2 SSH Special Interest Groups (SIGs)

IPE Affinity Group
Directors of SIM Centers
Anesthesiology
Critical Care
Emergency Medicine
Hospital-Based Centers
Nonphysician Providers
Nursing
OB/GYN
Serious Games-Virtual Learning Environments
Surgery
Technology Specialists
Pediatrics

Table 44.3 IMSH educational content tracks

Administration and program evaluation
Assessment using simulation
Curriculum development
Debriefing
Faculty development
Human factors
Interprofessional/team education
Patient Safety/quality improvement
Research
Technical operations
Other – specify

a curriculum of key simulation subjects, enabling learners to find the courses they need most (Table 44.3). These categories, identified through the needs assessment process, change annually as learners' needs change.

It is during this organizational phase that the IMSH chairpersons appoint the full planning committee (Table 44.4). A section chair is appointed to manage the content for each of the educational course and scientific content format types. In addition, several co-chairs for each section are added to comprise a total planning committee of well over 50 volunteers.

In March, the planning committee chairs select the plenary speakers and theme for the meeting. A preliminary budget for the meeting is developed. Society members receive the first of many announcements with information distributed via IMSH.

Each year on April 1st, the content submission database is opened for electronic entry of course proposals and scientific abstracts to be considered by the IMSH Planning Committee for inclusion in the meeting (Table 44.5; Figs. 44.1 and 44.2). The content comprising the final IMSH educational program is derived largely from these proposals submitted by practicing healthcare simulation professionals.

After each course proposal or abstract is registered in the system, all faculties and authors must complete an Author/Faculty Requirements Form (Fig. 44.3) before the proposal or abstract can be reviewed and/or considered for acceptance. Required documentation includes an attestation clause on

Table 44.4 IMSH session types

Educational course formats	Description
Debates in simulation	Large-group session that focuses on a key issue in simulation training. A moderator and panel members debate all sides of the topic. Audience participation is encouraged
Expert panel	Large-group session that focuses on a key issue in simulation. A moderator and panel members discuss all aspects of the chosen topic
Immersive courses	High-energy learning experience offering participants an opportunity to engage in a hands-on experiential activity. Group size is limited as the courses focus on all aspects of a clinical simulation experience: development, implementation, debriefing, and evaluation
Meet the SimPros roundtable discussion	Small groups of participants meet with recognized experts in an intimate and personal learning environment
Preconference course	Two- or four-hour courses offer participants an intensive comprehensive learning experience combining several learning formats
Podium presentation	Large-group didactic lectures presented on a wide array of simulation topics. Audience participation is not a feature of this session
Workshops	Compact and interactive sessions, which engage participants in hands-on learning to acquire and practice new skills and team development. Sessions have a high degree of interactivity among participants and faculty
Scientific content and professor rounds	
Program innovation abstracts	Focus on program development and practice in healthcare, education, industry, government, and other environments
Research abstracts	Quantitative, qualitative, or mixed designs that are based on a research question and report results and conclusions
Technology innovations abstracts	New technologies for healthcare simulation. Abstracts may involve substantial research but differ from the hypothesis-driven research submitted to the research abstract category.

society policy, a disclosure of financial interests, a brief biography, and an upload of a recent curriculum vitae (CV). All authors and faculties are required to complete this process in order for the site to accept the course proposal or abstract (Table 44.3).

Closes midnight of July 31st. The content submission process. Although faculties have 4 months to submit proposals, the majority of content is usually submitted in the last 2 weeks of that time period.

Table 44.5 IMSH content submission requirements

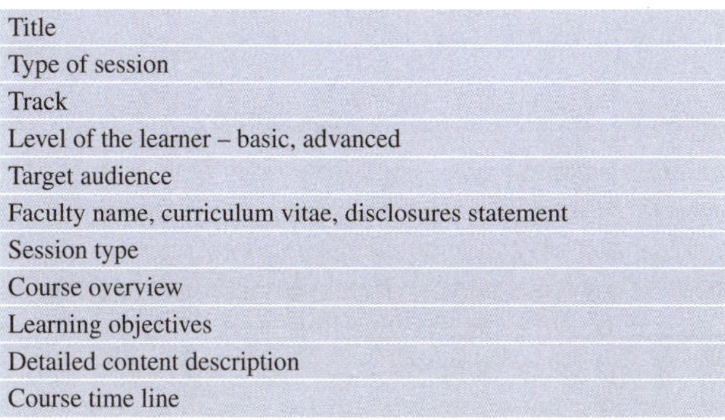

Title
Type of session
Track
Level of the learner – basic, advanced
Target audience
Faculty name, curriculum vitae, disclosures statement
Session type
Course overview
Learning objectives
Detailed content description
Course time line

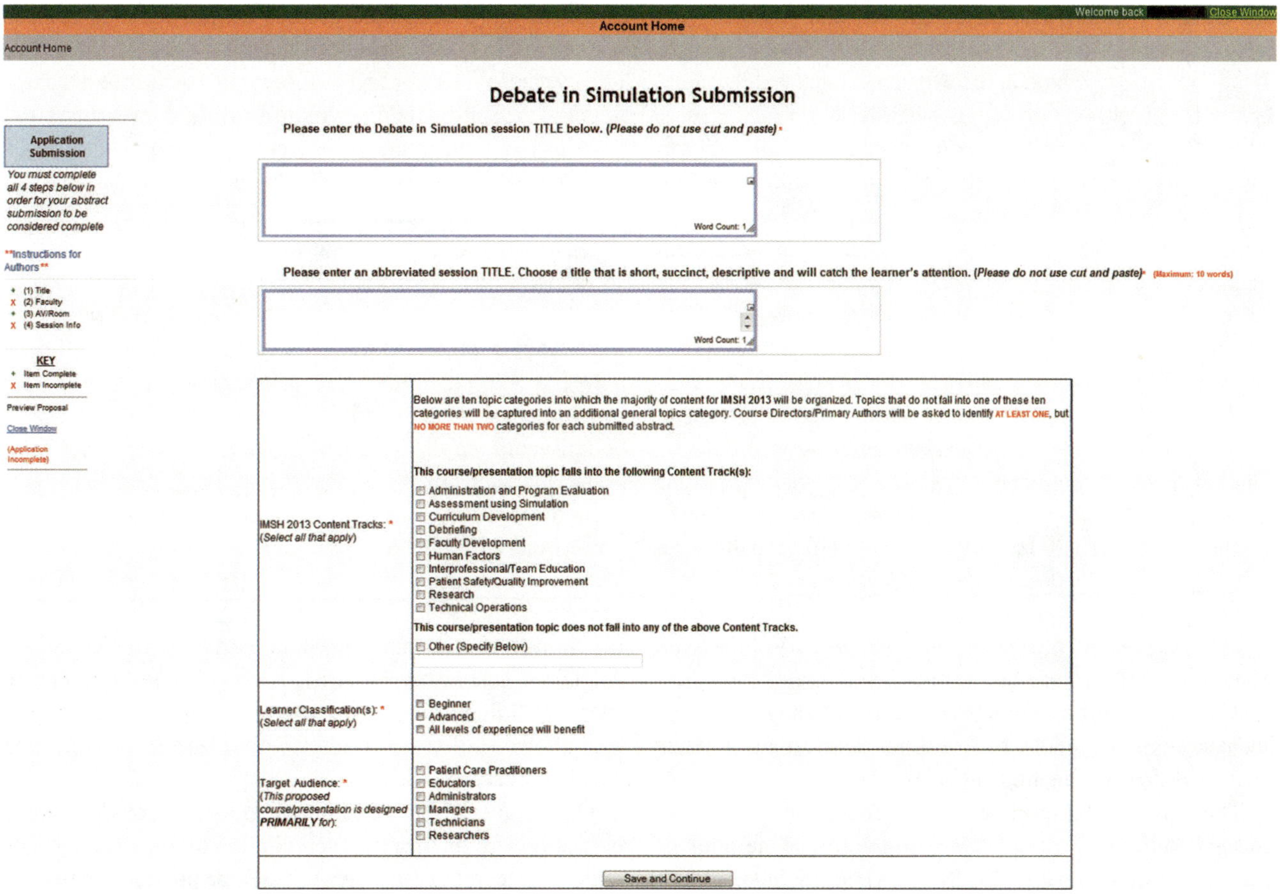

The content review process begins in early July and continues through late August. Each proposed course is peer reviewed by three reviewers and assessed for validity, rigor, and quality of content, independent from commercial bias, and effectiveness in learning and delivery format (Fig. 44.4). Members of the Education Committee and the SSH Director for Continuing Education review all proposed content for proper classification of topic and learner level, disclosure statements, and potential conflicts of interests.

In late August, the IMSH chairpersons discuss all completed review summaries and section team recommendations; at which time, final content is selected. As noted above, the needs assessment blueprint is used to guide the final acceptance process. If the planning committee determines and/or realizes that some content areas that were not submitted are needed by the healthcare simulation community, content experts in those areas will be invited to fill in the disparities.

Fig. 44.1 Screenshot of an educational content title page

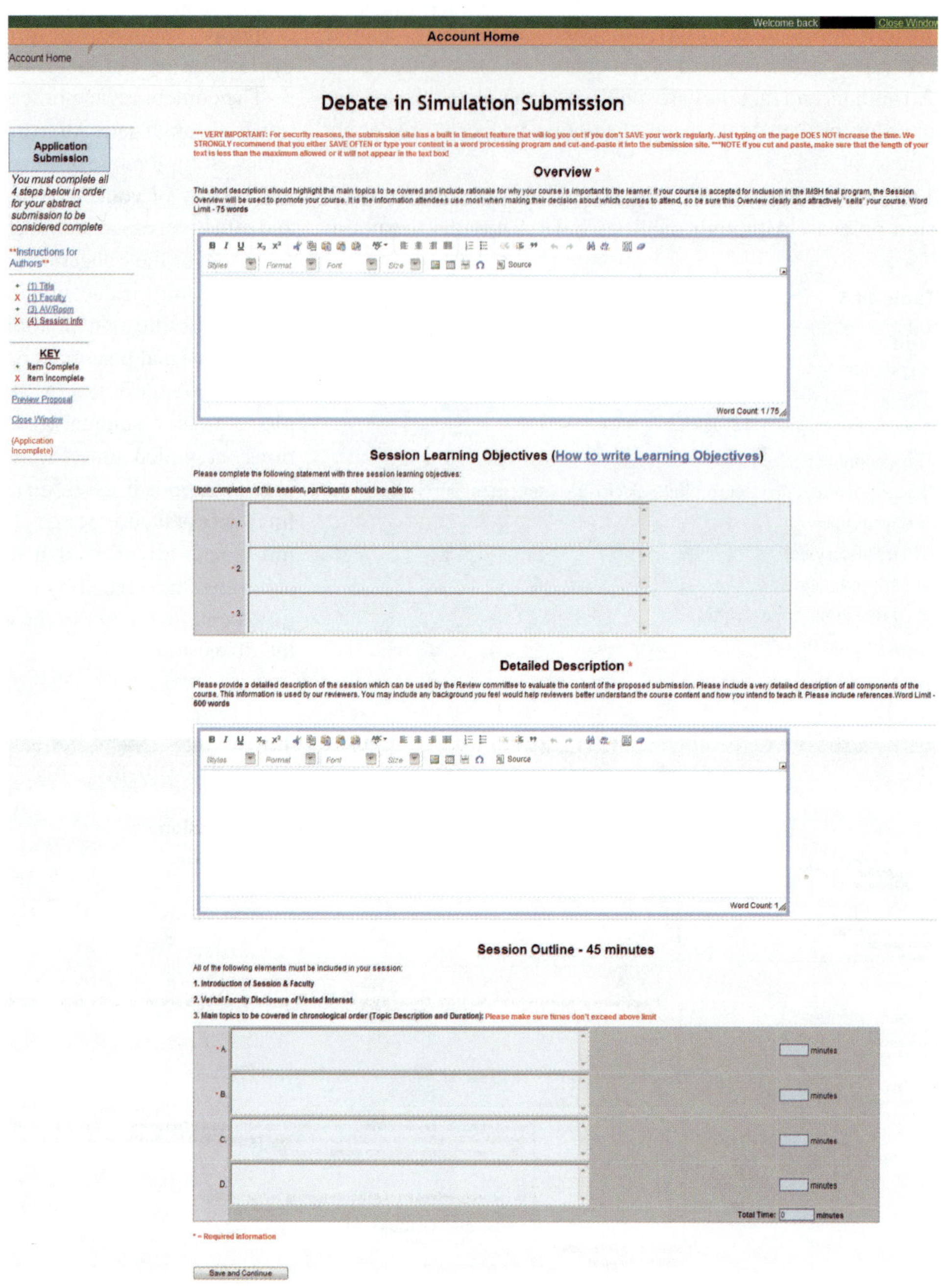

Fig. 44.2 Screenshot of the session information page from the content submission site

In September, all course directors and primary authors are notified as to the acceptance or rejection of their course proposals and scientific abstracts. If accepted, course directors and authors have 4 months to further develop and finalize their work for presentation at IMSH.

The SSH staff then begins the process of organizing and scheduling the large final program. The number of courses offered during the IMSH General Session has grown steadily in the past several years. At the time of this printing, nearly 300 courses are in the planning stages for IMSH 2013. At least 25 courses are held simultaneously, offering attendees a vast array of content from which to select.

Online registration is opened for the meeting in September. Attendees can reserve a seat in the courses they wish to attend well in advance of the meeting. This reservation process allows staff to more effectively plan the logistics and details for each course.

Once content is finalized, the SSH Director of Continuing Education will finalize the accreditation for the meeting. The society is accredited by the ACCME to provide continuing education for physicians and is applying to become an ANCC provider as well.

In late fall and early winter, SSH staff members confirm all faculty and AV needs, organize the scientific exhibition, determine final syllabus and program details, manage the

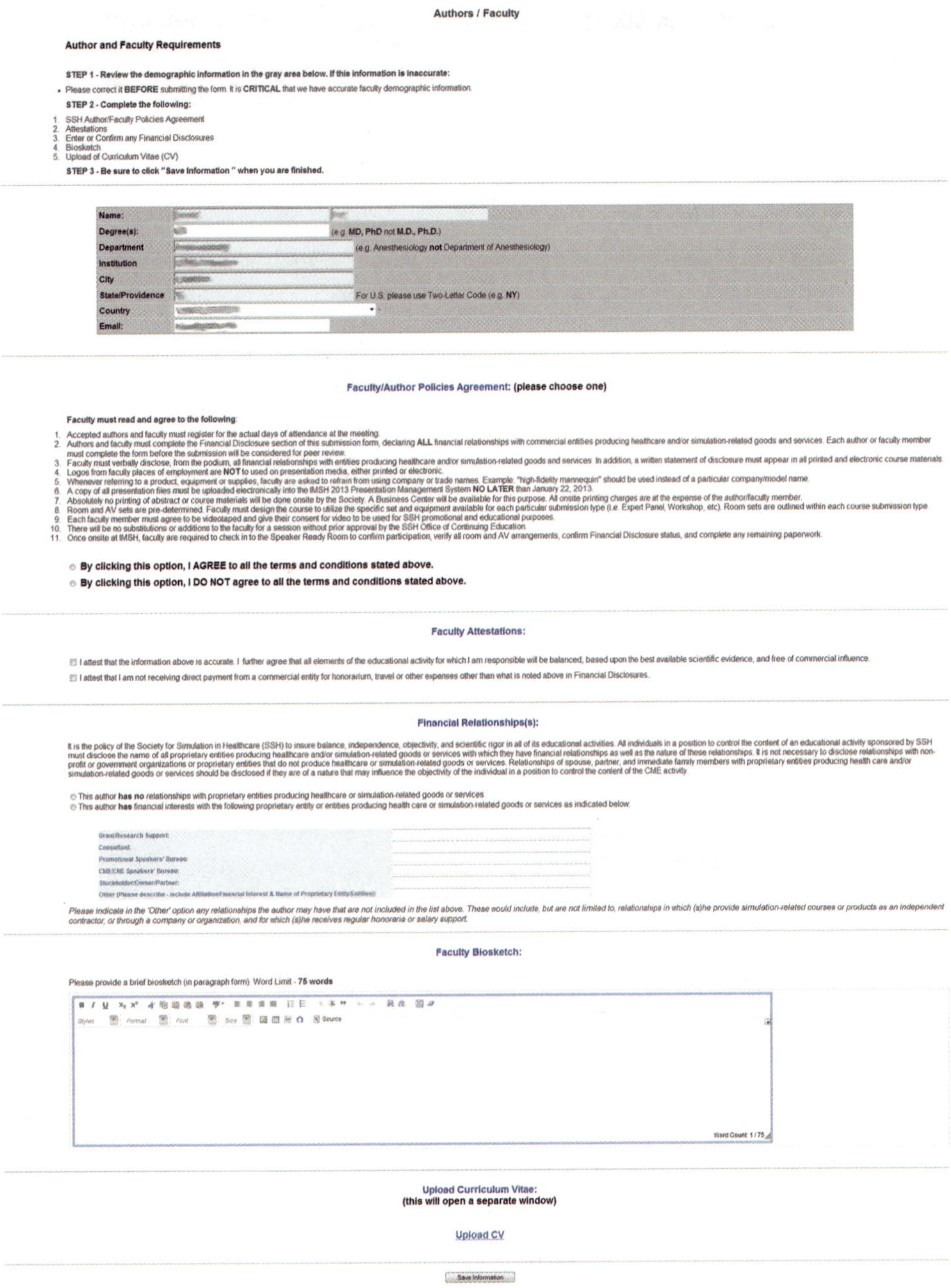

Fig. 44.3 Screenshot of the author/faculty disclosures form

Authors / Faculty

Author and Faculty Requirements

STEP 1 - Review the demographic information in the gray area below. If this information is inaccurate:

- Please correct it **BEFORE** submitting the form. It is **CRITICAL** that we have accurate faculty demographic information.

STEP 2 - Complete the following:

1. SSH Author/Faculty Policies Agreement
2. Attestations
3. Enter or Confirm any Financial Disclosures
4. Biosketch
5. Upload of Curriculum Vitae (CV)

STEP 3 - Be sure to click "Save Information" when you are finished.

Name:		
Degree(s):		(e.g. **MD, PhD** not **M.D., Ph.D.**)
Department		(e.g. Anesthesiology **not** Department of Anesthesiology)
Institution		
City		
State/Providence		For U.S. please use Two-Letter Code (e.g. **NY**)
Country		
Email:		

Faculty/Author Policies Agreement: (please choose one)

Faculty must read and agree to the following:

1. Accepted authors and faculty must register for the actual days of attendance at the meeting.
2. Authors and faculty must complete the Financial Disclosure section of this submission form, declaring **ALL** financial relationships with commercial entities producing healthcare and/or simulation-related goods and services. Each author or faculty member must complete the form before the submission will be considered for peer review.
3. Faculty must verbally disclose, from the podium, all financial relationships with entities producing healthcare and/or simulation-related goods and services. In addition, a written statement of disclosure must appear in all printed and electronic course materials.
4. Logos from faculty places of employment are **NOT** to used on presentation media, either printed or electronic.
5. Whenever referring to a product, equipment or supplies, faculty are asked to refrain from using company or trade names. Example: "high-fidelity mannequin" should be used instead of a particular company/model name.
6. A copy of all presentation files must be uploaded electronically into the IMSH 2013 Presentation Management System **NO LATER** than January 22, 2013.
7. Absolutely no printing of abstract or course materials will be done onsite by the Society. A Business Center will be available for this purpose. All onsite printing charges are at the expense of the author/faculty member.
8. Room and AV sets are pre-determined. Faculty must design the course to utilize the specific set and equipment available for each particular submission type (i.e. Expert Panel, Workshop, etc). Room sets are outlined within each course submission type.
9. Each faculty member must agree to be videotaped and give their consent for video to be used for SSH promotional and educational purposes.
10. There will be no substitutions or additions to the faculty for a session without prior approval by the SSH Office of Continuing Education.
11. Once onsite at IMSH, faculty are required to check in to the Speaker Ready Room to confirm participation, verify all room and AV arrangements, confirm Financial Disclosure status, and complete any remaining paperwork.

○ **By clicking this option, I AGREE to all the terms and conditions stated above.**

○ **By clicking this option, I DO NOT agree to all the terms and conditions stated above.**

Faculty Attestations:

☐ I attest that the information above is accurate. I further agree that all elements of the educational activity for which I am responsible will be balanced, based upon the best available scientific evidence, and free of commercial influence.

☐ I attest that I am not receiving direct payment from a commercial entity for honorarium, travel or other expenses other than what is noted above in Financial Disclosures.

Financial Relationships(s):

It is the policy of the Society for Simulation in Healthcare (SSH) to insure balance, independence, objectivity, and scientific rigor in all of its educational activities. All individuals in a position to control the content of an educational activity sponsored by SSH must disclose the name of all proprietary entities producing healthcare and/or simulation-related goods or services with which they have financial relationships as well as the nature of these relationships. It is not necessary to disclose relationships with non-profit or government organizations or proprietary entities that do not produce healthcare or simulation-related goods or services. Relationships of spouse, partner, and immediate family members with proprietary entities producing health care and/or simulation-related goods or services should be disclosed if they are of a nature that may influence the objectivity of the individual in a position to control the content of the CME activity.

○ This author **has no** relationships with proprietary entities producing healthcare or simulation-related goods or services.
○ This author **has** financial interests with the following proprietary entity or entities producing health care or simulation-related goods or services as indicated below.

Grant/Research Support:
Consultant:
Promotional Speakers' Bureau:
CME/CNE Speakers' Bureau:
Stockholder/Owner/Partner:
Other (Please describe - include Affiliation/Financial Interest & Name of Proprietary Entity/Entities):

Please indicate in the 'Other' option any relationships the author may have that are not included in the list above. These would include, but are not limited to, relationships in which (s)he provide simulation-related courses or products as an independent contractor, or through a company or organization, and for which (s)he receives regular honoraria or salary support.

Faculty Biosketch:

Please provide a brief biosketch (in paragraph form). Word Limit - **75 words**

Styles Format Font Size Source

Word Count: 1 / 75

Upload Curriculum Vitae:
(this will open a separate window)

Upload CV

Save Information

confirmation and scheduling process for faculty and authors, and organize the large conference support staff. The IMSH Presentation Archive is readied for faculty members to use in uploading their electronic presentations prior to the meeting. Course materials and onsite logistical guides are finalized for production.

The meeting occurs in the latter part of January. It takes the full IMSH Planning Committee, SSH staff, and hundreds of volunteer society members to ensure the meeting runs smoothly. Society members assist in the Speaker Ready Room, where final paperwork is completed and electronic presentation materials are screened by Education Committee reviewers one last time before being uploaded for final presentation and archival. Room hosts scan participant badges at the entrance to each course to verify attendance for continuing education documentation. The SSH Education Committee randomly monitors courses throughout the meeting, performing specific evaluations to assess quality of content and ensure independence for each session.

Following the meeting, both outgoing and incoming IMSH chairpersons meet with society leadership and staff to note successes and areas for additional improvement and development. Only 2 weeks following the meeting, final attendance data, evaluation summaries, budget figures, and specific course data are prepared for the first face-to-face meeting of the incoming IMSH chairpersons. The baton gets passed, and the continuing education content development process begins again.

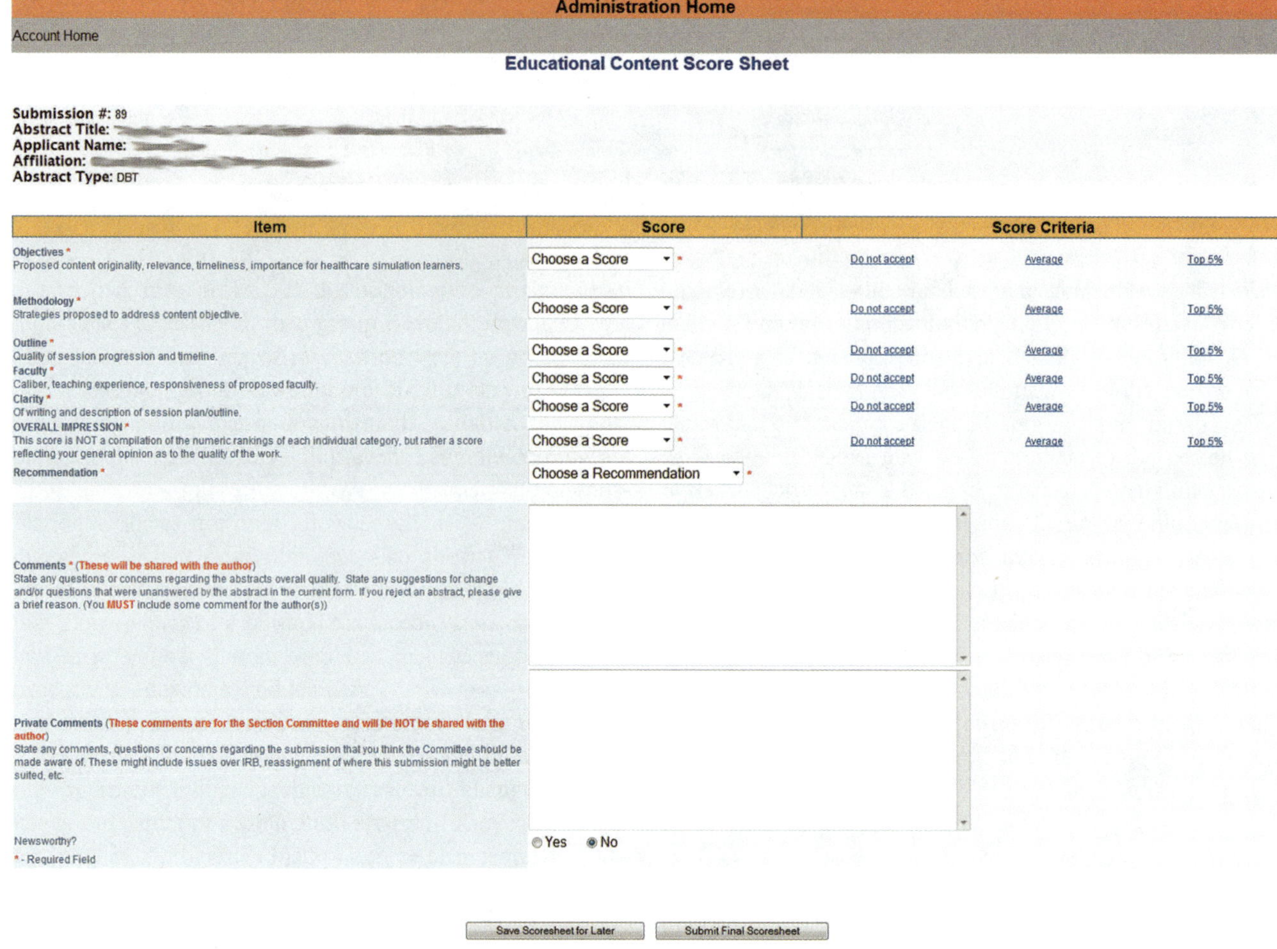

Welcome back Close Window

Administration Home

Account Home

Educational Content Score Sheet

Submission #: 89
Abstract Title:
Applicant Name:
Affiliation:
Abstract Type: DBT

Item	Score	Score Criteria		
Objectives * Proposed content originality, relevance, timeliness, importance for healthcare simulation learners.	Choose a Score *	Do not accept	Average	Top 5%
Methodology * Strategies proposed to address content objective.	Choose a Score *	Do not accept	Average	Top 5%
Outline * Quality of session progression and timeline.	Choose a Score *	Do not accept	Average	Top 5%
Faculty * Caliber, teaching experience, responsiveness of proposed faculty.	Choose a Score *	Do not accept	Average	Top 5%
Clarity * Of writing and description of session plan/outline.	Choose a Score *	Do not accept	Average	Top 5%
OVERALL IMPRESSION * This score is NOT a compilation of the numeric rankings of each individual category, but rather a score reflecting your general opinion as to the quality of the work.	Choose a Score *	Do not accept	Average	Top 5%
Recommendation *	Choose a Recommendation *			

Comments * (These will be shared with the author)
State any questions or concerns regarding the abstracts overall quality. State any suggestions for change and/or questions that were unanswered by the abstract in the current form. If you reject an abstract, please give a brief reason. (You MUST include some comment for the author(s))

Private Comments (These comments are for the Section Committee and will be NOT be shared with the author)
State any comments, questions or concerns regarding the submission that you think the Committee should be made aware of. These might include issues over IRB, reassignment of where this submission might be better suited, etc.

Newsworthy? Yes No

* - Required Field

Save Scoresheet for Later | Submit Final Scoresheet

Fig. 44.4 Screenshot of the reviewer score page form the content submission site

Conclusion

Healthcare simulation educators dedicate their efforts to the improvement of patient care by creating a learning environment that simulates day-to-day, practical learning experiences. The simulation environment is a unique stage from which to teach, with many nuances and characteristics often unavailable in more traditional settings. Continuing education (CE) offerings specific to this dynamic learning environment contribute not only to the advancement of knowledge and skills but also to a more comprehensive understanding and analysis of the unique and effective opportunities offered through simulation education. Rapid advances in healthcare strategies and technologies will continue to grow the demand for simulation education; thus, the demand for educators equipped to teach in this unique environment will also increase.

References

1. American Council for Continuing Medical Education. Available at: http://www.accme.org. Accessed 15 June 2012.
2. American Nurses Credentialing Center. Available at: http://www.nursecredentialing.org. Accessed 15 June 2012.
3. American Council for Pharmacy Education. Available at: http://www.acpe-accredit.org. Accessed 17 June 2012.
4. American Medical Association. Available at: http://www.ama-assn.org/resources/doc/med-ed-products/table16.pdf. Accessed 17 June 2012.
5. Wittich CM, Chutka DS, Mauck KF, Berger RA, Litin SC, Beckman TJ. Perspective: a practical approach to defining professional practice gaps for continuing medical education. Acad Med. 2012;87:582–5.
6. Standards for Disclosure and Commercial Support. Application Manual. Silver Springs: American Credentialing Center; 2009. p. B81–7.
7. Kirkpatrick DL, Kirkpatrick JD. The four levels: an overview. In: Kirkpatrick DL, Kirkpatrick JD, editors. Evaluating training programs. 3rd ed. San Francisco: Berrett-Koehler Publishers, Inc; 2006. p. 21–7.
8. International Nursing Association for Clinical Simulation and Learning. Available at: http://www.inacsl.org/INACSL_2010/. Accessed 23 June 2012.
9. International Pediatric Simulation Society. Available at: http://www.ipedsim.com/updatenews/simulation-news/43-ipsssociety. Accessed 23 June 2012.
10. Society in Europe for Simulation Applied to Medicine. Available at: http://www.sesam-web.org. Accessed 28 June 2012.
11. Association of Standardized Patient Educators. Available at: http://www.aspeducators.org. Accessed 28 June 2012.

Part V

Program Development in Simulation

Center Development and Practical Considerations

45

Michael Seropian, Bonnie Driggers, and Jesika Gavilanes

Introduction

Developing a simulation program is not a small task and is not for the faint of heart [1–3]. The thought and precision of the development process will directly impact the opportunities afforded to the learners and stakeholders alike [4]. This chapter will outline a variety of subject areas that should be considered. Not all areas will be applicable to every program. It is recommended that programs that are being developed or those already in operation should create a checklist that deliberately forces consideration of these key areas. The use of project timelines and deliverables will help developing programs remain on task and evaluate their progress. Consider the development of a simulation program as a journey that should leverage best accepted practice in several areas: simulation instruction, facility design, and instructor development, at a minimum. At times, evidence will be scarce, as the industry is still in its infancy, which will necessitate leveraging ideas from other industries that are similar (e.g., aviation). There is no one approach to simulation program development in general. Readers may appreciate that in certain circumstances, similar material is also covered in Chap. 46, "The Business of Simulation"; however, it is impossible to discuss one aspect of development without the other; therefore, this chapter will emphasize center design and planning and when pertinent will include relevant business and financial issues.

M. Seropian, MD (✉)
Department of Anesthesiology,
Oregon Health and Science University,
Portland, OR, USA
e-mail: seropian@ohsu.edu

B. Driggers, RN, MS, MPA
Department of Nursing,
Oregon Health and Science University,
Portland, OR, USA
e-mail: boncanby@aol.com

J. Gavilanes, Masters in Teaching
Statewide Simulation, Simulation and
Clinical Learning Center School of Nursing,
Oregon Health and Science University,
Portland, OR, USA
e-mail: gavilane@ohsu.edu

Project Management

Developing a simulation program can be a complex task. Depending on the size of the program it may involve one or many people involved in a variety of tasks. The use of project management principles to organize and assess progress is an important consideration. This may involve simple task lists to complex GANTT charts (a GANTT chart is a horizontal bar chart that was developed as a production control tool in 1917 by Henry L. Gantt and is frequently used in project management). Establishing clear lines of communications, team leaders, and deliverables is the cornerstone of successful implementation. Certain tasks will be dependent on the accomplishment of other prior or concurrent tasks, while some will not. For example, a contractor cannot build a facility until he receives construction documents from architects and engineers. Similarly, the purchase of equipment should follow curricular and instructional needs and should not be purchased beforehand.

Definition of a Simulation Center and Business Planning

Definitions

A center can be defined in many ways. It can represent a physical location, a variety of locations, a fiscal entity, or even a virtual concept. The use of the word "center" in itself encourages people to think of a physical location that houses specific activities. For the purpose of this chapter, a center

A.I. Levine et al. (eds.), *The Comprehensive Textbook of Healthcare Simulation*,
DOI 10.1007/978-1-4614-5993-4_45, © Springer Science+Business Media New York 2013

will signify a simulation program that may represent multiple stakeholders and a variety of locations. The program is larger than any one user group or location. This is an important distinction as it suggests that the "program" is more than a physical plant. Indeed, it embodies the very fabric of the program—all the elements that make it operationally viable. Operations are often misunderstood as relating to technical or administrative elements alone. They in fact represent the sum total of all the elements that make a program or entity function. This includes academic and nonacademic elements.

The Business Plan

A business plan is a written statement of your business (simulation program): what the program wants to achieve and the plan to achieve it. It should outline the structure of your business, the product(s) or service(s), the customer(s), the growth potential, and the financial statements.

In addition to identifying information about the business, the business plan should also inspire the program for future endeavors. It is a blueprint outlining the goals or benchmarks the program wants to achieve with a clear understanding of the methods intend to achieve them. It should not, however, act as a rigid prediction of every future occurrence. Programs cannot predict or control for all future circumstances nor can they anticipate outside circumstances that will have a significant impact on the direction of the program. A good business plan should at least give a clear direction for which to aim. Every business should have a plan whether it is just starting or whether it is expanding. It helps to define strategies, and if properly used, the plan will help involve and motivate key members of the staff.

The business plan can also facilitate success by helping avoid future failure by identifying potential pitfalls along the way. It should outline a realistic set of goals with timelines while being flexible in order to accommodate changes that are likely to occur. By generating a plan with targeted goals, one can monitor the program's progress and get the program back on track fairly quickly if anything goes wrong

Key Components of a Business Plan

Generating a business plan may seem like overkill and unimportant for those with smaller programs, but the underlying principles are critical and will help even the smallest simulation group clearly articulate the plan, starting with a clear identified mission and vision through implementation to mission realization. Many of the sections that follow are often found in a business plan.

Mission Versus Vision

The core of any plan must start with the mission and vision. A simple search on the Internet will show that the two terms are often confused with each other. The mission is often defined as the outward statement of your purpose. It is the statement (brief) that outlines, literally, your "mission." The vision on the other hand reflects how you are going to get there. Disney's vision is "To make people happy." This embodies the notion that to achieve Disney's mission, employees must "make people happy."

In simulation, it is important to clearly identify your mission so that your process and decisions can always tie back to this. Without a mission, a program will run the risk of making programmatic and fiscal decisions that may or may not be the best use of resources (people, time, and money). Even those with a mission must be cautious to avoid what is often called "mission creep" where a program extends beyond its stated mission and begins to involve itself in things that may not be a best use of personnel, time, or fiscal resources. Therefore, mission and vision discipline are critical.

Needs Assessment

A basic premise in any educational activity is that it should be based on a need [5]. When the word need is used, it suggests a problem is present. The need may in fact represent a problem or issue but may also simply reflect the specific "need" of your target stakeholder (e.g., a nursing student has a need for a thorough education in the field of nursing). The need drives the measurable objectives and goals, and the objectives and goals drive the strategy. The strategy in turn drives the equipment, space, time, and personnel needs. Essentially, the needs assessment drives the objectives. At times, the objectives may in fact be driven by a defined assessment. The needs of the program's stakeholders are paramount in determining what services to provide and to what degree. The term stakeholder refers to a heterogeneous group that includes everyone from the executive to the learner. Each stakeholder group must be considered. The services and programs offered must offer "substantive" value to the stakeholder [6]. Needs assessments may be as simple as reviewing curricular needs across specialties and disciplines or can be quite complex, entailing an in depth analysis of internal and external markets to determine met and unmet needs. Needs assessments can be conducted through surveys, in person interviews, SWOT analyses (Strengths, Weaknesses, Opportunities and Threats), and include a review of key data such as scores, outcomes, and risk management information [7].

Ultimately, the current and anticipated needs will drive your program. Failure to consider this basic principle will put even the best intended programs at risk of losing sight of their goals and failing to bring substantive value to stakeholders. While there is no firm rule of how often a formal needs assessment should be done, it is safe to say that a needs assessment is an ongoing process that must be a priority, as a business plan must be continually updated in the form of strategic planning. Strategic planning for organizations normally occur every 3–5 years or more often if the market and environment is unstable and rapidly changing.

Executive Buy-In

"No money…no mission and no mission…no money." This term is often used in business circles and has many meanings but put simply: A program cannot exist without money, and money will not flow to a program without a mission, political legitimacy, or substantive value. Executive buy-in refers to the acceptance and engagement of the executive (decision maker) in a given process. Buy-in can vary in level and may simply reflect support in principle or complete buy-in with financial support tied to key deliverables. Many simulation programs often have simple support with funding coming from soft sources or more limited sources controlled by intermediate level leadership. As programs expand and people change management positions, a program can find itself in jeopardy without substantive buy-in from both proximal and distal executives. The simulation program must be in alignment with executive interests and considerations. This brings into play not only financial issues but political ones as well.

There is no single rule or approach to executive buy-in. Informing and engaging the executive is not always easy. Access to these individuals is often considered the first step. Arguably, the first real step is having a solid understanding of what it is the program seeks to do, why it matters, and what it is that the program needs. All this must be presented in a brief format, as presentations to executives are often limited to 10–15 min. This is not to suggest that a plan should be brief but rather that the presentation (e.g. executive summary) must be brief, succinct, and to the point. It must, however, be backed by additional substantive detail upon request. Executive buy-in and engagement is a key business strategy in many industries. The transformational and cultural changes that simulation offers does require this level of support as simulation in healthcare enters into mass adoption.

Key Program Components

Human Resources

Educator Skillset and Expertise

Simulation in healthcare can be used in a variety of ways: education, assessment, research, and gap and system analysis. The use of simulation for education has become pervasive [8]. The very notion of education in healthcare is undergoing a transformative change. There will be a day when it will no longer be acceptable to simply receive your credential (e.g., MD) as a surrogate of the ability to teach. This standard of "credentialing" is without basis and is rooted in tradition. Educators will be required to understand the fundamentals of educational theory where courses are deliberate (see Chaps. 3 and 43). All courses should arguably be based on properly written learning objectives that meet the needs and skill level of the learner. These objectives must be measurable. With established learning objectives, an appropriate educational strategy is chosen. Finally, the activity and the learner performance are measured using assessment tool(s) that are coupled to the objectives and educational strategy used.

While this may seem outside the scope of this chapter and is actually discussed in great detail in another section of this book (see Chaps. 41, 42, 43, and 44), it underscores the need for properly trained educators as a core part of any program. Whether the program is small or large, the very same principles apply. Simulation is an educational strategy when used for training and assessment. It represents a tool that must be properly leveraged to gain its full potential. While simulation may entertain and has significant face validity, it is far too expensive to be used in a way that does not demonstrate real learner impact and downstream outcomes.

Simulation educators should have a solid education theory foundation and must understand the specifics of simulation as an educational, training, and assessment methodology. The educator needs to appreciate how to leverage the tool they are using. Does this imply that they must actually know how to use the technology? Some would argue that it does, and some would argue that it does not. The answer really resides in the middle and is situational. The need for an educator to understand how to operate the equipment they are leveraging depends on a variety of factors (Table 45.1).

An emerging standard is evolving where simulation educators will have access to a certification process. It remains to be understood the depth and breadth of this process at this time. It is the opinion of the authors that simulation educators should not only understand educational theory but should understand the use of the methodology and the equipment employed. This level of understanding will not only allow educators to choose the best strategy but also to use it to its fullest potential. It also avoids interdependence between skillsets that can become cost prohibitive and sluggish. Certifications may or may not include all three elements.

Educator Development

In the previous section, the need for educators to have a variety of skillsets was presented. A successful program should have an educator development pathway [9]. To move a novice educator to proficiency is not an act of chance but rather should be deliberate and based on sound educational strategies. The use of mastery learning, modeling, apprenticeship,

Table 45.1 Key considerations in equipment use

Simulation methodology used	There are many simulation methods that can be used, each having different operational requirements. A standardized patient versus a mannequin will require a different skillset. The same is true for procedural and task trainers. A simulation method may in fact use a variety of strategies that require the use of technology, actors, and appropriate environmental cues
The size of the program	A program with one person alone (no technical staff) will need to balance what educational strategies it uses and the understanding of how to dynamically utilize the technology (when applicable). Larger programs may leverage technical personnel to set up, run, and maintain the simulation equipment. Does this negate the need of the educator to understand what the equipment can do and how it works? From a purist standpoint, the answer should be no. The educators must be able to direct the technical personnel on how they wish the equipment to be used and how to dynamically adapt to different learning environments and situations. Simulation by definition is not a static activity. While automation of simulation equipment may represent a solution to this issue and is indeed emerging to be more reliable, it is far from perfect. Automation fails to adequately account for the single largest variable in a simulation: the learner. Predicting what a learner will do both temporally and physically is extremely difficult. This is likely true in professions that are not rule driven. Even within professions that are rule driven, as individuals progress along the path from novice to expert, they are much more likely to deviate from rules
How the simulation equipment is used	Simulation methods can be deployed in a variety of ways. The most complex equipment can be used in the most basic way. In the case where a complex mannequin is used to simply represent an inanimate body, the need to understand how it works is of diminished value. It could be argued that the use of such equipment in this way is an inadequate use of resources. Programs that are personnel poor and lack fundamental training are at risk of underutilizing and overbuying their equipment

and other educational techniques can collectively contribute to the overall development of a simulation educator. Like any learner, the simulation educator in training must have a clear understanding of the objectives and standards that they are trying to achieve. The objectives will depend on the type of simulation being used and the learner group that will ultimately be targeted. It is not yet understood whether there is one core skillset that spans all forms of simulation methodologies. This will likely be answered more comprehensively as simulation enters into the mass adoption phase. That notwithstanding, the need to develop simulation educators to a standard that represents current best accepted practice will allow a program to deliver more consistent educational opportunities for its target learners. The quality of a course should vary less when educators have been developed and trained with specific standards in mind. The question remains as to what educator standard should be used? There currently are no globally accepted standards that comprehensively describe a simulation educator. This does not, however, prevent a program from establishing its own standards. As long as the standards are defensible and based on sound principles, then they will likely provide some value if not consistency within the center.

Simulation education is rapidly evolving. Educators should be expected to maintain and update their skills to keep up with technologic and methodological changes and advancements. Programs should not only focus on new instructor development but continued professional development of existing educators. It is important that the simulation project timeline includes instructor development early in the process, as it takes time to develop competency prior to opening the doors of a simulation program.

The use of internal (e.g., educator debriefing) and external (e.g., conferences and trainer courses) development activities will help maintain a high level of quality. This also allows a program to develop a sense of value, purpose, and continual improvement.

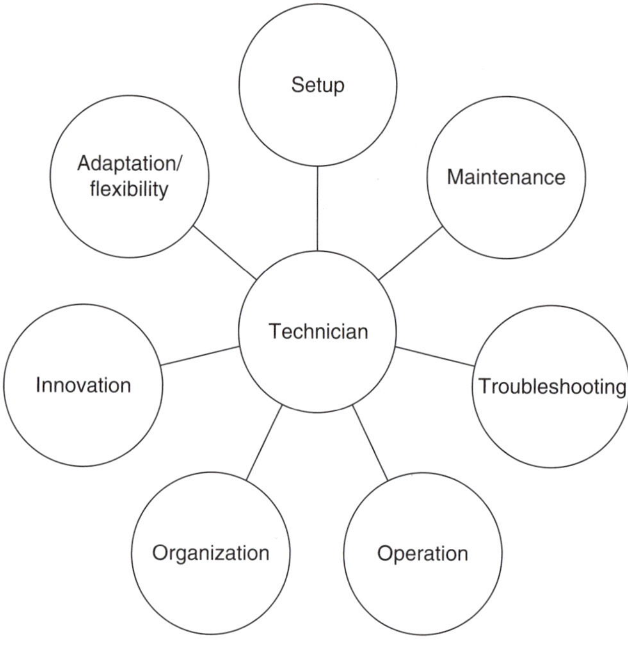

Fig. 45.1 Examples of technician skillset requirements

Technician Development and Skillset

The same principles (standards and development) described for simulation educators apply to simulation technicians as well. The technician must have a core understanding of their role (Fig. 45.1), the equipment they are using, the learner, and the purpose of the activity. In programs where a technician is not a possibility (e.g., due to financial constraints), the educator must assume the technician characteristics.

Table 45.2 Examples of standards across a variety of domains

Equipment	Hardware, software, interface, and documentation	Example: The face of a mannequin will allow for an easy and reliable seal with standard and readily available mask.
Educator	Skills, continuing education, behaviors	Example: An educator will use established basic pedogogical methods.
Technician	Skills, continuing education, behaviors	Example: The technician will operate equipment in a manner consistent with the educational activity and the equipments intent.
Assessment	Methods and development	Example: Assessment are to based on best practice. Assessment elements must be measurable and and perteninet to the area of study.
Train-the-trainer	Content, skills, certification	Example: All courses must cover core established content from referenceable material. Course instructors must carry certification as simulation educators and technicians.

Setup, maintenance, troubleshooting, and innovation are some key skills that are required in a simulation technician. The absence of these skills in a program will increase the likelihood that the program will languish and underutilize available simulation methods. The phenomenon of "mannequins remaining in a box" or "collecting dust" is real and represents a very poor use of limited resources as well as poor planning on the part of a program that did not anticipate their needs for properly trained staff. Like simulation educators, technician standards do not currently exist. Programs should use established business principles to appreciate the balance of skills needed (Fig. 45.1).

Standards

Standards may refer to many things. They may represent standards of conduct, standards of process, or standards of practice. All educational and healthcare institutions are held to certain standards that drive their activities, policies, and procedures. As has been implied in previous sections, simulation is currently standard poor, and there is no one set of accepted universal standards. While many programs have developed their own standards, there has yet to be one dominant standard to emerge. This lack of standards impacts simulation in healthcare (Table 45.2) in both variations in quality and return on investment. When an educator states they "simulate," what does that truly mean? It will become important to understand what underpins that statement to allow all individuals to have the same mental model.

Equipment manufacturers currently follow only basic standards that are not unique to simulation. They, however, do not follow a common set of standards that are more relevant to simulation applications. A good example of this is the variance of how simulated airways are developed and manufactured. The wide diversity in quality and reliability suggests a lack of standards. The application of standards and prerequisites for manufacturers will more closely couple form and function.

This also applies to simulation facility design. A variety of organizations have developed standards to help define specific key elements found in a simulation program. The Society for Simulation in Healthcare, the American Society of Anesthesiologists, and the American College of Surgeons are three examples [10]. These organizations have taken similar approaches to create general guidelines for simulation programs to establish core elements that are believed to be of high value in the success of a simulation program. Cross-referencing the program's development to these standards can be a useful exercise. The reader is referred to Chap. 48 for a detailed discussion of this topic and specific details on the individual accreditation processes.

Policies and Procedures

Whether one works in a hospital, outpatient setting, or school, they bear the responsibility to know and follow policies and procedures (so-called P&Ps). These are the very rules that allow an institution to follow regulatory and ethical requirements. They also serve a different purpose that is vital to any successful business—the ability to streamline processes and decision-making. Policies vary from addressing scheduling to confidentiality. These policies are underpinned by procedures that make them practical and applicable. In a simulation program, policies play an important role. Far too many institutions are late to establish their P&Ps in a formalized fashion. They are often boring to write and are considered by many as something that can be left for another day. If we critically look at the smallest to largest simulation program, we recognize that in fact we are applying policies all the time (whether written or not). Appendix includes a list of sample policy headings that any program should consider. For example, consider the situation where two key stakeholders want to schedule a course utilizing the same room on the same day (Table 45.3). Programs should anticipate such situations and preemptively generate polices that address these potentially difficult conflicts.

The solution to the example in Table 45.3 on the surface may seem intuitive on first read, but ultimately, the conflict will and should be resolved through the use of an established scheduling policy. Depending on what policy exists, group A

Table 45.3 Example of a typical scheduling scenario

	Group A	Group B
Group purpose	Teach about normal cardiovascular physiology as part of the circulation courses	Conduct a high-stakes assessment for an accelerated baccalaureate program
Group description	10 medical students	10 senior nursing students
Date space reservation made	Reserved 1 week before group B	Reserved 1 week after group A
Ownership stake	Same as group B	Same as group A
Date needed	Same as group B	Same as group A

or group B may prevail. If the policy gives preference to high-stakes assessment, then group B would prevail. On the other hand, if the time of reservation were by policy more important, then group A would prevail. It is easy to see how preexisting policy that is documented, available, and transparent to the stakeholders will prevent a simulation program from becoming mired in controversy, distrust, and dissatisfaction. Policies not only allow programs to create procedures for dispute resolution but also allow a program to create checks and balances that allow stakeholders to feel that they are part of a fair and balanced system. It is important to remember that stakeholders include everyone from executives, educators, and learners.

From a practical standpoint, it is often useful to work on P&Ps from a list (such as in Appendix) and recognize that they represent living documents that will change with the needs and nature of a simulation program. They can be written early in a program's history and be changed as the program evolves and matures. The policies need not be so rigid that they appear to restrict rather than promote order and innovation. They should change and be informed by unanticipated situations that improve future functionality.

Policies and procedures often dictate common approaches that are designed to make workflow and quality more reliable. The use of common curriculum development processes, common scenario templates, common databases are a few examples. These processes can help a simulation program create and maintain a system that is consistent and more likely to improve over time. The lack of standardization puts programs at risk and leads to potential ineffective use of time and resources. It is important to note that standardization of approach is not synonymous with squelching of innovation. A health simulation program not only has approaches and processes that invite innovation but also is frequently updated to reflect innovation.

Governance

Governance of a simulation program is perhaps one of the most contentious areas in many programs. Governance not only speaks to the organizational structure of a program but how decisions are made and by whom. Governance structures may be as simple as a faculty reporting to a Dean in a small community college, to a complex structure where multiple people report to a variety of intermediate management levels that eventually all report to an institution's CEO or President. What is interesting is that the person in the highest position on an organizational chart may not ultimately be the person who makes the day-to-day decisions. Moreover, the person who makes day-to-day decisions may be subordinate to the person who makes the larger annual budgetary decisions even if that person has little idea of the center's activities. Figure 45.2 illustrates two different institutional governance structure examples.

If this seems confusing, that is because it often can be. In institutions with complex executive and political relationships, it is important to clarify at each level of governance the relevant roles and responsibilities (Table 45.4). This is often described in bylaws, terms of reference, or policy. Irrespective of the size of a program, the exercise of delineating these issues is worthwhile and can insulate programs from variation and leadership changes.

There are many complex governance variations. At some point, the complexity can render decision-making authority ineffective and vague. This will vary by institution. Governance becomes particularly important when a program spans many disciplines, professions, and even institutions. Service line agreements and clear lines for decision-making are critical for success. The ability of an organization to operate efficiently and effectively is very much tied to its governance structure and governance discipline including respect for lines of communication. Governance structures should be identified early in the process of program development so as not to disrupt the success of a program.

The Physical Plant

The natural assumption is that all simulation programs have some sort of dedicated facility or physical plant. This is true in the absolute sense in that all simulation programs must have some physical plant where their simulation equipment is at a minimum housed. The physical plant may serve this sole purpose or may extend to house personnel or may be used to provide simulation-based services. Programs that are entirely point-of-care oriented may only require storage space, whereas programs that also provide simulation-facility-based simulation services will require considerably more space than the former.

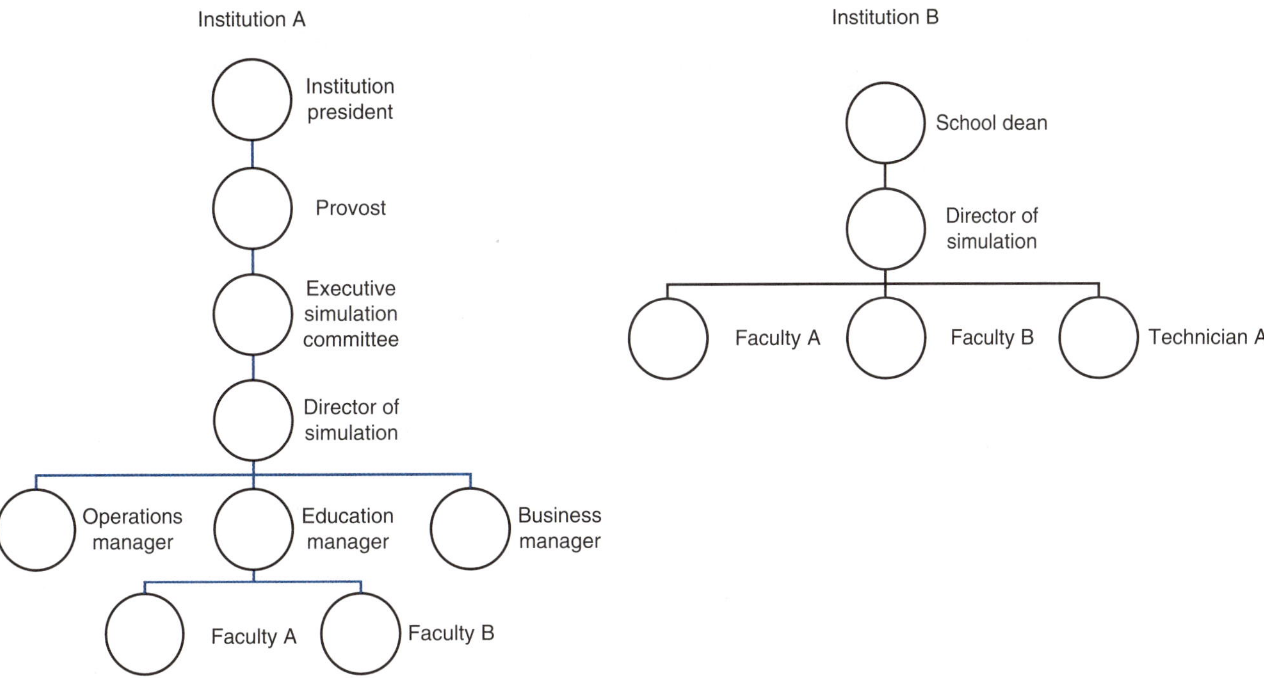

Fig. 45.2 Governance structure examples

Table 45.4 Example organizational scenarios/situations

	Institution A	Institution B
President	Delegates annual fiscal responsibility to provost	Not involved directly
Provost	Responsible for approving annual budget for simulation program	Not applicable
Executive simulation committee	Responsible for advancing an approving all budgetary considerations for presentation and final approval of the provost	Not applicable
School Dean	Involved at the executive simulation committee level or provides a delegate in their role	Responsible for approving annual budget for simulation program
Director of simulation	Responsible for creating, prioritizing, and justifying budgetary line items. Will sit with managers to evaluate overall budgetary needs. Will advance budget to executive simulation committee for approval	Responsible for creating, prioritizing, and justifying budgetary line items. Will advance budget to Dean for approval
Managers	Responsible for organizing budgetary requests and requirements specific to their domain (e.g., education)	Not applicable
Faculty	Will advance requests to managers for inclusion in budget	Will advance requests to Director of simulation for inclusion in budget

These two case examples are extremes of each other and have significant implications. Table 45.5 provides a useful comparison of the two models. Note that these are not the only models, and hybrids of the two exist and will have different considerations.

At the end of the day, the physical plant must meet the needs for storage, support, personnel, and ultimately the actual simulation learning or assessment activity. The construction and design of a dedicated simulation facility is a complex subject, as best practice is still being established. The basic premise that form must follow function, however, remains true, and any facility should be purpose-built. In the case where a dedicated facility is needed, then several space considerations come into play:

- Learning space(s)—classrooms, debrief rooms, simulation theaters, clinic rooms
- Control rooms—for mannequin, hybrid, and standardized patient (SP)-based simulation
- Storage—consumables and hard storage
- Offices—for permanent and temporary personnel
- Kitchen, break rooms, and copy rooms
- Bathrooms
- Utility rooms—gas tanks ("tank farms"), AV/IT server rooms, telephone/conference rooms
- Entry and reception areas

Table 45.5 Implications of the facility model

	Point-of-care only (A)	Point-of-care and facility based (B)
Space—storage	Hospital or off-site	Same as A and in simulation facility
Space—personnel	Will vary, may include dedicated hospital/off-site space or leverage space already allocated to personnel for their other responsibilities in the hospital	Will vary, may include (1) dedicated hospital/off-site space; (2) leverage space already allocated to personnel for their other responsibilities in the hospital; (3) use simulation facility space
Cost—utilities and space	Relative to space used (storage and personnel). Note: if personnel are leveraging space used for other responsibilities, then this cost is often absorbed by someone other than the simulation program	(1) Relative to space used (storage and personnel) in the hospital; (2) utilities related to the simulation facility; Note: if personnel are leveraging space used for other responsibilities, then this cost is often absorbed by someone other than the simulation program
Responsibility for space organization and maintenance	Organization limited to storage and office space used. Point-of-care location, the responsibility of the hospital? Excluding last-minute modifications related to simulation activity. Maintenance of fixed elements usually the full responsibility of the hospital	Same as A and full responsibility to organize and simulation facility. Maintenance of simulation-specific equipment (e.g., fixed audiovisual equipment), the responsibility of the simulation facility
Responsibility for stocking	Simulation supplies the responsibility of the simulation program; supplies relevant to point-of-care, the responsibility of the hospital	Same as A and the simulation program will have full responsibility for the stocking of consumable and nonconsumable supplies
Access	Will vary depending of patient census assuming patient care supersedes training space needs	Same as A and simulation facility access falls entirely under the control of the simulation program

While this list is somewhat general, it does illustrate the many considerations are involved when a simulation program either moves into a space or designs one. The program will either be defined by the space or the program will define the space. The latter is of course preferred but may not be an option for many programs that are given space with little budget and configurability. Even in this circumstance, it is possible for a program to take even the most inflexible space and make it suit its needs with a little innovation and patience.

As discussed in the section on policies and procedures, it is important that any dedicated facility be managed through the use of defendable and representative policies and procedures. Facilities are expensive to build and maintain. Maximizing utilization of any given space while retaining its functionality is an important consideration. When space is underutilized or misused, then programs run the risk of losing the space and/or funding.

Finances (Soft Versus Hard Money and Sustainability)

The subject of finances is complex. At the most basic level, finances can be broken down to capital and operational costs. Capital costs often refer to costs related to brick and mortar and equipment. Operational costs refer to costs related to operating a program on an ongoing basis—personnel, service agreements, utilities, equipment, etc. Good budgeting skills and a solid understanding of basic financial principles will help programs in the short and long term.

As programs become larger, they may need to develop financial pro forma that looks beyond just the next year but extend 3–5 years into the future. Many people have difficulty in developing these as they see them as guesswork. Developing a 3–5-year pro forma relies on making assumptions and applying those assumptions to establish expenses and income. The assumptions themselves should be based on historical and future considerations.

The origin of funds will vary by program. Many simulation programs are initially seeded by "soft" money. This refers to funding that is temporary and self-limited. Examples of this form of funding include grant and philanthropic funds. While this is a useful source for funding both initial startup and ongoing operations, they by their very nature are unreliable and leave a program vulnerable to reduction or even closure should the funding come to an end. The accountability with respect to soft funding is also different and may not be a rigorous as hard funding.

Hard funding refers to funding that comes from the institution as a line item (or several) for the purpose of conduction and delivering simulation services. This funding is generally more predictable and more closely tied to the mission and values of the organization. It is not without its risks as funding may fluctuate related to the overall priorities and condition of the institution. Changes in leadership will also impact this form of funding. The more "entrenched" a simulation program is, the more immune it will be to funding fluctuations or losses. This should not encourage complacence, and a program should always look outward and inward to evaluate its relevance—the unfortunate reality is that simulation often assumes a low priority at many institutions where budgeting is involved. Budgets for hard funding will follow the budgeting cycle of the source institution and will come under the regulations and scrutiny of the same.

Simulation programs are a resource to the institution and stakeholders they serve. They become a cost of business with a return on investment related to their activity. Programs must link their activities to definable outcomes so that they measure the cost of the activity to revenues generated. Recall though that in healthcare, the revenues generated may be in the form of cost saving, cost avoidance, or long-term risk reduction. Much as in the education and insurance world, the impact of an activity may not be realized for years. To take this from the abstract to the concrete: a nursing student who has superior training in part due to simulation will ultimately improve efficiency and effectiveness in the practice environment once they graduate and participate as licensed practitioners. This net gain is realized not only distal to the training intervention but may also be realized by an entirely different organization. The return on investment (ROI) and associated funding is a complex issue and will be driven by many factors and drivers. The more simulation programs make the case in real fiscal terms that simulation has a positive and relevant ROI, then the more likely an institution will be willing to provide hard and ongoing funding.

Utilization and Metrics

As students, learners, or other groups move through a simulation program, it is important to measure both the utilization of a program as well as the outcomes. Both of these concepts are quite complex but should be defined early in a program and revisited frequently. Utilization and outcomes are different and yet related concepts.

Utilization refers to the use of the program. It may reflect the learner hours (learners × hours spent in an activity) or may represent the room use in any given facility (room hours of use per day). There is no set standard currently for which metrics are of most use. The metric of most value will depend on many factors and will vary by institution. It is important to appreciate that if the data is not captured upfront, then the ability to create complete metrics will be difficult in the future. At a minimum, capturing key data points is important (Table 45.6). From these data, complex metrics can be calculated to assess program utilization. Utilization is important to understand as it defines the personnel, equipment, space, and time needs. It is difficult to predict future need as well as current issues without this data. At a most basic level, a program that is entirely facility bound can calculate the maximum number of room hours available in their facility if they know the number of rooms and the work hours.

Measuring outcomes from simulation-based education, training, research, and assessment is more complex. The level of evidence (Table 45.7) [11–13] will vary from the basic self-evaluation of the learner to complex outcomes that relate to the learners' impact on the market in which they practice. That is to say, as a person who has had a simulation-based intervention moves forward, they have an impact on a variety of people and systems. Patient outcome is an example of this as is system efficiency. These are complex issues that are multivariate. Estimating the impact of an intervention that is distal from the outcome must control for variables that are often outside of a simulation program's control. The application of standard healthcare outcome metrics may need to be reassessed to evaluate if measurement methods need to look to other industries on how to best evaluate outcomes. The education industry has developed sophisticated methods that estimate causal effect of interventions [14].

Table 45.6 Examples of core utilization metrics to capture

Metric
Number of unique learners per simulation course
Duration of simulation course
Number of simulation sessions per course
Time (duration) of each simulation session
Number of learners per session
Space used for each session
Equipment used per session
Personnel needed per session

Table 45.7 Levels of evidence

Level	Description
I	Systematic reviews (integrative/meta-analyses/clinical practice guidelines based on systematic reviews)
II	Single experimental study (randomized control trials)
III	Quasi-experimental studies
IV	Nonexperimental studies
V	Care report/program evaluation/narrative literature reviews
VI	Opinions of respected authorities/consensus panels

Mobile Simulation

The issue of mobility is increasingly becoming an issue. Does simulation need to be limited to a fixed facility? As we come to understand the multiple simulation modalities and learner/assessment needs, it is becoming apparent that simulation-based activities can in fact be carried out in a variety of locations including a fixed facility, traditional learning spaces (auditoriums), and actual patient care settings. Each of these locations offers different advantages and issues. To offer simulation-based services in multiple locations requires additional resources (personnel and equipment) and considerations. Ultimately demand, priorities, and resources will determine the availability for such services. Deciding to pursue a mobile program must be deliberate and often can leverage existing resources when demand is low.

Other Considerations: Equipment, Audiovisual, and Security

There are many other issues to consider when developing a simulation program. Some of these considerations are rooted in policy (program or organizational) as well as need. A systematic approach to these issues is helpful. Equipment, audiovisual, and security needs will also be determined by program needs balanced against budgetary considerations.

Equipment is driven by the education strategies used and by the volume of learners. All equipment will have a certain lifespan. The lifespan is determined by the absolute time a product can be expected to remain fully functional using recommended maintenance schedules. The lifespan can also refer to the natural product cycle time in which a product becomes outdated relative to market offerings. A product may not be serviceable after a certain amount of time due to manufacturer discontinuation, for example. Similarly, a product may not be useful as other technologies emerge and render that initial product irrelevant. Relative to other industries, the product life cycle in simulation has been relatively long, which is both good and bad for simulation programs. While it allows products to remain in service over longer period of time, the pace of innovation is slower which hinders progression within the industry as a whole. Equipment considerations can be summarized into four main categories: (1) simulation equipment (e.g., mannequin), (2) medical equipment (e.g., bed or pump), (3) consumables (e.g., syringes or office supplies), and (4) office equipment and furnishings.

The specifics of different AV and information/learning management systems are beyond the scope of this chapter alone. Audiovisual (AV) considerations in a simulation program can be broad and complex. The AV system must ultimately meet the needs of the educational activity and must be in alignment for security and policy requirements. For example, in some cultures, the filming of women is not considered acceptable. So the system must conform to needs as well as policies (internal and external) of a program. The AV system must be used to support operations, learning, and assessment. Educators (operations) and learners will use the AV system differently. Depending on the activity, the operations staff (technicians and faculty) may leverage the system to gather (and manipulate) information as well as deliver deliberate education to the learner (e.g. allowing learners to see specific cameras and views). The learner on the other hand is mainly gathering and integrating information. Lastly, the system should have the ability to archive materials for future review and cataloguing. This archive material may have utility to researchers, faculty, operations, and learners.

AV systems are rapidly moving to digital formats, although analog systems are very reliable and tested. The choice of the system will be determined by a variety of factors including budget, the expanse of the program, goals and objectives for the program, support for the equipment, and program skillset.

Security considerations in a simulation program relate to equipment, personal safety, as well as access to information. A simulation program must consider the level of security it needs. This may be as simple as a locked and keyed door to complex access systems that allow differential access to different levels of personnel and learners. This applies to space as well as information. The loss of mobile equipment can be costly to a program. Similarly, the political and safety considerations related to the theft of medications (whether fake or not) can be substantive and costly. The goals of a security system should be built around: (1) equipment and personnel security and (2) access control to consumables, equipment, and information. For simulation research, these guidelines and details are specifically outlined depending on the institutional research board protocols.

Logistics

Logistics is an important consideration for a successful simulation program. Robust and reliable scheduling, inventory, and maintenance protocols should be developed and put into place as a program evolves. Logistics needs to be based on policy, procedures, and guidelines. This allows for consistency but also inoculates a program from changes in personnel and shifts in funding. Programs that are larger may have the luxury of personnel dedicated to logistic considerations. There are examples where faculty and educators are entirely removed from logistic considerations. That is they arrive to teach and then they leave. While this may be an efficient mode of operation, it does leave a program vulnerable as groups lacked the cross-training to cover for each other especially in times where personnel may not be abundant.

Conclusion

The establishment of a simulation center can be a complex task that requires forethought and ongoing attention. Deliberate action will allow programs to manage what may on the surface seem unmanageable. This chapter has outlined a variety of considerations that will apply depending on circumstance. These elements come from some well establish business models that have been proven to be successful. It is important to consider each element to delineate their importance and priority in the process. Failure to do so can create downstream problems and obstacles. While it is tempting to create a rigid framework, it is important to consider that the structure of the center/program must incorporate flexibility to accommodate for future change and to remain relevant.

Appendix

POLICY & PROCEDURE CATEGORIES/LIST (partial)

General

- Mission statement
- Vision statement
- Values statement

Stakeholder definition

- Who are they (name them)
- Governance
- History of involvement
- Formal agreements
- Decision-making process
- Fiscal/funding sources

Instructors

- Skill categories
- Privileges (do they get to debrief, run sessions, etc...)
- Code of conduct
- Evaluation policy
- Development policy
- Confidentiality
- Travel
- Mentor policy

Personnel

- Operations Manager
- Business manager (if applicable)
- Simulation Technician
- Support staff & contact tree
- Overtime policy
- Scope of work/description for each personnel classification
- Org chart

Scheduling

- Process (intake and confirmation)
- Priority of use
- Facility use (what can or cannot be done in facility)
- Fee schedule if applicable
- Cancellation policy
- Recording of scheduling events (i.e. calendar structure and info)
- Final arbiter of scheduling needs policy

Equipment

- Loan out policy
- Acquisition policy and process – how to request, who makes the decision, etc...
- Maintenance & cleaning (type and frequency)
- Breakage and repair policy (internal and external))
- In-situ versus in-facility use

Supplies

- Acquisition
- Organization
- Inventory
- Budget source
- Usage and re-usage

Miscellaneous Policy - I

- Confidentiality
- Video recording policy
- Video distribution policy
- Video destruction policy

Miscellaneous Policy - II

- Observation of simulation policy for course participants
- Observation policy for non-participants
- Required disclaimers and pre-event statements
- Required event or course acknowledgements
- Simulation facility "Brand" use policy
- Publication policy

Fiscal

- required reporting, (type and frequency) and to who
- Annual budget reporting requirements
- Required fiscal year end documents
- Required documentation
- Purchase and acquisition procedure
- Reimbursement process

Meetings

- Meetings – going to meetings representing the center
- Reimbursement policy
- Covered expenses
- Priority scheduling in case of conflict

Research policy

- IRB policy
- General Guidelines if different from institutions
- Security
- Fiscal impact (overhead, etc....)

Scenarios

- Template use
- Structure and mandatory minimum components
- Authorship rules
- Storage rules
- When can a scenario be used – policy on validation

Operations Policy

- When scenarios are implemented what is the recommended procedure
- Turn-on process
- Turn-off process
- Security of information (video, scenarios, databases, files)
- Parking

Courses

- List of regular courses
- List of unacceptable courses
- Mandatory elements and documentation for each course
- CME, CE, recertification policy.
- Fee structure

Remediation

- Policy relating to how it must be done
- Documentation
- Policies to reduce liability for the center
- Ethical guidelines

Vendor relations policy

- Beta testing
- Gifts
- Events
- Showcases
- Grants
- Access to facility

Customer Relations Policy

- Dispute resolution process
- Marketing
- Web usage
- Information dissemination
- Official media policy

References

1. Seropian MA, Brown K, Gavilanes JS, Driggers B. Simulation: not just a mannequin. J Nurs Educ. 2004;43(4):164–9.
2. Seropian MA, Brown K, Gavilanes JS, Driggers B. An approach to simulation program development. J Nurs Educ. 2004;43(4):170–4.
3. Seropian MA. General concepts in full scale simulation: getting started. Anesth Analg. 2003;97(6):1695–705.
4. Murray DJ. Current trends in simulation training in anesthesia: a review. Minerva Anestesiol. 2011;77(5):528–33.
5. Tews MC, Hamilton GC. Integrating emergency medicine principles and experience throughout the medical school curriculum: why and how. Acad Emerg Med. 2011;18(10):1072–80.
6. Moore MH. Creating public value: strategic management in government. Cambridge: Harvard University Press; 1995.
7. Ahmed K, Amer T, Challacombe B, Jaye P, Dasgupta P, Khan MS. How to develop a simulation programme in urology. BJU Int. 2011;108(11):1698–702.
8. Passiment M, Sacks H, Huang G: Medical Simulation in Medical Education: Results of an AAMC Survey. Association of American Medical Colleges 2011. https://www.aamc.org/download/259760/data/medicalsimulationinmedicaleducationanaamcsurvey.pdf
9. Kim S, Ross B, Wright A, Wu M, Benedetti T, Leland F, et al. Halting the revolving door of faculty turnover recruiting and retaining clinician educators in an academic medical simulation center. Simul Healthc. 2011;6(3):168–75.
10. www.ssih.org,www.asahq.org,www.facs.org.
11. Harris RP et al. Current methods of the U.S. Preventive Services Task Force: a review of the process. Am J Prev Med. 2001;20(3 Suppl):21–35.
12. Melnyck BM, Fineout-Overholt E. Evidence-based practice in healthcare. Philadelphia: Lippincott; 2005.
13. Stetler CB, Morsi D, Rucki S, Broughton S, Corrigan B, Fitzgerald J, et al. Utilization-focused integrative reviews in a nursing service. Appl Nurs Res. 1998;11:195–206.
14. Schneider B, Carnoy M, Kilpatrick J, Schmidt WH. Estimating causal effects using experimental and observational designs: a think tank white paper prepared under the auspices of the American Educational Research Association Grants Program. Washington, D.C.: American Educational Research Association, 2007.

Business Planning Considerations for a Healthcare Simulation Center

46

Maria Galati and Robert Williams

...no industry in which human life depends on the skilled performance of responsible operators has waited for unequivocal proof of the benefits of simulation before embracing it. [1]

—*David Gaba, M.D.*

Introduction

Simulation-based training has been used for many years to manage risk and facilitate safety in hazardous professions outside of healthcare, especially in aviation. The use of simulation as a tool in medical education is relatively recent and follows the age-old medical tenet *primum non nocere* ("first, do no harm"). The use of simulation may also follow the more recent emphasis in the business of medicine on improving patient outcomes while reducing healthcare expenses. These demands for value and efficiency in an era of healthcare reform present both new opportunities and new challenges in justifying the investments required for the research and development of simulation to educate healthcare professionals. Although the readers will appreciate that similar material is covered in Chap. 45, for completeness, these chapters are intentionally left intact since it is impossible to discuss one without the other. This chapter will focus on the business and operational considerations in planning a healthcare simulation center and when appropriate will discuss center design concerns as they relate to the business of simulation.

Business Planning

The need to coordinate "vision-driven business planning" was identified as one of eight major themes in an effort to institutionalize and sustain simulation in healthcare by representatives from interested professional and regulatory organizations [2]. Business plans provide an organized construct for the presentation of a project or business, an analysis of the industry and marketplace in which the business will operate, and the strategic, management, and financial goals that are envisioned for the new entity. The depth and scope of a business plan will rest on several factors including the status of the entity as either an independent unit or as a component of an existing business, the scope of the entity's activities, and the type and amount of financial investment required.

In planning a healthcare simulation center, the decision of whether to establish a stand-alone facility or a center within a private or academic medical facility will rest on the mission and goals of the simulation center. The planned scope of simulation activities may include the use of standardized live patients, low-tech models or mannequins, and/or complex task trainers and realistic human patient simulators and may serve single-specialty or multispecialty purposes. The complexity of the simulation services offered will be reflected in the business planning process. Finally, the amount and source of funding required to finance the center will determine the complexity of the financial projections and will guide the planner in selecting the most appropriate metrics to define the investment's projected economic worth.

Three key elements of a business plan that should apply to healthcare simulation centers of all types and complexities are outlined and illustrated below. These include the formulation of (1) a mission statement, (2) an analysis of the market and strategic positions of the business, and (3) a financial overview of the plan. Other elements of a business plan may be included to illustrate and support the business case as is appropriate. A comprehensive listing of the elements of a business plan is shown in Table 46.1.

Mission Statement

Defining the mission and goals of a simulation center is an essential first step in the business planning process. A mission

M. Galati, MBA (✉)
Department of Anesthesiology,
Icahn School of Medicine at Mount Sinai,
1 Gustave L. Levy Place, Box 1010, New York, NY 10029, USA
e-mail: maria.galati@mssm.edu

R. Williams, MBA
Clinical Operations, Department of Anesthesiology,
The Mount Sinai Hospital, 1 Gustave L. Levy Place,
Box 1010, New York, NY 10029, USA
e-mail: bob.williams@mountsinai.org

A.I. Levine et al. (eds.), *The Comprehensive Textbook of Healthcare Simulation*,
DOI 10.1007/978-1-4614-5993-4_46, © Springer Science+Business Media New York 2013

Table 46.1 Elements of a business plan

I. Executive summary (a) General description of the business (b) Business mission and goals (c) Financial and operational resources
II. Company background and analysis (a) SWOT: Strengths, Weaknesses, Opportunities, Threats (b) Service offerings (c) Technology (d) Competitive position
III. Industry and market analysis (a) Scope (b) Barriers to entry (c) Demand (d) Market share (e) Customers/pricing plan (f) Marketing and promotional plan
IV. Strategic analysis (a) Mission and goals (b) Operating assumptions (c) Performance metrics (d) Time frames
V. Operations and management (a) Table of organization (b) Key personnel (c) Policies and procedures
VI. Financial analysis (a) Financial statements/forecasts (b) Capital and operating budgets (c) Supplemental justifications
VII. Conclusion
VIII. Appendices

Sources: Authors' compilation from: Finch [3] and Gerson [4]

statement is an internal document that communicates in a concise and specific way what the business is and what it proposes to do. It is typically constructed by answering a series of questions including:

1. What is the product or purpose of the entity?
2. Who are the entity's customers?
3. What are the entity's quality, human resources, and/or marketing-related goals?

An expanded mission statement may also incorporate goals of the business in a qualitative and/or quantitative manner and may set out timeframes or other specific objectives of the entity.

A mission statement for a healthcare simulation center may also reflect factors including its:

- Profit or nonprofit status or objective
- Scope of simulation services offered
- Range of medical specialties/groups of customers served
- Internal vs. external customer focus
- Educational, research, and/or clinical goals

The box shows an example of a mission statement for a medical school simulation center within an academic medical center.

Example: Medical school-based simulation center mission statement

"The mission of the Center is to provide state-of-the-art, realistic patient simulation to XYZ medical students residents and faculty with the goal of achieving excellence in medical education and assuring the highest standards of ethics, safety, and quality for the care of patients of the XYZ Medical Center."

Market Analysis and Competitive Strategy

A useful framework for analyzing a market and planning a competitive strategy has been described by Porter [5]. He described five forces that drive competition in an industry including the rivalry among existing firms, the bargaining power of both suppliers and buyers, the threat of new entrants, and the threat of substitute products or services.

Barriers to Entry: A Simulation Center in an Academic Medical Center

According to Porter, the threat of new entrants depends, in part, on the industry-specific barriers involving factors such as the economies of scale, capital requirements, product differentiation, switching costs, access to distribution channels, regulatory policy, and other cost advantages unrelated to scale, such as the learning or experience curve. The following is an example of how Porter's framework for competitive analysis may be utilized in planning a simulation center in an academic medical center.

Economies of scale accrue as a reduction in the unit cost of a product or operation as the output in a specific period of time increases. Scale economies accrue to a medical center that locates and organizes its simulation facilities for ease of use across several medical specialties. Capital investment advantages accrue to a medical center that leverages its existing physical plant, audiovisual and teaching lab equipment, and support staff in starting up a simulation center.

A simulation center may diversify its customer base to secure its competitive position. In its start-up period, the center may plan to target the medical students, residents, and faculty of the medical center. Later, this customer base may be expanded to include other community-based or affiliated trainees and faculty, ancillary healthcare personnel, and/or representatives of health-related industries to gain economies of scale.

A simulation center that is the first to enter a geographic market or that is the first to become known for quality services with a particular customer base secures loyalty and learning curve advantages and increases switching costs for customers who may be presented with new service provider options. These advantages may be bolstered by achieving certification and/or endorsement by professional organizations or regulatory bodies (see Chap. 48).

Academic healthcare training programs also control an important "distribution channel" of graduate trainees and alumni customers based on their long-standing relationships and/or reputation for quality education within these professional groups.

Finally, Porter identifies businesses that gain the most significant experience curve cost advantages as those with a high labor content when performing intricate tasks and/or complex assembly. Healthcare simulation centers require a major investment in human resources to design intricate clinical scenarios and execute sophisticated information technology tasks. Academic medical centers have a cadre of medical educators in place who are experienced in didactic and bedside clinical teaching methods that can be leveraged in the simulated education environment. These skills lend experience curve advantages that reduce costs by facilitating design and efficiency. Centers may also produce intellectual property that provides a source of supplemental revenue, reputational benefit, and product differentiation.

Financial Analysis

Financial projection and analysis of the investments required to initiate and maintain a new center are important business plan elements. The financial analysis section of a business plan must conform to the requirements of the business owners and investors. These requirements will vary by type of organization, size of project, availability of investment capital, and type of investor. Conformance to the business plan requirements alone, however, may not determine the success of the business plan. A study of the relation between the form and content of business planning documents and the funding decisions of venture capitalists found only a weak association and suggested that independent sources of information may be involved [6]. Business planners need to design a financial plan and analysis that presents the most robust cost/benefit projections and targets the needs and interests of the decision makers who will determine the fate of the proposal.

Figures of Merit

Capital investments are, by definition, costly and expected to endure over time. They are therefore best evaluated based upon the cash flows that are expected over the life of the project. Business planners must choose the appropriate "figure of merit" (a number that defines a capital investment's projected economic worth) to employ in the financial analysis. Given the long-range nature of capital investments, figures of merit typically incorporate the concept of the time value of money. The net present value (NPV) is one such figure of merit commonly used in business planning. It requires development of a set of assumptions that includes the amount and timing of cash outflows and inflows, and a discount rate, or the rate of return desired/expected on a particular investment.

In the case of a healthcare simulation center, the revenues from conducting training courses, certification programs, competency assessments, and other potential revenue-producing activities would constitute the expected cash inflow. Opportunities to reduce costs should also be counted in the cash flow analysis. Examples include the recapture by the center of continuing medical education fees paid to external providers or indirect savings derived from the avoidance of patient safety lapses and healthcare reimbursement penalties. In some cases, clinicians who participate in simulation-based training may be eligible under risk management incentive programs for reductions in malpractice premiums [7], and these should be included in financial projections, as applicable.

In healthcare, long-range investment decisions have traditionally been made based on medical or strategic needs with less of an emphasis on economic efficiency [8]. There are several reasons to avoid the exclusive use of traditional figures of merit such as NPV in business planning. These reasons stem from flaws in the methodology that lead to an underestimation of a business plan's benefits and a systematic bias against successful innovation [9]. These flaws include the fact that cash flows of the innovative project are compared against a default scenario in which no investment is made, and the assumption is, therefore, that the company's current success will persist in the absence of the investment.

Real Options Planning

Real options planning is a complementary approach used with traditional figures of merit for the financial analysis of capital investments. It has been described as a technique to "marry the theory of financial options to the foundational ideas in strategy, organizational theory, and complex systems" [10]. The technique shifts the focus of a business from how existing resources can be leveraged for long-term benefit to how an investment in the creation of new capabilities adds value.

Employing a real options approach in a business plan for a healthcare simulation center may involve modeling serial financial investments that will result in a staged implementation of the center. These models would pinpoint opportunities to modify the scale and complexity of the center's activities as the demand for services develops. This facilitates reduction of the initial capital investment, thereby maximizing chances for the success of the proposal when start-up funds are limited.

The real options approach for a simulation center would provide flexibility by accommodating the redirection of the scope, the specialty orientation, and even the location of the project after startup. This may be necessary and beneficial in responding to rapidly changing needs in the financial, educational, regulatory, or political environment in which the center operates.

A center may also incorporate plans to join with interested parties from industry to work in a joint venture arrangement. This arrangement, for example, could provide synergy in a project where a vendor needs a clinical partner to accomplish its product research and development goals and where an academic or clinical practice needs access to the vendor's equipment in order to further its medical education and clinical research goals. In this case, a legal review and documentation of the relationship would be required to avoid any potential conflicts of interest. Typically, a contract between the parties would serve to define the roles and responsibilities of the participants, assure compliance with all applicable laws, and define the ownership of any intellectual property and revenues that may result from the collaboration.

The Role of Philanthropy

Healthcare reform is bringing new uncertainties and new cash flow challenges to medical centers that will need to rely more than ever on their diminishing reserves and the debt markets to fund capital investments. This raises the importance of philanthropy as a supplemental source of funding for capital project needs. However, conditions in the economy can present confounding factors that limit access to capital in the debt markets and, at the same time, may influence donor behavior.

Limitations in the debt market followed the financial crisis of 2008 and nonprofit organizations experienced what may have been the effect of the broader market conditions on healthcare gifting in 2009. According to a report by the Association for Healthcare Philanthropy, gifts to healthcare organizations in 2009 fell 11% to $7.6 billion from $8.6 billion the previous year. At the same time, the return that organizations earned on fund-raising investments fell 9% [11]. This report also noted that in 2009, 8 out of 10 healthcare donors in the United States (US) were individuals with a personal connection to the institution and that 27% of all contributions funded construction and 18% funded investments in equipment.

Business plans for healthcare simulation centers should consider the opportunity and availability of funds from philanthropic sources to defray capital and/or operating costs. Fund-raising activities that provide the most efficient return (based on cost per dollar raised) are those that focus on obtaining major gifts and planned giving rather than on holding special events such as charity balls or benefits [12].

Simulation center activities may be an attractive investment for donors in the current climate of healthcare cost control and with the growing focus on patient safety. High-technology medical training methods present publicity opportunities that can be used to bolster a center's reputation in the community and to attract philanthropy. Business planners should include marketing and development office specialists as early as possible in the planning process to maximize the success of these opportunities.

Supplemental Justifications

The aim of the financial analysis section of a business plan is to show justification for the business's commitment of potentially scarce financial and operational resources to the new investment. In addition to the financial figures of merit chosen, important qualitative benefits of the planned investment may be included to supplement the financial analysis. Items to highlight in the case of healthcare simulation centers include the ethical, educational, and patient safety benefits of medical simulation.

Traditional clinical teaching methods employ live patients in the process of training healthcare professionals and in the general interest of promoting the safety and welfare of all patients. While some clinical experience with real live patients is essential and valuable, these traditional methods are difficult to standardize, inefficient, and create ethical concerns [13].

Centers with a limited patient population may argue for the use of medical simulation to augment live patient teaching methods and to ensure that all trainees receive a comprehensive, standardized, and efficient learning experience that covers the broadest scope of disease states, clinical presentations, and critical events. Simulation-based medical education also gives training programs the flexibility to determine and vary when, how, and for which types of patient interactions it may be appropriate and safe for trainees to participate in live patient care.

Patient safety has been a prominent focus in US healthcare since the release of the 1999 Institute of Medicine (IOM) report that attributed significant rates of mortality and inflation in healthcare and societal costs, measured in the billions of dollars per year, to medical errors [14]. Starting in 2003, regulatory agencies like the Joint Commission instituted programs to set national patient safety goals and governmental and private sector payers followed by linking reimbursement to the adoption and reporting of safety-related measures. The review of healthcare safety and efficiency continues to be an important focus and matter of concern in the US a decade after the IOM report. A 2009 report reviewing healthcare quality among nations found that the United States ranked last of 19 "developed" countries in avoiding preventable deaths [15]. Hospitals and physicians are increasingly incentivized via public reporting requirements and new reimbursement formulas under

Table 46.2 Project management team members and respective roles

Member	Description
Project manager	Responsible for overseeing all aspects of the endeavor. This individual is charged with monitoring its progress, keeping to a timeline, and monitoring expenses. The project manager will interact will all groups and generally keep the project organized
Architect	Provides architectural design expertise and works with the various team members and project groups to realize facility construction based on the scope and vision of the project
Administrator	This team member represents the institution's executive senior leadership and is responsible for assuring that the project satisfies the mission and financial expectations
Simulation expert(s)	May be internal faculty with expertise in simulation or contracted simulation consultants. This individual or group should ensure that the project's design will meet the goals of the simulation center. Experienced simulation instructors will have very valuable input in the design process
Contractor	The contractor should be selected and involved during the design phase of the project and work closely with the architects
Facilities management	Representative of the institution's Facilities Management should be involved to assure the construction meets the institution's standards. They are owner representatives focused on process as it relates to construction and engineering issues such as electrical, plumbing issues, and meeting building codes
IT and AV consultants	May be in-house or contracted. Role is to work with the simulation experts to ensure that defined IT and AV needs are met
Vendor representatives	Representatives from capital equipment vendors for simulation, operating room, and medical equipment should be involved to assure that design and installation requirements are met
Marketing/Development Office representatives	Depending upon the mission and funding plans for the center, representative from Marketing and Development may serve as ad hoc members or consultants to the team

health reform to facilitate compliance with health quality and outcome measures. By 2015, approximately 9% of all Medicare payments to hospitals are expected to be linked to the hospitals' ability to successfully reduce readmissions and hospital-acquired conditions and to publicly report medical errors [16].

Healthcare simulation centers can serve as the nexus for the introduction, practice, and maintenance of patient safety skills that facilitate success for hospitals in both the reimbursement and public reporting arenas. Business planners should consider how simulation training can benefit the organizations facing these challenges and should incorporate projections in the business planning process of the potential benefits of reducing costs and enhancing reimbursements.

Finally, organizations with a teaching mission can differentiate themselves with trainees, patients, prospective donors, and the community at large by highlighting the educational, patient safety, and ethical advantages of simulation-based training as a complement to traditional teaching methods.

Thus far, we have reviewed the considerations in developing a business plan for a healthcare simulation center based on the center's mission, including methods of financial and competitive analysis and other useful factors in justifying the investment. Successful business plans outline a clear mission, propose a strategy for competing in the marketplace, and meet the institutional or company "hurdle rate" for a return on the expected investment. The last step in the planning process is the presentation of the final business plan to key stakeholders and investors.

Estimating Expenses and Moving Beyond the Planning Phase

The remainder of the chapter will focus on elements of the business plan that help planners in outlining the projected expenses of the center and to begin to advance the project toward an implementation phase. Many of these steps are initiated in the course of business planning and can begin once the mission and scope of the center are defined and agreed upon by the stakeholders. Steps for projecting center costs and moving toward implementation include:

1. Selection of the project design and management team
2. Facility design
3. Development of a capital and operating budgets
4. Creation of a timeline and internal controls

Project Management Team

The project design and management team has the responsibility of overseeing the planning and design of the physical space, developing budgets, and monitoring the progress of each stage of the project. The team is typically supervised by the funders of the project. The design/management team should be well balanced and led by a knowledgeable and diligent project manager whose role is to keep the team focused [17]. Table 46.2 lists recommended team members and their respective roles. Collectively, the team will develop an architectural design based on the goals of the project and will select contractors and vendors to execute the plan using available funds. The team will also develop a realistic project timeline to assure that "go live" goals are achieved. Regular meetings to evaluate the project's progress are helpful in managing issues and problems as they arise. All team members should be motivated and possess superior communication skills. The team's ultimate goal is to guide the project from design phase to completion of construction and to ensure that everything is in place for the opening of the simulation center. After the construction phase has been completed, appropriate team members may function on a parallel track to ensure that processes are in place to support the planned curriculum.

Facility Design

The first step in a facility design project is to review the goals of the project and to justify the decision to move forward with a renovation, an expansion, or a commitment to new construction [18]. Goals of the project will dictate the scope of the architectural design. Starting new construction, renovating or expanding an existing educational operation is often subject to the availability of capital funding and the demonstration of financial viability [19]. New facility construction offers the significant advantage of beginning the project with a blank canvas. However, space and cost constraints make it likely that a medical simulation center will be created by renovating of existing space. In other cases, existing education programs will be expanded to include simulation, as it becomes the standard of practice in medical education. In any of these cases, key considerations in facility design include:

1. Fulfillment of the center's mission
2. An inventory of existing services and space/equipment resources
3. The assessment of need or demand for services to be provided
4. Plans for future expansion or increasing capacity

The next step is to review the program's planned or existing curriculum by quantifying the number of participants and programmatic offerings over a defined time period.

Physical space requirements for a simulation center will ideally consist of a suite of rooms including:

1. Simulation lab(s)
2. Control room(s)
3. Standardized patient examination room(s)
4. Conference room or class room
5. Debriefing space
6. Office space

Simulation centers should replicate the actual clinical environment as closely as possible. For example, a center with a surgical emphasis may include a replica of an operating room complete with anesthesia and surgical equipment setups. Depending on the complexity of the simulated environment, the space should be designed with input from physicians familiar with both the clinical environment and with the requirements of simulation education in order to create a realistic presentation. Simulation labs must accommodate hardware and ancillary materials that may include mannequins and patient conveyances, specialty-specific clinical work stations, supply carts, desk and counter space, and storage cabinets.

The number of trainers and trainees who will participate simultaneously in simulation scenarios is a factor in deciding the size and layout of the lab. Other space design considerations include designing the space to meet building, fire, and safety codes as well as structural requirements for the placement of furniture, the installation of medical gas supply systems, and the cabling for information technology (IT) and audiovisual (AV) systems.

Debriefing is an important aspect of simulation-based education and should be considered in facility design. The debriefing space is used as a place for trainers and trainees to review the simulation exercise, to engage in post-scenario discussion, and to reinforce learning objectives. Debriefing rooms should have the necessary AV equipment to view or review recorded simulation activities. Given space constraints, simulation labs or conference rooms may also function as debriefing space. Dedicated office space will be necessary in a stand-alone center. Alternatively, staff may use existing offices for these purposes.

Location of control rooms, size of the conference room, and the audiovisual setup should be based on input from the clinical educators as well as manufacturers' representatives. Simulation systems vendors and capital equipment manufacturers provide important information regarding structural requirements for extensive capital installations such as specialty lighting, ventilation, and medical gas systems. The final facility design should be based on collaboration of all team members, reflecting the needs of the simulation educators and their curriculum, and meet the financial constraints of the project.

The Capital Budget

Administrators or owners may have already determined the amount of funding that is available to be committed to a particular project. Alternatively, the cost of the project may be known and the institution may seek philanthropy or other funding sources to support the expenses. The process for development of the capital budget actually begins during the design phase and may impact or limit aspects of the new facility's design.

The capital budget for any project includes costs for space design, renovation and construction, building materials, and required equipment. Capital equipment is defined as nonexpendable equipment that is used to operate a business or

Table 46.3 Sample operating budget XYZ simulation center Annual operating budget: 20XX

	Quarter				
	1	2	3	4	Annual total
Salary expenses:					
Medical director (0.2 FTE)	$10,000	$10,000	$10,000	$10,000	$ 40,000
Instructor 1 (0.2 FTE)	$ 5,000	$ 5,000	$ 5,000	$ 5,000	$ 20,000
Instructor 2 (0.2 FTE)	$ 5,000	$ 5,000	$ 5,000	$ 5,000	$ 20,000
Administrator (0.2 FTE)	$ 6,000	$ 6,000	$ 6,000	$ 6,000	$ 24,000
Fringe benefits (25% salary)	$ 6,500	$ 6,500	$ 6,500	$ 6,500	$ 26,000
Total salary expenses:					$130,000
Non-salary expenses:					
Rent	$10,000	$10,000	$10,000	$10,000	$ 40,000
Utilities	$ 900	$ 900	$ 900	$ 900	3,600
Medical gases	$ 150	$ 150	$ 150	$ 150	$ 600
Preventive maintenance	$ 5,000	$ 5,000	$ 5,000	$ 5,000	$ 20,000
Repairs	$ 500	$ 500	$ 500	$ 500	$ 2,000
Clinical supplies	$ 150	$ 150	$ 150	$ 150	$ 600
Office supplies	$ 75	$ 75	$ 75	$ 75	$ 300
Total non-salary expenses:					$ 67,100
Total annual expenses:					$197,100

provide a service. Institutions have specific definitions in their policies for capital equipment. For example, any item costing more than $500 and/or with a useful life of more than 3 years may be considered capital. Capital equipment requirements for construction of a medical simulation center will vary with the organization's educational goals. Room furnishings, integrated simulation mannequin systems, anatomical training models, and IT/AV systems are examples of items that will appear in the capital budget. Additional items may include "props" such as medical equipment that would be found in the clinical setting. These may be specific to the course curriculum or targeted professional group. For example, equipment for an emergency medical technician training program will not be appropriate for a surgical residency training program.

The project management team should explore opportunities to seek in-kind support from vendors who may already have a relationship with the organization and may be able to donate capital equipment to the center. Alternatively, centers can consider equipping their simulation centers with capital equipment no longer suited for clinical use but with functionality adequate for simulations.

Most institutions have guidelines and requirements for capital acquisitions that include competitive bidding. Competitive bidding assures that vendors offer optimal pricing for the required capital investments. The project management team will be tasked with putting together a well thought-out and justified capital budget that will assure the best use of the scarce resources required to see the project through to completion.

The Operating Budget

An operating budget for a simulation center is a financial plan for the non-capital expenses of running the center for a specific period of time. It is typically projected on an annual basis and is normally subdivided showing expense projections for shorter monthly or quarterly intervals. These budget intervals provide managers with the ability to anticipate short-term cash flow requirements and to facilitate timely comparisons of actual expenses against the budgeted amounts. A comprehensive operating budget is developed and monitored by the responsible manager and forecasts all expenses for day-to-day operations. These usually include salaries and fringe benefits, fixed costs such as rent and utilities, as well as expenses for supplies, non-capital equipment, and preventive maintenance and repair. Table 46.3 shows a sample operating budget for a for a medical school-based simulation center. It assumes a work effort of 20% from existing employees of the medical school. Salaries are therefore prorated, reflecting the proportional work effort (0.20) of a full-time equivalent (FTE) employee. A stand-alone simulation center may not have the ability to share personnel, in which case the operating budget would reflect the expenses of the specific staffing plan.

Monitoring the Project

The project team is charged with the development of a project timeline. This step is critical to ensuring that the project stays on schedule and meets objectives as set out in the business plan. Many factors will influence the timeline and a careful review of these will enable the project team to create a timeline that is realistic. Key factors include:

- Meeting with stakeholders to develop the architectural plans
- Preparation of construction documents and obtaining permits
- Construction or renovation duration
- Schedule for equipment selection, purchase, installation, and testing

Variables such as lead time for equipment delivery, construction delays, or unplanned findings will complicate the project and affect the timeline. The project management team should meet regularly to review progress and deal with any issues so as to minimize delays. Coordination of equipment delivery and installation schedules to accommodate various phases of the construction process requires finesse and continual reassessment to prevent delays.

The project management team should also develop internal controls to periodically monitor the quality of the construction and work with vendors to monitor delays in delivery of supplies and equipment. They must also review expenses and reconcile any variances from the budget. Unplanned additional expenses must be brought to the attention of stakeholders and reincorporated into the planning process. As the facility project nears completion, the project manager and appropriate team members should shift their planning focus to preparation for the day-to-day operations.

Conclusion

This chapter presents the business planning concepts used to identify the operational requirements and justify the investments for the startup and maintenance of a healthcare simulation center. Demand for medical simulation educational programs will expand in response to regulatory, professional, and public interest pressures to optimize safety and efficiency in medical education and healthcare delivery. These basic planning concepts can be used to formulate a successful proposal for the initiation of a simulation-based healthcare education center.

References

1. Gaba D. Improving anesthesiologists' performance by simulating reality. Anesthesiology. 1992;76:491–4.
2. Sinz E. 2006 Simulation summit. Simul Healthc. 2007;2(1):33–8.
3. Finch B. Creating success: how to write a business plan. 3rd ed. London (GBR): Kogan Page Ltd.; 2010.
4. Gerson R. Writing and implementing a marketing plan: a guide for small business owners. Boston: Crisp Publications; 1991.
5. Porter ME. Competitive strategy techniques for analyzing industries and competitors. New York: Simon & Shuster Inc; 1980. p. 4.
6. Kirsch D, Goldfarb B, Gera A. Form or substance: the role of business plans in venture capital decision making. Strateg Manage J. 2009;30(5):487.
7. Gardner R, Walzer TB, Simon R, et al. Obstetric simulation as a risk control strategy: course design and evaluation. Simul Healthc. 2008;3(2):119–27.
8. Schafer EL. Financial Management for Long-Range Decisions. In: Ross A, Williams SJ, Schafer EL, editors. Ambulatory care management. 2nd ed. New York: Delmar Publishers; 1991. p. 130.
9. Christensen CM, Kaufman SP, Shih WC. Innovation killers. Harv Bus Rev. 2008;86(1):98–105.
10. Kogut B, Kulatilaka N. Capabilities as real options. Organ Sci. 2001;12:744.
11. Cohen T. U.S. Health-care Giving Ailing. Philanthropy Journal Website. www.philanthropyjournal.org/news. Accessed 14 Dec 2011.
12. McGinly WC. The maturing role of philanthropy in healthcare. Front Health Serv Manage. 2008;24(4):16.
13. Ziv A, Wolpe PR, Small SD, Glick S. Simulation-based medical education: an ethical imperative. Simul Healthc. 2006;1(4):252.
14. Kohn LT, Corrigan JM, Donaldson MS, editors. To err is human: building a safer health system. National Academy Press Website: http://www.nap.edu/books/0309068371/html/. Accessed 19 Dec 2011.
15. Docteur E, Berenson RA. How Does the Quality of U.S. Health Care Compare Internationally? Robert Wood Johnson Foundation and the Urban Institute; 2009. http://www.urban.org/uploadedpdf/411947_ushealthcare_quality.pdf. Assecced 13 Mar 2013.
16. Daly R. Special report. Sucker punched? Modern Healthcare. 20 June 2011. p. 20.
17. Seropian M, Lavey R. Design considerations for healthcare simulation facilities. Simul Healthc. 2010;5(6):339–40.
18. Kieburtz PA, Ross A. Facilities Design and Operations In: Ross A, Williams SJ, Schafer EL, editors. Ambulatory care management. 2nd ed. New York: Delmar Publishers; 1991. p.155–162.
19. Haluck RS, Satava RM, Fried G, et al. Establishing a simulation center for surgical skills: what to do and how to do it. Surg Endosc. 2007;21:1223–32.

Securing Funding for Simulation Centers and Research

47

Kanav Kahol

Introduction

While the benefits of simulation in medical education, establishment of best practices, and reduction of medical errors are undoubtedly being recognized, researchers and educators still struggle with establishing a viable business model for simulation centers (see Chaps. 45 and 46) and more importantly for innovations in simulation through research. Simulation centers primarily cater to residents and trainees and hence are part of the medical education division in most healthcare institutions. The misperception that a simulation center must focus only on training could preclude the significant impact simulation can have on patient safety and patient satisfaction.

While researchers have attempted to show the association between simulation-based training and increased patient satisfaction and patient safety, these studies have often lacked the scientific rigor to prove the obvious link [1–9]. This limits the advocacy and funding around the value of simulation in improving patient experience and safety. Within medical education too, simulation is seen as an add-on to traditional training and not as a required component of medical education worth funding. Further, existing centers are seen as a sink for hospital investment given the often sporadic and not fully translational nature of simulation-based education. Another factor that negatively impacts investment in simulation is the lack of affordable simulators. Simulation centers require significant investments in expensive virtual reality simulators as well as mannequins. Even in affluent nations and communities, the cost of simulation is often seen to far exceed the benefits.

This trifecta of (1) a lack of obvious link to patient safety and satisfaction, (2) a lack of complete integration of simulation into medical curricula, and (3) the high costs of simulation-based training together act as a major impediment to use, propagation, and funding of simulation. Given these obstacles, simulation programs struggle to develop sustainable revenue streams, particularly from entities outside their own institutions.

Since most simulation centers cater to their organization's internal educational and training needs, their funding generally comes from providing educational activities for the organization. While a revenue model of this nature is possibly sustainable, it limits the adoption of simulation for the purposes of research and technology development. Hence, there is a need to acquire external funding geared towards simulation research and simulator development. This external funding affords the opportunity to treat simulation as a true scientific enterprise worthy of research and development dollars; this is much needed considering the paucity of well-done scientific studies using simulation. In this chapter we will first outline methods by which a center can overcome the barriers identified and develop a multidimensional program that can seek funding from a variety of sources. We will also explore plausible and sustainable revenue streams for simulation programs with an emphasis on grant acquisition from the private and the public sectors.

Positioning a Center to Secure Funding

Seeking grant monies requires simulation programs to possess or develop certain elements. While the barriers presented above negatively impact fund generation for simulation centers, there are several possible strategies that can provide a systematic method to create a sustainable business model while supporting both research and education. Our simulation program has developed a successful multidimensional strategy towards financial sustainability: (1) integration of required simulation-based training and research into the curricula, (2) the use of simulation for "BEST PRACTICE" identification and training, (3) the use of simulation for

K. Kahol, PhD
Affordable Health Technologies, Public Health Foundation of India, ISID Campus, 4 Institutional Area, Vasant Kunj, New Delhi 110070, India
e-mail: kanav.kahol@phfi.org

A.I. Levine et al. (eds.), *The Comprehensive Textbook of Healthcare Simulation*,
DOI 10.1007/978-1-4614-5993-4_47, © Springer Science+Business Media New York 2013

national and international concerns, (4) the development of simulation-based research, and (5) the development of affordable simulator technologies. It should be apparent that these dimensions are not mutually exclusive and several can be accomplished using the same methodologies.

Integration of Simulation into Curricula

The first element of financial sustainability involves actively including simulation in required healthcare curricula. This not only maximizes the benefits for students, it also allows for successful demonstration of positive impact and may be responsible for improved resident recruitment [10]. In our institution the surgical curriculum was designed to focus on systems-based practice, a core competency identified by the Accreditation Council for Graduate Medical Education (ACGME) and adopted by the American College of Surgeons (ACS) [11]. The curriculum incorporated three types of mandatory, nonclinical educational activities, including simulation-based training, learning modules that focused on fiscal and operational training, and a research module. The key element in this rotation was to combine a research project with the simulation-based training. This required housestaff to engage in scientific study design, a literature review, and manuscript preparation. This arrangement not only allowed us to teach residents but also allowed us to mentor the residents while exponentially increasing the program's ability to generate research and publications. This strategy is one example of how simulation can be effectively integrated into the curriculum while fostering an environment that generates researchers and simulation-based research. This served to enrich our center's academic productivity and viability, making it a better candidate for funding.

Simulation and Best Practice

The second dimension of addressing the barriers to simulation buy-in focuses on best practices for hospitals. Simulation can prove to be a highly effective aid in experimenting with and deploying best practices. The advantage of focusing on best practices lies in their immediate impact on patient safety and satisfaction. This direct link between quality measures and the training imparted in simulation allows centers to address simulation distrust effectively. Several researchers have alluded to the impact simulation can have on best practices adoption and sustenance. By actively focusing simulation training on best practices, simulation centers can greatly increase the perceivable impact on quality measures. Again, this makes a center more likely to be funded given a track record of successful translation of simulation-based education to better patient outcomes. A key example of best practice was in central venous catheter placement. CVC insertion is a skill wherein simulation has been shown to have a positive impact [12]. CVC insertion skills translate into a measurable impact by hospitals in reduced infection rates and litigations. By direct measurement of the impact of simulation in improving skills, simulation centers can prove their contribution through the CVC best practice training.

Simulation for National and International Concerns

This third element is novel and lies around developing courses that address issues of national and international concern. Such programs may afford center opportunities for funding that were not likely considered during the center's inception. Often, simulation-based training is seen through the pigeonhole of skills training. However, simulation can be effective in large-scale team training and efforts such as disaster management. In the world health arena, simulation can be an effective aid in training healthcare workers. For example, a course that focuses on maternal and child health for healthcare workers would be extremely useful in attracting funding from the World Health Organization, United Nations, and several foundations. Once again, piecemeal work done in this direction has shown how simulation can revolutionize such type of efforts and also establish a revenue stream for simulation centers [13, 14].

Simulation Research

The fourth element towards generating a sustainable revenue stream for simulation programs is more traditional and lies in actively allocating funds for simulation-based research. Research and development should lie at the core of any simulation center's activities. There is no alternative to providing data on the applicability of simulation to improving skills and improving patient safety. In order for simulation as a discipline to stay relevant, research of this sort is necessary. Creating a solid program of research that produces publications is also a must to sustain interest and funding from the parent organization or funding agency. In terms of research, a few things must be emphasized. First, simulation centers should aim to produce multicenter research studies. Multicenter research studies whilst being rare in simulation are indeed very effective in gathering the required number of participants for publication in respected journals. They also lead to formation of consortia which are necessary to secure large-scale grant funding. Secondly, research should include multidisciplinary aspects. Often research in simulation is targeted towards a single specialty. While the benefits of such studies should not be underestimated, there is also major benefit in bringing together multiple disciplines and creating research programs that study teams. This is an effective way of implementing best practices and also maximizing the perceivable impact of simulation.

Simulator Technology Development

The final element in the strategy to address the barriers to simulation funding lies in developing novel and affordable simulation technology. Affordable customized solutions for simulation are necessary to reduce cost and increase applicability of simulation to a larger population. Creating affordable solutions requires interface with engineers and content experts such as nurses and physicians. Unfortunately, there is a built-in disconnect since the engineers are rarely medical experts and vice versa.

In a recently concluded event funded by the National Science Foundation, our group developed a doctoral consortium that brought together engineering students and clinical researchers participating in projects in medical simulation (http://www.nsf.gov/awardsearch/showAward.do?AwardNumber=0946781). We compared the publications of engineers pertaining to clinical simulations and the publications of clinicians pertaining to the same topics. We developed word clouds for aggregates of these publications wherein words that are repeated are rendered larger than the words that are less prominent. The word clouds in essence are a representation of concepts associated with clinical simulation, and one can compare the concepts covered by engineers and clinicians. Figures 47.1 and 47.2 show the word charts for clinicians and engineers, respectively.

The word clouds reveal a limited overlap between the concepts important to engineers and clinicians. This lack of common focus and vocabulary translates into limited interaction between the two communities even though a sustained exchange of ideas is necessary for development of effective, affordable solutions. A conclusion of the doctoral consortium was to encourage simulation centers to hire a part or full-time engineer to develop customized solutions. Such strategies are fundable as they generate true next-generation simulators which are both clinically applicable and affordable.

Using of the shelf Nintendo Wii®, our team of engineers and clinicians have developed several different simulators [15, 16]. These have been developed by a team of engineers working closely with clinicians and identifying needs of clinicians and finding technical affordable solutions. These were in some cases funded by grants through National Science Foundation and/or have been licensed for mass consumption by Simulab Corporation.

In conclusion, implementing these five strategies can greatly increase the chances of securing funding and

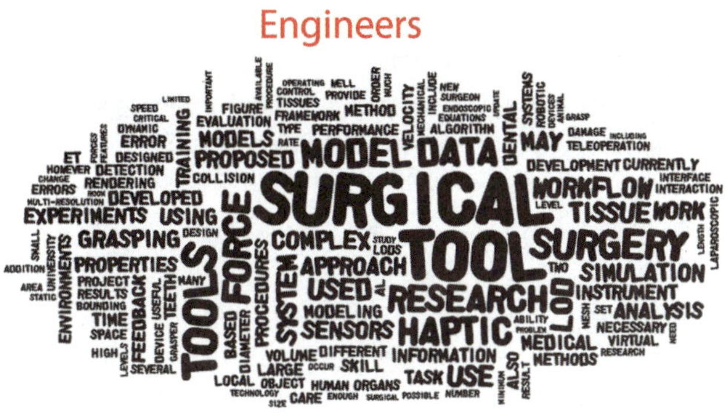

Fig. 47.1 Word cloud from publications on clinical simulations by engineer

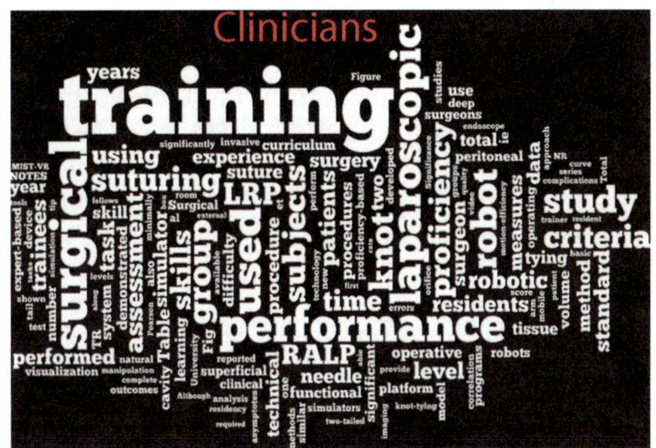

Fig. 47.2 Word cloud from publications by clinicians on clinical simulation

improving current funding situations for existing centers. It leads to an accountable organization in terms of a measurable impact and leads to an organization that commits to a culture of innovation, which is central to the concept of simulation and its uses in the healthcare community.

Innovation Plan for Simulation Centers

To address the needs of a simulation center, it is strongly recommended that simulation programs develop an innovation plan. Innovation plans are based on the five dimensions that address the simulation barriers above. In a simulation center being developed in India, an innovation plan outlined four areas of focus. These four areas were identified by documenting needs of the organization and established multidisciplinary collaborations in that area. We present excerpts from the innovation plan below as an example of how to create such a plan. This innovation plan outlines the overall strategy for one simulation center. It is presented to be used as a template for organizations to plan their innovation strategy towards higher funding levels.

Sample Innovation Plan

There are four focus areas of advanced medical education and learning where technology can play an important role and address gaps in our training capacity.

The *first focus area* lies in delivering *practical training and skills assessment* to the healthcare workforce. Skills such as IV insertion, suturing wounds, central venous catheter placement, cardiac stent placement, endoscopy, advanced cardiac life support, basic life support, blood pressure taking, and ECG monitoring, to name a few, are the basis of modern-day medical practice. Practicing these skills requires significant amount of time and resources. In addition to these technical skills, many skills are actually nontechnical such as team skills that require a healthcare workforce to function efficiently as a team. Traditionally these skills are practiced on patients, which is an extremely unsafe and inefficient method of acquiring such skills. Fortunately technology has been developed that allows for practicing such skills over and over again in a safe environment. Technology also exists for providing skills training on rare skills and rare treatments that enable the healthcare workforce to be prepared for any eventualities including disaster management. There are also provisions in technology for quantitative evaluation of skills that allows for development of benchmarks of examination and allows for competency-based training. This is critical in ensuring high-quality healthcare to the masses. Such technology centered on the core idea of medical simulation has matured rapidly in the past few decades and has been shown to translate to marked significant improvement in clinical skills and quality of care [1, 3, 9, 17–32]. Medical simulation refers to a suite of technologies available for healthcare professionals to practice skills in a variety of disciplines both individually and as a team. It is imperative to develop a coordinated approach to including simulation-based training in the medical education and training infrastructure.

Strategy: We will work with clinicians to identify low-hanging fruit in this area. We will also establish links with local and global engineering institutes to help realize the vision. Funds will be allocated for pilot projects in this domain, and the possible funding agencies will include Science Foundation (equivalent to NSF in USA). Clinicians may help point to direct impact on patient safety based on which institutes of Health (equivalent to NIH in USA) can be applied to. We will work with International Foundations by inviting them to visit the center and present to them skills relevant to their portfolio.

The *second focus area* lies in employing technology for *remote education and monitoring*. A key element of training the healthcare workforce is to contextualize the training to the sociotechnical condition of the environment. Traditionally this has been hard as such efforts require establishment of local infrastructure and local support system which is expensive. With the development of the information communication technology backbone, it is now possible to deliver didactic content and didactic training and examination remotely. The National Knowledge Network (http://www.nkn.in/) is an example of such efforts and displays an important example of leveraging ICT for education. In a similar vein we can deliver medical education and training remotely. There are however two additional opportunities that lie in further strengthening the mission of remote education and monitoring. The first lies in developing remote practice environments like the skills training systems described above so practical skills in addition to didactic material can be taught remotely. This is again possible with the technology of motion tracking, motion-based computing, and virtual reality. The second lies in using technology environments to create a personalized training module that is consistent with system practices of a region and its requirement. This can again be done through personalized content delivery and also by employing mobile units that deliver training through mobile systems.

Strategy: We will work with the telemedicine department to integrate our services with them. The content storage facilities of both the centers can be combined to achieve this goal.

The *third focus area* lies in delivering *best practices design, implementation, and training*. Best practices imbibed through guidelines, procedure checklists, and decision-making algorithms have become the corner stone of the quality drive in medical profession [33]. Training for best practices and implementing and designing best practices are however not trivial. Simple didactic training for best practices is not enough, and there is a need for a safe environment to practice implementation of best practices and adapting best practices to a particular sociotechnical system. There is also a need for a safe environment to design best practices. System-wide best practices and procedures can be designed and tested in a simulation environment, and such efforts have been shown to have a highly positive impact in improving clinical practice that is more significant than simply didactic training [34]. This is a golden opportunity for creating a culture of quality and safety in a system-wide sense.

Strategy: This is a high priority item. We will work with the quality department of our organization to identify metrics. Individual departments will be polled for impending rollout of best practices, and we will identify avenues where simulation can play a role. A joint committee would then be established for pursuing some best practice implementation. Funding can be obtained from Agency for Quality Research (equivalent to AHRQ in the USA). Funding for pilot project would be requested to our organization as it is a multidisciplinary effort.

The *fourth focus area* lies in practical training to ensure *optimal use of equipment and resources* for quality healthcare. An important part of training is to train usage of medical equipment, drug administration protocols, and optimal use of existing resources. Traditional training only serves as orientation training but does not allow for advanced usage. There are many features of equipment such as EKG monitors that are not used efficiently due to lack of training. Simulation environments allow interfacing medical simulators with equipment and provide the capability of designing training scenarios where equipment and resource usage can be taught.

Strategy: We will target equipment manufacturers and sales for this venture. Overall the vision would be to test medical devices in the simulation center. We will identify potential partners and work with them to showcase scenarios where the important points of the device are highlighted in practical use. Pilot funding will be obtained by industry collaboration. We will also keep the legal department in the loop for IP issues and transfer.

In order to develop viable solutions for these four focus areas, we need a comprehensive coordinated strategy to deliver skills education remotely and safely, allowing procedure standardization leading to best practices, objective measurement of skills and proficiency, and training for optimum usage of equipment and resources. With the availability of cheap computing infrastructure, readily available bandwidth, and growth of technologies such as medical simulation, virtual reality, movement analysis, computer graphics, persuasive technology, and mobile computing, it is possible to envision the future of advanced medical education that fully leverages the opportunities presented by these tools. There is a need to focus resources and develop these technologies for medical education and training for all levels of the healthcare workforce from senior physicians to paramedics. Such an effort will both lower the healthcare costs by decreasing medical errors and improving efficiency. We will develop a blueprint for 5 years for innovation.

Funding Sources and Strategies

Having discussed the core elements of a center pursuing funding and ways to prepare for this process, we now move onto a discussion of specific organizations funding simulation. Below we present several funding entities at the local, national, and international levels that have allocated resources towards simulation-based endeavors in the past.

Parent Institution

The core five ideas described above are the basis of securing funding from any source, including your parent institution. The success of the BannerHealth Phoenix (BHP) simulation center, one of the largest in the USA, has been due to tremendous support from the parent organization. This support was ultimately a result of a business plan that was in line with the needs of the organization. At BHP, our group developed an innovative educational program focused on the institution's need for a more efficient onboarding process. *Nurse onboarding* is an expensive process of orientation of new nurses to a new hospital. A plan was developed where simulation, not the traditional senior nurse mentorship model, would be used as the main training for new nurses. In the program, the simulation center proposed a reduction of nurse onboarding time from 4 to 3 weeks. This reduction was based on the assumption that the program would help nurses more efficiently achieve technical and nontechnical skills benchmarks using simulation. The budget proposal also included funding to support research that would investigate the use of simulation to reduce onboarding times while promoting patient safety and satisfaction.

The reduction of training time from 4 to 3 weeks not only allowed the hospitals to reduce cost and time of nurse onboarding, but the training provided a solid foundation for new nurses to improve their performance and participate in best practices implementation. This plan was very successful for our group and can serve as a template for other institutions. In this instance, the plan was targeted towards valued needs of the organization. When the organizational leaders perceived a simulation-based program as having value, they were amenable to funding the program. The overall budget for building the simulation center was approximately 12 million dollars and the projected break even was 4 years.

The National Institutes of Health

The National Institutes of Health (NIH) are the foremost research entities in the world that focus on health, with an annual budget approaching 32 billion dollars (www.nih.gov).

Within NIH, there are several institutes that focus on disease and organs like the National Cancer Institute and National Institute of Biomedical Imaging and Bioengineering. Unfortunately, a very small percentage of their funding is currently focused on simulation-driven initiatives. This could be attributed to several factors. A major factor however lies in the barriers presented earlier that prevent a direct link between patient safety and simulation. However, The National Institute of Biomedical Imaging and Bioengineering and the National Institute of General Medical Sciences are two prime organizations that fund simulation centers. Further, simulation centers can also be part of training initiatives and infrastructure projects that the NIH supports. The key again is to prove a measurable impact on patient safety attributable to simulation.

A related institute, the Agency for Healthcare Research and Quality (AHRQ), does have special calls related to simulation (see http://www.ahrq.gov/qual/simulproj11.pdf). Even in these calls, there is a requirement to directly impact and measure patient safety. Hence, the overall scope of any simulation-based research grant proposal should be towards developing protocols that impact patient safety or outcomes in general. The grant should include improvement of safety as a specific aim and highlight processes and methodologies to implement that plan.

The National Science Foundation

The National Science Foundation (NSF) is the premier organization that funds research in basic sciences and computation. Within the NSF, the directorate of Computer and Information Science and Engineering has funded several projects within the realm of medical simulation. Almost all of these projects are multidisciplinary in nature and include engineers and clinicians. A key factor for securing NSF funding lies in making contributions to the science of computation rather than simply creating a working simulator or demonstrating patient-related outcomes. For example, NSF is unlikely to fund a surgical simulator that uses off the shelf algorithms and technologies. On the other hand, NSF is likely to fund a project that involves new technologies and algorithms to make a surgical simulator. In comparison to the NIH, whose main interest lies in improving patient safety, the main interest of NSF lies in improving contributions to science. To seek NSF funding, it is important to work with engineers and develop a common vocabulary. There are several new algorithms being developed in computer science that could be effectively tested in clinical simulation environments. For example the use of Microsoft Kinect's tracking algorithms (www.microsoft.com/xbox) can greatly enhance surgical proficiency detection. Collaborative work with engineers can lead to major funding from NSF, and this is definitely one of the underutilized funding resources for the simulation community.

One area of funding that both NIH and NSF support are the small business grants and technology transfer grants. These grants provide funding that allows small businesses to work with educational and research institutes. These partnerships are very useful for developing novel simulation technologies. These grants in addition to scientific contributions also look at potential commercialization prospects. Successful applications need to demonstrate a clear business plan for simulator development and marketing.

Public Health Departments

Another underutilized stream of funding for simulation centers lies in the public health domain for training and education grants. Public health departments have a variety of training needs which may include disaster management, workshops for public health officials, and law enforcement professional training. Simulation can effectively support these ventures. Thus, it is important for centers interested in funding from these agencies to develop courses around areas of interest for public health officials and reach out to the local departments to understand their needs. Offering courses for emergency medical services (e.g., Advanced Trauma Life Support, Basic Life Support, Advanced Cardiac Life Support, and Pediatric Advanced Life Support) is another excellent and reliable way to generate revenue. The resources needed to conduct these courses are fairly modest, and the ability to conduct them for public health agencies can mean a relatively steady stream of fundable activities.

The Department of Defense

The Department of Defense (DoD) has been a source of major funding for design, development, and evaluation of clinical simulations and simulation technologies. Telemedicine and Advanced Technology Research Center (TATRC) (http://www.tatrc.org/) has been the primary funding body for DoD in clinical simulation. Other bodies include the Office of Naval Research and AirForce Laboratories. TATRC as a funding agency manages earmarked projects for the military in the broad area of telemedicine and simulation and also releases calls for proposals for specific projects of interest to the military. DoD's main aim is to improve healthcare but also to focus on design, development, and evaluation of novel technologies. A key concept in DoD funding lies in Technology Readiness Levels which is a scale to assess the maturity of evolving technologies (i.e., materials, components, devices) prior to incorporating these technologies into a system. It is critical to understand the importance of novel technologies and the applicability of these technologies to the military in order for a successful application for DoD funding.

DoD also releases several calls in which simulations may not have a direct role, but simulation centers can serve as effective testing facilities. For example, the DoD may be interested in experimenting with large datasets for rapid decision making. In these programs, the role of a simulation center as a testing ground can be quite important. Innovative and capable centers can capitalize on the DOD's need for such facilities.

Simulation Companies

Simulation companies often need to collaborate with clinicians in design, development, and evaluation of their products. These could be a suitable revenue source for simulation centers. In addition to product development, several simulation companies offer regular grants for curriculum design and implementation using their products. It is beyond the scope of this chapter to detail each company's program. However, most of these programs are available on company websites.

The key element in establishing a relationship with simulation companies lies in granting them access to clinical and engineering expertise. Clinical and engineering talent can help simulation companies design better products. Supporting this revenue stream naturally requires a base of intellectual property management skills within the simulation center. As simulation centers are designed to be cradles of knowledge generation, it is important for simulation centers to make investments into intellectual property management either as a skill set of directors/manager or as a dedicated human resource for the center.

International Agencies

International foundations like the MacArthur Foundation, Clinton Foundation, Bill and Melinda Gates Foundation, and organizations like United Nations, UNICEF, and The World Health Organization all have major programs that support the use of simulation products and resources. For example, maternal and child health programs supported by the organizations mentioned above are in need of novel technologies and integrated training programs for midwives and other healthcare workers in developing countries. Simulation centers often limit themselves to local contributions, which are important, but should not preclude development of programs that can support international health goals. Developing worldwide partnerships through outreach foundations and organizations is the key to initiating support from these international agencies. International agencies support several nongovernmental organizations which can benefit from courses in skills training (like birthing training, Basic Life Support training). Simulation centers should aggressively pursue these avenues for developing programs that could support patient safety worldwide as a viable and socially worthwhile endeavor.

Conclusions

Funding simulation centers and simulation research requires a dynamic approach that is inherently multidisciplinary in nature. Simulation centers should and must be seen as cradles of innovation. Innovation is necessary in order for centers to develop a sustainable business model. This chapter has provided foundational information on how to structure a simulation center for innovation and funding. While it is up to the reader to develop customized strategies that fulfill his or her center's mission, the elements highlighted in this chapter are universal. No matter what the setting or ultimate goal of the funding may be, cultivating a center's education, research, and development projects will facilitate financial well-being.

References

1. Aggarwal R, Black SA, Hance JR, Darzi A, Cheshire NJW. Virtual reality simulation training can improve inexperienced Surgeons' endovascular skills. Eur J Vasc Endovasc Surg. 2006;31(6):588–93.
2. Aggarwal R, Tully A, Grantcharov T, Larsen CR, Miskry T, Farthing A, et al. Virtual reality simulation training can improve technical skills during laparoscopic salpingectomy for ectopic pregnancy. BJOG. 2006;113(12):1382–7.
3. Anastakis DJ, Regehr G, Reznick RK, Cusimano M, Murnaghan J, Brown M, et al. Assessment of technical skills transfer from the bench training model to the human model. Am J Surg. 1999;177(2):167–70.
4. Andreatta PB, Woodrum DT, Birkmeyer JD, Yellamanchilli RK, Doherty GM, Gauger PG, et al. Laparoscopic skills are improved with LapMentor training: results of a randomized, double-blinded study. Ann Surg. 2006;243(6):854–60.
5. Hunt EA, Shilkofski NA, Stavroudis TA, Nelson KL. Simulation: translation to improved team performance. Anesthesiol Clin. 2007;25(2):301–19.
6. Mathis KL, Wiegmann DA. Construct validation of a laparoscopic surgical simulator. Simul Healthc. 2007;2(3):178–82.
7. Sutherland LM, Middleton PF, Anthony A, Hamdorf J, Cregan P, Scott D, et al. Surgical simulation: a systematic review. Ann Surg. 2006;243(3):291–300.
8. Verdaasdonk E, Dankelman J, Lange J, Stassen L. Transfer validity of laparoscopic knot-tying training on a VR simulator to a realistic environment: a randomized controlled trial. Surg Endosc. 2007;22(7):1636–42.
9. Voelker R. Virtual patients help medical students link basic science with clinical care. JAMA. 2003;290(13):1700–1.
10. Kahol K, Huston C, Hamann J, Ferrara JJ. Initial experiences in embedding core competency education in entry-level surgery

residents through a nonclinical rotation. J Grad Med Educ. 2011; 3(1):95–9.

11. Satava RM, Gallagher AG, Pellegrini CA. Surgical competence and surgical proficiency: definitions, taxonomy, and metrics. J Am Coll Surg. 2003;196(6):933–7.
12. Barsuk JH, McGaghie WC, Cohen ER, O'Leary KJ, Wayne DB. Simulation-based mastery learning reduces complications during central venous catheter insertion in a medical intensive care unit. Crit Care Med. 2009;37(10):2697–701. doi:10.1097/CCM.0b013e3181a57bc1.
13. Cowan ML, Cloutier MG. Medical simulation for disaster casualty management training. J Trauma. 1988;28(1 Suppl):S178–82.
14. Christie PMJ, Levary RR. The use of simulation in planning the transportation of patients to hospitals following a disaster. J Med Syst. 1998;22(5):289–300.
15. Bokhari R, Bollman-McGregor J, Kahol K, Smith M, Feinstein A, Ferrara J. Design, development, and validation of a take-home simulator for fundamental laparoscopic skills: using Nintendo Wii for surgical training. Am Surg. 2010;76(6):583–6.
16. Dommer P, Crismon H, Anand N, Kahol K, Harding S. 125: improving cardiopulmonary resuscitation training with the Nintendo Wii™. Ann Emerg Med. 2010;56(3):S42.
17. Broe D, Ridgway P, Johnson S, Tierney S, Conlon K. Construct validation of a novel hybrid surgical simulator. Surg Endosc. 2006;20(6):900–4.
18. Brydges R, Kurahashi A, Brümmer V, Satterthwaite L, Classen R, Dubrowski A. Developing criteria for proficiency-based training of surgical technical skills using simulation: changes in performances as a function of training year. J Am Coll Surg. 2008;206(2):205–11.
19. Buzink S, Koch A, Heemskerk J, Botden S, Goossens R, de Ridder H, et al. Acquiring basic endoscopy skills by training on the GI Mentor II. Surg Endosc. 2007;21(11):1996–2003.
20. Fernandez R, Parker D, Kalus JS, Miller D, Compton S. Using a human patient simulation mannequin to teach interdisciplinary team skills to pharmacy students. Am J Pharm Educ. 2007;71(3):1–7.
21. Fitch MT. Using high-fidelity emergency simulation with large groups of preclinical medical students in a basic science course. Med Teach. 2007;29(2/3):261–3. http://login.ezproxy1.lib.asu.edu/login?url=http://search.ebscohost.com/login.aspx?direct=true&db=aph&AN=26205736&site=ehost-live.
22. Grantcharov TP, Bardram L, Funch-Jensen P, Rosenberg J. Learning curves and impact of previous operative experience on performance on a virtual reality simulator to test laparoscopic surgical skills. Am J Surg. 2003;185(2):146–9.
23. Griner PF, Danoff D. Sustaining change in medical education. JAMA. 2000;283(18):2429–31.
24. Hravnak M, Beach M, Tuite P. Simulator technology as a tool for education in cardiac care. Cardiovasc Nurs. 2007;22(1):16–24.
25. Hutton IA, Kenealy H, Wong C. Using simulation models to teach junior doctors how to insert chest tubes: a brief and effective teaching module. Intern Med J. 2008;38(12):887–91.
26. Johnson L, Patterson MD. Simulation education in emergency medical services for children. Clin Pediatr Emerg Med. 2006;7(2):121–7.
27. Lathrop A, Winningham B, VandeVusse L. Simulation-based learning for midwives: background and pilot implementation. J Midwifery Womens Health. 2007;52(5):492–8.
28. Pugh CM, Heinrichs WL, Dev P, Srivastava S, Krummel TM. Use of a mechanical simulator to assess pelvic examination skills. JAMA. 2001;286(9):1021–3.
29. Stolz JL, Friedman AK, Arger PH. Breast carcinoma simulation. Mammography in congestive heart failure mimics acute mastitis and advanced carcinoma. JAMA. 1974;229(6):682–3.
30. Wheeler DW, Degnan BA, Murray LJ, Dunling CP, Whittlestone KD, Wood DF, et al. Retention of drug administration skills after intensive teaching. Anaesthesia. 2008;63(4):379–84.
31. Wright S, Lindsell C, Hinckley W, Williams A, Holland C, Lewis C, et al. High fidelity medical simulation in the difficult environment of a helicopter: feasibility, self-efficacy and cost. BMC Med Educ. 2006;6(1):49.
32. Young JS, DuBose JE, Hedrick TL, Conaway MR, Nolley B. The use of "war games" to evaluate performance of students and residents in basic clinical scenarios: a disturbing analysis. J Trauma. 2007;63(3):556–64.
33. Gorter S, Rethans J-J, Scherpbier A, van der Heijde D, Houben H, van der Vleuten C. Developing case-specific checklists for standardized-patient-based assessments in internal medicine: a review of the literature. Acad Med. 2000;75(11):1130–7.
34. Rosen MA, Salas E, Wilson KA, King HB, Salisbury M, Augenstein JS, et al. Measuring team performance in simulation-based training: adopting best practices for healthcare. Simul Healthc. 2008;3(1):33–41. doi:10.1097/SIH.0b013e3181626276.

Program and Center Accreditation

48

Rosemarie Fernandez, Megan Sherman, Christopher Strother, Thomas Benedetti, and Pamela Andreatta

Introduction

The use of simulation in healthcare is not new. Rather, if we are to adopt David Gaba's definition of simulation, that is, "…a technique, not a technology, to…evoke or replicate substantial aspects of the real world," then we must acknowledge that simulation-based training has been a part of healthcare education almost since its inception [1]. Over the past two decades, the use of simulation in healthcare education has increased markedly. This is likely the result of multiple factors, including decreased opportunity for real patient encounters, increased availability and accessibility of simulation-based technology, and an increased focus on patient safety and patient-centered healthcare. What has grown from this mix of demand for education, technological advances, and patient safety interests is a strong desire to understand and apply simulation-based training in a rational, evidence-based approach that matches learner needs with available training technology and delivery systems. In other words, there are likely best-practice approaches to simulation-based training.

Healthcare education organizations have begun to examine and, in some cases, implement accreditation processes as facilitators of growth and excellence in simulation-based education. This assumes that the establishment of an accreditation process will lead to more rigorous implementation of best practices. How (and if) this will occur in simulation is somewhat unclear. Certainly, the simple act of establishing credentialing standards and an accreditation process does not inherently ensure quality. Current accreditation and benchmarking programs are extremely diverse in their content, foci, and overall objectives. Additionally, several programs define standards over large programmatic areas, whereas other accreditation efforts focus on smaller areas of content or education delivery. Thus far, the benefits of an accreditation process in simulation have not been clearly demonstrated but have been postulated to include (1) externally referenced evidence of compliance with commonly accepted standards and best practices, (2) increased self-monitoring within accredited organizations, and (3) increased leveraging power for those seeking increased resources to comply with defined accreditation standards [2–4].

In this chapter, we offer some discussion about the benefits to accreditation processes as well as some of the potential ramifications. We discuss in general terms the differences in format of the four primary accreditation/benchmark efforts currently underway: (1) American College of Surgeons (ACS), (2) American Society of Anesthesiologists (ASA), (3) Society for Simulation in Healthcare (SSH), and (4) American College of Obstetricians and Gynecologists (ACOG). We then discuss in more detail each individual effort, process design, and result of efforts to date. While it is likely that other health professional organizations are also exploring an accreditation process for simulation-based efforts, this chapter focuses on these four, as they are

R. Fernandez, MD (✉)
Division of Emergency Medicine, Department of Medicine, University of Washington School of Medicine, Seattle, WA, USA
e-mail: fernanre@comcast.net

M. Sherman, BA
Department of Surgery, Institute for Simulation and Interprofessional Studies (ISIS), University of Washington, Seattle, WA, USA
e-mail: shermm@uw.edu

C. Strother, MD
Departments of Emergency Medicine and Pediatrics, Mount Sinai Hospital, New York, NY, USA
e-mail: christopher.strother@mountsinai.org

T. Benedetti, MD, MHA
Department of Obstetrics and Gynecology, University of Washington, Seattle, WA, USA
e-mail: benedeti@u.washington.edu

P. Andreatta, PhD
Department of Obstetrics and Gynecology, University of Michigan, 1500 East Medical Center Drive, G1105 Towsley Center, Ann Arbor, MI 48109-5201, USA
e-mail: pandreat@umich.edu

A.I. Levine et al. (eds.), *The Comprehensive Textbook of Healthcare Simulation*,
DOI 10.1007/978-1-4614-5993-4_48, © Springer Science+Business Media New York 2013

established, ongoing efforts at the time of this writing. By describing the underlying framework and processes involved in each program, we hope to give researchers, educators, and policy makers an understanding of the potential ways in which accreditation efforts can be adopted and assessed. We provide one caveat: the commentary here is based on review of current publicly available material and descriptions. The authors have made every attempt to accurately portray the scope and intent of each program; however, individuals interested in the most accurate and up-to-date information should contact individual accreditation organizations themselves.

Why Accreditation?

In the world of healthcare and healthcare education, providers are acutely aware of the impact of accreditation processes on practice. Curricula are rarely designed without an eye toward how they will be viewed by accrediting bodies such as the Accreditation Council for Graduate Medical Education or Liaison Committee on Medical Education. Hospital policy changes often center on Joint Commission recommendations. In each case, the presumed benefit is adherence to performance standards and external validation of quality. So, the question remains: Is this the place to take simulation?

First, it is important to define who or what would be the beneficiary of a simulation accreditation process. Both the ACS and the SSH state that advancing patient safety is a core objective driving their accreditation process [2, 5]. While this is a noble and important goal of any process, it is likely not the most immediate outcome. The immediate, direct beneficiaries of well-developed accreditation standards—adherence to best practices, adoption of evidence-based approaches, and implementation of solid organizational processes—are most likely the learners.

Beyond this direct effect, simulation program accreditation can positively impact the simulation program itself. Most accreditation processes are not trivial. Obtaining accreditation often requires the commitment of resources from the larger organization (e.g., medical school, hospital) to ensure that the simulation program meets the requirements of the accreditation process. As such, the accreditation process can be used by a simulation program to validate requests for resources such as capital and personnel to support ongoing programming and infrastructure. Simulation programs can also benefit by using accreditation as an external validation of quality. This could potentially translate into an increased client base, improved opportunity for funding, and ability to attract potential collaborators.

With such potential benefits, why not adopt accreditation processes? Well, there are several limitations and assumptions made in the above section. First, we are assuming that without an accreditation process to delineate and reward best practices, such excellence would not be achieved. While this may be true, it is equally possible that an organization would choose to place its energy and resources toward the pursuit of quality programming rather than toward the accreditation application process. Second, the ability of an accreditation process to "validate" quality depends greatly on stakeholder/consumer buy-in. Does the public recognize the need and value in simulation center accreditation? Are there significant numbers of high-quality simulation programs practicing without accreditation? Do funding agencies recognize accreditation as a measure of quality or simply as the ability to pay a fee? These questions illustrate that there is a perceived value metric that is difficult to assess yet directly impacts the level of benefit garnered from accreditation.

We again pose the question "Is accreditation the right thing for simulation-based training in healthcare?" Well, in many ways, this decision has already been made. Two groups (ACS and SSH) offer simulation accreditation programs with a broad institutional focus that encompass all forms of simulation [5–7]. At the time of the writing of this chapter the ACS lists 76 accredited centers, while SSH lists 27 accredited centers. The development and use of metrics to assess benefits to simulation programs, their learners, and, ultimately, patients will be helpful when determining the necessity of accreditation processes.

Overview of Accreditation Program Content and Design

Scope

The scope and breadth of criteria used in determining accreditation varies considerably among accreditation programs. Some (ASA, ACOG) take a specialty-based focus, with concentration on resources and programming dedicated to education in that specialty. Others (ACS, SSH) are broader in scope. Accreditation program scope can have a strong impact on educational institutions in terms of resource allocation, determination of stakeholders, and, potentially, learner access. The scope of an accreditation program is a clear reflection of the program's goals. In the following sections, each accreditation program's scope and overall objectives are reviewed.

Format

As with scope, the format of each accreditation program varies considerably. Currently there are three general approaches to accreditation criteria: (1) a single criteria-based system in which there is one set of criteria for standard accreditation met by all accredited programs [ACOG, ASA], (2) a multi-level system in which accreditation standards are defined at

Table 48.1 Society for Simulation in Healthcare Accreditation Core Standards and Criteria [5]

Standard	Criteria
Mission and governance	1. There exists a clear and publicly stated mission that specifically addresses the intent and functions of the simulation program
Organization and management	1. There is an organizing framework that provides adequate resources to support the mission of the program 2. There is a strategic plan designed to accomplish the mission of the program 3. There are written policies and procedures to assure the program provides high-quality services and meets its obligations and commitments
Facilities, application, and technology	1. There is an appropriate variety and level of technology and applications to support/achieve the activities of the program 2. The environment is conducive to accomplish its mission and activities
Evaluation and improvement	1. The program has a method to evaluate its overall program and services areas, as well as the individual educational, assessment, and/or research activities in a manner that provides feedback for continued improvement
Integrity	1. All activities, communications, and relationships demonstrate a commitment to the highest ethical standards
Expanding the field	1. The program demonstrates commitment to advocate for patients, simulation education, and contributes to the field of simulation.

Used with permission

two different levels across all content areas [ACS], and (3) a modular system [SSH] in which programs meet a core set of standards then chooses to seek accreditation in one or more content areas, such as assessment, education, and research. Each program's format and criteria (below) are discussed in the following sections.

Criteria and Standards

The four accreditation programs discussed here all have clearly defined benchmarks in four main areas: (1) curriculum, (2) instructor/personnel qualifications, (3) equipment and technology, and (4) organization and supporting infrastructure [8]. However, the level of emphasis given to each area varies by program. This is to be expected, considering widely variable programmatic goals and objectives. The criteria used to evaluate simulation programs and the standards required for attainment of accreditation will likely impact resource allocation more than any other factor of the accreditation process. In Tables 48.1, 48.2, and 48.3, we outline these criteria and discuss them in detail in the sections below.

Simulation Accreditation Programs by Organization

American College of Surgeons

Overview

In 2003, the American College of Surgeons Division of Education first proposed the idea of creating certification standards that were evidence based and focused on active learning techniques. The goal of such an accreditation program was to ensure consistency and rigorous application of education theory and operation to surgical educational programming. The result of these initial efforts has been the creation of a multilevel, comprehensive accreditation process that considers training of multiple types of healthcare learners in multiple types of institutions. This development process is described in the literature and remains a focus of the ACS Division of Education [2, 10]. The ACS Education Institutes' accreditation process was the first and, at the time of this writing, remains the largest effort focused on certifying simulation-based learning centers.

The application process for ACS accreditation requires a written application that is reviewed and, if appropriate, a site visit is conducted. Application costs total $5,250 for Level I ($2,850 for Level II) accreditation plus on-site surveyor costs. Applications are reviewed semiannually. Successful applicants receive accreditation for three years, contingent upon the completion of annual reports. Renewal at the end of three years requires a single surveyor on-site visit and renewal application. As of May 2013, there are 76 ACS Accredited Education Institutes [6].

Scope

The ACS Program for Accreditation of Education Institutes had several goals that helped define the scope and format of the program [7]. First, an accreditation program would help define a network of simulation centers that would support continuing professional education and resident training, thus promoting patient safety within surgical fields of practice. Second, the accredited centers would support training of medical students, nurses, and other health professionals with the goal of enhancing patient safety through interdisciplinary

Table 48.2 Brief summary of SSH simulation accreditation program characteristics [5]

Simulation areas	Personnel criteria	Curricular requirements	Hardware/infrastructure
Assessment	Instructors and staff are qualified by virtue of education and experience Instructors and staff are routinely evaluated to ensure competence Adequate technical support for data analysis is present Human factors, psychometric, and statistical support available when indicated	Processes are in place to assure that assessment methods and tools are appropriate, reliable, and valid	Facilities and technologies are appropriate for the individuals being assessed and the level of assessment IRB and data security needs are met and documented
Research	Instructors demonstrate a capability to perform research There is a designated director of research with roles delineated in the organizational structure and adequate support time There are instructors with specific research training and internal/external documentation of collaboration	There is evidence of publication and/or presentation of research findings in peer-reviewed forums There is documentation of mentoring simulation researchers	Program has an established record of research The mission statement includes a specific commitment to research Evidence of successful efforts to obtain research support exists Program uses a scholarly approach to training assessment Documentation of IRB adherence and data security protocol
Education	Program oversight is by an expert in simulation education Program facilitates professional development for instructors Instructors engage in certified ongoing training to improve skills Instructors are familiar with capabilities and limitations of simulation modalities	Offers comprehensive simulation-based learning Educational materials are evidence based, reliable, and valid Simulation modalities are appropriate for learning objectives Curriculum design process involves currently understood simulation education theory Program has the ability to offer CME	Educational activities are linked to the strategic plan Records are kept on all instructors and instructor's professional development Feedback incorporated into programming Program continually updates and improves its courses Record keeping supports evaluation, validation, and research of curriculum Records of learner, instructor, and coordinator activities are maintained
Systems integration and patient safety[a]	Simulation personnel are actively involved in performance improvement committees and activities	Process exists to identify and address opportunities for improvement within the organization that utilize principles of process engineering Program activities are influenced by risk management activities of the organization	Systems integration and patient safety activities are linked to the strategic plan Mission statement includes the desire to enhance individual, team, and organizational performance for improved patient outcomes

Used with permission

[a]Accreditation in systems integration and patient safety requires concomitant accreditation in one or more other areas

Table 48.3 Specialty-sponsored simulation program: a summary of characteristics

Sponsoring organization	Scope and model	Personnel criteria	Learner criteria	Curricular requirements	Hardware/infrastructure
ACS education institutes[a] [6]	Broad[b] Multilevel Level 1[a] Comprehensive Level 2 Basic	Institute director appointed for 3 years at 25% time protected Surgical director is FACS and has 10% time protected Administrator with 50% time for center Coordinator with 50% time	Must include surgeons plus 3 specialties/learner groups, for example: CME GME UME Allied health Nursing Other Must demonstrate the effectiveness of curriculum Must provide evidence of: Long-term follow-up of learners Maintenance of skills Research Interdisciplinary training Curriculum validation	Incorporates procedural and cognitive skills Curriculum development involves: Needs assessment Development of objectives Selection of instructional methods Creation of instructional materials Effective delivery Learner assessment Program assessment Assessment of effectiveness Educational programs are accredited by the LCME, ACGME, ACCME, or equivalent Faculty are appropriately trained	1,200 sq. ft contiguous with face to the public No less than 4,000 sq. ft. additional space for storage, lounge, etc. Can accommodate a minimum of 20 trainees at a time Has teleconferencing available Internet capable Has adequate space for administration Has adequate space for skills trainers Annual budget can support the activities of the institute Provides a mission statement Provides an organizational chart Establishes a steering committee or advisory board
ASA simulation endorsement [9]	Specialty-specific Single level	Must have an established mechanism for instructor training, evaluation, credentialing Program director should hold a doctoral degree and academic appointment at an accredited institution Course director should: Be credentialed as an instructor ASA member Hold appointment in the Department of Anesthesiology	UME, GME (optional)	Quality assurance program must be in place Methodologically sound program for curriculum development and assessment must be evident Sample curriculum and scenario required	Provides a mission statement Organization should maximize the likelihood that course quality will be maintained Document governance and financial model Program leadership and financial stability required Facilities should be sufficient for the coursework offered, including parking, and meals Written policies and procedures should exist Demonstrate necessary educational technology to conduct courses
ACOG simulation consortium	Specialty-specific	Not currently defined	GME Residents in approved OB/GYN programs All residencies can request access to consortium institutes for training of their residents	Simulation-based surgical skills education with patient safety focus Goal of developing a common curricula that can be taught by all Consortium institutions Goal of providing validated simulation-based education	Consortium institutions are defined as state-of-the-art surgical simulation centers States goal of developing standardized teaching methods that can be utilized by all consortium institutions

[a]Criteria listed reflect requirements for obtaining Level 1 (comprehensive) accreditation

[b]Programs with "broad" scopes are defined as those that seek to accredit programs with missions outside of a specific specialty. Those with "specialty-specific" focus are based entirely on performance and resources dedicated to training in one specialty or subspecialty

training. Third, learner assessment would help inform transfer of knowledge and assist with institutional credentialing processes. Finally, such a network of centers could support education-based research and evidence-based curriculum development via collaboration on multicenter studies.

With these goals in mind, the ACS approached its accreditation process with a relatively broad view of simulation training that includes additional guidance on programmatic components specific to surgical training. To ensure a focus on surgical training and expertise, the highest level of ACS accreditation requires that a simulation center appoint a director of surgical simulation at 10% protected time for educational and administrative responsibilities. Additionally, specific requirements for space and administrative staffing are clearly specified (Table 48.3). In setting such standards, the ACS has made an important comment on the need for faculty and resources necessary to build and sustain a successful simulation program. Such requirements have the potential to impact faculty recruitment and simulation center leadership decisions, academic promotions, and overall simulation strategies at institutions seeking accreditation [8].

Format and Criteria

The ACS format defines accreditation requirements at two different levels (Level I and Level II) across all content areas: (1) curricula and learners, (2) instructor/personnel requirements, (3) equipment and technology, and (4) organization and supporting infrastructure [6]. Table 48.3 outlines the criteria for Level 1 accreditation. While the majority of centers seeking accreditation apply for Level 1 accreditation, the presence of multiple levels of standards allows for the recognition of excellence within smaller, more narrowly focused simulation centers.

As stated above, the ACS accreditation program defines standards in four areas similar to criteria used by SSH and ASA. The ACS, more than any other program, specifies infrastructure and equipment requirements including minimum dedicated simulation and office space, teleconferencing capabilities, and availability of support facilities (locker rooms) to enable hands-on training for a minimum of 20 learners. The requirements for curriculum development and assessment are more loosely defined; however, the on-site visit allows surveyors to assess the presence of faculty and programmatic expertise necessary to support the mission of the ACS accreditation process [8].

Society for Simulation in Healthcare

Overview

The Society for Simulation in Healthcare (SSH) is a cross-disciplinary, cross-specialty international organization. As such, SSH currently holds a broad view of simulation and experiential learning utilizing multimodal simulation methodologies for education, assessment, and research. The organization's mission, "to lead in facilitating excellence in interprofessional healthcare education, practice, advocacy, and research through simulation modalities," is one of the primary driving forces behind the creation of the SSH's Council for Accreditation of Healthcare Simulation Programs (herein referred to as the Accreditation Council.) SSH defines a simulation program as one whose mission "is specifically targeted toward improving patient safety and outcomes through assessment, research, advocacy, and education using simulation technologies and methodologies." The goal of the accreditation process is to identify simulation programs that share such a mission as demonstrated through efforts in research, assessment, teaching, and healthcare systems integration.

SSH began its accreditation efforts by first defining standards and criteria for excellence in simulation. This was an iterative process with multiple reviews by appointed committee members as well as the membership at large. Applicants for accreditation submit a written application that is reviewed and followed by a 1-day on-site visit by an accreditation review team. Cost for the application process is $5,780. Successful applicants are granted accreditation for a 5-year period (originally it was for a 3-year period) conditional on the completion of yearly reports. Each yearly report review costs $250. In the first year (2010), seven programs received accreditation in one or more areas. At the time of this writing, there are 27 simulation programs that have been awarded SSH accreditation.

Scope

As a cross-disciplinary organization, SSH has proposed the broadest view of simulation and simulation-based education. Listed requirements for instructors, equipment, and processes are flexibly defined to include the wide variability in simulation programs and centers worldwide. Accreditation is not linked to performance in any one specialty or modality, and involvement of multiple types of learners from different specialties and disciplines is seen as a positive attribute. Standards and formatting (described below) reflect this broad approach and recognize that a "one size fits all" approach to simulation-based education is neither realistic nor optimal. Such a scope is aligned with SSH's objective of facilitating excellence in healthcare simulation across specialties and disciplines, both clinical and nonclinical.

Format

SSH utilizes a modular format within its accreditation process, separating assessment, teaching and education, research, and systems integration and patient safety into separate domains with individual requirements for accreditation. An applicant program must meet requirements for "Core Standards," then may select to apply for accreditation in one or more domain. Only the category of systems integration and patient safety requires concomitant accreditation in another domain (e.g., research).

Criteria

Accreditation criteria are somewhat complex and vary for each program depending upon the accreditation domains sought. All programs must meet a core set of standards regardless of the specific area in which they are applying for accreditation. Described in Table 48.1, these Core Standards are felt to be fundamental operational standards required for a successful program. Infrastructure and operational requirements exist for other accreditation processes. Unlike the explicit requirements in ACS accreditation process, SSH requires accreditation applicants to demonstrate resources, hardware, and infrastructure adequate for their simulation programming. This makes the process somewhat more flexible. However, less explicit requirements can also soften the external mandate for capital items, thus decreasing the leveraging power potentially associated with accreditation standards.

Beyond core requirements, SSH defines standards in four separate domains: (1) assessment, (2) teaching and education, (3) research, and (4) systems integration and patient safety. A program must achieve accreditation in one of the first three areas in order to also be considered for accreditation in the area of systems integration and patient safety. The standards for each domain are listed in Table 48.2. This domain-specific accreditation process is unique to SSH, especially those areas focused on research and system integration. The potential advantage of offering accreditation in specific domains is that smaller, more focused programs can still be recognized for excellent work. It is unclear how such standards and recognition will be adopted and integrated into the simulation culture and, if adopted, how they will influence the field of healthcare simulation.

American Society of Anesthesiologists

Overview

The American Society of Anesthesiologists (ASA) convened the Workgroup on Simulation Education in 2004 with the goal of defining the components of a simulation center essential to supporting high-quality, experiential continuing medical education (CME) [11]. This workgroup transitioned to become the ASA Committee on Simulation Education, which focused on the evaluation and endorsement of simulation programs capable of providing high-quality simulation-based CME programming. In an attempt to maintain a consistent membership over time. The committee transitioned to an editorial board in 2013. By design, such accredited simulation programs would form the ASA Simulation Network whose members would be certified to provide training for the completion of one of the American Board of Anesthesiology's (ABA) Maintenance of Certification in Anesthesiology (MOCA®) Part IV requirements.

The ASA had clear support of the American Board of Anesthesiology prior to establishing the role and scope of accreditation it would offer. This support is critical and has allowed the ASA's accreditation process to clearly highlight an advantage beyond those suggested by other accrediting groups, namely, the ability to provide courses that meets the requirements for MOCA®. Additionally, the ABA helped to defray costs for early accreditation applicants as a way to encourage applications [11]. Applicants must submit a written application along with a simulation-based scenario that would become part of the network's simulation bank if accreditation is awarded [9]. All accredited programs have access to this simulation bank. Application costs are $2,500 with a 3-year reaccreditation cycle and no on-site visit required. ASA requires all applications to be submitted via its online portal (https://simapps.asahq.org/). Currently there are 32 accredited programs nationwide.

Scope and Format

The scope of the ASA accreditation/endorsement program focuses on institutions providing anesthesia-based training and highlights offerings targeting licensed, practicing physicians. In line with its mission, the ASA Simulation Education Network accreditation application focuses heavily on current operations of the simulation program and the ability to facilitate evidence-based ABA MOCA® courses. ASA employs a single criterion accreditation design, with one set of standards defined for core accreditation [9]. Currently there are 2 additional endorsements for MOCA® specialties in pain management and critical care (MOCA® subs).

Criteria

Applicant centers for the ASA Simulation Education Network are required to demonstrate (1) ASA member value; (2) policies and procedures commensurate with high-quality educational offerings; (3) infrastructure that is consistent with the proposed/described services; (4) equipment and space that supports the educational objectives; (5) an evaluation process for the course, the instructors, and the program; (6) policies and procedures to provide ASA members with a confidential and secure environment; and (7) sound education process for course development and education. As suggested above, the requirements in each area are focused directly on what is necessary to support simulation-based MOCA® training courses. Applicants must also submit a detailed simulation-based scenario suitable for an anesthesiology CME course that would become part of a larger simulation case bank. Specific application components are briefly described in Table 48.3.

American Congress of Obstetricians and Gynecologists

Overview and Focus

The ACOG Simulation Consortium holds as its primary mission the development of consistent and substantive simulation-based curricula for graduate medical education and continuing medical education in obstetrics and gynecology. As a specialty-focused body, it shares similarities with the goals and objectives of the ASA Simulation Committee; however, its initial efforts have been targeted toward resident education rather than continuing medical education (ABA).

The consortium first convened in 2009 and consisted of 9 member institutions that were invited to participate by the Vice President of Education for the American College of Obstetricians and Gynecologists, Sterling Williams, MD, MS [12]. These institutions were selected after an in-depth screening process conducted by ACOG to include members who had established educationally sound simulation-based programs and that possessed expertise in using simulation for clinical training, assessment, and educational research. The number of participating institutions increased to 16 in 2010 and to 18 in early 2011, with a minimum of 24 total members planned [13]. Institutions who wish to join the consortium may contact Dr. Williams, who determines the basic qualifications and presents his recommendations to the consortium for approval. Applicants then complete a written application and host an on-site visit by a member of the consortium.

Consortium membership requires two representative delegates from each member institution. A consortium chair and cochair are selected from the representatives and serve a 2-year period. The consortium chair and cochair work in partnership with the ACOG staff and Dr. Williams to organize and lead quarterly meetings for the entire consortium. These meetings include two teleconferences and two in-person meetings at ACOG headquarters. There are currently five primary working committees, each of which is chaired by one or two delegates: obstetrics program, gynecology program, assessment, research, and models/simulators. Subcommittees work on specific needs, such as presenting our work at conferences, meetings, and ACOG publications. Committees and subcommittees work through e-mail and meet through teleconference as needed.

Future Directions

As the consortium has evolved, it became increasingly aware of the need and demand for high-quality and valid simulations for maintenance of certification, licensing and relicensing, and credentialing and re-credentialing of practicing physicians [12]. Active research efforts and simulation validation studies will support more robust simulation-based assessments in the future. However, as with most disciplines, the current data available on obstetric and gynecologic simulation does not satisfy requirements for high-stakes simulation.

Conclusion

The sections above provide a brief overview of current known efforts to further healthcare simulation via accreditation or endorsement programs. Each program is unique and closely linked to the goals and objectives of the parent organization. Clearly, the hope is to advance the science of simulation, whether specialty-specific or as it is broadly applied within healthcare. Development and implementation of measures will be important to study how such accreditation efforts impact simulation centers, healthcare/educational institutions, and the specialty of simulation.

References

1. Gaba DM. The future vision of simulation in health care. Qual Saf Health Care. 2004;13(1):i2–10.
2. Johnson KA, Sachdeva AK, Pellegrini CA. The critical role of accreditation in establishing the ACS education institutes to advance patient safety through simulation. J Gastrointest Surg. 2008;12(2):207–9.
3. D'Andrea G. Analyzing the value of accreditation: application of computer decision tools to a complex decision. Lippincotts Case Manag. 2006;11(5):249–52.
4. Gates S. Aligning strategic performance measures and results. The Conference Board, New York, 1999.
5. Society for Simulation in Healthcare Accreditation Committee. SSH Accreditation Process: A Pilot Study Accreditation Standards and Processes 2011. http://ssih.org/uploads/committees/membership%20committee/2011%20SSH%20Accreditation%20Informational%20Guide.pdf. Accessed 7 Nov 2011.
6. American College of Surgeons Division of Education. Accredited Education Institutes. 2008. http://www.facs.org/education/accreditationprogram/index.html. Accessed 7 Nov 2011.
7. Sachdeva AK, Pellegrini CA, Johnson KA. Support for simulation-based surgical education through American College of Surgeons - Accredited education institutes. World J Surg. 2008;32(2):196–207.
8. Fernandez R, Wang E, Vozenilek JA, et al. Simulation center accreditation and programmatic benchmarks: a review for emergency medicine. Acad Emerg Med. 2010;17(10):1093–103.
9. American Society of Anesthesiologists. ASA simulation program endorsement application. https://simapps.asahq.org/. Accessed 5 Dec 2011.
10. Pellegrini C, Sachdeva AK, Johnson KA. Accreditation of education institutes by the American College of Surgeons: a new program following an old tradition. Bull Am Coll Surg. 2006;91(3):8–12.
11. Steadman RH. The American Society of Anesthesiologists' national endorsement program for simulation centers. J Crit Care. 2008;23(2):203–6.
12. ACOG consortium advances: simulation training. ACOG Today. 2010. http://www.acog.org/~/media/ACOG%20Today/acogToday1110.ashx?dmc=1&ts=20111227T1546282381. Accessed 24 Dec 2011.
13. The American College of Obstetricians and Gynecologists 2010–2011 Donor Report. American College of Obstetricians and Gynecologists, Washington, D.C.; 2011.

A Future Vision

49

Adam I. Levine, Samuel DeMaria Jr., Andrew D. Schwartz, and Alan J. Sim

Nearly a decade ago many echoed David Gaba's predictions about the future of healthcare simulation: it would either be embraced, embedded, and extensively applied, or it would fail to meet expectations or improve patient outcomes and fall into obscurity.[1] Today it is clear which path simulation has taken (even this textbook is a testament to that), and we ask now, just how far and how widely healthcare simulation will spread and what its real impact will be. As editors, it has become apparent, having read each chapter in this book, that the application of simulation in the healthcare industry is limitless, and therefore, its impact cannot be overstated. With the assistance of many of the authors of this text, we frame this brief chapter as a future vision of simulation, contemplating the extent to which simulation will grow.

Simulation Saves Healthcare

With the next century comes tremendous change in healthcare education and delivery, and the impact of simulation will be widespread, transformative and will ultimately lead to the perseveration of this threatened industry. For this to occur, however, several phenomena will first take place.

Simulation Becomes Ubiquitous in Healthcare Education

Several confluent events occur during the early part of the twenty-first century that lead to an exponential proliferation of simulation-based education throughout healthcare. It is more widely determined and accepted that medical errors, patient harm, and poor patient outcomes can be traced back to inadequacies in healthcare education. Public outcry and outside political and financial forces demand that healthcare education becomes more accountable (much of this has already occurred). This gives rise to a healthcare educational system that is heavily regulated and where performance measures and outcomes are publically reported. Schools with graduates demonstrating persistently substandard performance become vulnerable to scrutiny and risk their accreditation, funding, and research opportunities. Mandated to stem the tide of error and patient harm, a paradigm shift in healthcare education is sought where fundamentals of teamwork, communication, and crisis resource management are introduced very early in practitioners' education.

> *"Team-based training utilizing simulation scenarios will expand to improve communication and teamwork in hospital settings. Medical students and residents will be expected to train with nursing students, physician assistants, pharmacists, and other health professional students. This training should lead to advances in patient safety and improve error recognition."*
> —Paul E. Ogden, MD, Courtney West, PhD, Lori Graham, PhD, Curtis Mirkes, DO, Colleen Y. Colbert, PhD

> *"There is no question to me that if we expect individual healthcare providers to work together effectively in interprofessional teams, we need to start training them together at all stages of education, from undergraduate training all the way through to continuing professional development. The last 20–30 years have seen us struggle with how to make this type of interprofessional training work...simulation will be the answer!"*
> —Vincent Grant, MD, FRCPC

> *"Simulation will evolve into more centralized centers to co-locate with learners in clinical spaces throughout health centers to allow for more frequent and multi-disciplinary training."*
> —James M. Cooke, MD

At the same time, older healthcare educators retire and are replaced with a new generation of innovative faculty. The longstanding barriers and opposition to the use of simulation for healthcare education dissipate as the "old guard" disappears from the workforce. Young educators, who have

A.I. Levine, MD (✉)
Departments of Anesthesiology, Otolaryngology, and Structural and Chemical Biology, Icahn School of Medicine at Mount Sinai, New York, NY, USA
e-mail: adam.levine@mountsinai.org

S. DeMaria Jr., MD • A.D. Schwartz, MD • A.J. Sim, MD
Department of Anesthesiology, Icahn School of Medicine at Mount Sinai, New York, NY, USA

A.I. Levine et al. (eds.), *The Comprehensive Textbook of Healthcare Simulation*,
DOI 10.1007/978-1-4614-5993-4_49, © Springer Science+Business Media New York 2013

experienced firsthand the virtue of simulation-based education, start to enthusiastically and creatively incorporate simulation throughout healthcare curricula in order to meet head-on the societal call for safer healthcare and a better healthcare workforce.

> *"Simulation will be recognized as a new approach to education, rather than a progression of technology."*
> —Mike Smith, MD, F.A.C.E.P.

Simulation becomes entrenched in the educational spectrum including allied health, nursing, dental, and medical arenas. The use of simulation becomes the standard by which healthcare professionals are educated to become master clinicians throughout their careers. The use of simulation is then recognized as critical for the assurance and development of healthcare providers who possess a superior and consistent body of knowledge and skills.

> *"Simulation will become an educational tool that is so ingrained into education that it is simply another tool that all educators use. The role of the dedicated simulation center and simulation "specialists" will wane as simulation becomes ubiquitous."*
> —Paula Craigo, MD and Laurence Torsher, MD

> *"Simulation techniques will spread further into clinical arenas, to allow for more frequent exposure of each learner with lower cost and thereby impact education and culture more broadly."*
> —Sara Goldhaber-Fiebert, MD

> *"In the future, healthcare simulation will be fully integrated into training, both initial and continuing, for all providers across a continuum."*
> —Marjorie Lee White, MD, MPPM, MEd

> *"Patient-dentist communication will become more critical and the virtual worlds will play an important role in training dental health care providers….emphasis on inter professional education will allow more opportunities for the oral health care provider to utilize the human simulator as part of the health care team."*
> —Riki Gottlieb, DMD, FAGD

> *"More medical schools will use virtual patients to improve clinical correlations in the preclinical years. Each student will be assigned a virtual patient or virtual family and will have assignments for care related to the area of study. For instance, during Anatomy, the student may get cases of trauma during musculoskeletal study, or students may be assigned cases directly related to the organ system they are studying. This would require the student to do a full history and physical, order tests, counsel patients, and do follow-up as part of their basic science studies. The virtual patients can be advanced during the clinical years to bring in ethical dilemmas, and other topics that are difficult for competency determination such as communication and systems issues. Virtual "environments," including medical "gaming" scenarios, will also be increasingly used, as they are in military training."*
> —Paul E. Ogden, MD, Courtney West, PhD, Lori Graham, PhD, Curtis Mirkes, DO, Colleen Y. Colbert, PhD

No longer are education and training time-based, but they are transformed to a competency-based model where students, residents, and even faculty attain and achieve milestones associated with the novice, the senior trainee, and the expert levels. Students and trainees are not expected to be taught for a specific number of years before they can graduate, only that their education will last as long as it takes to achieve competence. Simulation assumes its role as the cornerstone of the process of milestone attainment and achievement.

> *"Simulation will be used by medical schools and residencies as part of a "competency-based" promotion system that values standardized demonstration of skills over simply being present in enough rotations to be promoted."*
> —Christopher Strother, MD

> *"The challenge of time and chance is mitigated and learning curves are shifted in such a way that each practitioner and his/her team receive the best, individualized learning experience."*
> —Marjorie Lee White, MD, MPPM, Med

> *"Simulation will be incorporated more fully in the upcoming ACGME residency milestones for multiple medical and surgical specialties"*
> —James M. Cooke, MD

As simulation assumes a prominent role in milestone attainment, healthcare education becomes increasingly dependent on simulation, and the classic clinical apprenticeship model gives way to a simulation-based apprenticeship. The technology becomes so advanced that students, trainees, and practitioners can and must achieve levels of proficiency and attain competence in the simulated environment before actual patient encounters. As healthcare technology expands, practicing healthcare providers are mandated to first receive simulation-based training and assessment, demonstrating expertise before being allowed to apply new therapies or techniques on actual patients.

> *"There will be requirements, a certain number of simulated procedures must be done before being allowed to perform the procedure on real patients, and perhaps a simulation intern year or intern simulation block will be required for new trainees."*
> —Shekhar Menon, MD

> *"Simulation will be used to show procedural competence for hospital accreditation processes, taking precedence over 'procedure logs' "*
> —Christopher Strother, MD

Simulation Becomes Ubiquitous in Healthcare Assessment

During this rapid expansion and application of simulation for education, the entire healthcare educational system becomes more dependent on simulation, and educators and faculty become facile first with formative assessment and then with summative assessment, using simulation. Although checklists are used initially in this process, simulation-based assessment takes on a critical and high-stakes role in assuring student, resident, and practitioner competence throughout their careers, and global ratings become just as widely used and mastered by skilled educators and faculty.

Preadmission screening and the admission process incorporate simulation to identify and detect the most suitable students for the healthcare profession. While in training, simulation-based assessment is used to verify milestone attainment, and once graduated, simulation is a major component of licensure testing. Assessment is also frequent and regular during clinical training and practice. Once overall competence is achieved and confirmed with simulation, residency training is considered complete regardless of the time taken for completion, with certain restrictions placed on minimum and mandatory training intervals. Throughout the practitioners' careers, repetitive testing is made mandatory for Maintenance of Certification (MOC) processes. This complex and structured simulation-based assessment process proves critical to the wellness of the healthcare industry workforce, assuring true MOC.

> *"Surgical boards will require simulation, initially, as a component of the Maintenance of Certification process much like the new American Society of Anesthesiologists MOCA requirements"*
>
> —James M. Cooke, MD

> *"Board exams and MOC will have increased use of simulation in fields such as emergency medicine and intensive care."*
>
> —Christopher Strother, MD

> *"Simulation will become the norm for training and competency testing across medical specialties."*
>
> —Mike Smith, MD, F.A.C.E.P.

> *"Simulation will increasingly be used for national, standardized exams pertaining to clinical skills."*
>
> —Paul E. Ogden, MD, Courtney West, PhD, Lori Graham, PhD, Curtis Mirkes, DO, Colleen Y. Colbert, PhD

> *"There will be a push for safety and competency based training that will force all specialties to move more towards simulation. In some ways, these efforts will be easy in diagnostic radiology where imaging is digital and the images from real patients can be used to simulate the daily practice of radiologists."*
>
> —Alexander Towbin, MD

Simulation-Based Education and Assessment Improves Patient Care

As the integration of simulation becomes complete at the educational and assessment levels, multicenter studies are conducted that definitively demonstrate simulation-based education and assessment improves individual, team, institutional, and global healthcare industry performance. This takes several decades but provides the long-sought "holy grail" of evidence that simulation improves patient care, reduces injury due to medical error, and saves lives. The 2019 Institute of Medicine (IOM) report makes the claim that during the last 30 years, simulation has been transformative and has led to a reduction in medical errors as predicted. The report goes on to say that 60–90% of preventable deaths from medical errors have been averted through simulation-based programs and that the major risks to patients are now systems-based deficiencies. The IOM calls for greater use of simulation for systems processes given its widespread success at the individual and team levels.

> *"Institutions will progressively utilize simulations as internal organizational quality assessment tools (i.e. as a systems and/or process engineering tool)."*
>
> —William F. Dunn, MD

Simulation Leads to a Dramatic Decline in Healthcare Cost

Billions of dollars are saved due to a reduction in medical errors and healthcare-related deaths. Safer healthcare also saves billions of dollars annually in reduced malpractice rates resulting in a reduction in healthcare inflation. Improved healthcare performance causes patient discharge rates to dramatically improve as rebound admission rates drop. Overall, the cost of healthcare per person declines as life expectancy increases and infant mortality decreases. The savings provide a means to deliver healthcare more widely to the country while expanding healthcare research and technology funding. This affirmation regains the public trust in their healthcare provider and the medical industry.

> *"Residencies and fellowships will progressively require simulation training to performance standards facilitating patient safety."*
>
> —William F. Dunn, MD

Technology

In order for simulation to be widespread while also satisfying the new dependence on high-fidelity simulated environments for training and assessment, technologic advancement takes two paths. One is where simulation and simulators become affordable, portable, internet based, and more simplistic to program and operate, paving the way for mass utilization.

> *"Mobile, easy to use, screen-based technology that allows emotionally-charged practice of dynamic case management for various challenges – 'What If' verbal case scenarios will be greatly enhanced with simulated monitors providing realistic vital signs and pulse ox beeping."*
>
> —Sara Goldhaber-Fiebert, MD

"There will be a movement towards use of mobile devices in simulation. A modern smart phone is about as fast as a 5 year old laptop. Smart phones are adequately powered to run complex simulation scenarios."

—Kenneth Gilpin, MD

"Over the coming decade, diagnostic radiology will move out of the era of analog simulators and into the digital era. This move will accelerated by the move from an oral board exam to a computer-based exam. For years, radiology residents have prepared for the oral board exam by interpreting an unknown case shown to them by their attending in an effort to simulate the board experience. When the board exam moves to the computer, residents will employ new strategies to prepare for the exam. The corporate sector is already preparing for this change by placing content online and creating a mechanism for residents to review cases online."

—Alexander Towbin, MD

"Simulation technology will become simpler. The increased sophistication of simulation equipment over the last few years has brought incremental improvements in educational experience but large increases in unreliability, challenges in programing and cost."

—Paula Craigo, MD and Laurence Torsher, MD

The other path will have simulation moving toward the creation of Super Simulators and Super Simulated Virtual Environments (SSVE) used for the mandatory high-stakes assessments that are now part and parcel of healthcare. These sophisticated environments use physical and virtual technologies including robotics, artificial intelligence, holograms, and haptics to create a truly immersive, interactive, and fully autonomous experience. They are entirely manipulatable and can replicate any patient care environment from a single patient room and care suite to an entire hospital, an urban street corner, or even a battlefield. Individual institutions will be able to reproduce their own facility with exacting detail in the SSVE allowing for customized team training, system analysis, and system integration.

"There will be a trend towards virtualisation in simulation. Virtual solutions to engineering problems are cheaper than mechanical solutions (as they have a lower marginal cost). This movement towards virtual simulation may be driven by economic forces rather than best teaching practice per se."

—Kenneth Gilpin, MD

"Virtual environments will allow for just the right mix of fidelity and realism that translates into all patients receiving safe care."

—Marjorie Lee White, MD, MPPM, MEd

These super simulators are recognized as pivotal and critical for the development of fundamental and expert skills of individuals, teams, and institutions. As the dependence on these technologies for training and assessment becomes critical, SSVEs are identified as medical devices, and a governing body like the FDA oversees their fidelity to ensure public safety.

"There will be a validation of physiological models used in simulation. An international simulation organization will form, with input from medical colleges and resuscitation associations, which will aim to explicitly quantify the limitations in simulation models (both software and hardware) compared to real patients. Simulation companies will be obligated to objectively demonstrate the accuracy of their simulators to these organizations."

—Kenneth Gilpin, MD

The initial high cost of such simulation limits its access to centralized centers of excellence. The demand for SSVE training and assessment escalates, resulting in a dramatic reduction of cost due to mass production, and these environments are developed in every major healthcare facility and city as part of a federal initiative.

"Complacency needs to give way to some blue skies dreaming, since today's Model T (technology) simulation needs to move towards the Startrek Holodeck (Danger Room from X-Men) by 2030. This will take broad commitment from clinicians, computer scientists, human factors psychologists, clinical engineers and funding organizations. Real world anatomical scenarios, physiological processes, tissue deformation, fluid dynamics, instrument-tissue interactions; hey…you mean this isn't all real?"

—Derek Gould, FRCR, FRCP

"There will not be a quantum leap in simulator fidelity in the near future. The current limitations on simulator complexity are due to the economic cost of designing and validating complex simulation models (i.e. R&D), rather than the lack of computing power. The tumbling cost of processing power will not come to the rescue of the difficulties facing simulation."

—Kenneth Gilpin, MD

"Federal funding of simulation labs is found to be cost effective and leads to safer medical practice."

—Shekhar Menon, MD

The SSVE is later recognized as ideal for therapeutic and procedural rehearsal. Individual patient physiology and anatomy will be analyzed and downloaded into the environment where physicians and teams can conduct actual procedural rehearsal. Fine motor maneuvers will also be practiced, idealized, and mastered. The perfected moves will be downloaded and captured by intelligent robots, and it is these robots that will carry out the procedure with microsurgical perfection. Patients will now be able to undergo robotically facilitated, minimally invasive, endovascular and open procedures expertly "taught" by the world's top proceduralist without the need to travel long distances.

Taking the lead from psychiatry, the SSVE is used therapeutically for a variety of medical and psychiatric therapeutic interventions. The SSVE is proven to be a potent environment for the treatments of phobias, separation anxiety, post-traumatic stress syndrome. The military use of SSVE for deconditioning proves invaluable, and psychiatric and suicide rates are dramatically reduced for returning servicemen and women. Pediatricians use the SSVE to immerse patients and families into the clinical environment to prepare them for their planned procedures. The access to the environments becomes widespread and patients can "book" their own virtual tours of healthcare facilities or pre-experience their own proposed intervention.

SSVE proves to be invaluable for research and development. Computer-based simulations make dependence on tissue and animal models for experimentation obsolete and provide researchers a rich and reproducible platform to test new therapies. For example, computer-based simulators are used to test tumor responsiveness to chemotherapy. Individual patients with heart disease are benefited, since their own cardiovascular responsiveness to pharmacologic alterations of inotropy (contractility), chronotropy (heart rate), lusitropy (relaxation), and systemic vascular resistance can be tested using these computer-based simulations prior to therapeutic initiation.

By 2100 simulation proves to be indispensible. Training, assessment, and maintenance of competence are dependent on simulation for the individual, team, institution, and industry. No longer limited to healthcare provider training and assessment, therapeutic interventions take a quantum leap forward as simulation is used for treatment and rehearsal. Because of simulation, new and critical therapies, interventions, and pharmaceuticals will be able to be economically developed, tested, perfected, and introduced at accelerated rates affording more and more patients the benefit from remarkable and innovative technologies.

Finding a digital copy of "The Comprehensive Textbook of Healthcare Simulation," healthcare providers of the time will appreciate just how far they have come and contemplate the next extraordinary advances yet to be accomplished.

"A simulation center at every Starbucks!"
—Christopher Gallagher, MD

Back from the Future

Although we hope you enjoyed our (admittedly hyperbolic) journey to the future of simulation, we hope you appreciate that in the past few years, healthcare simulation has made an exponential transformation from a *best secret* to becoming a bona fide *best practice.* Few involved in its past could have imagined the speed, extent, and creative ways in which simulation has been applied in its present future. It's apparent that our only limitations are our imaginations. The future of healthcare simulation is here, bound in the pages of this text. It is our hope that by assembling this prestigious array of experts from around the world, their words and ideas will inspire others to make their own amazing contributions to healthcare simulation.

"The best way to predict the future is to create it."
—Peter Drucker (1909–2005),
Influential writer, consultant,
and social ecologist

Reference and Note About the Quotes

1. Gaba DM. The future vision of simulation in health care. Qual Saf Health Care. 2004;13:i2–10.

All quotes were provided via email.

Appendices

Appendix A: Simulation Center Sample Floorplans and Facility Pictures

> In this special section, we have included brief descriptions as well as sample floorplans and facilities pictures from several chapter authors' centers. We have specifically selected centers that represent a variety of design options from single discipline, one-room designs to multidisciplinary institutional-based centers. We hope that these virtual tours will provide the readers with ideas for their own center designs and upgrades.
>
> —*The Editors*

Children's Hospital of Philadelphia: Center for Simulation, Advanced Education, and Innovation

CPCE members utilize the resources provided by the Center for Simulation, Advanced Education and Innovation at CHOP, which operates within the division of anesthesiology and critical care medicine. The center facilitates the translation of scientific discoveries into practical implementation for both research and clinical care. The center is directed by Vinay Nadkarni, MD, and Evelyn Lengetti, RN, MSN, and is administered by Stephanie Tuttle, MBA.

The images included represent one component of our program. Known as OR 12, this small "in situ" complex is but one component of our virtual simulation center at CHOP.

Centralized classroom and skills lab training, satellite skills labs, and unit-based "virtual" lab exercises adjacent to patient care settings are routinely conducted.

The center is equipped with more than $500,000 of equipment in the form of:

- Flat-screen simulators
- Virtual reality technology
- Simulation mannequins with software
- Task trainers
- Defibrillators
- Video monitoring and programming equipment
- 10–12 PCs and monitors
- A network server with secure storage
- Video editing hardware and software
- Disposable supplies

In addition, there are collaborative links with the 7,000 ft^2 Brunner Technology Center at the Penn School of Nursing, which trains more than 8,000 simulation encounters annually, and the Measey Medical Simulation Center at the Penn School of Medicine. Both of these centers provide adjunctive expertise, equipment, and personnel to accomplish training and research objectives. These resources have been mobilized and committed to support the evolving Laerdal-funded CHOP Center of Excellence for Resuscitation Research (see Figs. A.1, A.2, A.3, and A.4).

A.I. Levine et al. (eds.), *The Comprehensive Textbook of Healthcare Simulation*,
DOI 10.1007/978-1-4614-5993-4, © Springer Science+Business Media New York 2013

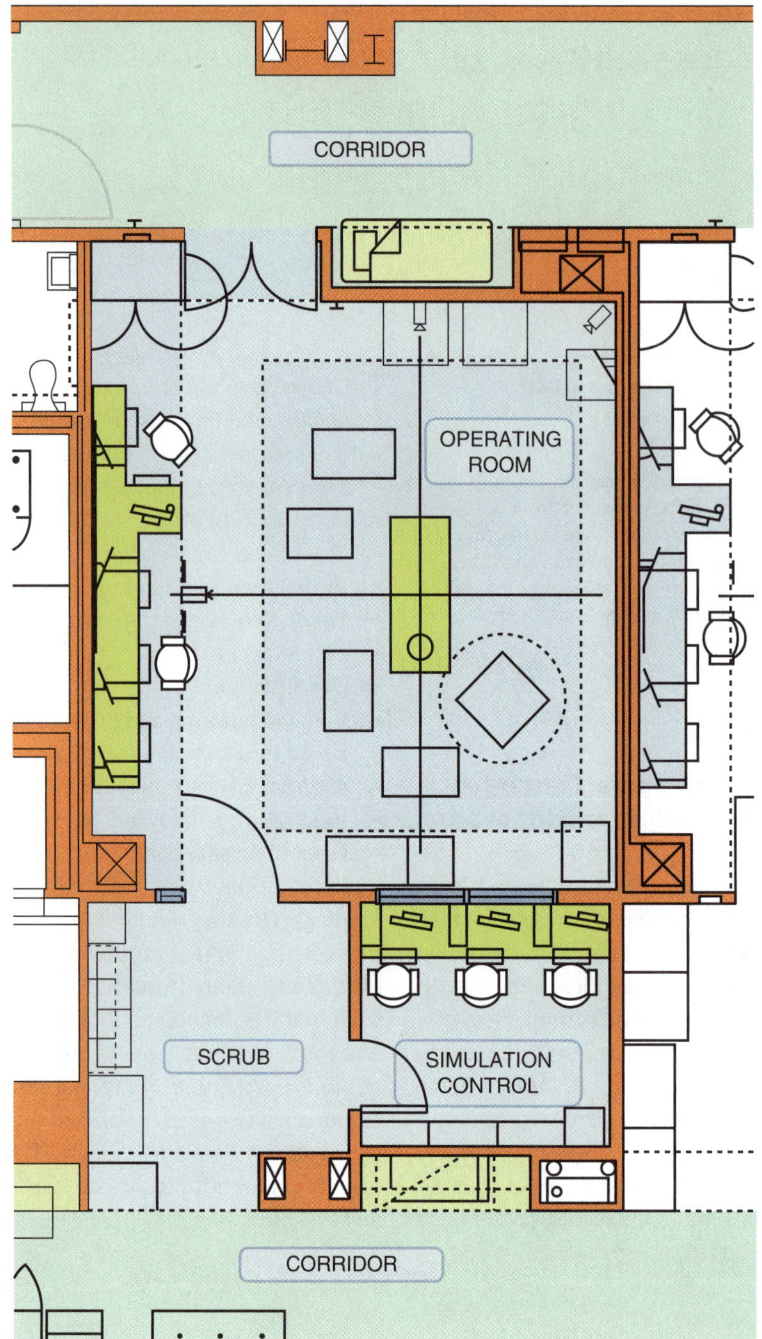
CORRIDOR
OPERATING ROOM
SCRUB
SIMULATION CONTROL
CORRIDOR
Diagram courtesy of The Children's Hospital of Philadelphia - Facilities Planning Department

Fig. A.1

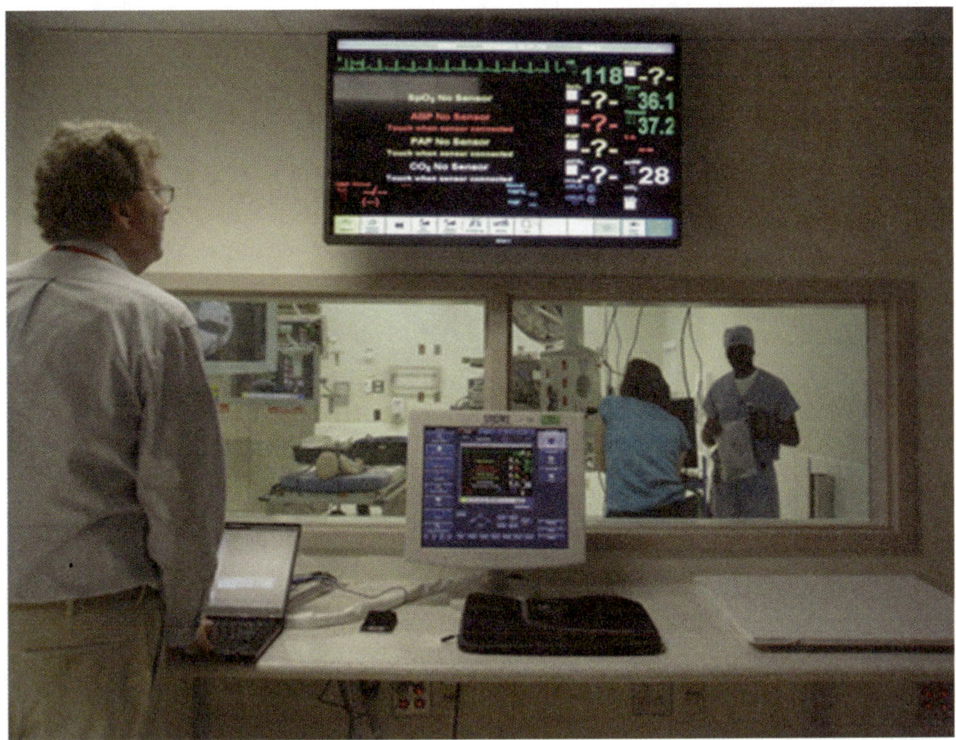
118
36.1
37.2
28

Fig. A.2

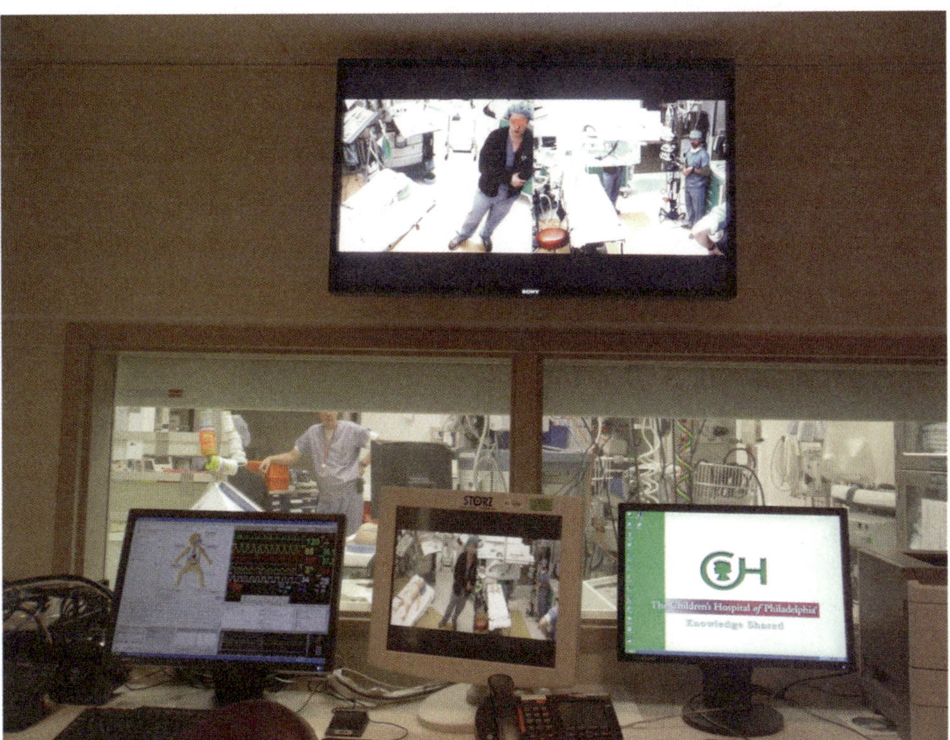
STORZ
The Children's Hospital of Philadelphia
Knowledge Shared

Fig. A.3

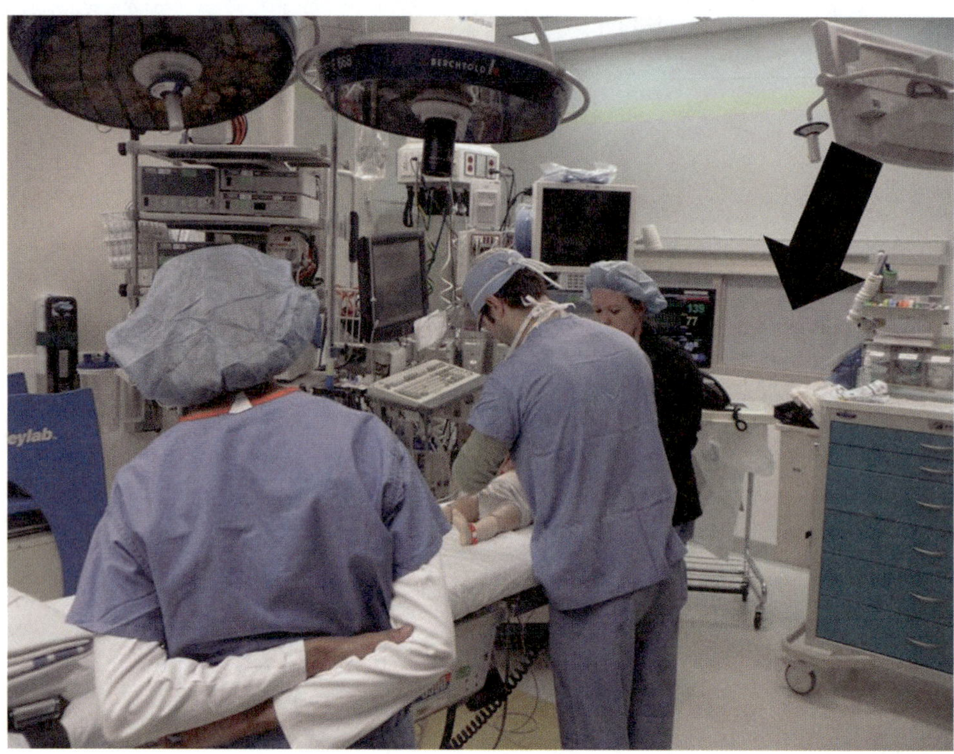

Fig. A.4

The Mount Sinai HELPS Center

The HELPS (Human Emulation, Education, and Evaluation Lab for Patient Safety) Center Program operates out of the state-of the-art HELPS Center which is owned and operated by the Department of Anesthesiology of the Mount Sinai School of Medicine. The program has been in operation since 1994, when the first simulator, based on the University of Florida's Anesthesia Simulator, was acquired. Although owned and operated exclusively by the Department of Anesthesiology, our target audience is multidisciplinary and includes all levels of training from students to board-certified physicians.

The Department of Anesthesiology's HELPS Center education complex is located in the department's office space. The center occupies approximately 1,500 ft^2 and features a large conference room (that seats approximately 40), a classroom (that seats approximately 20), and two fully functioning simulator rooms each capable of accommodating 15 students per room. Each simulator room is equipped with a dedicated CAE METI human patient simulator (HPS), patient monitor, computerized record keeper, and anesthesia delivery system. The center also houses two virtual reality bronchoscope/colonoscope simulators, a robotic intravenous placement trainer, a neuraxial anesthesia part-task trainer, and a transesophageal echocardiography simulator.

The HELPS Center is supported by a state-of-the-art integrated and custom-designed audiovisual system that includes four dedicated computers, one 65-in. plasma screen, and three wall-mounted 50-in. plasma screens each with overlaid "Smartboard" technology, enabling touch-screen capabilities. There is a dedicated ceiling-mounted LCD projector coupled with an automated projection screen. There are also multiple camera installations in each simulator rooms and a Polycom for teleconferencing.

Due to space limitations the AV system was designed so that every room in the center can have multiple functions; they can serve as a stand-alone classroom or be "linked" through a custom bidirectional intercom system to create a 1,500 ft^2 virtual classroom. Floor space conservation was also achieved by the omission of a control room (s). The AV system allows each room in the center to serve as a control room to any other room in the center, affording the operator the ability to wirelessly control the simulators and choose camera views and recording sources on the fly. The AV system also provides the ability to display and create video, CD, and DVD presentations. The custom-programmed touch-screen panels also enable local, national, and international telemedicine conferences from any location in the center (see Figs. A.5, A.6, A.7, A.8, A.9, A.10, and A.11).

DEPARTMENT OF ANESTHESIOLOGY

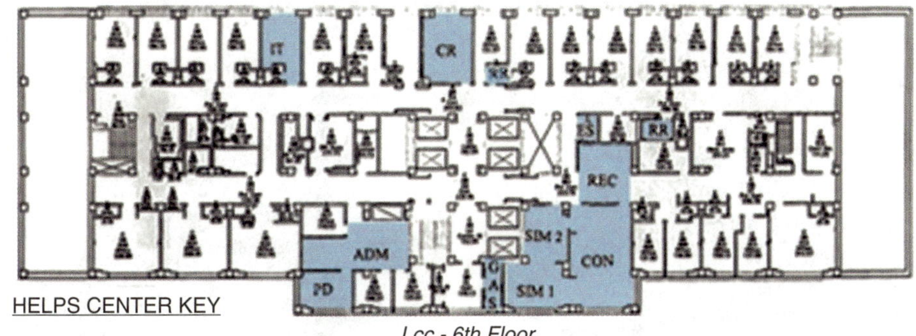

HELPS CENTER RECEPTION - REC
SIMULATOR ROOM 1 - SIM1
SIMULATOR ROOM 2 - SIM2
CONFERENCE ROOM - CON
IT SUPPORT - IT
CLASS ROOM - CR
GAS SUPPLY ROOM - GAS
EDUCATIONAL SUPPLY ROOM - ES
ADMINISTRATIVE OFFICE - ADM
PROGRAM DIRECTORS OFFICE - PD

Fig. A.5

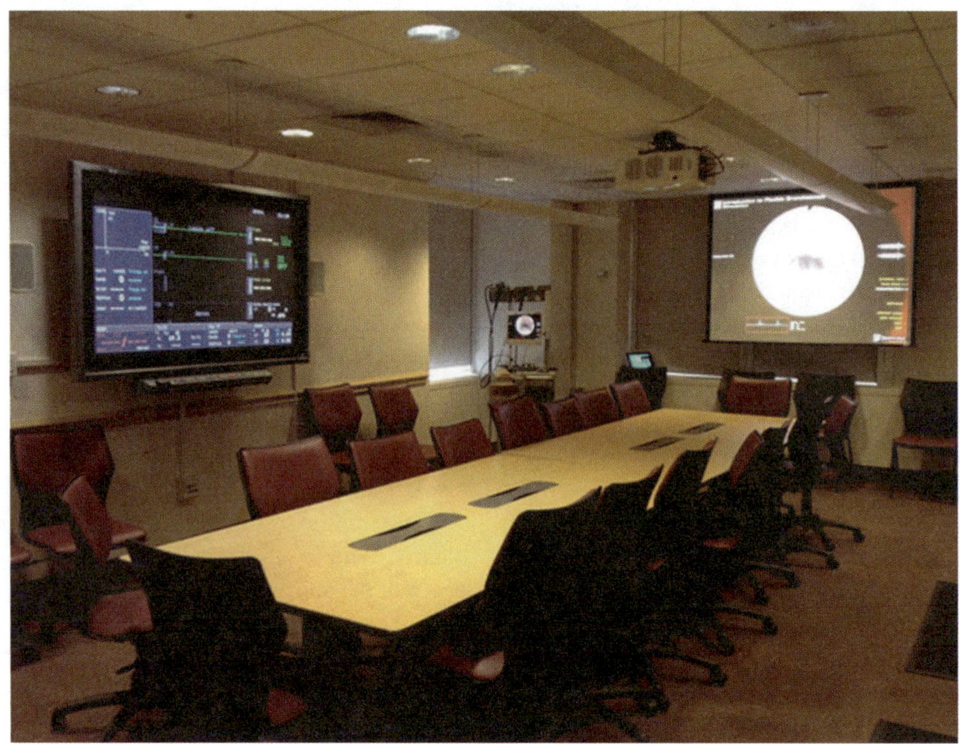

Fig. A.6

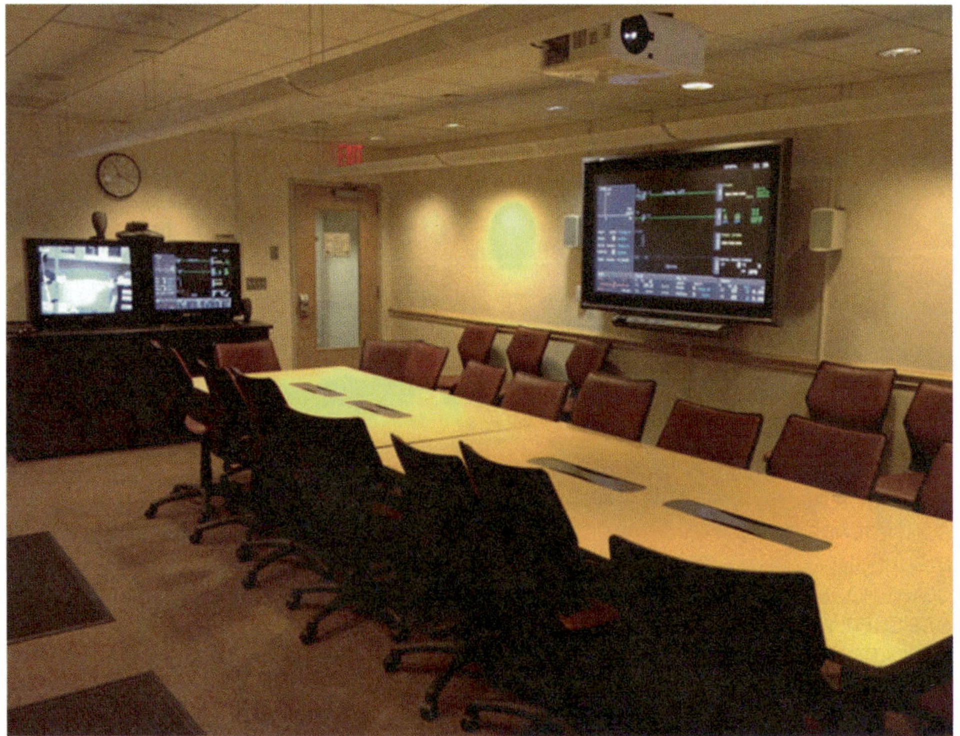

Fig. A.7

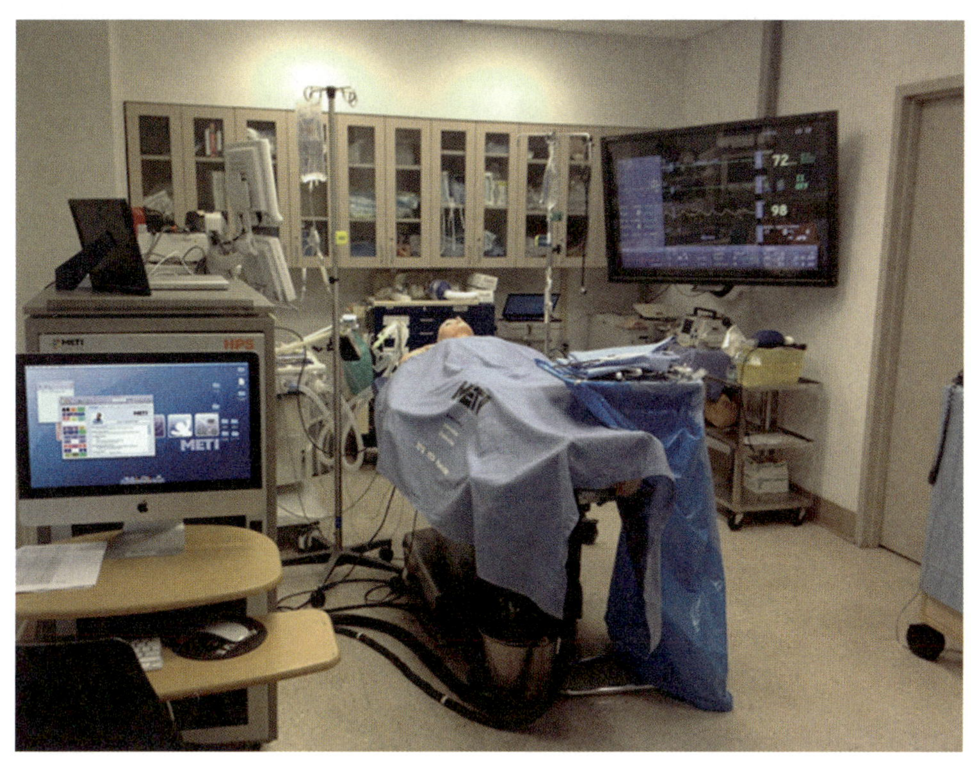

Fig. A.8

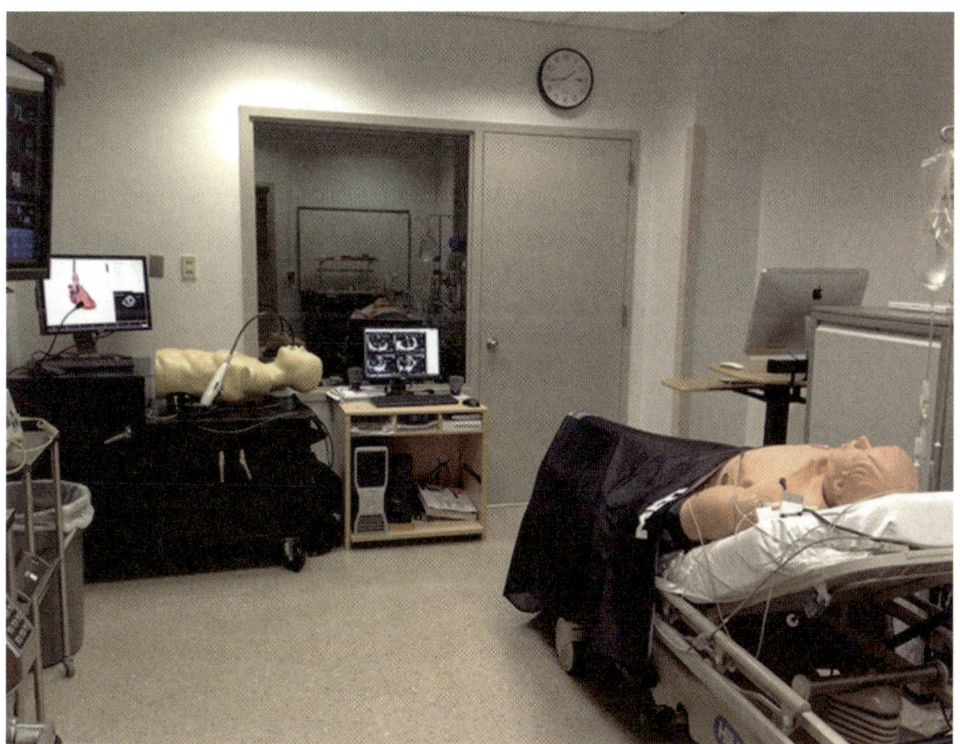

Fig. A.9

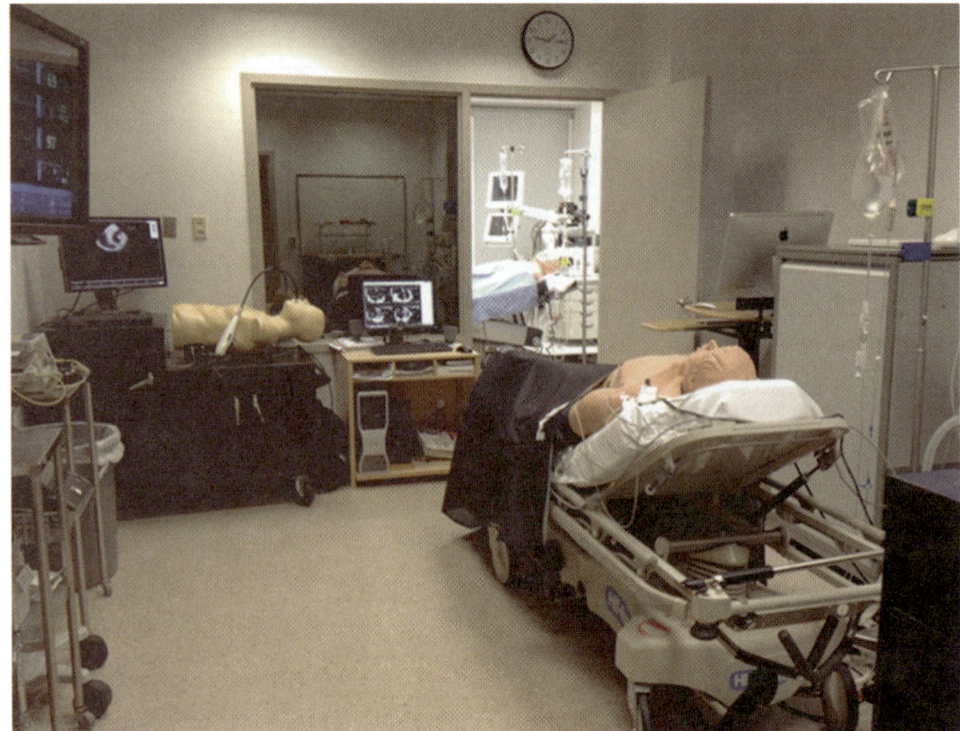

Fig. A.10

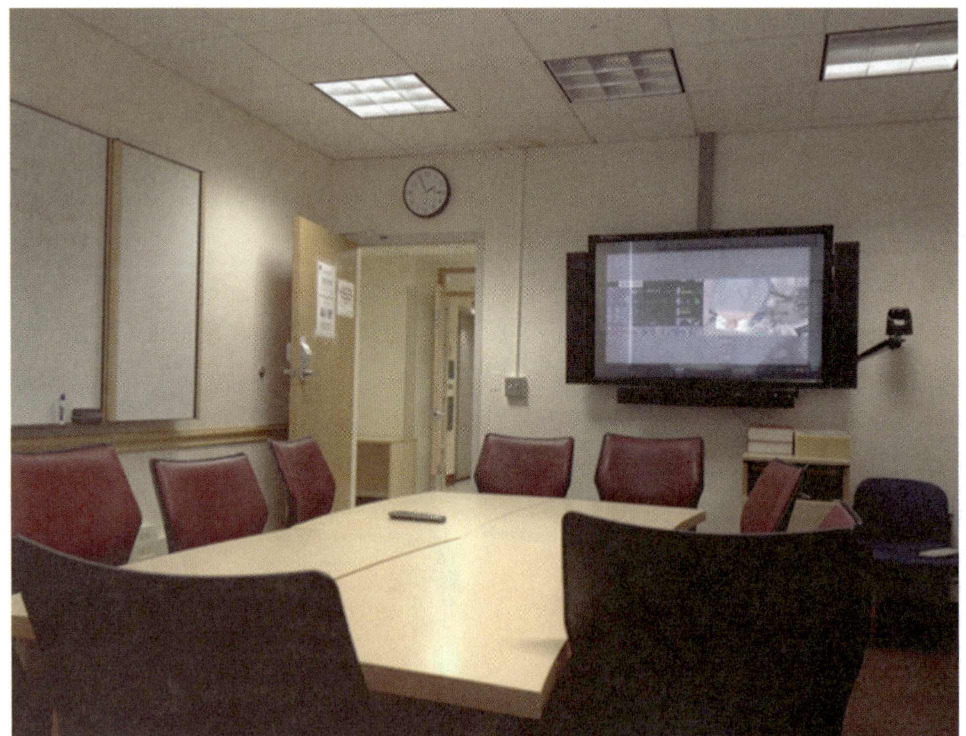

Fig. A.11

Children's Hospital University of Alabama Birmingham (UAB) Simulation Center

The Pediatric Simulation Center at Children's of Alabama is currently housed in four former patient rooms located in the main hospital facility just down the hall from patient care areas. One room has been adapted to be used as a conference/debriefing space, and the three other rooms house simulation activities. All rooms have cameras and the images can be viewed live in the conference room. Our center has provided learning opportunities for over 15,000 learners in its first 5 years both in this small facility and with in situ activities. We took a "low-budget" approach in which we placed the controller behind a curtain in the corner of each former patient room (instead of creating control booths in each room). Initially our nurse educator's desk was also located in our conference room. We have recently added simulation screens which have augmented this approach. We can run simultaneous simulations in each of our three rooms and we've even used the hallway for neonatal simulations when necessary! We've been able to expand to include two small offices and a storage area, but we make use of the hallway for daytime storage. We also find that our participants love our candy bowl (see Figs. A.12, A.13, A.14, A.15, A.16, A.17, A.18, and A.19).

(All photos were taken by Justine Cooper)

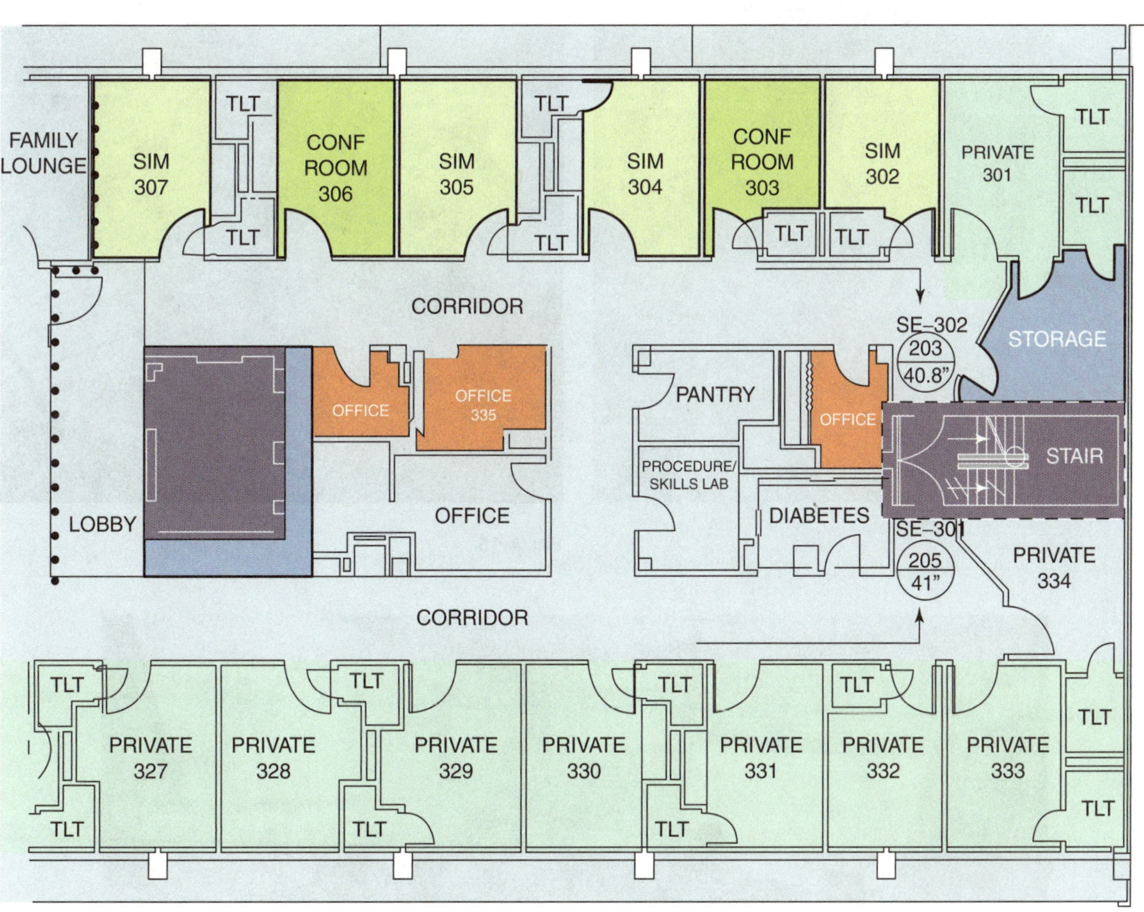

Fig. A.12

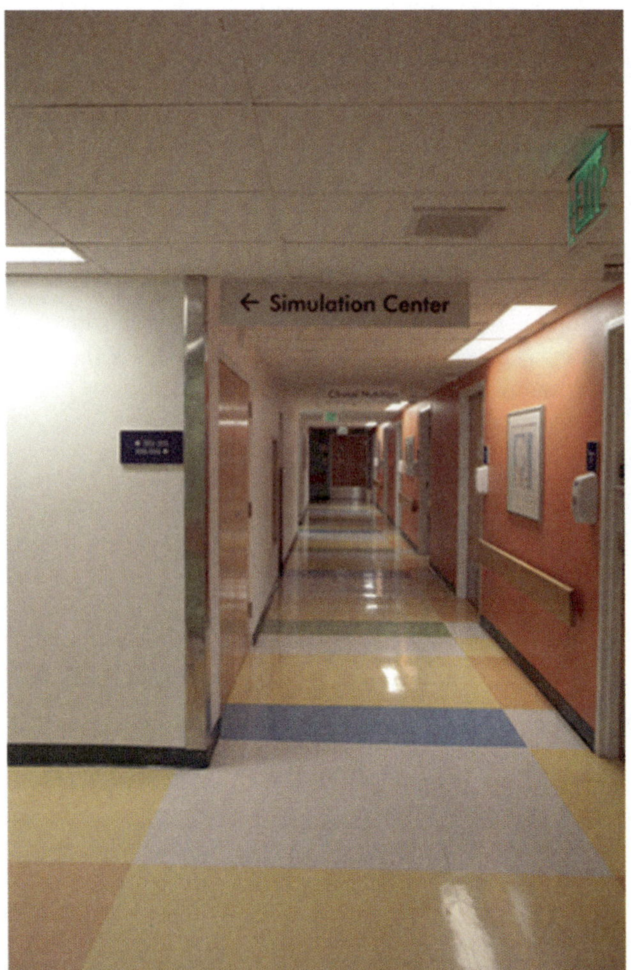

Fig. A.13

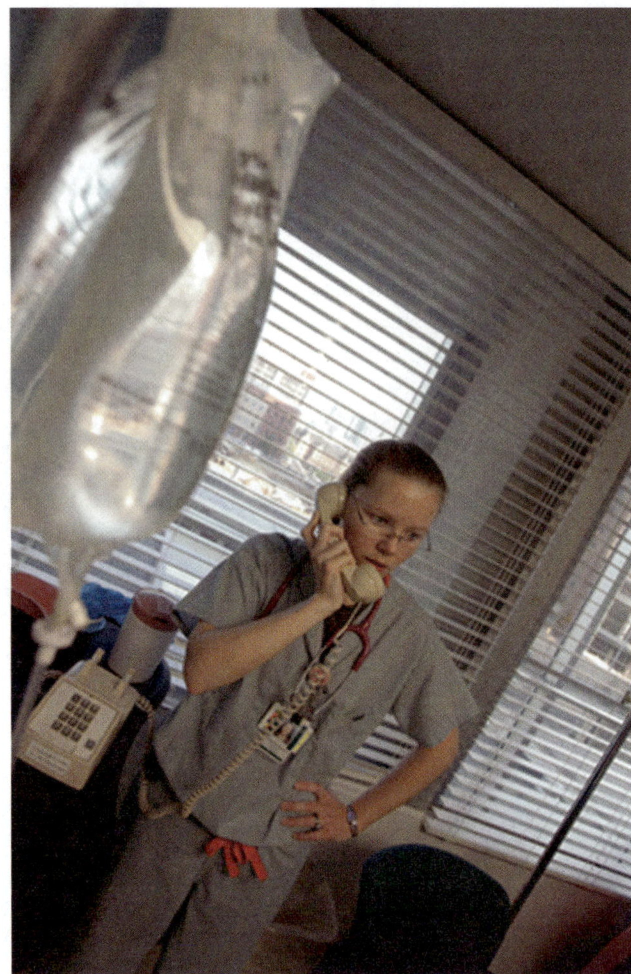

Fig. A.15

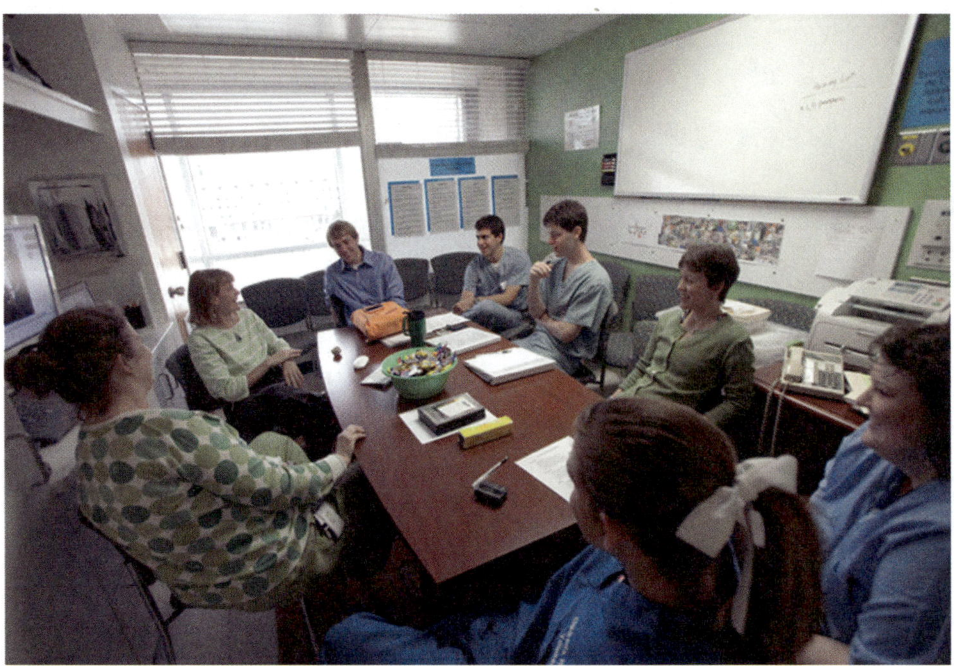

Fig. A.14

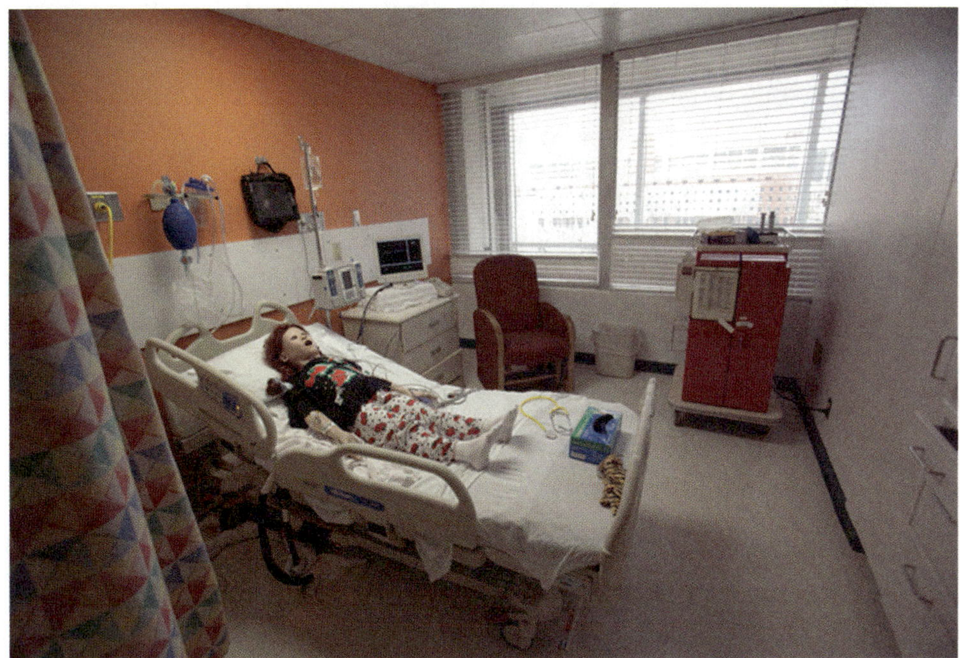

Fig. A.16

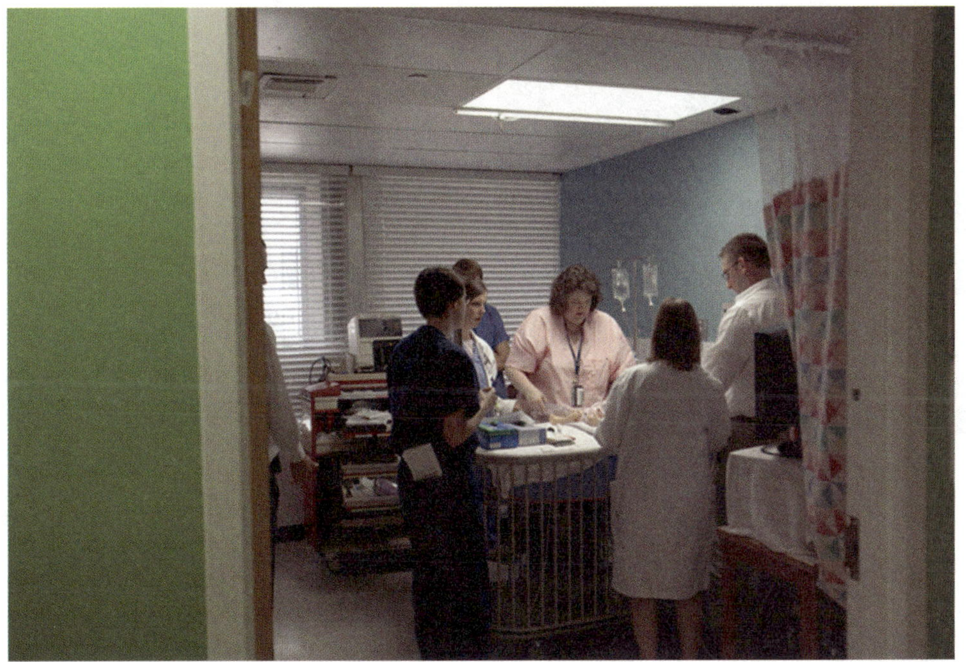

Fig. A.17

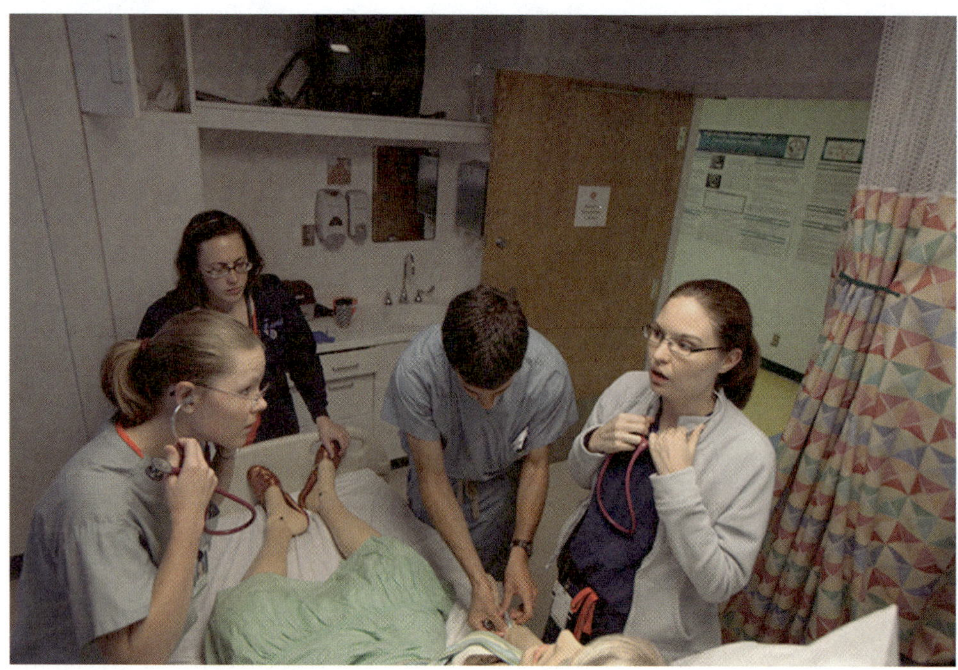

Fig. A.18

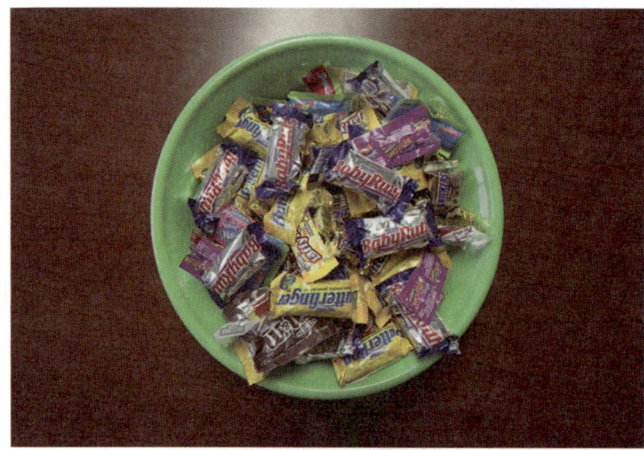

Fig. A.19

Virginia Commonwealth University (VCU) School of Dentistry

As part of the VCU Simulation Consortium, the VCU School of Dentistry joins VCU's other health sciences schools in incorporating a range of simulation practices into its curricula, regularly exposing students to lifelike scenarios that reinforce and enhance knowledge gained from classroom education.

Realizing the potential and the advantages of using the latest technologies available for teaching, the VCU School of Dentistry, like other leading dental schools worldwide, uses virtual reality-based technology to enhance and improve students' learning and performance. VCU dental students use this technology as part of their preclinical training, enabling them to treat patients earlier than in years past.

Virtual Reality Simulation Laboratory Layout

A schematic representation of the VCU virtual reality simulation laboratory. A total of 20 simulators are placed in a relatively small space, where each simulator and operator has enough room to work in. There are two hexagons and two quads. At VCU School of Dentistry, each class has about 100 students. We have created a schedule in which a total of five groups rotate through the lab in 1 week, and so 20 units work well with our curriculum. This layout also specifies the hand preference of the unit (L/R); however, each unit can be modified according to the student's preference. The instructor's station is location to the left of the main entrance (E). The instructor can access each of the individual simulation computers from one main computer (server), send and receive instant messages to and from the students, and view the students work in real time without leaving the instructor's station. Each procedure is also recorded in the system and may be reviewed by the student and/or the instructor following its completion, on any of the lab's computers.

Virtual Reality Simulation Laboratory Hexagon

This picture shows one hexagon in the VCU virtual reality simulation laboratory. The simulator includes an infrared camera, an Adec dental unit, a computer, and a monitor. It is important to position the simulators, so there is minimal chance of people accidentally moving the cameras or interfering with correct dental ergonomics. This setup has been working well.

Virtual Reality Simulation Laboratory

VCU School of Dentistry first year (D1) students practicing on the virtual reality simulator. The students use correct ergonomics, indirect vision, and follow OSHA guidelines while making cavity preparation in plastic teeth in a simulated head. The students receive immediate feedback from the computer about their work (in the form of 3D images, written comments, and individualized scores).

Mannequin Simulation Laboratory Layout

A schematic representation of the standard mannequin laboratory. There are 108 simulators that can be used for either right- or left-handed students (preferred locations for left-handed students are highlighted). The instructor's station is equipped with the latest audio visual technology that allows improved student engagement (e.g., projecting presentations, making demonstrations, and communicating with the students as the class is progressing).

Mannequin Simulation Laboratory

This is a picture of the VCU School of Dentistry standard mannequin laboratory. The simulators include a torso, head, and articulators. Plastic typodonts with plastic or sterilized extracted teeth are magnetically attached to the articulator. The simulated dental unit has the same clinical features as the unit used for patient care. At VCU, all students of one class participate in a lab session together (approximately 100 students in each year). The lab is divided into sections, and faculty members work with a group of 10–20 students per session (see Figs. A.20, A.21, A.22, A.23, A.24, A.25, A.26, and A.27).

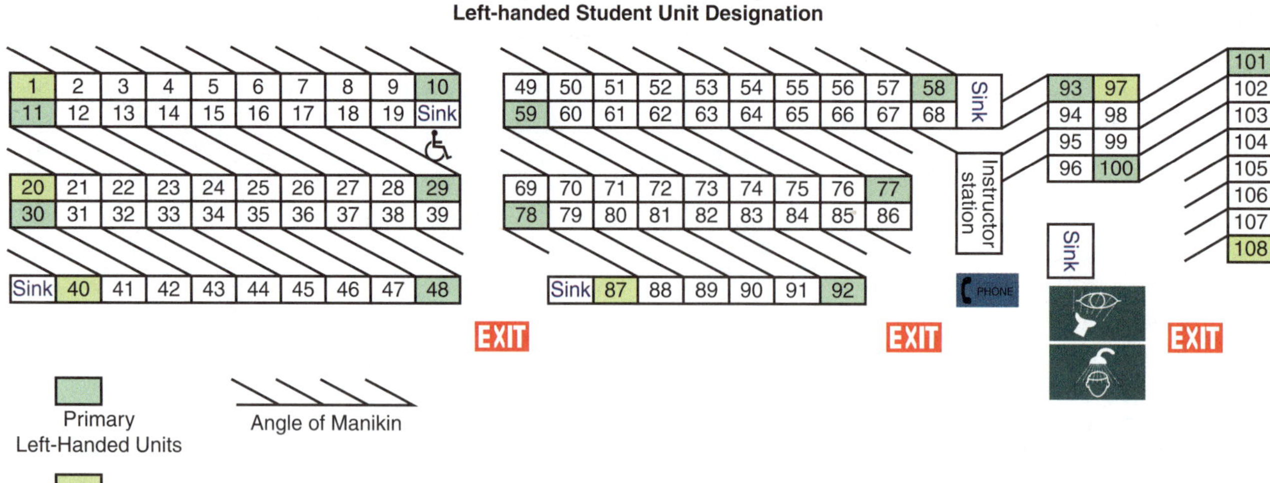

Fig. A.20

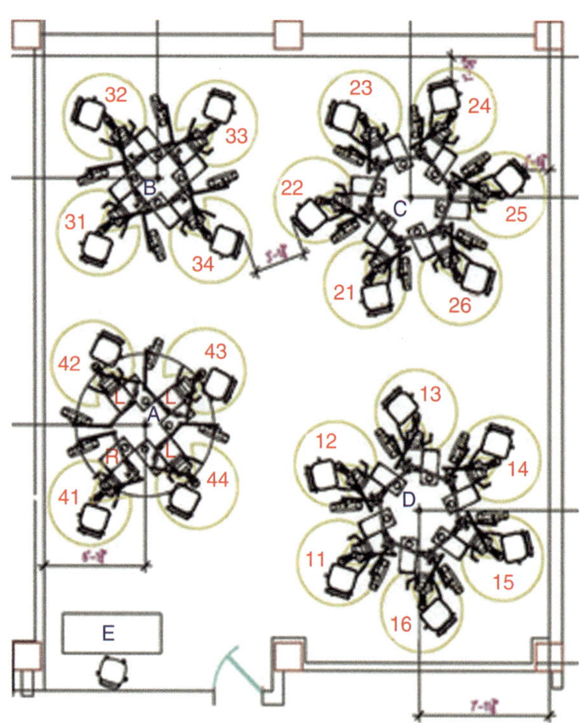

Fig. A.21

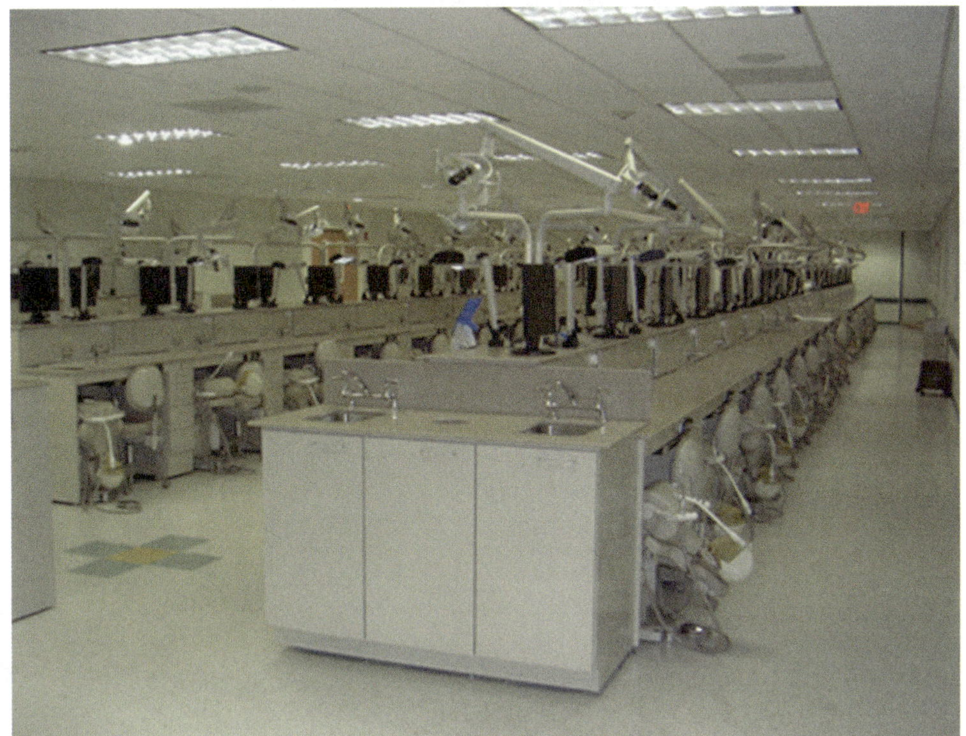

Fig. A.22

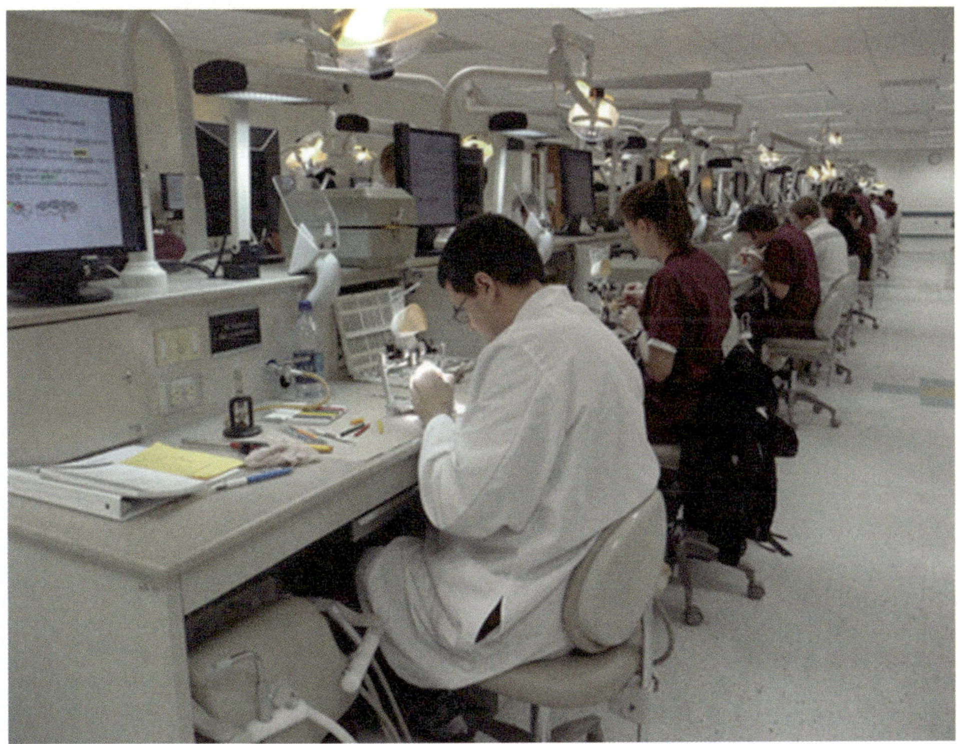

Fig. A.23

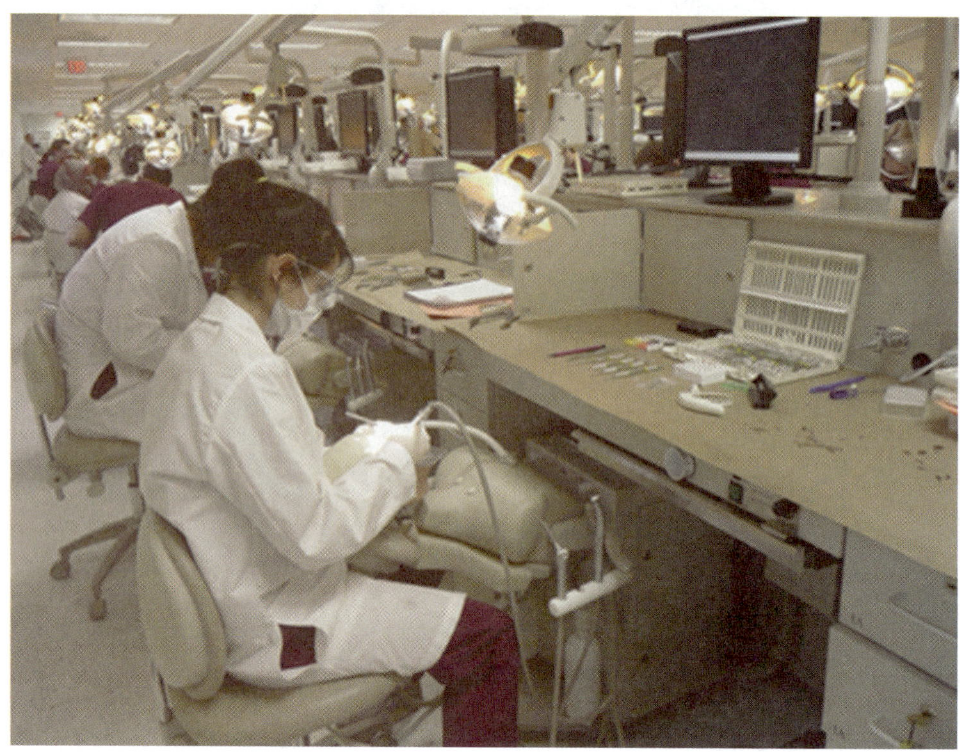

Fig. A.24

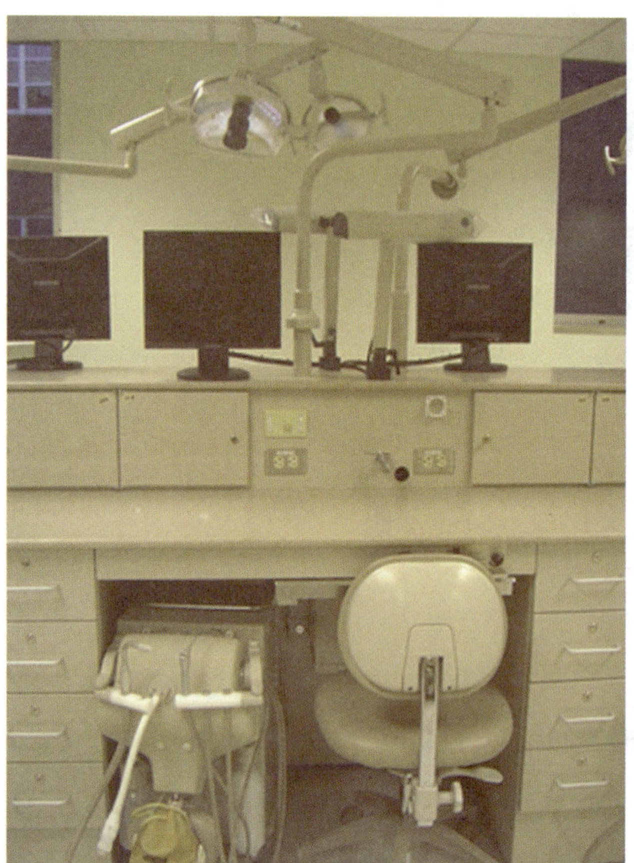

Fig. A.25

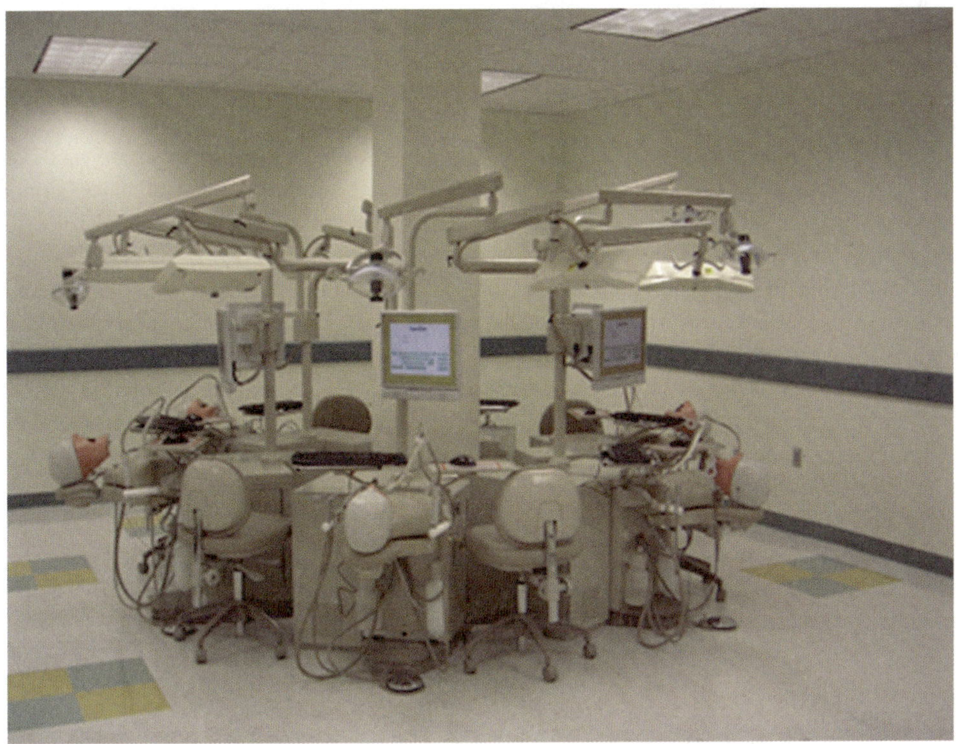

Fig. A.26

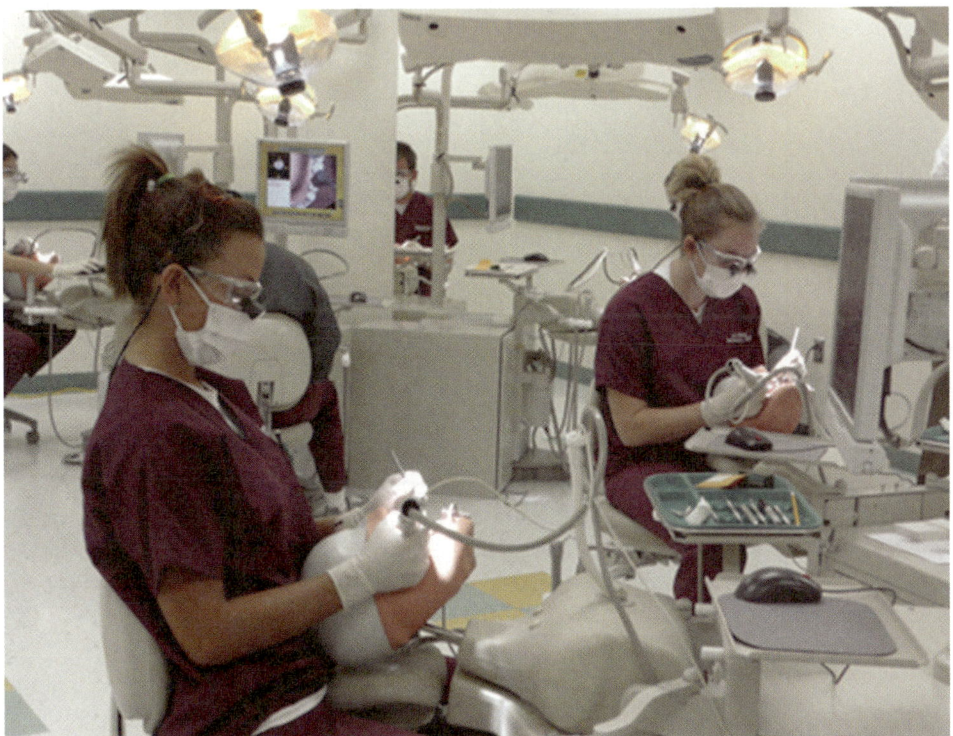

Fig. A.27

Mayo Clinic Florida Multidisciplinary Simulation Center

The Mayo Clinic Multidisciplinary Simulation Center transforms clinical medical education by helping educators to develop, implement, and evaluate experiential curricula that advance patient care.

Our simulation center represents a living collaborative between all specialties and health-care professions at Mayo Clinic, where the needs of the patient come first. It is through this lens—to best serve our patients—that our simulation center works to fully realize the benefits of simulation-based education and practice and research opportunities. Medical simulation has important lessons and applications for all involved in the risk-laden environment of health care. It provides the ideal environment for teaching health-care teams how to care for patients. By being allowed to make mistakes, learners can see the effects of those mistakes without harming patients. Simulation makes the learning environment come alive.

Medical centers of excellence must rise to the challenges of both demonstrated competence and scholarly analysis of efficacy via scientific methods, including the use of simulation in medical education.

Mayo Clinic has applied its renowned collaborative practice model to explore and advance simulation education across specialties and professional roles to better educate practitioners.

The Florida center spans 9,500 ft^2. There is a large lecture hall. There are two outpatient clinic rooms, a large ED suite, a large task training region, and a full-size OR. The OR can double as a radiographic simulation area (detailed picture available by request). There is a procedural skills lab for body parts that is fully endoscopically capable. There are two inpatient rooms or ICU rooms (they are the same in our hospital). The center is a direct replica of our hospital. It is very versatile and can be used in many settings. Each room has the capability of being flexible (see Figs. A.28, A.29, A.30, A.31, A.32, A.33, and A.34).

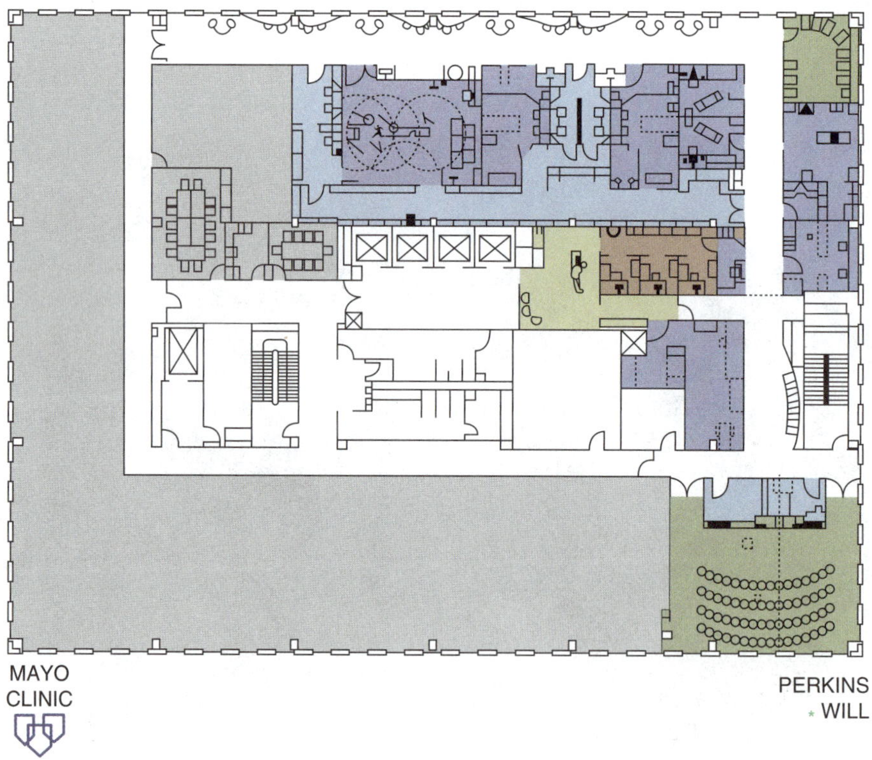

Fig. A.28

MAYO CLINIC

PERKINS
+WILL

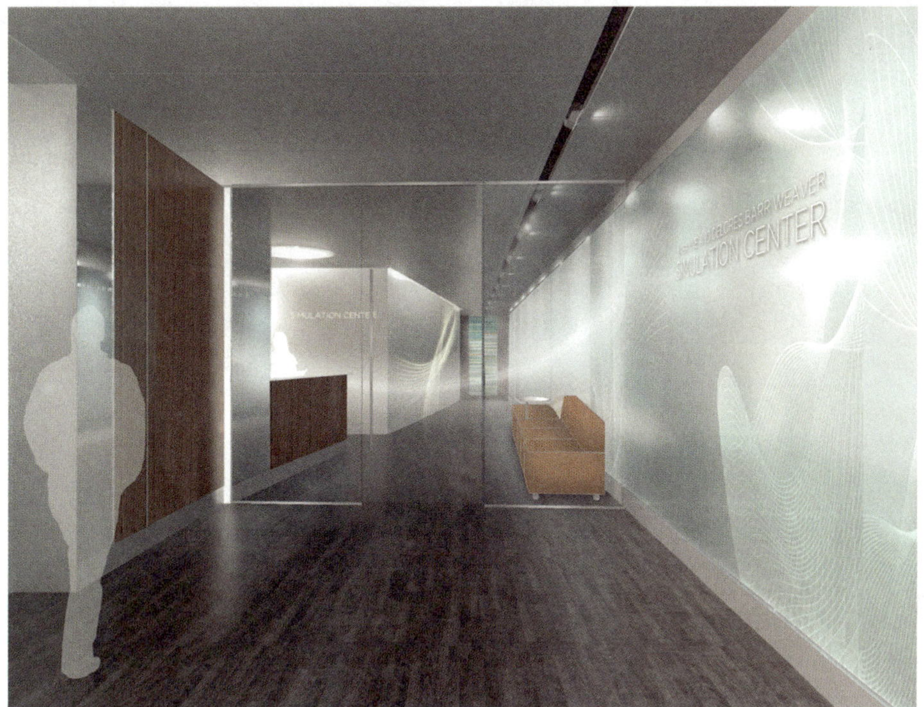

SIMULATION CENTER - LOBBY

07.17.2012

Fig. A.29

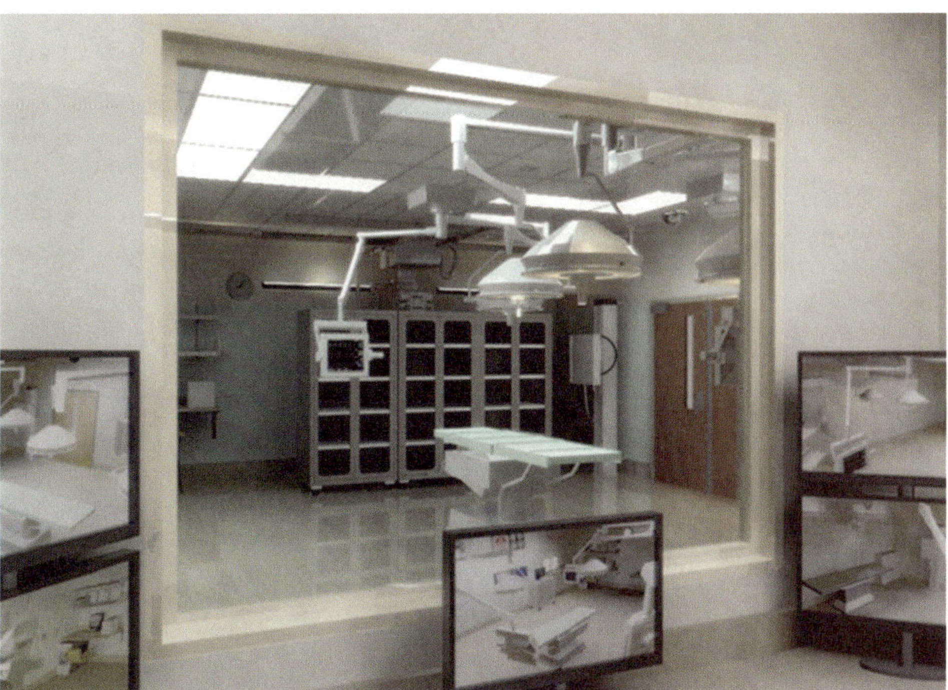

Fig. A.30

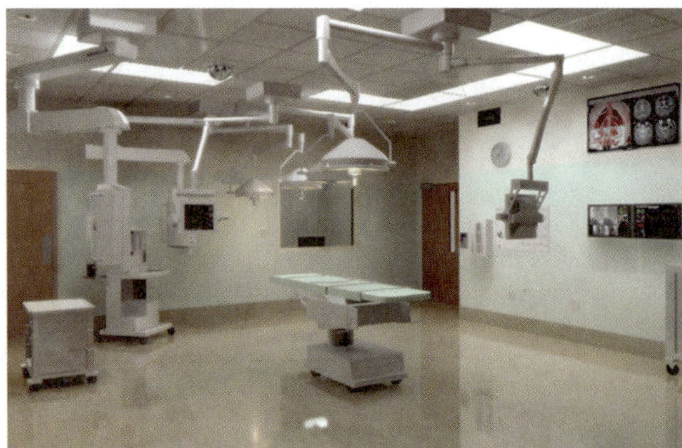

Fig. A.31

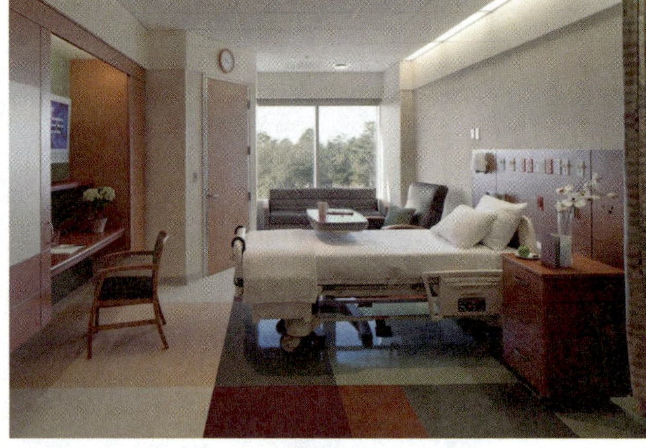

Fig. A.34

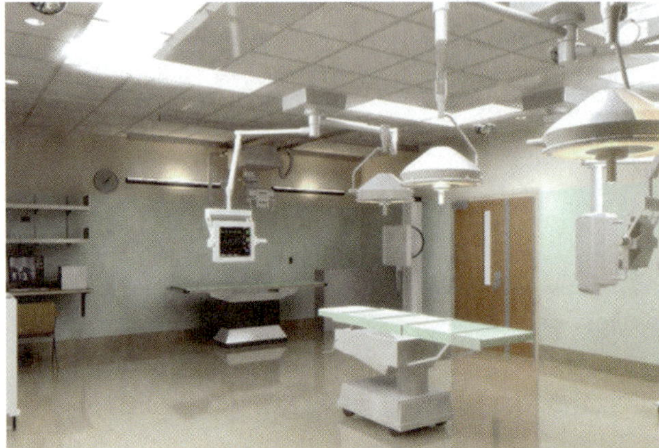

Fig. A.32

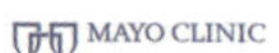

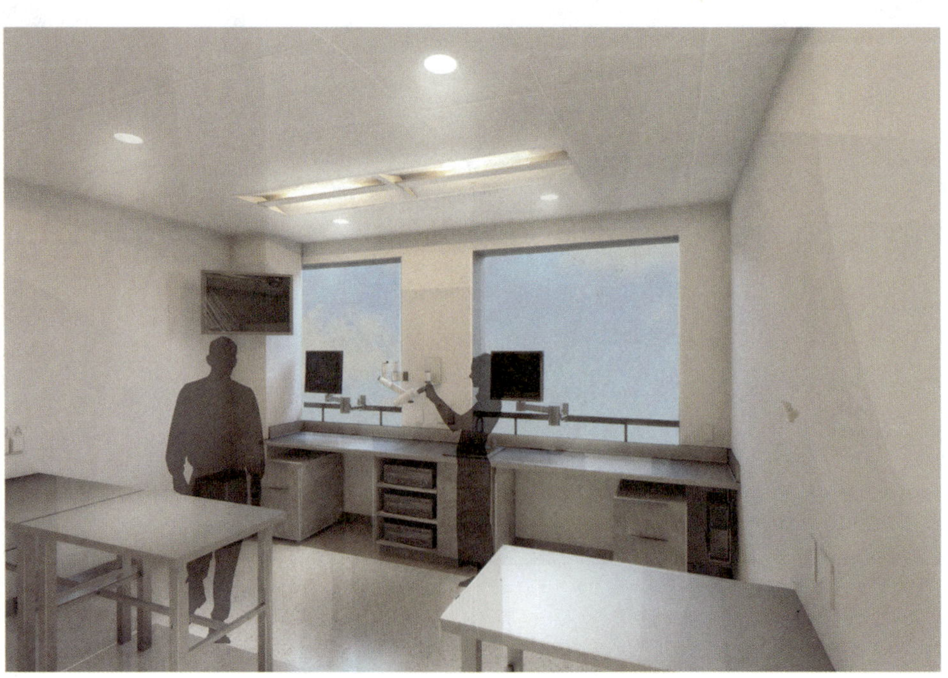

Fig. A.33

The New York Simulation Center for the Health Sciences

The mission of the New York Simulation Center for the Health Sciences (NYSIM) is to serve the academic needs of the health science schools and services of CUNY and NYU and to improve patient safety and quality of care. It is also our mission to provide simulation training for first responders to disasters in New York City. NYSIM is one of the most advanced facilities of this kind in the United States. It is being used actively by the NYU Langone Medical Center for training medical students and residents, by four nursing schools (Borough of Manhattan Community College, Hunter, NYU, and LaGuardia), by the Sophie Davis programs in Biomedical Sciences, by the NYU Langone Medical Center and Bellevue Hospitals for training nursing and medical staff, and by a host of allied health schools of the City University of New York including paramedic, physician assistant, and respiratory therapy training programs (see Figs. A.35, A.36, A.37, A.38, A.39, A.40, A.41, A.42, and A.43).

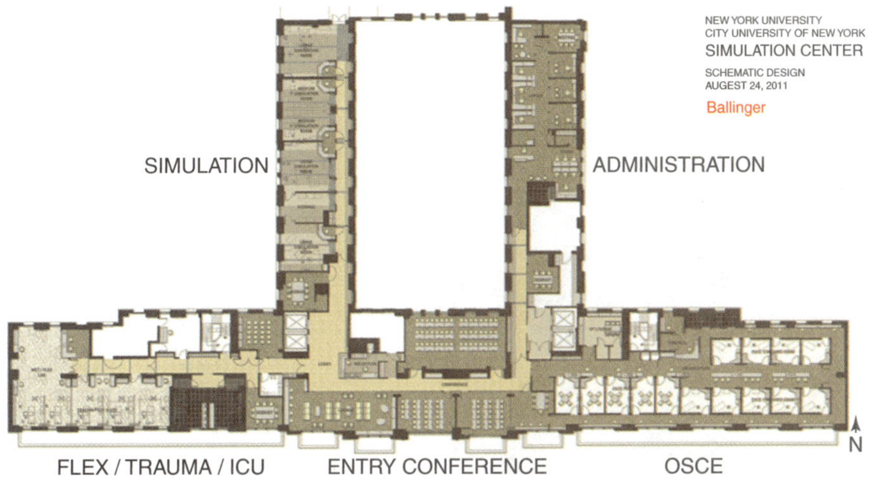

Fig. A.35

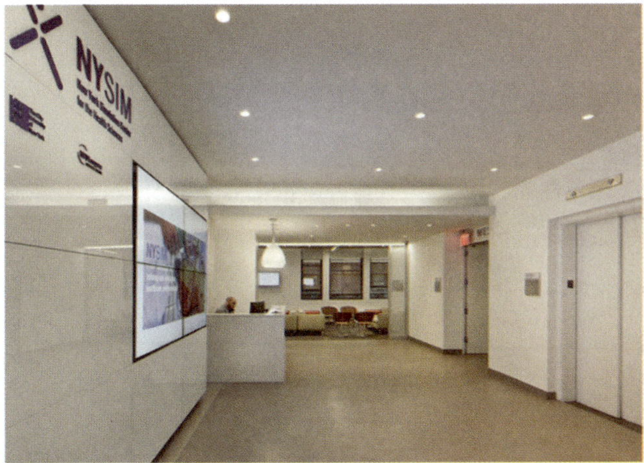

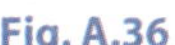
Fig. A.36

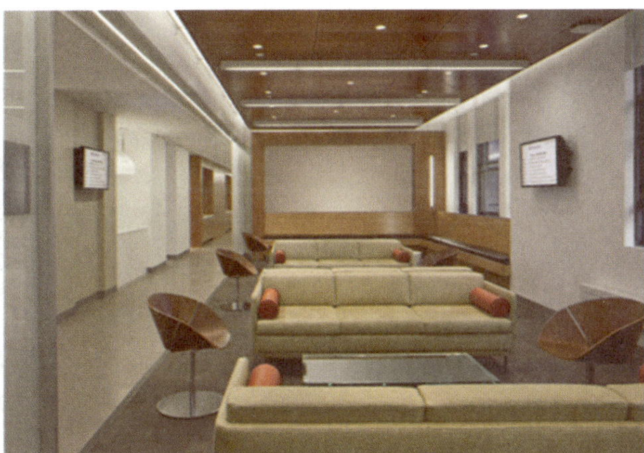

Fig. A.37

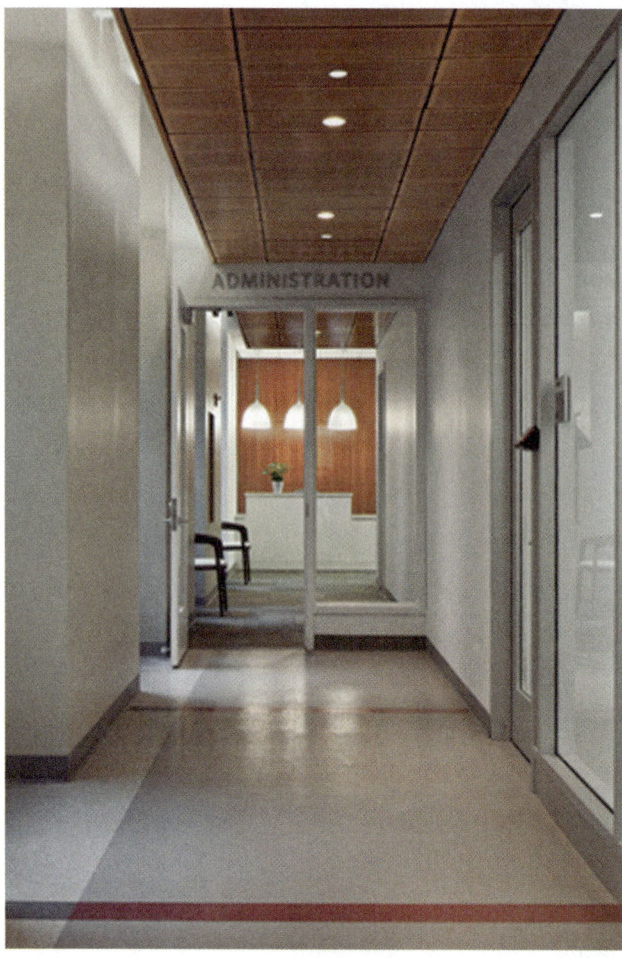

Fig. A.38

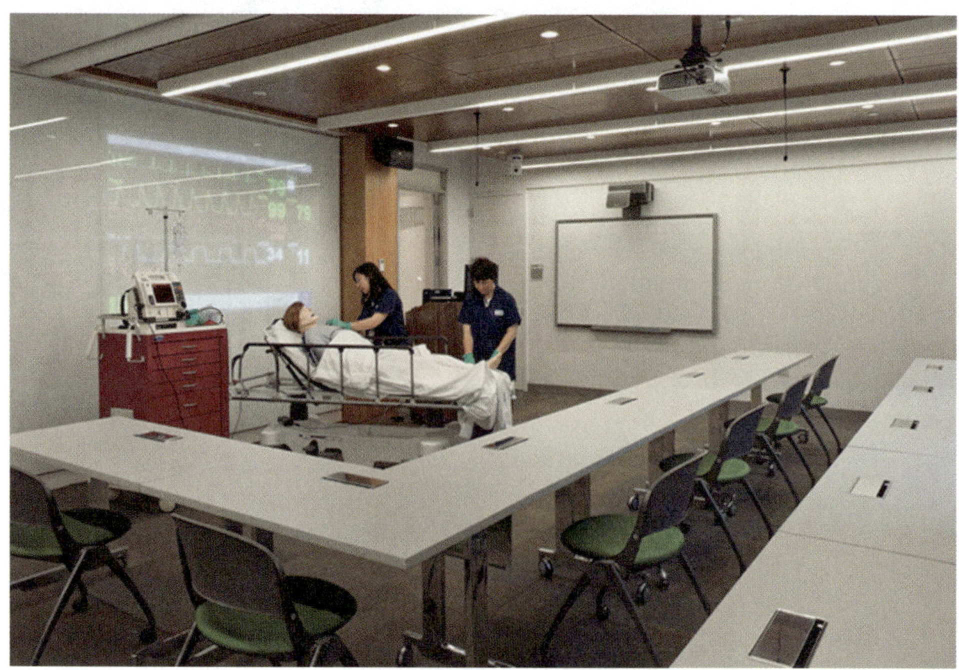

Fig. A.39

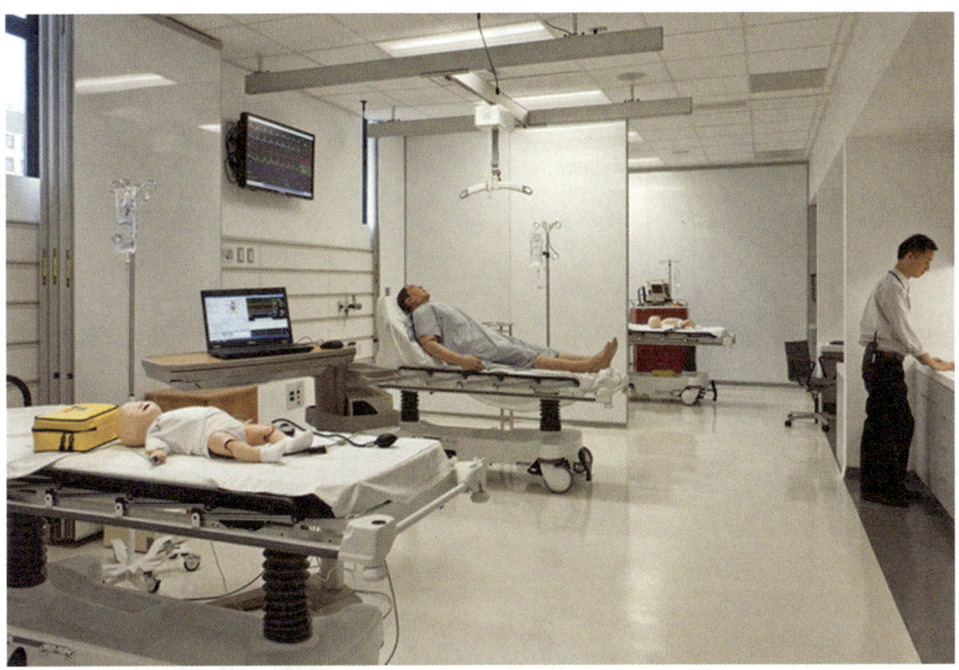

Fig. A.40

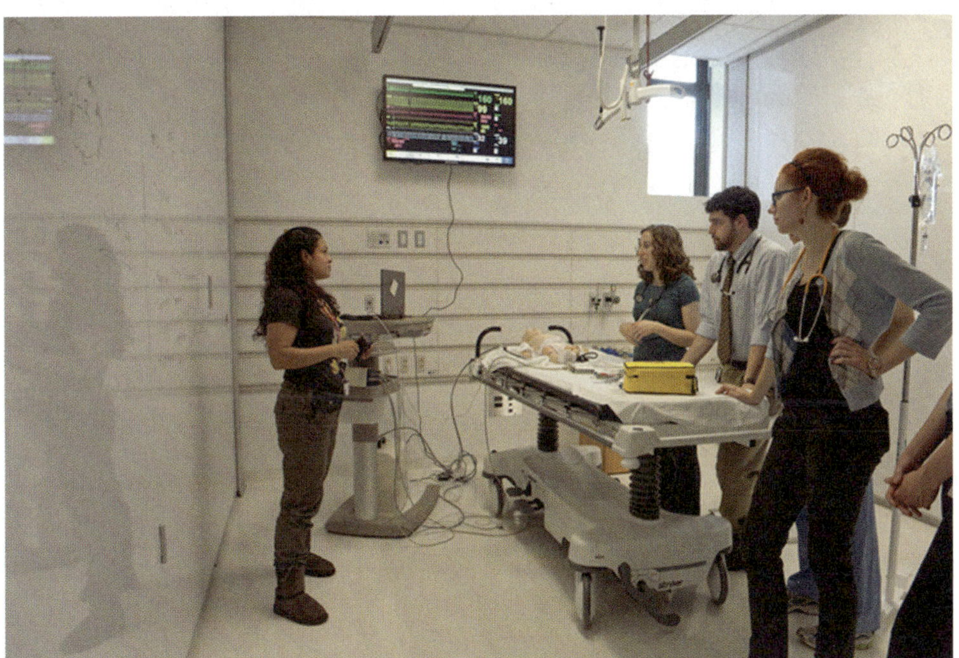

Fig. A.41

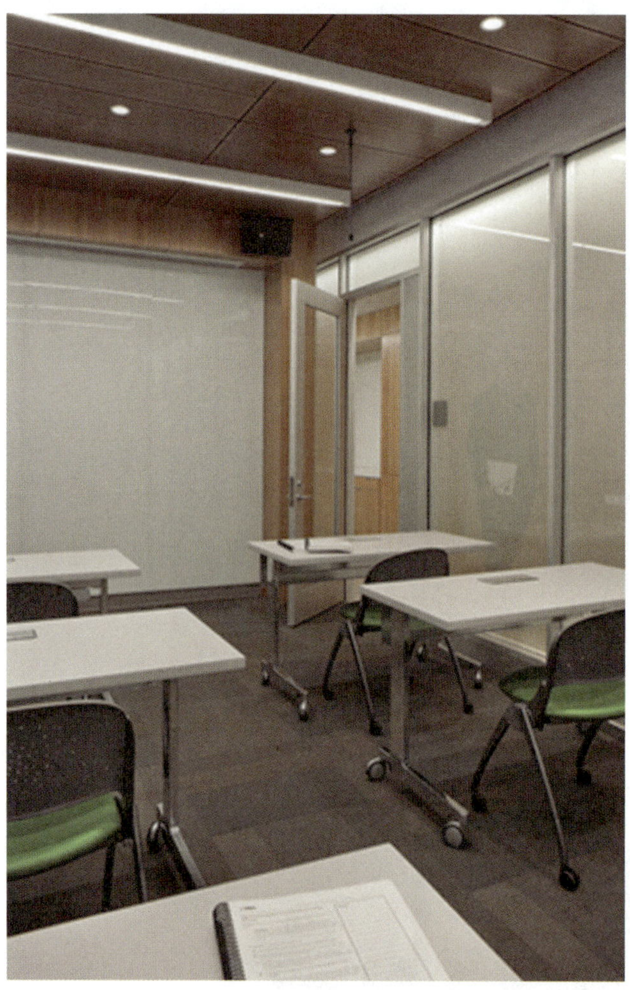

Fig. A.42

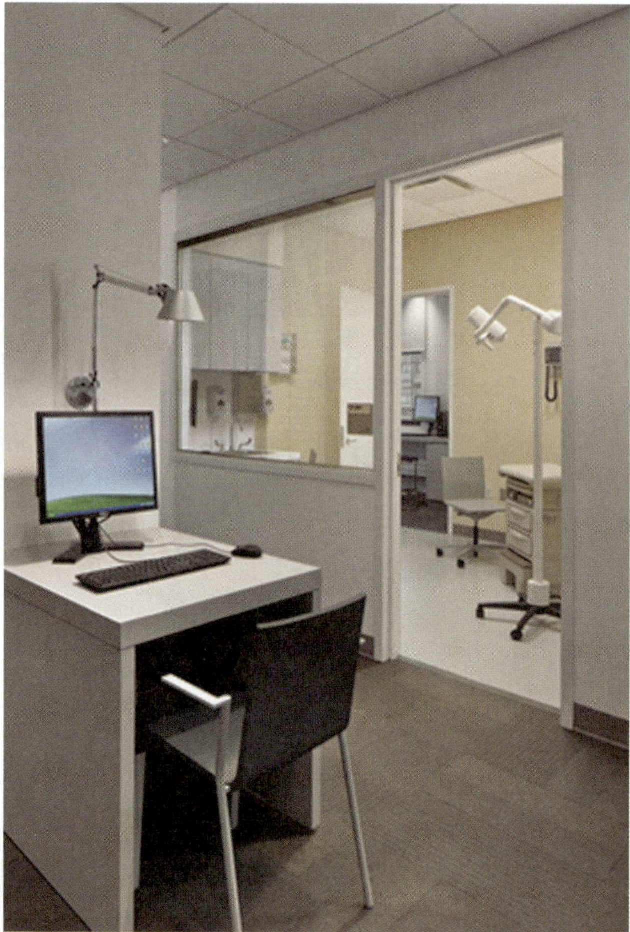

Fig. A.43

North Shore-Long Island Jewish: Patient Safety Institute, a Multidisciplinary Clinical Simulation Center

The health system advocates a zero-tolerance policy toward medical errors and infections and believes that better clinical education is key to bringing about this change. The Patient Safety Institute (PSI) features sophisticated, full-scale high-fidelity patient simulators with computer-based interactive technology. Faculty in control rooms with one-way mirrors manipulate the patient simulators to mimic diverse medical scenarios found in all areas of health care. PSI is adaptable to all clinical levels and allied health professions, and clinical teams from all over the health system have regularly scheduled sessions. Each program is customized in collaboration with each clinical team or discipline. Our programs integrate the aviation industry's Crew Resource Management (CRM) program for multidisciplinary clinical teams. Using the concept of deliberate practice, the high-fidelity medical simulators give clinicians an opportunity to practice their clinical and cognitive skills in a team environment without putting patients in danger; they can be programmed to simulate a variety of life-or-death scenarios. An important part of the process is the debriefing, where participants are guided to evaluate their recorded performance in a supportive and safe environment. The Patient Safety Institute is an important part of the curriculum for the new Hofstra North Shore-LIJ School of Medicine and in fact is referred to as part of the medical school's "west campus."

PSI features state-of-the-art medical simulators including adult, pediatric, neonate, endovascular, and obstetrical, to name a few. Numerous task trainers are also available and include heart/lung sounds, TEE, ultrasound, central line, etc.

The center itself is 45,000 ft^2 and is located off campus on two floors of a private building. It is comprised of several multimedia classrooms, 2 computer labs, 2 operating rooms/cardiac cath labs, 2 procedure rooms, a labor and delivery suite, 12 ICU-med/surge rooms, and 14 clinical skills exam rooms (standardized patient lab) (see Figs. A.44, A.45, A.46, A.47, A.48, A.49, A.50, A.51, A.52, A.53, A.54, A.55, A.56, and A.57).

Fig. A.44

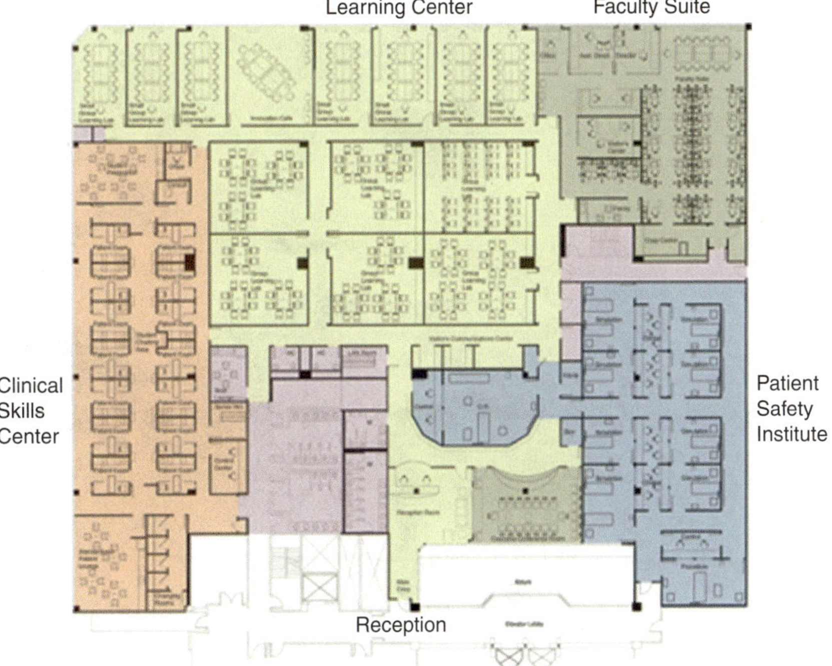

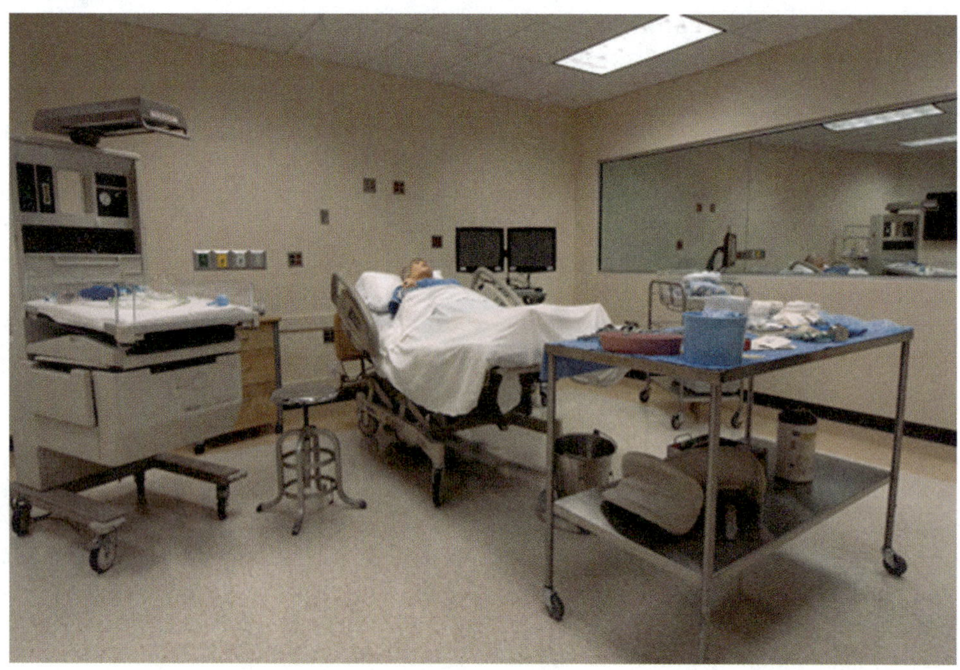

Fig. A.45

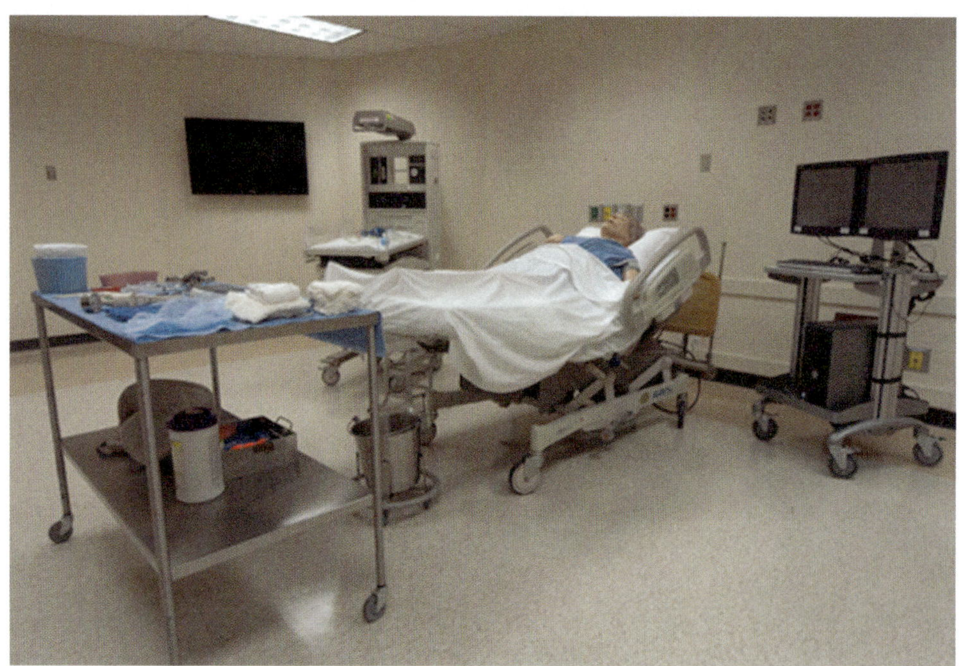

Fig. A.46

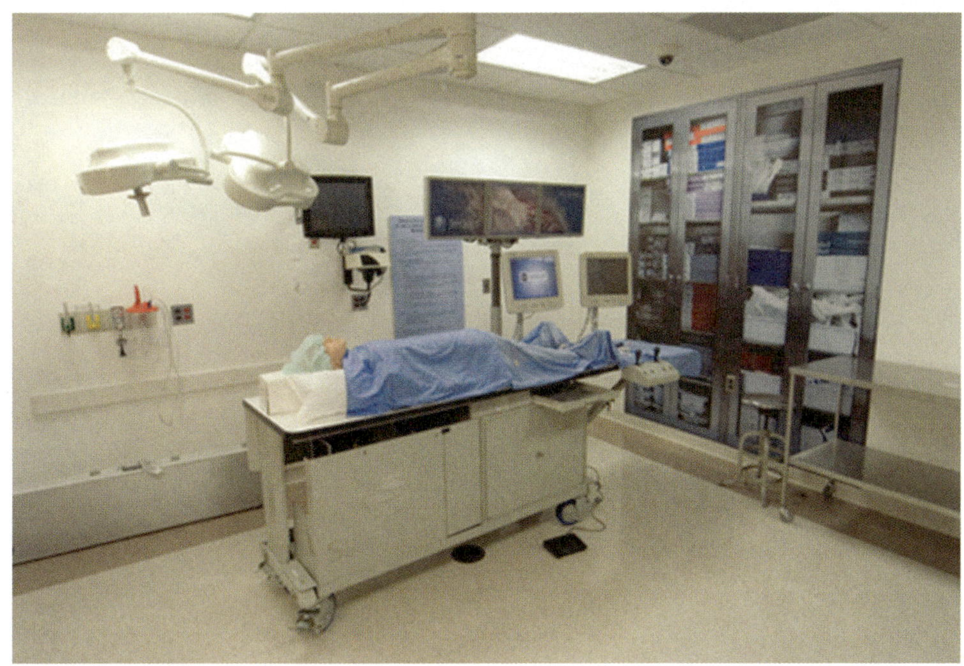

Fig. A.47

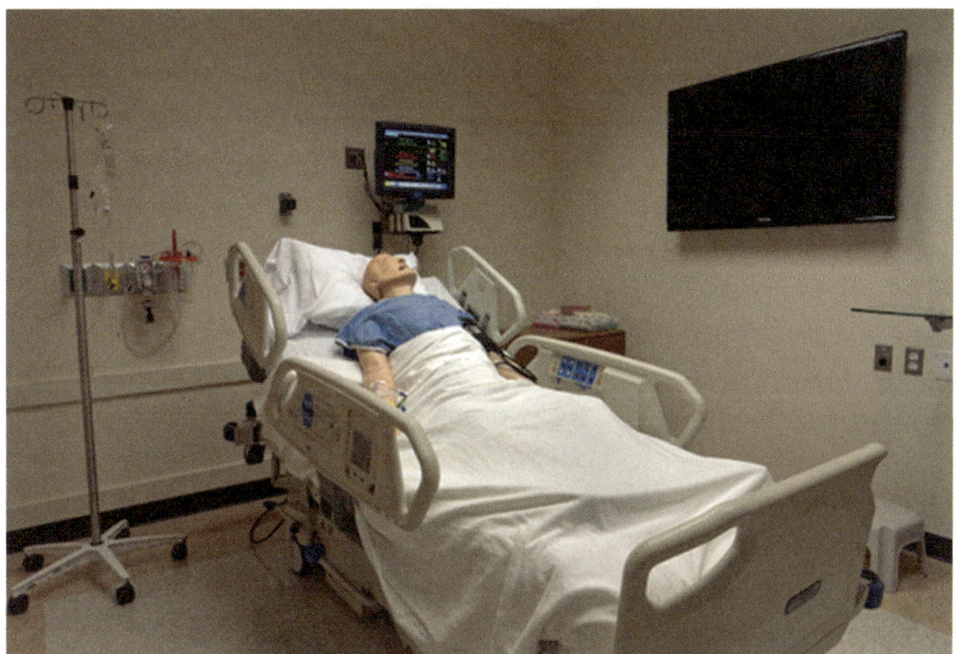

Fig. A.48

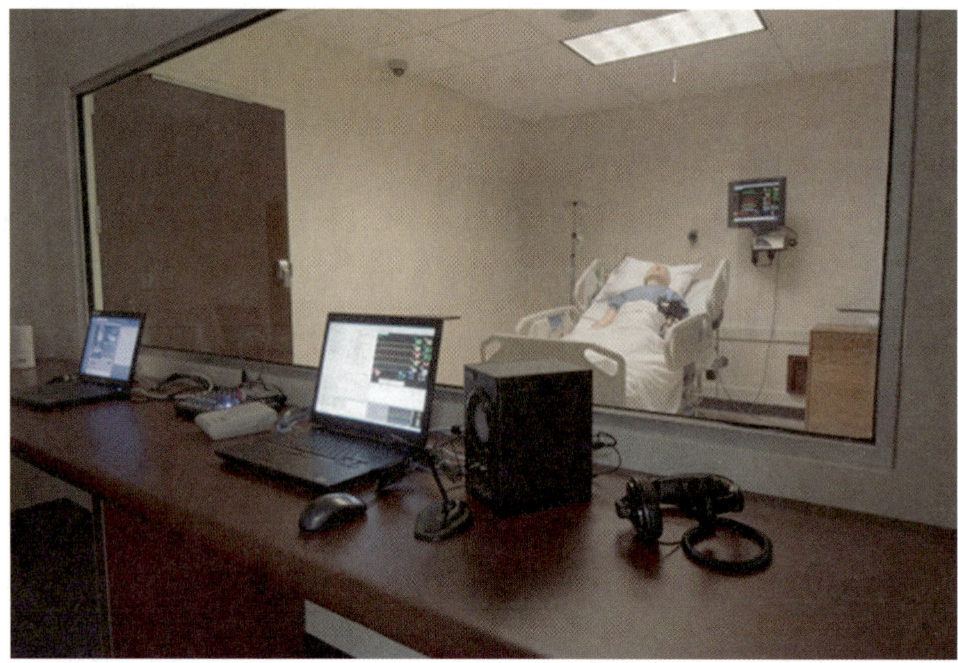

Fig. A.49

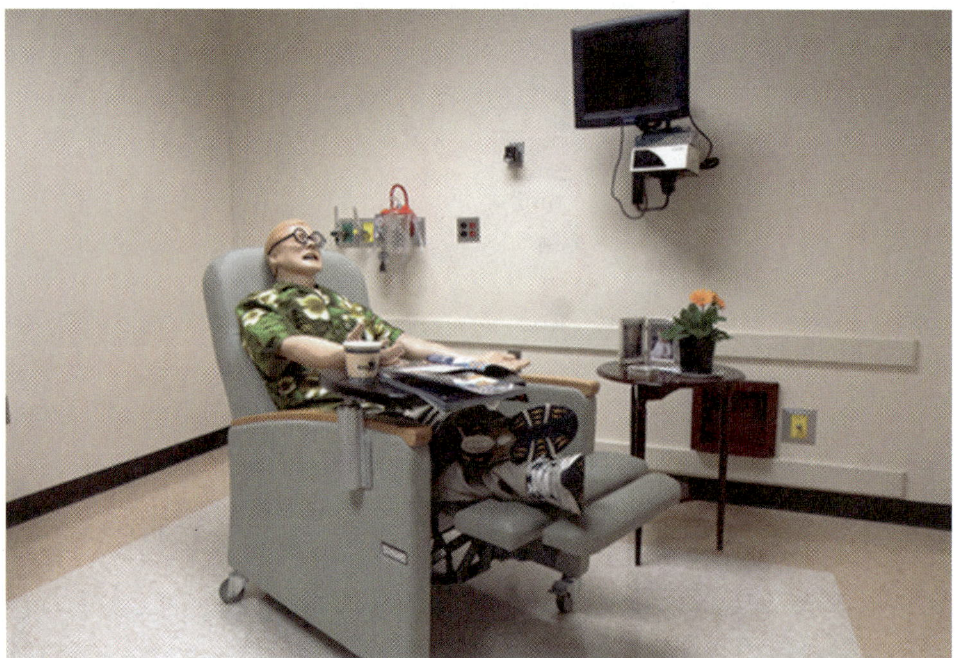

Fig. A.50

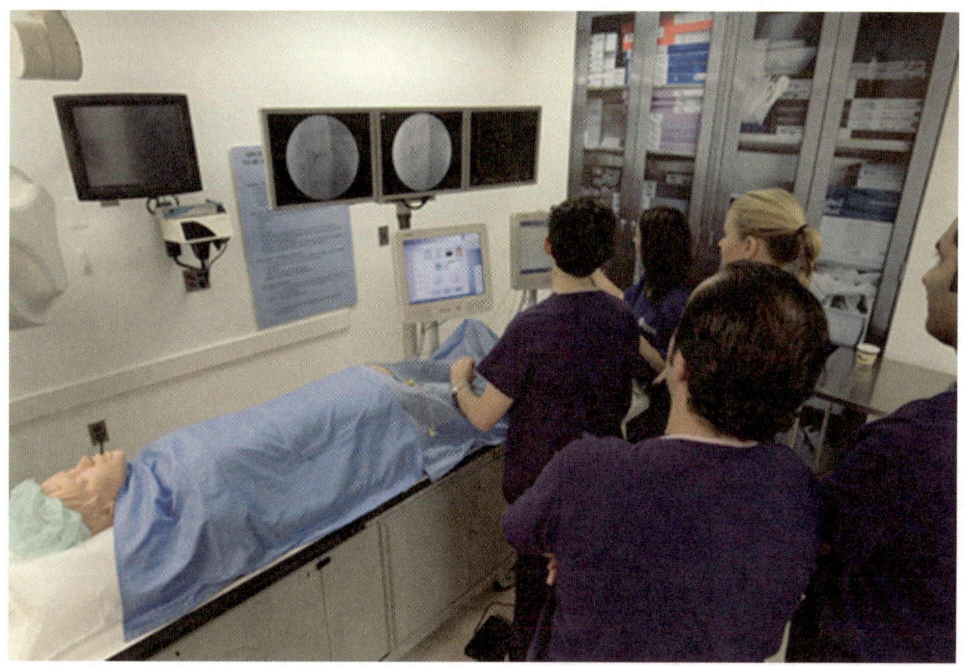

Fig. A.51

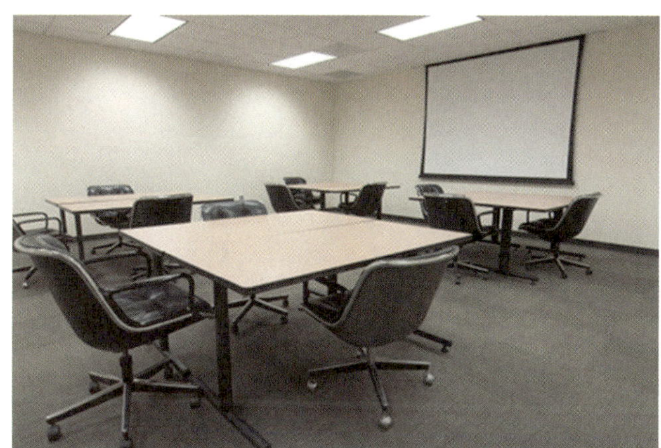

Fig. A.52

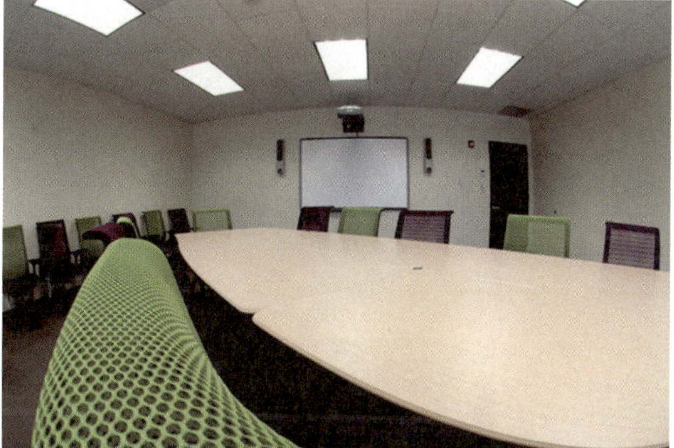

Fig. A.53

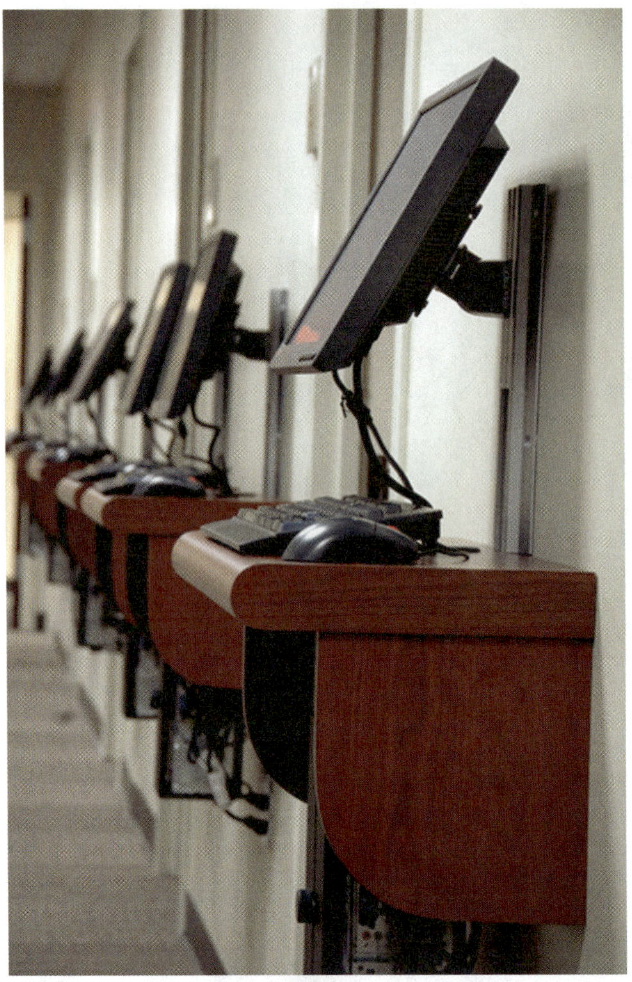

Fig. A.54

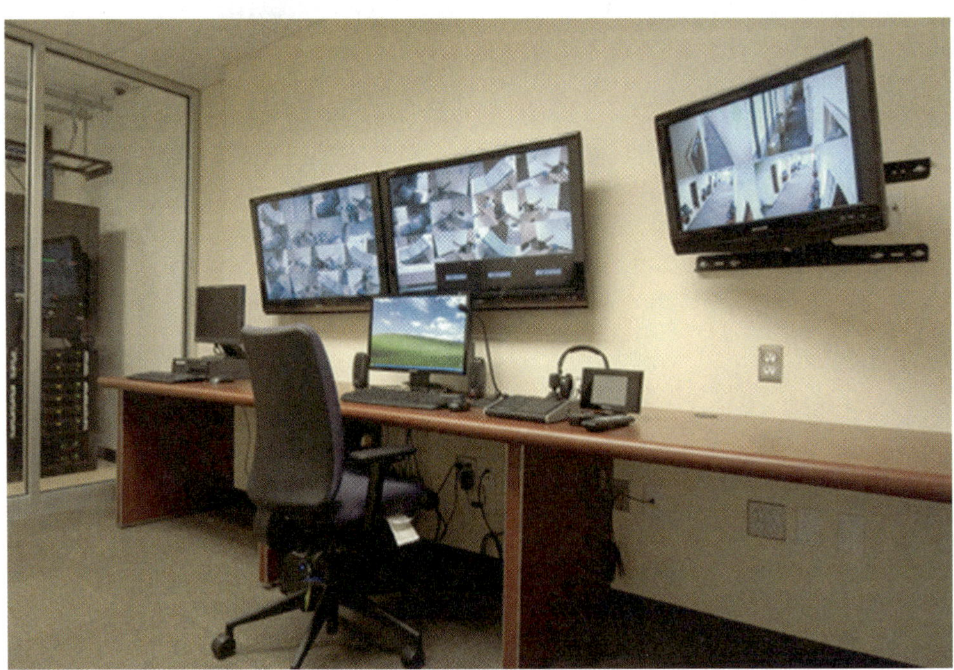

Fig. A.55

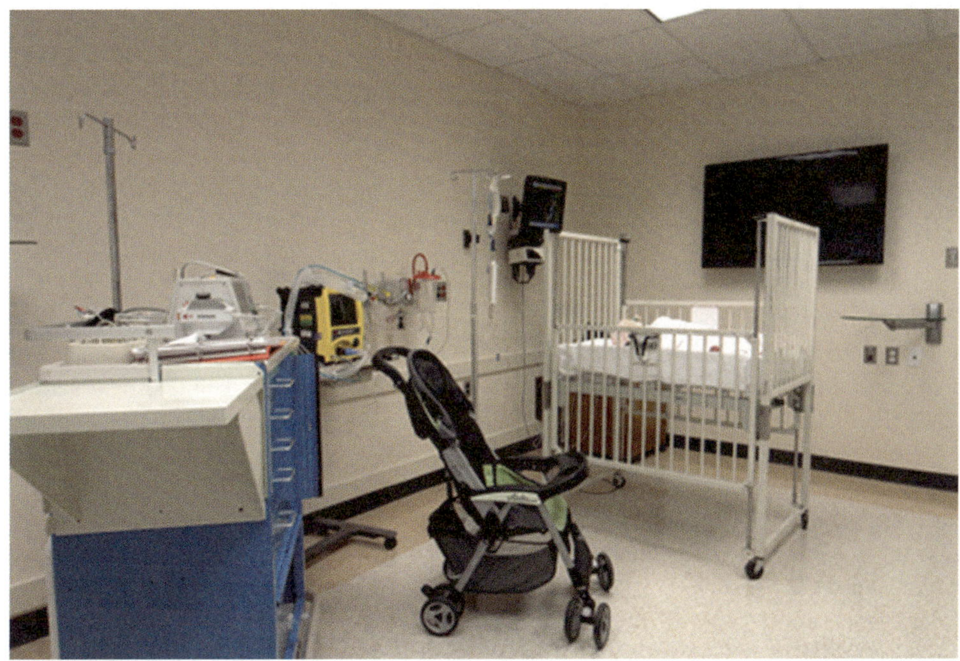

Fig. A.56

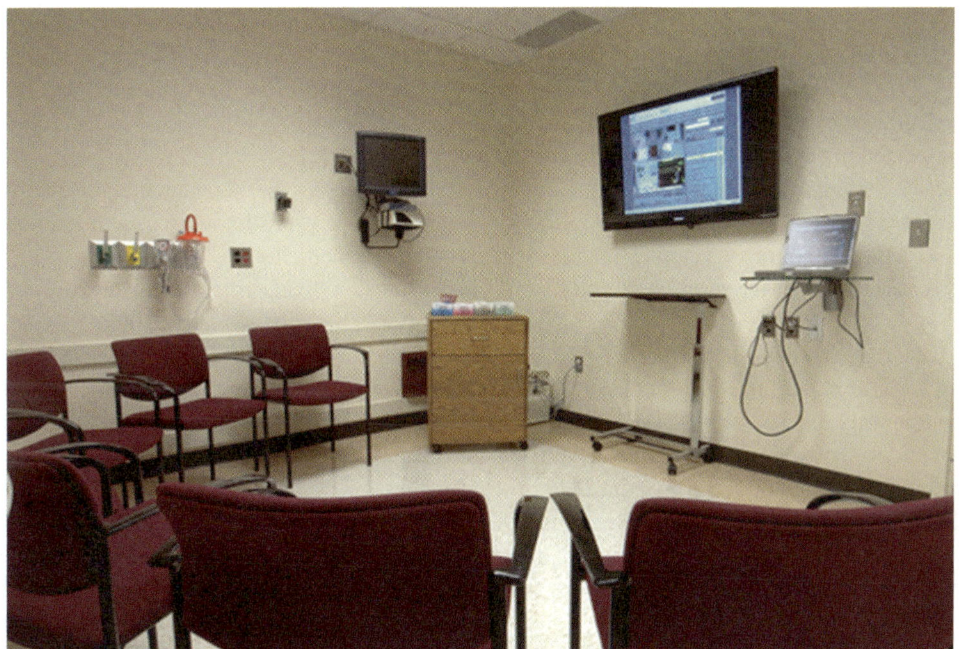

Fig. A.57

Appendix B: Terms and Terminology

Accreditation
a process in which a certification of competency, authority, or credibility is presented.

Accreditation Council for Continuing Medical Education (ACCME)
a nonprofit corporation based in Chicago, responsible for accrediting US institutions that offer continuing medical education (CME) to physicians and other healthcare professionals. ACCME also has a system for recognizing state medical societies as accreditors for local organizations offering CME. ACCME's mission is to identify, develop, and promote rigorous national standards for quality CME that improve physician performance and medical care for patients and their communities. ACCME's accreditation is a voluntary, self-regulatory system. ACCME's seven-member organizations are the American Board of Medical Specialties (ABMS), the American Hospital Association (AHA), the American Medical Association (AMA), the Association of American Medical Colleges (AAMC), the Association for Hospital Medical Education (AHME), the Council of Medical Specialty Societies (CMSS), and the Federation of State Medical Boards of the United States (FSMB).

Amygdala
almond-shaped groups of nuclei considered part of the limbic system located in the medial/temporal lobes of the brain in complex vertebrates, including humans. They have been indicated in serving a primary role in memory and emotional reactions, bridging the connection between emotions and the formation of long-term memories.

Anesthesia
derived from the Greek "without sensation" and traditionally associated with the condition of sensation (often noxious) that is temporarily blocked or removed. Recently, it has been defined as a more complex state of being in which the patient is pharmacologically induced into a reversible state of amnesia, analgesia, loss of responsiveness, loss of skeletal muscle reflexes, or decreased stress response, either simultaneously or separately.

Anesthesiology
traditionally defined as "the practice and study of anesthesia and anesthetic agents" but recently has been further defined as the study and practice of perioperative medicine, ensuring optimal analgesia and maintenance of physiologic homeostasis throughout the preoperative, intraoperative, and postoperative periods. Anesthesiologists may elect to subspecialize in anesthesia for particular types of surgery (cardiothoracic, obstetrical, neurosurgical, pediatric), regional anesthesia, acute or chronic pain medicine, or intensive care medicine.

Animal models
a living, nonhuman animal used during the research and investigation of human disease, for the purpose of better understanding the disease without the added risk of causing harm to an actual human being during the process. The animal chosen will usually meet a determined taxonomic equivalency to humans so as to react to disease or its treatment in a way that most closes resembles the necessary human physiology.

Anxiety
is a psychological and physiological state characterized by the displeasing feeling of fear and concern. It can be represented by a combination of somatic, emotional, cognitive, and behavioral components and can occur in the presence or absence of psychological stress. Increased anxiety serves the purpose of increased vigilance regarding potential threats in the environment as well as increased tendency to take proactive actions regarding such possible threats. It may also help an individual to deal with a demanding situation by prompting them to cope with it.

Arthroscopy
a minimally invasive surgical procedure in which an examination and sometimes treatment of damage of the interior of a joint is performed using an arthroscope, a type of endoscope that is inserted into the joint through a small incision.

Assessment
is the process of documenting, usually in measurable terms, a subject's knowledge, skills, attitudes, and beliefs.

Battlefield medicine
also called field surgery and later combat casualty care, is the treatment of wounded soldiers in or near an area of combat. Civilian medicine has been greatly advanced by procedures that were first developed to treat the wounds inflicted during combat. Battlefield medicine is a category of military medicine.

Business plan
a formal statement of a set of business goals, the reasons they are believed attainable, and the plan for reaching those goals. It may also contain background information about the organization or team attempting to reach those goals.

Cadaver
the body of a deceased human being, often for the purpose of dissecting for medical education.

Cardiovascular surgery
is surgery on the heart or great vessels performed by specialized surgeons. Frequently, it is done to treat complications of ischemic heart disease, correct congenital heart malformations, or treat valvular heart disease. It also includes heart transplantation surgery.

Cardiology
a specialty within medicine that deals with the study and treatment of various disorders of the heart such as congenital heart defects, coronary artery disease, heart failure, valvular heart disease, and electrophysiology.

Collaboration
the process where two or more people or organizations work together to realize shared goals, often with a deep, collective, determination to reach this identical objective.

Communication
is the exchange of thoughts, messages, or information, as by speech, visuals, signals, writing, or behavior.

Competency
having the state or quality of being adequately or well qualified to do a job properly. It can also be a set of defined behaviors that provide a structured guide enabling the identification, evaluation, and development of the behaviors in an individual's ability to perform a specific role.

Complex adaptive system
a system encompassing a complex, self-similar collection of interacting adaptive agents. *Complex* implies that they are dynamic networks of interactions and relationships not aggregations of static entities. They are *adaptive* in that their individual and collective behavior changes as a result of experience. Examples of complex adaptive systems include the stock market, social insect and ant colonies, the biosphere and the ecosystem, the brain and the immune system, manufacturing businesses, and social systems such as communities.

Complexity
many parts working in an intricate arrangement, often involving dynamic networks and relationships.

Computer simulation
is a computer program, or network of computers, that attempts to simulate an abstract model of a particular system. Computer simulations have become a useful part of mathematical modeling of many natural systems in physics, astrophysics, chemistry, and biology. It has also been applied to human systems in economics, social science, psychology, and engineering.

Confederate
is an individual other than the patient who is scripted in a simulation to provide realism, additional challenges, or additional information for the learner.

Construct validity
Construct validity refers to "the degree to which a test measures what it claims, or purports, to be measuring." In other words it occurs whenever a test is to be interpreted as a measure of some attribute or quality which is not operationally defined. In lay terms, construct validity examines the question: "Does the measure behave like the theory says a measure of that construct should behave?"

Content validity
Content validity (also known as logical validity) refers to the extent to which a measure represents all facets of a given social construct. For example, a depression scale may lack content validity if it only assesses the affective dimension of depression but fails to take into account the behavioral dimension. Content validity is different from face validity, which refers not to what the test actually measures, but to what it superficially appears to measure. Content validity requires the use of recognized subject matter experts to evaluate whether test items assess defined content and more rigorous statistical tests than does the assessment of face validity.

Continuing education
is an all-encompassing term within a broad spectrum of post-secondary learning activities and programs. The term is used mainly in the United States and Canada. Recognized forms of post-secondary learning activities within the domain include degree credit courses by nontraditional students, nondegree career training, workforce training, formal personal enrichment courses (both on-campus and online), self-directed learning (such as through Internet interest groups, clubs, or personal research activities), and experiential learning as applied to problem solving.

Continuing education provider
an organization or individual that offers an approved continuing education course and that is authorized by the contractor to offer the course to a licensee for credit toward the licensee's continuing education requirements.

Continuing medical education
a specific form of continuing education (CE) that helps those in the medical field maintain competence and learn about new and developing areas of their field. These activities may take place as live events, written publications, online programs, audio, video, or other electronic media. Content for these programs are developed, reviewed, and delivered by faculty who are experts in their individual clinical areas.

Cortisol
also known more formally as hydrocortisone, is a steroid hormone, more specifically a glucocorticoid, produced by the zona fasciculata of the adrenal gland. It is released in response to stress and a low level of blood glucocorticoids. Its primary functions are to increase blood sugar through gluconeogenesis, suppress the immune system, and aid in fat, protein, and carbohydrate metabolism.

Credentialing
is the process of establishing the qualifications of licensed professionals, organizational members or organizations, and assessing their background and legitimacy. The process is generally an objective evaluation of a subject's current licensure, training or experience, competence, and

ability to provide particular services or perform particular procedures.

Crisis resource management
: originally defined in the airline industry as "Crew Resource Management," and it promotes safety by addressing the behavioral and cognitive skills needed to effectively manage all available resources, especially during a crisis situation. This can be accomplished through the development of superior nontechnical skills such as communication, teamwork, situational awareness, and leadership.

Curriculum integration
: in many American medical schools, an integrated curriculum refers to a non-compartmentalized approach to basic science learning. As opposed to traditional medical curriculum, which separates subjects such as embryology, physiology, pathology, and anatomy, integrated curricula alternate lectures on these subjects over the course of the first 2 years. The course of study is instead organized around organ systems (such as "cardiovascular" or "gastrointestinal"). Another major component of the integrated medical curriculum is problem-based learning.

Cut suit
: a product created by Strategic Operations, Inc. (STOPS) that developed the Human Worn Partial Task Surgical Simulator (aka "Cut Suit") that supports two separate training requirements; the first is for tactical combat casualty care (TCCC) and the second as a surgical simulator. The Cut Suit used in realistic scenarios simulates the treatment of the three most common causes of preventable death on the battlefield: hemorrhage from extremity wounds, tension pneumothorax, and airway compromise.

Debriefing
: refers to conversational sessions that revolve around the sharing and examining of information after a specific event has taken place. Depending on the situation, debriefing can serve a variety of purposes. For example, these sessions can be used for military, psychological, or even academic purposes.

Deployment cycle
: that period of time from the commencement of one deployment to the commencement of the next deployment. Deployment is defined as the assignment of military personnel to tours of duty.

Echocardiography
: often referred to in the medical community as a cardiac ECHO or simply an ECHO, and is a sonogram of the heart. Also known as a cardiac ultrasound, it uses standard ultrasound techniques to image two-dimensional slices of the heart. The latest ultrasound systems now employ 3D real-time imaging. Echocardiography has become routinely used in the diagnosis, management, and follow-up of patients with any suspected or known heart diseases. It is one of the most widely used diagnostic tests in cardiology. It can provide a wealth of helpful information, including the size and shape of the heart (internal chamber size quantification), pumping capacity, and the location and extent of any tissue damage.

Education
: in its broadest, general sense is the means through which the aims and habits of a group of people lives on from one generation to the next [1]. Generally, it occurs through any experience that has a formative effect on the way one thinks, feels, or acts. In its narrow, technical sense, education is the formal process by which society deliberately transmits its accumulated knowledge, skills, customs, and values from one generation to another, for example, instruction in schools.

Educational theory
: refers to either speculative educational thought in general or to a theory of education as something that guides, explains, or describes educational practice.

Emergency medicine
: a medical specialty in which physicians care for patients with acute illnesses or injuries which require immediate medical attention. While not usually providing long-term or continuing care, emergency medicine physicians diagnose a variety of illnesses and undertake acute interventions to resuscitate and stabilize patients.

Emotional memory
: emotion can have a powerful impact on memory. Numerous studies have shown that the most vivid memories tend to be of emotional events, which are likely to be recalled more often and with more clarity and detail than neutral events. The activity of emotionally enhanced memory retention can be linked to human evolution; during early development, responsive behavior to environmental events would have progressed as a process of trial and error. Survival depended on behavioral patterns that were repeated or reinforced through life and death situations.

Endoscopy
: means looking inside and typically refers to looking inside the body for medical reasons using an endoscope, an instrument used to examine the interior of a hollow organ or cavity of the body. Unlike most other medical imaging devices, endoscopes are inserted directly into the organ.

Endoscopy simulation
: a simulator or device that allows for extensive training with an endoscope without using actual patients.

Experiential learning
: is the process of making meaning from direct experience. Simply put, experiential learning is learning from experience. The experience can be staged or left open.

Experiential learning is learning through reflection on doing, which is often contrasted with rote or didactic learning.

Face validity
Face validity is the extent to which a test is subjectively viewed as covering the concept it purports to measure. It refers to the transparency or relevance of a test as they appear to test participants. Face validity assesses whether the test "looks valid" to the examinees who take it, the administrative personnel who decide on its use, and other technically untrained observers. In simulation, the first goal of the simulation modeler is to construct a model that appears reasonable on its face to model users and others who are knowledgeable about the real system being simulated.

Facilitation
broadly used to describe any activity which makes tasks for others easy, or tasks that are assisted.

Facility design
architecture, exterior and interior design, and construction of facilities other than hospitals (e.g., dental schools, medical schools, ambulatory care clinics, and specified units of healthcare facilities). The concept also includes architecture, design, and construction of specialized contained, controlled, or closed research environments including those of space labs and stations.

Fellowship
the period of medical training in the United States and Canada that a physician may undertake after completing a specialty-training program (residency). During this time (usually more than 1 year), the physician is known as a fellow. Fellows are capable of acting as attending physician or consulting physician in the generalist field in which they were trained, such as internal medicine or pediatrics. After completing a fellowship in the relevant subspecialty, the physician is permitted to practice without direct supervision by other physicians in that subspecialty, such as cardiology or oncology.

Financial analysis
refers to an assessment of the viability, stability, and profitability of a business, sub-business, or project. It is performed by professionals who prepare reports using ratios that make use of information taken from financial statements and other reports. These reports are usually presented to top management as one of their bases in making business decisions.

Flight
the process by which an object moves, through an atmosphere (or air) or beyond it (as in the case of spaceflight), by generating aerodynamic lift, propulsive thrust, aerostatically by buoyancy, or by ballistic movement, without direct support from any surface.

Fracture
is the (local) separation of an object or material into two, or more, pieces under the action of stress. Often applied to the bones of living creatures, such as a bone fracture.

Full-scale simulation
a device or scenario that allows simulation of tasks related to applicable learners for a given operational requirement. It is capable of simulating the operational environment (e.g., audio, visual, and tactile) to achieve maximum realism and training effectiveness.

Funding agencies
are organizations that provide research funding in the form of research grants or scholarships.

Gastroenterology
is a branch of medicine focused on the digestive system and its disorders. Diseases affecting the gastrointestinal tract, which includes the organs from mouth to anus, along the alimentary canal, are the focus of this specialty.

General surgery
is a surgical specialty that focuses on abdominal intestines including esophagus, stomach, small bowel, colon, liver, pancreas, gallbladder and bile ducts, and often the thyroid gland. They also deal with diseases involving the skin, breast, soft tissue, and hernias.

Graduate medical education
refers to any type of formal medical education, usually hospital-sponsored or hospital-based training, pursued after receipt of the MD or DO degree in the USA. This education includes internship, residency, subspecialty and fellowship programs, and leads to state licensure and board certification.

Gynecology
is the medical practice dealing with the health of the female reproductive system (uterus, vagina, and ovaries). Literally, outside medicine, it means "the science of women."

Haptic
refers to the sense of touch (from Greek πτω = "I fasten onto, I touch"). It is a tactile feedback technology which takes advantage of the sense of touch by applying forces, vibrations, or motions to the user. This mechanical stimulation can be used to assist in the creation of virtual objects in a computer simulation, to control such virtual objects, and to enhance the remote control of machines and devices (telerobotics). Haptic devices may incorporate tactile sensors that measure forces exerted by the user on the interface.

Healthcare
is the diagnosis, treatment, and prevention of disease, illness, injury, and other physical and mental impairments in humans. Healthcare is delivered by practitioners in medicine, chiropractic, dentistry, nursing, pharmacy,

allied health, and other care providers. It refers to the work done in providing primary care, secondary care, and tertiary care, as well as in public health.

High-fidelity
is most commonly a term for the high-quality reproduction of sound or images. In simulation, it refers to the quality of the simulation as it pertains to reproducing actual events.

History
is the discovery, collection, organization, and presentation of information about past events.

Humor
is the tendency of particular cognitive experiences to provoke laughter and provide amusement. The term derives from the humoral medicine of the ancient Greeks, which taught that the balance of fluids in the human body, known as humors (Latin: humor, "body fluid"), controls human health and emotion.

Hyperrealistic environment
Strategic Operations Inc., on the lot of Stu Segall Productions, a full-service TV/movie studio, provides "Hyper-RealisticTM" training services and products for military, law enforcement, and other organizations responsible for homeland security. The company employs state-of-the-art Hollywood battlefield special effects, combat wound effects, role players, subject matter experts, combat training coordinators, and training scenarios to create training environments that are the most unique in the industry.

Innovation
is the creation of better or more effective products, processes, services, technologies, or ideas that are readily available to markets, governments, and society. Innovation differs from invention in that innovation refers to the use of better and, as a result, novel idea or method, whereas invention refers more directly to the creation of the idea or method itself.

Intensive care
is a branch of medicine concerned with the diagnosis and management of life-threatening conditions requiring sophisticated organ support and invasive monitoring.

Internal medicine
is the medical specialty dealing with the prevention, diagnosis, and treatment of adult diseases. Physicians specializing in internal medicine are called internists. They are especially skilled in the management of patients who have undifferentiated or multisystem disease processes. Internists care for hospitalized and ambulatory patients and may play a major role in teaching and research.

International Meeting on Simulation in Healthcare
(IMSH) is the world's largest annual conference dedicated to healthcare simulation learning, research, and scholarship. The program consists of approximately 300 sessions in various format styles and offers something for every simulation professional. From large plenary sessions to small, interactive immersive courses, attendees can expect to encounter a comprehensive array of learning forums and styles. Leading experts in the field of healthcare simulation are encouraged to attend and present on various topics in the field of simulation.

Laparoscopic urology training
is a rapidly evolving branch of urology and has replaced some open surgical procedures. Robot-assisted surgery of the prostate, kidney, and ureter has been expanding this field. Today, many prostatectomies and nephrectomies in the United States are carried out by laparoscopic or robotic assistance. As a result many residency training programs in urology place laparoscopic training as a high priority.

Laparoscopy
also called minimally invasive surgery (MIS), bandaid surgery, or keyhole surgery and is a modern surgical technique in which operations in the abdomen are performed through small incisions (usually 0.5–1.5 cm) as opposed to the larger incisions needed in laparotomy. The key element in laparoscopic surgery is the use of a laparoscope. There are two types: (1) a telescopic rod lens system that is usually connected to a video camera (single chip or three chip) or (2) a digital laparoscope where the charge-coupled device is placed at the end of the laparoscope, eliminating the rod lens system. Also attached is a fiber-optic cable system connected to a "cold" light source (halogen or xenon), to illuminate the operative field, inserted through a 5 or 10 mm cannula or trocar to view the operative field. The abdomen is usually insufflated, or essentially blown up like a balloon, with carbon dioxide gas. This elevates the abdominal wall above the internal organs like a dome to create a working and viewing space. CO_2 is used because it is common to the human body and can be absorbed by tissue and removed by the respiratory system. It is also nonflammable, which is important because electrosurgical devices are commonly used in laparoscopic procedures.

Leadership
is "organizing a group of people to achieve a common goal." The leader may or may not have any formal authority. Students of leadership have produced theories involving traits, situational interaction, function, behavior, power, vision and values, charisma, and intelligence, among others. Somebody whom people follow: somebody who guides or directs others. It has been described as "a process of social influence in which one person can enlist the aid and support of others in the accomplishment of a common task."

Learning
is acquiring new, or modifying existing, knowledge, behaviors, skills, values, or preferences and may involve synthesizing different types of information. The ability to learn is possessed by humans, animals, and some machines. Progress over time tends to follow learning curves. Learning is not compulsory, it is contextual. It does not happen all at once but builds upon and is shaped by what we already know. To that end, learning may be viewed as a process, rather than a collection of factual and procedural knowledge.

Maintenance of Certification (MOC)
is the process of keeping physician certification up to date through 1 of the 24 approved medical specialty boards of the American Board of Medical Specialties (ABMS). The Maintenance of Certification program provides an ongoing process designed to help physicians keep up to date in advances in their fields, develop better practice systems, and demonstrate lifelong learning. Several components must be met:

Professional standing: physicians must have a valid, unrestricted license to practice medicine and confirmation of good standing in their local practice community.

Lifelong learning and self-assessment: through examinations developed by ABMS member boards, physicians assess their clinical and practical knowledge. This component stimulates learning, requires that physicians document their learning, and ensures that physicians keep up with the rapidly evolving medical knowledge essential to quality patient care.

Cognitive expertise: physicians are required to pass a closed-book, proctored examination in their specialty area that assesses critical aspects of clinical knowledge and judgment in scenarios like those encountered in physician practice. This examination evaluates not only what physicians know but how they use what they know to promote health, diagnose, and treat illness effectively and efficiently.

Practice performance assessment: physicians use tools to self-assess their performance in medical practice, with an emphasis on patient care quality, measurement, and documented quality improvement. These assessment tools include various Practice Improvement Modules (PIMs) that evaluate physicians' performance in a clinical area relevant to their practice, compare their performance to clinical guidelines, help them to develop a plan to improve important aspects of their practice, and assess the impact of that improvement plan.

Maintenance of Certification for Anesthesiology
is the process of keeping physician certification up to date in the specialty of anesthesiology. The Maintenance of Certification program provides an ongoing process that was designed to help physicians keep abreast of advances in their fields, develop better practice systems, and demonstrate a commitment to lifelong learning. Physicians need to have—and maintain—the clinical judgment and skills upon which high-quality care depends. Each MOCA cycle is a 10-year period that includes ongoing *lifelong learning and self-assessment*, continual assessment of professional standing (medical licensure), periodic assessments of practice performance, and a decennial assessment of cognitive expertise. MOCA is an opportunity for physicians to improve their skills in six general competencies—medical knowledge, patient care, practice-based learning and improvement, professionalism, interpersonal and communication skills, and systems-based practice. ABA diplomats certified in 2000 or after hold a time-limited certificate and are enrolled in MOCA after initial board certification. This allows them the full 10-year period to meet all requirements. To avoid expiration of certification, all MOCA requirements must be completed within the 10-year period. Participation in MOCA by non-time-limited diplomates, those certified before 2000, is voluntary and encouraged.

Mannequin
is often an articulated doll used by artists, tailors, dressmakers, and others especially to display or fit clothing. The term is also used for life-sized dolls with simulated airways used in the teaching of first aid, CPR, and advanced airway management skills such as tracheal intubation and for human figures used in computer simulation to model the behavior of the human body. During the 1950s, mannequins were used in nuclear tests to help illustrate the effects of nuclear weapons on human beings. Mannequin comes from the French word mannequin, which had acquired the meaning "an artist's jointed model," which in turn came from the Middle Dutch word mannequin, meaning "little man, figurine."

Medical education
is education related to the practice of being a medical practitioner, either the initial training to become a doctor (i.e., medical school and internship), additional training thereafter (e.g., residency and fellowship), or physician assistant education. Medical education and training varies considerably across the world. Various teaching methodologies have been utilized in medical education, which is an active area of educational research.

Memory
is the processes by which information is encoded, stored, and retrieved. Encoding allows information that is from the outside world to reach our senses in the forms of chemical and physical stimuli. In this first stage we must change the information so that we may put the memory into the encoding process. Storage is the second memory stage or process. This entails that we maintain information over periods of time. Finally the third process is

retrieval. This is the retrieval of information that we have stored. We must locate it and return it to our consciousness. Some retrieval attempts may be effortless due to the type of information.

Mental health

describes a level of psychological well-being, or an absence of a mental disorder. From the perspective of "positive psychology" or "holism," mental health may include an individual's ability to enjoy life and create a balance between life activities and efforts to achieve psychological resilience. Mental health can also be defined as an expression of emotions and as signifying a successful adaptation to a range of demands.

Mentor

a term meaning someone who imparts wisdom to and shares knowledge with a less experienced colleague.

Mentoring

is a personal developmental relationship in which a more experienced or more knowledgeable person helps to guide a less experienced or less knowledgeable person. However, true mentoring is more than just answering occasional questions or providing ad hoc help. It is about an ongoing relationship of learning, dialog, and challenge. Mentoring is a process for the informal transmission of knowledge, social capital, and the psychosocial support perceived by the recipient as relevant to work, career, or professional development; mentoring entails informal communication, usually face to face and during a sustained period of time, between a person who is perceived to have greater relevant knowledge, wisdom, or experience (the mentor) and a person who is perceived to have less (the protégé)." The person in receipt of mentorship may be referred to as a protégé (male), a protégée (female), an apprentice, or, in recent years, a mentee.

Microsurgery

is a general term for surgery requiring an operating microscope. The most obvious developments have been procedures developed to allow anastomosis of successively smaller blood vessels and nerves (typically 1 mm in diameter) which have allowed transfer of tissue from one part of the body to another and reattachment of severed parts.

Mission

is a statement of the purpose of a company or organization. The mission statement should guide the actions of the organization, spell out its overall goal, provide a path, and guide decision-making.

Moulage

a French term to mean (1) a mold, as of a footprint, made for use in a criminal investigation, and (2) the making of such a mold or cast, as with plaster of Paris. For simulation it has meant to mean the makeup and molds applied to actors or mannequins used to portray lesions, skin findings, and bleeding and traumatized areas.

National organization

an organization or membership that is represented at a national level.

Neonatal

in medical contexts, newborn or neonate (from Latin, neonatus, newborn) refers to an infant in the first 28 days after birth; the term applies to premature infants, postmature infants, and full-term infants.

Neurosurgery

is the medical specialty concerned with the prevention, diagnosis, treatment, and rehabilitation of disorders which affect any portion of the nervous system including the brain, spinal cord, peripheral nerves, and extracranial cerebrovascular system.

Nursing education

consists in the theoretical and practical training provided to nurses with the purpose to prepare them for their duties as nursing care professionals. This education is provided to nursing students by experienced nurses and other medical professionals who have qualified or are experienced for educational tasks.

Obstetrics

(from the Latin obstare, "to stand by") is the medical specialty dealing with the care of all women's reproductive tracts and their children during pregnancy (prenatal period), childbirth, and the postnatal period.

Ophthalmic training programs

ophthalmologists are medical doctors (MD/MBBS or DO, not OD or BOptom) who have completed a college degree, medical school, and residency in ophthalmology. In many countries, ophthalmologists also undergo additional specialized training in one of the many subspecialties. Ophthalmology was the first branch of medicine to offer board certification, now a standard practice among all specialties.

Ophthalmic wet labs

surgical training laboratories (wet labs) have been shown to be an effective method for developing surgical proficiency. Wet labs provide a risk-free environment in which residents are introduced to the technical aspects of surgery. Wet labs are a particularly important training tool in helping residents develop competency in cataract surgery. The delicate nature of ocular tissue and the small scale of the eye's anatomical components result in a low tolerance for error. Wet labs typically use human cadaver, porcine, or manufactured eyes. Although porcine eyes are readily available, they differ significantly from human eyes, with the former having large anterior chambers, thick and more elastic anterior capsules, and large, soft lenses. Manufactured eyes from various materials can simulate portions of the procedure, such as nucleus removal, but are not as helpful for practicing other steps.

Objective structured assessment of technical skills (OSATS)
a multi-station examination with segments of six to eight stations performed on anatomical models. Candidates move from station to station marked by a qualified surgeon, who grades on two marking systems, task-specific checklists and global rating scales.

Part-task
refers to the parts of a concept or procedure and is often used in training particular skills separately or understanding incrementally in a context that allows them to understand how the part-tasks fit into the whole process or concept being studied.

Part-task trainer
task trainers are mechanical parts of the anatomy that simulate an individual skill. For example, an adult arm with an electronic trainer is used to teach nursing students how to take a person's blood pressure. According to Laerdal Medical's website, "Task trainers allow for repeated practice of individual skills while developing competency and confidence." Another advantage to using the task trainer is its relatively low cost. The disadvantage is that these trainers are low fidelity, so they should be used with beginning students.

Patient safety
a new healthcare discipline that emphasizes the reporting, analysis, and prevention of medical error that often leads to adverse healthcare events. The frequency and magnitude of avoidable adverse patient events was not well known until the 1990s, when multiple countries reported staggering numbers of patients harmed and killed by medical errors. Recognizing that healthcare errors impact one in every ten patients around the world, the World Health Organization calls patient safety an endemic concern.

Patient simulation
a branch of simulation technology related to education and training in medical fields of various industries. It can involve simulated human patients, educational documents with detailed simulated animations, casualty assessment in homeland security and military situations, and emergency response. Its main purpose is to train medical professionals to reduce accidents during surgery, prescription, and general practice. However, it is now used to train students in anatomy and physiology during their clinical training as allied health professionals. These professions include nursing, sonography, pharmacy assistants, and physical therapy.

Pediatrics
is the branch of medicine that deals with the medical care of infants, children, and adolescents. A medical practitioner who specializes in this area is known as a pediatrician, or paediatrician.

PHANTOM®
are specially designed objects that are scanned or imaged in the field of medical imaging to evaluate, analyze, and tune the performance of various imaging devices. These objects are more readily available and provide more consistent results than the use of a living subject or cadaver and likewise avoid subjecting a living subject to direct risk. Phantoms were originally employed for use in 2D x-ray-based imaging techniques such as radiography or fluoroscopy, though more recently phantoms with desired imaging characteristics have been developed for 3D techniques such as MRI, CT, ultrasound, PET, and other imaging methods or modalities.

Physical examination
is the process by which a doctor investigates the body of a patient for signs of disease. It generally follows the taking of the medical history—an account of the symptoms as experienced by the patient. Together with the medical history, the physical examination aids in determining the correct diagnosis and devising the treatment plan. This data then becomes part of the medical record.

Pioneer
one who opens up new areas of thought, research, or development.

Primary care
is the term for the health services by providers who act as the principal point of consultation for patients within a healthcare system. Such a professional can be a primary care physician, such as a general practitioner or family physician, or depending on the locality, health system organization, and patient's discretion, they may see a pharmacist, a physician assistant, a nurse practitioner, a nurse (such as in the UK), a clinical officer (such as in parts of Africa), or an Ayurvedic or other traditional medicine professional (such as in parts of Asia). Depending on the nature of the health condition, patients may then be referred for secondary or tertiary care.

Procedural trainers
trainers or simulators designed to help refine a learner's skills in performing a particular procedure. They are limited in scope and designed to obtain the same results under the same circumstances.

Procedure
is a set of actions or operations which have to be executed in the same manner in order to always obtain the same result under the same circumstances (e.g., emergency procedures).

Project management
is the discipline of planning, organizing, securing, managing, leading, and controlling resources to achieve specific goals.

Psychiatry
: is the medical specialty devoted to the study and treatment of mental disorders. These mental disorders include various affective, behavioral, cognitive, and perceptual abnormalities.

Pulmonary medicine
: is the medical specialty dealing with disease involving the respiratory tract. Pulmonology often involves managing patients who need life support and mechanical ventilation. Pulmonologists are specially trained in diseases and conditions of the chest, particularly pneumonia, asthma, tuberculosis, emphysema, and complicated chest infections.

Reflection
: is the capacity of humans to exercise introspection and the willingness to learn more about their fundamental nature, purpose, and essence. The earliest historical records demonstrate the great interest which humanity has had in itself. Human self-reflection invariably leads to inquiry into the human condition and the essence of humankind as a whole.

Research
: is creative work undertaken systematically to increase the stock of knowledge, including knowledge of humanity, culture, and society, and the use of this stock of knowledge to devise new applications. It is used to establish or confirm facts, reaffirm the results of previous work, solve new or existing problems, support theorems, or develop new theories. A research project may also be an expansion on past work in the field. To test the validity of instruments, procedures, or experiments, research may replicate elements of prior projects, or the project as a whole. The primary purposes of basic research (as opposed to applied research) are documentation, discovery, interpretation, or the research and development of methods and systems for the advancement of human knowledge.

Residency
: is a stage of graduate medical training. A resident physician or resident (also called a specialty registrar/ST doctor in the UK and several commonwealth countries) is a person who has received a medical degree (usually either a MD, or MBBS, MBChB, BMed) and who practices medicine under the supervision of fully licensed physicians, usually in a hospital or clinic. Residencies are also available, and may be required, for students graduating from pharmacy, physical therapy, and optometry schools. In the USA, the training of osteopaths, podiatrists, and dentists may also involve a residency period.

Review
: is an evaluation of a publication; a product; a service or a company such as a movie (a movie review), video game, musical composition (music review of a composition or recording), and book (book review); a piece of hardware like a car, home appliance, or computer; or an event or performance such as a live music concert, a play, musical theater show, or dance show. In addition to a critical evaluation, the review's author may assign the work a rating to indicate its relative merit.

Robotic surgery
: computer-assisted surgery and robotically assisted surgery are terms for technological developments that use robotic systems to aid in surgical procedures. Robotically assisted surgery was developed to overcome both the limitations of minimally invasive surgery and to enhance the capabilities of surgeons performing open surgery.

Salivary cortisol
: was first introduced to psychobiological stress research almost two decades ago. Among the pioneers to use this method, Stahl and Dorner (Stahl and Dorner, 1982) investigated changes in cortisol levels in response to medical diagnostic procedures in several patient populations. They were able to show that cortisol levels can increase manifold within short periods after onset of stimulation.

SawBones®
: a company offering "hands-on" anatomical workshop models for medical education, new product demonstration, sales training, and patient awareness.

Screen-based simulator
: screen-based or PC-based simulations are human-computer interactions that allow students to experience a variety of medical skills and procedures. This is best used with entry-level students. They can practice with basic skills at their own pace. The cost is relatively inexpensive—a computer and a CD. However, the simulation is low fidelity, meaning not very lifelike. It should not take the place of more realistic simulations or patient-student interactions.

Sedation
: is the reduction of irritability or agitation by administration of sedative drugs, generally to facilitate a medical procedure or diagnostic procedure.

Simulated clinical experience
: are based upon real-life clinical scenarios and utilize the simulated environment to provide a hands-on, safe clinical environment in which students have complete autonomy in providing patient care and decision-making. They are free to make mistakes, enabling them to see the real effects of any errors in interpretation of assessment findings.

Simulated participant
: the student or "learner" involved in the simulation or simulated event.

Simulated patient
: in healthcare, is an individual who is trained to act as a real patient in order to simulate a set of symptoms or problems. Simulated patients have been successfully used

in medical education, nursing education, evaluation, and research. Recent technology has allowed for the simulated patient to exist as a mannequin, robot, or Web- or computer-based avatar.

Simulation

is the imitation of the operation of a real-world process or system over time. The act of simulating something first requires that a model be developed; this model represents the key characteristics or behaviors of the selected physical or abstract system or process. The model represents the system itself, whereas the simulation represents the operation of the system over time. Simulation is used in many contexts, such as simulation of technology for performance optimization, safety engineering, testing, training, education, and video games. Training simulators include flight simulators for training aircraft pilots to provide them with a lifelike experience. Simulation is also used with scientific modeling of natural systems or human systems to gain insight into their functioning. Simulation can be used to show the eventual real effects of alternative conditions and courses of action. Simulation is also used when the real system cannot be engaged, because it may not be accessible, or it may be dangerous or unacceptable to engage, or it is being designed but not yet built, or it may simply not exist.

Simulation-based medical education (SBME)

is one form of medical education that allows students to learn via trial and error in a simulated environment. SBME works well with all forms of classroom learning such as lectures, problem solving, in hospital teaching, and other traditional forms of education. Several advantages appear while using this approach such as patient safety, higher knowledge retaining, teamwork, competence, and skill at the bedside.

Simulation center

an institution designed to conduct simulation, simulated events, debriefing, and educational activities.

Simulation funding

adequate funding is necessary to set up and run a successful simulation center. Grants and contributions from outside sources make up the majority of this funding.

Standardized patient

a simulated patient, standardized patient, or sample patient (SP) (also known as a patient instructor), in healthcare, is an individual who is trained to act as a real patient in order to simulate a set of symptoms or problems. Simulated patients have been successfully used in medical education, nursing education, evaluation, and research.

Stress

in psychology, stress is a concept about the condition that can be described as feeling of strain and pressure, feeling of anxiety and being overwhelmed, overall irritability, feeling of being insecure, nervousness, social withdrawal, loss of appetite, depression, panic attacks, exhaustion, high or low blood pressure, skin problems, insomnia, lack of sexual desire (sexual dysfunction), migraine, gastrointestinal problems (constipation or diarrhea), and for women menstrual problems, may cause more serious conditions like heart problems.

Stress inoculation

stress-inoculation training (or SIT) is a cognitive behavioral concept where the basic goal is to help people gain confidence in their ability to cope with anxiety and fear stemming from trauma-related reminders. In SIT, the teacher helps the learner become more aware of what things are reminders (also referred to as "cues") for fear and anxiety. In addition, students learn a variety of coping skills that are useful in managing anxiety, such as muscle relaxation and deep breathing. Participants learn how to detect and identify cues as soon as they appear so that they can put the newly learned coping skills into immediate action. In doing so, the participant can tackle the anxiety and stress early on before it gets out of control.

Structured and supported debriefing

a form of debriefing using structured and supported elements. Structured elements include three specific debriefing phases with related goals, actions, and time estimates. Supported elements include both interpersonal support and use of protocols, algorithms, and best evidence to inform debriefing statements/questions. A learner-centric process designed to standardize the instructor/student post-event interaction to assist learners in thinking about what they did, when they did it, how they did it, why they did it, and how they can improve.

Student

is a learner, or someone who attends an educational institution. In some nations, the English term (or its cognate in another language) is reserved for those who attend university, while a schoolchild under the age of 18 is called a pupil in English (or an equivalent in other languages). In its widest use, student is used for anyone who is learning.

Surgical simulation

refers to a virtual reality simulation of surgical procedures. Such simulations are used to practice often-dangerous surgical procedures without the need for an actual patient. The virtual reality simulation is used as an analog for the actual surgery where doctors can practice on a virtual patient before performing the surgery. Surgery simulation would give an objective evaluation of a surgeon's dexterity combined with a more intensive training activity. It would allow the simulation of rare pathological cases and could simulate the interaction with several organs. Complications can be introduced during the surgery testing the user on real-world scenarios. Virtually trained students may be more proficient and make fewer errors, and would thus be better prepared to assist during surgery.

Systems engineering
: is an interdisciplinary field of engineering focusing on how complex engineering projects should be designed and managed over their life cycles. Issues such as logistics, the coordination of different teams, and automatic control of machinery become more difficult when dealing with large, complex projects. Systems engineering deals with work processes and tools to manage risks on such projects, and it overlaps with both technical and human-centered disciplines such as control engineering, industrial engineering, organizational studies, and project management.

Systems integration
: in engineering, system integration is the bringing together of the component subsystems into one system and ensuring that the subsystems function together as a system. In information technology, systems integration is the process of linking together different computing systems and software applications physically or functionally, to act as a coordinated whole.

Teacher
: one who teaches or instructs; one whose business or occupation is to instruct others; an instructor; a tutor.

Teamwork
: in healthcare, teamwork is "those behaviors that facilitate effective team member interaction," with "team" defined as "a group of two or more individuals who perform some work-related task, interact with one another dynamically, have a shared past, have a foreseeable shared future, and share a common fate."

Technical skills
: technical job skills refer to the talent and expertise a person possesses to perform a certain job or task. Also called "hard skills," as opposed to soft skills, which refer to personality and character traits.

Thoracic surgery
: surgical specialty focused on the surgical treatment of diseases involving organs within the thorax, such as the lungs and great vessels; see also Cardiothoracic Surgery.

Training
: is the acquisition of knowledge, skills, and competencies as a result of the teaching of vocational or practical skills and knowledge that relate to specific useful competencies. Training has specific goals of improving one's capability, capacity, and performance.

Transrectal ultrasound simulation
: transrectal ultrasound creates an image of organs in the pelvis. The most common indication for transrectal ultrasound is for the evaluation of the prostate gland in men with elevated prostate-specific antigen or prostatic nodules on digital rectal exam. Ultrasound may reveal prostate cancer, benign prostatic hypertrophy, or prostatitis. Computerized imaging simulation exists to help train residents in obtaining better images without the use of patients.

Ureteroscopy training
: Ureteroscopy is an examination of the upper urinary tract, usually performed with an endoscope that is passed through the urethra, bladder, and then directly into the ureter. The procedure is useful in the diagnosis and the treatment of disorders such as kidney stones. Ureteroscopy trainers are haptics-based simulators which can help residents further hone their skills.

Virtual reality
: is a term that applies to computer-simulated environments that can simulate physical presence in places in the real world, as well as in imaginary worlds. Most current virtual reality environments are primarily visual experiences, displayed either on a computer screen or through special stereoscopic displays, but some simulations include additional sensory information, such as sound through speakers or headphones.

Virtual simulation
: the simulated environment can be similar to the real world in order to create a lifelike experience—for example, in simulations for pilot or combat training—or it can differ significantly from reality, such as in VR games. In practice, it is currently very difficult to create a high-fidelity virtual reality experience, due largely to technical limitations on processing power, image resolution, and communication bandwidth; however, the technology's proponents hope that such limitations will be overcome as processor, imaging, and data communication technologies become more powerful and cost effective over time.

Web-based simulation
: is the invocation of computer simulation services over the World Wide Web, specifically through a Web browser. Increasingly, the Web is being looked upon as an environment for providing modeling and simulation applications and, as such, is an emerging area of investigation within the simulation community.

Index

A.I. Levine et al. (eds.), *The Comprehensive Textbook of Healthcare Simulation*,
DOI 10.1007/978-1-4614-5993-4, © Springer Science+Business Media New York 2013

D

G

I

J

K

N

Y

Z

Printed in the United States of America